DRUG-INDUCED LIVER DISEASE

DRUG-INDUCED LIVER DISEASE

edited by

Neil Kaplowitz
Laurie D. DeLeve
University of Southern California
Los Angeles, California

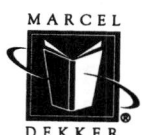

MARCEL DEKKER, INC.

NEW YORK · BASEL

To our loving families
and to the memory of Hy Zimmerman,
who inspired us with his intellect and dedication
in pioneering this field.
We are proud to follow in his footsteps.

ISBN: 0-8247-0811-3

This book is printed on acid-free paper.

Headquarters
Marcel Dekker, Inc.
270 Madison Avenue, New York, NY 10016
tel: 212-696-9000; fax: 212-685-4540

Eastern Hemisphere Distribution
Marcel Dekker AG
Hutgasse 4, Postfach 812, CH-4001 Basel, Switzerland
tel: 41-61-260-6300; fax: 41-61-260-6333

World Wide Web
http://www.dekker.com

The publisher offers discounts on this book when ordered in bulk quantities. For more information, write to Special Sales/Professional Marketing at the headquarters address above.

Preface

With the ever-increasing exposure to pharmaceuticals, more and more examples of drug-induced liver disease have been identified in recent years. At the same time, the basic science of hepatic pharmacology, toxicology, and immunology has exploded in the past decade, with exciting new developments and insights. At the beginning of the 21st century, we now have the opportunity to re-evaluate this important topic as we look to the promise of understanding, predicting, preventing, and healing a common problem that is of importance to all branches of clinical medicine and to anyone who prescribes pharmaceutical or alternative medications. Therefore, we believe that this authoritative, up-to-date volume—with contributions by experts in basic pathogenesis and clinical pathology, and coverage of various categories of agents—will be of great interest to a broad audience. In this regard we have drawn on worldwide expertise; one-third of the chapters were written by authors outside the United States.

Innovations in methodology have had a major impact on research in drug-induced liver injury, and this has led to a greater understanding of the mechanisms involved. A few examples should illustrate the progress that has been made and that is described in this book. The explosion of information on apoptosis has provided insight into the subtleties of drug-induced cell death (Chapter 2). The use of molecular biological techniques has permitted the cloning of numerous genes encoding for P450 isoenzymes. This has made possible the expression of recombinant P450 enzymes and specific P450 antibodies. The availability of recombinant enzymes and of specific inhibiting antibodies has facilitated studies to determine the contribution of individual P450 isoenzymes to the metabolism of specific drugs (Chapter 3). Until quite recently, cholestasis was thought to be due either to mechanical obstruction of bile flow or to cell toxicity which impeded the handling of bile. Improved techniques for isolating membrane vesicles and the cloning and characterization of hepatocyte membrane transporters have allowed the elucidation of a novel mechanism of cholestasis: drug-induced impairment of bile acid transporters in otherwise intact hepatocytes (Chapter 6). As more investigators have taken advantage of relatively new methods to isolate pure nonparenchymal cells, there have been rapid gains in information on the contribution of Kupffer cells, sinusoidal endothelial cells, and stellate cells to a variety of liver diseases, including drug- and toxin-induced liver injury (Chapter 10). The concept of the mitochondrion as a major target of drug-induced toxicity was raised only as recently as the early 1980s. Since then, toxicity of an ever-increasing number of drugs has been linked to selective toxicity in the mitochondrion (Chapter 4). Although reference is made in these examples to the chapters in Part I, on mechanisms in Section I, Part III will reiterate many of these processes in the context of individual drugs that have been linked to one of these modes of toxicity.

As noted, Part I examines hepatotoxicity from the perspective of the mechanisms, across categories of drugs, so that the principles involved can be explored in depth. Examples of drugs to which these mechanisms apply are provided, but the main focus is on the mechanism. Because the authors are experts who are writing about the state of the art in their own fields, this information will be useful both to clinicians who want to gain understanding of the fundamental principles as we understand them today and to knowledgeable clinicians and investigators who wish to read about the newest advances.

Part II provides a general outline of the clinical presentation and management of drug-induced hepatotoxicity. Chapter 11 systematically reviews the clinical presentation and pathological picture of the types of liver injury that can be induced by drugs and toxins. Chapter 12 reviews the factors that predispose an individual to drug toxicity, suggests strategies for monitoring patients at risk for toxicity, and provides information on preventive measures. The information provided in these chapters provide a basic framework for any clinician who might be confronted with xenobiotic-induced hepatotoxicity.

Part III systematically reviews specific toxins implicated in drug-induced hepatotoxicity. Each chapter examines the toxicity induced by drugs or toxins within a specific pharmacological class or by drugs used within a clinical specialty. The current understanding of the mechanism of toxicity, risk factors for developing toxicity, histological characteristics, clinical manifestations, and management are discussed for each category of drugs. This section will be of value to gastroenterologists and hepatologists who want a systematic review of drug-induced liver disease. It will also serve as a reference for clinicians in a variety of specialties who are confronted with a patient with liver disease that might be attributable to drug therapy.

Neil Kaplowitz
Laurie D. DeLeve

Contents

v

Contents

Contributors

Meena Bansal Department of Genetics, University of Pennsylvania School of Medicine, Philadelphia, Pennsylvania, U.S.A.

Leslie Z. Benet Department of Biopharmaceutical Sciences, University of California–San Francisco, San Francisco, California, U.S.A.

Alain Berson, M.D., Ph.D. INSERM Unit 481, Institut National de la Santé et de la Recherche Médicale, Clichy, France

Urs A. Boelsterli HepaTox Consulting and Institute of Clinical Pharmacy, University of Basel, Basel, Switzerland

Mauricio Bonacini, M.D. Department of Transplantation, California Pacific Medical Center, San Francisco, California, U.S.A.

Jean Marie Brogard Department of Internal Medicine, University Hospital, Strasbourg, France

Sam A. Bruschi Department of Medicinal Chemistry, University of Washington School of Pharmacy, Seattle, Washington, U.S.A.

Robert L. Carithers, Jr., M.D. Division of Gastroenterology–Hepatology, Department of Medicine, University of Washington School of Medicine, Seattle, Washington, U.S.A.

Felix A. de la Iglesia, M.D.   Department of Pathology, University of Michigan Medical School, Ann Arbor, Michigan, U.S.A.

Laurie D. DeLeve, M.D., Ph.D.   Division of Gastrointestinal and Liver Disease, and USC Research Center for Liver Diseases, Keck School of Medicine, University of Southern California, Los Angeles, California, U.S.A.

George Feuer, Ph.D.   Department of Clinical Biochemistry, University of Toronto, Toronto, Canada

Bernard Fromenty, Ph.D.   Institut National de la Santé et de la Recherche Médicale (INSERM), Clichy, France

Carol R. Gardner   Department of Pharmacology and Toxicology, Rutgers University, Piscataway, New Jersey, U.S.A.

Pramod Kumar Garg   Department of Gastroenterology, All India Institute of Medical Sciences, New Delhi, India

Jeffrey R. Haskins, Ph.D.   Cellomics, Inc., Pittsburgh, Pennsylvania, U.S.A.

Mary F. Hebert, Pharm.D.   Department of Pharmacy, University of Washington School of Pharmacy, Seattle, Washington, U.S.A.

Hartmut Jaeschke, Ph.D.   Department of Pharmacology and Toxicology, University of Arkansas for Medical Sciences, Little Rock, Arkansas, U.S.A.

Peter L. M. Jansen   Department of Gastroenterology and Hepatology, University of Gröningen, Gröningen, The Netherlands

Gary C. Kanel, M.D.   Department of Pathology, Keck School of Medicine, University of Southern California, Los Angeles, California, U.S.A.

Neil Kaplowitz, M.D.   Division of Gastrointestinal and Liver Disease, and USC Research Center for Liver Diseases, Keck School of Medicine, University of Southern California, Los Angeles, California, U.S.A.

J. Gerald Kenna   AstraZeneca Safety Assessment, Cheshire, England

Dominique Larrey, M.D., Ph.D.   Department of Hepatology and Gastroenterology, Hôpital Saint Eloi and Montpellier School of Medicine, Montpellier, France

Debra L. Laskin   Department of Pharmacology and Toxicology, Rutgers University, Piscataway, New Jersey, U.S.A.

William M. Lee   Department of Internal Medicine, University of Texas Southwestern Medical Center, Dallas, Texas, U.S.A.

J. Steven Leeder Division of Pediatric Pharmacology and Medical Toxicology, Children's Mercy Hospital, Kansas City, Missouri, U.S.A.

Wei Lei Department of Genetics, University of Pennsylvania School of Medicine, Philadelphia, Pennsylvania, U.S.A.

James H. Lewis, M.D. Division of Hepatology, Department of Medicine, Georgetown University Medical Center, Washington, D.C., U.S.A.

Chunze Li Department of Biopharmaceutical Sciences, University of California–San Francisco, San Francisco, California, U.S.A.

Stan Louie, Pharm.D., Ph.D. Departments of Pharmacy and Medicine, University of Southern California, Los Angeles, California, U.S.A.

Willis C. Maddrey Department of Internal Medicine, University of Texas Southwestern Medical Center, Dallas, Texas, U.S.A.

Michael Peter Manns Department of Gastroenterology and Hepatology, Hannover Medical School, Hannover, Germany

Abdellah Mansouri, Ph.D. Institut National de la Santé et de la Recherche Médicale (INSERM), Clichy, France

Michael Müller Department of Gastroenterology and Hepatology, University of Gröningen, and Wageningen University, Gröningen, The Netherlands

Muhammad Naeem, M.D. University of Texas Health Science Center at San Antonio, San Antonio, Texas, U.S.A.

Sidney D. Nelson Department of Medicinal Chemistry, University of Washington School of Pharmacy, Seattle, Washington, U.S.A.

Petra Obermeyer-Straub Department of Gastroenterology and Hepatology, Hannover Medical School, Hannover, Germany

George Ostapowicz Department of Hepatology, University of Texas Southwestern Medical Center, Dallas, Texas, U.S.A.

Georges-Philippe Pageaux, M.D., Ph.D. Department of Hepatology and Gastroenterology, Hôpital Saint Eloi and Montpellier School of Medicine, Montpellier, France

Dominique Pessayre, M.D. Institut National de la Santé et de la Recherche Médicale (INSERM), Clichy, France

Munir Pirmohamed Department of Pharmacology and Therapeutics, University of Liverpool, Liverpool, England

K. Rajender Reddy   Gastroenterology Division, Department of Medicine, University of Pennsylvania, Philadelphia, Pennsylvania, U.S.A.

Adrian Reuben   Division of Gastroenterology/Hepatology, Department of Medicine, Medical University of South Carolina, Charleston, South Carolina, U.S.A.

Kia Saeian   Division of Gastroenterology and Hepatology, Department of Medicine, Medical College of Wisconsin, Milwaukee, Wisconsin, U.S.A.

Steven Schenker, M.D.   Department of Gastroenterology and Nutrition, University of Texas Health Science Center at San Antonio, San Antonio, Texas, U.S.A.

John R. Senior, M.D.   Office of Drug Safety, Food and Drug Administration, Rockville, Maryland, U.S.A.

Rakesh Kumar Tandon   Department of Gastroenterology, All India Institute of Medical Sciences, New Delhi, India

Rebecca Taub   Department of Genetics, University of Pennsylvania School of Medicine, Philadelphia, Pennsylvania, U.S.A.

Shari L. Taylor, M.D.   GI Pathology Partners, P.C., Memphis, Tennessee, U.S.A.

Keith G. Tolman   Department of Gastroenterology, University of Utah School of Medicine, Salt Lake City, Utah, U.S.A.

Paul B. Watkins, M.D.   Department of Medicine, University of North Carolina at Chapel Hill, Chapel Hill, North Carolina, U.S.A.

Kevin Weissman, Pharm.D.   Pharmacy Department, King Drew Medical Center, Los Angeles, California, U.S.A.

Jean Frederic Westphal   Department of Internal Medicine, University Hospital, Strasbourg, France

DRUG-INDUCED LIVER DISEASE

1

Drug-Induced Liver Disorders: Introduction and Overview

NEIL KAPLOWITZ

University of Southern California, Los Angeles, California, U.S.A.

I. INTRODUCTION

Drug-induced liver disease represents an important problem for the following major reasons: (1) approximately 1000 drugs have been implicated in causing liver disease at least on rare occasion (1); (2) in the United States drug-induced liver disease is the most common cause of acute liver failure, accounting for one-third to one-half of cases (2,3); although acetaminophen accounts for the bulk of these, other drugs are still a more frequent cause of acute liver failure than viral hepatitis and other causes; (3) in addition, drug-induced liver disease represents an important diagnostic/therapeutic challenge for physicians caring for patients presenting with liver disorders, since it can mimic all forms of acute or chronic liver disease; (4) the frequency and economic impact of this problem is a major challenge for the pharmaceutical industry and regulatory bodies, especially since the toxic potential of some drugs is not evident in preclinical and phase 1–3 clinical testing.

Table 1   Spectrum of Hepatic Manifestations of Drug-Induced Liver Disease

Acute hepatitis	Acetaminophen, isoniazid, troglitazone, bromfenac
Chronic hepatitis[a]	Nitrofurantoin, methyldopa, diclofenac, minocycline, dantrolene
Acute cholestasis	Amoxicillin–clavulanic acid, erythromycins, sulindac, chlorpromazine, angiotensin–converting enzyme inhibitors
Mixed hepatitis/cholestasis or atypical hepatitis	Phenytoin, sulfonamides
Chronic cholestasis[a]	Chlorpromazine, numerous others on rare occasion
Nonalcoholic steatohepatitis	Amiodarone, tamoxifen
Fibrosis/cirrhosis	Methotrexate
Microvesicular fatty liver	Valproic acid, nucleoside reverse transcriptase inhibitors
Veno-occlusive disease	Busulfan, cyclophosphamide
Peliosis hepatitis	Azathoprine, hormones
Adenoma and hepatocellular carcinoma	Hormones

[a] Drugs that cause chronic disease more frequently cause acute disease.

II. CLINICAL OVERVIEW

Drug-induced liver diseases can mimic all forms of acute and chronic hepatobiliary diseases (4,5) (Table 1). However, the predominant clinical presentations resemble acute icteric hepatitis or cholestatic liver disease. The former is of grave significance as the mortality approximates 10% irrespective of the specific drug (1,4). This type of reaction is accompanied by systemic symptoms, jaundice, markedly elevated serum transaminases, ALT* $\times$ ULN/Alk. Ptase. $\times$ ULN $\geq$ 5, and, in the more severe cases, coagulopathy and encephalopathy indicative of acute (fulminant) liver failure. It is noteworthy that the height of the transaminases does not reliably predict severity except perhaps in the case of acute intrinsic toxins, e.g., acetaminophen. Cholestatic disease, although not usually life threatening, presents with jaundice, disproportionate increased serum alkaline phosphatase, ALT $\times$ ULN/Alk. Ptase. $\times$ ULN $\leq$ 2, and pruritus; cholestatic reactions tend to resolve very slowly (i.e., months vs. weeks for hepatitis) and on rare occasion lead to vanishing bile duct disease and biliary cirrhosis (6,7). Mixed injury patterns with intermediate ALT/Alk. Ptase. can resemble atypical hepatitis or granulomatous hepatitis. Individual drugs tend to exhibit a consistent pattern or clinicopathological signature of the reaction (Table 1) with characteristic latency and clinical presentation. However, some drugs may show several patterns: e.g., nimesulide can cause a short-latency, hypersensitivity-mediated cholestatic injury and a delayed idiosyncratic acute hepatitis-like reaction (8).

Drug-induced liver disease can be predictable (high incidence and dose related) or unpredictable (low incidence and may or may not be dose related). Unpredictable reactions can be viewed as either immune-mediated hypersensitivity or idiosyncratic reactions. Most potent predictable hepatotoxins are recognized in the animal testing or clinical phase of drug development. Those that slip through are almost always unpredictable. Latency between the initiation of therapy and the onset of liver disease is a component of the signature

---

* ALT = alanine aminotransferase; ULN = upper limit of normal; Alk. Ptase. = alkaline phosphatase.

of reactions to specific drugs and provides some clues as to the pathogenesis. Early onset within a few days (particularly if no previous exposure) is strong evidence for direct toxicity of the drug or its metabolite, which is characteristic of predictable reactions; acetaminophen overdose is an example (9).

Unpredictable reactions manifested as overt or symptomatic disease usually occur with intermediate (1–8 weeks) or long latency (up to 12 months). Intermediate latency is characteristic of hypersensitivity reactions. These tend to be associated with fever, rash, and eosinophilia and a rapid positive rechallenge (4,5). Hepatotoxicity of sulindac (10), phenytoin (11), and amoxicillin–clavulanic acid (12) are typical examples. Most cases of cholestatic liver injury and chronic hepatitis caused by drugs are of the hypersensitivity type. It is important to recognize that these reactions may occur up to 3–4 weeks after a 1–2 week course of medication (e.g., amoxicillin–clavulanic acid). In contrast, the long-latency type of reaction is characteristically not associated with features of hypersensitivity and the response to rechallenge is variable and delayed. Thus, one assumes that these events reflect some type of late-onset change in the metabolism of the drug or the response to injury (repair or regeneration). Drugs associated with variable, long latency include isoniazid (13) and troglitazone (14). This type of idiosyncratic reaction is extremely challenging with respect to understanding the pathogenesis and predicting the problem in individual cases. Table 2 provides a list of drugs that are associated with idiosyncratic reactions.

Low-frequency unpredictable reactions, either hypersensitivity or idiosyncratic, often occur on a background, higher rate of mild, asymptomatic, and usually transient liver injury, which is detected as abnormal biochemical tests, particularly serum ALT. Generally, the biochemical abnormality defined as ALT $> 3 \times$ ULN may occur 10–20 times more frequently than overt disease. In almost all instances, the ALT returns to normal despite continued drug use. Thus, in the majority of patients with increased ALT some type of adaptation or "tolerance" occurs and in the minority there is a failure to do so. This issue is further complicated by the uncertain explanation for the very long latency in some of the idiosyncratic reactions.

It should be emphasized that acute or chronic hepatitis induced by drugs subsides upon discontinuation of the drug without long-term sequelae with rare exception. A few reported cases of autoimmune hepatitis triggered by hypersensitivity drug reactions have

Table 2 Drugs Associated with Idiosyncratic Hepatitis

Benoxaprofen[a]	Labetalol
Bromfenac[a]	Nefazodone
Dantrolene	Pemoline
Diclofenac	Terbinafine
Disulfiram	Tolcapone
Felbamate	Troglitazone[a]
Flutamide	Trovafloxacin
Isoniazid	Valproic acid
Isotretinoin	Zafirlukast
Ketoconazole	Zileuton

[a] Withdrawn from marketing.

continued on without the drug, but it is questionable as to whether this was drug-induced liver disease or underlying autoimmune chronic hepatitis. Scarring may persist after severe subacute or chronic injury but is of little consequence after removal of the drug. Cholestatic reactions resolve very slowly after discontinuation of the offending drug, not infrequently associated with loss of interlobular bile ducts. However, the development of cirrhosis or effects on longevity are exceedingly rare.

III. PATHOGENESIS

Hepatotoxicity of drugs can be principally metabolism-dependent, parent drug–dependent, or a combination of both (Fig. 1). Metabolism takes place largely in the liver, which accounts for its susceptibility to drug-induced injury (5). The metabolites may be electrophilic chemicals or free radicals that deplete GSH, covalently bind to proteins, lipids, or nucleic acids, or induce lipid peroxidation. The consequences include hepatocellular necrosis, apoptosis, or sensitization to cytokines or inflammatory mediators produced by nonparenchymal cells. Alternatively, the reactive metabolites may covalently bind to or alter liver proteins such as CYPs leading to sensitization and immune-mediated injury. The immune phenomena nevertheless are metabolism dependent. Thus, the rare occurrence of immune-mediated liver disease is often superimposed on a higher frequency of mild injury (abnormal ALT) suggesting that the drug has a mild toxic potential (e.g., phenytoin or halothane) but in rare individuals this toxic potential leads to metabolism-dependent hypersensitivity. Perhaps in the case of certain drugs both immune and idiosyncratic reactions may develop from common upstream drug metabolism steps, but influenced by genetic and/or environmental factors that determine either an immune response or idiosyncratic reaction. Genetic polymorphisms of enzymes involving drug activation or detoxification have been implicated in the susceptibility to hypersensitivity reactions to sulfonamides (15,16), anticonvulsants (11,17), and tacrine (18). Presumably genetic polymorphisms of either MHC-I-dependent antigen presentation in hepatocytes or MHC-II-dependent antigen presentation in macrophages, which have scavenged necrotic or apoptotic hepatocytes directly killed by the drug, may further contribute to determining the rare occurrence of

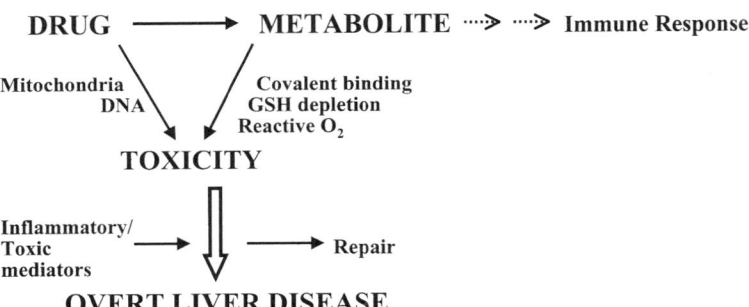

Figure 1 Pathogenesis of drug induced liver diseases. Upstream events in the hepatocytes affect viability of individual cells but sensitize to downstream processes leading to clinically overt organ damage. The latter involves a balance of effects of cytokines, chemokines, and inflammatory mediators, mainly produced by nonparenchymal cells and the effects on repair processes such as regeneration.

these hypersensitivity reactions (19) which most often have an incidence of 1:1000 or less. Parent drug–dependent toxicity occurs as a result of the properties of the parent drug (or metabolite) to accumulate in organelles [weak bases such as amiodarone accumulate in mitochondria (20), undergo nonspecific redox cycling (quinones cycle electrons from NADPH to O_2 generating O_2^-), or specifically inhibit enzymes or transporter (nucleoside reverse transcriptase inhibitors block mitochondrial DNA polymerase (21) or cyclosporin A inhibits canalicular transporters (22)]. In these cases, if the parent drug's chemical properties account for direct toxicity, factors that enhance its availability (decreased metabolism or export) may increase susceptibility.

Regardless of whether toxicity within a target liver cell (e.g., hepatocyte, sinusoidal endothelial cell, or bile duct cell) is parent drug- or metabolite-dependent, the ultimate severity of the liver disease in vivo may depend greatly on the subsequent downstream participation of toxic mediators released from various cell types and the recruitment of inflammatory cells as well as intracellular and tissue repair and regenerative responses. The toxic mediators include chemicals, such as NO and reactive oxygen metabolites, and the balance of cytokines that promote injury (e.g., TNFα, IL-1, IFNγ, IL-12, IL-18), or prevent injury (IL-4, IL-10, IL-13, MCP-1). Thus, toxin may somewhat injure hepatocytes but then sensitize to the effects of an imbalance in injurious versus protective cytokines (Fig. 2). For example, the toxicity of CCl_4 is abrogated in vivo by neutralizing TNF (23); the toxicity of acetaminophen is markedly enhanced in MCP-1 chemokine receptor knockouts associated with an enhanced TNFα response (24) and is abrogated by inactivating Kupffer cells (25). Thus, the direct and indirect influence of toxins on the production and balance of mediators and genetic polymorphisms in these responses may play a major role in unmasking the overt toxic potential of a drug culminating in overt idiosyncratic toxicity.

Another important factor that contributes to the extent of liver injury is the capacity of the liver to regenerate (Fig. 3). Thus, for example, TNFα will promote regeneration by acting on Kupffer cells (autocrine) to release IL-6, which will trigger, along with HGF, regeneration. Interference with IL-6 (knockout) worsens CCl_4 injury, and conversely, exogenous IL-6 treatment diminishes liver injury in wild-type mice (26). TNF also acts on hepatocytes through NF-κB signaling to promote survival gene transcription. If the toxin interferes with the latter pathway, TNFα-induced apoptosis may occur.

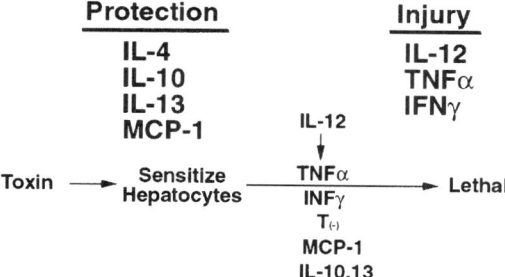

Figure 2 Role of cytokine balance in determining susceptibility to toxins. Drugs or metabolites may directly injure hepatocytes to a minor extent, but may markedly sensitize to the lethal effects of TNFα and IFNγ. The latter are modulated by cytokines that promote or inhibit their production or actions.

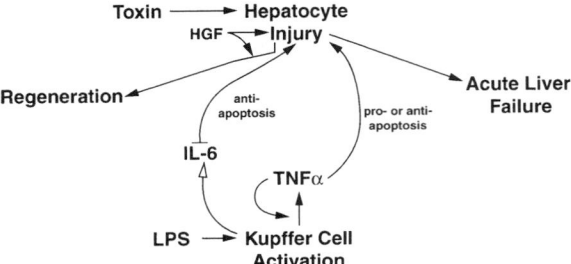

Figure 3   Role of cytokines and regeneration in toxin-induced liver disease. TNF activates NF-κB in nonparenchymal cells leading to IL-6 production, and in hepatocytes it promotes antiapoptotic survival gene expression. If the toxin interferes with the latter in hepatocytes or with the regenerative response, worsening of the overt injury will occur. IL-6, on the other hand, promotes survival and regeneration, minimizing overt liver injury.

IV.   RISK FACTORS

Regardless of whether hepatotoxicity is predictable (frequent) or unpredictable (rare), hypersensitivity-mediated or idiosyncratic, metabolism dependent or parent drug–dependent, the interplay of genetic and environmental risk factors influences susceptibility (Fig. 4) (27). Age, gender, concomitant drugs, and underlying diseases (e.g., HCV, HBV, HIV) have been most frequently identified. Table 3 lists examples of drugs and associated risk factors.

With the advent of new technologies in genomics and proteomics, one can anticipate that new insights into the mechanisms of susceptibility and liver injury from drugs will be forthcoming (28). Some of the genetic factors to consider are listed in Table 4. Polymorphisms (CYPs, cytokines, MHC, etc.) and rare heterozygous mutations (β-oxidation, BSEP) will need to be assessed.

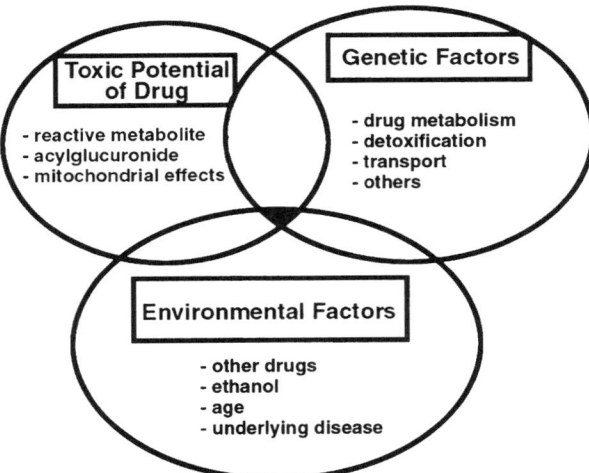

Figure 4   Risk of hepatotoxicity. The ultimate development of hepatotoxicity is determined by the interplay of the toxic potential of the drug or its metabolites and the susceptibility of the host as determined by genetic and environmental factors, both of which influence gene expression.

Table 3 Risk Factors for Drug-Induced Hepatotoxicity

Drug	Factors
Methotrexate	Chronic alcohol, obesity, diabetes, chronic hepatitis, psoriasis
Isoniazid	HBV, HCV, HIV, alcohol, older age, female, slow acetylator, rifampin, pyrazinamide
Acetaminophen	Chronic alcohol, fasting, isoniazid
Valproate	Young age, anticonvulsants, genetic defects of mitochondrial β-oxidation and respiratory chain enzymes
Diclofenac	Female, osteoarthritis
Anticonvulsants	Genetic defect in detoxification
Sulfonamides	HIV, slow acetylator, genetic defect in defense

V. DIAGNOSIS

Establishing a diagnosis of drug-induced liver disease in an individual case is mainly based upon circumstantial evidence aided by the signature type of reactions (if known) with respect to latency and clinical characteristics as well as exclusion of other more plausible alternative causes. Additional information can be gained from the response to removal of the drug—rapid improvement in cytotoxic reactions and slow improvement in cholestatic reactions. A rechallenge with recrudescence of liver abnormalities is the most definitive evidence, but hardly ever justified and not always positive in idiosyncratic cases. A practical approach is to consider the diagnosis probable/possible if the signature latency and pattern of disease fit and other causes are excluded (viral hepatitis, ischemic hepatitis, biliary disease). The remainder of cases are unlikely or unrelated depending on the completeness of the workup and the strength of the evidence in favor of an alternative diagnosis. This ad hoc approach is equivalent to diagnosing as yes, no, or maybe.

The presence of autoantibodies to specific forms of CYP has been associated with hypersensitivity reactions to certain drugs (19,29,30). Although of uncertain but intriguing significance with respect to pathophysiology, their presence may be helpful in the diagnosis of drug-induced liver disease in these special cases (Table 5). However, testing for these autoantibodies is mainly a research tool at present. Furthermore, sensitivity and specificity of the presence of these autoantibodies is uncertain.

Table 4 Possible Genetic Determinants of Risk

1. Drug metabolism (e.g., CYP polymorphisms)
2. Detoxification (e.g., GSH-related, epoxide hydrase)
3. Apoptosis and survival genes
4. Signal transduction (kinases and phosphatases)
5. MHC-I and -II
6. Cytokines/chemokines and receptors
7. Inflammatory mediators (Cox, NOS, etc.)
8. Regeneration/repair
9. Transporters (BSEP, MRP2, etc.)
10. Mitochondrial β-oxidation and respiratory chain
11. Structural integrity (e.g., cytokeratin 8/18)

Table 5 Autoantibodies in Drug-
Induced Liver Disease

Autoantibody target	Drug
CYP 2C9[a]	Tienilic acid
CYP 1A2[b]	Dihydralazine
CYP 3A[b]	Anticonvulsants
CYP 2E1	Halothane
mEH	Germander

[a] Also referred to as anti-LKM2 autoantibody.
[b] Also referred to as anti-LM autoantibody.
CYP, cytochrome P450; mEH, microsomal
epoxide hydrolase.

Several groups have attempted to generate quantitative systems designed to generate
a numerical score that reflects the probability of a drug as the cause for liver disease (31–
34). The RUCAM scoring system appears to be the most accurate (35,36) and puts numerical weight on the factors discussed above (Table 6) to generate a composite score that
reflects the probability that liver injury is drug-induced. The advantage is that this system
is less subjective than the ad hoc approach. This type of scoring system performs well
when validated against well-documented cases of drug-induced liver disease. Specialists,
the pharmaceutical industry, and regulatory bodies should be encouraged to use this scale.
It also would be reasonable to apply the scoring system to individual case reports submitted
to medical journals. Although it is not perfect and may not discriminate between multiple
concurrently used candidate toxins, it does provide consistency and focuses the attention
of the evaluator on most of the critical parameters that need to be considered in estimating
the probability of causality.

VI. DRUG DEVELOPMENT

Drug development involves a preclinical and clinical phase. Preclinical assessment is cen-
tered on animal testing using very high doses. Although animal testing is probably very
reliable in screening out potent, predictable toxins, it is far less reliable in identifying a
propensity for unpredictable toxicity. Experience has suggested that there are numerous
false positives and false negatives. A better understanding of the mechanisms of unpredict-

Table 6 Causality Assessment

1. Latency
2. Rate of resolution (dechallenge)
3. Risk factors (age, alcohol, pregnancy)
4. Exclusion of other causes (viral hepatitis, ischemia, biliary
   tract disease, alcohol)
5. Concomitant drugs
6. Track record (PDR, case reports)
7. Rechallenge

able hepatotoxicity, may eventually lead to the establishment of appropriate animal models that recapitulate the factors that determine susceptibility in humans. This will most likely be achieved with the use of transgenic and knockout mice to set up conditions that mimic human susceptibility. At present, some suggestion of hepatotoxicity at high doses in animals may at least warrant more careful or extensive assessment in the clinical phases of drug development.

During phases I–III of drug testing the likelihood of encountering overt hepatotoxicity (i.e., jaundice and high transaminases) depends on the frequency of the reaction. Most idiosyncratic reactions occur in 1 in 1000 or more individuals and acute liver failure in 1 in 10,000 or more. Typically in clinical development, drugs are tested in 1500–2500 individuals. Exclusion of an overt reaction with 95% confidence, if the true incidence is 1:1000, would require 3000 treated patients, assuming all were exposed for the appropriate duration (e.g., 6–9 months). This is usually not attained in clinical trials. Therefore, if one is not fortunate enough to identify overt hepatitis in one or two cases in the study population, the appearance of lesser signals needs to be the focus for scrutiny. It is very rare indeed to identify acute liver failure from idiosyncratic hepatotoxins in drug development. The rule of threes indicates that to identify acute liver failure with 95% confidence that has a true incidence of 1 in 10,000 would require 30,000 study patients.

Since the probability of identifying overt or life-threatening liver injury in clinical trials is so low, one must focus on the incidence of asymptomatic ALT and bilirubin elevations. The most sensitive parameter appears to be the incidence of ALT $> 3\times$ ULN in drug-treated versus placebo control–treated patients. Depending on the study population, the incidence of $3\times$ ALT in controls may vary from 0.1 to nearly 1.0%. Thus, an incidence of 2–3% in the drug-treated patients would be unequivocal cause for closer scrutiny. Although this is a sensitive indicator, it is not entirely specific since there are drugs, e.g., statins, tacrine, aspirin, etc., that are associated with an increased incidence of $3\times$ ALT, but have proved safe in postmarketing experience (?false-positive signal). More specificity is gained by examining the height of the transaminases. An ALT increase of eight-fold or greater is a more specific signal since this rarely occurs in controls. Even more specific is conjugated hyperbilirubinemia ($\geq$1.5-fold) associated with elevated ALT.

The experience with troglitazone exemplifies the issue of identification of a signal. In a cohort of 2500 study patients, ALT $> 3\times$ ULN occurred in 2% (vs. $<1\%$ in controls); ALT $> 8\times$ ULN occurred in 0.6% (vs. none of controls); and two cases with overt jaundice were observed (37). Thus, all the criteria for a hepatic signal were present at the time of approval of the drug. A similar premarketing experience was observed with bromfenac (38), which was also withdrawn postmarketing.

A critical issue is what is the appropriate regulatory response to the occurrence of a signal? In some cases, particularly when the drug is not crucial, approval is denied. If the drug is critical, warnings and education of physicians and patients are very important and there may be justification for recommending monitoring ALT (see below) and/or restrictions on the use of the drug.

VII. POSTMARKETING MONITORING

The background incidence of drug-induced mild, reversible liver injury provides the rationale for monitoring or surveillance. From this background of mild injury a minority of individuals will emerge with overt disease. Thus, by stopping the medications at the first sign of mild injury one should prevent serious consequences. Although this seems a logical approach, a number of problems must be considered. First, the approach applies only to delayed reactions. Hypersensitivity reactions occur relatively early and evolve rapidly so educating patients about symptoms is crucial in early cessation of the offending drug. Second, one is sacrificing potentially very important therapy to a much larger number of patients than would actually develop overt disease; third, compliance with such approaches is known to be very poor; fourth, the rate of development of overt disease from the first appearance of elevated ALT needs to be gradual for monthly monitoring to be efficacious in preventing life-threatening disease. Testing more frequently than monthly is not practical, although the future development of a finger-stick ALT test that could be applied in a fashion similar to monitoring glucose might change this by improving compliance and allowing more frequent monitoring. In any case, monthly monitoring for delayed idiosyncratic reactions is the best approach available, but the efficacy of the approach is assumed and not proven. Furthermore, this should not substitute for the need to educate patients about symptoms of hepatotoxicity, such as fever, rash, malaise, fatigue, anorexia, gastrointestinal complaints, abdominal pain, dark urine; jaundice, pruritus, etc., and the need to. report them to the physicians to insure expeditious cessation of offending agents. Despite monthly monitoring, some adverse events may appear rapidly in the few weeks after a normal test.

Ultimately, the most difficult challenge to the application of monitoring is cost effectiveness—monthly monitoring is expensive and one needs to weigh this quantitatively against the morbidity and mortality of adverse liver events. There is no clear answer to the question of what incidence of serious adverse idiosyncratic hepatitis warrants monitoring, how frequently it should be performed, and for how long. Furthermore, the postmarketing occurrence of adverse events must be weighed against the benefit of the drug. Risk/benefit assessment is ill-defined but ultimately becomes the crucial factor in recommending monitoring ALT versus removal of the drug from the market. In the case of the NSAID bromfenac, continued use of the drug in the face of infrequent, delayed idiosyncratic severe hepatotoxicity (38) could not be justified since many alternative treatments were available. In the case of troglitazone, the decision to withdraw was delayed and more complicated owing to the important and unique therapeutic properties of the drug in managing a serious medical condition, albeit with benefits that would not be evident for many years (i.e., the effect of long-term control of blood sugar on complications of diabetes). It was decided that the implementation of monthly monitoring would likely protect the users and the drug was continued. Although this strategy may have worked to some extent, the issue of compliance with monitoring and the possibility of occasional "rapid risers" meant that the population could not be completely protected. At the same time, several new drugs in this class were approved and after a year of postmarketing experience with the alternative new agents, it was concluded that these agents were probably less likely to induce severe hepatotoxicity, leading to the withdrawal of troglitazone.

A major issue in postmarketing surveillance is the frequency of serious adverse events compared to the background in the general population. Reliable data on the occurrence of hospitalization for idiopathic hepatitis and acute liver failure are very limited. However, several databases (Medicaid, HMO) suggest that hospitalization for cryptic acute hepatitis occurs in about 1:50,000–1:100,000 adult individuals in the general population each year (39–41). Acute liver failure is estimated to occur in up to 3000 individuals annually in the United States. About 10–20% of these cases are idiopathic with a resulting annual incidence of one to two cases per million individuals in the population. Thus, when a new drug is marketed and more than a few cases of unexplained acute liver failure are reported, concern should be raised. In the example of troglitazone, at least 30–40 cases of acute liver failure were reported to the FDA in the first year on the market from a population of about one million taking the drug. This was a much higher rate than predicted. Such a postmarketing signal may be less apparent when far fewer individuals are exposed. However, the current MedWatch system for reporting adverse events, with all its attendant problems regarding poor compliance and accurate causality assessment, has been reasonably successful in rapidly identifying problems with numerous drugs leading to withdrawal or severe restrictions of use.

VIII. CONCLUSIONS

The liver is a particular target for drugs because of its role in clearing and metabolizing chemicals. The parent drug or more frequently the metabolites may either affect critical functions, or sensitize to the effects of cytokines or inflammatory cells, or elicit an immune response. This often occurs in an unpredictable fashion, implying that environmental and genetic factors alter the susceptibility to these adverse events. A wide range of liver diseases can occur as adverse events but the individual drug tends to induce a characteristic signature reaction with respect to latency and clinicopathological manifestations. Hepatotoxicity from drugs poses a major challenge in drug development and postmarketing surveillance. The future identification of the pathogenesis of idiosyncratic reactions represents the major challenge in this field and will likely advance rapidly with the application of methods of toxicogenomics and pharmacogenomics in the preclinical and clinical arenas.

REFERENCES

1. Zimmerman H. Drug Hepatotoxicity. 2nd ed. Philadelphia: Lippincott, 1999.
2. Ostapowicz G, Fontana RB, Larson AM, et al. Etiology and outcome of acute liver failure in the USA: preliminary results of a prospective multi-center study (abstr). Hepatology 1999; 30(4):221A.
3. Shakil A, Kramer D, Mazariegos G, et al. Acute liver failure: clinical features, outcome analysis, and applicability of prognostic criteria. Liver Transplant 2000; 16:163–169.
4. Zimmerman H. Drug-induced liver disease. In: E Schiff, M Sorrell, W Maddrey, eds. Schiff's Diseases of the Liver. 8th ed. Philadelphia: Lippincott-Raven Publishers, 1999:973–1064.
5. Kaplowitz N. Drug metabolism and hepatotoxicity. In: N Kaplowitz, ed. Liver and Biliary Diseases. 2nd ed. Baltimore: Williams & Wilkins, 1996:103–120.
6. Desmet VJ. Vanishing bile duct syndrome in drug-induced liver disease. J Hepatol 1997; 26(suppl 1):31–35.
7. Degott C, Feldmann G, Larrey D, et al. Drug-induced prolonged cholestasis in adults: a histological semiquantitative study demonstrating progressive ductopenia. Hepatology 1992; 15: 244–251.
8. Van Steenberen W, Peeters P, DeBondt J, et al. Nimesulide-induced acute hepatitis: evidence from six cases. J Hepatol 1998; 29:135–141.
9. Pham T-V, Lu S, Kaplowitz N. Acetaminophen hepatotoxicity. In: Taylor, ed. Gastrointestinal Emergencies. 2nd ed. Baltimore: Williams & Wilkins, 1997:371–388.
10. Tarazi E, Harter JG, Zimmerman HJ, et al. Sulindac-associated hepatic injury. Analysis of 91 cases reported to the Food and Drug Administration. Gastroenterology 1993; 104:569–574.
11. Shear N, Spielberg S. Anticonvulsant hypersensitivity syndrome: in vitro assessment of risk. J Clin Invest 1988; 82:1826–1832.

12. Larrey D, Vial T, Micaleff A, et al. Hepatitis associated with amoxycillin-clavulanic acid combination. Report of 15 cases. Gut 1992; 33:368–371.
13. Thompson N, Caplin M, Hamilton M, et al. Anti-tuberculosis medication and the liver: dangers and recommendations in management. Eur Respir J 1995; 8:1384–1388.
14. Murphy E, Davern T, Shakil O, et al. Troglitazone-induced fulminant hepatic failure. Dig Dis Sci 2000; 45:549–553.
15. Rieder M, Uetrecht J, Shear N, et al. Diagnosis of sulfonamide hypersensitivity reactions by in vitro "rechallenge" with hydroxylamine metabolites. Ann Intern Med 1989; 110:286–289.
16. Rieder M, Shear N, Kanee A, et al. Prominence of slow acetylator phenotype among patients with sulfonamide hypersensitivity reactions. Clin Pharmacol Ther 1991; 49:13–17.
17. Gennis M, Vemusi R, Burns E, et al. Familial occurrence of hypersensitivity to phenytoin. Am J Med 1991; 91:631–634.
18. Becquemont L, Lecoeur S, Simon T, et al. Glutathione S-transferaseθ genetic polymorphism might influence tacrine in Alzheimer's patients. Pharmacogenetics 1997; 7:251–253.
19. Robin M, LeRoy M, Descatoire V, Pessayre D. Plasma membrane cytochromes P450 as neoantigens and autoimmune targets in drug-induced hepatitis. J Hepatol 1997; 26(1):23–30.
20. Berson A, DeBeco V, Letteron P, et al. Steatohepatitis-inducing drugs cause mitochondrial dysfunction and lipid peroxidation in rat hepatocytes. Gastroenterology 1998; 114:764–774.
21. Brinkman K, Hofstede H, Burger D, et al. Adverse effects of reverse transcriptase inhibitors: mitochondrial toxicity as common pathway. AIDS 1998; 12:1735–1744.
22. Kowdley K, Keefe E. Hepatotoxicity of transplant immunosuppressive agents. Gastroenterol Clin North Am 1995; 24:991–1001.
23. Czaja M, Xu J, Alt E. Prevention of carbon tetrachloride-induced rat liver injury by soluble tumor necrosis factor receptor. Gastroenterology 1995; 108:1849–1854.
24. Hogaboam C, Bone-Larson C, Steinhauser M, et al. Exaggerated hepatic injury due to acetaminophen challenge in mice lacking C-C chemokine receptor 2. Am J Pathol 2000; 156:1245–1252.
25. Laskin D, Gardner C, Price V, Jollow D. Modulation of macrophage functioning abrogates the acute hepatotoxicity of acetaminophen. Hepatology 1995; 21:1045–1050.
26. Cressman P, Greenbaum L, DeAngelis R, et al. Liver failure and defective hepatocyte regeneration in interleukin-6-deficient mice. Science 1996; 274:1379–1383.
27. DeLeve L, Kaplowitz N. Prevention and therapy of drug-induced hepatic injury. In: MM Wolfe, ed., GL Davis, section ed. Therapy of Digestive Disorders. Philadelphia: WB Saunders, Harcourt Brace & Company, 2000:334–348.
28. Nuwayser E, Bittner M, Trent J, et al. Microarrays and toxicology: the advent of toxicogenomics. Mol Carcinogen 1999; 24:153–159.
29. Beaune P, Lecoeur S. Immunotoxicology of the liver: adverse reactions to drugs. J Hepatol 1997; 26(suppl 2):37–42.
30. Neuberger J. Immune mechanisms in drug hepatotoxicity. Clin Liver Dis 1998; 2:471–482.
31. Maria V, Victorino R. Development and validation of a clinical scale for the diagnosis of drug-induced hepatitis. Hepatology 1997; 26:664–669.
32. Benichou C. Criteria of drug induced liver disorders: report of an international consensus meeting. J Hepatol 1990; 11:272–276.
33. Danan G, Benichou C. Causality assessment of adverse reactions to drugs. I. A. novel method based on the conclusions of international consensus meetings: application to drug-induced liver injuries. J Clin Epidemiol 1993; 46:1323–1330.
34. Benichou C, Danan G, Flahault A. Causality assessment of adverse reactions to drugs. II. An original model or validation of drug causality assessment methods: case reports with positive rechallenge. J Clin Epidemiol 1993; 46:1331–1336.
35. Lucena M, Camargo R, Andrade R, et al. Comparison of two clinical scales for causality assessment in hepatotoxicity. Hepatology 2001; 33:123–130.

36. Kaplowitz N. Causality assessment versus guilt by association in drug hepatotoxicity. Hepatology 2001; 33:308–310.

37. Watkins P, Whitcomb R. Hepatic dysfunction associated with troglitazone. N Engl J Med 1998; 338:916–917.

38. Moses P, Schroeder B, Alkhatib O, et al. Severe hepatotoxicity associated with bromfenac sodium. Am J Gastroenterol 1999; 94:1393–1396.

39. Walker A, Cavanaugh R. The occurrence of new hepatic disorders in a defined population. Post Marketing Surveill 1992; 6:107–117.

40. Carson J, Strom B, Duff A, et al. Safety of nonsteroidal anti-inflammatory drugs with respect to acute liver disease. Arch Intern Med 1993; 153:1331–1336.

41. Duh M-S, Walker A, Kronlund K. Descriptive epidemiology of acute liver enzyme abnormalities in the general population of central Massachusetts. Pharmacoepidemiol Drug Safety 1999; 8:275–283.

2

The Role of Cytochrome P450s in Drug-Induced Liver Disease

PAUL B. WATKINS

University of North Carolina at Chapel Hill, Chapel Hill, North Carolina, U.S.A.

I. INTRODUCTION

Chemical-induced liver injury usually does not result from the direct effects of the parent compound. Rather, toxicity generally results from conversion of the parent molecule to toxic metabolites within the liver (reviewed in refs. 1,2). This statement applies not just to drugs, but also to environmental chemicals, such as aflatoxins, bromobenzene, and carbon tetrachloride. The major family of liver enzymes implicated in generating potentially toxic metabolites from drugs are the cytochromes P450.

II. GENERAL PRINCIPLES OF DRUG METABOLISM

Most orally administered drugs have lipophilicity (fat solubility). This is because absorption of drugs from the gastrointestinal tract generally involves passive diffusion through

15

the brush border membranes of the small intestinal epithelial cells (enterocytes). Highly water-soluble compounds are generally poorly absorbed from the digestive tract and therefore pass out of the body in stool. Lipophilicity is also a desirable property for drugs once they have entered the body because most drugs must diffuse from the circulation through cell membranes to arrive at their therapeutic target. This usually essential property of lipophilicity creates a potential problem for the body, however. Lipophilic drugs tend to sequester into the body's fat stores. In plasma, lipophilic drugs bind to circulating proteins and therefore are not readily filtered in the kidney glomerulus and excreted into urine. If the lipophilic drugs are excreted in bile, they would tend to be reabsorbed from the digestive tract, thus undergoing enterohepatic cycling. Most drugs would, therefore, remain in the body for a very long period of time if the body did not have the ability to convert drugs into more water-soluble, and readily excreted, metabolites. Although many body tissues have some ability to metabolize drugs, the liver is far and away the major organ involved in drug metabolism.

III. DISCOVERY OF P450s

A major breakthrough promoting study of drug metabolism in the liver was the development of techniques to isolate the hepatocyte endoplasmic reticulum from whole pieces of liver. During this process, endoplasmic reticulum breaks up into small spheres called "microsomes." It was discovered that under certain experimental conditions, liver microsomes could produce most of the metabolites generated from drugs and other chemicals by the liver in vivo. Most of the reactions characterized involved insertion of an oxygen atom into the drug molecule (usually a hydroxylation) or covalent binding (conjugation) of the molecule to polar ligands such as glucuronic acid, sulfate, or glutathione. Many compounds had to first undergo hydroxylation to produce a reactive site on the molecule suitable for conjugation reactions. This frequent sequence of events led to the concept of dividing drug metabolism into two categories: phase I (predominantly hydroxylation reactions) and phase II (conjugation). It is now appreciated that most (but not all) of what was described as phase I microsomal drug metabolism is the result of the activity of a large family of enzymes termed "cytochromes P-450." This somewhat awkward name derived from the fact that when first isolated, these enzymes appeared to be chemically similar to mitochondrial cytochromes. The "P" is an abbreviation for "pigment," reflecting the fact that the enzymes are red in color (owing to the presence of heme in the molecule) and largely account for the reddish-brown color characteristic of microsomes. Finally, it was noted that under certain experimental conditions, these enzymes intensely absorbed light with 450-nm wavelength. The cytochromes P450 are now usually referred to simply as "P450s."

IV. P450s AND DRUG METABOLISM

The vast majority of drugs in clinical use today are metabolized by liver P450s. Although it was initially proposed that there might be hundreds or even thousands of different specific P450s, a recent realization is that there are relatively few P450s important for drug metabolism (3). Each P450 represents the product of a unique gene. The P450s involved in drug metabolism fall predominantly into three gene families, now termed CYP1, CYP2, and CYP3. Within each P450 family, there are subfamilies designated by capital letters. Each subfamily generally contains multiple members, designated by Arabic numbers usually reflecting the order in which they were discovered. In general, orthologous P450s (the equivalent form in different species) are given a different final Arabic number. For example, CYP3A4 is a human liver P450 and is not present in other animals, although each species examined to date has CYP3A enzymes (i.e., CYP3A2, CYP3A6, etc.).

It is widely believed that the P450s involved in drug metabolism evolved as a mechanism to protect the body from potentially harmful chemicals present in the environment, particularly in the diet (4). According to this theory, plants produce potentially toxic chemicals (xenobiotics) to render themselves inedible to insects and higher life forms. In addition, spoilage of food sources often involves bacteria and fungi capable of producing potentially toxic xenobiotics. The introduction into the environment of each new xenobiotic in turn created selection pressure for insects and animals to develop specific P450s capable of metabolizing and rapidly eliminating that xenobiotic (if the food source could not be easily avoided).

A list of the major P450s involved in human drug metabolism is shown in Table 1. The most abundant single P450 in human liver is CYP3A4, and it has been estimated that this specific P450 may be involved in the metabolism of over 50% of drugs used clinically (5). As previously stated, once a drug undergoes P450-mediated (phase I) metabolism, the resultant metabolite is often conjugated in a phase II reaction prior to elimination from the body. However, in most instances examined to date, P450-mediated metabolism is rate-limiting in the elimination of the drug (6). A simple schematic diagram illustrating principles of P450 metabolism is shown in Fig. 1. Drugs either passively diffuse, or are actively transported, into the liver during passage through sinusoidal blood. Once inside the liver, drugs probably passively diffuse to the particular P450s capable of metabolizing them. With some drugs, a single P450 is involved in the majority of the metabolism. This is illustrated in Fig. 1 by drug A, which is only capable of binding to, and being metabolized by, CYP2D6. The resulting metabolite generally then undergoes phase II conjugation and the conjugated metabolite is frequently excreted back into the space of Disse, now more water soluble and more readily eliminated by the kidneys. Alternatively, the metabolite can be sorted to the bile canaliculus (not shown in Fig. 1) to be excreted in bile into the small intestine, now less likely to undergo enterohepatic cycling.

Many drugs can be metabolized by more than one P450. In Fig. 1, drug B is shown as being capable of binding to, and being metabolized by, CYP3A4. However, it can be seen that the top portion of the molecule could fit into the binding site of CYP2D6 (if drug B were rotated 180°). Drug B could therefore undergo two phase I reactions, one catalyzed by CYP3A4, the other by CYP2D6.

There are large interindividual differences in the activity profile of the liver P450s, and in many instances, this variation appears to account for interpatient differences in the pharmacokinetics of medications (5). The variation among patients in the activities of specific P450s can reflect both genetic and nongenetic factors.

V. GENETIC FACTORS INFLUENCING P450 ACTIVITY

Genetic mutations in part explain why there are large interindividual differences in the activities of many of the P450s (7–10). For example, both CYP2D6 and CYP2C19 are termed "polymorphic" enzymes because the population can be divided into distinct groups based on the relative activity of these enzymes. Approximately 5% of Caucasians completely lack CYP2D6 activity and therefore are CYP2D6 "poor metabolizers." Patients who are CYP2D6 poor metabolizers have been shown to have increased sensitivity to

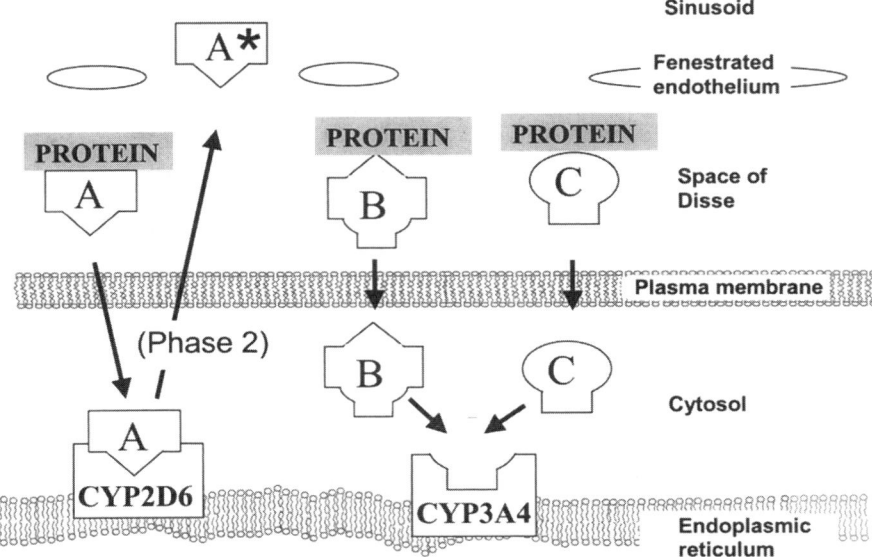

Figure 1 Handling of drugs by liver cytochromes P450. Illustrated are three hypothetical drugs, A, B, and C, which exist in blood bound to serum proteins. After the drugs enter the hepatocyte, they diffuse to the P450 they are capable of binding to, and being metabolized by. Refer to the text for a complete discussion of this process.

the effects of several drugs, including some medications commonly used to treat cardiac arrythmias, psychosis, and depression. The poor-metabolizer phenotype results from simultaneous inheritance of two of multiple known mutant CYP2D6 alleles (11). The incidence of CYP2D6 poor metabolizers varies substantially across different ethnic populations (12). For example, poor metabolizers are extremely unusual among Japanese (13).

The CYP2C19 poor-metabolizer phenotype also occurs in approximately 5% of Caucasians, but occurs in up to 20% of Asians (12). CYP2C19 poor metabolizers have been shown to have much higher blood levels of omeprazole than normal when treated with usual therapeutic doses (14). This appears to account for why CYP2C19 poor metabolizers have a higher cure rate for *Helicobacter* infection when treated with omeprazole-containing regimens (15). As is the case with CYP2D6, the poor-metabolizer phenotype also results from inheritance of two of several different mutant CYP2C19 alleles. In general, CYP2D6 and CYP2C19 poor-metabolizer phenotypes behave as autosomal recessive traits, with heterozygotes having metabolic capability that is intermediate between the normal and poor-metabolizer ranges.

Allelic mutations imparting diminished catalytic function have been described for other cytochromes P450, including CYP2C9 (16) and CYP2A6 (17), although individuals completely lacking these catalytically active enzymes have not yet been recognized. In addition, genetic mutations of unclear functional significance have been identified in CYP3A4 (18) and CYP2E1 (19) genes.

There is one example where genetic factors can cause abnormally high activity of a P450. Approximately 2% of Caucasians have gene duplication of CYP2D6 resulting in an "ultra rapid" metabolizer phenotype (9). These individuals exhibit unusually rapid

Table 1 Major Human Liver P450s

P450	Substrates	Inhibitors	Inducers
CYP1A2	Caffeine	Fluvoxamine	Omeprazole
	Clozapine	Furafylline[a]	Tobacco smoke
	Estradiol		
	Theophylline		
CYP2A6	Halothane	Methoxasalen[a]	—
	Nicotine		
CYP2C8	Rosiglitazone	—	Phenytoin
	Taxol		Rifampin
CYP2C9	Diclofenac	Sulfafenazole	Rifampin
	Ibuprofen		Secobarbital
	Tolbutamide		
	Warfarin		
CYP2C19	Omeprazole	Fluvoxamine	—
		Ketoconazole	
CYP2D6	Codeine	Fluoxetine	
	Chlorpromazine	Quinidine[a]	
	Despiramine		
	Dextromethorphan		—
	Encainide		
	Haloperidol		
	Metoprolol		
CYP2E1	Acetaminophen	Disulfiram[a]	Ethanol
	Halothane		Isoniazid
CYP3A4	Cyclosporin A	Delavirdine	Carbamazepine
	Estradiol	Erythromycin	Phenobarbital
	Indinavir	Grapefruit juice	Phenytoin
	Lovastatin	Ketoconazole	Rifampin
	Midazolam	Ritonavir	St. John's wort
	Nifedipine	Troleandomycin[a]	Troglitazone
	Quinidine		
	Docataxel		

[a] Used for selective inhibition in human studies.

clearance of at least some CYP2D6 substrates, and this can account for therapeutic failure of some medications. The incidence of ultrarapid metabolizers in non-Caucasian populations is currently under investigation.

VI. NONGENETIC FACTORS INFLUENCING P450 ACTIVITY

Concomitant disease and alterations in nutritional status can affect the activities of liver P450s (20). In addition, many drugs can alter the activities of P450s, resulting in drug interactions (21,22). Some drugs are known to inhibit the activity of specific P450s, reducing the elimination of drugs that require metabolism by that P450. Inhibition of cytochrome P450 activity can occur by a variety of mechanisms (23), but the most common form of inhibition reflects simple competition between two drugs for metabolism by the same P450. This is shown schematically in Fig. 1 where drugs B and C are each capable of binding to, and being metabolized by, CYP3A4. Hence, metabolism of drug B by CYP3A4 may be reduced in the presence of drug C, simply because drug C is physically interfering with drug B's ability to bind to the active site on CYP3A4. Of course, drug B could equally inhibit drug C's metabolism. Whether two drugs vying for metabolism by the same P450 will result in a clinically important interaction depends on a number of factors. These include the intracellular concentrations of each drug, the relative abundance of the P450, the importance of the P450 to the overall elimination of the drug, whether the metabolites generated by the P450 are pharmacologically active, and the relative safety (therapeutic index) of the drugs involved. Some clinically important interactions involving inhibition can be inferred from Table 1. For example, it is well known that cyclosporin A blood levels can rise to toxic levels in transplant recipients who receive concomitant treatment with erythromycin or ketoconazole, largely due to inhibition of CYP3A4 (24). Likewise, patients can develop toxicity from tricyclic antidepressants when they are concomitantly administered some selective serotonin reuptake inhibitors (SSRIs), owing to inhibition of CYP2D6 (25).

In addition to inhibition, a medication can sometimes result in an increase in the activity of a particular P450. In most cases, this "induction" in drug metabolism results from increased hepatocyte concentrations of a specific P450. Some medications that can induce P450s are shown in Table 1. Induction of P450 activity can occur by several mechanisms, but most commonly reflects an increase in the rate of transcription of the corresponding gene (26). In some instances, the cellular receptor involved in transcriptional activation has been identified. For example, induction of CYP3A4 by rifampin and antiseizure medications appears to involve a cytosolic receptor termed either the human pregnenolone-X receptor (hPXR) (27), or the steroid xenobiotic receptor (SXR) (28). The inducer binds the receptor, which then translocates to the nucleus, binding to the regulatory elements in the CYP3A4 gene. This results in increased transcription of the CYP3A4 gene, which in turn results in increases in the hepatocyte concentration of CYP3A4. It is currently unclear whether hPXR also mediates induction of CYP2C P450s by rifampin and certain antiseizure drugs. Induction of CYP1A2 involves a different receptor termed the arylhydrocarbon, or Ah, receptor (29). Aryl hydrocarbons in cigarette smoke, or the drug omeprazole, bind to the Ah receptor, mediating transcription of the CYP1A2 gene and increased production of the enzyme. Some P450s, such as CYP2D6 and CYP2A6, do not appear to be inducible.

Examples where induction causes clinically significant drug interactions can also be deduced from Table 1. When transplant recipients are treated with rifampin or certain antiseizure medications, blood levels of cyclosporin can fall to subtherapeutic levels due largely to induction of CYP3A4. These patients risk organ rejection unless their daily dose of cyclosporin is increased. Likewise, individuals treated with rifampin or antiseizure drugs risk therapeutic failure of oral contraceptives (CYP3A4) and warfarin (CYP2C9) (21,22).

VII. METHODS TO STUDY P450s IN THE LABORATORY

In general, the P450s involved in drug metabolism have been highly conserved in mammalian species. Orthologs to all of the major human liver P450s are found in the major animal species used in preclinical testing (mouse, rat, dog, and monkey). However, the catalytic specificity and regulation of orthologous forms are often not identical to their human counterparts (30). For example, rifampin is a very potent inducer of CYP3A4 in humans, whereas it is a weak inducer in the rat. Conversely, the synthetic steroid pregnenolone 16α-carbonitrile (PCN) is a highly effective inducer of CYP3A enzymes in the rat, but is only a very weak inducer in humans. These transspecies differences in CYP3A regulation have recently been explained by structural differences between the ligand-binding domains of the rodent and human PXR receptor. Transgenic techniques have recently been used to insert the human PXR receptor into PXR knockout mice (31). These mice show CYP3A induction after treatment with rifampin, but only weak induction after treatment with PCN (i.e., the inducer responsiveness pattern characteristic of humans and not mice).

In light of the above differences in catalytic activity and gene regulation, there is increasing disillusionment with the use of laboratory animals to predict drug metabolism and drug interactions in humans. Most pharmaceutical companies now have large programs using recombinant human P450s, human liver microsomes, and often cultured human hepatocytes to address these issues in a preclinical setting (32,33). These techniques can clearly demonstrate which P450s are capable of metabolizing a given drug. Extrapolating these results obtained in vitro to the in vivo situation has not been straightforward however, in large part because the concentrations of the drugs at the location of the P450 in vivo can rarely be estimated accurately from in vitro studies alone (34). As a result, there has been great interest in developing methods to study P450s in humans in vivo.

VIII. METHODS FOR STUDYING P450s IN MAN IN VIVO

It is now possible to use specific drugs as "probes" to monitor the activities of specific P450s in humans (35). Examples of some commonly used probes are shown in Table 2. For example, an individual's liver CYP3A4 activity can be assessed in a number of ways, including measuring the clearance of an intravenously injected dose of midazolam, or measuring the production of $^{14}CO_2$ in breath after an intravenous injection of [^{14}C N-methyl] erythromycin. Although considerable controversy still exists concerning the best probes to use in clinical studies, each of the listed probes has provided useful insight in

Table 2   P450-Specific Probes

P450	Test	Biomatrix
CYP1A2	Caffeine breath test	Breath
	Caffeine clearance	Plasma
	Caffeine MR	Urine
CYP3A4	Cortisol 6β-hydroxylation	Urine
	Erythromycin breath test	Breath
	Midazolam clearance	Plasma
CYP2C9	Tolbutamide clearance	Plasma
	Tolbutamide MR	Urine
CYP2C19	Mephenytoin S/R ratio	Urine
	Omeprazole clearance	Plasma
	Omeprazole hydroxylation index	Plasma
CYP2D6	Debrisoquine MR	Urine
	Dextromethorphan MR	Plasma, urine, saliva
CYP2E1	Chlorzoxazone clearance	Plasma

MR = metabolic ratio.

certain circumstances. For example, it is possible to determine whether a drug is an inducer or inhibitor of CYP3A4 activity by administering any of the CYP3A4 probes listed in Table 2 to subjects before and again after treatment with the drug. The parameter measured (i.e., breath $^{14}CO_2$ with the Erythromycin Breath Test, systemic clearance with midazolam, or urinary production of 6β-cortisol) will increase if the drug is an inducer of CYP3A4, and decrease if the drug is an inhibitor of CYP3A4. Another potential use of these probes is to guide dosing of drugs with narrow therapeutic indices. The probe-based test should predict the clearance of a drug if the P450 measured is rate-limiting in the elimination of the drug. For example, it has recently been shown that interpatient differences in the pharmacokinetics of taxotere correlate well with liver CYP3A4 activity as measured by the erythromycin breath test (36) or urinary 6β-cortisol (37).

It is also possible to utilize the inducers and inhibitors of specific P450s to gain insight into metabolism of a given drug. For example, if treatment of subjects with rifampin does not lead to accelerated clearance of a drug, this indicates that CYP3A4 and CYP2C enzymes are not rate-limiting in the elimination of that drug. Conversely, if treatment with ketoconazole does not reduce clearance of a drug, CYP3A4 cannot be an elimination-limiting pathway for metabolism of the drug. The best inhibitors to use in these studies are potent and selective for the target P450. In effect, these inhibitors create a temporary human equivalent of a P450 genetic "knockout" in mice. The contribution of a specific P450 can therefore be assessed in vivo by determining the pharmacokinetics of a drug in subjects before and again after that P450 has been chemically "knocked out." The most frequently used inhibitors of P450s are noted in Table 1. For example, administration of a single therapeutic dose of disulfiram results in greater than 90% inhibition of CYP2E1 activity, which lasts for hours (38). The effect of disulfiram is specific in that the catalytic activities of other major P450s are not affected [as measured by suitable probes (39)]. Another example is the antibiotic troleandomycin (TAO), which, when administered in the usual therapeutic dose, produces greater than 90% reduction in liver CYP3A4 activity that also persists for hours (40). Although less well studied in vivo than disulfiram, data obtained in human liver microsomes suggest that the effect of TAO is specific for CYP3A4 and other major P450s are not inhibited (41) Furafylline has also been used to chemically "knock out" CYP1A2 in humans (42), but this drug is not widely available. In addition, methoxsalen has been shown to significantly reduce CYP2A6 activity in vivo, but the specificity of the inhibition has not been established (43).

IX. ROLE OF P450s IN DRUG-INDUCED LIVER DISEASE

Most drugs that are capable of causing liver toxicity appear to do so through the generation of toxic metabolites in the liver. The critical role of metabolites in chemical-induced injury probably reflects the fact that in order to be absorbed into the body and reach the liver, chemicals must generally be lipophilic (fat soluble) and metabolically stable. Lipophilicity and metabolic stability are not typical properties of an intrinsic hepatotoxin. In the case of drugs, the role of metabolites probably also reflects the ability of routine preclinical animal testing to effectively screen parent molecules for intrinsic toxicity. If a drug produces liver toxicity in animals at doses close to those planned in humans, the drug is usually abandoned from further development. Toxicity resulting from metabolism of the drug in humans will be missed in preclinical studies if the animal species tested are not capable of generating toxic metabolites in sufficient quantity.

As discussed above, metabolism of drugs by P450s generally produces metabolites that are safely eliminated from the body. However, under certain circumstances P450s can generate reactive and potentially toxic metabolites. Indeed, the major enzymes implicated in the production of hepatotoxic metabolites are the P450s. The identical enzymes (Table 1) involved in the safe metabolism of drugs are also those that have been most implicated in the production of toxic metabolites. Species differences in P450 catalytic activities and regulation probably contribute to the imperfect ability of preclinical animal studies to identify human hepatotoxins.

X. SPECIFIC EXAMPLES

A. Acetaminophen

Acetaminophen is believed to cause toxicity in the liver owing to production of the *N*-acetyl benzoquinone amine metabolite (NAPQI). Studies with recombinant human liver enzymes suggested that this reactive metabolite could be produced by several P450s, including CYP2E1, CYP3A4, CYP1A2, and CYP2A6 (44–46). Investigators have approached addressing the relative importance of each of these enzymes in human studies using inducers and inhibitors of specific P450s. NAPQI formed from acetaminophen in the liver is conjugated to glutathione and eliminated as various thiol metabolites in urine. Hence, the total production of NAPQI can be estimated from the production of thiol metabolites eliminated in urine. It has been shown that urinary excretion of thiol metabolites is not increased in subjects who had been pretreated with omeprazole (47). As noted in Table 1, omeprazole treatment should have resulted in induction of CYP1A2 activity, especially since the investigators only studied subjects who were CYP2C19 poor metabolizers and who would therefore have had relatively high blood levels of omeprazole (14). The absence of an increase in NAPQI production after omeprazole treatment therefore suggests that CYP1A2 is not a substantial contributor to NAPQI production in humans receiving therapeutic doses of acetaminophen. Likewise, rifampin pretreatment did not produce a detectable increase in NAPQI production (48), indicating that CYP3A4 is likely to be at best a minor pathway for production of NAPQI from therapeutic doses of acetaminophen. However, pretreatment of subjects with the CYP2E1-specific inhibitor disulfiram resulted in a 69% reduction in production of NAPQI (48). Hence, although the in vitro studies indicated the potential involvement of multiple P450s, the in vivo studies in humans indicate that a single P450, CYP2E1, accounts for most of the NAPQI formed after therapeutic doses of acetaminophen. The enzymes responsible for production of the 30% of NAPQI formation uninhibited by disulfiram are currently unknown, but recent data suggest this may largely reflect CYP2A6 (46).

It should be noted that quite different conclusions regarding the role of P450s could be drawn from studies performed in rodents. For example, investigators have shown in rats that inhibition of CYP3A enzymes by TAO treatment substantially raises the LD_{50} (49) and treatment with inducers of CYP3A enzymes (50) lowers the LD_{50} of acetaminophen. These observations have been interpreted as implicating CYP3A enzymes as major contributors to NAPQI formation. These differences between rodents and humans probably in part reflect species differences in the catalytic activities P450s involved in NAPQI production (44). The differences may also reflect the very high doses of acetaminophen generally used in the rodent studies, whereas the human studies, by necessity, used nontoxic doses. It therefore remains possible that CYP3A4 could play a role in human toxicity produced by very large doses of acetaminophen.

Several case reports (51) exist of severe acetaminophen toxicity occurring in patients receiving treatment with various antiseizure medications, like phenytoin, that are known inducers of some P450s. These patients would not be expected to have induced CYP2E1 activity (Table 1). In one series of patients with acute liver failure (52), patients with acetaminophen liver injury who had been receiving treatment with antiseizure drugs appeared to have a worse outcome than other patients [although a more recent report (53) from the same institution did not verify these findings]. Three studies have directly addressed the effect of anti-seizure medications on production of NAPQI in humans (54–56). In each study, the total production of NAPQI (expressed as percent of administered dose) was not significantly increased by treatment with antiseizure drugs. However, the rate of elimination of acetaminophen was generally increased, and this appeared to be due to an increase in the rate of acetaminophen glucuronidation and sulfation. It is therefore likely that the antiseizure medications studied induce the phase II enzymes involved in the major pathway for elimination of acetaminophen, while having little effect on the aggregate activity of P450s involved in NAPQI production. These studies suggest that treatment with antiseizure drugs does not increase the risk of liver injury when acetaminophen is consumed as recommended. However, the increase in acetaminophen clearance caused by certain antiseizure drugs could result in more rapid wearing off of the analgesic effect of acetaminophen. A reasonable hypothesis to account for the association between antiseizure medications and acetaminophen liver toxicity is that treated epileptics unintentionally take more acetaminophen than recommended if they use symptom relief alone as the guide to dosing.

It is generally recognized that ethanol consumption can increase susceptibility to acetaminophen hepatotoxicity (57). Ethanol is a recognized inducer of CYP2E1 (Table 1), and ethanol induction of CYP2E1 provides an attractive explanation for incremental risks in ethanol consumers. Early animal (58,59) and human (60) studies attempting to directly show that ethanol consumption increases NAPQI production from acetaminophen have been unsuccessful. Indeed, these studies indicated that the presence of ethanol in the body actually reduces production of NAPQI. This paradoxical result has now been explained (61). Ethanol is a substrate for CYP2E1 and when ethanol is present in the body in substantial concentrations, a large proportion of the CYP2E1-binding sites in the liver are occupied by ethanol (62). Because ethanol has a high binding affinity for CYP2E1, the enzyme is less capable of metabolizing acetaminophen when ethanol is present, and hence the rate of production of NAPQI is reduced. This situation is directly analogous to the principle of competitive inhibition illustrated with drugs B and C in Fig. 1. An additional important finding is that when ethanol is bound to CYP2E1, the enzyme is stabilized against degradation, increasing its intracellular half-life (63). With prolonged intoxication, there is an accumulation of (ethanol-inhibited) CYP2E1. When ethanol is suddenly removed from the liver, the accumulated CYP2E1 becomes catalytically active, resulting in induced catalytic activity. The period of induction is relatively brief, however, since the uninhibited CYP2E1 degrades at its rapid baseline rate.

Slattery and co-workers (61,64) have developed mathematical models to describe the effect of "ligand binding" of substrates such as ethanol and isoniazid on CYP2E1 catalytic activity and accumulation within the liver. The model predicts that the magnitude of increase in CYP2E1 catalytic activity is a function of the blood concentration of the inducer/substrate as well as the total duration of exposure. In recent human studies, the model successfully predicted the magnitude of increase in rate of production of NAPQI from a test dose of acetaminophen after treatment with isoniazid (64) and ethanol (61). In the case of ethanol, an intravenous infusion to maintain a blood ethanol level at 100 mg/dL (a frequent legal limit of intoxification) for 6 h produced a mean 23% increase in NAPQI production immediately after ethanol was cleared from the body. This was close to the 21% increase predicted by the model. The ethanol exposure used in this study corresponds to the amount of ethanol present in roughly one six-pack of beer or one bottle of wine. Applying the model to additional ethanol consumption scenarios (61), the investigators predicted that the maximal increase in NAPQI production that could be produced by prolonged consumption of very large amounts of ethanol was 2.3-fold. The investigators also reported that the ethanol treatment had no effect on the activity of CYP3A4, as measured by the erythromycin breath test, verifying the specificity of ethanol's induction effects (61). This observation is at odds with data obtained in rodents and cultured human hepatocytes indicating that ethanol may induce CYP3A enzymes (67).

The model proposed by Slattery et al. (61,64) assumes that the entire inductive effect of ethanol on CYP2E1 is due to stabilization against degradation. However, it should be noted that ethanol in high concentrations has been shown to increase for CYP2E1 mRNA in rodent livers (68–70), and at least one report has indicated increased CYP2E1 mRNA levels in the livers of chronic human alcoholics (71). Nontheless, the approximate twofold increase in NAPQI production predicted by the model is similar to the twofold increase in CYP2E1 activity noted in chronic alcoholics (72).

B. Halothane

Halothane is known to undergo both reductive and oxidative metabolism in the liver (73). Reductive metabolism had been implicated in the low level of hepatocellular injury (serum ALT elevations) frequently observed following exposure to this anesthetic. The oxidative pathway of halothane metabolism has been implicated in producing the reactive metabolite [a trifluoroacetyl (TFA) intermediate], which can covalently bind to proteins in the liver cell. It is generally accepted that the rare life-threatening liver injury associated with halothane results from an immunogical response to the TFA proteins present on the liver cell (74).

Current evidence obtained in studies involving human liver microsomes and recombinant human liver P450s suggests that the oxidative pathway of halothane metabolism is catalyzed by CYP2E1 (75) whereas the reductive pathway is catalyzed by CYP2A6 and CYP3A4 (76). The role of CYP2E1 in halothane oxidative metabolism was confirmed in a clinical study (77) where the CYP2E1 specific inhibitor disulfiram was administered to patients prior to undergoing halothane anesthesia. The plasma and urine levels of fluoride (a by-product of the reductive pathway) were not significantly changed in patients receiving disulfiram, as would be expected if the reductive pathway is catalyzed by CYP2A6 and/or CYP3A4. However, disulfiram treatment resulted in a 70% inhibition in the plasma and urine levels of trifluoroacetic acid, the stable product of the oxidative pathway. In a subsequent study, inhibitors of CYP3A4 (TAO) and CYP2A6 (methoxasalen) were given to patients undergoing halothane anesthesia (78). A modest decrease in trifluoroacetic acid production was observed with methoxasalen, consistent with a minor role for CYP2A6 in the oxidative pathway.

C. Other Drugs

A variety of other studies have been performed to determine the role of specific P450s in liver disease produced by other drugs (79–81). In a few cases, positive results have been obtained. Five individuals who had completely recovered from liver toxicity due to perhexiline (an antianginal medication used in Europe) were administered debrisoquine to determine their CYP2D6 activity (Table 2) (82, 83). Four out of the five individuals were characterized as CYP2D6 poor metabolizers. This frequency was significantly greater than anticipated (5% in Caucasians). Perhexiline is believed to be metabolized by CYP2D6 and it is speculated that individuals deficient in CYP2D6 activity accumulate the drug in the liver. Toxicity could then either be produced by the parent drug or result from metabolites generated by alternate (non-CYP2D6) pathways of metabolism that must be relied upon in the CYP2D6 poor metabolizer.

Likewise, patients who have recovered from chlorpromazine-induced liver injury have been reported to have both a reduced ability to perform sulfoxidation of chlorpromazine (84) and an unusually high rate of hydroxylation of the drug (84). The enzymes involved in sulfoxidation of chlorpromazine are not known, but the hydroxylation pathway appears to be catalyzed by CYP2D6 (85). A logical, but as yet untested, hypothesis is that individuals predisposed to chlorpromazine-induced liver injury are both ultrarapid metabolizers of CYP2D6 (due to gene duplication) and poor sulfoxidators (reflecting polymorphism as an as-yet-unidentified gene). The impaired sulfoxidation hypothesis has been called into question because of methodological issues in phenotyping patients (85a).

In most instances to date, however, attempts to link susceptibility to liver toxicity to variation in activity of specific P450s have failed. For example, polymorphic expression of CYP2D6 has not appeared to correlate with susceptibility to liver toxicity due to several CYP2D6 substrates, including metoprolol, amitryptiline, or amodiaquine (86). Extensive studies with the anti-Alzheimer's treatment tacrine have also not yielded clear results. Tacrine treatment is associated with serum ALT elevations greater than three times the upper limit of normal in 25% of treated patients, and serum ALT levels greater than 20 times the upper limit of normal in 2% of treated patients (87). In vitro studies suggested that reactive metabolites, capable of covalent binding to proteins, were produced from tacrine by CYP1A2 (88). CYP1A2 activity in the population does not appear to be polymorphic (i.e., there are not distinct subpopulations with high or low activity). Nonetheless, the catalytic activity CYP1A2 has been shown to vary at least 40-fold among patients (89). These observations led to the hypothesis that patients with high CYP1A2 activity might be those at greatest risk for tacrine liver toxicity. To test this hypothesis, caffeine was administered as a probe of CYP1A2 activity to patients just before they received treatment with tacrine (90). No correlation was observed between CYP1A2 activity and the incidence or magnitude of serum ALT elevations. However, in a subsequent study, the CYP1A2 activity was shown to correlate reasonably well with the apparent oral clearance of tacrine (91). This is explained by the fact that the CYP1A2 catalyzes the major (nontoxic) pathways of metabolism of tacrine as well as production of the putative reactive metabolite(s).

The reason why there has been relatively little success applying our knowledge of P450s to the prediction of those at risk for drug-induced liver disease probably reflects multiple factors. First, the rate of production of a toxic metabolite by a given P450 is just one of many variables that are likely to determine whether toxicity actually occurs. In addition, most of the hypotheses that have been tested to date involve examination of the major P450 involved in the overall metabolism of the drug in question. Toxic metabolites are often the result of minor pathways of metabolism that have yet to be characterized. Indeed, a major problem is that the reactivity of toxic metabolites often makes them inherently difficult to "trap" and identify. An example of this may be diclofenac. Treatment with this NSAID is associated with serum ALT elevations in up to 15% of treated patients, and cases of liver failure have been attributed to the drug (92). The major pathway of metabolism of diclofenac (and most nonsteroidal anti-inflammatory drugs) is 4-hydroxylation catalyzed by CYP2C9 (93). A recent attempt to link functional mutations in CYP2C9 to risk of liver injury was unsuccessful (94). However, recent evidence indicates that the toxicity may be mediated by one of two 5-hydroxylated metabolites that appear to be produced by CYP2C19 (95). An untested hypothesis is that susceptibility to toxicity would be increased in those patients who are both deficient in CYP2C9 activity and relatively high in CYP2C19 activity.

D. Anti-P450 Antibodies

Liver disease due to several different drugs is associated with circulating antibodies to P450s (96,97). These antibodies were first detected by examining the ability of serum to react with mouse liver, stomach, and kidney slices placed on a single glass slide (this is a standard clinical laboratory assay used to detect other autoantibodies, including mitochondrial, smooth muscle, etc). Serum from patients with certain types of drug-induced liver disease reacted with endoplasmic reticulum in the liver and kidney cells, producing a characteristic fluorescent pattern. The antibodies detected were therefore termed liver kidney microsomal (LKM) antibodies. Some, but not all, LKM antibodies react with P450s. The current concept for formation of anti-P450 antibodies is that a very reactive metabolite is formed from the drug by the P450, and this metabolite binds covalently to the enzyme. In Fig. 1, this would occur if the metabolite of drug A generated by CYP2D6 reacted directly with the CYP2D6 protein (i.e., prior to phase II metabolism), generating an antigenic molecule. Anti-P450 antibodies generally recognize both the covalently modified P450 (protein with attached metabolite) and the unmodified (native) P450. Controversy remains over whether these antibodies actually mediate an immune attack on the liver, as no one has yet convincingly shown that they can cause liver disease in a living animal model. It remains possible that the antibodies are an epiphenomenon, resulting only after the antigens are released into circulation as hepatocytes are lysed by other mechanisms. However, several lines of evidence indicate that P450s are present in low abundance on the outside of the liver plasma membrane (96,97). Hence, these antigens may be presented to the immune system prior to hepatocyte lysis. Regardless of whether they mediate drug-induced liver disease, the presence of anti-P450 antibodies appears to indicate that P450s are producing metabolites reactive enough to covalently bind to liver proteins. In addition, these antibodies can be employed in immunochemical techniques to identify which specific human P450 is involved in generating the reactive metabolite, even if the structure of the reactive metabolite is unknown.

Halothane hepatitis is generally recognized to be immunologically mediated and is associated with circulating antibodies to both native and TFA-modified CYP2E1 (98). This is consistent with TFA intermediate production from halothane by CYP2E1. The fact that multiple other hepatocyte proteins (in addition to CYP2E1) are recognized by circulating antibodies (99) suggests that the TFA radical is sufficiently stable to diffuse away from the enzyme after it is produced to react with more distant proteins.

Anti-CYP2C9 antibodies are characteristically found in patients with tienilic acid–induced hepatitis (96). Autoantibodies to other liver proteins are typically absent. It has been shown that CYP2C9 produces a reactive metabolite from tienilic acid (believed to be a thiophene sulfoxide), which, once it leaves the P450 active site, will rapidly react with water to form 5-hydroxy tienilic acid. However, this metabolite can also covalently bind to CYP2C9, creating a new antigen. The absence of antibodies to other liver proteins (unlike those observed in halothane hepatitis) probably reflects the fact that the thiophene sulfoxide has a life span too short to allow its intact migration to proteins other than CYP2C9.

Anti-CYP1A2 antibodies are characteristically found in patients with liver injury due to dihydralazine (96). As expected, it has been shown that a reactive metabolite is produced from dihydralazine by CYP1A2. CYP1A2 is not present in the kidney, and this accounts for why the circulating antibodies only react with liver endoplasmic reticulum, creating LM antibodies.

It should also be noted that circulating antibodies to rat, but not human, P450s have been found in patients with liver injury due to several anticonvulsants (100). The reasons why these antibodies do not react with human P450s are unknown; it has been speculated that the human P450s may require modification by the reactive metabolite(s) to be recognized [101].

XI. OTHER P450-RELATED MECHANISMS FOR DRUG-INDUCED LIVER DISEASE

It has been shown that some P450s, particularly CYP2E1, are capable of generating reactive oxygen species simply as a function of their presence in the cells (102). Hence, induction of CYP2E1 as a consequence of isoniazid or ethanol treatment could lead to an increase in production of reactive oxygen species, oxidative stress, and liver injury without production of specific toxic metabolites.

It is also known that inducers of CYP3A4 are generally associated with liver toxicity in humans. Examples include phenytoin, carbamazepine, macrolide antibiotics, and troglitazone. It would be expected that induction of CYP3A4 would increase susceptibility to toxicity due to drugs converted to toxic metabolites by CYP3A4. Recent studies have suggested another mechanism whereby CYP3A4 inducers may cause liver disease. As discussed earlier, the cytoplasmic receptor hPXR (or SXR) has been shown to mediate drug induction of CYP3A4. In transgenic animals made to express an activated form of hPXR, liver disease was reported to be present in the absence of exposure to drugs or other chemicals (31). It is interesting to speculate that activation of SXR may mediate liver toxicity, perhaps through a mechanism independent of P450 induction.

REFERENCES

1. Gillette JR. Keynote address: man, mice, microsomes, metabolites, and mathematics 40 years after the revolution. Drug Metab Rev 1995; 27:1–44.
2. Pessayre D. Role of reactive metabolites in drug-induced hepatitis. J Hepatol 1995; 23:16–24.
3. Wrighton SA, VandenBranden M, Ring BJ. The human drug metabolizing cytochromes P450. J Pharmacokinet Biopharmaceut 1996; 24:461–473.
4. Nebert DW. Multiple forms of inducible drug-metabolizing enzymes: a reasonable mechanism by which any organism can cope with adversity. Mol Cell Biochem 1979; 27:27–46.
5. Benet LZ KD, Sheiner LB. Pharmacokinetics: the dynamics of drug absorption, distribution, and elimination. In JG Hardman, PB Molinoff, et al., eds. Goodman and Gilman's The Pharmacological Basis of Therapeutics. New York: McGraw-Hill, 1996:3–29.
6. Bertz RJ, Granneman GR. Use of in vitro and in vivo data to estimate the likelihood of metabolic pharmacokinetic interactions. Clin Pharmacokinet 1997; 32:210–258.

7. Tanaka E. Update: genetic polymorphism of drug metabolizing enzymes in humans. J Clin Pharm Ther 1999; 24:323–329.

8. Meyer UA, Zanger UM. Molecular mechanisms of genetic polymorphisms of drug metabolism. Ann Rev Pharmacol Toxicol 1997; 37:269–296.

9. Hasler JA. Pharmacogenetics of cytochromes P450. Mol Aspects Med 1999; 20:12–24, 25–137.

10. Evans WE, Relling MV. Pharmacogenomics: translating functional genomics into rational therapeutics. Science 1999; 286:487–491.

11. Marez D, Legrand M, Sabbagh N, et al. Polymorphism of the cytochrome P450 CYP2D6 gene in a European population: characterization of 48 mutations and 53 alleles, their frequencies and evolution. Pharmacogenetics 1997; 7:193–202.

12. Chida M, Yokoi T, Kosaka Y, et al. Genetic polymorphism of CYP2D6 in the Japanese population. Pharmacogenetics 1999; 9:601–605.

13. Bertilsson L. Geographical/interracial differences in polymorphic drug oxidation. Current state of knowledge of cytochromes P450 (CYP) 2D6 and 2C19. Clin Pharmacokinet 1995; 29:192–209.

14. Sohn DR, Kobayashi K, Chiba K, Lee KH, Shin SG, Ishizaki T. Disposition kinetics and metabolism of omeprazole in extensive and poor metabolizers of *S*-mephenytoin 4′-hydroxylation recruited from an Oriental population. J Pharmacol Exp Ther 1992; 262: 1195–1202.

15. Furuta T, Ohashi K, Kamata T, et al. Effect of genetic differences in omeprazole metabolism on cure rates for *Helicobacter pylori* infection and peptic ulcer. Ann Intern Med 1998; 129: 1027–1030.

16. Yamazaki H, Inoue K, Chiba K, et al. Comparative studies on the catalytic roles of cytochrome P450 2C9 and its Cys- and Leu-variants in the oxidation of warfarin, flurbiprofen, and diclofenac by human liver microsomes. Biochem Pharmacol 1998; 56:243–251.

17. Pelkonen O, Ratio A, Raunio H, Pasanen M. CYP2A6: a human coumarin 7-hydroxylase. Toxicology 2000; 144:139–147.

18. Sata F, Sapone A, Elizondo G, et al. CYP3A4 allelic variants with amino acid substitutions in exons 7 and 12: evidence for an allelic variant with altered catalytic activity. Clin Pharmacol Ther 2000; 67:48–56.

19. Wong NA, Rae F, Simpson KJ, Murray GD, Harrison DJ. Genetic polymorphisms of cytochrome p4502E1 and susceptibility to alcoholic liver disease and hepatocellular carcinoma in a white population: a study and literature review, including meta-analysis. Mol Pathol 2000; 53:88–93.

20. Morgan ET, Sewer MB, Iber H, et al. Physiological and pathophysiological regulation of cytochrome P450. Drug Metab Dispos 1998; 26:1232–1240.

21. Flockhart DA, Oesterheld JR. Cytochrome P450-mediated drug interactions. Child Adolesc Psychiatr Clin North Am 2000; 130–141.

22. Guengerich FP. Role of cytochrome P450 enzymes in drug-drug interactions. Adv Pharmacol (NY) 1997; 43:7–35.

23. Szklarz GD, Halpert JR. Molecular basis of P450 inhibition and activation: implications for drug development and drug therapy. Drug Metab Dispos 1998; 26:1179–1184.

24. Leichtman A, Watkins PB. The molecular basis of cyclosporin A metabolism, pharmacokinetics, and drug interactions. Organ Cell Transplant 1999; 2:177–182.

25. Greenblatt DJ, von Moltke LL, Harmatz JS, Shader RI. Drug interactions with newer antidepressants: role of human cytochromes P450 [see comments]. J Clin Psychiatry 1998; 59: 19–27.

26. Waxman DJ. P450 gene induction by structurally diverse xenochemicals: central role of nuclear receptors CAR, PXR, and PPAR. Arch Biochem Biophys 1999; 369:11–23.

27. Lehmann JM, McKee DD, Watson MA, Wilson TM, Moore JT, Kliewer SA. The human orphan nuclear receptor PXR is activated by compounds that regulate CYP3A4 gene expression and cause drug interactions. J Clin Invest 1998; 102:1016–1023.

28. Blumberg B, Sabbagh W, Jr., Juguilon H, et al. SXR, a novel steroid and xenobiotic-sensing nuclear receptor. Genes Dev 1998; 12:3195–3205.

29. Poellinger L. Mechanistic aspects—the dioxin (aryl hydrocarbon) receptor. Food Addit Contam 2000; 17:261–266.

30. Sharer JE, Shipley LA, Vandenbranden MR, Binkley SN, Wrighton SA. Comparisons of phase I and phase II in vitro hepatic enzyme activities of human, dog, rhesus monkey, and cynomolgus monkey. Drug Metab Dispos 1995; 23:1231–1241.

31. Xie W, Barwick JL, Downes M, et al. Humanized xenobiotic response in mice expressing nuclear receptor SXR. Nature 2000; 406:435–439.

32. Rodrigues AD. Integrated cytochrome P450 reaction phenotyping: attempting to bridge the gap between cDNA-expressed cytochromes P450 and native human liver microsomes. Biochem Pharmacol 1999; 57:465–480.

33. Li AP, Maurel P, Gomez-Lechon MJ, Cheng LC, Jurima-Romet M. Preclinical evaluation of drug-drug interaction potential: present studies of the application of primary human hepatocytes in the evaluation of cytochrome P450 induction. Chem Biol Interact 1997; 107:5–16.

34. Ito K, Iwatsubo T, Kanamitsu S, Nakajima Y, Sugiyama Y. Quantitative prediction of in vivo drug clearance and drug interactions from in vitro data on metabolism, together with binding and transport. Annu Rev Pharmacol Toxicol 1998; 38:461–499.

35. Streetman DS, Bertino JS, Jr., Nafziger AN. Phenotyping of drug-metabolizing enzymes in adults: a review of in-vivo cytochrome P450 phenotyping probes. Pharmacogenetics 2000; 10:187–216.

36. Hirth J, Watkins PB, Strawderman M, Schott A, Bruno R, Baker LH. The effect of an individual's cytochrome CYP3A4 activity on docetaxel clearance [see comments]. Clin Cancer Res 2000; 6:1255–1258.

37. Yamamoto N, Tamura T, Kamiya Y, Sekine I, Kunitoh H, Saijo N. Correlation between docetaxel clearance and estimated cytochrome P450 activity by urinary metabolite of exogenous cortisol. J Clin Oncol 2000; 18:2301–2308.

38. Kharasch ED, Thummel KE, Mhyre J, Lillibridge JH. Single-dose disulfiram inhibition of chlorzoxazone metabolism: a clinical probe for P450 2E1. Clin Pharmacol Ther 1993; 53:643–650.

39. Kharasch ED, Hankins DC, Jubert C, Thummel KE, Taraday JK. Lack of single-dose disulfiram effects on cytochrome P-450 2C9, 2C19, 2D6, and 3A4 activities: evidence for specificity toward P-450 2E1. Drug Metab Dispos 1999; 27:717–723.

40. Kharasch ED, Russell M, Mautz D, et al. The role of cytochrome P450 3A4 in alfentanil clearance. Implications for interindividual variability in disposition and perioperative drug interactions. Anesthesiology 1997; 87:36–50.

41. Newton DJ, Wang RW, Lu AY. Cytochrome P450 inhibitors. Evaluation of specificities in the in vitro metabolism of therapeutic agents by human liver microsomes. Drug Metab Dispos 1995; 23:154–158.

42. Sesardic D, Boobis AR, Murray BP, et al. Furafylline is a potent and selective inhibitor of cytochrome P450IA2 in man. Br J Clin Pharmacol 1990; 29:651–663.

43. Kharasch ED, Hankins DC, Taraday JK. Single-dose methoxsalen effects on human cytochrome P-450 2A6 activity. Drug Metab Dispos 2000; 28:28–33.

44. Patten CJ, Thomas PE, Guy RL, et al. Cytochrome P450 enzymes involved in acetaminophen activation by rat and human liver microsomes and their kinetics. Chem Res Toxicol 1993; 6:511–518.

45. Thummel KE, Lee CA, Kunze KL, Nelson SD, Slattery JT. Oxidation of acetaminophen to *N*-acetyl-*p*-aminobenzoquinone imine by human CYP3A4. Biochem Pharmacol 1993; 45:1563–1569.

46. Chen W, Koenigs LL, Thompson SJ, et al. Oxidation of acetaminophen to its toxic quinone imine and nontoxic catechol metabolites by baculovirus-expressed and purified human cytochromes P450 2E1 and 2A6. Chem Res Toxicol 1998; 11:295–301.

47. Sarich T, Kalhorn T, Magee S, et al. The effect of omeprazole pretreatment on acetaminophen metabolism in rapid and slow metabolizers of *S*-mephenytoin. Clin Pharmacol Ther 1997; 62:21–28.

48. Manyike PT, Kharasch ED, Kalhorn TF, Slattery JT. Contribution of CYP2E1 and CYP3A to acetaminophen reactive metabolite formation. Clin Pharmacol Ther 2000; 67: 275–282.

49. Sinclair JF, Szakacs JG, Wood SG, et al. Acetaminophen hepatotoxicity precipitated by short-term treatment of rats with ethanol and isopentanol: protection by triacetyloleandomycin, Biochem Pharmacol 2000; 59:445–454.

50. Walker BE, Kelleher J, Dixon MF, Losowsky MS. The effect of phenobarbitone pretreatment on paracetamol toxicity. Biomedicine 1973; 19:465–468.

51. Brackett CC, Bloch JD. Phenytoin as a possible cause of acetaminophen hepatotoxicity: case report and review of the literature. Pharmacotherapy 2000; 20:229–233.

52. Bray GP, Harrison PM, O'Grady JG, Tredger JM, Williams R. Long-term anticonvulsant therapy worsens outcome in paracetamol-induced fulminant hepatic failure [see comments]. Hum Exp Toxicol 1992; 11:265–270.

53. Makin AJ, Wendon J, Williams R. A 7-year experience of severe acetaminophen-induced hepatotoxicity (1987–1993). Gastroenterology 1995; 109:1907–1916.

54. Prescott LF, Critchley JA, Balali-Mood M, Pentland B, Effects of microsomal enzyme induction on paracetamol metabolism in man. Br J Clin Pharmacol 1981; 12:149–153.

55. Miners JO, Attwood J, Birkett DJ. Determinants of acetaminophen metabolism: effect of inducers and inhibitors of drug metabolism on acetaminophen's metabolic pathways. Clin Pharmacol Ther 1984; 35:480–486.

56. Tomlinson B, Young RP, Ng MC, Anderson PJ, Kay R, Critchley JA. Selective liver enzyme induction by carbamazepine and phenytoin in Chinese epileptics. Eur J Clin Pharmacol 1996; 50:411–415.

57. Zimmerman HJ, Maddrey WC. Acetaminophen (paracetamol) hepatotoxicity with regular intake of alcohol: analysis of instances of therapeutic misadventure [published erratum appears in Hepatology 1995; 22(6):1898]. Hepatology 1995; 22:767–773.

58. Sato C, Nakano M, Lieber CS. Prevention of acetaminophen-induced hepatotoxicity by acute ethanol administration in the rat: comparison with carbon tetrachloride-induced hepatoxicity. J Pharmacol Exp Ther 1981; 218:805–810.

59. Altomare E, Leo MA, Lieber CS. Interaction of acute ethanol administration with acetaminophen metabolism and toxicity in rats fed alcohol chronically. Alcoholism Clin Exp Res 1984; 8:405–408.

60. Banda PW, Quart BD. The effect of mild alcohol consumption on the metabolism of acetaminophen in man. Res Commun Chem Pathol Pharmacol 1982; 38:57–70.

61. Thummel KE, Slattery JT, Ro H, et al. Ethanol and production of the hepatotoxic metabolite of acetaminophen in healthy adults. Clin Pharmacol Ther 2000; 67:591–599.

62. Lieber C. Cytochrome P-4502E1: its physiological and pathological role. Physiol Rev 1997; 77:517–544.

63. Roberts BJ, Song BJ, Soh Y, Park SS, Shoaf SE. Ethanol induces CYP2E1 by protein stabilization. Role of ubiquitin conjugation in the rapid degradation of CYP2E1. J Biol Chem 1995; 270:29632–29635.

64. Chien JY, Thummel KE, Slattery JT. Pharmacokinetic consequences of induction of CYP2E1 by ligand stabilization. Drug Metab Dispos 1997; 25:1165–1175.

65. Murphy R, Swartz R, Watkins PB. Severe acetaminophen toxicity in a patient receiving isoniazid [published erratum appears in Ann Intern Med 1991; 114(3):253] [see comments]. Ann Intern Med 1990; 113:799–800.

66. Crippin JS. Acetaminophen hepatotoxicity: potentiation by isoniazid. Am J Gastroenterol 1993; 88:590–592.

67. Kostrubsky VE, Strom SC, Wood SG, Wrighton SA, Sinclair PR, Sinclair JF. Ethanol and

isopentanol increase CYP3A and CYP2E in primary cultures of human hepatocytes. Arch Biochem Biophys 1995; 322:516–520.

68. Kubota S, Lasker JM, Lieber CS. Molecular regulation of ethanol-inducible cytochrome P450-IIEI in hamsters. Biochem Biophys Res Commun 1988; 150:304–310.

69. Ronis MJ, Huang J, Crouch J, et al. Cytochrome P450 CYP 2E1 induction during chronic alcohol exposure occurs by a two-step mechanism associated with blood alcohol concentrations in rats. J Pharmacol Exp Ther 1993; 264:944–950.

70. Tsutsumi M, Lasker JM, Takahashi T, Lieber CS. In vivo induction of hepatic P4502E1 by ethanol: role of increased enzyme synthesis. Arch Biochem Biophys 1993; 304:209–218.

71. Takahashi T, Lasker JM, Rosman AS, Lieber CS. Induction of cytochrome P-4502E1 in the human liver by ethanol is caused by a corresponding increase in encoding messenger RNA. Hepatology 1993; 17:236–245.

72. Girre C, Lucas D, Hispard E, Menez C, Dally S, Menez JF. Assessment of cytochrome P4502E1 induction in alcoholic patients by chlorzoxazone pharmacokinetics. Biochem Pharmacol 1994; 47:1503–1508.

73. Ray DC, Drummond GB. Halothane hepatitis. Br J Anaesth 1991; 67:84–99.

74. Gut J, Christen U, Huwyler J. Mechanisms of halothane toxicity: novel insights. Pharmacol Ther 1993; 58:133–155.

75. Raucy JL, Kraner JC, Lasker JM. Bioactivation of halogenated hydrocarbons by cytochrome P4502E1. Crit Rev Toxicol 1993; 23:1–20.

76. Spracklin DK, Thummel KE, Kharasch ED. Human reductive halothane metabolism in vitro is catalyzed by cytochrome P450 2A6 and 3A4. Drug Metab Dispos 1996; 24:976–983.

77. Kharasch ED, Hankins D, Mautz D, Thummel KE. Identification of the enzyme responsible for oxidative halothane metabolism: implications for prevention of halothane hepatitis. Lancet 1996; 347:1367–1371.

78. Kharasch ED, Hankins DC, Fenstamaker K, Cox K. Human halothane metabolism, lipid peroxidation, and cytochromes P(450)2A6 and P(450)3A4. Eur J Clin Pharmacol 2000; 55: 853–859.

79. Park BK, Pirmohamed M, Kitteringham NR. The role of cytochrome P450 enzymes in hepatic and extrahepatic human drug toxicity. Pharmacol Ther 1995; 68:385–424.

80. Fontana RJ, Watkins PB. Genetic predisposition to drug-induced liver disease. Gastroenterol Clin North Am 1995; 24:811–838.

81. Larrey PG. Genetic predisposition to drug-induced hepatotoxicity. J Hepatol 1997; 26:12–21.

82. Morgan MY, Reshef R, Shah RR, Oates NS, Smith RL, Sherlock S. Impaired oxidation of debrisoquine in patients with perhexiline liver injury. Gut 1984; 25:1057–1064.

83. Satz N, Tauber M, Streuli R, Spycher MA, Maurer R. Perhexiline maleate–induced hepatitis. Hepato-Gastroenterology 1991; 38:314–316.

84. Watson RG, Olomu A, Clements D, Waring RH, Mitchell S, Elias E. A proposed mechanism for chlorpromazine jaundice—defective hepatic sulphoxidation combined with rapid hydroxylation. J Hepatol 1988; 7:72–78.

85. Brosen K, Gram LF. Clinical significance of the sparteine/debrisoquine oxidation polymorphism. Eur J Clin Pharmacol 1989; 36:537–547.

85a. Hofmann U, Eichelbaum M, Seefried S, Meese C. Identification of thiodiglycolic acid, thiodiglycolic acid sulfoxide, and (3-carboxymethyl-thio)lactic acid as major human biotransformation products of S-carboxymethyl-L-cysteine. Drug Metab Dispos 1990; 19:222–226.

86. Larrey D, Tinel M, Amouyal G, et al. Genetically determined oxidation polymorphism and drug hepatotoxicity. Study of 51 patients. J Hepatol 1989; 8:158–164.

87. Watkins PB, Zimmerman HJ, Knapp MJ, Gracon SI, Lewis KW. Hepatotoxic effects of tacrine administration in patients with Alzheimer's disease [see comments.] JAMA 1994; 271:992–998.

88. Spaldin V, Madden S, Pool WF, Woolf TF, Park BK. The effect of enzyme inhibition on

the metabolism and activation of tacrine by human liver microsomes. Br J Clin Pharmacol 1994; 38:15–22.

89. Shimada T, Yamazaki H, Mimura M, Inui Y, Guengerich FP. Interindividual variations in human liver cytochrome P-450 enzymes involved in the oxidation of drugs, carcinogens and toxic chemicals: studies with liver microsomes of 30 Japanese and 30 Caucasians. J Pharmacol Exp Ther 1994; 270:414–423.

90. Fontana RJ, Turgeon DK, Woolf TF, Knapp MJ, Foster NL, Watkins PB. The caffeine breath test does not identify patients susceptible to tacrine hepatotoxicity. Hepatology 1996; 23: 1429–1435.

91. Fontana RJ, deVries TM, Woolf TF, et al. Caffeine based measures of CYP1A2 activity correlate with oral clearance of tacrine in patients with Alzheimer's disease. Br J Clin Pharmacol 1998; 46:221–228.

92. Banks AT, Zimmerman HJ, Ishak KG, Hartner JG. Diclofenac-associated hepatotoxicity: analysis of 180 cases reported to the Food and Drug Administration as adverse reactions. Hepatology 1995; 22:820–827.

93. Miners JO, Birkett DJ. Cytochrome P4502C9: an enzyme of major importance in human drug metabolism. Brit J Clin Pharmacol 1998; 45:525–538.

94. Aithal GP, Leathart JBS, Daly AK. Relationship of polymorphism in CYP2C9 to genetic susceptibility to diclofenac-induced hepatitis. Pharmacogenetics 2000; 10:511–518.

95. Bort R, Ponsoda X, Jover R, Gomez-Lechon MJ, Castell JV. Diclofenac toxicity to hepatocytes: a role for drug metabolism in cell toxicity. J Pharmacol Exp Ther 1999; 288:65–72.

96. Robin MA, Le Roy M, Descatoire V, Pessayre D. Plasma membrane cytochromes P450 as neoantigens and autoimmune targets in drug-induced hepatitis. J Hepatol 1997; 26:23–30.

97. Manns MP, Obermayer-Straub P. Cytochromes P450 and uridine triphosphate-glucuronosyl-transferases: model autoantigens to study drug-induced, virus-induced, and autoimmune liver disease. Hepatology 1997; 26:1054–1066.

98. Eliasson E, Kenna JG. Cytochrome P450 2E1 is a cell surface autoantigen in halothane hepatitis. Mol Pharmacol 1996; 50:573–582.

99. Knight TL, Scatchard KM, Van Pelt FN, Kenna JG. Sera from patients with halothane hepatitis contain antibodies to halothane-induced liver antigens which are not detectable by immunoblotting [published erratum appears in J Pharmacol Exp Ther 1995 272(2):962]. Pharmacol Exp Ther 1994; 270:1325–1333.

100. Leeder JS, Riley RJ, Cook VA, Spielberg SP. Human anti-cytochrome P450 antibodies in aromatic anticonvulsant-induced hypersensitivity reactions. J Pharmacol Exp Ther 1992; 263: 360–367.

101. Leeder JS, Gaedigk A, Lu X, Cook VA. Epitone mapping studies with human anti-cytochrome P450 3A antibodies. Mol Pharmacol 1996; 49:234–243.

102. Goasduff T, Cederbaum AI. NADPH-dependent microsomal electron transfer increases degradation of CYP2E1 by the proteasome complex: role of reactive oxygen species. Arch Biochem Biophys 1999; 370:258–270.

3

Oxidative Stress, Antioxidant Defense, and Liver Injury

HARTMUT JAESCHKE

University of Arkansas for Medical Sciences, Little Rock, Arkansas, U.S.A.

I. INTRODUCTION

The liver, the bodies' largest solid internal organ, performs a substantial number of vital metabolic functions and is the main organ for drug and xenobiotic metabolism. These functions require an extensive aerobic metabolism to generate sufficient quantities of ATP in mitochondria. However, this metabolic activity causes a continuous formation of reactive oxygen species. In addition, drug metabolism and potential cell injury can dramatically increase the oxidant stress burden for each individual cell and the organ. This review will focus on the general discussion of reactive oxygen and nitrogen formation, description of antioxidant systems in different cellular and vascular compartments, and analysis of potential adverse consequences of excessive oxidant stress in the liver.

II. REACTIVE OXYGEN AND NITROGEN INTERMEDIATES

Molecular oxygen ($^3O_2$) can be reduced by one-electron steps to superoxide (O_2^-), hydrogen peroxide (H_2O_2), the hydroxyl radical ($OH^•$) and then water (Fig. 1). Superoxide is not very stable and dismutates rapidly to form hydrogen peroxide and singlet oxygen

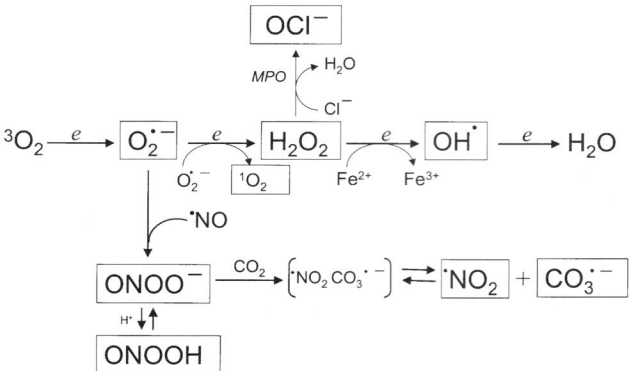

Figure 1 Reactive oxygen species generated by one-electron reduction steps of molecular oxygen ($^3O_2$). During the spontaneous dismutation of superoxide (O_2^-), singlet oxygen ($^1O_2$) is formed. If nitric oxide ($^•NO$) is present, superoxide reacts with NO and forms peroxynitrite ($ONOO^-$) and peroxynitrous acid (ONOOH). Peroxynitrite reacts with carbon dioxide to generate nitrating species such as the ($^•NO_2$) radical. Neutrophils release the enzyme myeloperoxidase to form hypochlorite (OCl^-).

($^1O_2$), another reactive oxygen species. However, in the presence of nitric oxide ($^•NO$), superoxide reacts preferably with NO to generate peroxynitrite ($ONOO^-$). The rate of peroxynitrite formation depends on the concentrations of both NO and superoxide (first-order kinetics) and this reaction is near diffusion controlled (1,2). With the ubiquitous presence of carbon dioxide (CO_2)/bicarbonate in vivo, peroxynitrite reacts rapidly with CO_2 to form reactive intermediates, which are highly effective oxidizing and nitrating species (1). In addition, peroxynitrite can be protonated to form peroxynitrous acid (ONOOH), which is a powerful oxidant. Hydrogen peroxide can be reductively cleaved to the extremely reactive hydroxyl radical in the presence of transition metals (Fenton reaction). However, if phagocytes release myeloperoxidase, hypochlorite (OCl^-), another potent oxidant, is generated. In addition to the described primary reactive intermediates (Fig. 1), a number of secondary radicals can be formed, e.g., alkyl ($R^•$), peroxy ($ROO^•$), and alkoxy ($RO^•$) radicals. In general, the secondary radicals are less reactive and more selective in their target. Formation and steady-state concentrations of any of these described reactive oxygen and nitrogen species in vivo are dependent on a number of factors including the formation rates of the precursors, detoxification reactions, pH, and availability of transition metals.

III. INTRACELLULAR AND VASCULAR SOURCES OF OXIDANTS

A. Mitochondria

Superoxide and hydrogen peroxide are the main initial reactive oxygen species generated in all liver cell types and the vascular space. A major continuous intracellular source of superoxide formation is the electron transport chain of mitochondria (3). Approximately 2% of total oxygen utilized in a cell is reduced to superoxide (4). NADH dehydrogenase (complex I) and ubiquinone–cytochrome b complex (complex III) release superoxide even under physiological conditions. The highest mitochondrial superoxide formation is observed during slow resting state 4 respiration, i.e., when the components of the respiratory chain are mainly in the reduced form (5). Mitochondrial superoxide can increase substantially when mitochondria are damaged. When superoxide is released from the electron transport chain, it can combine with NO, generated by a mitochondrial nitric oxide synthase (6), to form peroxynitrite within the mitochondrial matrix (7). In addition to the electron transport chain of the inner mitochondrial membrane, monoamine oxidases, which are located in the outer membrane, generate substantial amounts of hydrogen peroxide during the oxidative deamination of biogenic amines (8). Because of the localization, monoamine oxidases contribute to the oxidant stress in mitochondria and in the cytosol. A mitochondrial oxidant stress has been demonstrated in connection with mitochondrial dysfunction during hypoxia-reoxygenation (9), acetaminophen toxicity (10), chemical hypoxia (11), extracellular oxidant stress (12), and the toxicity of ethanol (13) and bile acids (14).

B. Microsomes

During phase I metabolism of xenobiotics, the microsomal P450 enzyme system can release activated oxygen intermediates. The formation of hydrogen peroxide and superoxide has been documented in isolated microsomes (15). However, during in vivo drug metabolism there is little, if any, evidence for increased oxidant stress (16,17), suggesting less leakage of ROS from cytochrome P450 enzymes in the intact cell than in isolated microsomes. Nevertheless, drug metabolism can lead to secondary oxidant stress in the liver, e.g., injury to mitochondria (10) and mobilization of transition metals (18). A severe oxidant stress can be generated by metabolism of redox-cycling agents such as diquat (19), paraquat (20), and menadione (21). These compounds are reduced by P450 reductase to a radical species, which can reduce oxygen to superoxide thereby regenerating the parent compound. Redox-cycling agents can undergo numerous cycles before they are excreted and create an enormous oxidant stress and cause severe liver damage (19).

C. Peroxisomes

These cell organelles contain a number of oxidases, e.g., fatty acyl CoA oxidase, amino acid oxidase, and urate oxidase, which generate hydrogen peroxide as a regular product (4). Owing to the very high levels of catalase in peroxisomes, the adverse effects are limited under physiological conditions. However, high-fat diet and drugs that are peroxisome proliferators cause an increase in fatty acyl CoA oxidase and potentiate the oxidant stress in this cell organelle (22,23).

D. Cytosol

Xanthine dehydrogenase is a major enzyme in the cytosol of all liver cells. Although the specific activity of this enzyme is the same in all three cell types, hepatocytes contain more than 85% of the total enzyme activity in the liver (24). Prolonged periods of ischemia (25) and certain drug toxicities (10) can cause a proteolytic cleavage of the enzyme resulting in loss of the capability to bind the cofactor NAD^+. Instead, the enzyme acts as an oxidase by using molecular oxygen as electron acceptor, which leads to formation of superoxide and hydrogen peroxide in the cytosol. Some time ago, xanthine oxidase (XO) was considered the main intracellular source of reactive oxygen formation during ischemia-reperfusion (reviewed in ref. 26). However, it is questionable whether XO can actually generate a quantitatively relevant oxidant stress in hepatocytes (27). The restricted availability of the substrates hypoxanthine or xanthine may be the limiting factor for the duration and extent of XO-mediated reactive oxygen formation (9). Recently, it was suggested that xanthine oxidase might be a relevant source of reactive oxygen in Kupffer cells (28) and, after release by hepatocytes and binding to endothelial cells, a major source of oxidant stress in vascular lining cells (28,29).

E. Vascular Oxidant Stress

Kupffer cell activation and hepatic neutrophil recruitment contributes to liver injury during drug metabolism (30–33), ischemia-reperfusion (34–36), endotoxemia/sepsis (37,38), and alcoholic hepatitis (39). A number of inflammatory mediators activate and prime Kupffer cells and neutrophils for enhanced superoxide formation including activated complement factors (40), TNFα (41), and platelet-activating factor (42). Kupffer cells are in a fixed position within the sinusoidal lining. Superoxide, generated by NADPH oxidase in Kupffer cells, is released into the sinusoidal lumen and space of Disse. Because of the close proximity to other cells, Kupffer cell–derived reactive oxygen can directly cause cell injury, which can be inhibited by vascular antioxidant enzymes (43). In contrast to Kupffer cells, neutrophils adherent to vascular endothelial cells release cytotoxic mediators only when excessively stimulated. However, this is rarely the case under realistic pathophysiological conditions in vivo. Injury occurs mainly after chemotactic stimulation, transmigration, and adherence of the neutrophil to hepatocytes (44,45). These processes require a number of adhesion molecules including β_2 integrins and intercellular adhesion molecule-1 (ICAM-1) (46). Upregulation of the β_2 integrin Mac-1 (CD11b/CD18) and the adhesion through this receptor (47) is critical for neutrophil-induced reactive oxygen formation. In support of this hypothesis, enhanced Mac-1 expression was shown in every model where neutrophils contribute to liver injury (48–51). In addition, antibodies against Mac-1 attenuated the postischemic oxidant stress by neutrophils and protected against neutrophil-induced liver injury (37,49).

Until recently, it was unclear whether or not reactive oxygen is directly involved in neutrophil-induced hepatocellular injury. Despite some evidence for reactive oxygen involvement in vivo, coculture systems consistently showed that activated neutrophils damage hepatocytes by protease release and not oxidant stress over a time frame of 15 h (52,53). Based on these data, it was concluded that reactive oxygen may be necessary for neutrophil cytotoxicity in vivo by inactivating antiproteases (reviewed in ref. 45). However, recent findings suggest that reactive oxygen generated by transmigrated and adherent neutrophils causes an oxidant stress not only in the vasculature but also intracellularly (37,54). The observation that glutathione peroxidase knockout mice are more susceptible to neutrophil cytotoxicity indicates that neutrophils can kill hepatocytes by reactive oxygen, a process that requires not more than 1 h after neutrophil attack (54). How can we explain the drastic differences between results of in vivo experiments and the coculture system in vitro? The most likely explanation for the opposite results is in the role of hepatocytes. In vivo, hepatocytes are exposed to the same inflammatory mediators as neutrophils, resulting in the upregulation of adhesion molecules such as ICAM-1 (48, 55,56) as well as the formation and release of CXC chemokines (57,58). Chemokines and ICAM-1 are important for neutrophil chemotaxis and adherence to hepatocytes (57), which is the final activating step for neutrophil degranulation and long-lasting adherence-dependent reactive oxygen formation. In contrast, all coculture experiments were done with control hepatocytes. Under these conditions, neutrophils do not firmly adhere (57) and the cytotoxicity is dependent on the excessive stimulation with inflammatory mediators. Reactive oxygen may be generated but not long enough and not in close proximity to hepatocytes. Therefore, the cytotoxicity in vitro is caused by slow proteolytic digestion, not the rapid killing by reactive oxygen.

IV. PATHOPHYSIOLOGICAL CONSEQUENCES OF OXIDANT STRESS

A. Lipid Peroxidation

Oxidant stress in the liver can cause lipid peroxidation (LPO), which is still a frequently hypothesized mechanism of cell injury. Two main observations suggest a role for LPO in pathogenesis: a significant increase in LPO and a cytoprotective effect of antioxidants in combination with reduced LPO (26,59). However, this association does not conclusively prove that LPO is the cause of cell injury. However, on a quantitative basis, the magnitude of LPO in vivo is mostly insufficient to directly cause cell death (60). Excessive intracellular superoxide formation alone does not kill hepatocytes by LPO even after depletion of glutathione (61). Extensive hepatic LPO in vivo was only observed when, in addition to reactive oxygen formation, the cellular antioxidants, e.g., vitamin E and GSH, were depleted (62,63), high levels of polyunsaturated fatty acids were present in membranes (63), and iron was mobilized from intracellular stores (18). If some of these factors come together, massive LPO with severe cell injury ensues.

However, under most realistic pathophysiological conditions LPO is minimal and is not likely to be responsible for cell damage. Does that mean LPO is not important? LPO products are potent chemotactic factors for neutrophils and can modulate superoxide formation (64). In addition, LPO products may enhance chemokine formation (65). These observations may explain the role of LPO products in maintaining an inflammatory response beyond the initial mediator formation (66). Furthermore, LPO products were shown to promote induction of collagen gene expression in activated stellate cells and contribute to fibrosis (67). Thus, LPO products can be important as signaling molecules under certain pathophysiological conditions.

B. Nitrotyrosine Formation

The reaction of peroxynitrite with carbon dioxide yields nitrating species, which react preferably with tyrosine (68). Nitrotyrosine residues were detected in the liver during hepatic ischemia-reperfusion injury (69,70) and acetaminophen toxicity (71). The pathophysiological relevance of enhanced peroxynitrite formation is not completely clear. After high doses of acetaminophen, an initial nitrotyrosine staining is observed in the vascular lining cells, followed by enzyme release and staining in hepatocytes (72). Inhibitors of Kupffer cells prevented nitrotyrosine staining and injury (73). In addition, allopurinol prevented mitochondrial dysfunction, oxidant stress, staining in hepatocytes, and injury after acetaminophen (72). These data suggest that vascular and hepatocellular peroxynitrite formation may be important for acetaminophen toxicity in the liver. Nevertheless, NO formation in the liver is also critical for maintenance of liver blood flow under various pathophysiological conditions (74,75). In most situations, peroxynitrite formation, especially in the presence of scavengers such as GSH and NADH, is less damaging than prolonged vasoconstriction and ischemia (75,76).

C. Reactive Oxygen and Cell Death

Reactive oxygen can cause hepatocellular necrosis without gross cell damage by lipid peroxidation. The mechanism of this necrotic cell death is linked to the opening of the mitochondrial membrane permeability transition (MPT) pore, which causes mitochondrial uncoupling and loss of the membrane potential (77). A significant oxidant stress causes oxidation of mitochondrial pyridine nucleotides and the formation of reactive oxygen species in mitochondria, both of which increase mitochondrial free Ca^{2+} (12). The MPT can be induced by an increase in mitochondrial Ca^{2+} directly (78) or through the activation of mitochondrial serine proteases (calpains) (79). Cytosolic calpains can induce membrane blebbing by degrading cytoskeletal proteins (80). These events lead to rapid necrotic cell death of hepatocytes within 1 h (12,77).

Reactive oxygen can also induce cell death through apoptosis (81). In the liver, apoptotic cell death induced or modulated by oxidant stress has been suggested for hepatocytes (82–84) and endothelial cells (84,85). However, the molecular mechanisms of reactive oxygen-induced apoptosis are not well described. Caspases, a family of cysteine proteases with essential sulfhydryl groups, are a potential target for reactive oxygen or reactive nitrogen species. Caspases can be activated by low concentrations of hydrogen peroxide (86). However, higher levels inhibit the enzyme presumably by oxidizing the essential sulfhydryl groups (86). This mechanism may be responsible for the delayed apoptosis of activated neutrophils at an inflammatory site (87). However, neither Fas antibody–induced nor TNF-induced apoptosis in the liver was affected in glutathione peroxidase knockout mice, suggesting no involvement of reactive oxygen species in the receptor-mediated apoptotic pathways in vivo (54). In addition to reactive oxygen species, NO and/or reactive nitrogen species can inactivate critical caspases and prevent apoptosis (88). Thus, reactive oxygen and nitrogen species can manipulate apoptotic cell death under certain conditions. However, the detailed mechanisms and the pathophysiological relevance need to be established.

D. Reactive Oxygen and Gene Transcription

The activation of several transcription factors including nuclear factor (NF)-κB and activating protein-1 (AP-1) can be induced or modulated by reactive oxygen species (89). A number of proinflammatory cytokines [e.g., TNFα, interleukin (IL)-1], chemokines (e.g., IL-8), adhesion molecules (e.g., ICAM-1, VCAM-1, and E-selectin), and stress genes (e.g., heme oxygenase (HO)-1) are regulated by these redox-sensitive transcription factors. Therefore, reactive oxygen can significantly enhance an inflammatory response, thereby indirectly contributing to cell damage. Despite extensive experimental data, the molecular mechanism of the redox sensitivity of these transcription factors is still unclear (90). It may involve a number of redox-sensitive targets and is certainly dependent on the nature of the activating mediator and the cell type (91). In the liver, TNFα formation can be modulated by oxidant stress. Antioxidants inhibited endotoxin-induced NF-κB activation and the formation of TNF mRNA and protein in isolated Kupffer cells (92). In support of these results, TNFα formation in vivo could be prevented by the radical scavenger dimethyl sulfoxide (93), and endotoxin-induced TNFα generation was three-times higher in glutathione peroxidase knockout mice (54). Furthermore, increased nonheme iron concentrations and increased reactive oxygen formation in hepatic macrophages isolated from alcohol-treated animals responded to endotoxin exposure with higher NF-κB activation and elevated transcription of cytokines and chemokines (94). Together these data clearly indicate that gene transcription in Kupffer cells can be modulated by reactive oxygen.

Stimulation with TNFα can induce an intracellular oxidant stress in hepatocytes (95). The radical scavenger dimethyl sulfoxide inhibited TNF-mediated NF-κB activation and ICAM-1 mRNA formation in the liver in vivo (93). In addition, several antioxidants attenuated the TNF-induced chemokine formation in HepG2 cells (96). Induction of HO-1 in hepatocytes during hemorrhagic shock and resuscitation is dependent on the activation of AP-1 (97). Because the activation of AP-1 and the induction of HO-1 could be inhibited by antioxidants (98), an oxidant stress can promote not only proinflammatory cytokine formation but also the induction of stress genes such as HO-1. This enzyme generates the antioxidant biliverdin and the vasodilator carbon monoxide, both of which may contribute to the hepatoprotective effect of HO-1 induction (98,99).

Stellate cells regulate sinusoidal blood flow and are, after transformation, the major source of extracellular matrix protein formation leading to fibrosis. There is considerable evidence that reactive oxygen and LPO can stimulate fibrogenesis (67,100). Reactive oxygen species induce or modulate transforming growth factor β_1-induced collagen α_1 (I) gene expression in vivo (101,102). Furthermore, reactive oxygen can stimulate chemokine transcription in stellate cells (103), thereby enhancing the inflammatory response.

V. ANTIOXIDANT DEFENSE SYSTEMS

The continuous formation of reactive oxygen and reactive nitrogen species during physiological functions of liver cells and the potential for a substantially increased oxidant stress under many pathophysiological conditions (Figure 1) require an effective defense system against these reactive intermediates. Because of the variety of oxygen and nitrogen metabolites formed and their different localization and reactivity, a sophisticated, multi-level network of antioxidant enzymes and small molecules is operative in every liver cell (Fig. 2).

A. Enzymatic Defense Mechanisms

Superoxide is removed by superoxide dismutases (SOD) in the major cellular compartments (104). Cu^{2+}/Zn^{2+}-SOD is located in the cytosol and nuclear matrix and Mn^{3+}-SOD is present in mitochondria (105). Superoxide first reduces the redox-active metal (Cu^{2+} or Mn^{3+}) that yields molecular oxygen; a second superoxide molecule is then reduced to hydrogen peroxide by the metal ion. The reaction of superoxide with SOD is diffusion limited. The high intracellular SOD levels (approx. 10 μM) keep the steady-state levels of superoxide in the range of 1–10 pM (2,4). Since superoxide is not a very toxic molecule by itself and the spontaneous dismutation has the same reaction products, why is it beneficial to have these high levels of SOD? In addition to the fact that SOD-catalyzed dismutation avoids the formation of singlet oxygen (Fig. 1), the main reason for the importance of SOD might be to limit peroxynitrite generation (1,2). Using the rate constants for the reaction of superoxide with SOD (2.4×10^9 $M^{-1}s^{-1}$) and NO (2×10^{10} $M^{-1}s^{-1}$), the rate of disappearance for superoxide is 20,000 s^{-1} with SOD (10 μM) and 200 s^{-1} with NO (estimated physiological concentration: 10 nM) (1). Thus, under physiological conditions, SOD prevents peroxynitrite formation. However, if the NO concentrations are in-

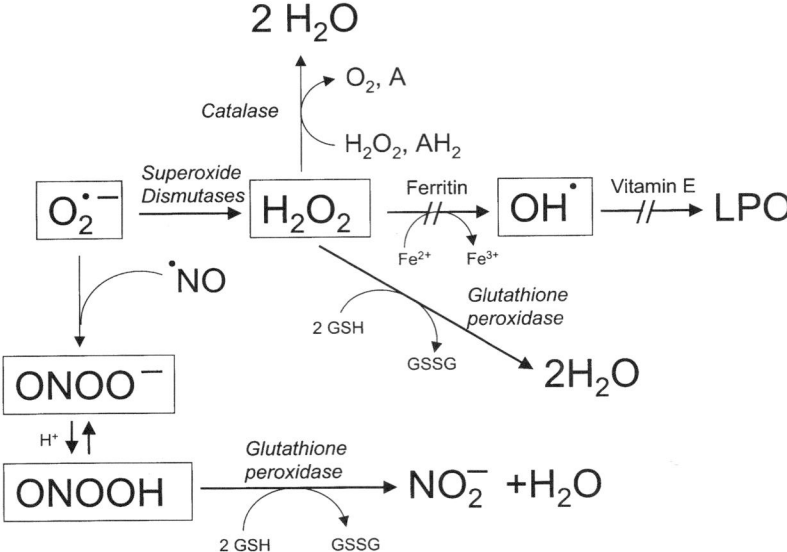

Figure 2 Cellular antioxidant defense mechanisms include enzymes for the rapid metabolism of reactive oxygen and nitrogen species, binding proteins for transition metals (e.g., ferritin), and chain-breaking antioxidants (e.g., vitamin E).

creased (10 μM), e.g., during an inflammatory response, the reaction with NO increases to 40,000 s^{-1} (1). This indicates that SOD cannot prevent intracellular peroxynitrite formation under inflammatory conditions. This situation is even more critical in the extracellular space, where SOD levels are much lower.

The hydrogen peroxide formed by SOD is degraded by catalase or glutathione peroxidase. Most of the catalase enzyme activity is located in peroxisomes. Mammalian catalase is a hemeprotein, which reduces hydrogen peroxide to water by utilizing electrons from either hydrogen peroxide (catalase reaction) or other small molecules such as ethanol or methanol (peroxidase reaction) (4). Catalase is inducible in the liver by caloric restrictions, phenobarbital, and hypolipidemic drugs, e.g., clofibrate (106). The main function of catalase is to metabolize hydrogen peroxide generated by oxidases in peroxisomes. Only under extreme conditions will any relevant amount of hydrogen peroxide escape peroxisomes or will significant amounts of cytosolic hydrogen peroxide be detoxified by catalase (107).

Glutathione peroxidase (GPx) is located in the cytosol (75%) and mitochondria (25%). The enzyme contains selenium in the form of selenocysteine, which is critical for the catalytic function (108). GPx can reduce peroxides, e.g., hydrogen peroxide and organic peroxides (108), and peroxynitrite (109). In contrast to its low specificity for peroxide substrates, the enzyme requires glutathione (GSH) as a cofactor. Glutathione disulfide (GSSG) is rapidly reduced back to GSH by glutathione reductase and NADPH. Because the reductase is the rate-limiting step of this cycle, GSSG accumulates to some degree and can be excreted into bile and plasma (16). The removal of GSSG either by the reductase (>95%) or export from hepatocytes (<5%) protects protein sulfhydryl groups from oxidation by high levels of GSSG. Mitochondria take up and release GSH but are not able to export GSSG (110). Consequently, reduction of GSSG within mitochondria is the only option to avoid GSSG accumulation. As in the case of acetaminophen toxicity, this cannot always be avoided (10).

A member of the glutathione-S-transferase family (GST-B) was identified as the enzyme responsible for the GPx activity in selenium-deficient mice (111,112). GST-B, which is inducible by selenium-deficiency (113), can only metabolize organic hydroperoxide but not hydrogen peroxide (114). However, despite this adaptation, selenium-deficient animals are more susceptible to reactive oxygen-induced liver injury (115). Another enzyme, a selenium-dependent phospholipid hydroperoxide glutathione peroxidase, which selectively uses lipid hydroperoxides as substrates, was identified (116). This enzyme is located in mitochondria, nuclei, and microsomes and is involved in metabolism of peroxidized lipids and therefore inhibits the propagation of LPO (117).

B.   Low-Molecular-Weight Antioxidants

Ascorbate (vitamin C), α-tocopherol (vitamin E), and glutathione (GSH) are examples of low-molecular-weight antioxidants. α-Tocopherol is the most effective chain-breaking compound in biological membranes (118). As for most antioxidants, the intracellular concentrations of α-tocopherol are not high enough to be a relevant hydroxyl radical scavenger. However, it effectively reduces peroxyl radicals (ROO$^{\bullet}$), one of the less reactive secondary radicals, to the lipid hydroperoxide, which can then be metabolized by the phospholipid hydroperoxide glutathione peroxidase (118). Thus, α-tocopherol prevents the propagation of the radical chain by avoiding the formation of new alkyl radicals. The α-tocopherol radical can be reduced by ascorbate and thiols such as GSH (119). Ascorbate is regenerated in the aqueous phase by a GSH-dependent dehydro-ascorbate reductase or a NADH-dependent semidehydro-ascorbate reductase (118). Thus, low-molecular-weight antioxidants act together to interrupt radical chain reactions and to divert radicals away from sensitive areas, e.g., hydrophobic membranes, to the aqueous phase (120). The critical importance of these compounds as defense systems to protect membranes has been shown in acetaminophen and allyl alcohol hepatotoxicity. In normal animals, LPO is not a relevant mechanism of cell injury for both of these compounds in vivo (121). However, in animals fed a vitamin E–deficient diet, LPO becomes the predominant injury mechanism with complete destruction of the liver within 1–4 h after administration of these compounds (62,63).

Glutathione is the most important water-soluble antioxidant. It is used as cofactor for glutathione peroxidases and S-transferases and it is important for maintenance of protein sulfhydryl groups. The key functional group of GSH is the cysteine sulfhydryl moiety, which is less susceptible to autoxidation than the same moiety in the isolated amino acid (122). GSH is synthesized intracellularly by two ATP-dependent enzymes, γ-glutamylcysteine synthetase and glutathione synthetase. Owing to its protease resistant γ-glutamyl bond, GSH cannot be degraded by intracellular proteases. Thus, for the cellular turnover, GSH has to be exported from the cell and is degraded by γ-glutamyltranspeptidase, which is present on the surface of epithelial cells in the kidney, lung, and intestine and also in the biliary tract (123). Sinusoidal and biliary transport proteins for GSH have been identified and characterized (124,125). The transport is electrogenic and does not require ATP (126). Approximately 90% of the GSH in plasma is supplied by the sinusoidal GSH release of hepatocytes (127). In contrast to the GSH transporter, a carrier for GSSG and GSH conjugates has only been clearly established for the canalicular membrane (128). Much less is known about a potential sinusoidal GSSG transporter (129). However, functional studies showed a release of GSSG into the sinusoids in the isolated perfused liver (27, 61,130) as well as in vivo (131). Quantitative estimations of GSSG formation and release even during severe oxidant stress indicated that 1–5% of all GSSG formed is exported and 95–99% is reduced by glutathione reductase (27,61). Approximately 80% of the exported GSSG is released into bile and 20% into the sinusoid (130). Thus, the biliary GSSG efflux is the most sensitive marker of intracellular oxidant stress.

GSH is present not only in the cytosol but also in other cellular compartments including mitochondria (15% of total hepatocellular GSH) (132). However, GSH is not synthesized in mitochondria but has to be taken up from the cytosol by a carrier different from the one on the plasma or canalicular membrane (133). An intact proton gradient is required to transport GSH into the mitochondrial matrix and keep it inside (134). A depletion of mitochondrial GSH impairs the detoxification mechanisms in this cell organelle and can lead to increased oxidative injury, loss of mitochondrial function, and cell death (135–137). Reactive oxygen escaping from mitochondria can induce NF-κB activation and promote gene transcription (137). On the other hand, any GSSG formed in mitochondria through the activity of GPx cannot be exported into the cytosol (110); GSSG has to be reduced or it will accumulate, as has been shown during acetaminophen toxicity (10).

C. Metal-Binding Proteins

Free radical processes such as LPO are dependent on the availability of redox-active transition metals. Therefore, another defense strategy is to keep metal ions such as Fe^{2+}/Fe^{3+} or Cu^+ tightly bound to transport or storage proteins. Metal-binding proteins include ferritin, transferrin, and lactoferrin for iron, caeruloplasmin for copper, and metallothionein for other metals (138). Because of its large number of cysteines, metallothionein may also act directly or indirectly as antioxidants (139).

VI. ANTIOXIDANT DEFENSE IN NONPARENCHYMAL CELLS

The previous paragraphs described various antioxidant strategies in the liver, i.e., hepatocytes. However, a limited number of studies suggest that similar systems are operative in nonparenchymal cells (140,141). In general, activities of SODs and selenium-dependent GPx are similar in nonparenchymal cells and in hepatocytes (140). Likewise, the GSH contents on a nmol/mg cellular protein basis are very similar in all cell types. However, owing to the much smaller cell size of nonparenchymal cells compared to hepatocytes, the total GSH content in nonparenchymal cells represents less than 5% of the liver GSH content (140). Thus, the detoxification capacity for reactive oxygen species is only a fraction of hepatocytes. Interestingly, Kupffer cells and endothelial cells adapt differently to an inflammatory stimulus. During endotoxemia, Kupffer cells modulate pro-oxidant pathways, resulting in increased superoxide formation (142). In contrast, endothelial cells upregulate SOD and GPx activities, the glucose transporter GLUT1, and key enzymes of the carbohydrate metabolism (141,142). This response supports the detoxification potential for reactive oxygen in endothelial cells and helps to maintain the integrity of the vascular lining cells.

VII. ANTIOXIDANT DEFENSE IN THE VASCULAR SPACE

Inflammatory cells can release reactive oxygen and nitrogen species into the vascular space and generate a substantial oxidant stress. Plasma antioxidants include albumin, transferrin, lactoferrin, ceruloplasmin, haptoglobin, urate, ascorbate, vitamin E, bilirubin, and extracellular SOD and GPx activities (reviewed in ref. 143). However, the main problems of plasma antioxidant systems are the low concentrations of the scavengers and the low activities of the enzymes, which make them much less effective than their intracellular counterparts. The exceptions are the metal transport proteins, which bind metals with high affinity and, therefore, virtually eliminate free iron from plasma (143). Extracellular Cu^{2+}/Zn^{2+}-SOD (eSOD) (144) and extracellular selenium-dependent GPx (eGPx) (145) are proteins distinct from the cellular enzymes. However, their biological relevance is not clear. ESOD can bind to surface proteoglycans on the endothelial cell surface (146). It can be speculated that this SOD may protect endothelial cells from a vascular oxidant stress induced by phagocytes and may limit peroxynitrite formation. Plasma eGPx is dependent on the cofactor GSH. In contrast to the mM K_m value of the enzyme (145), plasma GSH concentrations are generally in the $5–200$-μM range (147). Thus, it would be expected that eGPx is not very effective in removing peroxides from plasma. Nevertheless, a recent study showed that overexpressing plasma GPx protected against acetaminophen-induced liver injury (148), which is in agreement with a vascular oxidant stress by Kupffer cells as an initiating event in this model (31,73).

A more liver-specific antioxidant defense system has recently been recognized (147, 149). GSH can be oxidized in the vasculature during ischemia-reperfusion (35,149) and endotoxemia (147), reflecting a Kupffer cell–induced oxidant stress. In this situation, the plasma GSH levels are substantially increased ($100–200$ μM in the hepatic vein) owing to enhanced release of GSH from hepatocytes (147). These elevated levels, which may even be higher in the space of Disse, are sufficient to make GSH a fairly effective trapping agent for reactive oxygen species. In support of this conclusion, depletion of plasma GSH concentrations aggravated inflammatory liver injury (149) and an increase above baseline levels protected against injury (150). The oxidation of GSH occurred in the vascular space (35) and was not enzymatically catalyzed (151). In vitro studies showed that only H_2O_2 reacts with GSH and forms GSSG (150,151). Other relevant oxidants, i.e., hypochlorite and peroxynitrite, are trapped by GSH but generate mainly higher oxidation states such as sulfonic acid or sulfenic acid and very little GSSG (151). These data are supported by in vivo experiments, which showed that nitric oxide synthase inhibitors increased plasma GSH and GSSG levels during hepatic inflammation (75,76). In contrast, NO donors decreased GSH and GSSG concentrations in plasma (75). This suggests that when NO and superoxide are generated in the vascular space, at least some of these molecules react to form peroxynitrite, which can be trapped by GSH. If NO formation is prevented, less peroxynitrite is formed and less GSH is consumed by this detoxification reaction. At the same time, more superoxide dismutates to form hydrogen peroxide, which leads to more GSSG formation. On the other hand, if more NO is generated, higher peroxynitrite formation leads to GSH depletion and, because less hydrogen peroxide is formed, less GSSG is generated. Thus, GSH appears to be an important scavenger of reactive oxygen and nitrogen species in the vascular space under inflammatory conditions.

Another important antioxidant system in plasma is selenoprotein P (152). The plasma concentrations of this protein are in the range of $25–30$ mg/mL. The protein contains $7–10$ selenocysteine and 17 cysteine residues in each molecule (153). Thus, it should be able to function as a scavenger for reactive oxygen and peroxynitrite. Because many different organs can produce and release this protein, it was postulated that selenoprotein P acts as an antioxidant in the interstitial space (152). The importance of this selenoprotein P was demonstrated in experiments where the redox-cycling agent diquat or glutathione depletion with phorone induced lipid peroxidation and liver injury in selenium-deficient animals (154,155). Treatment of these animals with a dose of selenium, which was sufficient to restore selenoprotein P levels in plasma but did not affect the low levels of GPx in plasma or liver tissue, prevented LPO and liver injury (154,155). These observations suggest a significant role of selenoprotein P as antioxidant in plasma.

REFERENCES

1. Squadrito GL, Pryor WA. Oxidative chemistry of nitric oxide: The role of superoxide, peroxynitrite and carbon dioxide. Free Radic Biol Med 1998; 25:392–403.
2. Koppenol WH. The basic chemistry of nitrogen monoxide and peroxynitrite. Free Radic Biol Med 1998; 25:385–391.
3. Loschen G, Azzi A, Richter C, Flohe L. Superoxide radicals as precursors of mitochondrial hydrogen peroxide. FEBS Lett 1974; 18:68–72.
4. Chance B, Sies H, Boveris A. Hydroperoxide metabolism in mammalian organs. Pharmacol Rev 1979; 59:527–605.
5. Cadenas E, Davies KJA. Mitochondrial free radical generation, oxidative stress and aging. Free Radic Biol Med 2000; 29:222–230.
6. Tatoyan A, Giulivi C. Purification and characterization of a nitric-oxide synthase from rat liver mitochondria. J Biol Chem 1998; 273:11044–11048.
7. Valdez LB, Alvarez S, Arnaiz SL, Schopfer F, Carreras MC, Poderoso JJ, Boveris A. Reactions with peroxynitrite in the mitochondrial matrix. Free Radic Biol Med 2000; 29:349–356.
8. Hauptmann N, Grimsby J, Shih JC, Cadenas E. The metabolism of tyramine by monoamine oxidase A/B causes oxidative damage to mitochondrial DNA. Arch Biochem Biophys 1996; 335:295–304.
9. Jaeschke H, Mitchell JR. Mitochondria and xanthine oxidase both generate reactive oxygen species after hypoxic damage in isolated perfused rat liver. Biochem Biophys Res Commun 1989; 160:140–147.
10. Jaeschke H. Glutathione disulfide formation and oxidant stress during acetaminophen-induced hepatotoxicity in mice in vivo: the protective effect of allopurinol. J Pharmacol Exp Ther 1990; 255:935–941.
11. Gores GJ, Flarsheim CE, Dawson TL, Nieminen AL, Herman B, Lemasters JJ. Swelling, reductive stress, and cell death during chemical hypoxia in hepatocytes. Am J Physiol 1989; 257:C347–C354.
12. Nieminen AL, Byrne AM, Herman B, Lemasters JJ. Mitochondrial permeability transition in hepatocytes induced by t-BuOOH-NAD(P)H and reactive oxygen species. Am J Physiol 1997; 272:C1286–C1294.
13. Kukielka E, Dicker E, Cederbaum AI. Increased production of reactive oxygen species by rat liver mitochondria after chronic ethanol treatment. Arch Biochem Biophys 1994; 309: 377–386.
14. Sokol RJ, Winklhofer-Roob BM, Devereaux MW, McKim JM Jr. Generation of hydroperoxides in isolated rat hepatocytes and hepatic mitochondria exposed to hydrophobic bile acids. Gastroenterology 1995; 109:1249–1256.
15. Kuthan H, Ullrich V. Oxidase and oxygenase function of the microsomal cytochrome P-450 monooxygenase system. Eur J Biochem 1982; 126:583–588.
16. Lauterburg BH, Smith CV, Hughes H, Mitchell JR. Biliary excretion of glutathione and glutathione disulfide in the rat. J Clin Invest 1984; 73:124–133.
17. Smith CV, Jaeschke H. Effect of acetaminophen on hepatic content and biliary efflux of glutathione disulfide in mice. Chem Biol Interact 1989; 70:241–248.

18. Jaeschke H, Kleinwaechter C, Wendel A. NADH-dependent reductive stress and ferritin-bound iron in allyl alcohol-induced lipid peroxidation in vivo: the protective effect of vitamin E. Chem Biol Interact 1992; 81:57–68.

19. Smith CV, Hughes H, Lauterburg BH, Mitchell JR. Oxidant stress and hepatic necrosis in rats treated with diquat. J Pharmacol Exp Ther 1985; 235:172–177.

20. Brigelius R, Anwer MS. Increased biliary GSSG-secretion and loss of hepatic glutathione in isolated perfused rat liver after paraquat treatment. Res Commun Chem Pathol Pharmacol 1981; 31:493–502.

21. Di Monte D, Ross D, Bellomo G, Eklow L, Orrenius S. Alterations in intracellular thiol homeostasis during the metabolism of menadione by isolated rat hepatocytes. Arch Biochem Biophys 1984; 235:334–342.

22. Lazarow PB, De Duve C. A fatty acyl-CoA oxidizing system in rat liver peroxisomes: enhancement by clofibrate, a hypolipidemic drug. Proc Natl Acad Sci USA 1976; 73:2043–2046.

23. Conway JG, Neptun DA, Garvey LK, Popp JA. Role of fatty acyl coenzyme A oxidase in the efflux of oxidized glutathione from perfused livers of rats treated with the peroxisome proliferator nafenopin. Cancer Res 1987; 47:4795–4800.

24. Wiezorek JS, Brown DH, Kupperman DE, Brass CA. Rapid conversion to high xanthine oxidase activity in viable Kupffer cells during hypoxia. J Clin Invest 1994; 94:2224–2230.

25. Engerson TD, McKelvey TG, Rhyne DB, Boggio EB, Snyder SJ, Jones HP. Conversion of xanthine dehydrogenase to oxidase in ischemic rat tissues. J Clin Invest 1987; 79:1564–1570.

26. Jaeschke H. Reactive oxygen and ischemia/reperfusion injury of the liver. Chem Biol Interact 1991; 79:115–136.

27. Jaeschke H, Smith CV, Mitchell JR. Reactive oxygen species and ischemia-reflow injury in isolated perfused rat liver. J Clin Invest 1988; 81:1240–1246.

28. Yokoyama Y, Beckman JS, Beckman TK, Wheat JK, Cash TG, Freeman BA, Parks DA. Circulating xanthine oxidase: potential mediator of ischemic injury. Am J Physiol 1990; 258:G564–G570.

29. Houston M, Estevez A, Chumley P, Aslan M, Marklund S, Parks DA, Freeman BA. Binding of xanthine oxidase to vascular endothelium. J Biol Chem 1999; 274:4985–4994.

30. Laskin DL, Pilaro AM. Potential role of activated macrophages in acetaminophen hepatotoxicity. Toxicol Appl Pharmacol 1986; 86:204–215.

31. Laskin DL, Gardner CR, Price VF, Jollow DJ. Modulation of macrophage functioning abrogates the acute hepatotoxicity of acetaminophen. Hepatology 1995; 21:1045–1050.

32. Lawson JA, Farhood A, Hopper RD, Bajt ML, Jaeschke H. The hepatic inflammatory response after acetaminophen overdose: the role of neutrophils. Toxicol Sci 2000; 54:509–516.

33. Laskin DL, Robertson FM, Pilaro AM, Laskin JD. Activation of liver macrophages following phenobarbital treatment of rats. Hepatology 1988; 8:1051–1055.

34. Jaeschke H, Farhood A, Smith CW. Neutrophils contribute to ischemia/reperfusion injury in rat liver in vivo. FASEB J 1990; 4:3355–3359.

35. Jaeschke H, Farhood A. Neutrophil and Kupffer cell–induced oxidant stress and ischemia-reperfusion injury in rat liver in vivo. Am J Physiol 1991; 260:G355–G362.

36. Jaeschke H, Bautista AP, Spolarics Z, Spitzer JJ. Superoxide generation by Kupffer cells and priming of neutrophils during reperfusion after hepatic ischemia. Free Radic Res Commun 1991; 15:277–284.

37. Jaeschke H, Farhood A, Smith CW. Neutrophil-induced liver cell injury in endotoxin shock is a CD11b/CD18-dependent mechanism. Am J Physiol 1991; 261:G1051–G1056.

38. Molnar RG, Wang P, Ayala A, Ganey PE, Roth RA, Chaudry IH. The role of neutrophils

in producing hepatocellular dysfunction during the hyperdynamic stage of sepsis in rats. J Surg Res 1997; 73:117–122.

39. Bautista AP. Chronic alcohol intoxication induces hepatic injury through enhanced macrophage inflammatory protein-2 production and intercellular adhesion molecule-1 expression in the liver. Hepatology 1997; 25:335–342.

40. Jaeschke H, Farhood A, Bautista AP, Spolarics Z, Spitzer JJ. Complement activates Kupffer cells and neutrophils during reperfusion after hepatic ischemia. Am J Physiol 1993; 264: G801–G809.

41. Bautista AP, Schuler A, Spolarics Z, Spitzer JJ. Tumor necrosis factor-alpha stimulates superoxide anion generation by perfused rat liver and Kupffer cells. Am J Physiol 1991; 261: G891–G895.

42. Bautista AP, Spitzer JJ. Platelet activating factor stimulates and primes the liver, Kupffer cells and neutrophils to release superoxide anions. Free Radic Res Commun 1992; 7:195–209.

43. Bilzer M, Jaeschke H, Vollmar AM, Paumgartner G, Gerbes AL. Prevention of Kupffer cell-induced oxidant injury in rat liver by atrial natriuretic peptide. Am J Physiol 1999; 276: G1137–G1144.

44. Chosay JG, Essani NA, Dunn CJ, Jaeschke H. Neutrophil margination and extravasation in sinusoids and venules of the liver during endotoxin-induced injury. Am J Physiol 1997; 272: G1195–G1200.

45. Jaeschke H, Smith CW. Mechanisms of neutrophil-induced parenchymal cell injury. J Leukocyte Biol 1997; 61:647–653.

46. Jaeschke H. Cellular adhesion molecules: Regulation and role in the pathogenesis of liver disease. Am J Physiol 1997; 273:G602–G611.

47. Shappell SB, Toman C, Anderson DC, Taylor AA, Entman ML, Smith CW. Mac-1 (CD11b/CD18) mediates adherence-dependent hydrogen peroxide production by human and canine neutrophils. J Immunol 1990; 144:2702–2711.

48. Essani NA, Fisher MA, Farhood A, Manning AM, Smith CW, Jaeschke H. Cytokine-induced hepatic intercellular adhesion molecule-1 (ICAM-1) mRNA expression and its role in the pathophysiology of murine endotoxin shock and acute liver failure. Hepatology 1995; 21: 1632–1639.

49. Jaeschke H, Farhood A, Bautista AP, Spolarics Z, Spitzer JJ, Smith CW. Functional inactivation of neutrophils with a Mac-1 (CD11b/CD18) monoclonal antibody protects against ischemia-reperfusion injury in rat liver. Hepatology 1993; 17:915–923.

50. Witthaut R, Farhood A, Smith CW, Jaeschke H. Complement and tumor necrosis factor-α contribute to Mac-1 (CD11b/CD18) upregulation and systemic neutrophil activation during endotoxemia in vivo. J Leukocyte Biol 1994; 55:105–111.

51. Lawson JA, Burns AR, Farhood A, Bajt ML, Smith CW, Jaeschke H. Functional importance of E- and L-selectin for neutrophil-induced liver injury during endotoxemia in mice. Hepatology 2000; 32:990–998.

52. Mavier P, Preaux A-M, Guigui B, Lescs MC, Zafrani ES, Dhumeaux D. In vitro toxicity of polymorphonuclear neutrophils to rat hepatocytes: evidence for a proteinase-mediated mechanism. Hepatology 1988; 8:254–258.

53. Harbrecht BG, Biliar TR, Curran RD, Stadler J, Simmons RL. Hepatocyte injury by activated neutrophils in vitro is mediated by proteases. Ann Surgery 1993; 218:120–128.

54. Jaeschke H, Ho Y-S, Fisher MA, Lawson JA, Farhood A. Glutathione peroxidase-deficient mice are more susceptible to neutrophil-mediated hepatic parenchymal cell injury during endotoxemia: importance of an intracellular oxidant stress. Hepatology 1999; 29:443–450.

55. Essani NA, McGuire GM, Manning AM, Jaeschke H. Differential induction for mRNA of ICAM-1 and selectins in hepatocytes, Kupffer cells and endothelial cells during endotoxemia. Biochem Biophys Res Commun 1995; 211:74–82.

56. Farhood A, McGuire GM, Manning AM, Miyasaka M, Smith CW, Jaeschke, H. Intercellular adhesion molecule-1 (ICAM-1) gene expression and its role in neutrophil-induced ischemia-reperfusion injury in the liver. J Leukocyte Biol 1995; 57:368–374.

57. Nagendra AR, Mickelson JK, Smith CW. CD18 integrin and CD54-dependent neutrophil adhesion to cytokine-stimulated human hepatocytes. Am J Physiol 1997; 272:G408–G416.

58. Thornton AJ, Strieter RM, Lindley I, Baggiolini M, Kunkel SL. Cytokine-induced gene expression of a neutrophil chemotactic factor/IL-8 in human hepatocytes. J Immunol 1990; 144:2609–2613.

59. Jaeschke H. Mechanisms of oxidant stress-induced acute tissue injury. Proc Soc Exp Biol Med 1995; 209:104–111.

60. Mathews WR, Guido DM, Fisher MA, Jaeschke H. Lipid peroxidation as molecular mechanism of liver cell injury during reperfusion after ischemia. Free Radic Biol Med 1994; 16: 763–770.

61. Jaeschke H, Benzick EA. Pathophysiological consequences of enhanced intracellular superoxide formation in isolated perfused rat liver. Chem Biol Interact 1992; 84:55–68.

62. Wendel A, Jaeschke H, Gloger M. Drug-induced lipid peroxidation in mice II: Protection against paracetamol-induced liver necrosis by intravenous liposomally entrapped glutathione. Biochem Pharmacol 1982; 31:3601–3605.

63. Jaeschke H, Kleinwaechter C, Wendel A. The role of acrolein in allyl alcohol-induced lipid peroxidation and liver cell damage in mice. Biochem Pharmacol 1987; 36:51–57.

64. Curzio M, Esterbauer H, Di Mauro C, Cecchini G, Dianzani MU. Chemotactic activity of the lipid peroxidation product 4-hydroxynonenal and homologous hydroxyalkenals. Biol Chem Hoppe Seyler 1986; 367:321–329.

65. Jayatilleke A, Shaw S. Stimulation of monocyte interleukin-8 by lipid peroxidation products: a mechanism for alcohol-induced liver injury. Alcohol 1998; 16:119–123.

66. Liu P, Vonderfecht SL, McGuire GM, Fisher MA, Farhood A, Jaeschke H. The 21-aminosteroid tirilazad mesylate protects in a model of endotoxin shock and acute liver failure in rats. J Pharmacol Exp Ther 1994; 271:438–445.

67. Poli G, Parola M. Oxidative damage and fibrogenesis. Free Radic Biol Med 1997; 22:287–305.

68. Beckman JS. Oxidative damage and tyrosine nitration from peroxynitrite. Chem Res Toxicol 1996; 9:836–844.

69. Liu P, Yin K, Nagele R, Wong PY. Inhibition of nitric oxide synthase attenuates peroxynitrite generation, but augments neutrophil accumulation in hepatic ischemia-reperfusion in rats. J Pharmacol Exp Ther 1998; 284:1139–1146.

70. Skinner KA, Crow JP, Skinner HB, Chandler RT, Thompson JA, Parks DA. Free and protein-associated nitrotyrosine formation following rat liver preservation and transplantation. Arch Biochem Biophys 1997; 342:282–288.

71. Hinson JA, Pike SL, Pumford NR, Mayeux PR. Nitrotyrosine-protein adducts in hepatic centrilobular areas following toxic doses of acetaminophen in mice. Chem Res Toxicol 1998; 11:604–607.

72. Knight TR, Kurtz A, Bajt ML, Hinson JA, Jaeschke H. Vascular and hepatocellular peroxynitrite formation during acetaminophen toxicity: role of mitochondrial oxidant stress. Toxicol Sci 2001; 62:212–220.

73. Michael SL, Pumford NR, Mayeux PR, Niesman MR, Hinson JA. Pretreatment of mice with macrophage inactivators decreases acetaminophen hepatotoxicity and the formation of reactive oxygen and nitrogen species. Hepatology 1999; 30:186–195.

74. Nishida J, McCuskey RS, McDonnell D, Fox ES. Protective role of NO in hepatic microcirculatory dysfunction during endotoxemia. Am J Physiol 1994; 267:G1135–G1141.

75. Wang Y, Mathews WR, Guido DM, Jaeschke H. Inhibition of nitric oxide synthesis aggravates reperfusion injury after hepatic ischemia and endotoxemia. Shock 1995; 4:282–288.

76. Wang Y, Lawson JA, Jaeschke H. Differential effect of 2-aminoethyl-isothiourea, an inhibitor of the inducible nitric oxide synthase, on microvascular blood flow and organ injury in models of hepatic ischemia-reperfusion injury and endotoxemia. Shock 1998; 10:20–25.

77. Nieminen AL, Saylor AK, Tesfai SA, Herman B, Lemasters JJ. Contribution of the membrane permeability transition to lethal injury after exposure of hepatocytes to *t*-butylhydroperoxide. Biochem J 1995; 307:99–106.

78. Byrne AM, Lemasters JJ, Nieminen AL. Contribution of increased mitochondrial free Ca^{2+} to the mitochondrial permeability transition induced by tert-butylhydroperoxide in rat hepatocytes. Hepatology 1999; 29:1523–1531.

79. Aguilar HI, Botla R, Arora AS, Bronk SF, Gores GJ. Induction of the mitochondrial permeability transition by protease activity in rats: a mechanism of hepatocyte necrosis. Gastroenterology 1996; 110:558–566.

80. Miyoshi H, Umeshita K, Sakon M, Imajoh-Ohmi S, Fujitani K, Gotoh M, Oiki E, Kambayashi J, Monden M. Calpain activation in plasma membrane bleb formation during tert-butyl hydroperoxide-induced rat hepatocyte injury. Gastroenterology 1996; 110:1897–1904.

81. Sarafian TA, Bredesen DE. Is apoptosis mediated by reactive oxygen species? Free Radic Res 1994; 21:1–8.

82. Kurose I, Higuchi H, Miura S, Saito H, Watanabe N, Hokori R, Hirokawa M, Takaishi M, Zeki S, Nakamura T, Ebinuma H, Kato S, Ishii H. Oxidative stress-mediated apoptosis of hepatocytes exposed to acute ethanol intoxication. Hepatology 1997; 25:368–378.

83. Sanchez A, Alvarez AM, Benito M, Fabregat I. Apoptosis induced by transforming growth factor-β in fetal hepatocyte primary cultures: involvement of reactive oxygen intermediates. J Biol Chem 1996; 27:7416–7422.

84. Rauen U, Polzar B, Stephan H, Mannherz HG, de Groot H. Cold-induced apoptosis in cultured hepatocytes and liver endothelial cells: mediation by reactive oxygen species. FASEB J 1999; 13:155–168.

85. Motoyama S, Minamiya Y, Saito S, Saito R, Matsuzaki I, Abo S, Inaba H, Enomoto K, Kitamura M. Hydrogen peroxide derived from hepatocytes induces sinusoidal endothelial cell apoptosis in perfused hypoxic rat liver. Gastroenterology 1998; 114:153–163.

86. Hampton MG, Orrenius S. Dual regulation of caspase activity by hydrogen peroxide: implications for apoptosis. FEBS Lett 1997; 414:552–556.

87. Fadeel B, Ahlin A, Henter JI, Orrenius S, Hampton MB. Involvement of caspases in neutrophil apoptosis: regulation by reactive oxygen species. Blood 1998; 92:4808–4818.

88. Kim YM, Kim TH, Chung HT, Talanian RV, Yin XM, Billiar TR. Nitric oxide prevents tumor necrosis factor alpha-induced rat hepatocyte apoptosis by the interruption of mitochondrial apoptotic signaling through *S*-nitrosylation of caspase-8. Hepatology 2000; 32:770–778.

89. Schreck R, Albermann K, Baeuerle PA. Nuclear factor kappa B: an oxidative stress-responsive transcription factor of eukaryotic cells. Free Radic Res Commun 1992; 17:221–237.

90. Li X, Karin M. Is NF-κB the sensor of oxidative stress? FASEB J 1999; 13:1137–1143.

91. Janssen-Heininger YMW, Poynter ME, Baeuerle PA. Recent advances towards understanding redox mechanisms in the activation of nuclear factor κB. Free Radic Biol Med 2000; 28:1317–1327.

92. Bellezzo JM, Leingang KA, Bulla GA, Britton RS, Bacon BR, Fox ES. Modulation of lipopolysaccharide-mediated activation of rat Kupffer cells by antioxidants. J Lab Clin Med 1998; 131:36–44.

93. Essani NA, Fisher MA, Jaeschke H. Inhibition of NF-κB activation by dimethyl sulfoxide correlates with suppression of TNF-α formation, reduced ICAM-1 gene transcription and protection against endotoxin-induced liver injury. Shock 1997; 7:90–96.

94. Tsukamoto H, Lin M, Ohata M, Giulivi C, French SW, Brittenham G. Iron primes hepatic macrophages for NF-kappaB activation in alcoholic liver injury. Am J Physiol 1999; 277: G1240–G1250.

95. Adamson GM, Billings RE. Tumor necrosis factor induced oxidative stress in isolated mouse hepatocytes. Arch Biochem Biophys 1992; 294:223–229.

96. Dong W, Simeonova PP, Gallucci R, Matheson J, Fannin R, Montuschi P, Flood L, Luster MI. Cytokine expression in hepatocytes: role of oxidant stress. J Interferon Cytokine Res 1998; 18:629–638.

97. Rensing H, Jaeschke H, Bauer I, Patau C, Datene V, Pannen BHJ, Bauer M. Differential activation pattern of redox-sensitive transcription factors and stress-inducible dilator systems HO-1 and iNOS in hemorrhagic and endotoxin shock. Crit Care Med 2001; 29:1962–1971.

98. Rensing H, Bauer I, Peters I, Wein T, Silomon M, Jaeschke H, Bauer M. Role of reactive oxygen species for hepatocellular injury and heme oxygenase-1 gene expression following hemorrhage and resuscitation. Shock 1999; 12:200–308.

99. Pannen BHJ, Köhler N, Hole B, Bauer M, Clemens MG, Geiger KK. Protective role of endogenous carbon monoxide in hepatic microcirculatory dysfunction after hemorrhagic shock in rats. J Clin Invest 1998; 102:1220–1228.

100. Kaplowitz N, Tsukamoto H. Oxidative stress and liver disease. In: JL Boyer, RK Ockner, eds. Progress in Liver Diseases. Vol. 14. Philadelphia: WB Saunders, 1996:131–159.

101. Chojkier M, Houglum K, Lee KS, Buck M. Long- and short-term D-alpha-tocopherol supplementation inhibits liver collagen alpha1(I) gene expression. Am J Physiol 1998; 275:G1480–G1485.

102. Garcia-Trevijano ER, Iraburu MJ, Fontana L, Dominguez-Rosales JA, Auster A, Covarrubias-Pinedo A, Rojkind M. Transforming growth factor beta1 induces the expression of alpha1(I) procollagen mRNA by a hydrogen peroxide-C/EBPbeta–dependent mechanism in rat hepatic stellate cells. Hepatology 1999; 29:960–970.

103. Xu Y, Rojkind M, Czaja MJ. Regulation of monocyte chemoattractant protein 1 by cytokines and oxygen free radicals in rat hepatic fat-storing cells. Gastroenterology 1996; 110:1870–1877.

104. Fridovich I. Superoxide radical and superoxide dismutases. Annu Rev Biochem 1995; 64:97–112.

105. Slot JW, Geuze HJ, Freeman BA, Crapo JD. Intracellular localisation of the copper-zinc and manganese superoxide dismutases in rat liver parenchymal cells. Lab Invest 1986; 55:363–371.

106. Calabrese EJ, Canada AT. Catalase: its role in xenobiotic detoxification. Pharmacol Ther 1989; 44:297–307.

107. Oshino N, Chance B. Properties of glutathione release observed during reduction of organic hydroperoxide, demethylation of aminopyrine and oxidation of some substances in perfused rat liver, and their implications for the physiological function of catalase. Biochem J 1977; 162:509–525.

108. Flohe L. Glutathione peroxidase brought into focus. In: WA Pryor, ed. Free Radicals in Biology. Vol. V. New York: Academic Press, 1982:223–254.

109. Sies H, Sharov VS, Klotz LO, Briviba K. Glutathione peroxidase protects against peroxynitrite-mediated oxidations. J Biol Chem 1997; 272:27812–27817.

110. Olafsdottir K, Reed DJ. Retention of oxidized glutathione by isolated perfused rat liver mitochondria during hydroperoxide treatment. Biochim Biophys Acta 1988; 964:377–382.

111. Lawrence RA, Burk RF. Glutathione peroxidase activity in selenium-deficient rat liver. Biochem Biophys Res Commun 1976; 71:952–958.

112. Prohaska JR. The glutathione peroxidase activity of glutathione-S-transferases. Biochim Biophys Acta 1980; 611:87–98.

113. Hill KE, Burk RF, Lane JM. Effect of selenium depletion and repletion on plasma glutathione and glutathione-dependent enzymes in the rat. J Nutr 1987; 117:99–104.

114. Burk RF, Nishiki K, Lawrence RA, Chance B. Peroxide removal by selenium-dependent and selenium-independent glutathione peroxidases in hemoglobin-free perfused rat liver. J Biol Chem 1978; 253:43–46.

115. Burk RF, Lawrence RA, Lane JM. Liver necrosis and lipid peroxidation in the rat as the result of paraquat and diquat administration. J Clin Invest 1980; 65:1024–1031.

116. Ursini F, Maiorino M, Gregolin C. The selenoenzyme phospholipid hydroperoxide glutathione peroxidase. Biochim Biophys Acta 1985; 839:62–70.

117. Ursini F, Bindoli A. The role of selenium peroxidases in the protection against oxidation damage of membranes. Chem Phys Lipids 1987; 44:255–276.

118. Chow CK. Vitamin E and oxidative stress. Free Radic Biol Med 1991; 11:215–232.

119. Wefers H, Sies H. The protection by ascorbate and glutathione against microsomal lipid peroxidation is dependent on vitamin E. Eur J Biochem 1988; 174:353–357.

120. Sies H. Strategies of antioxidant defense. Eur J Biochem 1993; 215:213–219.

121. Mitchell JR, Smith CV, Lauterburg BH, Hughes H, Corcoran GB, Horning EC. Reactive metabolites and the pathophysiology of acute lethal cell injury. In: JR Mitchell, MG Horning, eds. Drug Metabolism and Drug Toxicity. New York: Raven Press, 1984:301–319.

122. Deleve LD, Kaplowitz N. Importance and regulation of hepatic glutathione. Semin Liver Dis 1990; 10:251–266.

123. Ookhtens M, Kaplowitz N. Role of the liver in interorgan homeostasis of glutathione and cyst(e)ine. Semin Liver Dis 1998; 18:313–329.

124. Ballatori N, Rebbeor JF. Roles of MRP2 and oatp1 in hepatocellular export of reduced glutathione. Semin Liver Dis 1998; 18:377–387.

125. Yi JR, Lu S, Fernandez-Checa J, Kaplowitz N. Expression cloning of the cDNA for a polypeptide associated with rat hepatic sinusoidal reduced glutathione transport: characteristics and comparison with the canalicular transporter. Proc Natl Acad Sci USA 1995; 92:1495–1499.

126. Fernandez-Checa JC, Ookhtens M, Kaplowitz N. Selective induction by phenobarbital of the electrogenic transport of glutathione and organic anions in rat liver canalicular membrane vesicles. J Biol Chem 1993; 268:10836–10841.

127. Lauterburg BH, Adams JD, Mitchell JR. Hepatic glutathione homeostasis in the rat: efflux accounts for glutathione turnover. Hepatology 1984; 4:586–590.

128. Oude-Elferink RPJ, Ottenhoff R, Liefting WGM, Schoemaker B, Groen AK, Jansen PLM. ATP-dependent efflux of GSSG and GS-conjugate from isolated rat hepatocytes. Am J Physiol 1990; 258:G699–G706.

129. Nicotera P, Moore M, Bellomo G, Mirabelli F, Orrenius S. Demonstration and partial characterization of glutathione disulfide-stimulated ATPase activity in the plasma membrane fraction from rat hepatocytes. J Biol Chem 1985; 260:1999–2002.

130. Jaeschke H. Glutathione disulfide as index of oxidant stress in rat liver during hypoxia. Am J Physiol 1990; 258:G499–G505.

131. Adams JD, Lauterburg BH, Mitchell JR. Plasma glutathione and glutathione disulfide in the rat: regulation and response to oxidative stress. J Pharmacol Exp Ther 1983; 227:749–754.

132. Reed DJ. Glutathione: Toxicological implications. Annu Rev Pharmacol Toxicol 1990; 30:603–631.

133. Garcia-Ruiz C, Morales A, Colell A, Roades J, Yi JR, Kaplowitz N, Fernandez-Checa JC. Evidence that the rat hepatic mitochondrial carrier is distinct from the sinusoidal and canalicular transporters for reduced glutathione. J Biol Chem 1995; 270:15946–15949.

134. Kurosawa K, Hayashi N, Sato N, Kamada T, Tagawa K. Transport of glutathione across the mitochondrial membranes. Biochem Biophys Res Commun 1990; 167:367–372.

135. Meredith MJ, Reed DJ. Depletion in vitro of mitochondrial glutathione in rat hepatocytes and enhanced lipid peroxidation by adriamycin and 1,3-bis(2-chloroethyl)-1-nitrosourea (BCNU). Biochem Pharmacol 1983; 32:1383–1388.

136. Colell A, Garcia-Ruiz C, Miranda M, Ardite E, Mari M, Morales A, Corrales F, Kaplowitz N, Fernandez-Checa JC. Selective glutathione depletion of mitochondria by ethanol sensitizes hepatocytes to tumor necrosis factor. Gastroenterology 1998; 115:1541–1551.

137. Garcia-Ruiz C, Colell A, Morales A, Kaplowitz N, Fernandez-Checa JC. Role of oxidative

stress generated from the mitochondrial electron transport chain and mitochondrial glutathione status in loss of mitochondrial function and activation of transcription factor nuclear factor-kappa B; studies with isolated mitochondria and rat hepatocytes. Mol Pharmacol 1995; 48:825–834.

138. Jaeschke, H. Antioxidant defense mechanisms. In: IG Sipes, CA McQueen, AJ Gandolfi, eds. Comprehensive Toxicology. Vol. IX. Oxford: Elsevier, 1997:181–197.

139. Hidalgo J, Campmany L, Borras M, Garvey JS, Armario A. Metallothionein response to stress in rats: role of free radical scavenging. Am J Physiol 1988; 255:E518–E524.

140. DeLeve LD. Glutathione defense in non-parenchymal cells. Semin Liver Dis 1998; 18:403–413.

141. Spolarics Z. Endotoxemia, pentose cycle, and the oxidant/antioxidant balance in the hepatic sinusoid. J Leukoc Biol 1998; 63:534–541.

142. Spolarics Z, Wu JX. Role of glutathione and catalase in H2O2 detoxification in LPS-activated hepatic endothelial and Kupffer cells. Am J Physiol 1997; 273:G1304–G1311.

143. Halliwell B, Gutteridge JMC. The antioxidants of human extracellular fluids. Arch Biochem Biophys 1990; 280:1–8.

144. Marklund SL. Human copper-containing superoxide dismutase. Proc Natl Acad Sci USA 1982; 79:7634–7638.

145. Takahashi K, Avissar N, Whitin J, Cohen H. Purification and characterization of human plasma glutathione peroxidase: a selenoglycoprotein distinct from the known cellular enzyme. Arch Biochem Biophys 1987; 256:677–686.

146. Karlsson K, Lindahl U, Marklund SL. Binding of human extracellular superoxide dismutase C to sulphated glycosminoglycans. Biochem J 1988; 256:29–33.

147. Jaeschke H. Enhanced sinusoidal glutathione efflux during endotoxin-induced oxidant stress in vivo. Am J Physiol 1992; 263:G60–G68.

148. Mirochnitchenko O, Weisbrot-Lefkowitz M, Reuhl K, Chen L, Yang C, Inouye M. Acetaminophen toxicity. Opposite effects of two forms of glutathione peroxidase. J Biol Chem 1999; 274:10349–10355.

149. Jaeschke H. Vascular oxidant stress and hepatic ischemia/reperfusion injury. Free Radic Res Commun 1991; 12–13:737–743.

150. Liu P, Fisher MA, Farhood A, Smith CW, Jaeschke H. Beneficial effect of extracellular glutathione against reactive oxygen-mediated reperfusion injury in the liver. Circ Shock 1994; 43:64–70.

151. Wang Y, Fisher MA, Jaeschke H. Detoxification of Kupffer cell-derived reactive oxygen and reactive nitrogen species by plasma glutathione during hepatic ischemia-reperfusion injury. In: E Wisse, DL Knook, C Balabaud, eds. Cells of the Hepatic Sinusoid. Vol. 6. Leiden: Kupffer Cell Foundation, 1997:205–206.

152. Burk RF, Hill KE. Selenoprotein P. A selenium-rich extracellular glycoprotein. J Nutr 1994; 124:1891–1897.

153. Read R, Bellew T, Yang JG, Hill KE, Palmer IS, Burk RF. Selenium and amino acid composition of selenoprotein P, the major selenoprotein in rat serum. J Biol Chem 1990; 265:17899–17905.

154. Burk RF, Hill KE, Awad JA, Morrow JD, Kato T, Cockwell KA, Lyons PR. Pathogenesis of diquat-induced liver necrosis in selenium-deficient rats: assessment of the roles of lipid peroxidation and selenoprotein P. Hepatology 1995; 21:561–569.

155. Burk RF, Hill KE, Awad JA, Morrow JD, Lyons PR. Liver and kidney necrosis in selenium-deficient rat depleted of glutathione. Lab Invest 1995; 72:723–730.

4

Hepatotoxicity Due to Mitochondrial Injury

**DOMINIQUE PESSAYRE, BERNARD FROMENTY,
ABDELLAH MANSOURI, and ALAIN BERSON**

*Institut National de la Santé et de la Recherche Médicale (INSERM), Clichy,
France*

I. INTRODUCTION

Three main mechanisms are responsible for drug-induced liver injury. The most frequent mechanism is the formation of reactive drug metabolites that can be directly toxic or cause immune reactions (1,2). Another is drug-induced impairment of mitochondrial function, which may decrease fat oxidation (causing steatosis) and/or energy production (causing cell dysfunction or cell death) (3–7). A third mechanism involves the opening of the mitochondrial permeability transition pore (MPTP), causing necrosis or apoptosis. Although this permeability transition can be triggered by direct or indirect effects of the parent drug on mitochondria (8,9), it is most frequently caused by the formation of reactive metabolites, which can trigger MPTP opening through either direct toxicity or immune reactions (8,9). Thus, even when hepatotoxicity is initially due to the formation of reactive metabolites, mitochondrial injury plays a major role in the final mechanism of cell death (8,9). Therefore, most forms of drug-induced liver lesions initially or secondarily involve mitochondrial injury (9).

II. ORIGIN AND STRUCTURE OF MITOCHONDRIA

Some 1.5–2 billion years ago, a precursor of present-day eukaryotes engaged in a parasitic/symbiotic partnership with a wild bacterium (10–12). This precursor allowed the bacterium to reside and divide within its cytoplasm. In exchange, the bacterium used the emerging oxygen atmosphere to completely degrade fuels into CO_2 and water, thus providing the host with considerable energy (11,12). Like their bacterial ancestors, mitochondria have two membranes. A circular outer membrane surrounds the intermembrane space, while an inner membrane with inner folds (the mitochondrial cristae) limits the mitochondrial matrix (12).

Although most of the initial bacterial genes have been transferred to the nucleus of the host, mitochondria have retained a small genome, located in the matrix (12). Each cell contains many copies of this circular, double-stranded genome, as there are several copies of mitochondrial DNA (mtDNA) in a single mitochondrion and many mitochondria per cell (10). mtDNA encodes 13 polypeptides of the respiratory chain, while the remaining respiratory polypeptides and all other mitochondrial proteins are encoded by nuclear DNA. These proteins are synthesized in the cytoplasm (usually with a mitochondrial-targeting presequence) and are then imported into the mitochondrial membranes or the matrix, where the presequence is cleaved (10).

Respiratory chain polypeptides are located in the inner membrane, except for cytochrome c, which is targeted to the intermembrane space (13). Although the initial shortening of very-long- and long-chain fatty acids is mediated by enzymes located in the inner membrane, most other enzymes involved in fatty acid β-oxidation and the tricarboxylic acid cycle are located in the mitochondrial matrix (10).

III. ROLES OF MITOCHONDRIA

A. Fat Oxidation and Energy Production

Mitochondria play a major role in fat oxidation and energy production. The entry of long-chain fatty acids into mitochondria is modulated by carnitine palmitoyl transferase I (Fig. 1). This outer membrane enzyme is inhibited by malonyl-CoA, which is the first step in the synthesis of fatty acids (14). This inhibition normally ensures a reciprocal relationship between fatty acid synthesis and the mitochondrial uptake and oxidation of fatty acids (14).

Once fatty acids are taken up by mitochondria, they are targeted toward oxidation (14). Fatty acyl-CoAs are split by β-oxidation cycles into acetyl-CoA subunits, which can either form ketone bodies or, like other fuels, be completely degraded to CO_2 by the tricarboxylic acid cycle (Fig. 1). The NADH and $FADH_2$ that are generated by both β-oxidation and the tricarboxylic acid cycle are then reoxidized by the mitochondrial respiratory chain (12). This regenerates the NAD^+ and FAD necessary for other cycles of fuel oxidation (Fig. 1), and also initiates the process of energy production (3).

NADH and $FADH_2$ transfer their electrons to the first complexes of the respiratory chain (12). Although a fraction of these electrons react with oxygen to form reactive oxygen species (ROS), as discussed later, most electrons migrate all the way along the respiratory chain, up to cytochrome c oxidase, where they safely combine with oxygen and protons to form water (Fig. 1). During this transfer of electrons along the respiratory chain, protons are extruded from the mitochondrial matrix into the intermembrane space (Fig. 1) (12). This creates a large electrochemical potential across the inner membrane whose potential energy is then used to generate ATP. When ADP is high, protons reenter

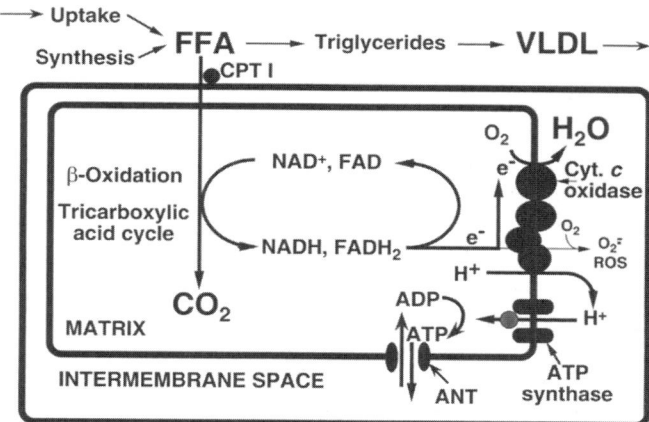

Figure 1 Fat metabolism in hepatocytes and mitochondria. Free fatty acids (FFA) are either synthesized in the liver or transferred from the intestine or adipose tissue. FFA either enter mitochondria, a step regulated by carnitine palmitoyl transferase I (CPTI), or are esterified into triglycerides that are stored in the cytoplasm or secreted as very-low-density lipoproteins. Inside mitochondria, FFA form acyl-CoA thioesters that are cut and oxidized by the β-oxidation and tricarboxylic acid cycles, generating NADH and FADH$_2$ that transfer electrons to the respiratory chain. Although part of these electrons react with oxygen to form the superoxide anion radical and other reactive oxygen species (ROS), most electrons migrate up to cytochrome c oxidase where they safely combine with oxygen and protons to form water. The transfer of electrons along the respiratory chain is associated with the extrusion of protons from the mitochondrial matrix into the intermembrane space. The reentry of protons in the matrix through ATP synthase transforms ADP into ATP, which is then extruded by the adenine nucleotide translocator (ANT), in exchange for cytosolic ADP.

the matrix through the F$_0$ portion of ATP synthase, causing the rotation of a molecular rotor in the F$_1$ portion of ATP synthase and conversion of ADP into ATP (Fig. 1). This ATP is then extruded by the adenine nucleotide translocator, in exchange for cytosolic ADP (12).

Thus mitochondria burn fat and other fuels into CO$_2$ and water, providing most of the cell's ATP. However, the price of this oxidative phosphorylation is a high formation rate of ROS (12).

B. Mitchondrial ROS Formation

A fraction of the electrons transferred to the first complexes of the respiratory chain by NADH and FADH$_2$ directly react with oxygen to form the superoxide anion radical and other ROS (Fig. 1) (12). Mitochondria are the main source of ROS in the cell (15).

Although mitochondria actively repair ROS-mediated mtDNA lesions (16), mtDNA is very sensitive to ROS-induced damage, owing to its proximity to the inner membrane (the main cellular source of ROS) and the absence of protective histones. ROS oxidize mtDNA bases, which causes errors during either mtDNA replication (17) or repair (18), leading to point mutations. ROS also cause mtDNA strand breaks, which can cause mtDNA deletions (19).

The mitochondrial theory of aging suggests that the accumulation of these mtDNA lesions eventually decreases mtDNA-encoded polypeptide synthesis and the transfer of

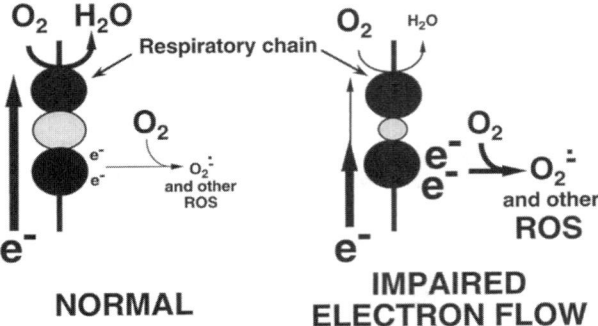

Figure 2   Impairment of respiration increases mitochondrial reactive oxygen species (ROS) formation. Even in the basal state, mitochondria are the most important sources of ROS in the cell. When the transfer of electrons is blocked, the respiratory chain components that are located upstream to the block become overly reduced and increasingly transfer their electrons to oxygen, forming larger amounts of the superoxide anion radical and other ROS.

electrons along the respiratory chain (15). Whenever the flow of electrons is blocked at some point along the respiratory chain, respiratory chain components located upstream become overly reduced and directly transfer their electrons to O_2, thus increasing the basal formation of ROS (Fig. 2) (20). This increased ROS formation further increases ROS-induced damage to mtDNA, causing more impairment of respiration and more ROS formation (10). This vicious circle could explain why mtDNA deletions (21), and some point mutations (22), which are uncommon before age 40, exponentially accumulate during old age. The high mitochondrial formation rate of ROS, and the oxidative damage it causes to mtDNA and nuclear DNA, is probably one important mechanism of aging (10,23).

Another role of mitochondria is to modulate cell death.

C.   Cell Survival and Cell Death

The partnership with parasitic bacteria may have been initially rather dangerous, because wild bacteria tend to proliferate when they are well fed (7,10). The problem was solved when the transcription and replication of the bacterial/mitochondrial genome were placed under the control of nuclear genes (24), thus transforming wild bacteria into tame mitochondria (10). Before this could occur, however, the host may have found ways to partially invalidate the proliferating bacteria, while bacteria may have disabled any mutant host that took advantage of this control mechanism (10). The present-day sequel to this double warfare is a shared decision-making process, in which both symbiotic partners play a role in regulating cell death (25).

Mitochondria are involved in this decision through either closure or opening of a pore in the inner membrane, called the MPTP (Fig. 3) (9,25). Pore closure allows the cell to survive, while pore opening causes cell death (Fig. 3) (9). Pore opening allows massive reentry of protons through the inner membrane, causing collapse of the mitochondrial membrane potential and interrupting mitochondrial ATP synthesis. If the pore opens quickly in all mitochondria, severe ATP depletion prevents apoptosis (an energy-requiring process) and causes necrosis (Fig. 3) (26). Pore opening also causes matrix expansion, rupture of the spherical outer membrane, herniation of the inner membrane and matrix

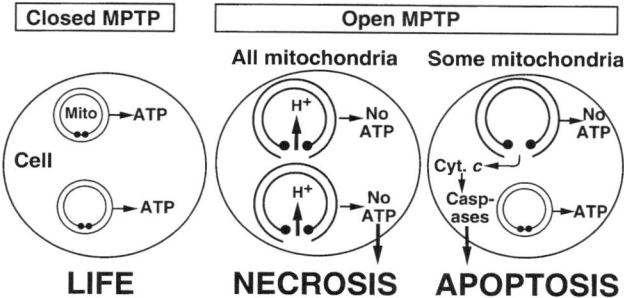

Figure 3   Regulation of life and death by the mitochondrial permeability transition pore (MPTP). Pore closure allows cell survival, whereas pore opening causes cell death. MPTP opening causes the reentry of protons into the mitochondrial matrix, thus bypassing ATP synthase and preventing ATP formation. Pore opening also causes matrix expansion, outer membrane rupture, and release of mitochondrial cytochrome c (cyt. c) from the intermembrane space into the cytosol. If the pore opens in all mitochondria, decreased ATP synthesis causes ATP depletion and necrosis. If the pore opens in only some mitochondria, unaffected mitochondria keep synthesizing ATP (thus avoiding necrosis), while permeabilized mitochondria release cytochrome c, which activates caspases, causing apoptosis.

through the outer membrane gap, and cytochrome c release from the intermembrane space into the cytosol (27,28). If the pore opens only in some mitochondria, unaffected mito- chondria keep synthesizing ATP, while permeabilized mitochodria release cytochrome c, which activates caspases in the cytosol, causing apoptosis (Fig. 3) (10,27,28).

IV. CONSEQUENCES OF IMPAIRED MITOCHONDRIAL FUNCTION

A. Primary Impairment of Fatty Acid Oxidation

Primary impairment of fatty acid oxidation causes hepatic steatosis (3). Mild inhibition is not enough—severe impairment is required (3). In this case, the free fatty acids, which are taken up by the liver or synthesized within the liver, are not oxidized by deficient mitochondria, but are esterified into triglycerides that accumulate within the cytoplasm of hepatocytes, causing hepatic steatosis (3).

Acute impairment of fatty acid β-oxidation typically causes microvesicular steatosis (3). In this peculiar form of steatosis, numerous tiny lipid vesicles leave the nucleus in the center of the cell and give the hepatocyte a "foamy," "spongiocytic" appearance. Mixed forms of steatosis can also occur when β-oxidation is more chronically impaired. Some hepatocytes are filled with tiny lipid vesicles, while others exhibit large fat vacuoles or both small vesicles and larger vacuoles. These associations and transitions suggest that tiny lipid vesicles can coalesce into larger vacuoles. Instead, prolonged causes of steatosis tend to cause macrovacuolar steatosis (3). In this form of steatosis, hepatocytes are dis- tended by a single, large vacuole of fat, displacing the nucleus to the cell periphery.

The acute onset (or sudden aggravation) of mitochondrial failure may leave no time for the progressive coalescence of small lipid vesicles into large vacuoles, explaining the microvesicular pattern of steatosis in acute mitochondrial diseases. Another mechanism could involve an emulsifying effect of free fatty acids (3). When mitochondrial β-oxidation is impaired, free fatty acids increase in the liver, and these amphiphilic compounds may form an emulsifying rim around lipid droplets, thus favoring the persistence of small fat vesicles (3).

Primary impairment of fatty acid oxidation also secondarily impairs mitochondrial energy production (3). Fatty acid oxidation represents the main cellular source of energy between meals, and subjects whose mitochondrial β-oxidation is impaired do not tolerate fasting (29). Fasting may trigger hypoglycemia in these patients (29), thus hampering energy production from this still oxidizable fuel in extrahepatic organs. Furthermore, fasting also causes massive adipocyte lipolysis, thus flooding the liver with free fatty acids, which are not oxidized by the deficient mitochondria and therefore accumulate in the liver (3). Free fatty acids and their dicarboxylic acid derivatives inhibit and uncouple mitocondrial respiration, further decreasing energy production (3). Although the energy deficit is not sufficient to cause cell death, it can cause cell dysfunction in different organs. These patients may develop mild liver failure (sometimes with renal failure and pancreatitis) and severe brain dysfunction, causing coma and death (29).

B. Primary Impairment of Mitochondrial Respiration

Impairment of mitochondrial respiration decreases energy formation and, depending on the severity of the deficit, can cause either cell dysfunction or cell death (3). Moderate impairment of respiration only causes cell dysfunction. Although there is no necrosis or apoptosis, this can nevertheless cause severe lactic acidosis and death (3). Severe impairment of respiration can cause liver cell necrosis, cholestasis, and fibrosis (30–32).

Impairment of respiration also blocks the transfer of electrons along the respiratory chain, causing overreduction of the respiratory chain components located upstream, which increases mitochondrial ROS formation (20). This increased ROS formation could contribute to the appearance of necroinflammation and fibrosis, as discussed later.

Finally, severe impairment of respiration secondarily impairs mitochondrial β-oxidation (33). Normally, the NADH formed by β-oxidation is reoxidized by the mitochondrial respiratory chain, thus regenerating the NAD^+ required for fatty acid β-oxidation. When respiration is severely impaired, NAD^+ regeneration is insufficient to sustain β-oxidation (33). This secondarily impairs β-oxidation and causes microvesicular steatosis (3).

C. Common Features

Thus primary impairment of β-oxidation causes both microvesicular steatosis and secondary energy deficiency (causing cell dysfunction), while primary impairment of respiration causes both energy deficiency (leading to cell dysfunction) and secondary impairment of β-oxidation (causing microvesicular steatosis). Thus, whatever the initial impairment, drug-induced mitochondrial dysfunction may associate features of both steatosis and cell dysfunction. However, each of these features may predominate according to the initial mechanism.

V. DIVERSITY OF MECHANISMS IMPAIRING MITOCHONDRIAL FUNCTION

Drugs may impair mitochondrial function by several mechanisms (3–9). They can degrade mtDNA, terminate or inhibit mtDNA replication, inhibit mtDNA transcription, inhibit or uncouple mitochondrial respiration, sequester CoA (which is required for fatty acid activation before their β-oxidation), directly inhibit β-oxidation enzymes, or inhibit both β-oxidation and respiration.

A. Degradation of mtDNA

1. Alcohol

Ethanol metabolism causes oxidative stress in the liver (34). Ethanol metabolism causes excess NADH formation, which can reduce ferric iron into ferrous iron (a potent generator of the hydroxyl radical) (35). Other ROS sources include increased levels of ROS-generating cytochrome P450 (CYP) 2E1 (36) and increased mitochondrial ROS formation (37). ROS cause oxidative damage to mitochondrial lipids (38), proteins (39), and DNA (40) in intoxicated animals.

A single, high dose of ethanol causes extensive mtDNA degradation and depletion within 2 h in mice (40). These effects are prevented by 4-methylpyrazole (blocking ethanol metabolism) or melatonin (an antioxidant) (40). Although damaged mtDNA molecules are quickly repaired or resynthesized de novo (40), the repetition of mtDNA strand breaks during chronic alcoholism can cause mtDNA deletions. The prevalence of mtDNA deletions is increased in alcoholics with microvesicular steatosis, but not in patients with alcoholic hepatitis or cirrhosis (41,42). The latter conditions increase liver cell turnover (43,44), which could eliminate mutated mtDNA genomes, if cells with a high proportion of mutated genomes fail to replicate and are progressively eliminated through apoptosis. When ethanol ingestion is stopped, alcohol-induced mtDNA deletions disappear quickly in white blood cells (45), which have a quick cell turnover.

Alcohol abuse can cause three primary types of liver lesions: macrovascular steatosis, microvesicular steatosis, and necroinflammation. Macrovacuolar steatosis seems to be mainly due to ROS-independent mechanisms. These include increased hepatic synthesis of fatty acids, decreased hepatic lipoprotein excretion, and impaired hepatic fatty acid oxidation due to the ethanol metabolism-mediated decrease in the $NAD^+/NADH$ ratio, which slightly inhibits mitochondrial β-oxidation and markedly inhibits the tricarboxylic acid cycle (46,47). Microvesicular steatosis is thought to be due to a combination of the mild inhibition of β-oxidation, and ROS-dependent damage to mitochondrial lipids, proteins, and DNA, which further impairs mitochondrial function (42). Necroinflammation seems to be mainly mediated by ROS. ROS cause lipid peroxidation, and also increase cytokine synthesis (10). Both effects cause necroinflammation and fibrosis, leading to alcoholic hepatitis and cirrhosis (10).

2. Topoisomerase Inhibitors

Topoisomerases play an important role in DNA replication and transcription (48). Type I topoisomerases act as monomers and cut one strand of DNA, while type II topoisomerases act as dimers or multimers and cut both strands of DNA. These enzymes cut the phosphodiester DNA backbone by forming a covalent bond between the liberated phosphorus and a tyrosine of the enzyme. Normally, this reaction is quickly reversible. These enzymes first cut DNA, thus allowing other DNA strand(s) to cross the gap, and then promptly reseal the DNA strand gap. Several antibacterial drugs (4-quinolones, novobiocine) or anticancer drugs (amsacrine, etoposide, anthracyclines, ellipticines, actinomycins) are topoisomerase inhibitors (48). Although the mechanisms of inhibition differ with different drugs, most inhibitors act by preventing the resealing of DNA, thus increasing the number of enzyme-bound cleaved DNA complexes (48). Mitochodria contain both type I topoisomerase and a bacterial-like type II topoisomerase (49).

The 4-quinolone antibiotics inhibit gyrase (the bacterial type II topoisomerase) and also the mitochondrial type II topoisomerase (50). Ciprofloxacin blocks the resealing of mtDNA breaks, causing accumulation of protein-linked double-strand mtDNA breaks (51). Ciprofloxacin and nalidix acid progressively decrease mtDNA in cultured mammalian cells, impairing mitochondrial respiration and cell growth (50). 4-Quinolone antibiotics can cause cholestasis, steatosis, and necrosis in humans (52,53), and trovafloxacin and alatrofloxacin were taken off the market because of an unacceptable risk of fulminant liver failure.

B. Inhibition of mtDNA Replication

1. 2′,3′-Dideoxynucleosides

Several 2′,3′-dideoxynucleosides are used in patients with the human immunodeficiency virus. These include 3′-azido-2′,3′-dideoxythymidine (zidovudine, AZT), 2′,3′-dideoxycytidine (zalcitabine, ddC), 2′,3′-dideoxyinosine (didanosine, ddI), 2′,3′-didehydro-3′-deoxythymidine (stavudine, D4T), and (−)-2′-deoxy-3′-thiacytidine (lamivudine, 3TC).

The normal 5′-hydroxyl group of deoxyribose is present in the sugar analog of these nucleosides, allowing formation of the triphosphate derivative and incorporation of the analog into a nascent chain of DNA (Fig. 4). However, the normal 3′-hydroxyl group of deoxyribose is absent in these analogs. Once a single molecule of the analog has been incorporated, the DNA molecule lacks a 3′-hydroxyl group. No other nucleotide can be incorporated, causing termination of DNA replication (Fig. 4) (54,55).

The effects of these dideoxynucleosides depend on the ability of various polymerases to incorporate them into DNA. The human immunodeficiency virus reverse transcriptase can perform this incorporation, impairing reverse transcription of the viral RNA (Fig. 4). In contrast, the DNA polymerase that act in the nucleus do not affect this incorporation, thus allowing the therapeutic use of these analogs (55). However, DNA polymerase

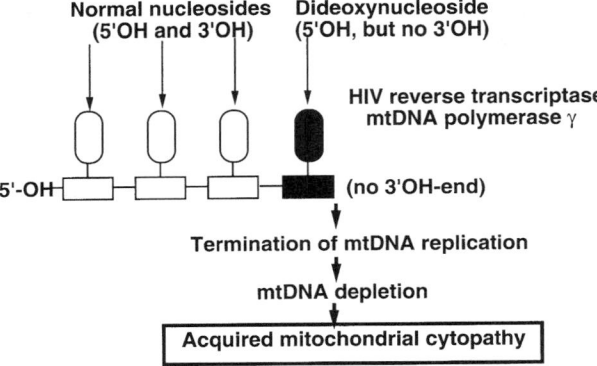

Figure 4 Termination of mtDNA replication by dideoxynucleosides. Once the human immunodeficiency virus (HIV) reverse transcriptase or mitochondrial DNA polymerase γ has incorporated a single molecule of dideoxynucleoside into a growing chain of DNA, the DNA now lacks a 3′ hydroxyl group, and no other nucleotide can be incorporated. In mitochondria, this can cause mtDNA depletion and an acquired mitochondrial cytopathy.

γ, which acts in mitochondria, also incorporates the dideoxynucleoside triphosphates into growing chains of mtDNA, which impairs mtDNA replication (Fig. 4) (56,57).

Even in postmitotic tissues, there is a constant turnover of mitochondria, requiring basal replication of mtDNA. When mtDNA replication is impaired, mtDNA levels may progressively decrease (Fig. 4). The different dideoxynucleosides have differential effects on mtDNA in diverse organs. In hepatic HepG2 cells, zalcitabine (ddC) markedly decreased mtDNA, while high doses of didanosine (ddI) caused a mild decrease, and stavudine (d4T) had no effect (58). Although zidovudine (AZT) also had no effect on mtDNA levels, it markedly increased lactate release (58). One possible explanation is that AZT also inhibits the adenine nucleotide translocator, thus impairing ATP release and blocking the flow of electrons along the respiratory chain (59). This may be one reason why lactate production may be decreased even though mtDNA levels are normal. Another reason may be increased ROS formation. Inhibition of the adenine nucleotide translocator can increase mitochondrial ROS formation, causing oxidative damage to mtDNA (60,61), and probably also other mitochondrial constituents. This oxidative damage could decrease mitochondrial function despite normal mtDNA levels (61).

Clinical manifestations of acquired (or inborn) mitochondrial cytopathies are extremely polymorphic. They include bone marrow suppression, pancreatitis, peripheral neuropathy, myopathy, and microvesicular steatosis of the liver, sometimes with fatal lactic acidosis and hepatic mtDNA depletion (62). Severe lactic acidosis has been mainly reported with zidovudine (AZT), followed by stavudine (d4T), didanosine (ddI), and lamivudine (3TC) (63).

2. Fialuridine

Clinical trials testing the efficacy of fialuridine in patients with chronic hepatitis B were abruptly interrupted after several patients developed microvesicular steatosis and unmanageable lactic acidosis, sometimes with pancreatitis, neuropathy, or myopathy (64).

This complication was unexpected because fialuridine possesses both a 5′-hydroxyl group and a 3′-hydroxyl group, so the incorporation of a single molecule of fialuridine into DNA should not immediately terminate mtDNA replication. However, when several adjacent molecules of fialuridine are successively incorporated, further activity of DNA polymerase γ is inhibited, decreasing mitochondrial DNA replication and mtDNA levels (65).

C. Inhibition of mtDNA Transcription by Interferon-α

Interferon-α is used in patients with chronic viral hepatitis B or C. In cultured cells, interferon-α inhibits the transcription of mitochondrial DNA into mitochondrial transcripts (66), thus decreasing mtDNA-encoded respiratory chain polypeptides and mitochondrial respiration (67). Some of the adverse effects of interferon-α, such as minor blood dyscrasias, myalgias, paresthesias, convulsions, and depression (68), resemble those observed in mild forms of inborn mitochondrial cytopathies. Interferon-α is usually administered thrice weekly, which may explain the mildness of the adverse effects. Mitochondrial transcripts may be restored on the days without interferon, and the transient decrease on treatment days may have a limited effect on mitochondrial proteins, whose half-life is long (69). Theoretically, high daily doses of interferon-α could have greater effects. They caused hepatic steatosis in a patient with chronic myelogenic leukemia (70). Although pegylated interferons also seem to result in sustained exposure, it is not yet known whether this modifies the incidence of adverse mitochondrial effects.

D. Sequestration of CoA and/or Direct Inhibition of β-Oxidation

1. Aspirin

Aspirin is quickly hydrolyzed into salicylic acid, which is activated into salicylyl-CoA on the outer mitochondrial membrane (71). Extensive salicylyl-CoA formation sequesters extramitochondrial CoA, leaving insufficient CoA to activate long-chain fatty acids and preventing their entry into mitochondria and β-oxidation (72).

Even though lethal overdoses of aspirin frequently cause microvesicular steatosis (73), therapeutic doses do not, although they can trigger Reye's syndrome in children with viral infections. Endogenous substances that impair mitochondrial function, such as interferon-α, tumor necrosis factor-α (TNFα), and nitric oxide, are released during viral infections. Interferon-α decreases mtDNA transcription and respiration (66,67). Nitric oxide reversibly inhibits mitochondrial respiration (74) and may open the MPTP (75). TNFα also inhibits respiration and opens the MPTP (8). Nevertheless, viral infections rarely cause Reye's syndrome, suggesting that these endogenous substances do not impair enough mitochondrial function to trigger the disease. However, if children take aspirin during a viral illness, the added effects of salicylate on mitochondrial function may sufficiently impair mitochondrial function to trigger the syndrome in some children. This potentiating effect of aspirin is based on the following evidence. In the past, 93% of children with Reye's syndrome had received aspirin during an acute viral illness (76), and children with Reye's syndrome had received aspirin more frequently than those with similar viral diseases not followed by Reye's syndrome (77). When aspirin use was advised against in feverish children, there was a corresponding decline in the use of aspirin and the incidence of Reye's syndrome in the United States (78). The few residual cases of Reye's syndrome now mainly occur in children with another potentiating factor, namely a latent genetic defect in mitochondrial β-oxidation enzymes (79).

Yet another effect of salicylate is to slightly uncouple mitochondrial respiration (72) and open the MPTP, as discussed later. This latter effect could be involved in the spotty liver cell death observed in patients receiving high therapeutic doses of aspirin (80) and could also contribute to Reye's syndrome.

2. Valproic Acid

Valproic acid is a branched-chain fatty acid used in several forms of seizures. Like natural short-chain fatty acid, valproic acid can enter mitochondria without undergoing previous activation. Inside mitochondria, valporic acid is extensively transformed into valproyl-CoA (81). The sequestration of intramitochondrial CoA inhibits the β-oxidation of long-, medium-, and short-chain fatty acids (Fig. 5) (81–83).

Several other effects contribute to the mitochondrial toxicity of valproate (Fig. 5). CYPs 2C9 and 2A6 desaturate the outer carbons of valproate, forming Δ_4-ene-valproate (84). This metabolite is activated into Δ_4-ene-valproyl-CoA inside mitochondria (85,86). The first dehydrogenation step of the β-oxidation cycle then forms Δ_2,Δ_4-diene-valproyl-CoA, which is a chemically reactive metabolite that may inactivate β-oxidation enzymes (85,86). This could explain why the hepatotoxicity of valproate is enhanced by the concomitant administration of antiepileptic drugs (87) that may induce CYP2A6, such as phenobarbital, phenytoin, and carbamazepine. Finally, valproic acid has an uncoupling effect, which favors MPTP opening (Fig. 5), as discussed later.

An asymptomatic increase in serum aminotransferase activity, which normalizes with either dose reduction or drug discontinuation, is frequent during administration of

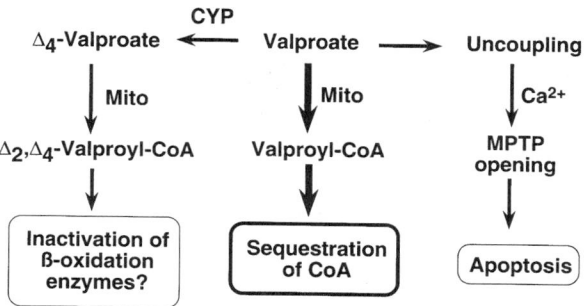

Figure 5 Mitochondrial effects of valproate. Valproate is extensively transformed into valproyl-CoA in mitochondria, thus sequestering intramitochondrial CoA and impairing mitochondrial fatty acid β-oxidation. Valproate is also desaturated by cytochrome P450 (CYP) into Δ_4-ene-valproate, which forms Δ_4-ene-valproyl-CoA in mitochondria, and then Δ_2,Δ_4-diene-valproyl-CoA, an electrophilic metabolite that may inactivate β-oxidation enzymes. Finally, valproic acid uncouples mitochondrial respiration, thus favoring Ca^{2+}-induced opening of the mitochondrial permeability transition pore (MPTP), thus triggering apoptosis.

this antiepileptic agent (87). A much less frequent side effect is a Reye's-like syndrome (88), which occurs mainly (but not exclusively) in very young children and between the first and fourth month of treatment. Histologically, centri- and midzonal microvesicular steatosis is associated with centrizonal necrosis, and sometimes cirrhosis (88). This combination of microvesicular fat and liver cell death may be related to the dual effect of valproic acid, which both inhibits mitochondrial β-oxidation and opens the MPTP (7).

Valproate toxicity might be enhanced in patients with inborn mitochondrial cytopathies, although the evidence is limited to a few case reports (89–91).

3. Tetracyclines

Tetracycline itself and the various tetracycline derivatives produce extensive microvesicular steatosis of the liver in experimental animals (92,93). This is due to the dual effect of these antibiotics, which inhibit both the mitochondrial β-oxidation of fatty acids (92,93) and the hepatic secretion of very-low-density lipoproteins (93). The latter effect occurs at doses that do not inhibit protein synthesis, suggesting impairment of the assembly and/or vesicular transport of these lipoproteins (94).

At presently administered oral doses, tetracycline may produce minor degrees of hepatic steatosis of no clinical severity in humans. However, severe microvesicular steatosis has occurred in the past during the intravenous administration of high doses of tetracycline (95). Predisposing factors included impaired renal function (which may decrease tetracycline elimination) and pregnancy (which may impair mitochondrial function, as discussed later). The syndrome usually appeared after 4–10 days of tetracycline infusion. Microvesicular steatosis has also been observed after intravenous administration of several other tetracycline derivatives (3,95).

4. Nonsteroidal Anti-inflammatory Drugs

Several nonsteroidal anti-inflammatory drugs are 2-arylpropionate derivatives. Hepatic injury due to these drugs consists of hepatitis and/or microvesicular steatosis of the liver.

The latter condition has been observed with pirprofen, naproxen, ibuprofen, and ketoprofen (96–99).

2-Arylpropionates have an asymmetrical carbon and exist as either S(+)- or R(−)-enantiomers. Only the S(+)-enantiomer inhibits prostaglandin synthesis, whereas only the R(−)-enantiomer is converted into the acyl-CoA derivative. Nevertheless, both the S(+)-enantiomer and the R(−)-enantiomer of ibuprofen inhibit the β-oxidation of medium- and short-chain fatty acids (100). Inhibition of β-oxidation has also been observed with pirprofen, tiaprofenic acid, and flurbiprofen (101).

5. Amineptine and Tianeptine

These antidepressant drugs have a tricyclic moiety and a heptanoic side chain. They may rarely cause immunoallergic hepatitis, due to the formation of reactive metabolites by P450 (102,103). Rarely, they can also cause microvesicular steatosis, due to impaired β-oxidation (3). Both amineptine and tianeptine are metabolized by the β-oxidation of their heptanoic side chain, forming the five-carbon and three-carbon derivatives (104,105). In the presence of these drugs, mitochondria are thus exposed to C7, C5, and C3 analogs of natural fatty aids. These analogs reversibly inhibit the β-oxidation of medium- and short-chain fatty acids (106,107).

6. Female Sex Hormones

About one in 13,000 pregnant women develop microvesicular steatosis during the last trimester of pregnancy (108). Untreated, the disease progresses to coma, kidney failure, and hemorrhage, and leads to the death of the mother and child in 75–85% of cases. In contrast, rapid termination of pregnancy results in delivery of a healthy child and rapid resolution of the mother's disease in most cases (109). Both pregnancy and the administration of estradiol and progesterone alter mitochondrial ultrastructure and function in mice (110,111). However, these effects are mild; β-oxidation is only slightly impaired and microvesicular steatosis does not develop in these mice (110,111). Similarly, most human pregnancies do not cause acute fatty liver. Therefore, additional factors are probably required to trigger this syndrome.

Partial deficiency of long-chain 3-hydroxyacyl-CoA dehydrogenase (LCHAD), which is part of the trifunctional membrane-bound enzyme, has been reported in some women with acute fatty liver of pregnancy (112). Mothers with a single defective LCHAD allele who are unlucky enough to marry a heterozygous carrier and then to conceive a fetus with two defective alleles develop the disease (112), whereas those who bear an unaffected child usually have uncomplicated pregnancies. These observations, however, do not reflect the real prevalence of this association in an unselected series of acute fatty liver of pregnancy. We did not detect the most prevalent LCHAD mutation in any of 14 consecutive women with histologically confirmed acute fatty liver of pregnancy (113). These findings suggest that the LCHAD deficiency is an uncommon cause of acute fatty liver of pregnancy in unselected cases. Furthermore, although one in 70 French persons is heterozygous for the A985G medium-chain acyl-CoA dehydrogenase (MCAD) mutation (114), which accounts for 89% of all deficient MCAD alleles, none of the 14 women with acute fatty liver of pregnancy carried the A985G MCAD mutation (113).

These observations should not prevent screening for various defects in mitochondrial β-oxidation in women with acute fatty liver of pregnancy (particularly those with recurrent disease or with a stillborn or unhealthy child). However, together with epidemiological data, they do suggest that such defects are rarely involved. Indeed, with few exceptions, when pregnancy is terminated early, the child is healthy and the acute fatty liver of pregnancy does not recur in subsequent pregnancies. Drugs, food, stress, infections, and auto-immune reaction triggered by the foreign child, or placental ischemia associated with preeclampsia may perhaps trigger the syndrome in different women.

7. Glucocorticoids

Glucocorticoids inhibit acyl-coenzyme A dehydrogenases and produce microvesicular steatosis of the liver in mice (115). Glucocorticoids can cause macrovacuolar steatosis (95) and steatohepatitis (116) in humans, and we have observed some patients with microvesicular steatosis during treatment with high doses of glucocorticoids.

8. Calcium Hopantenate

Calcium hopantenate has caused several cases of Reye's-like syndrome in Japan (117). Pantothenic acid is a constituent of CoA, and calcium hopantenate may decrease CoA and inhibit mitochondrial β-oxidation (117).

E. Inhibition of Both β-Oxidation and Respiration: Role in Steatohepatitis

1. Amiodarone, 4,4′-Diethylaminoethoxyhexestrol, and Perhexiline

Amiodarone, 4,4′-diethylaminoethoxyhexestrol, and perhexiline are cationic amphiphilic compounds. They have a lipophilic moiety and an amine function that can become protonated (and thus positively charged). This structure is responsible for the two liver lesions that occur with these drugs, namely lysosomal phospholipidosis and steatohepatitis (7).

The uncharged, lipophilic form of these drugs crosses the lysosomal membrane (118). In the acidic lysosomal milieu, the unprotonated drug molecule is protonated and trapped, since it cannot cross back through the lysosomal membrane. It reaches high intralysosomal concentrations and forms noncovalent but tight complexes with phospholipids, thus hampering the action of intralysosomal phospholipases (118). Phospholipids are not degraded, and the phospholipid-drug complexes progressively accumulate as myelin-like figures in enlarged lysosomes (118). Although phospholipidosis is frequent and may be constant in patients receiving these drugs, it appears to have no clinical consequence, since it often occurs without clinical symptoms or biochemical disturbances (119).

However, the cationic amphiphilic structure of these drugs also causes impaired mitochondrial function (Fig. 6) (120–124). The unprotonated, lipophilic form easily crosses the mitochondrial outer membrane and is protonated in the acidic intermembranous space (120–124). This positively charged, protonated form is "pushed" inside mitochondria by the high electrochemical potential existing across the inner mitochondrial membrane and thus reaches high intramitochondrial concentrations (120–124). It remains unknown whether this transport occurs through inner membrane transporters or directly through the lipid bilayer. These high intramitochondrial concentrations inhibit β-oxidation (causing steatosis) and also block the transfer of electrons along the respiratory chain (120–124). Respiratory chain components become overly reduced and increasingly transfer their electrons to oxygen to form the superoxide anion radical and other ROS (124). This increased ROS formation causes lipid peroxidation (124), and, like ethanol (10), could also increase cytokine production (10). Both lipid peroxidation and cytokines can cause steatohepatitis lesions (10).

Prolonged administration of these three drugs can cause typical steatohepatitis

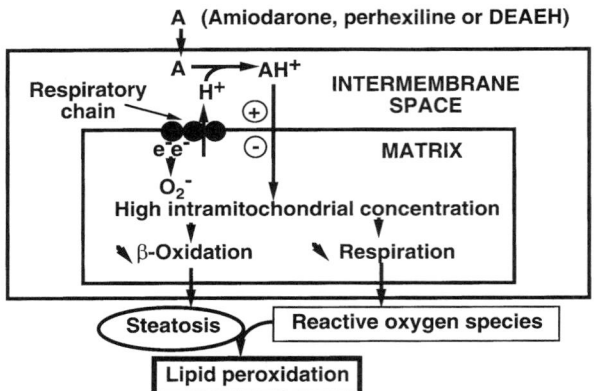

Figure 6   Effects of amphiphilic cationic drugs on mitochondrial function. After crossing the outer membrane, the uncharged tertiary or secondary amine (A) of amiodarone, perhexiline, or diethylaminoethoxyhexestrol (DEAEH) is protonated in the intermembranous space. This positively charged molecule (AH$^+$) is "pushed" by the mitochondrial membrane potential into the matrix. High intramitochondrial concentrations inhibit both β-oxidation (causing steatosis) and oxidative phosphorylation (increasing the formation of reactive oxygen species). The latter may oxidize fat deposits, causing lipid peroxidation, which, together with ROS-induced cytokine production, could cause steatohepatitis.

lesions, with steatosis, necrosis, Mallory bodies, a mixed inflammatory cell infiltrate (containing neutrophils), fibrosis, and even cirrhosis (125–130).

2.   Tamoxifen

Steatohepatitis has been also reported in many patients treated with tamoxifen (131,132). This is also a cationic amphiphilic drug that could inhibit both β-oxidation and respiration, like the above-mentioned drugs.

3.   Buprenorphine

This morphine analog is used as a substitution drug in heroin addicts. The sublingual route is used, to partly prevent extensive first-pass metabolism in the liver. At high concentrations, buprenorphine inhibits both mitochondrial β-oxidation and respiration in rat hepatocyte mitochondria (133). Much lower concentrations are observed in humans, and the drug is usually well tolerated. However, cytolytic hepatitis and steatosis have been observed in a few patients (134). Predisposing factors could include intravenous buprenorphine misuse (resulting in higher concentrations) and concomitant exposure to viruses, other drugs, or ethanol (which impair mitochondrial function) (134).

F.   Uncoupling of Mitochondrial Respiration by Protonophoric Drugs

Several drugs can translocate protons from the intermembrane space into the mitochondrial matrix (Fig. 7). This occurs with either cationic or carboxylic compounds. Cationic drugs, such as amiodarone, 4,4′-diethylaminoethoxyhexestrol, perhexiline, tacrine, and buprenorphine, have an amine function (A) that is protonated (AH$^+$) in the acidic intermembrane space. This positively charged molecule is pushed by the membrane potential across the

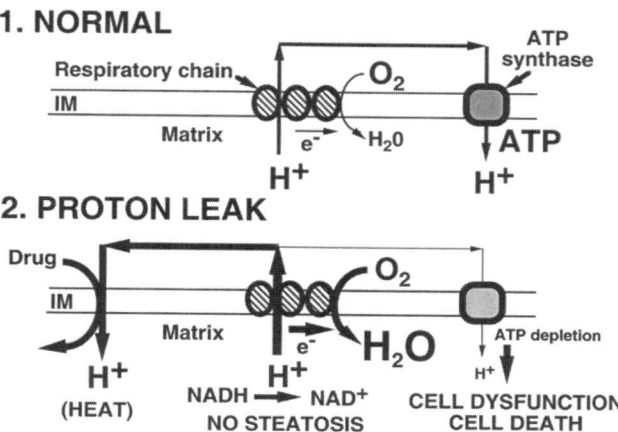

Figure 7 Opposite effects of uncouplers on mitochondrial respiration and ATP formation. Uncouplers translocate protons across the inner membrane (IM). The reentry of protons into the mitochondrial matrix decreases the membrane potential, unleashing the flow of electrons in the respiratory chain and increasing basal mitochondrial respiration. However, ATP synthase is bypassed, and this increased respiration produces heat instead of ATP, which may cause cell dysfunction or cell death. The increased respiration also increases the reoxidation of NADH into NAD^+, thus stimulating fatty acid β-oxidation. Steatosis is not observed, unless the drug has other mitochondrial effects (such as mitochondrial permeability transition, or inhibition of respiration or β-oxidation).

inner membrane (124,134). It releases its proton in the alkaline matrix, thus reforming the uncharged molecule (A), which may cross back through the inner membrane lipid bilayer, to be protonated again in the intermembrane space, ready for another cycle of proton translocation (124,134). Carboxylic compounds cross the inner-membrane lipid bilayer in the uncharged form (R-COOH), release H^+ in the alkaline matrix, and then the anionic form ($RCOO^-$) is pulled by the membrane potential into the intermembrane space. This second crossing of the inner membrane occurs through anion transporters (135). Inside the acidic intermembrane space, the uncharged acid (COOH) is formed again, ready for another cycle of proton translocation.

The reentry of protons into the intermembrane space increases basal respiration (Fig. 7). As explained above, the flow of electrons along the respiratory chain is coupled with the extrusion of protons from the mitochondrial matrix into the intermembranous state (Fig. 1). Once a high membrane potential is achieved, it blocks the flow of electrons in the respiratory chain. Uncouplers cause the reentry of protons into the mitochondrial matrix and decrease the mitochondrial membrane potential (136), unleashing the flow of electrons in the respiratory chain and increasing basal oxygen consumption (Fig. 7). However, ATP synthase is bypassed, and this increased respiration occurs in vain, to produce heat instead of ATP. Severe uncoupling decreases cell ATP and can cause cell dysfunction or cell death (136).

Unlike respiratory chain inhibitors, which impair the reoxidation of NADH into NAD^+ and may secondarily inhibit mitochondrial β-oxidation (which requires NAD^+), uncouplers increase respiration, the regeneration of NAD^+, and mitochondrial β-oxidation (Fig. 7) (122). Steatosis does not occur, unless the drug has other effects on mitochondrial function.

G. Induction of Uncoupling Protein 2

Another mechanism that could uncouple respiration is induction of the uncoupling protein 2 (UCP2). When UCP2 is highly expressed in yeast cells, this inner mitochondrial membrane protein has an uncoupling effect (137). UCP2 could sustain the cycling of free fatty acids across the inner membrane, by permitting the transport of the charged anionic form (RCOO$^-$) from the mitochondrial matrix into the intermembrane space, where RCOO$^-$ is protonated to RCOOH, which can cross the lipid bilayer to translocate one proton into the matrix (138). The UCP2 messenger RNA is expressed in hepatocytes and increased by free fatty acids, ROS, lipopolysaccharide, TNFα, interleukin-1, and peroxisome proliferator-activated receptor agonists in rodents (139,140). It is still unclear, however, whether the UCP2 protein is also sufficiently expressed to significantly uncouple respiration in hepatocytes (139,140). Any uncoupling due to UCP2 is probably too mild to cause deleterious pathological changes, although it might accelerate hepatic fatty acid β-oxidation, and also potentiate the toxicity of ATP-depleting drugs (139).

VI. MITOCHONDRIAL PERMEABILITY TRANSITION

Some drugs cause direct MPTP opening, while other drugs form reactive metabolites, which open the MPTP due to either direct toxicity or immune reactions.

A. Parent Drug

1. Salicyclic Acid, Valproic Acid, and Other Carboxylic Drugs

Carboxylic drugs often have a mild uncoupling effect, which tends to decrease the mitochondrial membrane potential, favoring MPTP opening (141). Salicylic acid, valproic acid, and several carboxylic acids potentiate the MPTP opening caused by calcium (142). The fact that an increase in cell calcium is a prerequisite may explain why these drugs rarely have a cytopathic effects in clinical use. Nevertheless, they can trigger liver cell death in some patients, as previously discussed.

2. Betulenic Acid and Lonidamide

Betulenic acid is a pentacyclic triterpene proposed as an anticancer drug. It opens the MPTP in isolated mitochondria, even without added calcium, and causes apoptosis in treated cells (143). Lonidamide is another investigational antineoplastic agent, which also opens the MPTP in the absence of added calcium and causes apoptosis (144).

B. Direct Toxicity of Reactive Metabolites

The most frequent mechanism of drug-induced hepatitis is the formation of chemically reative metabolites (1). Free radials cause lipid peroxidation, while electrophilic metabolites react with glutathione or covalently bind to hepatic macromolecules. When only small amounts of electrophilic metabolites are formed, they are detoxified by glutathione, and direct toxicity does not occur. When large amounts of electrophilic metabolites are formed, direct toxicity can occur (1).

1. Necrosis or Apoptosis

Although it was initially thought that the direct toxicity of electrophilic drug metabolites causes only liver cell necrosis (145), it is now clear that it can also cause apoptosis. Several

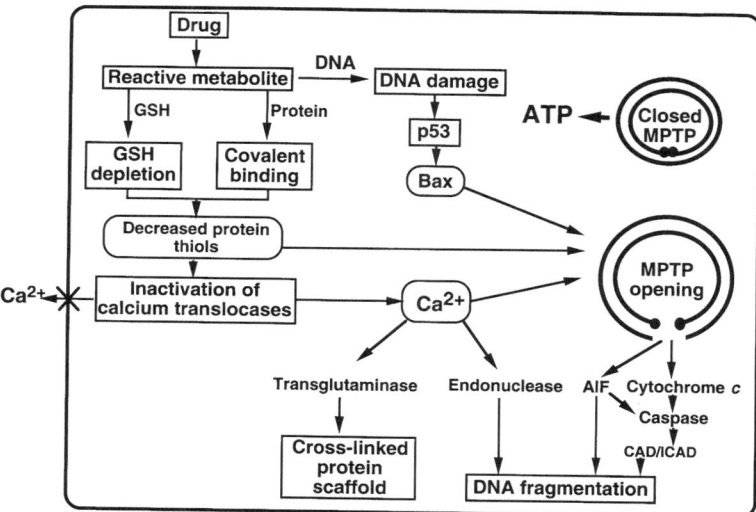

Figure 8 Involvement of mitochondria in reactive metabolite-mediated direct toxicity. The extensive formation of reactive metabolites may cause glutathione (GSH) depletion, covalent binding to protein thiols, and also DNA damage, leading to p53 and Bcl-2-associated x protein (Bax) overexpression. GSH depletion and covalent binding decrease protein thiols and inactivate calcium translocases. The increase in cell Ca^{2+} activates Ca^{2+}-dependent tissue transglutaminase (forming a crosslinked protein scaffold) and endonucleases (causing DNA fragmentation). The overexpression of Bax, the oxidation of protein thiols, causing disulfide bond formation in the mitochondrial permeability transition pore (MPTP) protein structure, and the increase in intramitochondrial Ca^{2+} open the MPTP in some mitochondria. Unaffected mitochondria keep synthesizing ATP, while permeabilized mitochondria release cytochrome c, which activates caspases. MPTP opening also releases apoptosis-inducing factor (AIF), which cuts DNA into large fragments, while caspase 3 cuts the inhibitor of caspase-activated deoxyribonuclease (ICAD), allowing this nuclease (CAD) to enter the nucleus and further fragment nuclear DNA.

compounds transformed into reactive metabolites (e.g., acetaminophen, dimethylnitrosamine, cocaine) have been shown to cause internucleosomal DNA fragmentation in hepatocytes (146–148). This type of DNA fragmentation (which results in a DNA ladder on agarose gels) is typically associated with apoptosis, whereas necrosis results in diffuse DNA fragmentation (and a diffuse smear on agarose gels). The extensive formation of reactive metabolites has been shown to cause morphological lesions of apoptosis, necrosis, or both (149–152). Dimethylnitrosamine administration mainly causes hepatocyte apoptosis in mice (149). The administration of carbon tetrachloride (which is transformed into a free radical) causes both hepatic necrosis and apoptosis in rats (150). Finally, reactive metabolites from germander diterpenoids cause liver cell necrosis in vivo (151), but hepatocyte apoptosis in vitro (152).

2. Mechanisms of Cell Death

The initial cellular mechanisms causing metabolite-mediated hepatocyte apoptosis (Fig. 8) were studied with germander (152). This medicinal plant was marketed for use in weight control diets (153). This popular indication and the natural-medicine fad led to large-scale utilization and an epidemic of hepatitis in France (153). Germander contains furano *neo-*

clerodane diterpenoids, which are responsible for the in vivo hepatotoxicity of germander in mice (151). In vitro, these furano diterpenoids are activated by CYP3A into electrophilic metabolites (154). Extensive formation of glutathione conjugates exceeds the capacity of hepatocyctes to resynthesize glutathione (154). The resulting glutathione depletion causes oxidation of protein thiols, and protein thiols are further decreased by the covalent binding of the metabolite (154). Protein thiol oxidation decreases the activity of plasma membrane calcium translocases, whose role is the constant extrusion of calcium from hepatocytes (145), thus increasing cytosolic Ca^{2+} (Fig. 8) (152). Increased cell Ca^{2+} activates Ca^{2+}-dependent tissue transglutaminase (forming a cross-linked protein scaffold) and Ca^{2+}-dependent endonucleases (causing internucleosomal DNA fragmentation) (152).

The final cellular events in metabolite-mediated apoptosis were studied with skullcap (28). This medicinal plant also contains diterpenoids transformed into reactive metabolites by CYP3A (28). In addition to the effects mentioned above, effects on the MPTP were also studied. MPTP opening was observed, probably due to three mechanisms (Fig. 8) The oxidation of protein thiols can form disulfide bonds within the MPTP structure, causing MPTP opening. The increase in cytosolic Ca^{2+} increases intramitochondrial Ca^{2}, a potent stimulus for pore opening. Finally, reactive metabolites may also damage DNA. This DNA damage increases p53, a transcriptional activator of the Bcl-2-associated $\times$ protein (Bax), which translocates to michondria and opens the MPTP (28).

MPTP opening in some mitochondria caused matrix expansion, outer mitochondrial membrane rupture, and release of mitochondrial cytochrome c from the intermembrane space into the cytosol (Fig. 8) (28). Cytosolic cytochrome c has been shown to associate with apoptosis protein activating factor (apaf-1), causing activation of procaspase 9 (11). The latter activates effector procaspases, including procaspase 3 (11). Caspases cut cytosolic, cytoskeletal, and nuclear proteins, contributing to the ultrastructural lesions of apoptosis (155). Although it was not documented in the skullcap study (28), outer-membrane rupture also releases apoptosis inducing factor (AIF), causing large-sized DNA fragmentation (156), while caspase 3 cuts the inhibitor of caspase-activated deoxyribonuclease (ICAD), allowing caspase-activated deoxyribonuclease (CAD) to enter the nucleus and cause further DNA fragmentation (Fig. 8) (157)

In support of the sequence of events suggested in Fig. 8, the internucleosomal DNA fragmentation and apoptotic cell death caused by skullcap diterpenoids were decreased by acting on either one of these successive steps (28). Apoptotic cell death was prevented when metabolic activation was inhibited by a CYP3A inhibitor, when the depletion of cellular thiols was attenuated by GSH precursors, or when the activation of Ca^{2+}-dependent enzymes and Ca^{2+}-induced MPTP opening were inhibited by a calcium/calmodulin inhibitor (28). Cyclosporin A, a direct inhibitor of MPTP opening, prevented cytochrome c release, caspase 3 activation, and cell death (28). Finally, aurintricarboxylic acid, an endonuclease and caspase inhibitor, and Ac-DEVD-CHO, a caspase 3 inhibitor, also prevented apoptosis (28).

C. Immune Reactions

Drugs that form small amounts of reactive metabolites do not cause direct toxicity (1,2). These drugs can nevertheless cause hepatitis in some patients, due to immune reactions (1,2).

1. Mechanism of Immunization

The immune system recognizes proteins that differ from those of the individual (9). Peptides derived from both self- and foreign proteins are transported to the cell surface, where

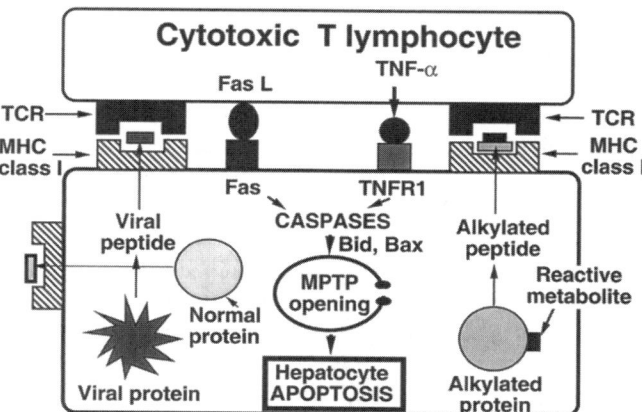

Figure 9 Involvement of mitochondria in reactive metabolite-mediated immunoallergic hepatitis. In viral hepatitis, the T-cell receptor (TCR) of cytotoxic T lymphocytes recognizes viral peptides presented by major histocompatibility complex (MHC) class 1 molecules. In drug-induced immunoallergic hepatitis, chemically reative metabolites alkylate self-proteins, which may lead to the presentation of alkylated peptides. Cytotoxic T lymphocytes express Fas ligand (Fas L) on their surface, and express or release TNF-α. The interaction of Fas L with Fas and that of TNF-α with its receptor (TNFR1) activate caspases, causing Bid (BH3 interacting domain death agonist) truncation and Bid mitochondrial translocation. Truncated Bid also causes a conformational change in Bax (Bcl-2-associated x protein) allowing Bax mitochondrial translocation. Opening of the mitochondrial permeability transition pore (MPTP) further activates caspases, causing hepatocyte apoptosis.

major histocompatibility complex (MHC) class II molecules present them to helper T lymphocytes (9). Somatic clonal mutations of the T-cell receptor (TCR) provide a vast array of different lymphocytes. The helper T lymphocytes that recognize normal peptides are deleted or rendered anergic. Only the helper T lymphocytes whose receptor recognizes something else remain active. Some of these lymphocytes can recognize a viral peptide and start the immunization process. The drawback to this system is that a self-protein modified by the covalent binding of a reactive metabolite will also differ from the normal self, which, in some subjects, can trigger immune reactions directed against the modified protein (1,2,9).

2. Mechanisms of Cell Death

Hepatocytes express MHC class I molecules that present peptides for possible recognition by cytotoxic T lymphocytes (Fig. 9). When only normal peptides are presented, no cytotoxic T lymphocytes recognize these peptides (since autoreaction T lymphocytes are normally deleted or inactivated). In viral hepatitis, viral peptides are presented, and recognized by the TCR of cytotoxic T lymphocytes (Fig. 9) (158,159). Similar mechanisms are probably involved in drug-induced immunoallergic hepatitis (9). Owing to the alkylation of proteins by reactive metabolites, hepatocytes may express alkylated peptides on their MHC class I molecules (Fig. 9) (9). These modified self-peptides differ from normal peptides and may be recognized by the TCR of cytotoxic T lymphocytes (Fig. 9) (9).

Cytotoxic lymphocytes practice euthanasia: they help their diseased targets commit suicide (Fig. 9) (9). They express Fas ligand on their surface and express or release TNFα at contact sites with their cellular targets (158,159). Binding of Fas ligand causes activation of Fas (Fig. 9) (160), which recruits a protein called FADD (Fas-associated protein with death domain) and pro-caspase 8 (160). Pro-caspase 8 is an initiator caspase with autocatalytic activity. When pro-caspase 8 is oligomerized by binding to FADD molecules, one molecule of pro-caspase 8 may cut another pro-caspase 8 molecule, forming the active caspase 8 tetramer. The latter then cuts and activates effector caspases, such as caspases 3 and 7 (160). The binding of TNFα to its receptor (TNFR1) has similar effects. The activated TNFR1 first associates with TRADD (TNFR1-associated death domain), with recruits FADD (the same molecule that binds to activated Fas). FADD recruits pro-caspase 8, causing effector caspase activation as described above (160).

Both caspase 3 and caspase 8 cleave Bid (BH3 interacting domain death agonist) (161,162). The C-terminal fragment of truncated Bid translocates to mitochondria and causes mitochondrial membrane permeabilization (162). This C-terminal Bid fragment also causes a conformational change in Bax (163,164), which translocates to mitochondria (165) to open the MPTP (166). In vivo, Fas-mediated MPTP opening causes matrix expansion, outer-membrane rupture, and release of cytochrome c from the intermembrane space into the cytosol (27). Cyclosporin A (an inhibitor of MPTP opening) prevents these mitochondrial effects, caspase activation and apoptosis, showing that MPTP opening plays a major role in Fas-mediated apoptosis in vivo (27).

Similar effects occur in TNFα-induced cell death, and MPTP opening again plays a major role (167,168). Thus, immunoallergic drug-induced hepatitis, like viral hepatitis, involves mitochondrial effects in the final mechanism of cell death (Fig. 9) (9).

VII.   CONCLUSIONS

Drugs or their reactive metabolites can open the MPTP and cause either necrosis (due to ATP depletion) or apoptosis (due to caspase activation). Necrosis can also be due to drug-induced uncoupling or inhibition of mitochondrial respiration (causing ATP depletion).

Drugs may also inhibit β-oxidation and cause microvescular steatosis. Drugs can sequester coenzyme A (aspirin, valproic acid), inhibit mitochondrial β-oxidation enzymes (tetracyclines, 2-arylpropionate anti-inflammatory drugs, amineptine and tianeptine, glucocorticoids, amiodarone, and perhexiline), impair mitochondrial structure and function (female sex hormones), inhibit either mitochondrial DNA replication (dideoxynucleosides, fialuridine) or its transcription (interferon-α), or cause structural damage to mtDNA and mtDNA depletion (alcohol, topoisomerase II inhibitors) (7). In the three latter instances, oxidative phosphorylation is first impaired and this, in turn, secondarily inhibits β-oxidation. A single drug (e.g., valporic acid) may have several different effects on mitochondrial function, and several factors (e.g., aspirin and viral infection) may add their deleterious effects on mitochondrial function.

When β-oxidation is impaired, fatty acids are poorly oxidized by mitochondria, and are instead esterified into triglycerides, which mainly accumulate as small lipid vesicles. Impaired energy production due to the inability to oxidize fatty acids, as well as the mitochondrial toxicity of free fatty acids and dicarboxylic acids, explains the severity of microvesicular steatosis, which can cause liver failure, coma, and death (7).

These mechanisms of drug-induced toxicity have only been described recently, and are rarely investigated during the preclinical development of new drug molecules. However, cases of microvesicular steatosis have led to the recall of diethylaminoethoxyhexestrol, the discontinuation of clinical trials with fialuridine, a limited use of perhexiline or tacrine, as well as early therapeutic misadventures with tetracyclines and valproic acid.

We suggest that new drug molecules should be screened for possible mitochondrial effects before they are released on the market.

REFERENCES

1. Pessayre D. Role of reactive metabolites in drug-induced hepatitis. J Hepatol 1995; 23(suppl 1):16–24.
2. Robin MA, Le Roy M, Descatoire V, Pessayre D. Plasma membrane cytochromes P450 as neoantigens and autoimmune targets in drug-induced hepatitis. J Hepatol 1997; 26(suppl 1): 23–30.
3. Fromenty B, Pessayre D. Inhibition of mitochondrial beta-oxidation as a mechanism of hepatotoxicity. Pharmacol Ther 1995; 67:101–154.
4. Fromenty B, Pessayre D. Impaired mitochondrial function in microvesicular steatosis. Effects of drugs, ethanol, hormones, and cytokines. J Hepatol 1997; 26(suppl 2):43–53.
5. Fromenty B, Berson A, Pessayre D. Microvesicular steatosis and steatohepatitis: role of mitochondrial dysfunction and lipid peroxidation. J Hepatol 1997; 26(suppl 1):13–22.
6. Pessayre D, Mansouri A, Haouzi D, Fromenty B. Hepatotoxicity due to mitochondrial dysfunction. Cell Biol Toxicol 1999; 15:367–373.
7. Pessayre D, Fromenty B, Mansouri A. Drug-induced steatosis and steatohepatitis. In: JJ Lemasters, AL Niemenen, eds. Mitochondria in Pathogenesis. New York: Plenum Press, 2001: 489–517.
8. Pessayre D, Feldmann G, Haouzi D, Fau D, Moreau A, Neuman M. Hepatocyte apoptosis triggered by natural substances (cytokines, other endogenous substances and foreign toxins). In: RG Cameron, G Feuer, eds. Apoptosis and Its Modulation by Drugs. Heidelberg: Springer Verlag, Handbook Exp Pharmacol 2000; 142:59–108.
9. Pessayre D, Haouzi D, Frau D, Robin MA, Mansouri A, Berson A. Withdrawal of life support, altruistic suicide, fratricidal killing and euthanasia by lymphocytes: different forms of drug-induced hepatic apoptosis. J Hepatol 1999; 31:760–770.
10. Pessayre D, Berson A, Fromenty B, Mansouri A. Mitochondria in steatohepatitis. Semin Liver Dis 2001; 22:57–69.
11. Green DR, Reed JC. Mitochondria and apoptosis. Science 1998; 281:1309–1312.
12. Wallace DC. Mitochondrial disease in man and mouse. Science 1999; 283:1482–1488.
13. Saraste M. Oxidative phosphorylation at the fin de siècle. Science 1999; 283:1488–1493.
14. McGarry JD, Foster DW. Regulation of hepatic fatty acid oxidation and ketone body production. Annu Rev Biochem 1980; 49:395–420.
15. Shigenaga MK, Hagen TM, Ames BN. Oxidative damage and mitochondrial decay in aging. Proc Natl Acad Sci USA 1994; 91:10771–10778.
16. LeDoux SP, Driggers WJ, Hollensworth BS, Wilson GL. Repair of alkylation and oxidative damage in mitochondrial DNA. Mutat Res 1999; 434:149–159.
17. Kuchino Y, Mori F, Kasai H, Inoue H, Iwai S, Miura K, Ohtsuka E, Nishimura S. Misreading of DNA templates containing 8-hydroxydeoxyguanosine at the modified base and adjacent residues. Nature 1987; 327:77–79.
18. Pinz KG, Shibutani S, Bogenhagen DF. Action of mitochondrial DNA polymerase γ at sites of base loss or oxidative damage. J Biol Chem 1995; 270:9292–9206.
19. Berneburg M, Grether-Beck S, Kürten V, Ruzicka T, Briviba K, Sies H, Krutmann J. Singlet oxygen mediates the UVA-induced generation of the photoaging-associated mitochondrial common deletion. J Biol Chem 1999; 274:15345–15249.
20. Esposito LA, Melov S, Panov A, Cottrell BA, Wallace DC. Mitochondrial disease in mouse results in increased oxidative stress. Proc Natl Acad Sci USA 1999; 96:4820–4825.
21. Cortopassi GA, Shibata D, Soong NW, Arnheim N. A pattern of accumulation of a somatic deletion of mitochondrial DNA in aging human tissues. Proc Natl Acad Sci USA 1992; 89: 7370–7374.

22. Michikawa Y, Mazzucchelli F, Bresolin N, Scarlato G, Attardi G. Aging-dependent large accumulation of point mutations in the human mtDNA control region for replication. Science 1999; 286:774–779.

23. Sohal RS, Weindruch R. Oxidative stress, caloric restriction, and aging. Science 1996; 273: 59–63.

24. Wiesner RJ. Adaptations of mitochondrial gene expression to changing cellular energy demands. News Physiol Sci 1997; 12:178–183.

25. Kroemer G, Reed JC. Mitochondrial control of cell death. Nature Med 2000: 6:513–519.

26. Leist M, Single B, Castoldi AF, Kühnle S, Nicotera P. Intracellular adenosine triphosphate (ATP) concentration: a switch in the decision between apoptosis and necrosis. J Exp Med 1997; 185:1481–1486.

27. Feldmann G, Haouzi D, Moreau A, Durand-Scheider AM, Bringuier A, Berson A, Mansouri A, Fau D, Pessayre D. Opening of the mitochondrial permeability transition pore causes matrix expansion and outer membrane rupture in Fas-mediated hepatic apoptosis in mice. Hepatology 2000; 31:674–683.

28. Haouzi D, Lekehal M, Moreau A, Moulis G, Feldmann G, Robin MA, Lettéron P, Fau D, Pessayre D. Cytochrome P450-generated reactive metabolites cause mitochondrial permeability transition, caspase activation and apoptosis in rat hepatocytes. Hepatology 2000; 32: 303–311.

29. Saudubray JM, Martin D, de Lonlay P, Touati G, Poggi-Travert F, Bonnet D, Jouvet P, Boutron G, Slama A, Vianey-Saban C, Bonnefont JP, Rabier D, Kamoun P, Brivet M. Recognition and management of fatty acid oxidation defects: a series of 107 patients. J Inher Metab Dis 1999; 22:488–502.

30. Morris AAM. Mitochondrial respiratory chain disorders and the liver. Liver 1999; 19:357–368.

31. Morris AAM, Taanman JW, Blake J, Cooper JM, Lake BD, Malone M, Love S, Clayton PT, Leonard JV, Schapira AHV. Liver failure associated with mitochondrial DNA depletion. J Hepatol 1998; 28:556–563.

32. Bioulac-Sage P, Parrot-Roulaud F, Mazat JP, Lamireau T, Coquet M, Sandler B, Demarquez JL, Cormier V, Munnich A, Carré M, Balabaud C. Fatal neonatal liver failure and mitochondrial cytopathy (oxidative phosphorylation deficiency): a light and electron microscopic study of the liver. Hepatology 1993; 18:839–846.

33. Watmough NJ, Bindoff LA, Birch-Machin MA, Jackson S, Bartlett K, Ragan CI, Poulton J, Gardner RM, Sherratt HSA, Turnbull DM. Impaired mitochondrial β-oxidation in a patient with an abnormality of the respiratory chain. Studies in skeletal muscle mitochondria. J Clin Invest 1990; 85:177–184.

34. Lettéron P, Duchatelle V, Berson A, Fromenty B, Fisch C, Degott C, Benhamou JP, Pessayre D. Increased ethane exhalation, an in vivo index of lipid peroxidation, in alcohol abusers. Gut 1993; 34:409–414.

35. Kukielka E, Cederbaum AI. NADH-dependent microsomal interaction with ferric complexes and production of reactive oxygen species. Arch Biochem Biophys 1989; 275:540–550.

36. Dai Y, Rashba-Step J, Cederbaum AI. Stable expression of human cytochrome P450 2E1 in HepG2 cells: characterization of catalytic activities and production of reactive oxygen intermediates. Biochemistry 1993; 32:6928–6937.

37. Kukielka E, Dicker E, Cederbaum AI. Increased production of reactive oxygen species by rat liver mitochondria after chronic ethanol treatment. Arch Biochem Biophys 1994; 309: 377–386.

38. Nordmann R, Ribière C, Rouach H. Implication of free radial mechanisms in ethanol-induced cellular injury. Free Radic Biol Med 1992; 12:219–240.

39. Wieland P, Lauterburg BH. Oxidation of mitochondrial proteins and DNA following administration of ethanol. Biochem Biophys Res Commun 1995; 213:815–819.

40. Mansouri A, Gaou I, De Kerguenec C, Amsellem S, Haouzi D, Berson A, Moreau A, Feld-

mann G, Lettéron P, Pessayre D, Fromenty B. An alcoholic binge causes massive degradation of hepatic mitochondrial DNA in mice. Gastroenterology 1999; 117:181–190.

41. Fromenty B, Grimbert S, Mansouri A, Beaugrand M, Erlinger S, Rötig A, Pessayre D. Hepatic mitochondrial DNA deletion in alcoholics: association with microvesicular steatosis. Gastroenterology 1995; 108:193–200.

42. Mansouri A, Fromenty B, Berson A, Robin MA, Grimbert S, Beaugrand M, Erlinger S, Pessayre D. Multiple hepatic mitochondrial DNA deletions suggest premature oxidative aging in alcoholic patients. J Hepatol 1997; 27:96–102.

43. Hillan KJ, Logan MC, Ferrier RK, Bird GLA, Bennett GL, McKay IC, MacSween RNM. Hepatocyte proliferation and serum hepatocyte growth factor levels in patients with alcoholic hepatitis. J Hepatol 1996; 24:385–390.

44. Ballardini G, Groff P, Zoli M, Bianchi GP, Giostra F, Francesconi R, Lenzi M, Zauli D, Cassani F, Bianchi F. Increased risk of hepatocellular carcinoma development in patients with cirrhosis and with high hepatocellular proliferation. J Hepatol 1994; 20:218–222.

45. Tsuchishina M, Tsustumi M, Shiroeda H, Yano H, Ueshima Y, Shimanaka K, Takase S. Study of mitochondrial DNA deletion in alcoholics. Alcohol Clin Exp Res 2000; 24:12S–15S.

46. Leiber CS. Hepatic, metabolic and toxic effects of ethanol: 1991 update. Alcohol Clin Exp Res 1991; 15:573–592.

47. Grunnet N, Kondrup J. The effect of ethanol on the β-oxidation of fatty acids. Alcohol Clin Exp Res 1986; 10:64S–68S.

48. Schneider E, Hsiang YH, Liu LF. DNA topoisomerases as anticancer drug targets. Adv Pharmacol 1990; 21:149–183.

49. Taanman JW. The mitochondrial genome: structure, transcription, translation and replication. Biochim Biophys Acta 1999; 1410:103–123.

50. Lawrence JW, Darkin-Rattray S, Xie F, Neims AH, Rowe TC. 4-Quinolones cause a selective loss of mitochondrial DNA from mouse LK1210 leukemia cells. J Cell Biochem 1993; 51:165–174.

51. Lawrence JW, Claire DC, Weissig V, Rowe TC. Delayed cytotoxicity and cleavage of mitochondrial DNA in ciprofloxacin-treated mammalian cells. Mol Pharmacol 1996; 50:1178–1188.

52. Labowitz JK, Silverman WB. Cholestatic jaundice induced by ciprofloxacin. Dig Dis Sci 1997; 42:192–194.

53. Lopez-Navidad A, Domingo P, Cadafalch J, Farrerons J. Norfloxacin-induced hepatotoxicity. J Hepatol 1990; 11:277–278.

54. Mitsuya H, Broder S. Inhibition of the in vitro infectivity and cytopathic effect of human T-lymphotrophic virus type III/lymphadenopathy-associated virus (HTLV-III/LAV) by 2′,3′-dideoxynucleosides. Proc Natl Acad Sci USA 1986; 83:1911–1915.

55. Yarchoan R, Mitsuya H, Myers CE, Broder S. Clinical pharmacology of 3′-azido-2′,3′-dideoxythymidine (zidovudine) and related dideoxynucleosides. N Engl J Med 1989; 321:726–738.

56. Chen CH, Cheng Y C. Delayed cytotoxicity and selective loss of mitochondrial DNA in cells treated with the anti-human immunodeficiency virus compound 2′,3′-dideoxycytidine. J Biol Chem 1989; 264:11934–11937.

57. Lewis W, Dalakas MC. Mitochondrial toxicity of antiviral drugs. Nature Med 1995; 1:417–422.

58. Pan-Zhou XR, Cui L, Zhou XJ, Sommadossi JP, Darley-Usmar VM. Differential effects of antiretroviral nucleoside analogs on mitochondrial function in HepG2 cells. Antimicrob Agents Chemother 2000; 44:496–503.

59. Barile M, Valenti D, Passarella S, Quagliariello E. 3′-Azido-3′-deoxythymidine uptake into isolated rat liver mitochondria and impairment of ADP/ATP translocator. Biochem Pharmacol 1997; 53:913–920.

60. de la Asuncion JG, del Olmo ML, Sastre J, Millan A, Pellin A, Pallardo FV. AZT treatment induces molecular and ultrastructural oxidative damage to muscle mitochondria. Prevention by antioxidant vitamins. J Clin Invest 1998; 102:4–9.

61. Skuta G, Fisher GM, Janaky T, Kele Z, Szabo P, Tozser J, Sumegi B. Molecular mechanism of the short term cardiotoxicity caused by 2′,3′-dideoxycytidine (ddC): modulation of reactive oxygen species levels and ADP-ribosylation reactions. Biochem Pharmacol 1999; 58:1915–1925.

62. Chariot P, Drogou I, de Lacroix-Szmania I, Eliezer-Vanerot MC, Chazaud B, Lombès A, Schaeffer A, Zafrani ES. Zidovudine-induced mitochondrial disorder with massive liver steatosis, myopathy, lactic acidosis and mitochondrial DNA depletion. J Hepatol 1999; 30: 156–160.

63. Mégarbane B, Brivet F, Guérin JM, Baud FJ. Acidose lactique et défaillance multiviscérale secondaire aux thérapeutiques anti-rétrovirales chez les patients infectés par le VIH. Presse Med 1999; 28:2257–2264.

64. McKenzie R, Fried MW, Sallie R, Conjeevaram H, Di Biseglie AM, Park Y, Savarese B, Kleiner D, Tsokos M, Luciano C, Pruett T, Stotka JL, Straus SE, Hoofnagle JH. Hepatic failure and lactic acidosis due to fialuridine (FIAU), an investigational nucleoside analogue for chronic hepatitis B. N Engl J Med 1995; 333:1099–1105.

65. Lewis W, Levine ES, Griniuviene B, Tankersley KO, Colacino JM, Sommadossi JP, Watanabe KA, Perrino FW. Fialuridine and its metabolites inhibit DNA polymerase γ at sites of multiple adjacent analog incorporation, decrease mtDNA abundance, and cause mitochondrial structural defects in cultured hepatoblasts. Proc Natl Acad Sci USA 1996; 93:3592–3597.

66. Shan B, Vazquez E, Lewis JA. Interferon selectively inhibits the expression of mitochondrial genes: a novel pathway for interferon-mediated responses. EMBO J 1990; 9:4307–4314.

67. Lewis JA, Huq A, Najarro P. Inhibition of mitochondrial function by interferon. J Biol Chem 1996; 22:13184–13190.

68. Okanoue T, Sakamoto S, Itoh Y, Minami M, Yasui K, Sakamoto M, Nishioji K, Katagishi T, Nakagawa Y, Tada H, Sawa Y, Mizuno M, Kagawa K, Kashima K. Side effects of high-dose interferon therapy for chronic hepatitis C. J Hepatol 1996; 25:283–291.

69. Hare JF, Hodges R. Turnover of mitochondrial inner membrane proteins in hepatoma monolayer cultures. J Biol Chem 1982; 257:3575–3580.

70. Castéra L, Kalinsky E, Bedossa P, Tertian G, Buffet C. Macrovacuolar steatosis induced by interferon alfa therapy for chronic myelogenous leukemia. Liver 1999; 19:259–260.

71. Killenberg PG, Davidson ED, Webster LT. Evidence for a medium-chain fatty acid coenzyme A ligase (adenosine monophosphate) that activates salicylate. Mol Pharmacol 1971; 7:260–268.

72. Deschamps D, Fisch C, Fromenty B, Berson A, Degott C, Pessayre D. Inhibition by salicyclic acid of the activation and thus oxidation of long-chain fatty acids. Possibly role in the development of Reye's syndrome. J Pharmacol Exp Ther 1991; 259:894–904.

73. Partin JS, Daugherty CC, McAdams AJ, Partin JC, Schubert WK. A comparison of liver ultrastructure in salicylate intoxication and Reye's syndrome. Hepatology 1984; 4:687–690.

74. Borutaité V, Brown GC. Rapid reduction of nitric oxide by mitochondria, and reversible inhibition of mitochondrial respiration by nitric oxide. Biochem J 1996; 315:295–299.

75. Susin SA, Zamzami N, Kroemer G. Mitochondria as regulators of apoptosis: doubt no more. Biochim Biophys Acta 1998; 1366:151–165.

76. Hurwitz ES, Barrett MJ, Bregman D, Gunn WJ, Schonberger LB, Fairweather WR, Drage JS, Lamontagne JR, Kaslow RA, Burlington DB, Quinnan GV, Parker RA, Phillips K, Pinsky P, Dayton D, Dowdle WR. Public health service study on Reye's syndrome and medications. Report of the pilot phase. N Engl J Med 1985; 313:849–857.

77. Forsyth BW, Horwitz RI, Acampora D, Shapiro ED, Viscoli CM, Feinstein AR, Henner R, Holabird NB, Jones BA, Karabelas ADE, Kramer MS, Miclette M, Wells JA. New epidemio-

logic evidence confirming that bias does not explain the aspirin/Reye's syndrome association. JAMA 1989; 261:2517–2524.

78. Remington PL, Rowley D, McGee H, Hall WN, Monto AS. Decreasing trends in Reye syndrome and aspirin use in Michigan, 1979 to 1984. Pediatrics 1986; 77:93–98.

79. Rowe PC, Valle D, Brusilow SW. Inborn errors of metabolism in children referred with Reye's syndrome; a changing pattern. JAMA 1988; 260:3167–3170.

80. Zimmerman HJ. Effects of aspirin and acetaminophen on the liver. Arch Intern Med 1981; 141:333–342.

81. Ponchaut S, Van Hoof F, Veitch K. In vitro effects of valproate and valproate metabolites on mitochondrial oxidations. Relevance of CoA sequestration to the observed inhibitions. Biochem Pharmacol 1992; 43:2435–2442.

82. Turnbull DM, Bone AJ, Bartlett K, Koundakjian PP, Sherratt HSA. The effects of valproate on intermediary metabolism in isolated rat hepatocytes and intact rats. Biochem Pharmacol 1983; 32:1887–1892.

83. Bjorge SM, Baillie TA. Inhibition of medium-chain fatty acid β-oxidation in vitro by valproic acid and its unsaturated metabolite, 2-*n*-propyl-4-pentenoic acid. Biochem Biophys Res Commun 1985; 132:245–252.

84. Sadeque AJM, Fisher MB, Korzekwa KR, Gonzalez FJ, Rettie AE. Human CYP2C9 and CYP2A6 mediate formation of the hepatotoxin 4-ene-valproic acid. J Pharmacol Exp Ther 1997; 283:698–703.

85. Kassahun K, Farrell K, Abbott F. Identification and characterization of the glutathione and *N*-acetylcysteine conjugates of (E)-2-propyl-2,4-pentadienoic acid, a toxic metabolite of valproic acid, in rats and humans. Drug Metab Dispos 1991; 19:525–535.

86. Kassahun K, Hu P, Grillo MP, Davis MR, Jin L, Baillie TA. Metabolic activation of unsaturated derivatives of valproic acid. Identification of novel glutathione adducts formed through coenzyme A-dependent and -independent mechanisms. Chem Biol Interact 1994; 90:253–275.

87. Farrell G. Drug-induced Liver Disease. London: Churchill-Livingstone, 1994.

88. Zimmerman HJ, Ishak KG. Valproate-induced hepatic injury: analyses of 23 fatal cases. Hepatology 1982; 2:591–597.

89. Chabrol B, Mancini J, Chretien D, Rustin P, Munnich A, Pinsard N. Valproate-induced hepatic failure in a case of cytochrome *c* oxidase deficiency. Eur J Pediatr 1994; 153:133–135.

90. Lam CW, Lau CH, Williams JC, Cahn YW, Wong LJC. Mitochondrial myopathy, encephalopathy, lactic acidosis and stroke-like episodes (MELAS) triggered by valproate therapy. Eur J Pediatr 1997; 156:562–564.

91. Krähenbühl S, Brandner S, Kleinle S, Liechti S, Straussmann D. Mitochondrial diseases represent a risk factor for valproate-induced fulminant liver failure. Liver 2000; 20:346–348.

92. Fréneaux E, Labbe G, Lettéron P, Le Dinh T, Degott C, Genève J, Larrey D, Pessayre D. Inhibition of the mitochondrial oxidation of fatty acids by tetracycline in mice and in man: possible role in microvesicular steatosis induced by this antibiotic. Hepatology 1988; 8:1056–1062.

93. Labbe G, Fromenty B, Fréneaux E, Morzelle V, Kettéron P, Berson A, Pessayre D. Effects of various tetracycline derivatives on in vitro and in vivo β-oxidation of fatty acids, egress of triglycerides from the liver, accumulation of hepatic triglycerides, and mortality in mice. Biochem Pharmacol 1991; 41:638–641.

94. Deboyser D, Goethals F, Krack G, Roberfroid M. Investigation into the mechanism of tetracycline-induced steatosis: study in isolated hepatocytes. Toxicol Appl Pharmacol 1989; 97:473–479.

95. Zimmerman HJ. Hepatotoxicity: The Adverse Effects of Drugs and Other Chemicals on the Liver. New York: Appleton-Century-Crofts, 1978.

96. Bravo JF, Jacobson MP, Mertens BF. Fatty liver and pleural effusion with ibuprofen therapy. Ann Intern Med 1997; 87:200–201.

97. Victorino RM, Silveira JC, Baptista A, de Moura MC. Jaundice associated with naproxen. Prostgrad Med J 1980; 56:368–370.

98. Danan G, Trunet P, Bernuau J, Degott C, Babany G, Pessayre D, Rueff B, Benhamou JP. Pirprofen-induced fulminant hepatitis. Gastroenterology 1985; 89:210–213.

99. Dutertre JP, Bastides F, Jonville AP, De Muret A, Sonneville A, Larrey D, Autret E. Microvesicular steatosis after ketoprofen administration. Eur J Gastroenterol Hepatol 1991; 3: 953–954.

100. Fréneaux E, Fromenty B, Berson A, Labbe G, Degott C, Lettéron P, Larrey D, Pessayre D. Stereoselective and nonstereoselective effects of ibuprofen enantiomers on mitochondrial β-oxidation of fatty acids. J Pharmacol Exp Ther 1990; 255:529–535.

101. Genève J, Hayat-Bonan B, Labbe G, Degott C. Lettéron P, Fréneaux E, Le Dinh T, Larrey D, Pessayre D. Inhibition of mitochondrial β-oxidation of fatty acids by pirprofen: role in microvesicular steatosis due to this nonsteroidal anti-inflammatory drug. J Pharmacol Exp Ther 1987; 242:1133–1137.

102. Genève J, Larrey D, Amouyal G, Belghiti J, Pessayre D. Metabolic activation of the tricyclic antidepressant amineptine by human liver cytochrome P-450. Biochem Pharmacol 1987; 36: 2421–2424.

103. Larrey D, Tinel M, Lettéron P, Maurel P, Loeper J, Belghiti J, Pessayre D. Metabolic activation of the new tricyclic antidepressant tianeptine by human liver cytochrome P-450. Biochem Pharmacol 1990; 40:545–550.

104. Sbarra, C, Castelli MG, Noseda A, Fanelli R. Pharmacokinetics of amineptine in man. Eur J Drug Metab Pharmacokin 1981; 6:123–126.

105. Grislain L, Gelé P, Bertrand M, Luijten W, Bromet N, Salvadori C, Kamoun A. The metabolic pathways of tianeptine, a new antidepressant, in healthy volunteers. Drug Metab Dispos 1990; 18:804–808.

106. Le Dinh T, Fréneaux E, Labbe G, Lettéron P, Degott C, Genève J, Berson A, Larrey D, Pessayre D. Amineptine, a tricyclic antidepressant, inhibits the mitochondrial oxidation of fatty acids and produces microvesicular steatosis of the liver in mice. J Pharmacol Exp Ther 1988; 247:745–750.

107. Fromenty B, Fréneaux E, Labbe G, Deschamps D, Larrey D, Lettéron D, Pessayre D. Tianeptine, a new tricyclic antidepressant metabolized by β-oxidation of its heptanoic side chain, inhibits the mitochondrial oxidation of medium and short chain fatty acids in mice. Biochem Pharmacol 1989; 38:3743–3751.

108. Kaplan MM. Acute fatty liver of pregnancy. N Engl J Med 1985; 313:367–370.

109. Ebert EC, Sun EA, Wright SH, Decker JP, Librizzi RJ, Bolognese RJ, Lipshutz WH. Does early diagnosis and delivery in acute fatty liver of pregnancy lead to improvement in maternal and infant survival? Dig Dis Sci 1984; 29:453–455.

110. Grimbert S, Fromenty B, Fisch C, Lettéron P, Berson A, Durand-Schneider AM, Feldmann G, Pessayre D. Decreased mitochondrial oxidation of fatty acids in pregnant mice: possible relevance to development of acute fatty liver of pregnancy. Hepatology 1993; 17:628–637.

111. Grimbert S, Fisch C, Deschamps D, Berson A, Fromenty B, Feldmann G, Pessayre D. Effects of female sex hormones on liver mitochondria in non-pregnant female mice: possible role in acute fatty liver of pregnancy. Am J Physiol 1995; 268(Gastrointest Liver Physiol 31): G107–G115.

112. Ibdah JA, Bennett MJ, Rinaldo P, Zhao Y, Gibson B, Sims HF, Strauss AW. A fetal fatty-acid oxidation disorder as a cause of liver disease in pregnant women. N Engl J Med 1999; 140:1723–1731.

113. Mansouri A, Fromenty B, Durand F, Degott C, Bernuau J, Pessayre D. Assessment of the prevalence of genetic metabolic defects in acute fatty liver of pregnancy. J Hepatol 1996; 25:781.

114. Fromenty B, Mansouri A, Bonnefont JP, Courtois F, Munnich A, Rabier D, Pessayre D.

Most cases of medium-chain acyl-CoA dehydrogenase deficiency escape detection in France. Hum Genet 1996; 97:367–368.

115. Lettéron P, Brahimi-Bourouina N, Robin MA, Moreau A, Feldmann G, Pessayre D. Glucocorticoids inhibit mitochondrial matrix acyl-CoA dehydrogenases and fatty acid β-oxidation. Am J Physiol 1997; 272(Gastrointest Liver Physiol 35):G1141–G1150.

116. Itoh S, Igarashi M, Tsukada Y, Ichinoe A. Non-alcoholic fatty liver with alcoholic hyalin afer long-term glucocorticoid therapy. Acta Hepato-Gastroenterol 1977; 24:415–418.

117. Noda S, Umezaki H, Yamamoto K, Araki T, Murakami T, Ishii N. Reye-like syndrome following treatment with the pantothenic acid antagonist, calcium hopantenate. J Neurol Neurosurg Psychiatry 1988; 51:582–585.

118. Kodavanti UP, Mehendale HM. Cationic amphiphilic drugs and phospholipid storage disorder. Pharmacol Rev 1990; 42:327–354.

119. Guigui B, Perrot S, Berry JP, Fleury-Feith J, Martin N, Métreau JM, Dhumeaux D, Zafrani ES. Amiodarone-induced hepatic phospholipidosis: a morphological alteration independent of pseudoalcoholic liver disease. Hepatology 1988; 8:1063–1068.

120. Fromenty B, Fisch C, Labbe G, Degott C, Deschamps D, Berson A, Lettéron P, Pessayre D. Amiodarone inhibits the mitochondrial β-oxidation of fatty acids and produces microvesicular steatosis of the liver in mice. J Pharmacol Exp Ther 1990; 255:1371–1376.

121. Fromenty B, Fisch C, Berson A, Lettéron P, Larrey D, Pessayre, D. Dual effect of amiodarone on mitochondrial respiration. Initial photonophoric uncoupling effect followed by inhibition of the respiratory chain at the levels of complex I and complex II. J Pharmacol Exp 1990; 255:1377–1384.

122. Fromenty B, Lettéron P, Fisch C, Berson A, Deschamps D, Pessayre D. Evaluation of human blood lymphocytes as a model to study the effects of drugs on human mitochondria: effects of low concentrations of amiodarone on fatty acid oxidation, ATP levels and cell survival. Biochem Pharmacol 1993;46:421–432.

123. Deschamps D, De Beco V, Fisch C, Fromenty B, Guillouzo A, Pessayre D. Inhibition by perhexiline of oxidative phosphorylation and the β-oxidation of fatty acids: possible role in pseudoalcoholic liver lesions. Hepatology 1994; 19:948–961.

124. Berson A, De Beco V, Lettéron P, Robin MA, Moreau C, El Kahwaji J, Verthier N, Feldmann G, Fromenty B, Pessayre D. Steatohepatitis-inducing drugs cause mitochondrial dysfunction and lipid peroxidation in rat hepatocytes. Gastroenterology 1998; 114:764–774.

125. Simon JB, Manley PN, Brien JF, Armstrong PW. Amiodarone hepatotoxicity simulating alcoholic liver disease. N Engl J Med 1984; 311:167–172.

126. Poucell S, Ireton J, Valencia-Mayoral P, Downar E, Larratt L, Patterson J, Blendis L, Phillips MJ. Amiodarone-associated phospholipidosis and fibrosis of the liver. Light, immunohistochemical, and electron microscopic studies. Gastroenterology 1984; 86:926–936.

127. Lewis JH, Ranard RC, Caruso A, Jackson LK, Mullick F, Ishak KG, Seef LB, Zimmerman HJ. Amiodarone hepatotoxicity: prevalence and clinicopathologic correlations among 104 patients. Hepatology 1989; 9:679–685.

128. De La Inglesia FA, Feuer G, Takada A, Matsuda Y. Morphologic studies on secondary phospholipidosis in humans. Lab Invest 1974;4:539–549.

129. Shikata T, Kanetaka T, Endo Y, Nagashima K. Drug-induced generalized phospholipidosis. Acta Pathol Jpn 1972; 22:517–531.

130. Pessayre D, Bichara M, Feldmann G, Degott C, Potet F, Benhamou JP. Perhexiline maleate-induced cirrhosis. Gastroenterology 1979; 76:170–177.

131. Cortez-Pinto H, Baptista A, Camilo MA, de Costa EB, Valente A, de Moura MC. Tamoxifen-associated hepatitis—report of three cases. J Hepatol 1995; 23:95–97.

132. Oien KA, Moffat D, Curry GW, Dickson J, Habeshaw T, Mills PR, MacSween RNM. Cirrhosis with steatohepatitis after adjuvant tamoxifen. Lancet 1999; 353:36–37.

133. Berson A, Fau D, Fornacciari R, Degove-Goddard P, Sutton A, Descatoire V, Haouzi D, Lettéron P, Moreau A, Feldmann G, Pessayre D. Mechanism for experimental buprenorphine

hepatotoxicity: major role of mitochondrial dysfunction versus metabolic activation. J Hepatol 2001; 34:261–269.

134. Berson A, Gervais A, Cazals D, Boyer N, Durand F, Bernuau J, Marcellin P, Degott C, Valla D, Pessayre D. Hepatitis afer buprenorphine misuse in heroin addicts. J Hepatol 2001; 34: 346–350.

135. Wieckowski MR, Wojtczak L. Involvement of the dicarboxylate carrier in the protonophoric action of long-chain fatty acids in mitochondria. Biochem Biophys Res Commun 1997; 232: 414–417.

136. Berson A, Renault S, Lettéron P, Robin MA, Fromenty B, Fau D, Le Bot MA, Riché C, Durand-Schneider AM, Feldmann G, Pessayre D. Uncoupling of rat and human mitochondria: a possible explanation for tacrine-induced liver dysfunction. Gastroenterology 1996; 110:1878–1890.

137. Fleury C, Nererova M, Collins S, Raimbault S, Champigny O, Levi-Meyrueis C, Bouillaud F, Seldin MF, Surwit RS, Ricquier D, Warder CH. Uncoupling protein-2: a novel gene linked to obesity and hyperinsulinemia. Nature Genet 1997; 15:269–272.

138. Jaburek M, Varecha M, Gimeno RE, Dembski M, Jezek P, Zhang M, Burn P, Tartaglia LA, Garlid KD. Transport function and regulation of mitochondrial uncoupling proteins 2 and 3. J Biol Chem 1999;274:26003-26007.

139. Cortez-Pinto H, Lin HZ, Yang SQ, Da Costa SOD, Diehl AM. Lipids up-regulate uncoupling protein 2 expression in rat hepatocytes. Gastroenterology 1999; 116:1184–1193.

140. Fleury C, Sanchis D. The mitochondrial uncoupling protein-2: current status. Int J Biochem Biophys 1999; 31:1261–1278.

141. Lemasters JJ. Mechanisms of hepatic toxicity V. Necrapoptosis and the mitochondrial permeability transition: shared pathways to necrosis and apoptosis. Am J Physiol 1999; 276(Gastrointest Liver Physiol): G1–G6.

142. Trost LC, Lemasters JJ. The mitochondrial permeability transition: A new pathophysiological mechanism for Reye's syndrome and toxic liver injury. J Pharmacol Exp Ther 1996; 278: 1000–1005.

143. Fulda S, Scaffidi C, Susin SA, Krammer PH, Kroemer G, Peter ME, Debatin KM. Activation of mitochondria and release of mitochondrial apoptogenic factors by betulinic acid. J Biol Chem 1998; 273:33942–33948.

144. Ravagnan L, Marzo I, Costantini P, Susin SA, Zamzami N, Petit PX, Hirsh F, Goulbern M, Poupon MF, Micolli L, Xie Z, Reed JC, Kroemer G. Lonidamide triggers apoptosis via a direct, Bcl-2-inhibited effect on the mitochondrial permeability transition pore. Oncogene 1999; 18:2537–2546.

145. Bellomo G, Orrenius S. Altered thiol and calcium homeostasis in oxidative hepatocellular injury. Hepatology 1985; 5:876–882.

146. Ray SD, Kamendulis LM, Gurule MW, Yorkin RD, Corcoran GB. Ca^{2+} antagonists inhibit DNA fragmentation and toxic cell death induced by acetaminophen. FASEB J 1993; 7:453–463.

147. Kamendulis LM, Corcoran GB. DNA as a critical target in toxic cell death: enhancement of dimethylnitrosamine cytotoxicity by DNA repair inhibitors. J Pharmacol Exp Ther 1994; 271:1694–1698.

148. Cascales M, Alvarez A, Gasco P, Fernandez-Simon L, Sanz N, Bosca L. Cocaine-induced liver injury in mice exhibits specific changes in DNA ploidy and induces programmed death of hepatocytes. Hepatology 1994; 20:992–1001.

149. Oyaizu T, Shikata N, Senzaki H, Matsuzawa A, Tsubura A. Studies on the mechanism of dimethynitrosamine-induced liver injury in mice. Exp Mol Pathol 1997; 49:375–380.

150. Shi J, Aisaki K, Ikawa Y, Wake K. Evidence of hepatocyte apoptosis in rat liver after the administration of carbon tetrachloride. Am J Pathol 1998; 153:515–525.

151. Loeper J, Descatoire V, Lettéron P, Moulis C, Degott C, Dansette P, Fau D, Pessayre D. Hepatotoxicity of germander in mice. Gastroenterology 1994; 106:464–472.

152. Fau D, Lekehal M, Farrell G, Moreau A, Moulis C, Feldmann G, Haouzi D, Pessayre D. Diterpenoids from germander, a herbal medicine, induce apoptosis in isolated rat hepatocytes. Gastroenterology 1997; 113:1334–1346.

153. Larrey D, Vial T, Pauwels A, Castot A, Biour M, David M, Michel H. Hepatitis after germander (*Teucrium chamaedrys*) administration: another instance of herbal medicine hepatotoxicity. Ann Intern Med 1992; 117:129–132.

154. Lekehal M, Pessayre D, Lereau JM, Moulis C, Fourasté I, Fau D. Hepatotoxicity of the herbal medicine, germander. Metabolic activation of its furano diterpenoids by cytochrome P450 3A depletes cytoskeleton-associated protein thiols and forms plasma membrane blebs in rat hepatocytes. Hepatology 1996; 24:212–218.

155. Evan G, Littlewood T. A matter of life and death. Science 1998; 281:1317–1322.

156. Susin SA, Lorenzo HK, Zamzami N, Marzo I, Snomw BE, Brothers GM, Mangion J, Jacotot E, Costantini P, Loeffler M, Larochette N, Goodlett DR, Aebersold R, Siderovski DP, Penninger JM, Kroemer G. Molecular characterization of mitochondrial apoptosis-inducing factor. Nature 1999; 397:441–446.

157. Sakahira H, Enari M, Magata S. Cleavage of CAD inhibitor in CAD activation and DNA degradation during apoptosis. Nature 1998; 391:96–99.

158. Kondo T, Suda T, Fukuyama H, Adachi M, Nagata S. Essential roles of the Fas ligand in the development of hepatitis. Nature Med 1997; 3:409–413.

159. Ando K, Hiroishi K, Kaneko T, Moriyama T, Muto Y, Kayagaki N, Yagita H, Okumura K, Imawari M. Perforin, Fas/Fas ligand, and TNF-α pathways as specific and bystander killing mechanisms of hepatitis C virus-specific human CTL. J Immunol 1997; 158:5283–5291.

160. Nagata S. Apoptosis by death factor. Cell 1997; 88:355–365.

161. Bossy-Wetzel E, Green DR. Caspases induce cytochrome *c* release from mitochondria by activating cytosolic factors. J Biol Chem 1999; 274:17484–17490.

162. Li H, Zhu H, Xu C, Yuan J. Cleavage of BID by caspase 8 mediates the mitochondrial damage in the Fas pathway of apoptosis. Cell 1998; 94:491–501.

163. Desagher S, Osen-Sand A, Nichols A, Eskes R, Montessuit S, Lauper S, Maundrell K, Antonson B, Martinou JC. Bid-induced conformational change of Bax is responsible for mitochondrial cytochrome c release during apoptosis. J Cell Biol 1999; 144:891–901.

164. Murphy KM, Streips UN, Lock RB. Bcl-2 inhibits a Fas-induced conformational change in the Bax N terminus and Bax mitochondrial translocation. J Cell Biol 2000; 275:17225–17228.

165. Murphy KM, Streips UN, Lock RB. Bax membrane insertion during fas (CD95)-induced apoptosis precedes cytochrome *c* release and is inhibited by Bcl-2. Oncogene 1999; 18:5991–5999.

166. Narita M, Shimizu S, Ito T, Chittenden T, Lutz RJ, Matsuda H, Tsujimoto Y. Bax interacts with the permeability transition pore to induce permeability transition and cytochrome *c* release in isolated mitochondria. Proc Natl Acad Sci USA 1998; 95:14681–14686.

167. Angermüller S, Kunstle G, Tiegs G. Pre-apoptotic alterations in hepatocytes of TNFα-treated galactosamine-sensitized mice. J Histochem Cytochem 1998; 46:1175–1183.

168. Tafani M, Schneider TG, Pastorino JG, Farber JL. Cytochrome *c*-dependent activation of caspase-3 by tumor necrosis factor requires induction of the mitochondrial permeability transition. Am J Pathol 2000; 156:2111–2121.

5

Mechanisms of Cell Death and Relevance to Drug Hepatotoxicity

NEIL KAPLOWITZ

University of Southern California, Los Angeles, California, U.S.A.

I. INTRODUCTION

The purpose of this chapter will be to provide a brief overview of the subject of cell death and then to focus on what is known about the role of apoptosis and necrosis in drug hepatotoxicity.

II. OVERVIEW OF CELL DEATH

It is currently recognized that the demise of cells reflects the triggering of the activation of a death program either by death receptor signaling or as a source of intracellular stress leading to apoptosis versus the massive loss of cell integrity from overwhelming stress leading to necrosis (1,2). The former involves shrinkage and nuclear disassembly (apoptosis) and the latter involves swelling and lysis (necrosis). The type of cell death and the susceptibility to death-inducing stimuli vary greatly from cell type to cell type and from transformed cells to normal cells. In the liver, death of hepatocytes is the major event leading to organ failure but in special circumstances the sinusoidal endothelial cells (e.g., veno-occlusive disease) (3) or bile duct epithelium (vanishing duct syndrome) (4) may be a key target. Hepatocyte death accounts for the key findings in drug-induced hepatitis, namely elevated serum AST, ALT, and functional disorders such as jaundice and coagulopathy.

A. Apoptotic Cell Death

Apoptosis is a form of cell death that involves the shrinkage and disassembly of the nucleus and cytoskeleton so that the cell is broken down into small fragments (Councilman bodies seen in histology of liver), which undergo rapid clearance by phagocytosis by surrounding cells or professional phagocytes. Apoptotic cell death (unless massive) tends not to elicit inflammation and is therefore a mechanism for "quiet" removal. The entire "machinery" of apoptosis is listed in Table 1. The process of dismantling involves the participation of proteolytic enzymes, caspases, which are present in zymogen forms and are activated in a cascade from initiator to executioner members of this class (5). The trigger for the activation process to begin occurs either at the cell surface, where a death receptor binds a ligand, or from an intracellular stress that initiates the process independent of death receptors (Fig. 1). Death receptors of major significance in liver include TNF-R1 and Fas, which bind TNFα and FasL (on T cells), respectively. When ligand binds, it causes aggregation of receptors leading to conformational changes on the cytoplasmic side so that adaptor or scaffolding proteins associate with the receptor, i.e., TRADD, FADD. These then bind procaspase 8 causing it to self-activate by cleavage to release caspase 8. In some cell types, sufficient initiator caspase 8 is released to activate procaspase 3 to produce sufficient caspase 3 (executioner) to carry out the actual apoptosis. However, in hepatocytes the death receptor–induced formation of caspase 8 is insufficient to activate caspase 3 directly and an amplification mechanism is required, which involves the participation of mitochondria with the release of intermembrane proteins such as cytochrome c leading to the assembly on a cytoplasmic scaffold (apaf-1) of cytochrome c, procaspase 9, and ATP (apoptosome) (6). Self-cleavage releases caspase 9, an initiator caspase, which

Table 1   The Machinery of Apoptosis

1. Key participants
     Death receptors (Fas, TNF-R1)
     Caspases (Initiators—caspase 8,9,10) (Executioners—caspase 3,6,7)
     Bid, Bax, Bak
     Mitochondrial proteins (cytochrome c, AIF, Smac/Diablo), ?MPT
2. Other factors
     p53
     Ceramide
     Oxidative stress
     ER stress
     Cathepsins
     Granzyme
     JNK, p38 kinases
3. Survival factors
     NF-κB (IAPs etc)
     PI-3-Kinase
     IAPs
     HSP
     $NO + O_2^{\cdot-}$
     Bcl_2, $Bcl-X_L$

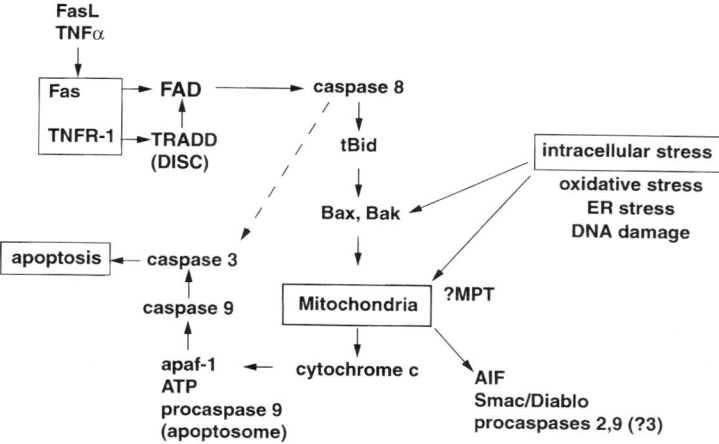

Figure 1   Apoptosis cascade: death receptor and intracellular stress pathways emphasizing the central role of mitochondria.

then cleaves procaspase 3 to release its active form. Caspase 3 then cleaves a number of specific proteins as well as procaspase 7 and 2, which may have their respective specific targets (7).

Mitochondria participate in apoptosis in many cell types. With death receptor signaling, the generation of activated caspase 8 cleaves a Bcl_2 family member, Bid, to form tBid. tBid causes Bax to insert in mitochondria and Bak to self-aggregate (6,8). Either Bax or Bak or both cause the outer mitochondrial membrane to become permeable, leading to the release of cytochrome c. The intermembrane space contains other proteins that may participate, including some pro-caspases, AIF, and Smac/Diablo. The latter binds apoptosis inhibitors, such as IAP_1, IAP_2, and XIAP. IAPs are cytoplasmic proteins that inhibit caspases so the release of Smac/Diablo incapacitates these caspase inhibitors allowing apoptosis to proceed (9,10).

Considerable controversy and uncertainty centers around the precise mechanism of release of intermembrane proteins with regard to the role of the mitochondrial permeability transition (MPT). This is a pore, composed of inner- and outer-membrane proteins, which is normally closed but when opened causes depolarization and release of proteins. The pore consists of the outer-membrane-voltage-dependent anion channel (VDAC), and peripheral benzodiazepine receptor, inner membrane adenine nucleotide translocase (ANT), matrix cyclophin (which binds cyclosporin A), and cytosol hexokinase and creatine kinase. Pro-apoptotic Bcl_2 members such as Bax promote opening of the pore and antiapoptotic members such as Bcl_2 and $Bcl-X_L$ inhibit opening. The pore contains functional vicinal thiols so that it is responsive to changes in the thiol-disulfide status of the milieu; i.e., disulfide formation opens the pore (11). Opening is inhibited by cyclosporin A and promoted by atractyloside and brongkrekic acid binding to ANT.

Apoptosis may also be triggered by events within the cell that occur downstream of death receptors, caspase 8, and/or t-Bid. This usually involves some type of stress— oxidative stress, DNA damage, ER stress, etc. Drug toxicity might cause any of these phenomena to occur. The resultant stress usually leads to participation of mitochondria but the precise mechanisms leading to their participation are not well established but could include alterations in the balance of Bcl$_2$ members, the participation of p53, or direct effects on the MPT pore.

A number of factors serve to inhibit apoptosis. Some are under the control of the transcription factor, NF-κB (12), and include the IAPs (9) and iNOS (13) (NO inhibits caspases). Stress kinases, such as JNK and p38, have been associated with pro and anti-apoptotic effects (14). HSP can inhibit caspases (15). Hepatocytes are extremely resistant to lethal actions of TNFα because TNFα not only activates the apoptosis cascade, but also activates NF-κB leading to upregulation of survival genes. The resistance to TNFα can be overcome by inhibition of transcription (16) or depletion of GSH (17,18). The former blocks the production of survival gene products, whereas the mechanism for the latter is less certain, but may include increased susceptibility of mitochondria to oxidative stress or alterations in redox control of kinases and transcription factors (tipping the balance toward proapoptotic events).

B. Necrotic Cell Death

Necrosis is a lytic cell death that usually involves cell swelling and rupture due to loss of the ability to maintain ion gradients and active transport as a consequence of profound ATP depletion. Thus, loss of mitochondrial function plays a key role. The determination of whether cells will die by apoptosis or necrosis appears to depend on how severely impaired mitochondria become. Some critical level of ATP is required for the function of the apoptosome (19). Furthermore, if extensive reactive oxygen species (ROS) or NO production occurs, mitochondria may release cytochrome c but the ROS and NO may inactivate caspases leaving the cell to progressively swell and lyse owing to loss of mitochondrial electron transport.

Thus, depending on the triggering phenomenon, cells may be committed to die as a result of effects on mitochondria and the mode of death depends on the status of ATP and the extent of inhibition of caspases. In other circumstances, the effects on mitochondria may be only sufficient to cause apoptosis or may be so profound as to lead to rapid necrosis. Other unusual phenomena that overlap apoptosis and necrosis have been described in special circumstances and have been described as aponecrosis, paraptosis, and caspase-independent apoptosis (20–24). These are not well understood but underscore the concept that cell death may not simply occur as apoptosis or necrosis, but may represent a continuum or spectrum.

III. CELL DEATH IN DRUG HEPATOTOXICITY

Surprisingly little is known about the role of apoptosis versus necrosis in drug hepatotoxicity. It seems reasonable to assume that immune hypersensitivity reactions directed at the liver involve apoptosis. The histological picture of mononuclear cell infiltration and spotty "necrosis" of individual hepatocytes (Councilman bodies), resembling the histological picture of viral hepatitis, supports this view; viral hepatitis mainly induces apoptotic death of liver cells. The immune-mediated killing is directed at hepatocytes through antigen recognition (MHC1) and the likely participation of either FasL binding or the porin-dependent delivery of granzyme to the cytoplasm. Granzymes can directly cleave procaspase 8 upstream of mitochondria or perhaps procaspase 3 downstream (25). The potential for the participation of the Fas pathway is evident from the fact that agonistic monoclonal antibody to Fas can induce fulminant hepatic failure in mice as a consequence of massive

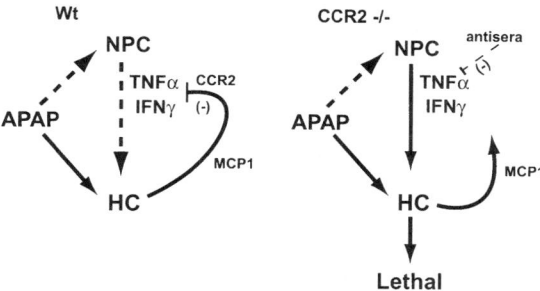

Figure 2 Mechanism for increased acetaminophen hepatotoxicity in chemokine c receptor 2 (CCR2) null mice compared to wild type (Wt). Acetaminophen (APAP) acts on hepatocytes (HC) to sensitize to the lethal actions of TNFα and IFNγ while upregulating monocyte chemoattractant protein-1 (MCP-1). MCP-1 acting via CCR2 on nonparenchymal cells (NPC), particularly Kupffer cells, downregulates the cytokines. In null mice, MCP-1 does not have a receptor leading to augmented TNFα and IFNγ production and lethal effects on the sensitized hepatocytes.

hepatocellular apoptosis (16). The role of apoptosis in the action of direct hepatotoxins such as CCl₄ or acetaminophen has been investigated, whereas the role in idiosyncratic delayed reactions is not known.

As noted in the chapter by Laskin in this volume, activation of Kupffer cells plays an important role in direct toxicity of CCl₄ and acetaminophen. In the case of CCl₄, the role of TNFα produced by Kupffer has been well established in that toxicity is abrogated by immunoneutralization of TNFα (26) or use of TNF-R1 knockouts (27). In the case of acetaminophen, some controversy exists. Although macrophage inhibitors protect against acetaminophen (28), TNFα knockout mice are not protected (29). However, the susceptibility to acetaminophen is enhanced in C-C chemokine receptor 2 (CCR2) knockouts, an effect that can be attenuated by immunoneutralization of TNFα or IFNγ (30); CCR2 expression thus is protective through regulation of cytokine generation by MCP-1 (Fig. 2). Furthermore, others have shown that neutralization of TNFα seems to slow the development of acetaminophen-induced injury and speed its resolution (31,32). Recently, IL-10 knockout has been shown to sensitize to acetaminophen (59). Limited data are available with other hepatotoxicants. LPS enhances allyl alcohol toxicity by a mechanism independent of TNFα but abrogated by pentoxifylline (33). As discussed below, hepatotoxicants may be directly lethal to hepatocytes or may sensitize hepatocytes to the lethal actions of TNFα. In either case, there is considerable uncertainty as to the mode of cell death.

A. Carbon Tetrachloride (CCl₄)

When rats were administered a modest dose of CCl₄, a mixture of apoptosis and necrosis was observed. Although TUNEL staining may not be completely reliable in distinguishing apoptosis from necrosis in situ, the TUNEL staining was correlated with characteristic cellular morphological changes of apoptosis as well as DNA laddering (34). It is difficult to quantitate the extent of apoptosis since these cells are rapidly phagocytized. However, apoptosis was appreciable. It is speculated that the dose of CCl₄ may be a factor with massive exposure leading to overwhelming necrosis and lesser exposure leading to a mixture of necrosis and apoptosis. It is uncertain but certainly plausible that the apoptosis, and perhaps the necrosis, are triggered by TNFα in the CCL₄-sensitized hepatocytes.

B.   Acetaminophen

Considerable controversy has existed concerning the mode of liver cell death induced by acetaminophen and its mechanism. The classic view is that covalent binding of NAPQI to critical proteins mediates the lethal toxicity but it should be recognized that covalent binding does not occur until all the cell GSH has been depleted, including mitochondrial GSH for covalent binding in this organelle (which correlates with killing). Thus, profound GSH depletion itself may exert a lethal action owing to the loss of the defense against endogenous reactive oxygen species normally produced in mitochondria (and possibly enhanced by the action of TNF) leading to lethal oxidative stress. In cultured mouse hepatocytes the suspectibility to acetaminophen killing is potentiated by BCNU inhibition of GSSG reductase and abrogated by iron chelators (35,36). Liposome-encapsulated SOD protects rats against acetaminophen-induced liver injury without altering covalent binding or GSH depletion (37). Similar results have been observed with an SOD mimic (38) and intravenous SOD itself (39).

Although oxidative stress appears to play a major role in acetaminophen-induced liver injury, the contribution of apoptosis versus necrosis is less certain. Earlier histological evaluation suggested the appearance of apoptotic hepatocytes at the proximal edge of the necrotic zone (40). Subsequent studies in the rat have suggested that nearly half the dead cells are apoptotic by morphological criteria with confirmation by the appearance of electrophoretic DNA laddering (41). Others have confirmed these findings more recently using TUNEL staining and increased caspase 9 and 3 activities (38). In contrast, Jaeschke and co-workers have observed that caspases are inhibited after acetaminophen treatment (? direct arylation or inhibitory effects of reactive oxygen or nitrogen species) (42) so appearance of TUNEL positive cells and DNA fragmentation in the liver after acetaminophen administration suggests a role for Ca^{2+}-activated endonuclease and a necrotic cell death (43,44). Indeed, prevention of acetaminophen-induced increased cell calcium protects against DNA fragmentation (45). Thus, the bulk of evidence favors the view that acetaminophen-induced profound GSH depletion leads to lethal oxidative stress with the mode of cell death being caspase-independent and therefore presumably necrotic. The appearance of TUNEL-positive cells and DNA fragmentation in this case are features of necrotic cell death, underscoring the lack of specificity of these phenomena. However, it remains possible that a significant contribution of cytokine-induced apoptosis in acetaminophen-sensitized hepatocytes occurs, particularly at lower doses of acetaminophen or in midzonal cells not overwhelmed by the production of NAPQI or that the mode of cell death involves an overlap or caspase-independent apoptosis.

C.   Role of GSH in Susceptibility to FasL and TNFα

Fas-mediated apoptotic killing of hepatocytes in vivo was prevented by phorone-induced profound GSH depletion, an effect associated with inhibition of caspase 3 activation (46). Antioxidants could not replace GSH, suggesting a direct effect of GSH on caspase activity, i.e., redox maintenance of protein thiols critical for enzymatic activity. On the other hand, chronic GSH depletion sensitized the liver to Fas-mediated apoptosis (47). This effect correlated with GSH depletion-induced upregulation of p53 (presumably via oxidative stress) and consequent upregulation of Bax. However, it is unclear whether the increase in Bax or other effects of decreased GSH mediate the increased susceptibility.

The effect of GSH depletion in sensitizing to the lethal actions of TNFα has received considerable attention. Intracellular signaling following the binding of TNFα to TNF-R1 leads to increased reactive oxygen metabolite production in mitochondria (17). It has been proposed that this involves the activation of acidic sphingomyelinase and the release of ceramide and its products, which then act on mitochondria to block electron transport at the complex III–ubiquinone cycle leading to auto-oxidation of O_2 from the buildup of electrons (48). Goosens et al. were the first to demonstrate this in a murine fibrosarcoma cell; they showed that depletion of mitochondrial GSH markedly enhanced the TNFα-induced oxidative stress and killing, whereas lesser depletion of mainly cytosol GSH was ineffective (49). A critical point in their studies was that GSH depletion had to be delayed for several hours after administration of TNFα to avoid the suppression of TNFα signaling, hinting at the critical nature of the timing. Fernandez-Checa, Kaplowitz, and co-workers subsequently observed that the selective depletion of mitochondrial GSH by chronic ethanol feeding rendered hepatocytes susceptible to TNFα killing, but the killing was mainly in the form of necrotic cell death (17). Subsequently, it was found that profound depletion of GSH by diethylmaleate sensitized hepatocytes to TNFα-induced apoptotic cell death (50). Thus, it appears that depletion of mitochondrial GSH sensitizes to TNFα-induced oxidative stress and lethal actions but the mode of cell death depends on the condition: chronic ethanol appears to interfere with the apoptotic machinery in some fashion.

Conflicting results have been published on the effect of GSH depletion on the hepatotoxicity of LPS (or TNFα) + galactosamine. Aside from the issue of acute verus chronic GSH depletion mentioned above, gradual GSH depletion with BSO pretreatment sensitized the liver (47) and hepatocytes (18), or protected in another study (52), whereas acute depletion sensitized in one study (51) or protected in several studies (47,52,53). However, in our own work, we have observed sensitization of mouse hepatocytes to TNFα-induced apoptosis by acute GSH depletion (50). Similar results have been reported by Fausto and co-workers using a well-differentiated, nontransformed mouse hepatocyte cell line (18).

D. Role of NF-κB

Galactosamine, actinomycin D, and α-amanitin induce a transcriptional arrest, which markedly sensitized to TNFα either directly administered, stimulated by exogenous LPS, or endogenously produced (54). Transcriptional arrest in hepatocytes interferes with TNFα-induced NF-κB dependent survival gene expression while leaving unopposed TNFα-induced apoptotic signaling via DISC, caspase 8, and tBid or ceramide leading to effects on mitochondria (Fig. 3). The role of stress kinases is less certain, i.e., pro- versus antiapoptotic effects. However, NF-κB responsive genes inhibit JNK (60,61).

Since GSH depletion also sensitizes to TNFα at least under some experimental conditions, it is of interest to understand the effect of GSH depletion on NF-κB activation and transactivation. In Molt-4 cells, GSH depletion inhibited NF-κB activation and GSSG inhibited DNA binding (55). GSH depletion has also been shown to inhibit NF-κB-dependent transcription in response to oxidative stress in Jurkat cells (56). In contrast, GSH depletion stimulated JNK activation, which then phosphorylates c-jun leading to increased AP-1 transactivation of antioxidative stress genes, including GSH-S-transferases (GST) and γ-glutamylcysteine synthetase. Thiol-disulfide control of the stress kinase pathway has been shown to be exerted at the level of ASK-1 (a kinase upstream of JNK and p38) by redox-responsive thioredoxin (57) and at the level of JNK by GST-Pi monomer (58). Thus, at present the mechanism by which GSH depletion sensitizes to TNFα-induced

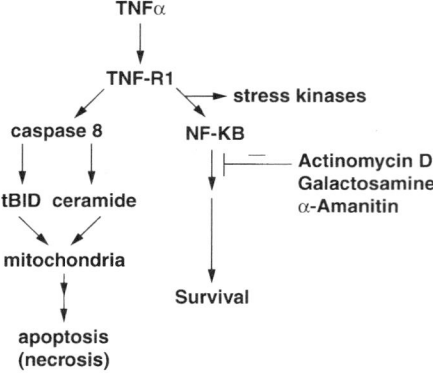

Figure 3 Opposing pathways of death and survival induced by TNFα.

apoptosis/necrosis is not entirely clarified and may include decreased defense against mitochondrial oxidative stress, inhibition of NF-κB activation or transactivation, or increased activation of stress kinases.

IV. CONCLUSIONS

Hepatotoxicity of drugs and chemicals involves lethal effects on hepatocytes or other cell types in the liver. Hepatotoxicants may illicit an immune response leading to apoptosis or affect liver cells in one of two ways: direct killing or sensitization to cytokines. The mode of cell death in these circumstances may involve apoptosis, necrosis, or a mixture of the two.

REFERENCES

1. Kaplowitz N. Cell death at the millennium: implications for liver diseases. Clin Liver Dis 2000; 4:1–23.
2. Kaplowitz N. Mechanisms of liver cell injury. J Hepatol 2000; 32:39–47.
3. DeLeve L, Wang X, Kuhlenkamp J, Kaplowitz N. Toxicity of azathioprine and monocrotaline in murine sinusoidal endothelial cells and hepatocytes: the role of glutathione and relevance to hepatic venoocclusive disease. Hepatology 1996; 23:589–599.
4. Odin JA, Huebert RC, Casciola-Rosen L, LaRusso N, Rosen N. Bcl-2-dependent oxidation of pyruvate dehydrogenase-E2, a primary biliary cirrhosis autoantigen, during apoptosis. J Clin Invest 2001; 108:223–232.
5. Thornberry NA, Lazebnik Y. Caspase: enemies within. Science 1998; 281:1312–1316.
6. Zhao Y, Li S, Childs E, et al. Activation of pro-death Bcl-2 family proteins and mitochondria apoptosis pathway in TNFα-induced liver injury. J Biol Chem 2001; 276:27432–27440.
7. Slee EA, Adrain C, Martin SJ. Executioner caspase-3, -6, and -7 perform distinct, nonredundant roles during the demolition phase of apoptosis. J Biol Chem 2001; 276:7320–7326.
8. Wei MC, Zong WX, Chang E, et al. Pro-apoptotic BAX and BAK: a requisite gateway to mitochondrial dysfunction and death. Science 2001; 292:727–730.
9. Goyal L. Cell death inhibition: keeping caspases in check. Cell 2001; 104:805–808.
10. Chauhan D, Hideshima T, Rosen S, Reed JC, Kharbanda S, Anderson KC. Apaf-1/cytochrome c-independent and Smac-dependent induction of apoptosis in multiple myeloma cells. J Biol Chem 2001; 276:24453–24456.

11. Zamzani N, Marzo I, Susin S, et al. Thiol crosslinking agent diamide overcomes the apoptosis-inhibitory effect of Bcl-2 by enforcing mitochondrial permeability transition. Oncogene 1998; 16:1055–1063.

12. Aggarwal B. Apoptosis and nuclear factor-kB: a tale of association and dissociation. Biochem Pharm 2000; 60:1033–1039.

13. Kim Y-M, Talanian RV, Billiar TR. Nitric oxide inhibits apoptosis by preventing increases in caspase-3-like activity via two distinct mechanisms. J Biol Chem 1997; 272:31138–31148.

14. Kyriakis J, Banerjee P, Nilolakaki E, et al. The stress-activated protein kinase subfamily of c-Jun kinases. Nature 1994; 369:156–160.

15. Masser DD, Antoine C, Bourget L, et al. Role of the human heat shock protein hsp 70 in protection against stress-induced apoptosis. Mol Cell Biol 1997; 17:5317–5327.

16. Feng G, Kaplowitz N. Colchicine protects mice from the lethal effect of agonistic anti-Fas antibody. J Clin Invest 2000; 105:329–339.

17. Colell A, Garcia-Ruiz C, Miranda M, et al. Selective depletion of mitochondrial GSH by ethanol sensitizes to TNFα. Gastroenterology 1998; 115:1541–1551.

18. Pierce RH, Campbell JS, Stephenson AB, et al. Disruption of redox homeostasis in tumor necrosis factor-induced apoptosis in a murine hepatocyte cell line. Am J Pathol 2000; 157: 221–236.

19. Leist M, Single A, Castoldi A, et al. Intracellular adenosine triphosphate (ATP) concentration, a switch in the decision between apoptosis and necrosis. J Exp Med 1997; 185:1481–1486.

20. Dèas O, Dumont C, MacFarlane M, et al. Caspase-independent cell death induced by anti-CD2 or staurosporine in activated human peripheral T lymphocytes. J Immunol 1998; 161: 3375–3383.

21. Formigli L, Papucci L, Tani A, et al. Aponecrosis: morphological and biochemical exploration of a syncretic process of cell death sharing apoptosis and necrosis. J Cell Physiol 2000; 182: 41–49.

22. Sperandio S, deBelle I, Bredesen DE. An alternative, nonapoptotic form of programmed cell death. Proc Natl Acad Sci USA 2000; 97:14376–14381.

23. Ruefli AA, Smyth MJ, Johnstone RW. HMBA induces activation of a caspase-independent cell death pathway to overcome P-glycoprotein-mediated multidrug resistance. Blood 2000; 95:2378–2385.

24. Hamatake M, Iguchi K, Hirano K, Ishida R. Zinc induces mixed types of cell death, necrosis, and apoptosis, in Molt-4-cells. J Biochem 2000; 128:933–939.

25. Pinkoski MJ, Waterhouse NJ, Heibein JA, et al. Granzyme B-mediated apoptosis proceeds predominantly through a Bcl-2-inhibitable mitochondrial pathway. J Biol Chem 2001; 276: 12060–12067.

26. Czaja M, Xu J, Alt E. Prevention of carbon tetrachloride-induced rat liver injury by soluble tumor necrosis factor receptor. Gastroenterology 1995; 108:1849–1854.

27. Morio LA, Chiu H, Sprowles KA, et al. Distinct roles of tumor necrosis-α and nitric oxide in acute liver injury induced by carbon tetrachloride in mice. Toxicol Appl Pharm 2001; 172: 44–51.

28. Laskin DL, Gardner CR, Price VF, Jollow DJ. Modulation of macrophage functioning abrogates the acute hepatotoxicity of acetaminophen. Hepatology 1995; 21:1045–1050.

29. Boess F, Bopst M, Althaus R, et al. Acetaminophen hepatotoxicity in tumor necrosis factor/lymphotoxin-α gene knockout mice. Hepatology 1998; 27:1021–1029.

30. Hogaboam CM, Bone-Lasron CL, Steinhauser ML, et al. Exaggerated hepatic injury due to acetaminophen challenge in mice lacking c-c chemokine receptor 2. Am J Pathol 2000; 156: 1245–1252.

31. Blazka ME, Wilmer JL, Holladay SD, et al. Role of proinflammatory cytokines in acetaminophen hepatotoxicity. Toxicol Appl Pharmacol 1995; 133:43–52.

32. Blazka ME, Elwell MR, Holladay SD, et al. Histopathology of acetaminophen-induced liver

changes. Role of interleukin 1α and tumor necrosis factor α. Toxicol Pathol 1996; 24:181–189.

33. Sneed RA, Buchweitz JP, Jean PA, Ganey PE. Pentoxifylline attenuates bacterial lipopolysaccharide-induced enhancement of allyl alcohol hepatotoxicity. Toxicol Sci 2000; 56:203–210.

34. Shi J, Aisaki K, Ikawa Y, Wake K. Evidence of hepatocyte apoptosis in rat liver after the administration of carbon tetrachloride. Am J Pathol 1998; 153:515–525.

35. Adamson GM, Harman AW. Oxidative stress in cultured hepatocytes exposed to acetaminophen. Biochem Pharm 1993; 145:2289–2294.

36. Arnaiz SL, Lesuy S, Cutrin JC, Boveris A. Oxidative stress by acute acetaminophen administration in mouse liver. Free Radic Biol Med 1995; 19:303–310.

37. Nakae D, Yamamoto K, Yoshiji H, et al. Liposome-encapsulated superoxide dismutase prevents liver necrosis induced by acetaminophen. Am J Pathol 1990; 136:787–795.

38. Ferret P-J, Hammoud R, Tulliez M, et al. Detoxification of reactive oxygen species by a nonpeptidyl mimic of superoxide dismutase cures acetaminophen-induced acute liver failure in the mouse. Hepatology 2001; 33:1173–1180.

39. Mirochnitchenko O, Weisbrot-Lefkowitz M, Reuhl K, et al. Acetaminophen toxicity: opposite effects of two forms of glutathione peroxidase. J Biol Chem 1999; 274:10349–10355.

40. Dixon MF, Dixon B, Aparicio SR, Loney DP. Experimental paracetamol-induced hepatic necrosis. A light and electron microscope, and histochemical study. J Pathol 1975; 116:17–29.

41. Ray SD, Mumaw VR, Raje RR, Fariss MW. Protector of acetaminophen-induced hepatocellular apoptosis and necrosis by cholesteryl hemisuccinate pretreatment. J Pharmacol Exp Ther 1996; 279:1470–1483.

42. Lawson JA, Fisher MA, Simmons CA, et al. Inhibition of a Fas receptor (CD95)-induced hepatic caspase activation and apoptosis by acetaminophen in mice. Toxicol Appl Pharmacol 1999; 156:179–186.

43. Ray SD, Sorge CL, Raucy JL, Corcoran GB. Early loss of large genomic DNA in vivo with accumulation of Ca^{2+} in the nucleus during acetaminophen-induced liver injury. Toxicol Appl Pharmacol 1990; 106:346–351.

44. Shen W, Kamendulis LM, Ray SD, Corcoran GB. Acetaminophen-induced cytotoxicity in cultured mouse hepatocytes: Correlation of nuclear Ca^{2+} accumulation and early DNA fragmentation with cell death. Toxicol Appl Pharmacol 1991; 111:242–254.

45. Ray SD, Kamendulis LM, Gurule MW, et al. Ca^{2+} antagonists inhibit DNA fragmentation and toxic cell death induced by acetaminophen. FASEB J 1993; 7:453–463.

46. Hentze H, Kunstle G, Volbracht C, et al. CD95-mediated murine hepatic apoptosis requires an intact glutathione status. Hepatology 1999; 30:177–185.

47. Haouzi D, Lekehal M, Tinel M, et al. Prolonged, but not acute, glutathione depletion promotes Fas-mediated mitochondrial permeability transition and apoptosis in mice. Hepatology 2001; 33:1181–1188.

48. Fernandez-Checa J, Kaplowitz N, Garcia-Ruiz C, et al. GSH transport in mitochondria: defense against TNF-induced oxidative stress and alcohol-induced defect. Am J Physiol 1997; 273:G7–17.

49. Goosens V, Grooten J, DeVos K, Fiers W. Direct evidence for tumor necrosis factor–induced mitochondrial reactive oxygen intermediates and their involvement in cytotoxicity. Proc Natl Acad Sci USA 1995; 92:8115–8119.

50. Nagai H, Matusmaru K, Feng G, Kaplowitz N. GSH depletion causes oxidative stress-dependent necrosis and sensitization to TNFα-induced, oxidative stress-independent apoptosis in cultured mouse hepatocytes. Hepatology. Submitted 2001.

51. Xu Y, Jones BE, Neufeld DS, Czaja MJ. Glutathione modulates rat and mouse hepatocyte sensitivity to tumor necrosis factor α toxicity. Gastroenterology 1998; 115:1229–1237.

52. Jones JJ, Fan J, Nathens AB, et al. Redox manipulation using the thiol-oxidizing agent diethylmaleate prevents hepatocellular necrosis and apoptosis in a rodent endotoxemia model. Hepatology 1999; 30:714–724.

53. Hentze H, Gantner F, Kolb SA, Wendel A. Depletion of hepatic glutathione prevents death receptor-dependent apoptotic and necrotic liver injury in mice. Am J Pathol 2000; 156:2045–2056.

54. Leist M, Gantner F, Naumann H, et al. Tumor necrosis factor-induced apoptosis during the poisoning of mice with hepatotoxins. Gastroenterology 1997; 112:923–934.

55. Mihm S, Galter D, Droge W. Modulation of transcription factor NF-kB activity by intracellular glutathione levels and by variations of the extracellular cysteine supply. FASEB J 1995; 9: 246–252.

56. Ginne-Pease ME, Whisler RL. Optimal NF-kB mediated transcriptional responses in Jurkat T cells exposed to oxidative stress are dependent on intracellular glutathione and costimulatory signals. Biochem Biophys Res Commun 1996; 226:695–702.

57. Sitoh M, Nishitoh H, Fuju M, et al. Mammalian thioredoxin is a direct inhibitor of apoptosis signal-regulating kinase (ASK)-1. EMBO J 1998; 17.

58. Adler V, Yin Z, Fuchs S, et al. Regulation of JNK by GSTp. EMBO J 1999; 18:1321–1334.

59. Bourdi M, Masubuchi Y, Reilly TP, et al. Protection against acetaminophen-induced liver injury and lethality by interleukin-10: role of inducible nitric oxide synthase. Hepatology 2002; 35:289–298.

60. De Smaele E, Zazzeroni F, Papa S, et al. Induction of gadd45(beta) by NF-(kappa)B down-regulates pro-apoptotic JNK signalling. Nature 2001; 414:308–312.

61. Tang G, Minemoto Y, Dibling B, et al. Inhibition of JNK activation through NF-(kappa)B target genes. Nature 2001; 414:313–317.

6

The Role of Membrane Transport in Drug-Induced Hepatotoxicity and Cholestasis

PETER L.M. JANSEN

University of Gröningen, The Netherlands

MICHAEL MÜLLER

University of Gröningen and Wageningen University, Gröningen, The Netherlands

I. INTRODUCTION

Since the liver plays such a central role in drug metabolism it is not surprising that this organ often is a target of adverse drug reactions. Despite extensive and rigorous testing of drugs in animals, hepatotoxicity in premarketing trials is a frequent cause of termination of a drug-development program. The fialuridine story is a recent example. Fialuridine was a promising drug for treatment of hepatitis B virus–associated chronic hepatitis yet proved to be extremely toxic in a phase II trial. The drug caused multisystem toxicity characterized by lactic acid acidosis, neuropathy, myopathy, and pancreatitis (1). Patients died of hepatic failure characterized by microvesicular steatosis, glycogen depletion, bile duct proliferation, and cholestasis (2). Hepatic toxicity was probably amplified by the enterohepatic cycling, which caused unpredicted high intrahepatic drug concentrations (3). The drug appeared to affect mitochondrial DNA. Thus successful animal tests do not always preclude toxicity in humans. An increasing number of drugs are taken off the market because of adverse drug reactions (4). Unexpected untoward effects are often due to drug-drug interactions or to prolonged use of a drug. Drug reactions may be rare but when these drugs are used in large populations, rare events may become relevant. An example is bromfenac with an incidence of hepatotoxicity of $1:20,000$ when used longer than 10 days. To find this in premarketing trials, the test population would have to be 100,000 persons on prolonged use. Also, diseases may change the behavior of a drug, in particular liver and renal diseases. The problem should not be underestimated as adverse drug reactions are estimated to rank among the top 10 causes of death in the United States and costs to the community vary between $30 and 130 billion annually (5,6). It would be of great benefit to patients, health care providers, and industry if tests could be developed that would detect a potential hepatotoxicity risk. A thorough knowledge of the way drugs are handled by the liver is a good starting point.

Hepatic drug reactions can be acute and reversible but also chronic and irreversible. When mitochondrial or nuclear DNA is involved, drug reactions may be delayed. Delayed and chronic drug reactions are less easily detected since time and effect relationships are less clear. In practice it often occurs that a drug is dismissed as the cause of liver disease but interrupting its use does not lead to resolution of the liver disease. This may be the cause of a considerable underestimation of drug-related adverse effects and drug-related hepatotoxicity.

In the liver, drug-metabolizing enzymes convert drugs to metabolites. Some of these metabolites are unstable and reactive. For a given drug the pattern of drug metabolism may be complex, with involvement of a number of enzymes. Many drug reactions are unpredictable and idiosyncratic. This should not lead to the misconception that in those situations drug metabolism does not play a role. A drug metabolite, for instance, can form a neo-antigen upon covalent linkage to a protein and this can be the basis of an allergic type of adverse drug reaction. The cytochrome P450 system plays a key role in many of these metabolic conversions. Subsequent conjugation reactions make drugs fit for biliary secretion.

There are many examples of drug interactions at the level of cytochrome P450. For instance, erythromycin, ketoconazole, mibefradil, simvastatin, tacrolimus, and cyclosporin A are all metabolized by CYP3A4. Combining these drugs may lead to toxic levels with severe adverse reactions for the drugs with the narrowest therapeutic range, such as tacrolimus, cyclosporin (both nephrotoxic), and simvastatin (rhabdomyolysis) (7,8). Certain drugs, such as phenothiazines, barbiturates, rifampicin, and alcohol, induce isoenzymes of the cytochrome P450 system thus increasing the synthesis of potentially toxic drug metabolites such as paracetamol and isoniazid (9–12). Therefore, the risk for hepatotoxic adverse drug reactions in patients on antiepileptic drugs or alcoholics is increased. This is usually explained by an altered drug metabolism in these patients.

Before a drug is metabolized in the liver it has to be taken up in hepatocytes and this occurs via one of many recently cloned uptake solute carrier proteins. Whether these uptake systems are involved in hepatotoxicity is unclear. In analogy to the cytochrome P450 system, uptake carrier proteins are induced by drugs. This may increase the intra-hepatocellular concentration of a potential toxic drug. Uptake carrier genes may contain barbiturate-responsive elements. Some solute carriers are downregulated (13), others are upregulated (Oatp2) or unchanged (Oatp1, Oatp4, Ntcp) by phenobarbital (14). As for inhibition of hepatic uptake, it has to be realized that there is a considerable redundancy of hepatic uptake carriers. For example, the sodium-dependent bile salt transporter NTCP (Na^+/taurocholate cotransporting protein) is downregulated by high bile salt concentrations (15,16). In contrast, prolactin and cyclic AMP have been reported to increase Ntcp expression in rats (17,18). This would increase the intracellular bile salt concentration. However, hepatocytes can deal with considerable bile salt loads as long as their secretion capacity is unimpaired.

The main solute carrier proteins in the hepatocyte are the ones that actively pump drugs and metabolites out of the cell. They predominantly belong to the superfamily of ATP-binding cassette (ABC) proteins and to a minor extent also to the family of P-type ATPases. Members of the ABC superfamily are ubiquitous in nature and are present in prokaryotes, worms, and eukaryotes, including yeasts and mammalian cells. These proteins primarily function as drug efflux pumps and prevent the untoward intracellular accumulation of drugs. In cancer cells these pumps are often overexpressed and, as such, cause a multidrug-resistance phenotype. One type of multidrug resistance is attributed to overexpression of P-glycoproteins. These are transporters of a wide range of hydrophobic cationic anticancer agents including anthracyclines and vinca alkaloids (19). Another type is associated with overexpression of the multidrug resistance–associated protein (MRP1) and some homologs (20).

Mitochondrial damage is an important determinant of hepatotoxicity. The hepatotoxicity of diclofenac, cocaine, ethanol, aspirin, valproic acid, ibuprofen, and zidovudine is attributed to inhibition of mitochondrial β-oxidation, interference with mitochondrial DNA, or a direct effect on mitochondrial respiration (21–23). Mitochondria are generators of reactive oxygen species and oxidative stress may cause apoptosis through release of cytochrome c from mitochondria. Thus the relation between plasma membrane transporters and mitochondria may be twofold: plasma membrane transport helps in reducing the intracellular concentration of toxic drugs and may help in protecting the cells against oxidative stress. The glutathione conjugate of 4-hydroxynonenal, for example, is a substrate for MRP1 (ABCC1) (24). In view of the central role of mitochondria in cell metabolism, and perhaps also because of their evolutionary background, mitochondria probably have their own set of drug efflux transporters. Indeed, recently mitochondrial ABC transporters have been identified (25–29).

II. UPTAKE SOLUTE CARRIERS

Plasma membrane solute carriers in the liver allow uptake and secretion of useful, but also of potentially toxic, agents. To perform this task hepatocytes contain a great number of plasma membrane solute carriers. The uptake carriers in human and rodent hepatocytes are shown in Tables 1 and 2. NTCP/Ntcp, in humans and rodents, respectively, has a limited substrate specificity and is a specialized carrier for the Na^+-dependent hepatic uptake of bile salts (30). Although neither the endothelin antagonist BQ-123 nor indomethacin is a substrate of Ntcp, both significantly inhibit Na^+-dependent bile salt transport (31). Many other organic anions, such as steroid conjugates, bumetanide, furosemide, and verapamil, also inhibit Ntcp-mediated bile salt uptake (32). The only non–bile salt substrate of Ntcp discovered thus far is estrone-3-sulfate (33).

It is estimated that under normal physiological conditions Ntcp is responsible for about 80% of taurocholate and for about 40% of cholate uptake in the liver (30). However, reduced Ntcp expression does not seem to lead to a decreased bile salt uptake (34). The OATP/Oatp's (solute carrier family 21: SLC21/slc21) have considerable bile salt transport capacity and may be able to partially compensate for reduced Ntcp expression.

Ntcp expression is subject to transcriptional and posttranslational regulation. Cell swelling causes a cAMP-mediated translocation to the basolateral plasma membrane in isolated rat (35). Delivery and insertion of Ntcp into the plasma membrane is microtubule- and microfilament-dependent (36). Prolactin causes increased expression of Ntcp and this

Table 1 Human Liver Uptake Transporters: The Human Liver NTCP/OATP/OCT Family (46,130,131)

	NTCP SLC10A1	OATP-A SLC21A3	OATP-B SLC21A9	OATP-C SLC21A6	OATP8 SLC21A8	PGT SLC21A2	OCT1 SLC22A1
Alternative names		OATP1		LST-1, OATP2			
Substrates							
Bromosulfophthalein	−	++	+	+	++		
Taurocholate	++	+	−	+	+		
Estrone-3-sulfate	−	+	+	+	+		
Estradiol-17β-glucuronide	−	+	−	+	+		
Dehydroepiandrosterone sulfate	−	++	+	+	+		
Ouabain	−	+	−	−	+		
Digoxin	−	−	−	−	+		
Pravastatin				+			
N-methyl quinine	−	+++		−	−		
Leukotriene C4	−	−		+	+		
Prostaglandin E2	−	+		+	−	++	
T3,T4	−	+	−	+	+		
Small organic cations[a]							+
Polarity	Basolateral	Basolateral	Basolateral	Basolateral	Basolateral	Basolateral	Basolateral
Tissue distribution	H	B	H,B	H	H	W	H > K,He,M
Chromosome (human)	14q24.1-24.2	12p12	11q13	12		3q21	6q26

[a] Small organic cations are N-1-methylnicotinamide, tetraethylammonium and 1-methyl-4-phenylpyridinium (48).
H, hepatocytes; B, brain; W, wide tissue distribution; He, heart; M, muscle.

Table 2 Rat Liver Uptake Transporters: Rat Liver ntcp/oatp/oct Family (30–32,45,47,50,132–134)

	Ntcp	Oatp1 Slc21a1	Oatp2 Slc21a5	Oatp4 Slc21a10	Oct1
Alternative names				Lst-1	
Substrates					
Bromosulfophthalein	−	+	−	+	
Taurocholate	+ +	+	+	+	
Estrone-3-sulfate	+	+	+	+	
Estradiol-17βglucuronide		+ +	+ +	+	
Dehydroepiandrosterone sulfate		+			
Ouabain	−	±	+		
Digoxin			+ +		
Pravastatin		−	+ +		
Ochratoxin A		+	+		
T3,T4		+	+		
Bilirubin monoglucuronide		+	−		
Endothelin receptor antagonist, BQ-123		−	+ +		
Small organic cations					+ +
Bulky organic cations[a]		+			
Polarity	Basolateral	Basolateral	Basolateral	Basolateral	Basolateral
Tissue distribution	H	H,K	H,K,B	H	H,K
Chromosome (rat)	6q24	XA3-A5			1q11-12

[a] Bulky organic cations are ajmalinium and rocuronium (50).
H, hepatocytes; K, kidney; B, brain.

is mediated by Stat-5-regulated increased transcription (37). Phenobarbital induces the mRNA expression of Oatp2 but not the expression of Oatp1, Oatp4, Mrp2, and Bsep (14). A recently identified basolateral methotrexate-transporting protein is downregulated by phenobarbital treatment (13).

Low bile salt concentrations enhance Ntcp expression (38). High bile salt concentrations, on the other hand, appear to reduce Ntcp expression. For instance, Ntcp is reduced in cholestasis (15,39) and this may be mediated by high bile salt concentrations. Also, in two noncholestatic mice models, i.e., mice with erythropoietic protoporphyria and Mdr2−/− mice, both with very high serum bile salt levels, Ntcp is significantly downregulated (34,40). Endotoxin, TNFα, IL-1β, and IL-6 inhibit bile salt uptake and downregulate Ntcp expression (41,42). The cytokines probably result in a downregulation of nuclear hormone receptors such as RXR, RAR, and HNF$_1$ that bind to response element in the promotor region of the *Ntcp* gene (42,43). Bile salts interfere with *Ntcp* gene transcription by inducing the transcription of the so called small heterodimer partner, shp, that inhibits the binding of RXR/RAR to the *Ntcp* gene (44). OATP-C (LST-1) and Oatp4 (rLst-1) have been proposed as important backup systems for bile salt uptake (45,46). These proteins, however, are also downregulated under cholestatic (bile duct ligation) and septic (cecal puncture) conditions (45,46). Thus the downregulation of NTCP/Ntcp as well as proteins belonging to the OATP/Oatp class of membrane transporters may be responsible for the decreased bile salt uptake during sepsis and cholestasis. As we will see below, some of the efflux transporters are also downregulated under these conditions. Thus the reduced expression of the uptake carriers may be considered to be cytoprotective.

Bromosulfophthalein and its glutathione conjugate are widely used model substrates in transport studies and indeed are substrates for a number of uptake transporters (Tables 1 and 2). For taurocholate and other bile salts NTCP/Ntcp may be the principal carrier proteins but bile salts are substrates for a great number of human and rodent uptake transporting proteins. Also, the thyroid hormones, T4 and T3, are transported by a number of uptake carriers. From a toxicological point of view ochratoxin A is of interest. Ochratoxin A is a widespread mycotoxin occurring on moldy foodstuffs. Once ingested it has a very long biological half-life. It is nephrotoxic and possibly also carcinogenic and teratogenic. Ochratoxin A is a substrate for both Oatp1 and Oatp2 (47).

The OCT/Oct family of transporters have organic cations as their substrates. They are particularly active in the kidney. OCT1/Oct1 in the liver is responsible for the uptake of small molecular organic cations such as N-1-methylnicotinamide, tetraethylammonium and 1-methyl-4-phenylpyridinium (48,49). The more bulky organic cations, ajmalinium and rocuronium, are substrates for oatp1 in the rat (50). These carriers are of particular importance during anesthesia since many anaesthetic drugs are organic cations.

III. DRUG EFFLUX PUMPS

Before excretion into the bile, drugs have to exit the liver via the canalicular membrane of the hepatocyte. Drugs, which first are metabolically converted in the liver and are then secreted via the kidneys, leave the hepatocyte via the basolateral membrane. To perform these functions the canalicular and basolateral membranes contain ATP-dependent drug efflux pumps. Most of these pumps belong to the ABC superfamily of transporter proteins. These pumps are summarized in Tables 3 and 4. Human MDR1, MDR3, and BSEP, and the rat orthologs Mdr1a and 1b, Mdr2 and Bsep, are P-glycoproteins that are constitutively expressed in the canalicular membrane. MDR3 (Mdr2) and BSEP (Bsep) are liver-specific whereas MDR1 (Mdr1a/1b) occurs in many cells and in cancer plays an important role in multidrug resistance. In the intestine MDR1 acts as a reverse drug pump lowering serum levels of orally absorbed drugs. For example, the bioavailability of digoxin is profoundly influenced by the intestinal expression of MDR1: high intestinal MDR1 expression is associated with low digoxin plasma levels (51).

The canalicular bile salt export pump BSEP (ABCB11) is of paramount importance for bile formation and liver function. BSEP appears to be the principal driving force in the enterohepatic cycle of bile salts. Also, the bile-salt-dependent fraction of bile flow depends on BSEP. Bile salts are the major, if not the only, substrates of BSEP. Rat, mouse, and human *BSEP* genes have been cloned recently (52–55). Natural mutations and knockout models provide the clearest proof of the function of this pump and show the consequences of disturbed BSEP function. Examples are given in Table 5. Progressive familial intrahepatic cholestasis is a group of diseases characterized by congenital cholestasis. PFIC type 2 is caused by mutations of the *BSEP* gene (56,57). These patients have severe cholestasis from birth and a low serum γ-glutamyltransferase activity. The liver in these diseases shows the consequences of bile-salt-induced hepatotoxicity.

MDR3 (ABCB4; Mdr2 in rodents) is a translocator of phosphatidylcholine. MDR3 acts as a flippase and translocates phospholipids from the cytosolic to the outer leaflet of the canalicular membrane (58). Bile salt micelles are needed to extract or dissolve phospholipids from the membrane into the bile (59). Thus, phospholipid secretion depends on bile salt secretion. Therefore, bile of patients with a *BSEP* gene mutation contains little phospholipids (57). In contrast, bile of patients with a *MDR3* gene mutation has a normal bile salt concentration (60,61). In the absence of phospholipids, bile salts are highly cyto-

Table 3 Multidrug Resistance-Associated Proteins in the Liver

	MRP1 ABCC1	MRP2 ABCC2	MRP3 ABCC3	MRP6 ABCC6
Alternative names		CMOAT		
Substrates				
Glutathione (GSH)	+	+		
Glutathione disulfide (GSSG)	+	+		
Leukotriene C$_4$	+	+		
S-glutathionyl 2,4,-dinitrobenzene	+	+		
S-glutathionyl prostaglandin A$_1$	+	+		
S-glutathionyl prostaglandin A$_2$	+			
S-glutathionyl ethacrynic acid	+	+		
S-glutathionyl N-ethylmaleimide	+	+		
S-glutathionyl 4-hydroxynonenal	+			
S-glutathionyl aflatoxin B1	+			
Monoglucuronosyl bilirubin	+	+		
Bisglucuronosyl bilirubin	+	+		
Estradiol 17-β-D-glucuronide	+	+	+	
Glucuronosyl etoposide	+			
Taurocholate			+	
Glycocholate			+	
3α-Sulfotaurochenodeoxycholate			+	
6α-Glucuronosyl hyodeoxycholate	+			
3α-Sulfotaurolithocholate	+		+	
Ochratoxin A		+		
Methotrexate	+	+	+	
BQ-123				+
Polarity	Basolateral	Canalicular	Basolateral	Basolateral, canalicular
Tissue distribution	H,E,B	H,I,K	H,C	H
Chromosome (human)	16p13.1	10q24	17q21.3	16p13.1

For MRP1, MRP2, and MRP3 this table is modified from ref. 135. MRP4 and MRP5 are not important for the liver. Estradiol 17-β-D-glucuronide (136), bile salt transport by Mrp3 (76,108) transport of methotrexate by Mrp1 and Mrp2 (137).

H, hepatocytes; C, cholangiocytes; E, erythrocytes; K, kidney; B, brain; I, intestine.

toxic. This became clear upon the generation of mdr2−/− knockout mice. The liver of these mice shows biliary fibrosis, bile duct proliferation, and eventually malignancy. These changes are even more pronounced when the mice are fed a cholate-containing diet (62). From these studies one can conclude that drugs capable of inhibiting MDR3 may be able to cause biliary disease. Drugs are poor substrates for MDR3 but they nevertheless could be able to inhibit its function (63).

MRP2 (ABCC2; Mrp2 in rodents) belongs to the family of multidrug-resistance-associated proteins and is a canalicular efflux pump for organic anions. This protein is not confined to the liver in its expression; it is also expressed in intestine and kidneys (64–66). Its role in these latter organs is not clear. In the liver it functions as the efflux pump for many organic anions most of which are products of phase II drug metabolism. Bilirubin mono- and diglucuronide are clear examples (67). Genetic deficiency of MRP2 in humans leads to the Dubin-Johnson syndrome, characterized by hyperbilirubinemia

Table 4 P-Glycoproteins in Human Liver

	MDR1 ABCB1	BSEP ABCB11	MDR3 ABCB4
Alternative names		SPGP	
Substrates, inhibitors			
Cyclosporin A	+		
Tacrolimus, FK 506	+		
Rhodamine	+		
Digoxin	+		+
Vinblastine	+	+	+
Doxorubicine	+		
Paclitaxel	+		+
Fexofenadine	+		
Tributylmethyl ammonium	+		
Azidoprocainamide methoiodide	+		
Tamoxifen	+		
Vecuronium	+		
Dexamethasone	+		
Talinolol	+		
Erythromycin	+		
Verapamil	+		
Itraconazole	+		
Taurocholate		+	
Glycocholate		+	
Cholate		+	
Taurolithocholate		+	
Taurochenodeoxycholate		+	
Taurodeoxycholate		+	
Tauroursodeoxycholate		+	
Phosphatidylcholine			+
Polarity	Canalicular	Canalicular	Canalicular
Tissue distribution	Widely	L	L
Chromosome	7q21	2q24	7q21

References to human MDR1- and murine Mdr1a-mediated transport of paclitaxel (Taxol) (138); Bsep (Spgp) has a transport function toward bile salts, vinblastine and calcein-acetoxymethyllester but not toward the MDR1 substrates vincristine, daunomycin, paclitaxel, digoxin, and rhodamine (54); erythromycin (a MDR1 substrate) increases the oral availability of cyclosporin A, digoxin, and the beta-blocker Talinolol, suggesting that these all are MDR1 substrates (139); MDR1-mediated transport of vinblastine, daunorubicin, and doxorubicin is inhibited by itraconazole, suggesting that itraconazole also is a MDR1 substrate (140).

(68,69). The TR− rat is an animal model in which the disease is caused by a single nucleotide deletion (70).

To complete the picture of hepatic ABC transporters, MRP1 (ABCC1) and MRP3 (ABCC3) (Mrp1 and Mrp3 in rodents) have to be mentioned. They are expressed in the basolateral membrane of the hepatocyte but only under special conditions: Mrp1 during liver regeneration and endotoxin-mediated cholestasis (71,72) and Mrp3 during cholestasis and hyperbilirubinemia (73–75). These pumps function as reverse transporters. They help

Table 5 Genetic Defects of Hepatobiliary Transport

Disease	Chromosome	Gene	Gene function	Phenotype	Animal model
Progressive familial intrahepatic cholestasis type 1	18q21	FIC1	Aminophospholipid flippase	Congenital cholestasis, low gamma GT	
Benign recurrent intrahepatic cholestasis	18q21	FIC1	Aminophospholipid flippase	Recurrent cholestasis, low gamma GT	
Progressive familial intrahepatic cholestasis type 2	2q24	BSEP ABCB11	Canalicular bile salt transport	Congenital cholestasis, low gamma GT	Bsep−/−mouse
Progressive familial intrahepatic cholestasis type 3	7q21	MDR3 ABCB4	PC translocase	Congenital cholestasis, high gamma GT	Mdr2−/−mouse
Intrahepatic cholestasis of pregnancy	e.g. 7q21	MDR3 ABCB4	PC translocase	Cholestasis during pregnancy	
Dubin-Johnson syndrome	10q24	MRP2 ABCC2	Canalicular anion transport	Conjugated hyperbilirubinemia	TR−/EHBR rats

Gamma GT, gamma glutamyltransferase; PC translocase, phosphatidylcholine translocase. For references see text.

to reduce the intracellular metabolite concentration when secretion via the canalicular route is impaired. MRP3 is mainly a pump for monovalent glucuronides and MRP1 for glutathione S-conjugates (76). They also play a role in multidrug resistance in cancer cells (77,78).

The multispecificity of these transporters allows for drug-drug interactions at the transporter level: transport of one drug can competitively inhibit the transport of another drug by the same transporter. Since these transporters also mediate the transport of endogenous compounds, interference with export of bilirubin glucuronides (MRP2) or bile salts (BSEP) is possible. However, drug-induced hyperbilirubinemia or cholestasis will only occur upon prolonged inhibition of transport. Some of these transporters can be inhibited either from the cytosolic, or "*cis*," side or canalicular, or "*trans*," side. For instance Bsep-mediated transport, in vitro, is inhibited by cyclosporin A, rifamycin, rifampicin, and glibenclamide on the *cis* side while estradiol-17β-glucuronide is a *trans* inhibitor. *Trans* inhibition requires that a drug first is transported into the bile canaliculus before it can exert its inhibitory effect. Transport of estradiol-17β-glucuronide is mediated by Mrp2. Thus for estradiol-17β-glucuronide-mediated Bsep inhibition two transporters are required, Mrp2 as transporter and Bsep as target of the inhibitory action (79).

For most cholestatic drugs the exact mechanism of drug-induced cholestasis is unknown. Possibilities are competitive or noncompetitive inhibition of transport, interference with transcription, interference with signal transduction, and interference with the intracellular targeting of the transporter protein. Single nucleotide polymorphisms or heterozygosity for null alleles of transporter genes may enhance the probability of adverse drug reactions. For instance, within families with the PFIC type 3 trait (mutations of the MDR3 gene) females may be susceptible to intrahepatic cholestasis of pregnancy (60,80). Oral contraceptive use in these females may also lead to cholestasis.

Drugs may cause pure intrahepatic cholestasis, inflammatory cholestasis, or ductopenic cholestasis. Some of these drugs are summarized in Table 6. This list is not exhaustive. Some drugs may be so highly concentrated in bile that their precipitation represents a physical mechanism of cholestasis. This mechanism has been proposed for chlorpromazine-induced cholestasis. Ceftriaxone, a MRP2 substrate that is highly concentrated in bile, may cause biliary sludge, cholelithiasis, and even cholestasis (81,82).

Table 6 Drugs Causing Cholestasis

Cholestasis	Cholestatic hepatitis	Ductopenic cholestasis
Estradiol 17-betaglucuronide	Phenothiazines	Ajmaline
Cyclosporin A	Amoxicillin-clavulanic acid	Carbamazepine
Rifamycin	Sulfonylureas	Chlorpromazine
Rifampicine	Propylthiouracil	Chlorpropamide
Glibenclamide	Erythromycine estolate	C-trimoxazole
Azathioprine		Cyproheptadine
6-Mercaptopurine		Flucloxacillin
Busulfan		Haloperidol
		Thiabendazole
		Tolbutamide
		Tricyclic antidepressants

IV. REGULATION OF HEPATIC ABC-TRANSPORTER GENE TRANSCRIPTION

The expression of hepatic ABC transporters varies widely under different conditions. Experimentally cholestasis has been tested in endotoxin-treated and bile-duct-ligated rats. Also, liver regeneration, as a very common phenomenon in liver injury, has been studied. Results are summarized in Table 7. It is clear that transcriptional and posttranscriptional mechanisms must be in operation here. These changes are also of relevance for drug-induced hepatotoxicity: drugs can interfere with regulatory mechanisms, in particular with gene transcription where drugs and hormones may act as ligands.

As explained, MDR1, MRP2, BSEP, and MDR3 have very different functions. Therefore, it can be assumed that regulation and transcriptional control of the expression of their genes will be different. BSEP and MDR3 are liver-specific transporters and thus need control mechanisms to allow for the hepatocyte-specific expression of their genes. The expression of canalicular MDR1 and MRP2 and basolateral MRP1 and MRP3 appears to respond to various conditions including inflammation-induced stress and differences in substrate concentrations. MRP2, MRP1, and MRP3 appear to be regulated more or less inversely: when MRP2 expression is reduced, the expression of either MRP1 or MRP3 is enhanced. With identification of molecules involved in intracellular signaling, and the cloning and characterization of transporter genes and their 5′-flanking DNA regions, insight into the molecular mechanisms of transcriptional regulation of transporter gene expression is progressing.

Gene expression by transcription of mRNA by RNA polymerase II can be regulated at least at five potential control points (83): (1) activation of the gene structure; (2) initia-

Table 7 Regulation of the Hepatic Transporters in Rat Liver

Transporter	Endotoxin treatment (96)	Bile duct ligation (74,95,144)	Partial hepatectomy (72,97)	Other regulatory events
Mdr1a	↔	↔	↑	—
Mdr1b	↑	↑	↑↑	↑ by ROS, TNFα, insulin, statins (125,141–143)
Mdr2	↔	↔	↑	↑ by fibrates, statins, bile salts (122–126) ↓ by cholesterol, during chronic bile diversion (124)
Bsep	↓	↓	↔	↓ during EE-induced cholestasis (95)
Mrp1	↑	n.d.	↑	↑ by ROS, in cultured hepatocytes (103, 141)
Mrp2	↓	↓	↔	↑ by dexamethasone, PCN (145) ↑ (mRNA) 2-acetylaminofluorene, cisplatin, cyclohexamide (99)
Mrp3	↑[a]	↑	↑*	↑ in EHBR, Gunn rats (73,74) ↑ by phenobarbital, bilirubin, α-naphthylisothiocyanate (74)

↔, little or no change in expression; ↑, upregulation; ↓, downregulation, n.d., not done.
[a] Unpublished data.
EE, ethinyl estradiol; PCN, pregnenolone-16-α carbonitrile.

Table 8 Transcription Factors and Their
Target Transporter Genes (88,120,146–149)

Name	Dimer with	Target genes
PPARα NR1C1	RXR	Mdr2
LXRα	RXR	ABCA1 ABCG1 ABCG5/8
NR1H3		
FXR	RXR	BSEP MRP2
NR1H4		
PXR	RXR	MDR1 MRP2 Oatp2
NR1I2		
CARα NR1I3	RXR	MRP2
RAR NR1B1	RXR	Mrp2
SP1	—	MRP1 MRP2 Mdr1b Mdr2
c-JUN	c-FOS	Mdr1b
HNF3β	HNF3s	MRP2
NF-κB	p50/p65	Mdr1b
P53	tetramer	Mdr1b MRP1

For the nuclear hormone receptors (NHRs) the official nomenclature is also given.

tion of transcription (for most genes the major control point); (3) processing the transcript; (4) transport to cytoplasm; and (5) translation of RNA. Many factors act together with RNA polymerase II: in addition to factors of the basal transcription apparatus and other nonregulated DNA-binding proteins, other factors that are inducible, or that can be activated, have regulatory functions. These transcription factors bind to so-called responsive elements (RE). Activity of transcription factors may be controlled by protein synthesis (C/EBP), covalent modification of the protein (c-JUN), ligand binding (nuclear hormone/ orphan receptors such as FXR, LXRα, PPARs), cleavage to release the active factor (SREBPs), release after breakdown of an inhibitor (NF-κB), or change of partner (MYC). Some of these transcription factors are known to bind to bona fide REs in transporter gene promoter sequences and modulate gene transcription activity (Table 8).

A. The Nuclear Ligand-Activated Receptors

Nuclear hormone or orphan receptors (NHR) comprise a large superfamily of ligand-modulated transcription factors that, in part, mediate response to steroids, retinoids, and thyroid hormones and play key roles in development and physiology (84–88). Of major interest are the RARs (9-*cis* retinoic acid receptors), RXRs (retinoid X receptors), PPARs (peroxisome proliferator-activated receptors), FXRs (farnesoid X receptors), and LXRs (liver X receptors). These NHRs and several others such as PXR (pregnane X receptor) and CAR (constitutively activated receptor) require heterodimerization with RXR for high-affinity DNA binding (Table 8). Furthermore, most of the factors possess the feature of activating target genes only when bound by specific ligands. The preferred organization of the NHR responsive elements is direct repeats (DR) of AGTTCA or AGGTCA separated by one (DR-1) to five (DR-5) nucleotides. Shortly after their isolation, the strategy of "reversed endocrinology" was used to identify orphan ligands of these NHRs. This has led to the identification of physiological ligands. Many of the recently identified "orphans" are not hormones in the classic sense. For FXR the endogenous ligands appear to be bile salts (89–91) and PPARs bind, e.g., eicosanoids and certain unsaturated fatty acids (92).

B. Disturbance in Transcriptional Control of Hepatocanalicular Transporter Gene Expression as Cause of Liver Disease

High-affinity ligands of these NHRs are substrates for members of the ABC transporter superfamily and their activities are interdependent. This relationship is important for the physiological regulation of ABC transporter genes and other NHR target genes in vivo. However, during liver disease this regulatory cross-talk may be disturbed because of the acute-phase response-coupled downregulation of NHRs and their target genes. Infection, inflammation, and trauma induce a wide array of metabolic changes in the liver that constitute the acute-phase response, mediated by cytokines, particularly TNFα, IL-1β, and IL-6. In fulminant hepatic failure, for example, serum levels of TNFα and TNF receptors are significantly increased. In the liver of patients with fulminant hepatic failure, infiltrating mononuclear cells express high amounts of TNFα and hepatocytes overexpress TNF receptor 1 (TNF-R1) (93). Acute-phase response is associated with a decrease in mRNAs coding for certain NHR proteins such as RXRα, RXRβ, RXRγ, LXRα, PPARα, and PPARγ expression levels, resulting in an overall decreased binding activity to regulatory elements (93). It can be hypothesized that the reduction in RXR levels, along with levels of other nuclear hormone receptors in the liver, could be a mechanism for downregulation of a large number of genes including ABC transporter genes during the acute-phase response (94). Downregulation of specific hepatic nuclear factors, such as HNF1 and HNF4, during acute-phase response likely plays a key role in the regulation of certain negative acute-phase proteins. For example, a decrease in HNF1 is thought to be responsible for the reduced transcription of albumin or Ntcp. The acute-phase response results in marked alterations in lipid metabolism in the liver. Many of the enzymes and transporters involved in these metabolic changes are known to be regulated by PPARα or LXRα. It is possible that during the acute-phase response, the reduced availability of RXR protein and possibly of NHRs represents a mechanism to coordinately regulate these metabolic changes in the liver. Additionally, it has recently been recognized that the NHRs PXR and CAR form heterodimers with RXR and modulate drug metabolism by regulating the expression of CYP2 and CYP3 P450 enzymes. A decrease in RXR could by itself explain the well-characterized decrease in P450 enzymes and inhibition of drug metabolism that occurs during the acute-phase response.

The importance of RXRs for liver gene expression has been demonstrated in a recent study using cre-mediated recombination to disrupt the mouse RXRα gene specifically in hepatocytes (94). Biochemical parameters indicate that PPARα, CARβ, PXR, LXR, and FXR coupled metabolic pathways in the liver were compromised in the absence of RXRα. Thus, RXRα is integrated into a number of diverse physiological pathways as a common regulatory component of cholesterol, fatty acid, bile salt, steroid, and xenobiotic metabolism and homeostasis.

C. Regulation of BSEP

From animal models some information is available on the expression of rat *Bsep* under conditions of endotoxin treatment (95,96), bile duct ligation (95), and ethinylestradiol-induced cholestasis (95). In cholestatic and stress models the reduction of *Bsep* mRNA and protein expression is minor when compared to the marked downregulation of Ntcp and Mrp2 (42,95–97). Thus Bsep may continue to secrete bile salts, although at impaired rates. Remarkably, also after partial hepatectomy the mRNA level of *Bsep* is only slightly decreased and its protein level is unaffected. This contrasts with a marked reduction of Ntcp expression (72,97). This may explain why after partial hepatectomy the remnant liver is not cholestatic. In the regenerating liver other basolateral transport systems such Oatp1 and Oatp2 remain active in mediating the uptake of bile salts. Furthermore, due to the 10-fold increase of serum bile salts, hepatocytes of the entire acinus, instead of only the periportal hepatocytes, will contribute to bile salt secretion.

Recently, we have cloned the promoter sequence of the human *BSEP* gene. It contains several potential REs for CCAAT enhancer binding protein (C/EBP) β and hepatocyte nuclear factor (HNF) 3β (Table 7) as well as a RE for FXR/RXR (98). The presence and functionality of these REs may explain the liver-specific expression of BSEP and the response of *BSEP* gene expression to variations in intracellular bile salt concentrations.

D. Regulation of the MRPs

The anionic conjugate transporter MRP2 (ABCC2) contributes to bile formation by transporting GSH, a major driving force for bile-salt-independent bile flow (Fig. 1). In addition, MRP2 has also a major role in anionic phase II–conjugate transport across the canalicular membrane. A dose- and time-dependent induction of *Mrp2* expression was observed in isolated rat hepatocytes, cultured in the presence of vincristine, tamoxifen, or the PXR ligand rifampicin (99). This indicates that *Mrp2* gene transcription may respond to substrates of MRP2 and phase I and II enzymes. The promoter regions of the human *MRP2* and the rat *Mrp2* genes have been isolated (100,101). Sequence analysis of the human *MRP2* promoter showed a number of putative consensus binding sites for both ubiquitous and liver-enriched transcription factors, including activating protein AP1, SP1, HNF1, and HNF3β (100–102) (Fig. 2). From studies with various deletion constructs it appears that important elements are localized in the −431/−258 region that controls expression in HepG2 cells. This region contains a putative binding site for C/EBPβ and mutations in this site result in a 50% decrease of promoter activity. Thus C/EBPβ likely has an important role in the transcriptional control of *MRP2* gene expression, at least in HepG2 cells (101).

A major question is still unanswered: Why is rat Mrp2 so rapidly downregulated under conditions of endotoxin treatment? Recently, an important role of RXR and RAR has been suggested (41), as discussed above (Fig. 2). Similar to the bile salt uptake transporter Ntcp, *Mrp2* is rapidly downregulated via reduction in gene transcription. *Ntcp* suppression by endotoxin in vivo is caused by downregulation of transactivators including the footprint B

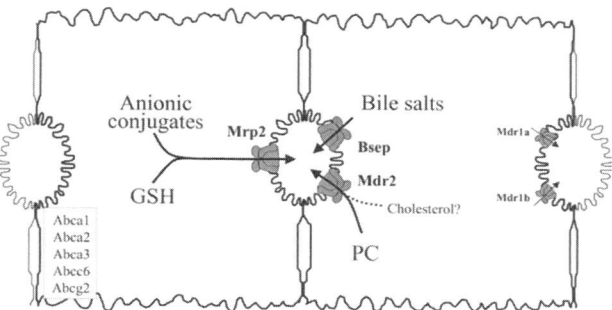

Figure 1 Hepatic ABC transporter proteins in normal cells. Transporter proteins located in the canalicular membrane are responsible for the coupled biliary secretion of bile salts, PC, cholesterol, and GSH, on the one hand, and for the excretion of potentially toxic compounds, on the other hand (150–152). These transporter proteins comprise the bile salt transporter Bsep, the PC translocator Mdr2, the anionic conjugate transporter Mrp2, and the multidrug transporters Mdr1a and Mdr1b (in humans MDR1). Little is known about the function, localization, and regulation of the recently described hepatic ABC transporters ABCA1, ABCA2, ABCA3 (153), ABCG1 (154), and MRP6/ABCC6 (155,156). They are not discussed in this chapter. For a recent overview on human ABC transporter proteins and the official nomenclature see http://nutrigene.4t.com/humanabc.htm.

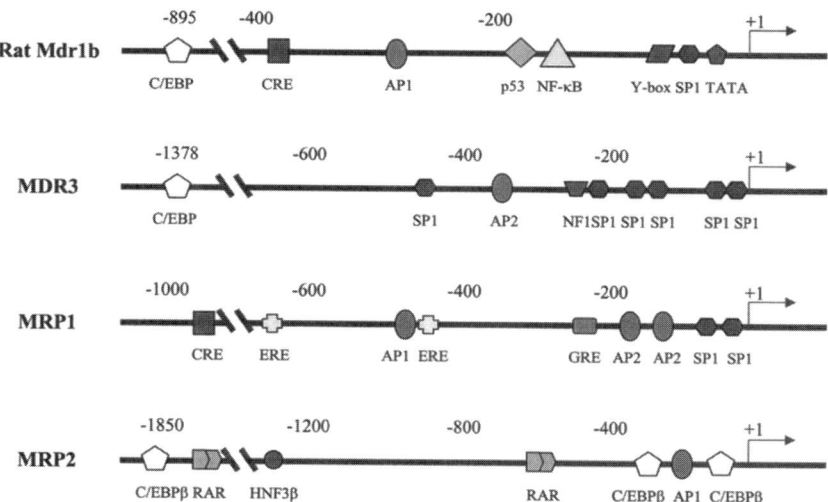

Figure 2 Potential responsive elements in the 5′-untranslated regions of rat *Mdr1b*, human *MDR3*, *MRP1*, and *MRP2*. The potential binding sites for C/EBPβ, RAR, HNF3β, AP1, AP2, SP1, NF1 (nuclear factor 1), CRE (cyclic AMP RE), ERE (estrogen RE), GRE (glucocorticoid RE) in the promoter regions of *Mdr1b* (143,157), *MDR3* (158), *MRP1* (106,107,159), and *MRP2* (160) are shown.

binding protein (41). Both the *Ntcp* footprint B binding protein RE and the *Mrp2* promoter contain potential RXR-responsive elements. Taurochenodeoxycholate and chenodeoxy-cholate, ligands for FXR (89–91), but not the nonligand tauroursodeoxycholate, inhibited activation by retinoids, specifically through the RXR/RAR-responsive element.

The levels of Mrp1 (Abcc1) mRNA and protein are considerably increased after endo-toxin administration (96) (Table 7) whereas Mrp2 is strongly downregulated. Furthermore, MRP1 mRNA and protein levels were increased in HepG2 cells and SV40 large T antigen-immortalized human hepatocytes (103). These results suggest that MRP1/Mrp1 expression and function may be associated with cell proliferation. Indeed, we recently reported that in isolated rat hepatocytes that have entered the cell cycle, Mrp1 expression is induced while expression of Mrp2 is decreased (103). This switch in expression occurred in the mid-G1 phase of the cell cycle, and appeared associated with a decrease in cell polarity.

Mrp1 is induced when rat hepatoma H4IIE cells are exposed to compounds that generate reactive oxygen species (104) (Table 7). This is coupled to an increased expres-sion of γ-glutamylcysteine synthetase (γGCS), a rate-limiting enzyme in the biosynthesis of GSH. GSH is an important factor in Mrp1 function as well as in the defense against metabolites generated by oxidative stress (104). Based on these results, it is proposed that the expression of *Mrp1* as well as γ*GCS* is, at least partially, mediated by the intracellular reduction-oxidation (redox) status (104). A parallel expression pattern of *MRP1* and γ*GCS* has been reported for many drug-resistant cell lines, colon tumors from patients, and nor-mal mouse tissues (105). Analysis of the promoter region of the *MRP1* gene has identified consensus binding sites for numerous transcription factors including the activator proteins AP1 and AP2, SP1, cyclic AMP RE, estrogen RE, and glucocorticoid Res (106,107) (Fig. 2). At present, the mechanisms underlying redox-mediated regulation of *MRP1* expression are unknown. Several oxidative stress-responsive-like sequences located upstream from the promoter of *MRP1* have been noted; however, whether these sites can function as authentic oxidative stress RE (ORE) remains to be demonstrated (104).

MRP3 (ABCC3) mediates basolateral export of organic anions and bile salts from hepatocytes (76,108). Interestingly, Mrp3 is upregulated in the Mrp2-deficient EHBR rat and in bile-duct-ligated cholestatic rats (73,109–111) (Table 2). Also, increased amounts of MRP3 are detected in livers of Dubin-Johnson patients (111). Considering the cellular localization of Mrp3, its upregulation during cholestasis, and its substrate specificity, it is hypothesized that Mrp3 may play a significant role in the basolateral export of organic anions under conditions in which Mrp2 (or Bsep) is downregulated. The inducible nature of the rat Mrp3 has recently been investigated (74). An increase in Mrp3 expression was observed in Gunn rats exhibiting hyperbilirubinemia due to a defect of UDP-glucuronosyl transferase. In addition, the elevated level of Mrp3 observed after bile duct ligation was associated with an elevated level of unconjugated bilirubin and bilirubin glucuronides (74). These compounds were shown to induce the hepatic expression of Mrp3. Recently, also the human MRP3 promoter has been cloned and several putative binding sites for transcription factors, including AP1, AP2, and SP1, have been identified (102,111). How-ever, future experiments have to clarify which transcription factors, ligands, and respon-sive elements are responsible for the compensatory upregulation of Mrp3/MRP3 in hepa-tocytes under conditions wherein Mrp2/MRP2 (and BSEP) function is disturbed.

E. Regulation of MDR1

In vitro studies reveal that expression of the human *MDR1* (*ABCB1*) gene is induced by a variety of toxic agents, ultraviolet irradiation (112), and heat shock (113), implying that

MDR1 promoter activation may be part of a general stress response in many cells. The human *MDR1* promoter contains an inverted CCAAT box (-82 to -73), which is known as a core sequence of the Y-box, a GC element (-56 to -42), and a number of putative recognition sites for transcription factors, including those for AP1, NF-Y, and Y-box-binding protein (YB) 1 (114,115). Recently, an important role for both NF-Y and SP1 in the transcriptional activation of the *MDR1* gene after genotoxic stress was demonstrated. NF-Y and SP1 interact with the Y box and the GC-rich region, respectively. In contrast, YB-1, which has been identified by others as important for the UV-response in *MDR1* upregulation (114,115), was found not to be sufficient to mediate this activation (113).

The impact of *MDR1/Mdr1a* expression on the drug-induced expression of CYP3A has been tested in human and mouse samples (116). This has been demonstrated for rifampicin. This is an excellent inducer of *CYP3A* and a substrate for MDR1 and its rodent homologs. Consequently, cells with increased levels of MDR1 need higher rifampicin concentrations to cause CYP3A induction. MDR1 and CYP3A (and other CYPs) likely are complementary systems to detoxify hydrophobic compounds. Decreased MDR1 levels result in increased CYP expression, and under conditions of suppressed CYP-expression (e.g., under cytokine-induced stress) *Mdr1b* expression is increased (116).

More recently, the impact of hepatic Mdr1a/Mdr1b-expression on CYP expression in the liver was studied (117). Mdr1a($-/-$) and Mdr1a/Mdr1b($-/-$) mice (118,119) were used to demonstrate that these proteins have distinct functional roles in influencing expression of CYPs. Mdr1a appears to be the major regulator of hepatic CYP expression (117). Somewhat surprisingly, the strong effects on CYP expression were almost exclusively seen in mice housed in the Amsterdam animal house and not in U.S.-housed animals (117). Different contents of inducing agents in the diet such as pesticides, endogenous steroids, or phytoestrogens may be the underlying cause. These compounds are efficient stimulators of the NHR PXR (see above) (120,121) and upregulate many CYPs, phase II enzymes, and possibly also drug efflux transporters. However, the cellular bioavailability of PXR ligands will be largely affected by MDR1 and functionally related transporter proteins. This concept will have consequences for human drug therapy because individual differences in expression of MDR1 (and other drug-transporting ABC transporter proteins) will consequently result in individual differences in the expression of CYPs (phase I), phase II–conjugating enzymes and ABC transporter proteins (phase III).

F. Regulation of MDR3

Secretion of PC, cholesterol, and bile salts are closely coupled and regulated processes that are mainly controlled by MDR3 (ABCB4; in rodents Mdr2) and BSEP (ABCB11) activities (Fig. 1). Expression of the PC translocase Mdr2 in rodent liver appears to be unaltered under most conditions of cellular stress (Table 7). *Mdr2* expression was not affected after endotoxin treatment (96), and was only slightly enhanced after partial hepatectomy (72). Recent studies with fibrates (122), bile salts (123,124), and statins (125,126), however, provide evidence that *Mdr2* expression is "controlled" by its substrates cholesterol, PC, and bile salts (as "cosubstrates" in PC secretion).

When mice were fed a diet supplemented with the peroxisome proliferators ciprofibrate or clofibrate, increased Mdr2 mRNA and protein levels and increased PC secretion were observed (122), suggesting a potential involvement of PPARα in *Mdr2* gene expression. In mice fed a diet supplemented with the hydrophobic bile salt cholate, *Mdr2* mRNA levels were found to be induced, which was functionally reflected in a concomitant increase of the maximal PC secretion capacity (123). Feeding the (relatively) hydrophilic bile salt ursodeoxycholate did not influence *Mdr2* mRNA levels or the maximal PC output capacity (123). These latter findings imply that the type of bile salt in plasma may influence the expression level of *Mdr2* and therefore the rate of PC secretion. The finding that plasma bile salt concentrations may influence Mdr2 expression may also explain increased *Mdr2* levels found in regenerating rat livers after 70% partial hepatectomy (72). In these animals a 10-fold increased plasma bile salt level was found. In recent studies with isolated rat hepatocytes further evidence was provided for regulatory functions of hydrophobic bile salts and cholesterol on Mdr2 expression (124). Taurocholate and taurodeoxycholate both increased *Mdr2* mRNA levels in a time-and-concentration-dependent manner. Squalestatin, an inhibitor of cholesterol biosynthesis, increased *Mdr2* mRNA levels by sevenfold in primary hepatocyte cultures. In contrast, cholesterol feeding and chronic bile diversion decreased *Mdr2* mRNA significantly (124).

Continuous exposure of rats to the statins simvastatin or pravastatin, inhibitors of 3-hydroxy-3-methylglutaryl-coenzyme A (HMGCoA) reductase, resulted in decreased levels of liver cholesterol and increased biliary PC output (125,126). This was accompanied by increased levels of *Mdr2* mRNA and protein (125,126). These studies further show that statins increase the expression of *Mdr1b* in rat liver (Table 7). For an effect on *Mdr2* expression continuous exposure to statins was necessary. *Mdr2* mRNA returned to control levels within 9–12 h after drug withdrawal. However, during this rebound phase, Mdr2 protein levels remained elevated and, accordingly, biliary phospholipid secretion remained increased in both continuously fed and rebound rats. In contrast, *Mdr1b* mRNA levels remained increased in the rebound group, indicating different mechanisms of induction of *Mdr2* and *Mdr1b* gene expression or differences in mRNA stability. In this model NF-κB may be activated by statins, as demonstrated for other xenobiotics. Alternatively, NF-κB activation may be the result of stress signals from the endoplasmic reticulum caused by overexpression of HMGCoA reductase (127).

The finding that biliary cholesterol/PC ratios in continuously fed and control animals were identical, despite suppression of cholesterol synthesis in the first group, suggests that PC secretion per se is an important regulatory factor for cholesterol secretion (Fig. 1). Data from diosgenin-treated rats demonstrate that hypersecretion of cholesterol can occur independently of Mdr2 induction and that cholesterol hypersecretion per se does not cause induction of Mdr2 (125).

Mdr2 is localized in periportal hepatocytes in control as well as in statin-treated livers. This zonal distribution is very similar to the reported distribution of HMGCoA reductase and HMGCoA synthase before and after statin treatment, which suggests that the factors controlling the expression of these proteins may be similar (125).

Until now, SP1 is the only transcription factor identified to functionally interact with the promoter of the *MDR3/Mdr2* gene (Fig. 2). SP1 seems necessary for basal expression (128). We have hypothesized from our study with statin-induced Mdr2 expression that transcriptional control of *Mdr2* gene expression might, at least partially, be mediated via SREBPs. The 5′-flanking region of the *Mdr2* gene contains elements that are possibly recognized by SREBPs (129). We have recently tested this hypothesis. Exposure of freshly isolated rat hepatocytes to statins [simvastatin, lovastatin, or atorvastatin (0.1–100 μM) for 24 or 48 h] caused a strong increase in mRNA levels of the gene encoding for HMGCoA reductase and *Srebp2*, whereas *Mdr2* mRNA levels were moderately increased. *Srebp1* mRNA levels were not significantly affected by statin treatment. Transient transfection studies with HepG2 cells revealed that statins stimulated *Mdr2* promoter activity up to 10-fold, whereas cotransfection with a nuclear-SREBP1 expression plasmid enhanced *Mdr2* promoter activity more than 10-fold. We conclude from these preliminary studies that *Mdr2* gene expression is, at least partially, under control of Srebps. These findings further demonstrate the importance of the hepatic PC translocator Mdr2 in the regulation of cholesterol homeostasis (Fig. 1).

V. CONCLUSION

Compared to the extensive literature on drug-metabolizing systems, the pharmacology of drug transporters is still in its infancy. Emphasis has been on the role of P-glycoproteins and MRPs in multidrug resistance in cancer chemotherapy, but it appears that these same transporters are also important for uptake, secretion, and bioavailability of drugs. In analogy to the drug-metabolizing enzymes, called phase II drug metabolism, the drug transporters can be considered as part of a phase III drug metabolism. Since some of these transporters are important for bile formation and inhibition or impairment of expression, these transporters may lead to cholestasis. However, impairment of transporter function can also lead to increased intracellular substrate concentrations and to cytotoxicity. Thus, although cholestasis comes to mind as a first and obvious consequence of impaired transport in the liver, noncholestatic hepatotoxic reactions may also occur when drug efflux pumps are not functioning properly. An even more complex picture may arise when BSEP and MDR3 activity becomes unbalanced, for instance by drug inhibition of one but not the other transporter. The production of cytotoxic bile and bile duct injury may be the result. It is even imaginable that neoantigens are uncovered in this situation and autoimmunity is triggered. This may seem speculative but is not an unlikely scenario for some drug reactions.

There is evidence that the intestinal MDR1 expression is subject to genetic variation (51); similar genetic variations may occur in the liver. This may have consequences for drug metabolism. Some adverse drug reactions may result from inappropriate drug dosing in patients with unexpectedly low hepatic transporter expression. This falls within the realm of pharmacogenomics. Variations of cytochrome P450 expression and variations of transporter expression need to be charted and, when existent, taken into consideration.

REFERENCES

1. Honkoop P, Scholte HR, de Man RA, Schalm SW. Mitochondrial injury. Lessons from the fialuridine trial. Drug Safety 1997; 17(1):1–7.
2. Kleiner DE, Gaffey MJ, Sallie R, Tsokos M, Nichols L, McKenzie R, Straus SE, Hoofnagle JH. Histopathologic changes associated with fialuridine hepatotoxicity. Mod Pathol 1997; 10(3):192–199.
3. Schmid R. Fialuridine toxicity [letter]. Hepatology 1997; 25(6):1548.
4. Friedman MA, Woodcock J, Lumpkin MM, Shuren JE, Hass AE, Thompson LJ. The safety of newly approved medicines: do recent market removals mean there is a problem? [see comments]. JAMA 1999; 281(18):1728–1734.
5. Lazarou J, Pomeranz BH, Corey PN. Incidence of adverse drug reactions in hospitalized patients: a meta-analysis of prospective studies [see comments]. JAMA 1998; 279(15):1200–1205.
6. Johnson JA, Bootman JL. Drug-related morbidity and mortality. A cost-of-illness model. Arch Intern Med 1995; 155(18):1949–1956.

7. Krahenbuhl S, Menafoglio A, Giostra E, Gallino A. Serious interaction between mibefradil and tacrolimus. Transplantation 1998; 66(8):1113–1115.

8. Schmassmann-Suhijar D, Bullingham R, Gasser R, Schmutz J, Haefeli WE. Rhabdomyolysis due to interaction of simvastatin with mibefradil [letter]. Lancet 1998; 351(9120):1929–1930.

9. Thummel KE, Slattery JT, Ro H, Chien JY, Nelson SD, Lown KE, Watkins PB. Ethanol and production of the hepatotoxic metabolite of acetaminophen in healthy adults. Clin Pharmacol Ther 2000; 67:591–599.

10. Vermeulen NP, Bessems JG, Van de Straat R. Molecular aspects of paracetamol-induced hepatotoxicity and its mechanism-based prevention. Drug Metab Rev 1992; 24(3):367–407.

11. Durand F, Jebrak G, Pessayre D, Fournier M, Bernuau J. Hepatotoxicity of antitubercular treatments. Rationale for monitoring liver status. Drug Safety 1996; 15(6):394–405.

12. Schluger LK, Sheiner PA, Jonas M, Guarrera JV, Fiel IM, Meyers B, Berk PD. Isoniazid hepatotoxicity after orthotopic liver transplantation. Mt Sinai J Med 1996; 63(5–6):364–369.

13. Honscha W, Dotsch KU, Thomsen N, Petzinger E. Cloning and functional characterization of the bile acid-sensitive methotrexate carrier from rat liver cells. Hepatology 2000; 31(6): 1296–1304.

14. Hagenbuch N, Reichel C, Streger B, Cattori V, Fattinger KE, Landmann L, Meier PJ, Kullak-Ublick GA. Effect of phenobarbital on the expression of bile salt and organic anion transporters in the liver. J Hepatol 2001; 34(6):881–887.

15. Gartung C, Ananthanarayanan M, Rahman MA, Schuele S, Nundy S, Soroka CJ, Stolz A, Suchy FJ, Boyer JL. Down-regulation of expression and function of the rat liver Na+/bile acid cotransporter in extrahepatic cholestasis. Gastroenterology 1996; 110(1):199–209.

16. Karpen SJ, Sun AQ, Kudish B, Hagenbuch B, Meier PJ, Ananthanarayanan M, Suchy FJ. Multiple factors regulate the rat liver basolateral sodium-dependent bile acid cotransporter gene promoter. J Biol Chem 1996; 271(25):15211–15221.

17. Ganguly TC, Liu Y, Hyde JF, Hagenbuch B, Meier PJ, Vore M. Prolactin increases hepatic Na+/taurocholate co-transport activity and messenger RNA post partum. Biochem J 1994; 303(Pt 1):33–36.

18. Mukhopadhayay S, Ananthanarayanan M, Stieger B, Meier PJ, Suchy FJ, Anwer MS. cAMP increases liver Na^+-taurocholate cotransport by translocating transporter to plasma membranes. Am J Physiol 1997; 273(4 Pt 1):G842–G848.

19. Ling V. Multidrug resistance: molecular mechanisms and clinical relevance. Cancer Chemother Pharmacol 1997; 40 Suppl:S3–S8.

20. Cole SPC, Deeley RG. Multidrug resistance mediated by the ATP-binding cassette transporter protein MRP. BioEssays 1998; 20(11):931–940.

21. Pessayre D, Mansouri A, Haouzi D, Fromenty B. Hepatotoxicity due to mitochondrial dysfunction. Cell Biol Toxicol 1999; 15(6):367–373.

22. Bort R, Ponsoda X, Jover R, Gomez-Lechon MJ, Castell JV. Diclofenac toxicity to hepatocytes: a role for drug metabolism in cell toxicity. J Pharmacol Exp Ther 1999; 288(1):65–72.

23. Boess F, Ndikum-Moffor FM, Boelsterli UA, Roberts SM. Effects of cocaine and its oxidative metabolites on mitochondrial respiration and generation of reactive oxygen species. Biochem Pharmacol 2000; 60(5):615–623.

24. Renes J, De Vries EE, Hooiveld GJ, Krikken I, Jansen PL, Muller M. Multidrug resistance protein MRP1 protects against the toxicity of the major lipid peroxidation product 4-hydroxynonenal. Biochem J 2000; 350(Pt 2):555–561.

25. Allikmets R, Raskind WH, Hutchinson A, Schueck ND, Dean M, Koeller DM. Mutation of a putative mitochondrial iron transporter gene (ABC7) in X-linked sideroblastic anemia and ataxia (XLSA/A). Hum Mol Genet 1999; 8(5):743–749.

26. Csere P, Lill R, Kispal G. Identification of a human mitochondrial ABC transporter, the functional orthologue of yeast Atm1p. FEBS Lett 1998; 441(2):266–270.

27. Shirihai OS, Gregory T, Yu C, Orkin SH, Weiss MJ. ABC-me: a novel mitochondrial trans-

porter induced by GATA-1 during erythroid differentiation. EMBO J 2000; 19(11):2492–2502.

28. Zhang F, Hogue DL, Liu L, Fisher CL, Hui D, Childs S, Ling V. M-ABC2, a new human mitochondrial ATP-binding cassette membrane protein. FEBS Lett 2000; 478(1–2):89–94.

29. Hogue DL, Liu L, Ling V. Identification and characterization of a mammalian mitochondrial ATP-binding cassette membrane protein. J Mol Biol 1999; 285(1):379–389.

30. Kouzuki H, Suzuki H, Ito K, Ohashi R, Sugiyama Y. Contribution of sodium taurocholate co-transporting polypeptide to the uptake of its possible substrates into rat hepatocytes. J Pharmacol Exp Ther 1998; 286(2):1043–1050.

31. Kouzuki H, Suzuki H, Stieger B, Meier PJ, Sugiyama Y. Characterization of the transport properties of organic anion transporting polypeptide 1 (oatp1) and Na(+)/taurocholate co-transporting polypeptide (Ntcp): comparative studies on the inhibitory effect of their possible substrates in hepatocytes and cDNA-transfected COS-7 cells. J Pharmacol Exp Ther 2000; 292(2):505–511.

32. Zimmerli B, Valantinas J, Meier PJ. Multispecificity of Na+-dependent taurocholate uptake in basolateral (sinusoidal) rat liver plasma membrane vesicles. J Pharmacol Exp Ther 1989; 250(1):301–308.

33. Schroeder A, Eckhardt U, Stieger B, Tynes R, Schteingart CD, Hofmann AF, Meier PJ, Hagenbuch B. Substrate specificity of the rat liver Na(+)-bile salt cotransporter in Xenopus laevis oocytes and in CHO cells. Am J Physiol 1998; 274(2 Pt 1):G370–G375.

34. Meerman L, Koopen NR, Bloks V, Van Goor H, Havinga R, Wolthers BG, Kramer W, Stengelin S, Muller M, Kuipers F, Jansen PL. Biliary fibrosis associated with altered bile composition in a mouse model of erythropoietic protoporphyria. Gastroenterology 1999; 117(3):696–705.

35. Webster CR, Blanch CJ, Phillips J, Anwer MS. Cell swelling-induced translocation of rat liver Na+/Taurocholate cotransport polypeptide is mediated via the phosphoinositide 3-kinase signaling pathway. J Biol Chem 2000; 275(38):29754–29760.

36. Dranoff JA, McClure M, Burgstahler AD, Denson LA, Crawford AR, Crawford JM, Karpen SJ, Nathanson MH. Short-term regulation of bile acid uptake by microfilament-dependent translocation of rat ntcp to the plasma membrane. Hepatology 1999; 30(1):223–229.

37. Ganguly TC, O'Brien ML, Karpen SJ, Hyde JF, Suchy FJ, Vore M. Regulation of the rat liver sodium-dependent bile acid cotransporter gene by prolactin. Mediation of transcriptional activation by Stat5. J Clin Invest 1997; 99(12):2906–2914.

38. Konieczko EM, Ralston AK, Crawford AR, Karpen SJ, Crawford JM. Enhanced Na+-dependent bile salt uptake by WIF-B cells, a rat hepatoma hybrid cell line, following growth in the presence of a physiological bile salt. Hepatology 1998; 27(1):191–199.

39. Dumont M, Jacquemin E, D'Hont C, Descout C, Cresteil D, Haouzi D, Desrochers M, Stieger B, Hadchouel M, Erlinger S. Expression of the liver Na+-independent organic anion transporting polypeptide (oatp-1) in rats with bile duct ligation. J Hepatol 1997; 27(6):1051–1056.

40. Koopen NR, Wolters H, Voshol P, Stieger B, Vonk RJ, Meier PJ, Kuipers F, Hagenbuch B. Decreased Na+-dependent taurocholate uptake and low expression of the sinusoidal Na+-taurocholate cotransporting protein (Ntcp) in livers of mdr2 P-glycoprotein-deficient mice. J Hepatol 1999; 30(1):14–21.

41. Denson LA, Auld KL, Schiek DS, McClure MH, Mangelsdorf DJ, Karpen SJ. Interleukin-1β suppresses retinoid transactivation of two hepatic transporter genes involved in bile formation. J Biol Chem 2000; 275(12):8835–8843.

42. Trauner M, Arrese M, Lee H, Boyer JL, Karpen SJ. Endotoxin downregulates rat hepatic ntcp gene expression via decreased activity of critical transcription factors. J Clin Invest 1998; 101(10):2092–2100.

43. Beigneux AP, Moser AH, Shigenaga JK, Grunfeld C, Feingold KR. The acute phase response is associated with retinoid X receptor repression in rodent liver. J Biol Chem 2000; 275(21): 16390–16399.

44. Denson LA, Sturm E, Echevarria W, Zimmerman TL, Makishima M, Mangelsdorf DJ, Karpen SJ. The orphan nuclear receptor, shp, mediates bile salt-induced inhibition of the rat bile acid transporter, ntcp. Gastroenterology 2001; 121(1):218–220.

45. Kakyo M, Unno M, Tokui T, Nakagomi R, Nishio T, Iwasashi H, Nakai D, Seki M, Suzuki M, Naitoh T, Matsuno S, Yawo H, Abe T. Molecular characterization and functional regulation of a novel rat liver-specific organic anion transporter rlst-1. Gastroenterology 1999; 117(4):770–775.

46. Abe T, Kakyo M, Tokui T, Nakagomi R, Nishio T, Nakai D, Nomura H, Unno M, Suzuki M, Naitoh T, Matsuno S, Yawo H. Identification of a novel gene family encoding human liver-specific organic anion transporter LST-1. J Biol Chem 1999; 274(24):17159–17163.

47. Kontaxi M, Echkardt U, Hagenbuch B, Stieger B, Meier PJ, Petzinger E. Uptake of the mycotoxin ochratoxin A in liver cells occurs via the cloned organic anion transporting polypeptide. J Pharmacol Exp Ther 1996; 279(3):1507–1513.

48. Gorboulev V, Ulzheimer JC, Akhoundova A, Ulzheimer-Teuber I, Karbach U, Quester S, Baumann C, Lang F, Busch AE, Koepsell H. Cloning and characterization of two human polyspecific organic cation transporters. DNA Cell Biol 1997; 16(7):871–881.

49. Zhang L, Dresser MJ, Gray AT, Yost SC, Terashita S, Giacomini KM. Cloning and functional expression of a human liver organic cation transporter. Mol Pharmacol 1997; 51(6):913–921.

50. van Montfoort JE, Hagenbuch B, Fattinger KE, Muller M, Groothuis GM, Meijer DK, Meier PJ. Polyspecific organic anion transporting polypeptides mediate hepatic uptake of amphipathic type II organic cations. J Pharmacol Exp Ther 1999; 291(1):147–152.

51. Hoffmeyer S, Burk O, von Richter O, Arnold HP, Brockmoller J, Johne A, Cascorbi I, Gerloff T, Roots I, Eichelbaum M, Brinkmann U. Functional polymorphisms of the human multidrug-resistance gene: multiple sequence variations and correlation of one allele with P-glycoprotein expression and activity in vivo. Proc Natl Acad Sci USA 2000; 97(7):3473–3478.

52. Childs S, Yeh RL, Georges E, Ling V. Identification of a sister gene to P-glycoprotein. Cancer Res 1995; 55(10):2029–2034.

53. Gerloff T, Stieger B, Hagenbuch B, Madon J, Landmann L, Roth J, Hofmann AF, Meier PJ. The sister of P-glycoprotein represents the canalicular bile salt export pump of mammalian liver. J Biol Chem 1998; 273(16):10046–10050.

54. Lecureur V, Sun D, Hargrove P, Schuetz EG, Kim RB, Lan LB, Schuetz JD. Cloning and expression of murine sister of P-glycoprotein reveals a more discriminating transporter than MDR1/P-glycoprotein. Mol Pharmacol 2000; 57(1):24–35.

55. Green RM, Hoda F, Ward KL. Molecular cloning and characterization of the murine bile salt export pump. Gene 2000; 241(1):117–123.

56. Strautnieks SS, Bull LN, Knisely AS, Kocoshis SA, Dahl N, Arnell H, Sokal E, Dahan K, Childs S, Ling V, Tanner MS, Kagalwalla AF, Nemeth A, Pawlowska J, Baker A, Mieli-Vergani G, Freimer NB, Gardiner RM, Thompson RJ. A gene encoding a liver-specific ABC transporter is mutated in progressive familial intrahepatic cholestasis. Nat Genet 1998; 20(3):233–238.

57. Jansen PL, Strautnieks SS, Jacquemin E, Hadchouel M, Sokal EM, Hooiveld GJ, Koning JH, De Jager-Krikken A, Kuipers F, Stellaard F, Bijleveld CM, Gouw A, Van Goor H, Thompson RJ, Muller M. Hepatocanalicular bile salt export pump deficiency in patients with progressive familial intrahepatic cholestasis. Gastroenterology 1999; 117(6):1370–1379.

58. Smit JJ, Schinkel AH, Oude ER, Groen AK, Wagenaar E, van Deemter L, Mol CA, Ottenhoff R, van der Lugt NM, van Roon MA. Homozygous disruption of the murine mdr2 P-glycoprotein gene leads to a complete absence of phospholipid from bile and to liver disease. Cell 1993; 75(3):451–462.

59. Crawford AR, Smith AJ, Hatch VC, Oude ER, Borst P, Crawford JM. Hepatic secretion of phospholipid vesicles in the mouse critically depends on mdr2 or MDR3 P-glycoprotein expression. Visualization by electron microscopy. J Clin Invest 1997; 100(10):2562–2567.

60. de Vree JM, Jacquemin E, Sturm E, Cresteil D, Bosma PJ, Aten J, Deleuze JF, Desrochers M, Burdelski M, Bernard O, Oude ER, Hadchouel M. Mutations in the MDR3 gene cause progressive familial intrahepatic cholestasis. Proc Natl Acad Sci USA 1998; 95(1):282–287.

61. Deleuze JF, Jacquemin E, Dubuisson C, Cresteil D, Dumont M, Erlinger S, Bernard O, Hadchouel M. Defect of multidrug-resistance 3 gene expression in a subtype of progressive familial intrahepatic cholestasis. Hepatology 1996; 23(4):904–908.

62. Van Nieuwkerk CM, Elferink RP, Groen AK, Ottenhoff R, Tytgat GN, Dingemans KP, van den Bergh Weerman MA, Offerhaus GJ. Effects of Ursodeoxycholate and cholate feeding on liver disease in FVB mice with a disrupted mdr2 P-glycoprotein gene. Gastroenterology 1996; 111(1):165–171.

63. Smith AJ, van Helvoort A, van Meer G, Szabo K, Welker E, Szakacs G, Varadi A, Sarkadi B, Borst P. MDR3 P-glycoprotein, a phosphatidylcholine translocase, transports several cytotoxic drugs and directly interacts with drugs as judged by interference with nucleotide trapping. J Biol Chem 2000; 275(31):23530–23539.

64. Keppler D, Konig J. Hepatic canalicular membrane 5: Expression and localization of the conjugate export pump encoded by the MRP2 (cMRP/cMOAT) gene in liver. FASEB J 1997; 11(7):509–516.

65. van Aubel RA, Peters JG, Masereeuw R, van Os CH, Russel FG. Multidrug resistance protein Mrp2 mediates ATP-dependent transport of classic renal organic anion p-aminohippurate. Am J Physiol Renal Physiol 2000; 279(4):F713–F717.

66. van Aubel RA, Hartog A, Bindels RJ, van Os CH, Russel FG. Expression and immunolocalization of multidrug resistance protein 2 in rabbit small intestine. Eur J Pharmacol 2000; 400(2–3):195–198.

67. Kamisako T, Leier I, Cui Y, Konig J, Buchholz U, Hummel-Eisenbeiss J, Keppler D. Transport of monoglucuronosyl and bisglucuronosyl bilirubin by recombinant human and rat multidrug resistance protein 2. Hepatology 1999; 30(2):485–490.

68. Paulusma CC, Kool M, Bosma PJ, Scheffer GL, ter-Borg F, Scheper RJ, Tytgat GN, Borst P, Baas F, Oude ER. A mutation in the human canalicular multispecific organic anion transporter gene causes the Dubin-Johnson syndrome. Hepatology 1997; 25(6):1539–1542.

69. Kartenbeck J, Leuschner U, Mayer R, Keppler D. Absence of the canalicular isoform of the MRP gene-encoded conjugate export pump from the hepatocytes in Dubin-Johnson syndrome. Hepatology 1996; 23(5):1061–1066.

70. Paulusma CC, Bosma PJ, Zaman GJ, Bakker CT, Otter M, Scheffer GL, Scheper RJ, Borst P, Oude ER. Congenital jaundice in rats with a mutation in a multidrug resistance-associated protein gene. Science 1996; 271(5252):1126–1128.

71. Vos TA, Hooiveld GJ, Koning H, Childs S, Meijer DK, Moshage H, Jansen PL, Muller M. Up-regulation of the multidrug resistance genes, Mrp1 and Mdr1b, and down-regulation of the organic anion transporter, Mrp2, and the bile salt transporter, Spgp, in endotoxemic rat liver. Hepatology 1998; 28(6):1637–1644.

72. Vos TA, Ros JE, Havinga R, Moshage H, Kuipers F, Jansen PL, Muller M. Regulation of hepatic transport systems involved in bile secretion during liver regeneration in rats. Hepatology 1999; 29(6):1833–1839.

73. Hirohashi T, Suzuki H, Ito K, Ogawa K, Kume K, Shimizu T, Sugiyama Y. Hepatic expression of multidrug resistance-associated protein-like proteins maintained in eisai hyperbilirubinemic rats. Mol Pharmacol 1998; 53(6):1068–1075.

74. Ogawa K, Suzuki H, Hirohashi T, Ishikawa T, Meier PJ, Hirose K, Akizawa T, Yoshioka M, Sugiyama Y. Characterization of inducible nature of MRP3 in rat liver. Am J Physiol Gastrointest Liver Physiol 2000; 278(3):G438–G446.

75. Konig J, Rost D, Cui Y, Keppler D. Characterization of the human multidrug resistance protein isoform MRP3 localized to the basolateral hepatocyte membrane. Hepatology 1999; 29(4):1156–1163.

76. Hirohashi T, Suzuki H, Sugiyama Y. Characterization of the transport properties of cloned

rat multidrug resistance-associated protein 3 (MRP3). J Biol Chem 1999; 274(21):15181–15185.

77. Renes J, de Vries EGE, Jansen PLM, Müller M. The (patho)physiological functions of the MRP family. Drug Resistance Updates 2000.

78. Borst P, Evers R, Kool M, Wijnholds J. A family of drug transporters: the multidrug resistance-associated proteins. JNCI 2000; 92(16):1295–1302.

79. Stieger B, Fattinger K, Madon J, Kullak-Ublick GA, Meier PJ. Drug- and estrogen-induced cholestasis through inhibition of the hepatocellular bile salt export pump (Bsep) of rat liver. Gastroenterology 2000; 118(2):422–430.

80. Dixon PH, Weerasekera N, Linton KJ, Donaldson O, Chambers J, Egginton E, Weaver J, Nelson-Piercy C, Swiet M, Warnes G, Elias E, Higgins CF, Johnston DG, McCarthy MI, Williamson C. Heterozygous MDR3 missense mutation associated with intrahepatic cholestasis of pregnancy: evidence for a defect in protein trafficking. Hum Mol Genet 2000; 9(8):1209–1217.

81. Ko CW, Sekijima JH, Lee SP. Biliary sludge. Ann Intern Med 1999; 130(4 Pt 1):301–311.

82. Zinberg J, Chernaik R, Coman E, Rosenblatt R, Brandt LJ. Reversible symptomatic biliary obstruction associated with ceftriaxone pseudolithiasis. Am J Gastroenterol 1991; 86(9):1251–1254.

83. Lewin B. Genes VII. 7th ed. London: Oxford University Press, 2000.

84. Di Croce L, Okret S, Kersten S, Gustafsson JA, Parker M, Wahli W, Beato M. Steroid and nuclear receptors. Villefranche-sur-Mer, France, May 25–27, 1999. EMBO J 1999; 18(22):6201–6210.

85. Mangelsdorf DJ, Evans RM. The RXR heterodimers and orphan receptors. Cell 1995; 83(6):841–850.

86. Willy PJ, Mangelsdorf DJ. Nuclear orphan receptors: the search for novel ligands and signaling pathways. In: BW O'Malley, ed. Hormones and Signaling. San Diego, CA: Academic Press, 1998:307–358.

87. Waxman DJ. P450 gene induction by structurally diverse xenochemicals: central role of nuclear receptors CAR, PXR, and PPAR. Arch Biochem Biophys 1999; 369(1):11–23.

88. Giguere V. Orphan nuclear receptors: from gene to function. Endocr Rev 1999; 20(5):689–725.

89. Parks DJ, Blanchard SG, Bledsoe RK, Chandra G, Consler TG, Kliewer SA, Stimmel JB, Willson TM, Zavacki AM, Moore DD, Lehmann JM. Bile acids: natural ligands for an orphan nuclear receptor. Science 1999; 284(5418):1365–1368.

90. Makishima M, Okamoto AY, Repa JJ, Tu H, Learned RM, Luk A, Hull MV, Lustig KD, Mangelsdorf DJ, Shan B. Identification of a nuclear receptor for bile acids. Science 1999; 284(5418):1362–1365.

91. Wang H, Chen J, Hollister K, Sowers LC, Forman BM. Endogenous bile acids are ligands for the nuclear receptor FXR/BAR. Mol Cell 1999; 3(5):543–553.

92. Xu HE, Lambert MH, Montana VG, Parks DJ, Blanchard SG, Brown PJ, Sternbach DD, Lehmann JM, Wisely GB, Willson TM, Kliewer SA, Milburn MV. Molecular recognition of fatty acids by peroxisome proliferator-activated receptors. Mol Cell 1999; 3(3):397–403.

93. Streetz K, Leifeld L, Grundmann D, Ramakers J, Eckert K, Spengler U, Brenner D, Manns M, Trautwein C. Tumor necrosis factor alpha in the pathogenesis of human and murine fulminant hepatic failure. Gastroenterology 2000; 119(2):446–460.

94. Wan YJ, An D, Cai Y, Repa JJ, Hung-Po CT, Flores M, Postic C, Magnuson MA, Chen J, Chien KR, French S, Mangelsdorf DJ, Sucov HM. Hepatocyte-specific mutation establishes retinoid X receptor alpha as a heterodimeric integrator of multiple physiological processes in the liver. Mol Cell Biol 2000; 20(12):4436–4444.

95. Lee JM, Trauner M, Soroka CJ, Stieger B, Meier PJ, Boyer JL. Expression of the bile salt export pump is maintained after chronic cholestasis in the rat. Gastroenterology 2000; 118(1):163–172.

96. Vos TA, Hooiveld GJEJ, Koning H, Childs S, Meijer DKF, Moshage H, Jansen PLM, Müller M. Up-regulation of the multidrug resistance genes, mrp1 and mdr1b, and down-regulation of the organic anion transporter, mrp2, and the bile salt transporter, spgp, in endotoxemic rat liver. Hepatology 1998; 28(6):1637–1644.

97. Gerloff T, Geier A, Stieger B, Hagenbuch B, Meier PJ, Matern S, Gartung C. Differential expression of basolateral and canalicular organic anion transporters during regeneration of rat liver. Gastroenterology 1999; 117(6):1408–1415.

98. Plass JR, Mol O, Heegsma J, Geuken M, Faber KN, Jansen PL, Müller M. Farnesoid X receptor and bile salts are involved in transcriptional regulation of the gene encoding the bile salt export pump. Hepatology 2002; 35(3):589–596.

99. Kauffmann HM, Keppler D, Kartenbeck J, Schrenk D. Induction of cMrp/cMoat gene expression by cisplatin, 2-acetylaminofluorene, or cycloheximide in rat hepatocytes. Hepatology 1997; 26(4):980–985.

100. Tanaka T, Uchiumi T, Hinoshita E, Inokuchi A, Toh S, Wada M, Takano H, Kohno K, Kuwano M. The human multidrug resistance protein 2 gene: Functional characterization of the 5'-flanking region and expression in hepatic cells. Hepatology 1999; 30(6):1507–1512.

101. Kauffmann HM, Schrenk D. Sequence analysis and functional characterization of the 5'-flanking region of the rat multidrug resistance protein 2 (mrp2) gene. Biochem Biophys Res Commun 1998; 245(2):325–331.

102. Stockel B, Konig J, Nies AT, Cui Y, Brom M, Keppler D. Characterization of the 5'-flanking region of the human multidrug resistance protein 2 (MRP2) gene and its regulation in comparison with the multidrug resistance protein 3 (MRP3) gene. Eur J Biochem 2000; 267(5): 1347–1358.

103. Roelofsen H, Hooiveld GJ, Koning H, Havinga R, Jansen PL, Muller M. Glutathione S-conjugate transport in hepatocytes entering the cell cycle is preserved by a switch in expression from the apical MRP2 to the basolateral MRP1 transporting protein. J Cell Sci 1999; 112(Pt 9):1395–1404.

104. Yamane Y, Furuichi M, Song R, Van NT, Mulcahy RT, Ishikawa T, Kuo MT. Expression of multidrug resistance Protein/GS-X pump and gamma-glutamylcysteine synthetase genes is regulated by oxidative stress. J Biol Chem 1998; 273(47):31075–31085.

105. Kuo MT, Bao J, Furuichi M, Yamane Y, Gomi A, Savaraj N, Masuzawa T, Ishikawa T. Frequent coexpression of MRP/GS-X pump and gamma-glutamylcysteine synthetase mRNA in drug-resistant cells, untreated tumor cells, and normal mouse tissues. Biochem Pharmacol 1998; 55(5):605–615.

106. Zhu Q, Center MS. Cloning and sequence analysis of the promoter region of the MRP gene of HL60 cells isolated for resistance to adriamycin. Cancer Res 1994; 54(16):4488–4492.

107. Zhu QC, Center MS. Evidence that SP1 modulates transcriptional activity of the multidrug resistance-associated protein gene. DNA and Cell Biol 1996; 15:105–111.

108. Hirohashi T, Suzuki H, Takikawa H, Sugiyama Y. ATP-dependent transport of bile salts by rat multidrug resistance-associated protein 3 (Mrp3). J Biol Chem 2000; 275(4):2905–2910.

109. Kiuchi Y, Suzuki H, Hirohashi T, Tyson CA, Sugiyama Y. cDNA cloning and inducible expression of human multidrug resistance associated protein 3 (MRP3). FEBS Lett 1998; 433(1–2):149–152.

110. König J, Nies AT, Cui Y, Leier I, Keppler D. Conjugate export pumps of the multidrug resistance protein (MRP) family: localization, substrate specificity, and MRP2-mediated drug resistance. Biochim Biophys Acta 1999; 1461(2):377–394.

111. Fromm MF, Leake B, Roden DM, Wilkinson GR, Kim RB. Human MRP3 transporter: identification of the 5'-flanking region, genomic organization and alternative splice variants. Biochim Biophys Acta 1999; 1415(2):369–374.

112. Hu Z, Jin S, Scotto KW. Transcriptional activation of the MDR1 gene by UV irradiation. Role of NF-Y and Sp1. J Biol Chem 2000; 275(4):2979–2985.

113. Chin KV, Tanaka S, Darlington G, Pastan I, Gottesman MM. Heat shock and arsenite increase

expression of the multidrug resistance (MDR1) gene in human renal carcinoma cells. J Biol Chem 1990; 265(1):221–226.

114. Ohga T, Koike K, Ono M, Makino Y, Itagaki Y, Tanimoto M, Kuwano M, Kohno K. Role of the human Y box-binding protein YB-1 in cellular sensitivity to the DNA-damaging agents cisplatin, mitomycin C, and ultraviolet light. Cancer Res 1996; 56(18):4224–4228.

115. Ohga T, Uchiumi T, Makino Y, Koike K, Wada M, Kuwano M, Kohno K. Direct involvement of the Y-box binding protein YB-1 in genotoxic stress-induced activation of the human multidrug resistance 1 gene. J Biol Chem 1998; 273(11):5997–6000.

116. Schuetz EG, Schinkel AH, Relling MV, Schuetz JD. P-glycoprotein: A major determinant of rifampicin-inducible expression of cytochrome P4503A in mice and humans. Proc Natl Acad Sci USA 1996; 93:4001–4005.

117. Schuetz EG, Umbenhauer DR, Yasuda K, Brimer C, Nguyen L, Relling MV, Schuetz JD, Schinkel AH. Altered expression of hepatic cytochromes P-450 in mice deficient in one or more mdr1 genes. Mol Pharmacol 2000; 57(1):188–197.

118. Schinkel AH, Smit JJM, van Tellingen O, Beijnen JH, Wagenaar E, van Deemter L, Mol CAAM, van der Valk MA, Robanus-Maandag EC, te Riele HPJ, Berns AJM, Borst P. Disruption of the mouse mdr1a p-glycoprotein gene leads to a deficiency in the blood-brain barrier and to increased sensitivity to drugs. Cell 1994; 77:491–502.

119. Schinkel AH, Mayer U, Wagenaar E, Mol CA, van Deemter L, Smit JJ, van der Valk MA, Voordouw AC, Spits H, van Tellingen O, Zijlmans JM, Fibbe WE, Borst P. Normal viability and altered pharmacokinetics in mice lacking mdr1-type (drug-transporting) P-glycoproteins. Proc Natl Acad Sci USA 1997; 94(8):4028–4033.

120. Blumberg B, Evans RM. Orphan nuclear receptors—new ligands and new possibilities. Genes Dev 1998; 12(20):3149–3155.

121. Blumberg B, Sabbagh W, Jr., Juguilon H, Bolado J, Jr., van Meter CM, Ong ES, Evans RM. SXR, a novel steroid and xenobiotic-sensing nuclear receptor. Genes Dev 1998; 12(20): 3195–3205.

122. Miranda S, Vollrath V, Wielandt AM, Loyola G, Bronfman M, Chianale J. Overexpression of mdr2 gene by peroxisome proliferators in the mouse liver. J Hepatol 1997; 26(6):1331–1339.

123. Frijters CM, Ottenhoff R, van Wijland MJ, Van Nieuwkerk CM, Groen AK, Oude Elferink RP. Regulation of mdr2 P-glycoprotein expression by bile salts. Biochem J 1997; 321(Pt 2): 389–395.

124. Gupta S, Todd SR, Pandak WM, Müller M, Vlahcevic ZR, Hylemon PB. Regulation of multidrug resistance 2 P-glycoprotein expression by bile salts in rats and in primary cultures of rat hepatocytes. Hepatology 2000; 32(2):341–347.

125. Hooiveld GJEJ, Vos TA, Scheffer GL, van Goor H, Koning H, Bloks V, Loot AE, Meijer DK, Jansen PLM, Kuipers F, Müller M. 3-Hydroxy-3-methylglutaryl-coenzyme A reductase inhibitors (statins) induce hepatic expression of the phospholipid translocase mdr2 in rats. Gastroenterology 1999; 117(3):678–687.

126. Carrella M, Feldman D, Cogoi S, Csillaghy A, Weinhold PA. Enhancement of mdr2 gene transcription mediates the biliary transfer of phosphatidylcholine supplied by an increased biosynthesis in the pravastatin-treated rat. Hepatology 1999; 29(6):1825–1832.

127. Pahl HL. Signal transduction from the endoplasmic reticulum to the cell nucleus. Physiol Rev 1999; 79(3):683–701.

128. Brown PC, Silverman JA. Characterization of the rat mdr2 promoter and its regulation by the transcription factor Sp1. Nucleic Acids Res 1996; 24(16):3235–3241.

129. Hooiveld GJEJ, Heegsma J, Silverman JA, Groothuis GMM, Jansen PLM, Meijer DKF, Kuipers F, Müller M. Induction of hepatic Mdr2 expression by cholesterol synthesis inhibitors (statins) is mediated via Srebps. Hepatology 1999; 30[4]:428A.

130. Konig J, Cui Y, Nies AT, Keppler D. Localization and genomic organization of a new hepatocellular organic anion transporting polypeptide. J Biol Chem 2000; 275(30):23161–23168.

131. Hsiang B, Zhu Y, Wang Z, Wu Y, Sasseville V, Yang WP, Kirchgessner TG. A novel human hepatic organic anion transporting polypeptide (OATP2). Identification of a liver-specific human organic anion transporting polypeptide and identification of rat and human hydroxy-methylglutaryl-CoA reductase inhibitor transporters. J Biol Chem 1999; 274(52):37161–37168.

132. Eckhardt U, Schroeder A, Stieger B, Hochli M, Landmann L, Tynes R, Meier PJ, Hagenbuch B. Polyspecific substrate uptake by the hepatic organic anion transporter Oatp1 in stably transfected CHO cells. Am J Physiol 1999; 276(4 Pt 1):G1037–G1042.

133. Reichel C, Gao B, Van Montfoort J, Cattori V, Rahner C, Hagenbuch B, Stieger B, Kamisako T, Meier PJ. Localization and function of the organic anion-transporting polypeptide Oatp2 in rat liver. Gastroenterology 1999; 117(3):688–695.

134. Noe B, Hagenbuch B, Stieger B, Meier PJ. Isolation of a multispecific organic anion and cardiac glycoside transporter from rat brain. Proc Natl Acad Sci USA 1997; 94(19):10346–10350.

135. Suzuki H, Sugiyama Y. Excretion of GSSG and glutathione conjugates mediated by MRP1 and cMOAT/MRP2. Semin Liver Dis 1998; 18(4):359–376.

136. Morikawa A, Goto Y, Suzuki H, Hirohashi T, Sugiyama Y. Biliary excretion of 17beta-estradiol 17beta-D-glucuronide is predominantly mediated by cMOAT/MRP2. Pharm Res 2000; 17(5):546–552.

137. Bakos E, Evers R, Sinko E, Varadi A, Borst P, Sarkadi B. Interactions of the human multidrug resistance proteins MRP1 and MRP2 with organic anions. Mol Pharmacol 2000; 57(4):760–768.

138. Smith AJ, Mayer U, Schinkel AH, Borst P. Availability of PSC833, a substrate and inhibitor of P-glycoproteins, in various concentrations of serum. JNCI 1998; 90(15):1161–1166.

139. Schwarz UI, Gramatte T, Krappweis J, Oertel R, Kirch W. P-glycoprotein inhibitor erythro-mycin increases oral bioavailability of talinolol in humans. Int J Clin Pharmacol Ther 2000; 38(4):161–167.

140. Takara K, Tanigawara Y, Komada F, Nishiguchi K, Sakaeda T, Okumura K. Cellular pharma-cokinetic aspects of reversal effect of itraconazole on P-glycoprotein-mediated resistance of anticancer drugs. Biol Pharm Bull 1999; 22(12):1355–1359.

141. Thevenod F, Friedmann JM, Katsen AD, Hauser IA. Up-regulation of multidrug resistance P-glycoprotein via nuclear factor-kappaB activation protects kidney proximal tubule cells from cadmium- and reactive oxygen species-induced apoptosis. J Biol Chem 2000; 275(3): 1887–1896.

142. Ros JE, Schuetz JD, Geuken M, Streetz K, Moshage H, Kuipers F, Manns MP, Jansen PLM, Trautwein C, Müller M. Induction of Mdr1b expression by tumor necrosis factor-alpha in rat liver cells is independent of p53 but requires NF-kappaB signaling. Hepatology 2001; 33(6):1425–1431.

143. Zhou G, Kuo MT. NF-kappaB-mediated induction of mdr1b expression by insulin in rat hepatoma cells. J Biol Chem 1997; 272(24):15174–15183.

144. Trauner M, Arrese M, Soroka CJ, Ananthanarayanan M, Koeppel TA, Schlosser SF, Suchy FJ, Keppler D, Boyer JL. The rat canalicular conjugate export pump (Mrp2) is down-regu-lated in intrahepatic and obstructive cholestasis. Gastroenterology 1997; 113(1):255–264.

145. Courtois A, Payen L, Guillouzo A, Fardel O. Up-regulation of multidrug resistance-associ-ated protein 2 (MRP2) expression in rat hepatocytes by dexamethasone. FEBS Lett 1999; 459(3):381–385.

146. Collingwood TN, Urnov FD, Wolffe AP. Nuclear receptors: coactivators, corepressors and chromatin remodeling in the control of transcription. J Mol Endocrinol 1999; 23(3):255–275.

147. Desvergne B, Wahli W. Peroxisome proliferator-activated receptors: nuclear control of me-tabolism. Endocr Rev 1999; 20(5):649–688.

148. Doyle DF, Mangelsdorf DJ, Corey DR. Modifying ligand specificity of gene regulatory proteins. Curr Opin Chem Biol 2000; 4(1):60–63.

149. Grober J, Zaghini I, Fujii H, Jones SA, Kliewer SA, Willson TM, Ono T, Besnard P. Identification of a bile acid-responsive element in the human ileal bile acid-binding protein gene. Involvement of the farnesoid X receptor/9-cis-retinoic acid receptor heterodimer. J Biol Chem 1999; 274(42):29749–29754.

150. Muller M, Jansen PL. Molecular aspects of hepatobiliary transport. Am J Physiol 1997; 272: G1285–G1303.

151. Müller M, Jansen PLM. The secretory function of the liver: New insights in hepatobiliary transport. J Hepatol 1998; 28(2):344–354.

152. Klein I, Sarkadi B, Varadi A. An inventory of the human ABC proteins. Biochim Biophys Acta 1999; 1461(2):237–262.

153. Broccardo C, Luciani M, Chimini G. The ABCA subclass of mammalian transporters. Biochim Biophys Acta 1999; 1461(2):395–404.

154. Klucken J, Buchler C, Orso E, Kaminski WE, Porsch-Ozcurumez M, Liebisch G, Kapinsky M, Diederich W, Drobnik W, Dean M, Allikmets R, Schmitz G. ABCG1 (ABC8), the human homolog of the drosophila white gene, is a regulator of macrophage cholesterol and phospholipid transport I. Proc Natl Acad Sci USA 2000; 97(2):817–822.

155. Kool M, van der LM, de Haas M, Baas F, Borst P. Expression of human MRP6, a homologue of the multidrug resistance protein gene MRP1, in tissues and cancer cells. Cancer Res 1999; 59(1):175–182.

156. Madon J, Hagenbuch B, Landmann L, Meier PJ, Stieger B. Transport function and hepatocellular localization of mrp6 in rat liver. Mol Pharmacol 2000; 57(3):634–641.

157. Zhou G, Kuo MT. Wild-type p53-mediated induction of rat mdr1b expression by the anticancer drug daunorubicin. J Biol Chem 1998; 273(25):15387–15394.

158. Smit JJM, Mol CAAM, van Deemter L, Wagenaar E, Schinkel AH, Borst P. Characterization of the promoter region of the human MDR3 p-glycoprotein gene. Biochem Biophys Acta–Gene Struct Express 1995; 1261:44–56.

159. Zhu QC, Center MS. Cloning and sequence analysis of the promoter region of the MRP gene of HL60 cells isolated for resistance to adriamycin. Cancer Res 1994; 54:4488–4492.

160. Tanaka T, Uchiumi T, Hinoshita E, Inokuchi A, Toh S, Wada M, Takano H, Kohno K, Kuwano M. The human multidrug resistance protein 2 gene: Functional characterization of the 5′-flanking region and expression in hepatic cells. Hepatology 1999; 30(6):1507–1512.

7

Immunological Mechanisms in Liver Injury

PETRA OBERMAYER-STRAUB
and MICHAEL PETER MANNS

Hannover Medical School, Hannover, Germany

I. INTRODUCTION

Liver injury by drugs may be caused by direct toxicity of a drug, which is dependent on the structure and the metabolic properties of the drug itself and leads to damage of cellular compounds such as proteins, lipids, or DNA. Direct toxicity of a drug occurs in the majority of patients and may be reproducible in animal models. In a small percentage of patients, however, severe adverse drug reactions are noted that are either mediated by the immune system or due to metabolic idiosyncrasies direct toxicity in rare susceptible individuals. We will focus on immunopathogenetic reactions. These adverse reactions often affect the liver and are mediated by activation of the drug to reactive metabolites that modify liver proteins, mostly the cytochrome P450 (CYP) that generate them. An immune reaction

125

directed against modified and native CYPs results in an immune-mediated attack on hepatocytes that causes severe, sometimes life-threatening hepatitis. Mechanisms involved in drug-induced hepatitis will be discussed with tienilic acid–induced hepatitis, dihydralazine hepatitis, halothane hepatitis, anticonvulsant hepatitis, and diclofenac hepatitis as examples. Since the prevalence of drug-induced hepatitis is 1:10,000 or less, adduct formation alone will not result in drug-induced hepatitis. Defects and polymorphisms in immunoregulatory genes that facilitate autoimmune reactions have to be postulated.

Recently, an autoimmune regulator (*AIRE*) gene has been cloned. This gene seems to be involved in the induction and maintenance of tolerance, and defects in the *AIRE* cause a syndrome characterized by multiple autoimmune diseases, such as hepatitis. *AIRE* and related genes are good candidates to describe genetic polymorphisms in drug-induced hepatitis. While adduct formation is the basic pathogenetic mechanism in drug-induced hepatitis and the *AIRE* gene defect causes the autoimmune polyendocrine syndrome type 1, little is known about the factors involved in autoimmune hepatitis type 2 (AIH-2). However in AIH-2, enzymes of phase I and phase II drug metabolism are also autoantigens and there is a genetic background that predisposes to autoimmune diseases. Further research is necessary to investigate whether parallels to drug-induced hepatitis and APS-1 exist by chance or whether these parallels highlight similar pathogenetic mechanisms.

Metabolism and detoxification of a wide variety of chemically unrelated xenobiotics is performed in the liver and in the intestinal mucosa. Detoxification is achieved by a two-phase process (Fig. 1). In phase I detoxification, xenobiotic compounds are hydroxylated by the multigene family of cytochrome P450 enzymes (CYPs). Phase II consists of conjugation with water-soluble compounds. Enzymes active in phase II detoxification are UDP-glucuronosyltransferases (UGTs), glutathione-*S*-transferases, *N*-acetyltransferases and sulfotransferases. After conjugation, products are water soluble and may be excreted via urine

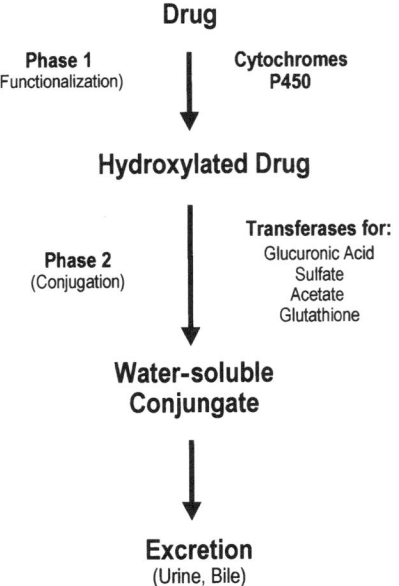

Figure 1   Enzymes active in phase I and phase II detoxification. (From ref. 117.)

or bile. Detoxification reactions are usually beneficial. However sometimes one of these reactions transforms a xenobiotic substance into a reactive metabolite. This metabolite may bind directly to the active center of the enzyme that created it. Alternatively, it may leave the active center and bind to other proteins and to cellular compounds (Fig. 2). Adduct formation may interfere with metabolic reactions of the cell and cause direct toxicity. Chemical modifications of DNA may result in either apoptosis or carcinogenesis. In very few patients, adduct formation with cellular proteins will induce an immune reaction and result in a severe, sometimes life-threatening, immune-mediated disease. Since the liver is one of the main organs of detoxification, drug-induced immune responses are frequently directed against hepatic-drug-metabolizing enzymes and other liver proteins, resulting in severe, sometimes life-threatening, hepatitis. Such an idiosyncratic reaction is called immune-mediated drug-induced hepatitis. The disease may go along with typical signs of an immune reaction such as fever, eosinophilia, and rash. Autoantibodies may be generated, which are directed either against the modifying hapten domain alone, against a hapten-protein domain, or against native unmodified proteins.

In immune-mediated drug-induced hepatitis, adduct formation has been established as a pathogenetic mechanism. However, this mechanism alone cannot explain the low prevalence of 1:10,000 patients. Therefore, it is assumed that there is a genetic predisposition for the development of immune-mediated drug-induced hepatitis. Candidates are polymorphisms and defects in two defense systems: drug-metabolizing enzymes and the immune system. A model disease for a defect in immune regulation is the autoimmune polyglandular syndrome type 1 (APS-1). Caused by defects in a single gene, APS-1 is characterized by a broad spectrum of organ-specific autoimmune diseases. One of these

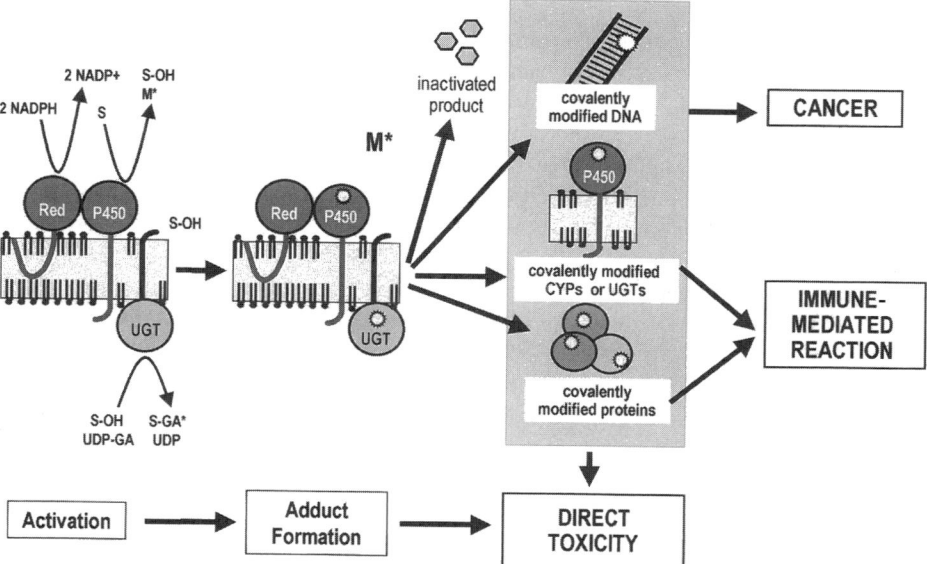

Figure 2 Formation of reactive metabolites and protein adducts is the initial step in the induction of direct toxicity and immune-mediated toxicity of drugs. S, substrate; S-OH, hydroxylated substrate; M*, reactive metabolite; GA, glucuronic acid; CYP or P450, cytochrome P450; UGT, UDP-glucuronosyltransferase; Red, reductase.

autoimmune diseases is hepatitis, featuring autoantibodies directed against CYP 1A2 and CYP 2A6. Furthermore, in the adrenal and ovarian autoimmune manifestations of APS-1, autoantibodies are detected that are directed against CYPs active in steroid biosynthesis. The mechanism of autoantibody induction in APS-1 is not known. However, adduct formation during CYP-mediated hydroxylation might pinpoint these enzymes as targets for an immune system that is defective in downregulatory mechanisms.

In contrast to drug-induced hepatitis and APS-1, little is known about the pathogenesis of autoimmune hepatitis type 2 (AIH-2). However, it is intriguing that in AIH-2, enzymes of both phase I and phase II detoxification are targets of autoimmunity. AIH-2 has been shown to be triggered by interferon treatment in several patients with chronic viral infections, indicating that either molecular mimicry with viral proteins or the presence of inflammatory cytokines may play a pathogenic role.

II. ADDUCT FORMATION AS A PATHOGENIC MECHANISM IN IMMUNE-MEDIATED DRUG-INDUCED HEPATITIS

A. Hepatitis Induced by Tienilic Acid

1. Clinical Features

Tienilic acid (Ticrynafen) is an uricosuric diuretic that was used in the treatment of hypertension. Tienilic acid was withdrawn from the market because of severe hepatitis that developed in 0.1–0.7% of patients treated (1). Eighty-five percent of patients with tienilic acid–associated hepatitis developed jaundice and about 10% of the icteric patients died. In general, equal numbers of males and females were affected. Tienilic acid–induced hepatitis shows several features typical for immune-mediated drug-induced hepatitis:

1. There is a latency period between the beginning of drug treatment and the manifestation of hepatitis. This latency period in tienilic acid–induced hepatitis ranges between 2 and 35 weeks (1).
2. Upon rechallenge with the drug, hepatitis recurs. The latency period upon rechallenge tends to be shorter than on initial exposure. For tienilic acid–induced hepatitis, one patient was reported who experienced four successive episodes of tienilic acid administration with progressive shortening of the latency period (3 months, 12 days, 3 days, 6 hours) (2).
3. Severity of hepatitis is independent of the amount of drug administered and discontinuation of treatment results in recovery from hepatitis.
4. In some cases, typical signs of an immunological reaction are seen, e.g., fever, rash, or eosinophilia. A viral-like disease was recorded in 8% of cases of tienilic acid–induced hepatitis, rash in 3%, and eosinophilia in 1.5% (1).

2. Autoantibodies

In sera of patients with tienilic acid–induced hepatitis, antibodies were found that are directed against liver and kidney microsomes and were named LKM-2 autoantibodies (3). These autoantibodies are not detected in healthy patients treated with the drug. In indirect immunofluorescence, LKM-2 autoantibodies stain the centrilobular region of the liver and recognize a protein of about 50 kDa. The LKM-2 autoantibody specifically recognizes cytochrome P450 2C9 (CYP 2C9) (4,5). LKM-2 autoantibodies are very specific. In spite of significant sequence homology with other CYPs, no cross-reactivity was detectable with recombinant CYP 3A4, CYP 1A1, CYP 1A2, or CYP 2C18 (6).

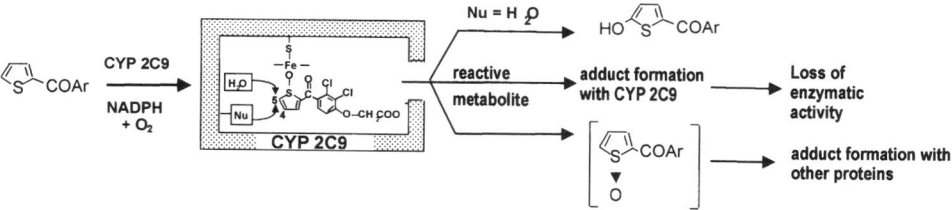

Figure 3   Structure of tienilic acid, and a hypothesis for suicide inactivation of CYP 2C9 by tienilic aid and adduct formation with other proteins. [Modified according to Beaune et al. (25).]

3.   Mechanism of Induction—A Hypothesis

CYP 2C9 is the major tienilic acid metabolizing enzyme in human liver (6). In vitro, incubation of human or rat microsomes leads to formation of 5-OH tienilic acid, which is the major excretion product of tienilic acid in human urine (Fig. 3) (7,8). During 5-hydroxylation of tienilic acid, reactive metabolites are formed that bind covalently to the active center of CYP 2C9 and inactive this enzyme (4,5,8,9). In the presence of glutathione only monoadducts of tienilic acid with CYP 2C9 are detected, while diadducts and adducts with other hepatic proteins are present in the absence of glutathione (4,5,10). There is evidence that suggests that the activated metabolite of tienilic acid is a sulfoxide (8,9).

LKM-2 autoantibodies are a marker of tienilic acid–induced hepatitis. They were shown to be directed against both the native and the modified CYP 2C9 protein. On the native protein, LKM-2 autoantibodies recognize a three-dimensional epitope (11,12). Pessayre has proposed a hypothesis, on the induction of autoantibodies directed against the native protein (Fig. 4) (13). Low numbers of autoreactive B cells are detectable in humans (14). These B cells will remain quiescent since they are not activated by helper T cells. Mild direct toxicity of tienilic acid may lead to a release of alkylated CYP 2C9 from

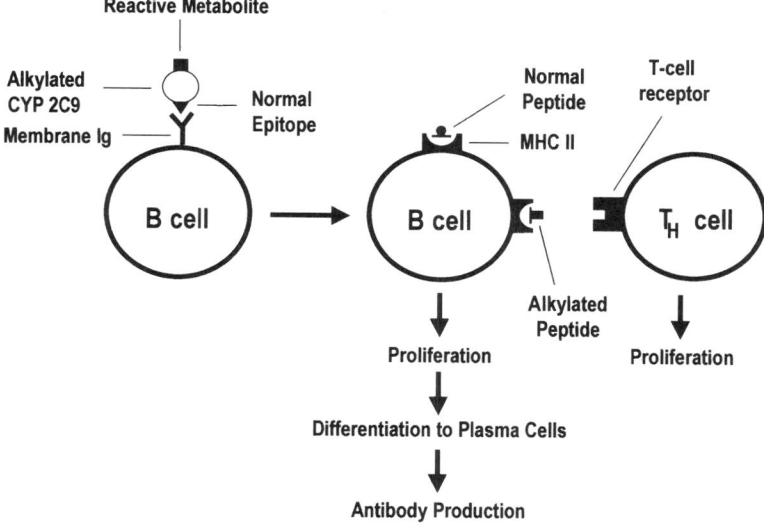

Figure 4   A hypothetial mechanism for the induction of the LKM-2 autoantibody. [Modified according to Pessayre (13).]

hepatocytes. Alkylated CYP 2C9 may bind to the surface IgM of an autoreactive quiescent B cell, which most likely recognizes a native epitope on the surface of CYP 2C9. After binding, CYP 2C9 is internalized and digested into small peptides. These peptides are bound to MHC class II molecules and presented on the B-cell surface. In the absence of autoreactive T cells, this process will have no consequences. However, owing to covalent binding of tienilic acid, one of the peptides will be modified by a tienilic acid metabolite. In contrast to native peptides, this "modified self-peptide" may be recognized by T_H cells and lead to activation and proliferation of both the autoreactive B cell and the interacting T cell (Fig. 4). Some autoreactive B cells will differentiate to plasma cells and produce anti-CYP 2C9 autoantibodies. These antibodies most likely will be directed against the native CYP. Owing to increased numbers of autoreactive cells and to the earlier appearance of circulating autoantibodies, the system is now more sensitive. If modified CYP 2C9 is produced for prolonged periods, this process will enhance itself over time, IgG will be produced, and a dangerous overshooting immune reaction may develop, which is known as tienilic acid induced–hepatitis.

B. Dihydralazine Hepatitis

1. Clinical Features

Long-term treatment with the vasodilatory drug dihydralazine resulted in the induction of severe hepatitis in many patients. Females were overrepresented among hepatitis patients (female:male ratio 3:1) and most patients were slow acetylators (15). Hepatitis occurred with a delay of 2–48 weeks after the beginning of treatment. Severity of dihydralazine hepatitis was independent of the dosage of dihydralazine administered (16). After termination of dihydralazine treatment a complete recovery was noted in most patients, but fatal cases were reported (17). Rechallenge with dihydralazine led to recurrence of disease with a shorter latency period than during initial exposure (18,19). One patient was reported with six successive episodes of fever and heaptitis, with progressive shortening of the interval between onset of treatment and recurrence of symptoms (18).

2. Autoantibodies

Biopsies of patients with dihydralazine hepatitis revealed centrolobular necrosis with an inflammatory infiltrate (20). In many patients antibodies were detected that showed a centrilobular staining pattern on liver sections (21,22). Since the antibodies did not react in the kidney, the antibodies were called anti-liver-microsome (anti-LM) antibodies. LM autoantibodies disappeared after recovery (21). Anti-LM autoantibodies recognize an unmodified protein of 54 kDa. The molecular target of anti-LM autoantibodies was identified as cytochrome P450 1A2 (CYP1 A2) (22). Anti-LM autoantibodies are highly specific. They do not cross-react with the closely related CYP 1A1, which shares more than 80% sequence identity with CYP 1A2 (23). LM antibodies inhibit the enzymatic activity of CYP 1A2 and are directed against a three-dimensional epitope (24).

3. Mechanism of Induction: Environmental and Genetic Factors May Modulate the Risk

It is believed that upon oxidative metabolism of dihydralazine a reactive metabolite is produced (25). Experimental evidence suggests that dihydralazine is activated by CYP 1A2 and that the reactive metabolite binds to the active center of CYP 1A2, generating a modified self-protein (26). The modified CYP 1A2 may be presented to the immune

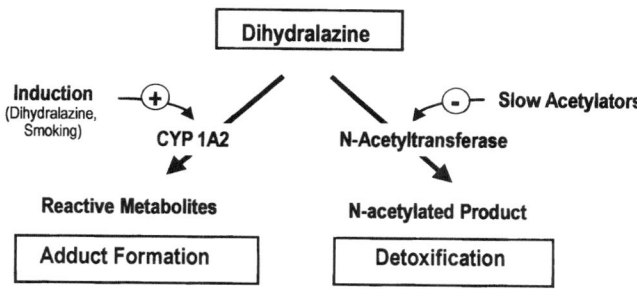

Figure 5 The risk for dihydralazine hepatitis is modulated by genetic and environmental factors. [Modified according to Beaune et al. (25).]

system as small modified peptides via MHC receptors or by transport of the uncleaved protein to the plasma membrane (11,27,28). In susceptible patients, presentation of the modified CYP 1A2 to the immune system results in an immune response with formation of anti-CYP 1A2 (anti-LM) autoantibodies.

A second metabolic pathway exists for the detoxification of dihydralazine. This second pathway is an *N*-acetylation reaction and is not associated with adduct formation (Fig. 5). Owing to a polymorphism of *N*-acetyltransferase, about 50% of Caucasians are deficient in *N*-acetylation, the so-called "slow acetylator" phenotype (29,30). In accordance with the hypothesis of adduct formation as a critical event for the induction of drug-induced hepatitis, slow acetylators are overrepresented in the patient population (25). Furthermore, this result indicates that environmental factors that change the balance between beneficial and harmful metabolic pathways may influence the personal risk for drug-induced hepatitis (Fig. 5).

C. Hepatitis Induced by Halothane and Related Compounds

1. Clinical Features

Even today halothane and chemically related compounds are commonly used anesthetics. Intrinsic toxicity of halothane, which results in mild tissue damage and modest increases in transaminase values, may be detected in about 20% of patients (31). Severe, often fulminant, hepatitis will develop in about 1 in 10,000 patients treated with halothane. Halothane-induced hepatitis is characterized by jaundice, fever, high transaminase values, and severe centrilobular necrosis. Hepatic encephalopathy may occur, resulting in a high rate of mortality (14–67% of cases). Risk factors are female gender (male/female 1:2), obesity, HLA A11 (32), and multiple exposures. An average latency period of 12 days is noted between first exposure and the first signs of halothane hepatitis. The latency period decreases to 7 days after the second and to 5 days after the third exposure (33). Frequent manifestations of hypersensitivity are fever (70%), eosinophilia (40%), and rash (10%). Usually an inflammatory infiltrate of mononuclear cells, neutrophils, and, sometimes, eosinophils is present (33).

2. Autoantibodies and Mechanisms of Induction

Halothane was reported to be metabolized by several CYPs, resulting in two different pathways of metabolism, an oxidative and a reductive pathway (Fig. 6) (34,35). The reduc-

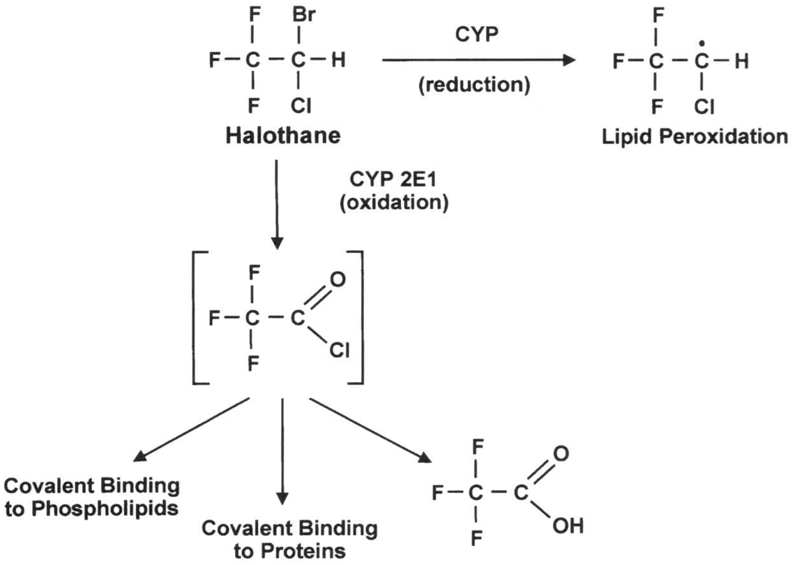

Figure 6 Halothane metabolism. (Modified according to ref. 118.)

tive pathway is believed to be responsible for the mild form of hepatic injury. In contrast, an oxidative pathway, mediated by CYP 2E1, is believed to generate a highly reactived trifluoroacetylchloride (TFA), the key component in the pathogenesis of halothane hepatitis (36–40). The majority of reactive metabolites are believed to leave the active center of CYP 2E1 and to modify ε-amino goups of lysines, which are present in many proteins (41). Many TFA adducts are generated with molecular weights between 50 kDa and 170 kDa (Table 1). Analysis of purified proteins by ELISA showed that autoantibodies not

Table 1 Known Autoantigens in Halothane Hepatitis

Protein	MW (kDa)
UDP-glucose: glycoprotein glucosyltransferase	170
Erp99	100
BiP/GRP78	82
ERp72	80
Calreticulin	63
Carboxylesterase	59
Isomerase	58
Protein disulfide isomerase	57
CYP 2E1	50
Epoxidhydrolase	50

Source: Data from this table were derived from refs. 50 and 118.

only bound to TFA-modified domains, but were also able to detect conformational epitopes on native proteins (42–46). A pathological relevance of these autoantibodies is suggested by the presence of TFA conjugates on the surface of hepatocytes, which were able to induce a cytotoxic reaction in vitro (37,47).

3. Hepatitis Induced by Enflurane, Isoflurane, and Desflurane

Further evidence that adduct formation may be the critical event for induction of halothane-induced hepatitis comes from a major effort to decrease toxicity of anesthetics. New compounds were generated that show a uch lower degree of metabolism and adduct formation (48,49). Metabolism decreased from halothane (20%) to enflurane (2.4%), isoflurane (0.2%), and desflurane (0.01%) (48). Adducts generated by these new compounds are either cross-reactive (enfluorane) or identical (desflurane and isoflurane) to those adducts generated by halothane (Fig. 7). Metabolism correlates with the numbers of reported patients who experienced toxicity: 900 patients with halothane hepatitis, 15–24 patients with enflurane hepatitis, five patients with isoflurane hepatitis, and one case of desflurane hepatitis (50). The patient with desflurane-induced hepatitis was exposed twice previously to halothane, indicating that the initial immunization of this patient was due to previous halothane exposures (51).

4. Hepatitis Induced by Incidental Exposure to Hydroxyfluorocarbons

Hydrofluorocarbons (HCFC) have an even higher rate of metabolism than halothane. These compounds are used as ozone-sparing substitutes for chlorofluorocarbons in industrial settings (52). Upon contact HCFCs are detoxified by a mechanism similar to halothane, resulting in TFA intermediates and TFA adducts. Repeated accidental exposure of nine industrial workers to a mixture of 1,1-dichloro-2,2,2-trifluoroethane (HCFC 123) and

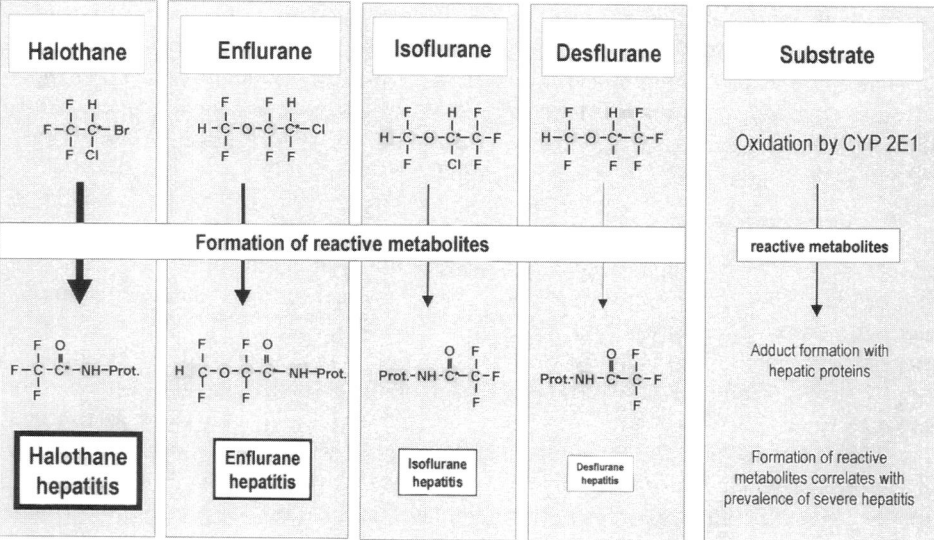

Figure 7   The prevalence of hepatitis induced by the fluorinated inhalation anesthetics halothane, enflurane, isoflurane, and desflurane is dependent on the rate of metabolism. (Modified from ref. 50.)

1-chloro-1,2,2,2-tetrafluoroethane (HCFC 124) was reported (53). Two of nine workers developed acute hepatitis and all workers exposed showed some degree of hepatic abnormality. TFA adducts were detected in the liver of a worker with severe hepatitis. Furthermore, in the serum of six workers autoantibodies were detected that were directed against CYP 2E1 and protein disulfide isomerase. These results demonstrate that repeated exposure of humans to HCFCs 123 and 124 may cause serious liver injury in a high proportion of people (53). The high incidence of adverse reactions to HCFCs upon repeated, subchronic exposure is in good acordance with the hypothesis that adduct formation with reactive metabolites generated during detoxification reactions may induce immune-mediated drug-induced hepatitis.

D.   Antiepileptic Drug Hypersensitivity Syndrome

1.   Clinical Features

Aromatic anticonvulsants, namely phenobarbital, phenytoin, and carbamazepine, may induce life-threatening systemic reactions, called the antiepileptic drug hypersensitivity syndrome (AHS) (54). AHS is characterized by fever, rash, and single or multiorgan involvement (e.g., hepatitis, blood dyscrasias, nephritis) (55). Upon first use, skin reactions occur with a prevalance of about 3 : 10,000 patients (56). Males and females are equally affected (female/male ratio 1 : 1). The latency period between the beginning of drug treatment and the onset of symptoms ranges between 2 weeks and 2 months (55). Upon rechallenge, the length of the latency period decreases (55,57). No correlation between drug dosage and severity of symptoms was detectable.

    Familial occurrence of AHS indicates that genetic factors may predispose for AHS (58). As patients with AHS were found to exhibit increased toxicity by in vitro drug metabolite challenge of lymphocytes, part of this genetic predisposition for AHS may be an abnormal metabolism of aromatic anticonvulsants. Interestingly, previously unexposed family members of AHS patients were found to exhibit increased toxicity by in vitro drug metabolite challenge of lymphocytes (58,59). Reactions to phenytoin, phenobarbital, and carbamazepine share similar clinical characteristics (55). Some patients who were exposed successively to two or all three anticonvulsants showed adverse reactions to each of them (55,57). When cross-sensitivity was assessed by the in vitro rechallenge assay, cross-reactivity was found in 80% of patient sera (55).

2.   Autoantibodies

In nine of 24 patients with anticonvulsant-induced idiosyncratic reactions, autoantibodies were detected that were directed against a 53-kDa hepatic protein. Protein targets that react with these antibodies are rat CYP 3A1 and rat CYP 2C11 (57). However, when an array of recombinant human CYPs was tested, neither human CYP 1A1, CYP 1A2, CYP 2A6, CYP 2B6, CYP 2D6, CYP 2E1, nor CYP 3A4 was recognized by these autoantibodies. Furthermore, in Western blot tests with human liver proteins only three weak signals were detected at 50–55 kDa. In contrast, a strong signal was recognized in liver proteins derived from a patient who died from hepatitis after phenytoin/phenobarbital therapy (57). The identity of the target protein is still unknown. In an effort to elucidate the identity of the molecular target of anticonvulsant hepatitis, a gene bank of fusion proteins with partial sequences of rat CYP 3A1 was screened for recognition sequences. Positive clones overlapped at a consensus sequence of amino acids 355–367 of rat CYP 3A1 (60). This epitope was recognized by sera of all patients with idiosyncratic reactions to anticonvulsants. This epitope differs from the respective sequence of human CYP 3A4 by a V361L substitution. If this substitution is introduced into the rat enzyme, binding activity is lost (60). Therefore, the molecular target of antibodies in anticonvulsant hepatitis remains unknown; however, it is believed that oxidation via CYPs results in the formation of an epoxide that may be the reactive metabolite. Therefore, it was suggested that epoxide hydrolase activity may play a critical pathogenetic role in detoxification of reactive epoxides. However, no differences in epoxide hydrolase activity were detectable between carbamazephine hypersensitive patients and normal controls (61).

E. Diclofenac Hepatitis

1. Clinical Features

Diclofenac is a member of the arylalkanoic subgroup of nonsteroidal anti-inflammatory drugs (NSAIDS). Several members of this chemical subgroup of NSAIDS have shown significant hepatotoxicity previously and have been withdrawn from the market, namely alclofenac, fenclofenac, zomepirac, benoxaprofen, suprofen, and piriprofen (62). Several other NSAIDS have been suggested to cause hepatic injury; however, a striking variability in the incidence of adverse reactions exists. Ibufenac was found to cause adverse reactions in approximately 5% of individuals (63,64). In contrast, idiosyncratic reactions to diclofenac, naproxen, or piroxicam range from 0.05% to 0.001% (65). Here we will focus on idiosyncratic reactions to diclofenac, since extensive studies were performed both on the clinical features of diclofenac hepatitis and on the mechanisms involved.

Diclofenac is used worldwide as a therapeutic agent against rheumatoid arthritis, osteoarthritis, or ankylosing spondylitis. Despite its widespread use, two types of reactions have been reported: (1) borderline increases in serum transaminases in approximately 15% of patients, and (2) diclofenac-induced hepatitis, which was estimated to occur in about 1–4 per 1,000,000 patients treated (66). Females show a twofold increased risk of developing diclofenac hepatitis (66–68). An increased suceptibility to diclofenac hepatitis seems to exist in patients with osteoarthritis. Seventy-two percent of patients affected by diclofenac hepatitis suffered from osteoarthritis, yet only 20% of prescriptions were for this condition (67). These findings indicate that diclofenac hepatitis may occur in a patient population with a genetic disposition, which may facilitate the development of autoimmune problems. The molecular mechanisms underlying diclofenac hepatitis are not understood. Symptoms such as fever, rash, and eosinophilia were reported in some patients and point to a hypersensitivity reaction (68). However, a dose dependence of toxicity was demonstrated, suggesting that direct toxicity of the drug may also play a role in the pathogenesis of the disease (66). Toxicity occurs with a latency period of less than 3 months in 63%, 3–12 months in 34%, and even longer in 3% of patients (67). In most patients the disease improves upon withdrawal of the drug (66,68). The average recovery period was 6 weeks (68). Two patients were reported who had to be maintained on steroid therapy after withdrawal of the drug, indicating that diclofenac had triggered autoimmune hepatitis (69–71). Also, recurrence of disease was demonstrated upon rechallenge with diclofenac (68).

A latency period until development of toxicity is consistent with the hypothesis that diclofenac may accumulate in patients with impaired clearance of the drug. A spectrum of severity was evident among patients, ranging from minor disturbances to 40-fold increases in transaminase activity. Interestingly, the cumulative diclofenac dose correlated well with peak aspartate transaminase (AST) and alanine transaminase (ALT) values after withdrawal of the drug (66). Furthermore, experiments with diclofenac and isolated hepatocytes demonstrated direct toxicity of diclofenac (72). Therefore, both toxic and immunological mechanisms may play a role in diclofenac hepatitis.

2. Biotransformation of Diclofenac: Adduct Formation is Mediated by CYPs and UGTs

Diclofenac exposure leads to formation of protein adducts in rat liver and in isolated hepatocytes (73). One of the protein adducts of diclofenac is located in the microsomal membrane. It has a molecular weight of about 50 kDa and its formation is dependent on diclofenac hydroxylation by CYPs. Inhibitor studies with human liver microsomes and with recombinant CYPs expressed in the baculovirus system revealed CYP 3A4 as a major diclofenac-metabolizing enzyme and as a major target of adduct formation (74). Most of the protein adducts, however, were generated by the formation of unstable acylglucuronides by UGTs (73). Kretz-Rommel and Boelsterli reported a major adduct of 60 kDa and, to a lesser extent, adducts of 50 kDa, 80 kDa, and 126 kDa molecular weight in rat hepatocytes (75). The major 60-kDa adduct was present not only in liver, but also in lung and spleen (76). As illustrated in Fig. 8, glucuronidation of diclofenac by UGTs results in an unstable acylglucuronide. This acylglucuronide may mediate adduct formation with UGTs and other hepatic proteins by two different mechanisms:

1. A nucleophilic displacement of glucuronic acid may lead to an adduct, in which diclofenac is directly bound to the protein.
2. An imine mechanism may include both diclofenac and the glucuronic aid moiety in the adduct. The imine mechanism may explain the existence of a broad cross-reactivity between adverse reactions of aromatic nonsteroidal drugs. All these drugs might form adducts via the imine mechanism (77).

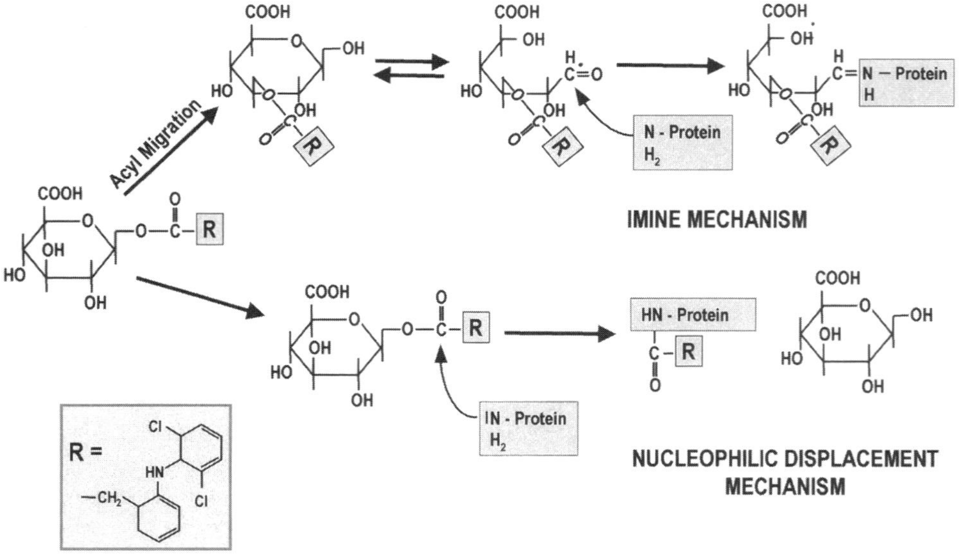

Figure 8 Activation of nonsteroidal antiinflammatory drugs by UGTs follows two different mechanisms. (Modified according to ref. 77.)

The imine mechanism shows that by glucuronidation of drugs, adducts may be formed that contain a carbohydrate moiety with a structure that is different from the ring structure of glucuronic acid. Such a novel glucuronic acid–derived domain could lead to immunological cross-reactivity between drug adducts derived from reactions with chemically different drugs.

III. HEPATITIS IN APS-1: A SINGLE GENE DEFECT CAUSES IMMUNE-MEDIATED HEPATITIS AND OTHER AUTOIMMUNE DISEASES

A. Clinical Features

APS-1 is a rare autosomal recessive disorder that is caused by mutations in a single gene, called autoimmune regulator (AIRE) (78,79). Absence of a functional AIRE protein results in a complex syndrome called APS-1 with mucocutaneous candidiasis and multiple autoimmune diseases in a single patient (Table 2) (80,81). Frequently, autoimmune manifestations affect endocrine glands such as parathyroids, adrenals, or ovaries. Ectodermal disease components, such as hypoplasia of the dental enamel, nail dystrophy, keratopathy, alopecia, and vitiligo, are found with a high prevalence (82). Less frequent, but severe, are the manifestations that affect the gastrointestinal tract, e.g., malabsorption and hepatitis. Hepatitis is found in 12–20% of APS-1 patients and may range from mild disease to fulminant hepatitis with lethal outcome (80,83,84).

B. CYPs Are Frequent Target Proteins in APS-1

Hepatitis in APS-1 is associated with autoantibodies directed against CYP 1A2 (85). In Finnish patients anti-CYP 1A2 autoantibodies were found in four of seven APS-1 patients

Table 2 Disease Components in APS-1

Disease component	Prevalence (%)
Endocrine components	
Hypoparathyroidism	79
Adrenal failure	12
IDDM	12
Parietal cell atrophy	13
Hypothyroidism	4
Ovarian failure in females (13 years and older)	60
Testicular failure in males (16 years and older)	14
Nonendocrine components	
Candidiasis	100
Alopecia	29
Vitiligo	13
Keratopathy	35
Hepatitis	12
Intestinal malabsorption	18
Enamel hypoplasia	77
Tympanic membrane calcification	33
Nail dystrophy	52

Source: Data for this table were derived from ref. 80.

with hepatitis, whereas none of the 61 APS-1 patients without hepatitis developed this autoantibody. In the absence of APS-1, anti-CYP 1A2 autoantibodies are detected only in patients with dihydralazine hepatitis. Anti-CYP 1A2 autoantibodies are not detected in healthy controls, in patients with other autoimmune liver diseases, or in patients with chronic HCV oir HBV infections (86). These findings suggest that anti-CYP 1A2 autoantibodies are very specific for hepatitis in APS-1 (87). Another autoantigen in APS-1 is CYP 2A6 (88). This autoantigen was detected in three of seven Finnish APS-1 patients with hepatitis; however, it was also present in 12% of APS-1 patients without hepatitis.

About 70% of APS-1 patients develop adrenal failure. Interestingly, autoantibodies directed against three different CYPs are detected in patients with adrenal failure in APS-1, namely, anti-CYP 21, anti-CYP 11 and anti-CYP 17 (reviewed in ref. 81). All three enzymes are involved in steroid biosynthesis. CYP 21 is also an autoantigen in idiopathic adrenal failure (called Addison's disease).

C. Defects in the *AIRE* Gene Cause APS-1

The *AIRE* gene is located on the long arm of chromosome 21 (89). About 20 different mutations in the *AIRE* gene have been described, and APS-1 occurs when both *AIRE* alleles code for mutated proteins (Fig. 9). These mutations are scattered along the whole coding sequence of *AIRE* and most of them result in premature translational stops (reviewed in ref. 90). The *AIRE* gene codes for a protein of 545 amino acids. The AIRE protein shows two PHD ring finger motifs and several other domains which indicates a function in transcriptional regulation (Fig. 9) (78,79,91). Cellular localization of AIRE shows a distribution along microtubular cytoskeletal elements and in nuclear dots (92,93). AIRE is not expressed in the target organs of autoimmunity, but in rare cells of lymphoid

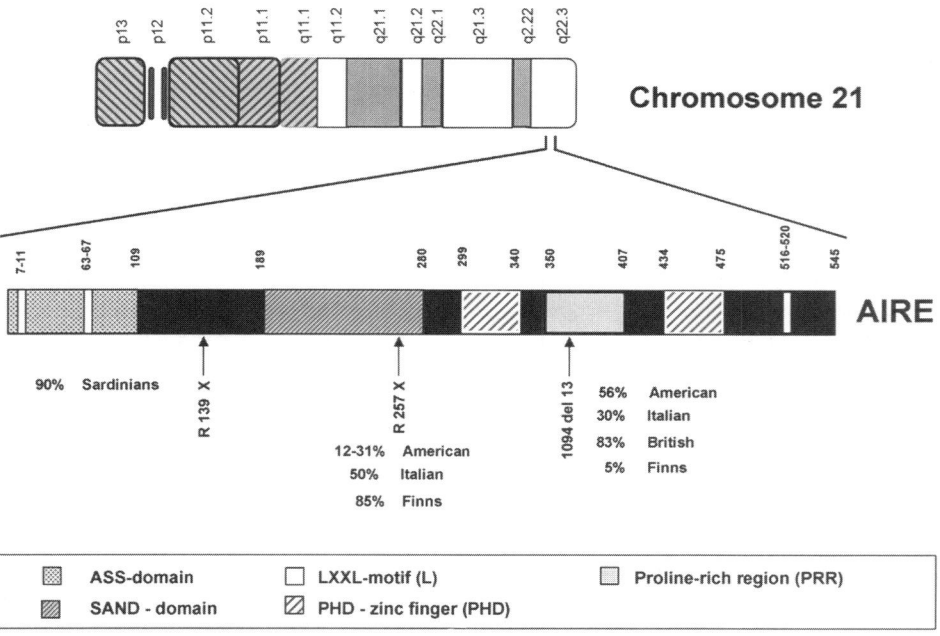

Figure 9   *AIRE,* a gene defect in a putative transcription factor, causes APS-1.

tissues, e.g., thymus medulla, lymph nodes, spleen, and the fetal liver. In thymus, 90% of AIRE-positive cells are of epithelial origin and 5–10% are derived from the dentritic lineage (93). All AIRE-positive cells strongly express HLA DR (93). Thymic medullary epithelial cells are believed to be involved in clonal deletion of a subset of high-affinity T cells and in the induction of anergy in low-affinity subsets. These results and the disease spectrum seen in APS-1 indicate that *AIRE* may be involved in the establishment and maintenance of tolerance (93).

APS-1 demonstrates that defects in genes that are unrelated to CYP expression and to the target organs of autoimmunity may induce autoimmune diseases with autoantibodies directed against specific hepatic, adrenal, or ovarian CYPs. Therefore, CYPs themselves seem to be attractive targets for immune reactions. The *AIRE* gene defect may lead to an immune system with impaired tolerance mechanisms, resulting in multiple autoimmune reactions with targets that are attractive to the immune system and therefore similar to the molecular targets in idiopathic autoimmune diseases and APS-1. The question is: what are the features that make CYPs attractive to the immune system? Most likely the answer is function. Hydroxylation by CYPs involves activation of molecular oxygen in the active center and the production of energy-rich reaction intermediates. Therefore, chemical modifications and adduct formation with CYP substrates may not be a rare finding. The immune system may continuously be challenged with CYP-derived modified self-peptides. In patients with a normal immune system, reactions below a certain threshold level may be tightly suppressed. In APS-1 patients, however, suppressive mechanisms may be defensive, resulting in self-perpetuating pathogenetic processes that overcome the immunoregulatory controls and result in overshooting autoimmune destruction.

IV. AUTOIMMUNE HEPATITIS TYPE 2

A. Clinical Findings

Autoimmune hepatitis type 2 (AIH-2) is a disease of unknown pathogenesis that affects predominantly young females (female:male ratio 8:1). Patients are characterized by high levels of serum aminotransferases, γ-globulins (>30 g/L), and circulating antibodies against liver and kidney microsomes (LKM) and/or liver cytosolic proteins type 1 (LC-1) (94). About 25% of patients show a fulminant onset of disease (95). Untreated AIH has a poor prognosis with a 5-year survival rate of 50%. AIH-2 may be treated by immunosuppressive therapy, either with prednisone or prednisolone alone or with a combination therapy of prednisolone and azathioprine (96–98).

It is believed that patients with AIH-2 have a genetic predisposition for autoimmune diseases, since about 30% of all patients with AIH-2 and 30% of their first-degree relatives are affected by other autoimmune diseases, e.g., autoimmune thyroiditis, diabetes mellitus or vitiligo (94,95). Interestingly, the prevalence for AIH-2 shows geographic differences. While AIH-2 comprises about 10% of all patients with autoimmune hepatitis in southern Europe, AIH-2 is practically unknown in Sweden and is rare in the United States. These geographic differences may suggest that environmental factors may be important for the development of AIH-2 (99,100).

B. Autoantibodies

LKM-1 autoantibodies are the serological markers of AIH-2 (3,101,102). By indirect immunofluorescence LKM-1 autoantibodies show an even cytoplasmic staining of the entire liver lobule and the exclusive staining of the proximal renal tubules. Western blots with hepatic and renal microsomes reveal a protein band at 50 kDa. Cytochrome P450 2D6 (CYP 2D6) is the major antigen of LKM-1 autoantibodies (103–105). Anti-CYP 2D6 autoantibodies are found in 95–100% of patients with AIH-2 (104–106). LKM-1 autoantibodies inhibit the enzymatic activity of CYP 2D6 (107,108).

CYP 2D6 is active in phase I of detoxification and is involved in the detoxification of at least 40 different drugs (29). A significant polymorphism exists for CYP 2D6 in the Caucasian population, where 10% of people lack CYP 2D6 enzymatic activity, resulting in a slow metabolizer phenotype for all CYP 2D6 substrates, e.g., debrisoquine or sparteine (109). Studies with sparteine as a test substrate in patients permit measurements of CYP 2D6 activity in vivo. All patients with LKM-1 antibodies tested were of the extensive metabolizer phenotype, expressing functionally intact CYP 2D6 protein (107). Hence an adequate expression of CYP 2D6 seems to be a prerequisite for the development of LKM-1 autoantibodies.

LKM-3 autoantibodies are detected in 10% of patients with AIH-2, where they may be detected either alone or in combination with LKM-1 autoantibodies (110). LKM-3 autoantibodies are directed against family 1 UDP-glucuronosyltransferases (UGT1) (110,111).

C. Cytokines and Virus Infections as Potential Triggers of AIH

Autoantibodies to CYP 2D6 and UGT1 are seen not only in patients with AIH-2, but also in patients infected with hepatotropic viruses. Antibodies directed against CYP 2D6 are seen in up to 4% of patients with chronic hepatitis C and anti-UGT autoantibodies are detected in 13% of patients with chronic hepatitis D (112). HCV infections are currently treated with interferon-α in combination with ribavirin. Interestingly, in about 10% of patients with LKM-1-positive hepatitis C, hepatitis is exacerbated and will respond favorably to immunosuppressive treatment (113–116). Furthermore there are reports of induction of autoimmune thyroiditis and diabetes by interferon treatment in chronic hepatitis C. These findings indicate that preexisting autoimmune processes induced by chronic viral infections may be unmasked by aggressive immune attacks by proinflammatory cytokines. Such subclinical autoimmune processes may also exist in many patients with a genetic predisposition for autoimmune diseases. Viral infections that induce inflammatory cytokines may boost a subclinical autoimmune reaction above a critical level and start a self-perpetuating clinical disease.

V. CONCLUSIONS

Three types of immune-mediated liver injury have been discussed: drug-induced hepatitis, hepatitis in APS-1, and autoimmune hepatitis type 2. All three diseases are characterized by circulating autoantibodies directed against drug-metabolizing enzymes (Fig. 10). In drug-induced hepatitis adduct formation was identified as the initiating pathogenetic process (Fig. 11). As seen in halothane hepatitis, the rate of metabolism of the causative agent correlates with the prevalence of hepatitis induced by halothane and related compounds. Similarly in dihydralazine hepatitis, genetic defects in a competitive beneficial pathway increase the risk of developing the disease. Similarly, environmental influences such as smoking, fasting, and drug therapies may change the balance detoxification and adduct formation. Only very few individuals develop drug-induced hepatitis in response to therapy with adduct-inducing drugs, indicating that an immune response to drug adducts is

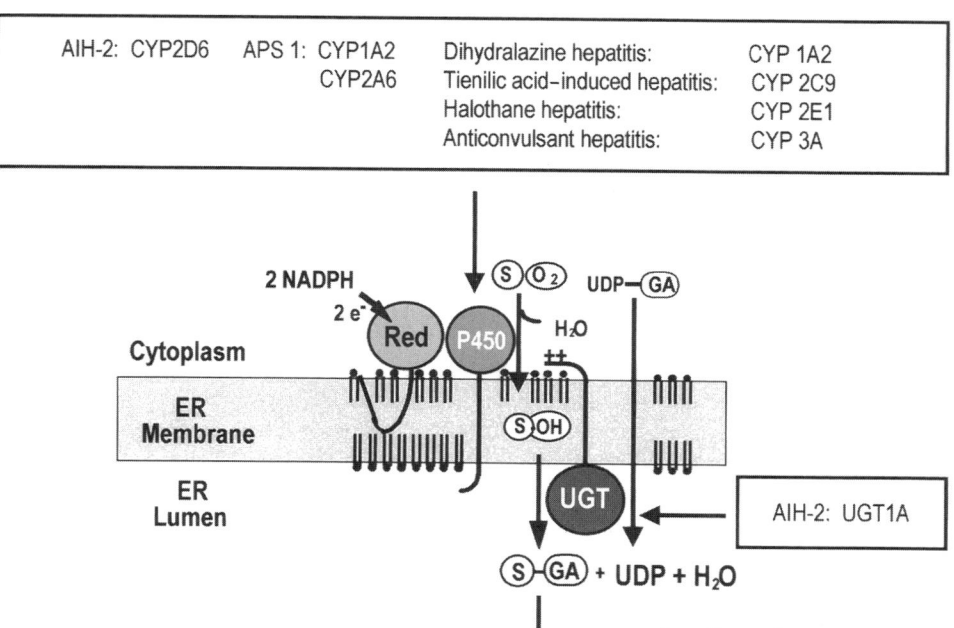

Figure 10 Phase I and phase II drug-metabolizing enzymes are known targets in hepatic autoimmunity.

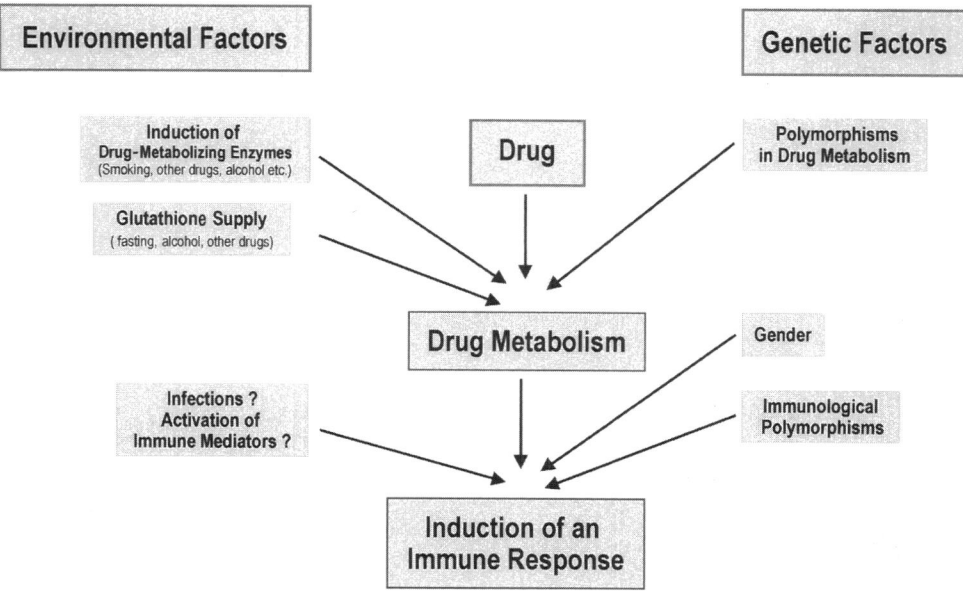

Figure 11 Genetic and environmental factors may contribute to drug-induced hepatitis.

downregulated in the vast majority of people. Therefore, a genetic predisposition must exist that affects immune regulation. Except for a correlation of certain idiosyncratic reactions with specific HLA alleles and sometimes a predisposition of females, nothing is known about the role of immune regulatory polymorphisms in drug-induced heapitis.

With AIRE, a gene defect has been identified for the first time that causes organ-specific autoimmune diseases (Fig. 9). Ninety percent of Finnish patients with alleles predisposing to APS-1 share one single mutation (R257X), resulting in a patient population that is very homogeneous for this single gene defect. Despite this genetic homogeneity, APS-1 is a very heterogeneous syndrome, resulting in a spectrum of more than 15 different autoimmune diseases (Table 2). The predisposition does not predict the organ affected, but confers a very high risk for certain autoimmune diseases, among them a subtype of autoimmune hepatitis. Since one single gene defect causes both autoimmune endocrinopathies and autoimmune hepatitis, mechanisms involved in endocrine and hepatic autoimmunity may be similar. Among autoantigens in APS-1, multiple CYPs are targets of autoimmunity (Fig. 10). Since hydroxylation by CYPs is an energy-consuming process that involves activation of molecular oxygen and the generation of energy-rich reaction intermediates, adduct formation of CYPs with endogeneous and exogeneous metabolites may not be an unusual event and may predispose this multigene family to recognition by the immune system. Furthermore, CYPs active in steroid biosynthesis and active in detoxification are expressed in a restricted number of tissues, facilitating breakage of tolerance. AIRE is believed to be involved in the induction and maintenance of tolerance and will help to identify biochemical pathways important in drug-induced hepatitis and organ-specific autoimmune diseases.

Little information is available on autoimmune hepatitis type 2 (Fig. 12). Interestingly, phase I and phase II drug-metabolizing enzymes are targets of autoimmune reactions

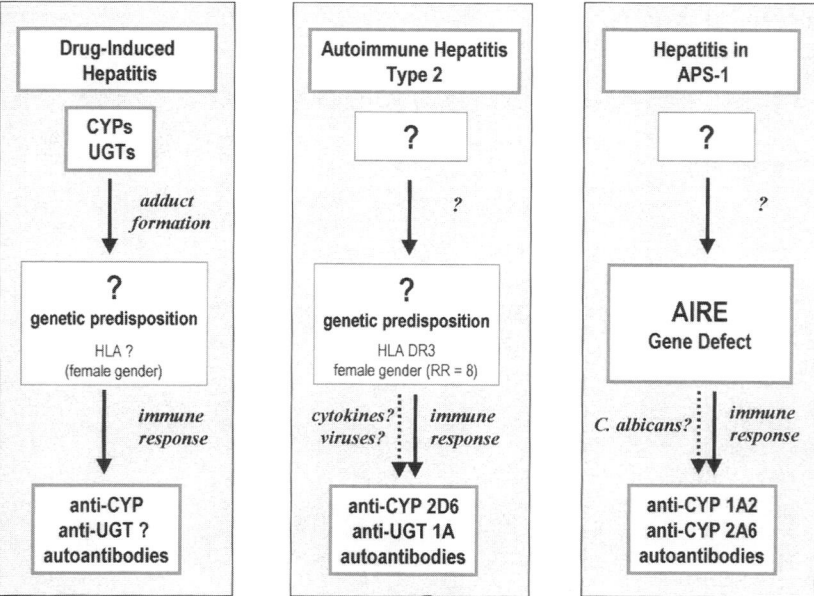

Figure 12   Hypothetical etiology of different forms of immune-mediated hepatitis.

in AIH-2. Induction of "chronic active hepatitis" by dihydralazine and by diclofenac has been reported several times, indicating that drugs may cause chronic hepatitis. In the absence of a known inducer, these cases would fulfill the criteria for "autoimmune hepatitis." For autoimmune hepatitis viral infections and inflammatory cytokines have been suggested to have a promoting role. When patients with LKM-1-positive chronic hepatitis C receive interferon-α therapy, about 10% of patients show exacerbation of hepatitis and may be treated successfully, with immunosuppression. It is assumed that subclinical autoimmune processes were active in these patients and were prompted by interferon-α to full-blown autoimmune disease. Further research is necessary to establish the nature of these preexisting subclinical processes.

ACKNOWLEDGEMENT

This work was supported by a grant of the Deutsche Forschungsgemeinschaft: SFB 244-C11.

REFERENCES

1. Zimmerman HJ, Lewis JH, Ishak KG, Maddrey W. Ticrynafen-associated hepatic injury: analysis of 340 cases. Hepatology 1984; 4:315–323.
2. Bernuau J, Mallet L, Benhamou JP. Hepatotoxicite due a l'acide teinilique. Gastroenterol Clin Biol 1981; 5:692–693.
3. Homberg JC, Andre C, Abuaf N. A new anti-liver/kidney-microsome antibody (anti-LKM2) in tienilic acid–induced hepatitis. Clin Exp Immunol 1984; 55:561–570.
4. Beaune P, Dansette PM, Mansuy D, Kiffel L, Finck M, Amar C, Leroux JP, Homberg JC. Human anti-endoplasmic reticulum autoantibodies appearing in a drug-induced hepatitis are directed against a human liver cytochrome P-450 that hydroxylates the drug. Proc Natl Acad Sci USA 1987; 84:551–555.
5. Lecoeur S, Bonierbale E, Challin D, Gatier JC, Valadon P, Dansette PM, Catinot R, Ballet F, Mansuy D, Beaune PH. Specificity of in vitro covalent binding of tienilic acid metabolites to human liver microsomes in relationship with the type of hepatotoxicity: comparison with two directly hepatotoxic drugs. Chem Res Toxicol 1994; 7:434–442.
6. Lopez-Garcia MP, Dansette PM, Valadon P, Amar C, Beaune PH, Guenguerich FP, Mansuy D. Human liver P450s expressed in yeast as tools for reactive-metabolite formation studies: oxidative activation of tienilic acid by cytochrome P450 2C9 and P450 2C10. Eur J Biochem 1993; 213:223–232.
7. Mansuy D, Dansette P, Foures C, Jaouen M, Moinet G, Bayer N. Metabolic hydroxylation of the thioprene ring: Isolation of 5-hydroxytienilic acid as the major urinary metabolite in rat and man. Biochem Phamacol 1984; 33:1429–1435.
8. Dansette PM, Amar C, Smith C, Pons C, Mansuy D. Oxidative activation of the thiophene ring by hepatic enzymes. Hydroxylation and formation of electrophilic metabolites during metabolism of tienilic acid and its isomer by rat liver microsomes. Biochem Pharmacol 1990; 39:911–918.
9. Lopez-Garcia MP, Dansette PM, Mansuy D. Thioprene derivatives as new mechanism-based inhibitors of cytochromes P450: Inactivation of yeast expressed human liver cytochrome P450 2C9 by tienilic acid. Biochemistry 1994; 33:166–175.
10. Koenigs LL, Peter RM, Hunter AP, Haining RL, Rettoe AE, Friedberg T, Pritchard MP, Shou M, Rushmore TH, Trager WF. Electrospray ionization mass spectrometric analysis of intact cytochrome P450: identification of tienilic acid adducts to P450 2C9. Biochemistry 1999; 38:2312–2319.

11. Robin M-A, Marat M, Le Roy M, Le Breton F-P, Bonierbale E, Dansette P, Ballet F, Mansuy D, Pessayre D. Antigenic targets in tienilic acid hepatitis: both cytochrome P450 2C11 and 2C11-tienilic acid adducts are transported to the plasma membrane of rat hepatocytes and recognized by human sera. J Clin Invest 1996; 98:1471–1480.

12. Lecoeur S, Andre C, Beaune PH. Tienilic acid-induced autoimmune hepatitis: anti-liver and -kidney microsomal type 2 autoantibodies recognize a three-site conformational epitope on cytochrome P4502C9. Mol Pharmacol 1996; 50:326–333.

13. Pessayre D. Toxic and immune mechanisms leading to acute and subacute drug induced liver injury. In: JP Miguet, D Dhumeaux, eds. Progress in Hepatology. Paris: John Libbey Eurotext, 1993:23–39.

14. Guilbert B, Dighiero G, Avrameas S. Naturally occurring antibodies against nine common antigens in normal humans. I. Detection, isolation, and characterization. J Immunol 1982; 28:2779–2783.

15. Siegmund W, Franke G, Biebler KE, Donner I, Kawellis R, Kairies M, Scherber A, Huller H. The influence of the acetylator phenotype on the clinical use of dihydralazine. Int J Clin Pharmacol Ther Toxicol 1985; 23:74–78.

16. Roschlau G, Baumgarten R, Fengler JD. Dihydralazine hepatitis. Morphologic and clinical criteria for diagnosis. Zentralbl Allg Pathol 1990; 136:127–134.

17. Machnik G, Bergert A, Justus J, Kunze P. Müller R, Reinhardt M, Schulz H, Stein G, Thiele R. Arzneimittelhepatitis nach Dihydralazin mit tödlichem Verlauf. Zentralbl Allg Pathol Pathol Anat 1988; 134:164–177.

18. Baumgarten R, Binus R, Fengler JD, Roschlau G. Zur Pathogenese der Dihydralazin-Hepatitis. Dt Gesundh Wesen 1984; 39:952–956.

19. Reinhardt M, Machnik G, Krombholz B, Jashn H. Die sogenannte Dihydralazin-Hepatitis. Ein Beitrag zur Pathogenese. Dt Ztschr Verdauungs-und Stoffwechselkrankh 1985; 45:283–294.

20. Roschlau G. Hepatitis mit konfluierenden Nekrosen durch Dihydralazin (Depressan). Ztrlblt Allg Pathol 1983; 127:385–393.

21. Nataf J, Bernuau J, Larrey D, Guillin MC, Rueff B, Benhamou J-P. A new anti-liver microsome antibody: a specific marker of dihydralazine-induced hepatitis. Gastroenterology 1986; 90:1751.

22. Bourdi M, Larrey D, Nataf J, Bernuau J, Pessayre D, Iwasaki M, Guengerich FP, Beaune PH. Anti-liver endoplasmic reticulum antibodies are directed against human cytochrome P-450IA2: a specific marker of dihydralazine hepatitis. J Clin Invest 1990; 85:1967–1973.

23. Bourdi M, Gautier JC, Mircheva J, Larrey D, Guillonzo A, Andre C, Belloc C, Beaune P. Anti-liver microsomes autoantibodies and dihydralazine induced hepatitis: specificity of autoantibodies and inductive capacity of the drug. Mol Pharmacol 1992; 42:280–285.

24. Belloc C, Gauffre A, Andre C, Beaune PH. Epitope mapping of human CYP1A2 in dihydralazine-induced autoimmune hepatitis. Pharmacogenetics 1997; 7:181–186.

25. Beaune PH, Pessayre D, Dansette P, Mansuy D, Manns MP. Autoantibodies against cytochromes P450: role in human diseases. Adv Pharmacol 1994; 30:199–245.

26. Bourdi M, Tinel M, Beaune PH, Pessayre D. Interactions of dihydralazine with cytochromes P450 1A: a possible explanation for the appearance of anti-cytochrome P450 1A2 autoantibodies. Mol Pharmacol 1994; 45:1287–1295.

27. Robin MA, Maratrat M, Loeper J, Durand-Schneider AM, Tinel M, Ballet F, Beaune P, Feldman G, Pessayre D. Cytochrome P4502B follows a vesicular route to the plasma membrane in cultured rat hepatocytes. Gastroenterology 1995; 108:1110–1123.

28. Neve EPA, Eliasson E, Pronzato MA, Albano E, Marinari U, Ingelman-Sundberg M. Enzyme-specific transport of rat liver cytochrome P450 to the golgi apparatus. Arch Biochem Biophys 1996; 333:459–465.

29. Meyer UA, Zanger UM. Molecular mechanisms of genetic polymorphisms of drug metabolism. Annu Rev Pharmacol Toxicol 1997; 37:269–296.

30. Bock KW. Metabolic polymorpshisms affecting activation of toxic and mutagenic aryl-amines. Trends Pharmacol 1992; 13:223–226.

31. Wright R, Eade OE, Chisholm M, Hawksley M, Lloyd B, Moles TM, Gardner MJ. Controlled prospective study of the effect on liver function of multiple exposures to halothane. Lancet 1975: 1:817–820.

32. Eade O, Grice D, Krawitt EL, Trowell J, Albertini S, Fesenstein H, Wright R. HLA A and B locus antigens in patients with unexplained hepatitis following halothane anesthesia. Tissue Antigens 1981; 17:428–432.

33. Zimmerman HJ. The Adverse Effects of Drugs and Other Chemicals on the Liver. In: HJ Zimmerman, ed. Hepatotoxicity. New York: Appleton Century Crofts, 1978.

34. Sipes IG, Gandolfi J, Pohl LR, Krishna G, Brown BR. Comparison of the biotransformation and hepatotoxicity of halothane and deuterated halothane. J Exp Ther 1980; 214:716–720.

35. Spracklin DK, Thummel KE, Kharasch ED. Hukman reductive halothane metabolism in vitro is catalyzed by cytochrome. P450 2A6 and 3A4. Drug Metab Dispos 1996 24:976–983.

36. Brown RM, Guenguerich FP, Wood M. Halothane microsomal oxidation is inhibited by diethyldithiocarbamate, an inhibitor of CYP2E1. Anesth Analg 1995; 80:60.

37. Eliasson E, Kenna G. Cytochrome P450 2E1 is a cell surface autoantigen in halothane hepatitis. Mol Pharmacol 1996; 50:573–582.

38. Madan A, Parkinson A. Characterization of the NADPH-dependent covalent binding of [14C]halothane to human liver microsomes: a role for cytochrome P4502E1 at low substrate concentrations. Drug Metabol Dispos 1996; 24:1307–1313.

39. Kharasch ED, Hankins D, Mautz D, Thummel KE. Identification of the enzyme responsible for oxidative halothane metabolism: implications for prevention of halothane hepatitis. Lancet 1996; 347:1367–1371.

40. Spracklin DK, Hankins DC, Fisher JM, Thummel KE, Kharasch ED. Cytochrome P450 2E1 is the principal catalyst of human oxidative halothane metabolism in vitro. J Pharmacol Exp Ther 1997; 281:400–411.

41. Kenna JG, Martin JL, Satoh H, Pohl LR. Purification o f trifluoroacetylated protein antigens from livers of halothane-treated rats. Eur J Pharmacol 1990; 183:1139–1140.

42. Martin JL, Kenna JG, Martin BM, Thomassen D, Reed GF, Pohl LR. Halothane hepatitis patients have serum antibodies that react with protein disulfide isomerase. Hepatology 1993; 18:858–863.

43. Pumford NR, Martin BM, Thomassen D, Burris JA, Kenna JG, Martin JL, Pohl LR. Serum antibodies from halothane hepatitis patients react with the rat endoplasmic reticulum protein ERp72. Chem Res Toxicol 1993; 6:609–615.

44. Ma Y, Peakman M, Lobo-Yeo A, Wen L. Lenzi M, Gaken J, Farzaneh F, Mieli-Vergani G, Bianchi FB, Vergani D. Differences in immune recognition of cytochrome P4502D6 by liver kidney microsomal (LKM) antibody in autoimmune hepatitis and chronic hepatitis C virus infection. Clin Exp Immunol 1994; 97:94–99.

45. Smith GCM, Kenna JC, Harrison DJ, Tew D, Wolf CR. Antibodies to hepatic microsomal carboxylesterase in halothane hepatitis. Lancet 1993; 342:963–964.

46. Bourdi M, Chen W, Peter RM, Martin JL, Buters JT, Nelson SD, Pohl LR. Human P4502E1 is a major autoantigen associated with halothane hepatitis and the epitopes are conformational. Chem Res Toxicol 1996; 9:1159–1166.

47. Vergani D, Mieli-Vergani G, Alberti A, et al. Antibodies to the surface of halothane-altered rabbit hepatocytes in patients with severe halothane-associated hepatitis. N Engl J Med 1985; 303:66–71.

48. Christ DD, Satoh H, Kenna JG, Pohl LR. Potential metabolic basis for enflurane hepatitis and the apparent cross-sentization between enflurane and halothane. Drug Metab Dispos 1988; 16:135–140.

49. Christ DD, Kenna JG, Kammerer W, Satoh H, Pohl LR. Enflurane metabolism produces

covalently bound liver adducts recognized by antibodies from patients with halothane hepatitis. Anesthesiology 1988; 69:833–838.

50. Pohl LR, Pumford NR, Martin JL. Mechanisms, chemical structures and drug metabolism. Eur J Haematol 1996; 57:98–104.

51. Martin JL, Plevak DJ, Flannery KD, Charlton M, Poterucha JJ, Humphreys CE, Derfus G, Pohl LR. Hepatotoxicity after desflurane anesthesia. Anesthesiology 1995; 83:1125–1129.

52. Yin H, Anders M, Korzewa K. Designing safer chemicals: predicting the rates of metabolism of halogenated alkanes. Proc Natl Acad Sci USA 1995; 92:11076–11080.

53. Hoet P, Graf MLM, Bourdi M, Pohl LRD, Chen W, Peter RM, Nelson SD, Verlinden N, Lison D. Epidemic of liver disease caused by hydrofluorocarbons used as ozone-sparing substitutes of chlorofluorocarbons. Lancet 1997; 350:556–559.

54. Schlienger RG, Shear NH. Antiepileptic drug hypersensitivity syndrome. Epilepsia 1998; 39:S3–S7.

55. Shear NH, Spielberg SP. Anticonvulsant hypersensitivity syndrome: In vitro assessment of risk. J Clin Invest 1988; 82:1826–1832.

56. Tennis P, Stern RS. Risk of serious cutaneous disorders after initiation of use of phenytoin, carbamazepine, or sodium valproate: a record linkage study. Neurology 1997; 49:542–546.

57. Leeder JS, Riley RJ, Cook VA, Spielberg SP. Human anti-cytochrome P450 antibodies in aromatic anticonvulsant-induced hypersensitivity reactions. J Pharmacol Exp Ther 1992; 263: 360–367.

58. Gennis MA, Vermuri R, Burns EA, Hill JV, Miller MA, Spielberg SP. Familial occurrence of hypersensitivity to phenytoin. Am J Med 1991; 91:631–634.

59. Spielberg SP, Gordon GB, Blake DA, Mellitis ED, Bross DS. Anticonvulsant toxicity in vitro: possible role of arene oxids. J Pharmacol Exp Ther 1981; 217:386–389.

60. Leeder S, Gaedigk A, Lu X, Cook VA. Epitope mapping studies with human anti-cytochrome P450 3A autoantibodies. Mol Pharmacol 1996; 49:234–243.

61. Davis CD, Pirmohamed M, Park BK. Analysis of lymphocyte microsomal epoxide hydrolase activity in carbamazepine hypersensitive patients using ^{3}H-cis-silbene oxide. Br J Clin Pharmacol 1994; 39:539P–588P.

62. Zimmerman HJ. Update of hepatotoxicity due to classes of drugs in common clinical use: non-steroidal drugs, anti-inflammatory drugs, antibiotics, antihypertensives, and cardiac and psychotropic agents. Semin Liver Dis 1990; 109:322–328.

63. Hart FD, Boardman PL. Ibufenac (4-isobutylphenylacetic acid). Ann Rheum Dis 1965; 24: 61–65.

64. Thomson M, Stephenson P, Percy JS. Ibufenac in the treatment of arthritis. Ann Rheum Dis 1964; 23:397–404.

65. Jick H, Derby LE, Rodriguez LAG, Jick SS, Dean AD. Liver disease associated with diclofenac, naproxen, and piroxicam. Pharmacotherapy 1992; 12:207–212.

66. Purcell P, Henry D, Melville G. Diclofenac hepatitis. Gut 1991; 32:1381–1385.

67. Banks AT, Zimmerman HJ, Ishak KG, Harter JG. Diclofenac-associated hepatotoxicity: analysis of 180 cases reported to food and drug administration as adverse reactions. Hepatology 1995; 22:820–827.

68. Scully LJ, Clarke D, Barr RJ. Diclofenac induced hepatitis: three cases with features of autoimmune chronic active hepatitis. Dig Dis Sci 1993; 38:744–751.

69. Mazeika PK, Ford MJ. Chronic active hepatitis associated with dichlofenac sodium therapy. Br J Clin Proc 1989; 43:125–126.

70. Sallie RW, McKenzie T, Reed WD, Quinlan MF, Shilkin KB. Diclofenac hepatitis. NZ J Med 1991; 21:151–255.

71. Iveson TJ, Ryley NG, Kelly PMA, Trowell JM, McGee OD, Chapman RWG. diclofenac associated hepatitis. J Hepatol 1990; 10:85–90.

72. Schmitz G, Stauffert I, Sippel H, Lepper H, Estler CJ. Toxicity of diclofenac in isolated hepatocytes. J Hepatol 1992; 14:408–409.

73. Kretz-Rommel A, Boelsterli UA. Diclofenac covalent protein binding is dependent on acyg-lucuronide formation and is inversly related to P450-mediated actue cell injury in cultured rat hepatocytes. Toxicol Appl Pharmacol 1993; 120:151–155.

74. Shen S, Marchick MR, Davis MR, Doss GA, Pohl LR. Metabolic activation of diclofenac by human cytochrome P4503A4: role of 5-hydroxydiclofenac. Chem-Res Toxicol 1999; 12: 214–222.

75. Kretz-Rommel A, Boelsterli UA. Selective protein adducts to membrane proteins in cultured rat hepatocytes exposed to diclofenac: radiochemical and immunochemical analysis. Mol Pharm 199; 45:237–244.

76. Kretz-Rommel A, Boelsterli UA. Liver, lung and spleen as target tissues for protein adduct formation associated with metabolism of the nonsteroidal antiinflammatory drug diclofenac. Toxicologist 1994; 14:425–431.

77. Kretz-Rommel A, Boelsterli UA. Mechanism of covalent adduct formation of diclofenac to rat hepatic microsomal proteins. Retention of the glucuronic acid moiety in the adduct. Drug Metab Dispos 1994; 22:956–961.

78. Nagamine K, Peterson P, Scott HS, Kudoh J, Minoshima S, Heino M, Krohn KJE, Lalioti MD, Mullis PE, Antonarakis SE, Kawasaki K, Asakawa S, Ito F, Shimiziu N. Positional cloning of the APECED gene. Nature Genet 1997; 17:393–398.

79. Consortium TF-GA. An autoimmune disease, APECED, caused by mutations in a novel gene featuring two PhD-type zinc finger domains. Nature Genet 1997; 17:399–403.

80. Ahonen P, Myllärniemi S, Sipilä I, Perheentupa J. Clinical variation of autoimmune polyen-docrinopathy-candidiasis-ectodermal dystrophy (APECED) in a series of 68 patients. N Engl J Med 1990; 322:1829–1836.

81. Obermayer-Straub P, Manns MP. The autoimmune polyglandular syndromes. Baillieres Clin Gastroenterol 1999; 12:293–315.

82. Perheentupa J. Autoimmune polyendocrinopathy-candidiasis-ectodermal dystrophy (APECED). Horm Metab Res 1996; 28:353–356.

83. Neufeld M, Maclaren NK, Blizzard RM. Two types of autoimmune Addison's Disease asso-ciated with different polyglandular autoimmune (PGA) syndromes. Medicine 1980; 60:355–362.

84. Betterle C, Greggio NA, Volpato M. Autoimmune polyglandular syndrome type 1. Clin En-docrinol Metab 1998; 83:1049–1055.

85. Clemente MG, Obermayer-Straub P, Meloni A, Strassburg CP, Arangino V, Tukey RH, De Virgiliis S, Manns MP. Cytochrome P450 1A2 is a hepatic autoantigen in autoimmune poly-glandular syndrome type 1. J Clin Endocrinol Metab 1997; 82:1353–1361.

86. Dalekos GN, Obermayer-Straub P, Maeda T, Tsianos EV, Manns MP. Antibodies against cytochrome P4502A6 (CYP2A6) in patients with chronic viral hepatitis are mainly linked to hepatitis C virus infection. Digestion 1998; 59:S36.

87. Obermayer-Straub P, Braun S, Grams B, Loges S, Clemente MG, Lüttig B, Perheentupa J, Manns MP. Different liver cytochromes P450s are autoantigens in patients with autoimmune hepatitis and with autoimmune polyglandular syndrome type 1 (APS1). Hepatology 1996; 24:429.

88. Clemente MG, Meloni A, Obermayer-Straub P, Frau F, Manns MP, DeVirgiliis S. Two cyto-chromes P450 are major hepatocellular autoantigens in autoimmune polyglandular syndrome type 1. Gastroenterology 1998; 114:324–328.

89. Aaltonen J, Börses P, Sandkuijl L, Perheentupa J, Peltonen L. An autosomal locus causing autoimmune disease: autoimmune polyglandular disease type I assigned to chromosome 21. Nature Genet 1994; 8:83–87.

90. Obermayer-Straub P, Manns MP. Autoimmunity in the autoimmune polyglandular syndrome type 1 after the discovery of the gene. In: MP Manns, G Paumgartner, U Leuschner, eds. Proceedings of the Falk Symposium 102 "Immunology and the liver," Held in Basel, Switzer-land, October 20–21 1999. Dodrecht, Boston, London: Karger, 2000.

91. Gibson TJ, Ramu C, Gemund C, Aasland R. AIRE-1 involved in the polyglandular autoimmune syndrome APECED, contains the SAND domain and is a probable DNA-binding transcription factor. Trends Biochem Sci 1998; 23:242–244.

92. Bjorses P, Pelto-Huikko M, Kaukonen J, Aaltonen J, Peltonen L, Ulmanen I. Localization of the APECED protein in distinct nuclear dots. Hum Mol Genet 1999; 8:259–266.

93. Heino M, Peterson P, Kudoh J, Nagamine K, Lagerstedt A, Ovod V, Ranki A, Rantala I, Nieminen M, Tuukkanen J, Scott HS, Antonarakis SE, Shimizu N, Krohn K. Autoimmune regulator is expressed in the cells regulating immune tolerance in thymus medulla. Biochem Biophys Res Commun 1999; 257:821–825.

94. Homberg JC, Abuaf N, Bernard O, Islam S, Alvarez F, Khalil SH, Poupon R, Darnis F, Levy VG, Grippon P. Chronic active hepatitis associated with anti-liver/kidney microsome type 1: a second type of "autoimmune" hepatitis. Hepatology 1987; 7:1333–1339.

95. Gregorio GV, Portman B, Reid F, Donaldson PT, Doherty DG, McCartney M, Vergani D, Mieli-Vergani G. Autoimmune hepatitis in childhood: a 20-year experience. Hepatology 1997; 25:541–547.

96. Cook GC, Mulligan R, Sherlock S. Controlled protective trial of corticoid therapy in active chronic hepatitis. Q J Med 1971; 40:159–185.

97. Murray-Lyon IM, Stern RB, Williams R. Controlled trial of prednisone and azathioprine in active chronic hepatitis. Lancet 1973; I:735–737.

98. Summerskill WHJ, Korman MG, Ammon HV, Baggenstoss AH. Prednisone for chronic active liver disease: dose titration, standard dose and combination with azathioprine compound. Gut 1975; 16:876–883.

99. Lindgren S, Braun HB, Michel G, Nemeth A, Nilsson S, Thome-Kromer B, Eriksson S. Absence of LKM-1 antibody reactivity in autoimmune and hepatitis-C-related chronic liver disease in Sweden. Swedish Internal Medicine Liver Club. Scand J Gastroenterol 1997; 32: 175–178.

100. Czaja AJ, Carpenter HA, Manns MP. Antibodies to soluble liver antigen, P450IID6, and mitochondrial complexes in chronic hepatitis. Gastroenterology 1993; 105:1522–1528.

101. Johnson PJ, McFarlane IG. Meeting report: International autoimmune hepatitis group. Hepatology 1993; 18:998–1005.

102. Desmet VJ, Gerber M, Hoofnaagle JH, Manns M, Scheuer PJ. Classification of chronic hepatitis: diagnosis, grading and staging. Hepatology 1994; 19:1513–1520.

103. Manns MP, Johnson EF, Griffin KJ, Tan EM, Sullivan KF. Major antigen of liver kidney microsomal antibodies in idiopathic autoimmune hepatitis is cytochrome P450db1. J Clin Invest 1989; 83:1066–1072.

104. Ma Y, Gregorio G, Gäken J, Muratori L, Bianchi FB, Mieli-Vergani G, Vergani D. Establishment of a novel radioligand assay using eukaryotically expressed cytochrome P450 2D6 for the measurement of liver kidney microsomal type 1 antibody in patients with autoimmune hepatitis and hepatitis C virus infection. J Hepatol 1997; 26:1396–1402.

105. Yamamoto AM, Johanet C, Duclos-Vallee JC, Bustarret FA, Alvarez F, Homberg JC, Bach JF. A new approach to cytochrome CYP2D6 antibody detection in autoimmune hepatitis type-2 (AIH-2) and chronic hepatitis C virus (HCV) infection: a sensitive and quantitative radioligand assay. Clin Exp Immunol 1997; 108:396–400.

106. Obermayer-Straub P, Sugimura T, Braun S, Lüttig B, Loges S, Kayser A, Durazzo M, Strassburg CP, Manns MP. Definition of a novel CYP2D6 epitope in autoimmune hepatitis type 2 and in chronic hepatitis C [abstract]. J Hepatol 1998; 28(suppl 1):139.

107. Zanger UM, Hauri HP, Loeper J, Homberg JC, Meyer UA. Antibodies against human cytochrome P-450db1 in autoimmune hepatitis type 2. Proc Natl Acad Sci USA 1988; 85:8256–8260.

108. Manns M, Zanger U, Gerken G, Sullivan KF, Meyer zum Büschenfelde KH, Meyer UA, Eichelbaum M. Patients with type II autoimmune hepatitis express functionally intact cyto-

chrome P450 db1 that is inhibited by LKM1 autoantibodies in vitro but not in vivo. Hepatology 1990; 12:127–132.

109. Gonzalez FJ, Skoda RC, Kimura S, Umeno M, Zanger UM, Nebert DW, Gelboin HV, Hardwick JP, Meyer UA. Characterization of the common genetic defect in debrisoquine metabolism. Nature 1988; 331:442–449.

110. Strassburg C, Obermayer-Straub P, Alex B, Durazzo M, Rizzetto M, Tukey RH, Manns MP. Autoantibodies against glucuronosyltransferases differ between viral hepatitis and autoimmune hepatitis. Gastroenterology 1996; 11:1582–1592.

111. Philipp T, Durazzo M, Trautwein C, Alex B, Straub P, Lamb JG, Johnson EF, Tukey RH, Manns MP. Recognition of uridine diphosphate glucuronosyl transferases by LKM-3 antibodies in chronic hepatitis D. Lancet 1994; 344:578–581.

112. Manns MP, Obermayer-Straub P. Cytochromes P450 and UDP-Glucuronosyltransferases: Model autoantigens to study drug-induced, virus-induced and autoimmune liver disease. Hepatology 1997; 26:1054–1066.

113. Todros L, Touscoz G, D'Urso N, Durazzo M, Albano E, Poli G, Baldi M, Rizzetto M. Hepatitis C virus-related chronic liver disease with autoantibodies to liver-kidney microsomes (LKM). Clinical characterization from idiopathic LKM-positive disorders. J Hepatol 1991; 13:128–131.

114. Duclos-Vallee J-C, Nishioka M, Hosomi N, Arima K, Leclerc A, Bach J-F, Yamamoto AM. Interferon therapy in LKM-1 positive patients with chronic hepatitis C: follow-up by a quantitative radioligand assay for CYP2D6 antibody detection. J Hepatol 1998; 28:965–970.

115. Dalekos GN, Wedemeyer H, Obermayer-Straub P, Kayser A, Barut A, Frank H, Manns MP. Epitope mapping of cytochrome P4502D6 autoantigen in patients with chronic hepatitis C during α-interferon treatment. J Hepatol 1999; 30:366–375.

116. Muratori L, Lenzi M, Ma Y, Cataleta M, Mieli-Vergani G, Vergani D, Bianchi FB. Heterogeneity of liver/kidney microsomal antibody type 1 in autoimmune hepatitis and hepatitis C virus related liver disease. Gut 1995; 37:406–412.

117. Obermayer-Straub P, Manns MP. Cytochromes P450 and UDP-glucuronosyltransferases as hepatocellular autoantigens. Baillieres Clin Gastroenterol 1996; 10:501–532.

118. Van Pelt F, Straub P, Manns M. Molecular basis of drug-induced immunological liver injury. Semin Liver Dis 1995; 15:283–300.

8

Mechanistic Role of Acyl Glucuronides

CHUNZE LI and LESLIE Z. BENET

University of California–San Francisco, San Francisco, California, U.S.A.

I. INTRODUCTION

Only a few years ago, it was generally recognized by pharmaceutical scientists that phase II metabolites of drugs, such as acyl glucuronide conjugates, are readily excreted following their formation in the body and that these metabolites are neither active nor reactive. We and others have shown that this is not generally true (1,2). Acyl glucuronide conjugates are, in fact, reactive metabolites, capable of undergoing hydrolysis, intramolecular acyl migration, and covalent binding to proteins, both in vitro and in vivo. This newly recognized reactivity has an important, but still poorly defined, bearing on biological distribution and metabolism of a widely prescribed class of drugs. It may also be directly associated with the perplexing toxicity of many carboxylic acid–containing drugs (3,4). It is striking that of 47 drugs withdrawn from U.S., British, and Spanish markets from 1964 through 1993 owing to severe toxicity (3,4), 10 are carboxylic acids, all of which are metabolized by humans to acyl glucuronides.

Conjugation with glucuronic acid is the major route for the elimination of xenobiotic and endogenous compounds with a carboxylic acid function (1). These acyl-linked glucuronides are chemically reactive electrophiles (2) and have been shown to be susceptible to hydrolysis, to transacylation by methanol (5), ammonia (6), ethanethiol (7), and glutathione (8,9), and to reaction with chemical nucleophiles such as 4-(p-nitrobenzyl)pyridine (NBP) (10). Acyl-linked glucuronides have been observed to undergo intramolecular nucleophilic substitution reactions with the hydroxyl groups on the glucuronic acid moiety resulting in intramolecular migration of the xenobiotic moiety from the 1-O-β-position to the 2-, 3-, 4-position of the glucuronic acid ring (Fig. 1). Such intramolecular acyl migration and hydrolysis may occur during biological sample handling and, of particular relevance, also under the pH and temperature conditions found in vivo. Earlier studies not employing correct sample stabilization procedures yielded inaccurate measures of the pharmacokinetics of carboxylic acid–containing drugs as well as their glucuronides.

In addition to hydrolysis and intramolecular acyl migration, acyl glucuronides also readily react with the nucleophiles on proteins, both in vivo and in vitro. Covalent modification of cellular proteins by acyl glucuronides has been suggested to mediate the rare, but potentially fatal, idiosyncratic hypersensitivity associated with carboxylic acids (1). The mechanisms responsible for the initiation of such immune-type toxic side effects, including anaphylaxis and drug-induced liver injury (11), remain poorly understood. A current explanation for the different types of hypersensitivity reactions caused by drugs or other small molecules is the "hapten hypothesis" (12). Small foreign molecules such as drugs are not immunogenic in themselves, but may become so after covalent attachment to endogenous carrier proteins (such as albumin), which facilitate recognition by the immune system. In general, the extent of the exposure of the organism or an organ to the potential immunogen is one possible determinant for the occurrence of adverse reaction, as depicted schematically in Fig. 2.

This chapter will focus on the chemical reactivity of acyl glucuronides. We will summarize the general properties and newer aspects of formation and degradation of acyl glucuronides, and their reversible and irreversible binding to plasma and tissue proteins in vitro and in vivo. The selective modification of tissue proteins by acyl glucuronides and their potential drug-induced organ toxicity (especially liver) will also be discussed.

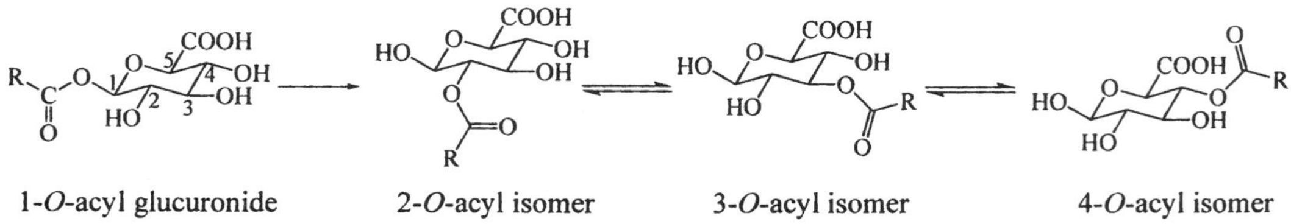

1-O-acyl glucuronide   2-O-acyl isomer   3-O-acyl isomer   4-O-acyl isomer

Figure 1   Migration of the acyl group of the β-1-O-acyl glucuronide from C1 to C2, C3, and C4 of the glucuronic acid ring. The rearrangement is reversible with one exception: the C1-isomer is not formed from the C2-isomer. (Modified from Ref. 2.)

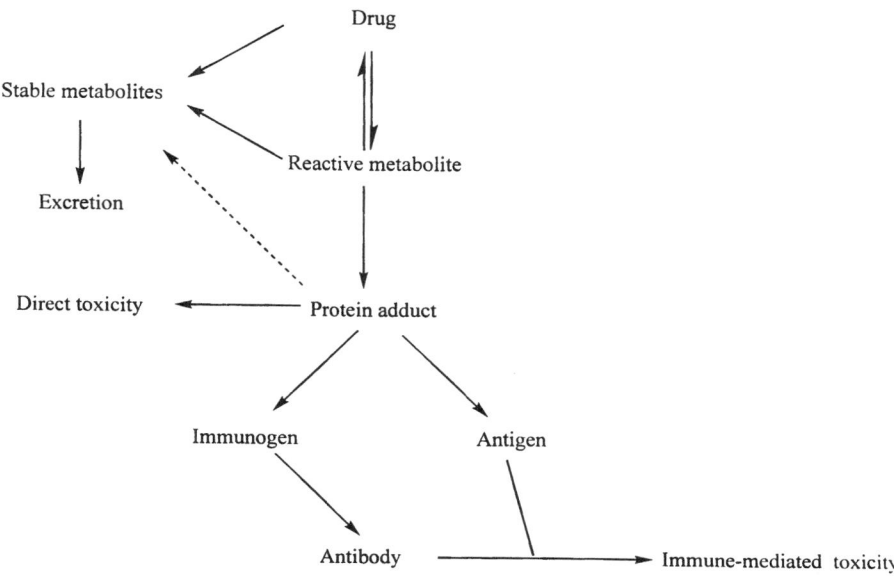

Figure 2 Interrelationship between immune response and disposition of the drug ("hapten hypothesis"). (Modified from Ref. 2.)

II. BIOCHEMICAL ASPECTS OF ACYL GLUCURONIDATION

Conjugation with glucuronic acid is the major route for the biotransformation and elimination of carboxylic acid–containing drugs (1,2). Under normal condition, acyl glucuronides are formed primarily in the liver and excreted predominantly through the urine in humans (Fig. 3).

The formation of acyl glucuronides is catalyzed by a membrane-bound enzyme, uridine 5′-diphosphate (UDP)-glucuronosyltransferase (UGT, EC 2.4.1.17), which transfers the glucuronic acid from UDP-glucuronic acid (UDPGA) to the carboxyl group of the aglycone, resulting in ester-linked glucuronides. The mechanism of the reaction catalyzed by UGT is a S_N2-type reaction. The anomeric center undergoes inversion during the enzymatic transfer of α-D-glucuronic acid in UDPGA to the acceptor substrate, resulting in the formation of the β-configuration (Fig. 3). UGT is a family of closely related isoenzymes mainly located in the endoplasmic reticulum and exhibiting different, but overlapping, substrate specificities (13). Studies with Gunn rats, which are genetically deficient in bilirubin glucuronidation, revealed that the isoform(s) involved in glucuronidation of carboxylic acid-containing drugs was different from those responsible for bilirubin acyl conjugation, at least for the arylpropionic acids (14). Recently, several human liver UGTs have been cloned and the cDNAs expressed in heterologous cell lines. This technological advance has allowed assessment of the functional specificity of these UGTs. Of these, UGT1A9 and UGT2B7 appear to be key isoforms in the glucuronidation of a wide range of xenobiotic carboxylic acids (13).

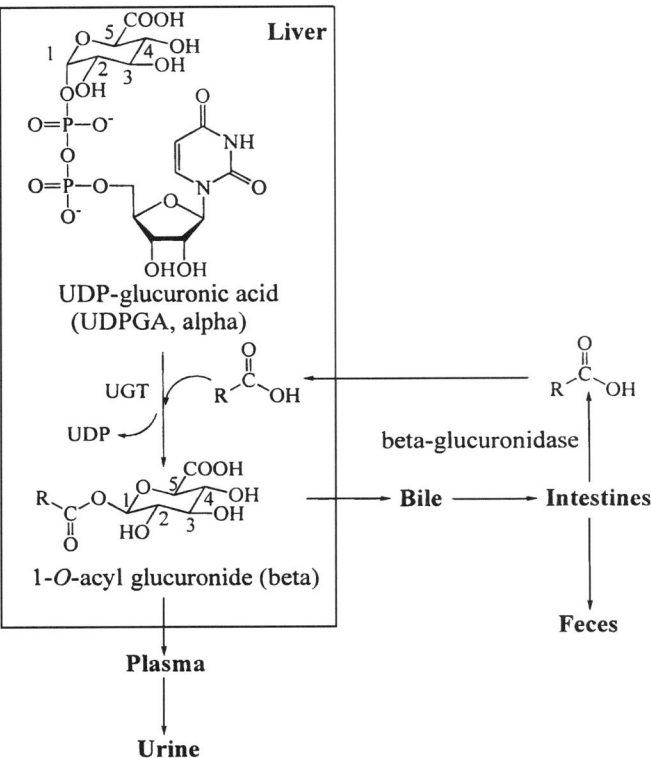

Figure 3 The formation and elimination of β-1-*O*-acyl glucuronide.

III. SYNTHESIS, ISOLATION, AND CHARACTERIZATION OF ACYL GLUCURONIDES

A. Biosynthesis of Acyl Glucuronides

Owing to the difficulty and expense of synthesizing the labile acyl glucuronides by chemical methods (1,15), alternative biosynthetic methods are preferable for the preparation of acyl glucuronides.

Acyl glucuronide metabolites may be synthesized in vitro using crude enzyme mixtures derived from animal tissue (e.g., liver microsomes) or using in vitro purified enzyme systems (e.g., immobilized enzymes). Many investigators have successfully utilized these two methods to obtain small quantities of acyl glucuronides. Ruelius et al. (16) synthesized oxaprozin glucuronide by combining labeled oxaprozin aglycone and UDPGA using a crude enzyme preparation from a rhesus monkey liver homogenate, which resulted in 7.5% conversion of the parent aglycone to 1-*O*-acyl glucuronide. A similar incubation with sheep liver microsomes by the addition of inhibitors of hydrolytic enzymes (e.g., esterases and β-glucuronidase) was utilized to prepare zomepirac-[^{14}C]glucuronide, with an improved yield of 10.1% (17). Grubb et al. (18) also successfully biosynthesized fenofibric and clofibric [^{14}C]-glucuronides by incubation of aglycone and radiolabeled UDPGA with rabbit and human hepatic microsomes, leading to 14% and 36% conversion of UDP[^{14}C]GA to the glucuronides, respectively. High yield of tolmetin glucuronide (>60%

of aglycone) with freshly prepared sheep liver microsomes (20 mg protein/mL) has been achieved in our laboratory (Ojingwa and Benet, unpublished results) with the following concentrations: 1 mM aglycone, 10 mM UDPGA, 10 mM $MgCl_2$ in 100 mM Tris-HCl buffer pH = 6.9 containing the enzyme inhibitor phenylmethylsulfonyl fluoride (2 mM) and 1,4-saccharic acid lactone (20 mM), and the detergent Triton X-100 (0.2%).

Immobilized UGT, covalently bound to cyanogen bromide–activated agarose (19) or Sepharose (20), has been used for the preparation of a variety of glucuronide conjugates. Using partially purified immobilized liver UGT, van Breeman and Fenselau (21) were able to synthesize a series of aglycone-labeled 1-O-acyl glucuronides. The yields obtained were benoxaprofen glucuronide, 2%; clofibric glucuronide, 3%; flufenamic glucuronide, 7%; and indomethacin glucuronide, 28%. Using similar immobilized UGT preparations, Bradow et al. (22) also synthesized small quantities of 1-O-acyl glucuronides of salicylic acid, S-benoxaprofen, and Δ^9-11-carboxy-tetrahydrocannabinol.

The above two in vitro enzymatic biosynthetic methods are fairly useful for the preparation of small quantities of acyl glucuronides, particularly for the glucuronides radiolabeled in either the drug or glucuronic acid moieties (1). However, for preparation of larger quantities, in vivo biosynthesis has significant advantages. Mostly, this has been accomplished by harvesting glucuronides from the urine of drug-dosed humans or animals. In 1981, the isolation of probenecid acyl glucuronide from urine by ethyl acetate extraction and HPLC purification was described by Eggers and Doust (23). Such extraction and purification methods from human urine dosed with the parent drugs have been successfully used to prepare the acyl glucuronides of a number of carboxylic acids, including zomepirac (24), tolmetin (25), diflunisal (26), beclobric acid (27), carprofen (28), etodolac (29), suprofen (30), ibuprofen (31), furosemide (32), and mefenamic acid (33). Relatively large-scale preparations of clofibric glucuronide and fenofibric glucuronides (18) were also achieved from the urine of rabbits dosed with the corresponding carboxylic acids, and of salicylic acid (34), valproic acid (35), and zomepirac (36) from rat urine and bile.

B. Separation and Quantification of Acyl Glucuronides

Two classes of analytical methods, indirect and direct, are available to quantify acyl glucuronides. The indirect methods, which were used almost exclusively before the early 1980s, involve enzymatic and alkaline hydrolysis of the ester bond, leading to release of the parent aglycone. Since only 1-O-acyl glucuronide can be hydrolyzed by β-glucuronidase and both 1-O-acyl glucuronides and its β-glucuronidase-resistant isomers are labile in alkaline solution, a differentiation between 1-O-acyl glucuronide and its positional isomers is possible by fractional hydrolysis.

With the improvement of HPLC techniques, the development of direct HPLC methods for glucuronides allowed investigators to chromatographically separate the different components in the glucuronide fraction and then to study the chemical properties (such as stability) of acyl glucuronides under different conditions. Compared to indirect methods, the direct procedures are more convenient and sensitive. Sinclair and Caldwell (37) reported one of the first HPLC separations of different glucuronide isomers of clofibric acid. Zomepirac, its β-1-O-acyl glucuronide, and four isomers were assayed on a reversed-phase (C_{18}) HPLC column utilizing a mixture of methanol and sodium acetate buffer as the mobile phase (24). A similar HPLC condition, including an ion-pairing reagent, tetrabutyl ammonium (TBA), was successfully applied to tolmetin, allowing simultaneous quantification of all the glucuronide conjugates (38).

Because of the various forms of isomerism, the analytical problems may, depending on the nature of the glucuronide conjugate, become rather complex. Isomerization is possible not only via intramolecular rearrangement by acyl migration (2-, 3-, and 4-*O*-isomers), but also via isomerization of the sugar group, yielding furanose as opposed to pyranose structures. Except for the C-1 position (β-1-*O*-acyl glucuronides), α- and β-anomeric forms may occur in addition to open-chain forms and lactones (39). As a consequence, numerous isomers of the enzymatically formed β-1-*O*-acyl glucuronide may occur. Several authors have reported the presence of more than three isomers in addition to the β-1-*O*-acyl glucuronides. Hansen-Moller et al. (40) isolated and identified the α- and β-anomers of three positional isomers of diflunisal glucuronide. Dickinson et al. (34) separated six structural isomers of salicylic acid glucuronide and speculated on the presence of α- and β-anomers of the three 2-, 3- and 4-*O*-isomers. Eight isomeric peaks of furosemide glucuronide other than 1-*O*-acyl glucuronide and the free acid were observed utilizing gradient HPLC by our group (41).

Resolution of the diastereomeric (*R*)- and (*S*)-glucuronides of 2-arylpropionic acids could also be achieved by HPLC on octadecylsilane (ODS) stationary phases. We described the resolution of diastereomeric naproxen glucuronides as well as the glucuronides of various other 2-arylpropionic acids [e.g., flunoxaprofen (42), benoxaprofen (43), carprofen (28), and fenoprofen (44)] on Ultrasphere ODS using a gradient of acetonitrile (ACN) in 9 or 10 mM TBA buffer (pH 2.5) with elution order (*S*)- before (*R*)-glucuronide. Fournel-Gigleux et al. (45) used a Lichrosorb Hibar RT column and ACN/trifluoroacetic acid (TFA)/water (19:0.04:81) to resolve the diastereomeric conjugates of 2-phenylpropionic acid (elution order (*R*)- before (*S*)-glucuronide). El Mouelhi et al. (46) employed different ACN/ammonium acetate or phosphate buffer systems to resolve the stereoisomeric conjugates of naproxen, ibuprofen, and benoxaprofen on an Ultrasphere ODS column with elution order (*S*)- before (*R*)-conjugate for all compounds. HPLC separation of (*R*)- and (*S*)-carprofen glucuronides, using Lichrosorb RP18 column and ACN/water/TFA (40:60:0.04) system, were also reported by Georges et al. (47), with the elution order (*R*) before (*S*). Additional analytical studies with naproxen glucuronide were published by Buszewski et al. (48) and with ketoprofen glucuronides by Chakir et al. (49). The HPLC conditions for the separation of acyl glucuronides of various carboxylic acids are summarized in Table 1.

C. Structural Characterization of Acyl Glucuronides

General procedures for the structural elucidation of glucuronides were summarized by Heirwegh and Compernolle (50). Different analytical methods have been used to identify the structures of acyl glucuronides and their isomers, including mass spectrometry and nuclear magnetic resonance spectrometry (NMR). Compernolle et al. (51) utilized gas chromatography/mass spectrometry in their determination of the structures of bilirubin glucuronide isomers. The structures of furosemide glucuronide and its isomerization products were confirmed by negative-ion thermospray liquid chromatography/mass spectrometry by Rachmel et al. (32). These scientists detected the abundant (M-1)$^-$ ion at mass 505, the aglycone fragment at m/z 329, and the characteristic sugar fragment ion of mass 175 in the spectra of the β-1-*O*-acyl glucuronide and the isomers, whereas an ion at m/z 221 was noted only in the case of the β-1 conjugate.

Eggers and Doust (23) have used ^{13}C-NMR studies to confirm the isomerization of probenecid glucuronide. Smith and Benet (52), using ^{1}H-NMR, confirmed that the four

Table 1 HPLC Conditions for Acyl Glucuronides of Xenobiotic Carboxylic Acids

Compound	Detection	Column	Running buffer	Ref.
Benoxaprofen (+)	254 nm	ODS	ACN/0.05 M KH_2PO_4, pH = 4.5	22
Benoxaprofen (R/S)	254 nm	ODS	ACN/0.01 M phosphate buffer, pH = 6.5	46
	313/365 nm	ODS	ACN/0.01 M TBA, pH = 2.5	43
Carprofen (R/S)	290/365 nm	ODS	ACN/9 mM TBA	68
	245 nm	ODS	ACN/water/TFA (40:60:0.04)	47
Clofibric acid (+)	226 nm	ODS	MeOH/water/TFA (40:60:0.1)	37
	226 nm	ODS	ACN/5 mM TBA	18
Diclofenac (+)	280 nm	ODS	MeOH/0.05 M ammonium acetate, pH = 4.5 (50:50)	57
Diflunisal (+)	226 nm	ODS	MeOH/0.01 M Na_2HPO_4, pH = 2.7, 4% (w/v) Na_2SO_4 (54:46)	123
Etodolac	280 nm	ODS	MeOH/0.01 M TFA (47:53 v/v)	29
Fenofibric acid	290 nm	Octyl	ACN/10 mM phosphate buffer, 5 mM TBA, pH = 7.5 (45:55)	18
Fenoprofen (R/S)	272 nm	ODS	ACN/10 mM TBA, pH = 2.5	44
Flufenamic acid (+)	254 nm	ODS	ACN/0.05 M KH_2PO_4, pH = 4.5	22
Flunoxaprofen (R/S)	313/365 nm	ODS	ACN/0.01 M TBA, pH = 2.5	42
Furosemide (+)	233/289 nm	ODS	ACN/0.08 M phosphoric acid (30:70)	32
Gemfibrozil (+)	284/316 nm	Cyano	ACN/10 mM TBA, pH = 3.5	124
Ibufenac	214 nm	ODS	MeOH/0.01 M TFA, pH = 2.2 (55:45)	31
Ibuprofen	214 nm	ODS	MeOH/0.01 M TFA, pH = 2.2 (57:43)	31
Isoxepac	254 nm	ODS	ACN/phosphoric acid (0.2%)	55
Ketoprofen (R/S)	254 nm	ODS	ACN/10 mM TBA, 1 mM potassium phosphate, pH = 4.3	49
Mefenamic acid	280 nm	Octyl	ACN/0.05 M ammonium acetate, pH = 4.5 (30:70)	33
Naproxen (R/S)	275/355 nm	ODS	ACN/66 mM ammonium acetate, pH = 6.0 (25:75)	64
Oxaprozin (+)	280 nm	Octyl	ACN/0.05 M phosphate buffer (26:74)	16
2-Phenylpropionic acid (R/S)	254 nm	ODS	ACN/TFA/water (19:0.04:81)	45
Probenecid	254 nm	Octyl	MeOH/water/acetic acid (50:50:1), 40 mM TBA	84
Salicylic acid (+)	240 nm	ODS	MeOH/0.1 M sodium phosphate buffer, pH = 2.7	34
Suprofen	295 nm	ODS	MeOH/0.01 M sodium acetate, pH = 5.1 (37.5:62.5)	30
Tolmetin (+)	313 nm	Octyl	MeOH/0.01 M TBA, 0.05 M sodium acetate, pH = 4.5	38
Zomepirac (+)	313 nm	ODS	MeOH/0.01 M sodium acetate, pH = 5.1	24

+ denotes the simultaneous assay of isomeric conjugates resulting from acyl migration; R/S, the separation of diastereomeric glucuronides. MeOH, methanol; ACN, acetonitrile; TBA, tetrabutyl ammonium sulfate; TFA, trifluoroacetic acid; ODS, octadecylsilane.
Source: Partially from Ref. 2.

fractions that could be separated by HPLC were positional isomers of zomepirac glucuronide. The structural assignments for flufenamic acid and (*S*)-benoxaprofen (22) were also confirmed by ¹H-NMR. In 1988, Hansen-Moller et al. (40) described a simultaneous separation of the α- and β-anomers of three positional isomers of diflunisal glucuronide, in addition to the β-1-*O*-acyl glucuronide. Using two-dimensional NMR spectrometry they were able to identify these six different α- and β-anomers. Similarly, the α- and β-isomers of flufenamic acid glucuronide were also found by ¹H-NMR, and their structures were confirmed by a series of successive decoupling experiments (22). The available data suggest that anomerization is a general phenomenon for C2–C4 isomers of all acyl glucuronides.

IV. STABILITY OF ACYL GLUCURONIDES

Acyl glucuronides are generally less stable than other glucuronides (2). Hydrolysis and intramolecular acyl migration are two major reactions contributing to this instability.

A. Hydrolysis of Acyl Glucuronides

Hydrolysis of an acyl glucuronide leads to regeneration of the pharmacologically active parent drug. Potential catalysts include hydroxide ion, β-glucuronidases, serum albumin, and esterases. Rates of hydrolysis are dependent on pH and temperature, with more rapid degradation of the enzymatically formed β-1-*O*-acyl glucuronide at higher pH, also at physiological pH, than at a more acidic level. Hydrolysis of an acyl glucuronide conjugate occurs readily in biological samples, for example in urine and plasma, in vitro under laboratory conditions, and during storage. The rate of chemical hydrolysis decreases significantly in cold and acidic conditions (pH 3–4), but hydrolysis may still occur slowly during freezing and especially during thawing (53). This may result in substantial increase in the concentration of the parent compound and may be responsible for some of the variation in the apparent extent of the amount excreted unchanged in the urine of some drugs as reported by different investigators. Acyl glucuronides can undergo substantial hydrolysis to the parent aglycone in vivo and this may be due to enzymatic cleavage by β-glucuronidase or nonspecific esterases under physiological conditions. Degradation of the conjugates in bile and intestines will contribute to the enterohepatic recirculation of the parent compound (Fig. 3).

B. Intramolecular Acyl Migration of Acyl Glucuronides

Intramolecular acyl group rearrangement is a well-established reaction in carbohydrate chemistry (54) and is mechanistically related to alkaline hydrolysis. Migration of the acyl moiety occurs from the 1-carbon hydroxyl group to the neighboring 2-, 3-, and 4-hydroxyl groups of the glucuronyl moiety (Fig. 1). This results in the formation of β-glucuronidase-resistant glucuronic acid esters that exhibit chromatographic properties different from the β-1-*O*-acyl glucuronide. Intramolecular acyl migration was first demonstrated for bilirubin glucuronide. Studies with endogenous bilirubin-IXα-glucuronides collected from bile demonstrated a sequential migration of the original biosynthetic 1-*O*-acyl glucuronide to 2-, 3-, and 4-*O*-isomers (51). Subsequently, studies of acyl glucuronides of various xenobiotic carboxylic acids have shown intramolecular acyl migration to be a general phenomenon for acyl glucuronides (1).

The mechanism of acyl migration is well established and proceeds via nucleophilic attack on the neighboring hydroxyl group and formation of an ortho-ester intermediate (22,54). In situ mechanistic studies with ¹H-NMR spectroscopy of HPLC-purified isomers have determined the order of migration to be from the biosynthetic glucuronide to the 2-O-isomer followed by formation of the 3- and 4-O-isomers. Migration between the three positional isomers is reversible but reformation of the parent 1-O-β-acyl glucuronide is very unlikely owing to the mutarotation at C-1 after movement of the acyl group. The studies of Bradow et al. (22) indicated that there is no evidence for rearrangements beyond nearest-neighbor hydroxyl groups.

C. Factors that Influence the Degradation of Acyl Glucuronides

The loss of 1-O-acyl glucuronides (including hydrolysis and acyl migration) follows apparent first-order kinetics over the measurable concentration range. Subsequent loss of the rearranged isomers is generally much slower than that of 1-O-acyl glucuronide. The disappearance of zomepirac 1-O-acyl glucuronide and the formation of isomers and parent zomepirac in vitro at pH 7.4 and 37°C is depicted in Fig. 4, which demonstrates that intramolecular acyl migration under physiological conditions is the predominating reaction in the early stages of the in vitro incubations, whereas hydrolysis of 1-O-acyl glucuronide and its isomers becomes the more important reaction at later times or under alkali conditions (24).

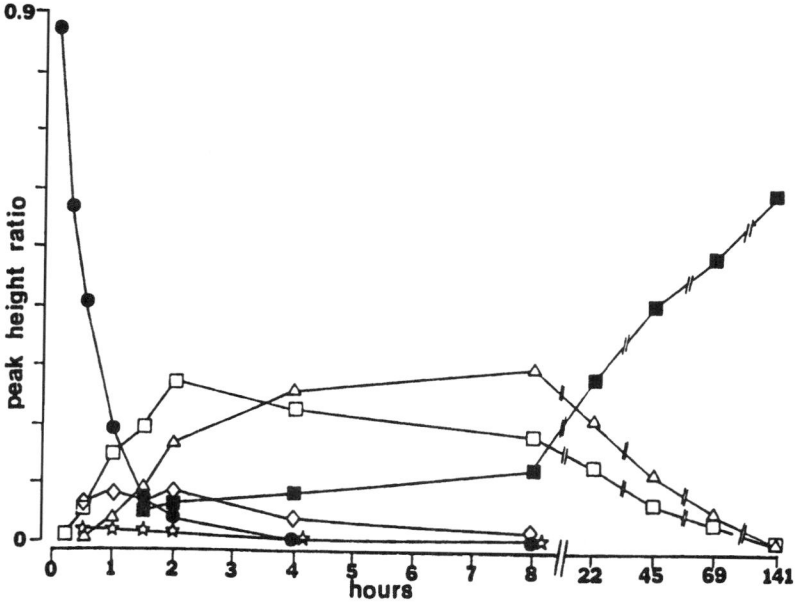

Figure 4   Time-dependent degradation of zomepirac glucuronide (Zgl) to its isomeric conjugates (2-, 3-, 4-O-iso) and hydrolysis to zomepirac (Z) in 0.1 M phosphate buffer, pH 7.4, 37°C. (2-, 3-, and 4-iso represents the α/β-2-O-, α/β-3-O-, α/β-4-O-acyl isomers). Solid circles = Zgl; solid squares = Z; open diamonds = 2-O-iso; open squares = 3-O-iso; open triangles = 4-O-iso; open stars = an unidentified product. (From Ref. 24.)

The rate of acyl migration and hydrolysis varies among different compounds and is influenced by many factors. Both hydrolysis and rearrangement are accelerated at alkaline pH and with increasing temperature. Hasegawa et al. (24) described an apparent first-order pH-dependent degradation (including acyl migration and hydrolysis) of zomepirac glucuronide with minimal isomerization occurring at pH 5, similar to what was reported for isoxepac (55), valproic acid (56), and furosemide (32,41). Degradation half-lives for the β-1-O-acyl glucuronides for various compounds in the physiological pH range are summarized in Table 2. Large variation has been noted in the degradation of acyl glucuronides, from highly labile glucuronides like that of diclofenac (57) and tolmetin (25) (no substitution at the alpha carbon), to most stable species like gemfibrozil (58) (disubstitution at the alpha carbon) and valproic acid (35) (highly steric-hindered dipropyl substitution at the alpha carbon). More interestingly, a single replacement of a chloro group (a better

Table 2 Apparent First-Order Degradation Half-Lives of β-1-O-acyl Glucuronides at pH 7.0–7.5 at 37°C

Compound	pH	Buffer type/medium	$t_{1/2}$(h)	Ref.
Beclobric acid	7.4	Phosphate buffer, 150 mM	25.7 (+), 22.7 (−)	27
Benoxaprofen	7.4	Tris-HCl buffer, 50 mM	2.0 (R), 4.1 (S)	43
Carprofen	7.4	Phosphate buffer (0.067 M)	2.5 (R), 3.5 (S)	47
	7.4	Kreb-Ringer phosphate buffer	1.7 (R), 2.9 (S)	75
Clofibric acid	7.4	Phosphate buffer	7.3	125
	7.0	Tris/maleate (0.1 M)	7.0[a]	18
	7.5	Phosphate buffer (50 mM)	3.0[a]	8
Diclofenac	7.4	Phosphate buffer	0.47	57
Diflunisal	7.4	Phosphate buffer (100 mM)	0.60	65
Etodolac	7.4	Phosphate buffer (150 mM)	20.0	29
Fenoprofen	7.4	Sodium phosphate	0.99 (R), 1.95 (S)	62
Flufenamic acid	7.4	Phosphate buffer	7.0	125
Flunoxaprofen	7.4	Tris-HCl buffer, 50 mM	4.5 (R), 8.0 (S)	42
Furosemide	7.4	Tris maleate, 50 mM	5.289	32
Gemfibrozil	7.4	Phosphate buffer (0.1 M)	44	58
Ibufenac	7.4	Phosphate buffer (0.15 M)	1.1	31
Ibuprofen	7.4	Phosphate buffer (0.15 M)	3.3	31
Indomethacin	7.4	Phosphate buffer	1.4	125
Isoxepac	7.0	Urine	0.29[a]	155
Ketoprofen	7.4	Phosphate buffer	0.66 (R), 1.26 (S)	126
Mefenamic acid	7.4	Phosphate buffer	16.5	33
Naproxen	7.4	Sodium phosphate (0.1 M)	0.92 (R), 1.75 (S)	64
Oxaprozin	7.4	Phosphate buffer (0.1 M)	1.3	127
Probenecid	7.4	Phosphate buffer (0.2 M)	0.4	84
Salicylic acid	7.4	Phosphate buffer	1.55	34
Suprofen	7.4	Phosphate buffer (150 mM)	1.4	30
Tolmetin	7.4	Phosphate buffer	0.26	25
Valproic acid	7.4	Phosphate buffer (0.1 M)	60[a]	35
Wy-18,251	7.4	Phosphate buffer (0.1 M)	0.38	127
Wy-41,770	7.4	Phosphate buffer (0.1 M)	14	127
Zomepirac	7.4	Phosphate buffer (0.1 M)	0.45	24

[a] Half-life was calculated from the data given in the reference.
Source: References prior to 1992 from Spahn-Langguth and Benet (2).

electron-withdrawing group than fluoro) on benoxaprofen by a fluoro group, which becomes flunoxaprofen, leads to a marked increase of stability of the acyl glucuronides. The half-lives of (R)- and (S)-benoxaprofen glucuronides are 2.0 h and 4.0 h, respectively (43), whereas, the half-lives of acyl glucuronides of (R)- and (S)-flunoxaprofen are 4.5 and 8.8 h, respectively (42). It appears that the degradation rate of acyl glucuronide at physiological conditions is predictable based on the chemical structure of the acid and depends on: (1) the degree of substitution at the alpha carbon to the carboxylic acid (59), and (2) electron-withdrawing or donating groups at the alpha carbon or on the conjugated aromatic ring. Considering both steric hinderance and electronic effect on the chemical reactivity of acyl glucuronide gives a better understanding of the marked differences in degradation rates of structurally diverse carboxylic acid–containing drugs.

Degradation rates of acyl glucuronides depend not only on the pH and temperature, but also on the nature of the solution (e.g., buffer, organic solvent, plasma, blood, urine, bile). Furosemide glucuronide (128) was shown to degrade much faster in bile ($t_{1/2}$ = 19.5 min) and a supernatant solution of a duodenal homogenate from rabbits ($t_{1/2}$ = 1.2 min) than in buffer (pH = 7.4, $t_{1/2}$ = 5.3 h). Degradation of zomepirac glucuronide in blood and plasma was found to be faster than in buffer (60). Ruelius et al. (16) also found accelerated degradation of oxaprozin glucuronide in human serum albumin (HSA) and plasma. Indeed, they showed that albumin was catalytic for all three reactions (intramolecular acyl migration, hydrolysis, and covalent binding). Reports in literature suggest that the effects of albumin or plasma on the stability of acyl glucuronide conjugates and their isomers vary with the drugs studied. HSA has been shown to enhance the degradation rates of acyl glucuronides of many carboxylic acid–containing drugs, including zomepirac (60), oxaprozin (16,61), fenoprofen (62), etodolac (29), ketoprofen (63), naproxen (64), clofibric acid (18), gemfibrozil (58), and diclofenac (57). An opposite (stabilizing) effect of HSA was observed for tolmetin glucuronide, but bovine serum albumin (BSA) causes an increase in the rate of hydrolysis (25). In the presence of HSA, degradation of diflunisal (65), salicylic acid (34), mefenamic acid (33), and furosemide (66) glucuronides in albumin solution was retarded in comparison to that found in buffer alone, while no significant change in the degradation rate of ibufenac glucuronide was observed with or without HSA.

These data suggest that the effect of HSA toward acyl glucuronides is strongly dependent on the chemical structure of the aglycone moiety. To explain the accelerated degradation of oxaprozin glucuronide in the presence of HSA, Ruelius et al. (16) hypothesized that the degradation reaction of oxaprozin glucuronide in HSA proceeds through the formation of a reversible complex of oxaprozin glucuronide with HSA at the benzodiazepine-binding site [site II, as classified by Sudlow et al. (67)]. Located within this site is a reactive tyrosine, which appears to be the nucleophile responsible for mediating all the reactions, including hydrolysis, acyl migration, and covalent binding. Support for this hypothesis was obtained when other agents, like naproxen, decanoic acid, and oxaprozin itself, that strongly bind to the benzodiazepine site inhibited both hydrolysis and acyl migration (16,61). Watt and Dickinson (65) proposed a similar mechanism to explain the protective effect of albumin on the degradation of acyl glucuronide, by introducing two binding sites: one a reversible binding site and the other the primary site catalyzing degradation of acyl glucuronide (catalytic site). If the reversible binding site happens to be the catalytic site, albumin may accelerate the degradation of acyl glucuronides, like oxaprozin. Otherwise, it may retard the degradation rate of acyl glucuronides, such as diflunisal and salicylic acid. The correctness of such speculation clearly requires further investigation.

V. REVERSIBLE BINDING OF ACYL GLUCURONIDES TO PROTEINS

As mentioned above, by introducing the reversible binding of oxaprozin glucuronide to HSA, Ruelius et al. (16) could well explain the catalytic effect of HSA on the hydrolysis and acyl migration of acyl glucuronides. They also hypothesized that a correlation exists between reversible binding and irreversible (covalent) binding to plasma proteins, with reversible binding acting as a preliminary or an intermediate step (16,61). Measurements of reversible plasma protein binding of glucuronide conjugates, however, are rare. With respect to acyl glucuronides, the lack of data mainly results from experimental difficulties, since the studies need to be carried out under physiological conditions (37°C, pH = 7.4), that is, the conditions at which acyl glucuronides are not stable. By rapid ultrafiltration, reversible binding of acyl glucuronides to HSA has been studied for carprofen (47,68), zomepirac (69), tolmetin (69), ketoprofen (63), fenoprofen (70), naproxen (64), and furo-semide (66). Interestingly, significant binding to HSA was found for the β-1-O-acyl glucuronides as well as for their positional isomers (69). Stereoselective reversible binding of (R)- and (S)-glucuronides of carprofen, naproxen, fenoprofen, and ketoprofen to HSA was also observed. (S)-glucuronides of carprofen (47,68) and fenoprofen (70) had a higher affinity to HSA than the (R)-glucuronides. An opposite result, (R)-glucuronide having a higher affinity than the (S)-diastereomer, was observed for naproxen glucuronide (64).

Presumably, reversible binding of acyl glucuronides to proteins acts as a preliminary step for irreversible (covalent) binding. Studies of reversible binding might help us better understand the mechanism of covalent binding and the HSA effect on the stability of acyl glucuronides.

VI. COVALENT BINDING OF ACYL GLUCURONIDES TO PROTEINS

Hydrolysis and intramolecular acyl migration of acyl glucuronide conjugates of carboxylic acid–containing compounds have been extensively documented in recent years (1,2). A third reaction manifesting the inherent chemical electrophilicity of acyl glucuronides involves their capacity to act as substrates for the covalent binding of the aglycone to tissue proteins, notably albumin. Covalent binding, first described for bilirubin in 1966 (71), was demonstrated to be dependent on the presence of bilirubin acyl glucuronides in vitro and in vivo. Van Breeman and Fenselau (21) reported covalent binding of flufenamic acid, indomethacin, clofibric acid, and benoxaprofen to bovine serum albumin (BSA), when acyl glucuronides were incubated with the protein in vitro, and suggested that the mechanism involved transacylation with the free sulfhydryl group of cysteine residues. Ruelius and co-workers (16,61) documented the in vitro covalent binding of oxaprozin to HSA via acyl glucuronide, and concluded, on the basis of extensive inhibition studies, that the site of covalent binding to HSA was a tyrosine residue located within the benzodiazepine binding site (transacylation with the hydroxyl group of tyrosine). We have demonstrated that such covalent binding occurs in vivo in humans, as well as in vitro, for zomepirac (72), tolmetin (25,73,74), carprofen (75), fenoprofen (62), beclobric acid (27), naproxen (64), and diclofenac (57), while McKinnon and Dickinson have shown such binding for diflunisal and probenecid (76), William et al. for valproic acid (35), and more recently Sallustio et al. for clofibric acid (77) and gemfibrozil (58).

A. Procedures to Assay Covalent Binding

Generally, the extent of covalent binding is quantified as the amount of aglycone that remains bound to proteins after an exhaustive washing procedure, which is then liberated after treatment with strong base (78). Proteins are usually precipitated by addition of, for example, ice-cold isopropanol and acidic acetonitrile (ACN) or an ACN/ethanol mixture. The protein pellet obtained after centrifugation is washed several times (at least 5–10 times) with methanol/diethylether (3:1; vortexing and sonication, followed by centrifugation) to remove the reversibly bound aglycone and conjugates from the proteins. Aglycone-protein adducts are then dissolved in sodium hydroxide solution at 70–80°C overnight, to release the bound aglycone. The liberated aglycone can be either quantified by scintillation counting if the aglycone is radiolabeled, or quantified by HPLC for nonradiolabeled aglycone (72). The extent of covalent binding, determined by such an indirect assay, is usually expressed as picomoles or nanomoles of covalently bound aglycone per milligram of protein. This indirect procedure could be applied for both in vitro and in vivo covalent binding studies and the bound aglycone (drug) can be assayed specifically, even stereospecifically, by HPLC; however, these methods cannot differentiate the individual proteins to which aglycone binds.

The aglycone-modified protein targets could be identified by SDS-PAGE and fluorography, if radiolabeled aglycone is available. Because of the limited availability of radiolabeled compounds, recently, immunochemical methods have been developed and have become the preferred methods to detect and identify xenobiotic covalent bound proteins. The immunochemical methods involve the production of highly selective polyclonal antibodies by immunization of animals (e.g., rabbits) with aglycone-linked immunogenic protein. Via these methods, the protein covalent binding can be determined both quantitatively and qualitatively. Western blots permit detection of individual proteins targeted by the reactive metabolite and ELISA techniques permit quantification of protein adducts in tissues and subcellular fractions (79). In addition, immunohistochemical analysis permits assessment of distribution of covalent adducts among tissues and localization within individual cell types (80). The immunochemical methods have been successfully utilized to investigate the mechanisms of tissue toxicity of halothane, acetaminophen, diclofenac (81), and a variety of other chemicals. The results produced by such methods, however, are highly variable between laboratories: sometimes, a completely different pattern of protein adducts is detected, mainly due to the different specificity of polyclonal antibodies produced among different laboratories.

B. In Vitro Covalent Binding of Acyl Glucuronides to Proteins

As a consequence of the chemical reactivity of acyl glucuronides, a large number of carboxylic acid–containing drugs have been demonstrated to covalently bind to plasma proteins, especially albumin in vitro, including nonsteroidal anti-inflammatory drugs [benoxaprofen (21), indomethacin (21), flufenamic acid (21), oxaprozin (16), zomepirac (72), tolmetin (25), carprofen (75), fenoprofen (62), naproxen (64), diclofenac (57), diflunisal (65), salicylic acid (34), etodolac (29), suprofen (30), ibuprofen (31), ibufenac (31), ketoprofen (83), and mefenamic acid (33)], the uricosuric drug probenecid (84), the antihyperlipoproteinemic reagents [clofibric acid (18,21), fenofibric acid (18,82), gemfibrozil (58), and beclobric acid (27)], the diuretic agent furosemide (66), and the antiepileptic drug valproic acid (35).

From these in vitro studies, the extent of covalent binding was found to be clearly dependent on time (21,61), pH (25,30,72), glucuronide concentration (83), and origin of albumin (25,65). For oxaprozin glucuronide (16,61), the highest yield of protein adduct was obtained after the glucuronide and HSA were incubated at pH 7 for approximately 1 h at 37°C. Similarly, maximum covalent binding to HSA for zomepirac glucuronide occurred after 1-h incubation at pH 9, although the level of protein adducts decreased rapidly after this time owing to the instability of the adducts at this pH. High concentrations of adduct were also observed after 6-h incubation of zomepirac glucuronide and HSA at pH 7 and 8 at 37°C (72). The in vitro covalent binding of suprofen glucuronide to HSA was shown to increase with increasing pH at 37°C and to be time-dependent (30). The extent of covalent binding of ketoprofen glucuronide (83) to albumin was proportional to acyl glucuronide concentration over the range studied (from 11.62 to 69.72 μM). Watt and Dickinson (65) showed that covalent binding of diflunisal glucuronide was greater with fatty-acid-free HSA than with rat plasma albumin (RSA) and human and rat plasma proteins, and suggested that the different animal origins and the state of purity of albumin might be important for the stability and covalent binding of acyl glucuronides. Similar findings were also reported for tolmetin glucuronide (25). The extent of covalent binding of tolmetin glucuronide with BSA was much less than, but the rate of adduct formation was the same as, that with HSA.

In addition to 1-O-acyl glucuronide, the isomeric conjugates could also form covalent protein adducts. Isomeric conjugates of zomepirac glucuronide (17,72) were found to covalently bind to HSA, at somewhat decreased extents as compared to the β-1-O-acyl glucuronide itself (% bound: C1 > C2 > C4 > C3). Reports in the literature suggest that certain isomeric conjugates were even more reactive toward proteins than the β-1-O-acyl glucuronide. Isomers of suprofen glucuronide exhibited time-dependent covalent binding and this binding was 38% higher than that of the β-1-O-acyl glucuronide (30). Similarly, protein adduct formation of valproic acid (35), salicylic acid (34), etodolac (29), and diflunisal (91) was shown to be much more rapid and extensive from isomeric glucuronide conjugates than from the β-1-O-acyl glucuronides. However, not all of the isomeric conjugates are important for the covalent binding. Ruelius et al. (16) reported that only the β-1-O-acyl glucuronide of oxaprozin, not the isomers, led to significant irreversible binding.

Studies performed by Dubois et al. (83), as well by our laboratory (85), suggest that HSA is the major binding protein with respect to covalent binding to plasma proteins; for example, no covalent binding was detected with fibrinogen and γ-globulins, and only 0.14% of ketoprofen was bound to α- and β-globulins after a 3-h incubation. However, covalent binding is not restricted to albumin. Bailey et al. (86) have shown that zomepirac glucuronide and its isomers covalently modified microtubular protein in a dose-dependent manner and suggested that perturbation of the tubulin/microtubulin dynamics might contribute to the hepatotoxicity of certain acidic drugs. In vitro studies of covalent binding of tolmetin glucuronide to tissue homogenates from rat and sheep indicated that the extent of tissue covalent binding was comparable to that detected with albumin and plasma proteins (85). Similarly, incubation of rat liver microsomes with [^{14}C]-diclofenac showed that diclofenac covalently bound to hepatic microsome proteins varied as a function of exposure time and the concentration of the cofactor, UDPGA (87). Hepatic microsomes incubated with [^{14}C]-UDPGA and nonradiolabeled diclofenac resulted in similar covalent binding of the radiolabeled compound to microsomal protein, which was significantly decreased in the presence of 7,7,7-triphenylheptyl-UDP, a specific inhibitor of UGT.

C. Mechanism of Covalent Binding of Acyl Glucuronides to Proteins

The mechanism of the irreversible binding of acyl glucuronide to proteins has been investigated extensively. Basically, two pathways have been proposed, each resulting in a different type of adduct (Fig. 5). The first is a nucleophilic displacement reaction whereby

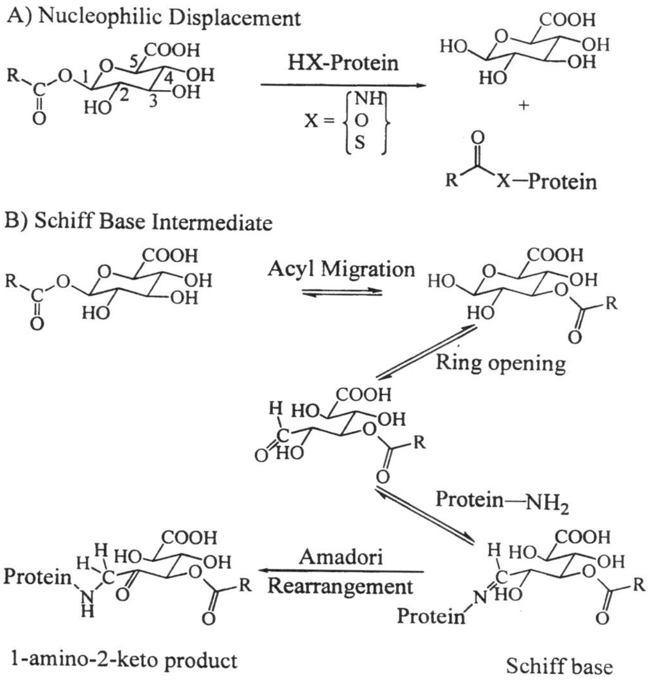

Figure 5 Proposed mechanism for covalent binding of acyl glucuronides to proteins. (From Ref. 74.)

protein nucleophiles, including sulfhydryl, hydroxyl, and amine groups, react with the facile carbonyl-carbon of the acyl glucuronide. This mechanism leads to the acylation of proteins giving rise to thioester-, oxygen ester-, and amide-linked conjugates. The consequence of this reaction would be the direct covalent linkage of the drug to the target protein without the glucuronic acid moiety. Evidence of the involvement of nucleophilic groups such as -SH of cysteine residues (21), -OH of tyrosine residues (61), and -NH$_2$ of lysine residues (88,89) in the formation of covalent adducts between protein and various acyl glucuronides has been documented.

The second mechanism of covalent binding of acyl glucuronides to proteins is analogous to the nonenzymatic glycosylation of albumin (90) and requires prior acyl migration of the drug moiety away from the biosynthetic β-1-O-acyl glucuronide to permit ring opening of the sugar. The reactive aldehyde group so exposed can then reversibly form an imine (Schiff's base) with an amine group on protein. Subsequent Amadori rearrangement could then yield a stable ketoamine derivative. Thus, in contrast to the trans-acylation mechanism, both drug and glucuronic acid moieties (still linked together by an ester group) become bonded to proteins. This mechanism was first proposed for the covalent binding of zomepirac to plasma protein (72). In covalent binding studies with zomepirac and tolmetin glucuronides, imine trapping agents (cyanide or cyanoborohydride) significantly increased the extent of covalent binding of the drug, supporting this mechanism. Furthermore, isomeric glucuronide conjugates released after extensive washing and subsequent acid treatment (17,72), gave evidence that the glucuronic acid moiety is part of the adduct. In vitro studies with clofibryl and fenofibryl glucuronides (18) showed that covalent binding of ^{14}C to proteins was markedly higher after incubation of HSA with clofibryl or fenofibryl glucuronide labeled with ^{14}C on the glucuronyl moiety, compared with the label on the aglycone. Binding of ^{14}C to HSA was 14.9-fold (24-h incubation) higher for clofibryl glucuronide and 5.9-fold (24-h incubation) higher for fenofibryl glucuronide when labeled on the glucuronyl moiety than on the aglycone (18). This is consistent with the proposed Schiff's base mechanism, in which the glucuronyl moiety becomes covalently bound to proteins.

The two mechanisms proposed for adduct formation contrast sharply. The simpler transacylation mechanism involves nucleophilic attack at the ester group by -SH, -OH, or $-NH_2$ groups on protein. The drug moiety itself thus becomes directly linked to the protein via a thioester, ester, or amide bond, and glucuronic acid is lost. Under physiological pH conditions, relative facile transacylation reactions might be expected of the 1-*O*-acyl glucuronide itself, but not of its 2-, 3-, or 4-isomers, since only in the β-1-*O*-acyl glucuronide is the carboxyl group of the drug linked to the glucuronic acid moiety via an acetal. Conversely, the Schiff's base mechanism for adduct formation requires prior migration of the drug moiety away from the 1-position of the glucuronic acid ring and thus is operative for the isomers but not the 1-*O*-acyl glucuronide itself. According to this mechanism, the glucuronic acid moiety, still bearing the ester-linked drug, becomes bound to an amine group on protein via an imine (Schiff's base).

Because the reversibility of acyl migration does not include reformation of the parent acyl glucuronide (Fig. 1), the two mechanisms of adduct formation are theoretically distinguishable on the basis of whether the glucuronide or its isomers are the better substrate. The isomeric conjugates of some xenobiotic carboxylic acids, such as diflunisal (91), valproic acid (35), and salicylic acid (34), have been shown to be more reactive toward protein than the corresponding β-1-*O*-acyl glucuronide, supporting the Schiff's base (glycosylation) mechanism. On the other hand, Ruelius et al. (16) presented strong evidence favoring a transacylation mechanism for covalent binding of oxaprozin to HSA. After incubation of radiolabeled oxaprozin glucuronide with HSA at pH 7 for 1 h, 22% of the radioactivity became attached to HSA, but only 0.6% when the label was in the glucuronic acid moiety. Furthermore, only 2.1% attachment of label to HSA occurred after incubation with the 2-isomer of $[^{14}C]$-oxaprozin glucuronide. Smith et al. (17,72) showed that zomepirac-HSA adduct formation from zomepirac acyl glucuronide was roughly comparable to that from its purified 2-isomer and greater than that from its purified 4- and 3-isomers, over a 45-min incubation with HSA at pH 7.4 and 37°C. Munafo et al. (25) found that the rate of covalent binding of tolmetin to HSA was 10 times greater for tolmetin glucuronide than for a mixture of its isomers (predominantly the 3-isomers, generated in situ from tolmetin glucuronide by preincubation in albumin-free buffer). All of these researchers suggested that more than one mechanism was operative. Mass spectrometric analysis of tryptic digests of albumin adducts (92,93) provided direct evidence that the in vitro binding of tolmetin glucuronide to HSA occurs via both mechanisms. Similar findings have recently been reported for benoxaprofen glucuronide (94). It is possible that both mechanisms occur concurrently in vivo.

D. In Vivo Covalent Binding of Acyl Glucuronides to Proteins

1. In Vivo Plasma Protein Binding

Unlike many reactive metabolites that may never leave the organ of synthesis, acyl glucuronides are stable enough to reach the circulation and subsequently be excreted into the urine. The in vivo formation of covalently bound plasma protein adducts by acyl glucuronides has now been demonstrated in humans for a large number of compounds, including beclobric acid (27), clofibric acid (77), carprofen (75), diclofenac (57), diflunisal (76), fenoprofen (62), gemfibrozil (101), ketoprofen (83), probenecid (76), salicylic acid (34), tolmetin (73,74), valproic acid (35), and zomepirac (72).

From these in vivo studies, the extent of protein binding of acyl glucuronides in vivo was found to correlate well with the extent of the exposure of acyl glucuronides, which is measured as the area under the curve (AUC). Increase in plasma glucuronide concentrations leads to higher covalent binding. Increased adduct formation can thus be expected during chronic dosage or with decreased renal clearance of the glucuronide as in renal failure or resulting from a drug-drug interaction. Indeed, adduct concentrations in elderly patients treated with tolmetin were significantly higher than those in the control group of elderly patients given a single dose (73). Significant accumulation of protein adducts of tolmetin has also been observed in healthy human volunteers after a 10-day multiple dosing regimen of tolmetin. The bound levels after administration of multiple doses were approximately 10 times higher than those after a single dose was given to the same subjects (74). Valproic acid adducts were measurable in the plasma of epileptic patients on chronic drug therapy (35). Coadministration of probenecid and zomepirac resulted in an increase in the amount of covalent binding and an increase in exposure to zomepirac glucuronide plasma concentrations (95). Covalent binding of diflunisal and probenecid has been investigated after administration of multiple doses of each drug. After a 6-day regimen in healthy human volunteers of oral diflunisal with concomitant administration of oral probenecid during the last 2 days, measurable covalent binding of both drugs via their acyl glucuronide metabolite has been observed (76).

2. In Vivo Tissue Protein Binding

In contrast to the well-documented adduct formation of xenobiotic carboxylic acid–containing drugs to plasma proteins, fewer studies have investigated the intracellular adduct formation in organs exposed to the drugs or their glucuronides. The in vivo formation of covalent adducts with tissue proteins was demonstrated for diflunisal in liver, kidney, skeletal muscle, and small and large intestine of rats given the drug (96,97), as well as urinary bladder tissue proteins (98). Following daily diflunisal dosing, the adduct concentration increased in all tissues over time and declined slowly after cessation of drug administration with a half-life of approximately 20 h (98). Similarly, chronic dosing of rats with clofibric acid over a 21-day period resulted in higher concentrations of clofibric acid covalently bound to liver proteins. Concentration of tissue protein adducts seemed to increase linearly with time, with no indication of steady state having been achieved by 21 days (77). In vivo covalent binding of carboxylic acids to tissue proteins has also been documented for diclofenac, sulindac, and ibuprofen in mice liver (99), and for zomepirac and valproic acid in rat liver (100).

3. Stability of Protein Adducts

At present, very little is known about the pharmacokinetics of the covalently bound protein adducts formed by carboxylic acid drugs in plasma and tissues, although the in vivo stability (half-life) of the formed adduct may be important for the potential immunogenic effects of a hapten (11). From the currently available data, it is evident that the plasma protein adducts are long-lived, with half-lives much greater than those of their parent carboxylic acids and acyl glucuronide conjugates. Tolmetin-protein adducts persisted in plasma beyond the period when concentrations of tolmetin and its glucuronide were measurable (74). Specifically, tolmetin-plasma protein adducts exhibited an average half-life of approximately 4.8 days, whereas tolmetin and its glucuronide had a half-life of 5 h (73). McKinnon and Dickinson (76) have reported terminal half-lives for the plasma protein adducts of diflunisal and probenecid in humans of 10 and 13.5 days, respectively. The half-lives of (−)- and (+)-beclobric acid plasma protein adducts in humans were reported to be 1.75 and 2.9 days, respectively (27). These values are significantly shorter than the half-life of albumin in humans (17–23 days) and may represent clearance of adducts formed with plasma proteins other than albumin, or may be caused by the breakdown of relatively unstable adducts, independent of the longer turnover rates for the protein itself. In vitro studies of diflunisal glucuronide (91) with HSA revealed a biphasic decline with an apparent terminal half-life of about 28 days. Kitteringham et al. (102) have also demonstrated that the clearance of dinitrobenzene-albumin adducts was dependent on the degree of substitution of the albumin, with clearance increasing as epitope density was increased, which may be another factor contributing to the elimination of plasma adducts formed from acyl glucuronides. Owing to the long-lived protein adduct, steady-state adduct concentrations may not be achieved until months after the commencement of chronic dosing, with significant accumulation at steady state. These long-lived adducts may lead to enhanced uptake by antigen-presenting cells (e.g., macrophages), resulting in greater possibilities to be processed and presented to the immune system.

E. Selectivity of Covalent Binding of Acyl Glucuronides to Tissue Proteins

Evidence has accumulated to show that the protein covalent binding via acyl glucuronides is not random, but rather selective with respect to the proteins targeted. Selective binding to specific cellular target proteins may correlate better with toxicity than total protein covalent binding. Using a fluorescence detection technique, covalently bound flunoxaprofen and benoxaprofen (103) were associated with a 39-kDa and a 62-kDa protein in a rat hepatic microsome system in the presence of UDPGA. Similarly, immunochemical detection of diclofenac adducts in mouse liver homogenates, after oral treatment of mice with diclofenac, revealed a dose-dependent formation of four major protein adducts with apparent molecular masses of 50, 70, 110, and 140 kDa (81). Dose- and time-dependent covalent modifications of hepatic proteins by diclofenac were also detected in rats given diclofenac (104). Subcellular fractionation of rat liver homogenate from diclofenac-treated rats showed that a 50-kDa microsomal protein and 110-, 140-, and 200-kDa plasma membrane proteins were preferentially modified by diclofenac. Hargus et al. (104) presented evidence implicating UGT-dependent glucuronidation in the formation of the 110-, 140-, and 200-kDa diclofenac protein adducts in vitro in rat liver homogenate, while the formation of the 50-kDa microsome protein was shown to be cytochrome-P450-dependent. Using immunofluorescence and immunohistochemistry, the majority of the diclofenac adducts were detected on the plasma membrane and localized within the bile canalicular membrane (104).

On the other hand, studies undertaken by Kretz-Rommel and Boelsterli (105) have reported immunochemical identification of 50-, 60-, 80-, and 126-kDa adducts, which were expressed in cultured rat hepatocytes exposed to diclofenac in vitro, and of 60- and 80-kDa adducts expressed in vivo in livers of rats given diclofenac. The 60-kDa protein was also detected by fluorography in a UGT-dependent microsomal incubation of diclofenac and UDPGA, with radiolabel on either diclofenac or UDPGA (87). Furthermore, Gil and co-workers (106) have reported detection of a major 60-kDa adduct generated in vitro when rat and human hepatocytes were cultured with diclofenac. The reasons for the different patterns found in the different laboratories are unclear at present, but contributing factors could include differences in the model system (in vivo/in vitro rat, mouse, and cultured hepatocytes), samples (liver homogenate and subcellular fractions), and specificity of antisera.

A similar pattern of covalent binding was found with other carboxylic acid–containing drugs using drug-specific antibodies. Diflunisal and zomepirac (100) were shown to produce major 110-, 140-, and 200-kDa hepatic protein adducts in vivo, similar to the results found with diclofenac. A different pattern of protein modification was detected in the livers of clofibric acid– and valproic acid–treated rats (100). A 70-kDa protein adduct was detected in clofibric acid–treated rats, while a 140-kDa protein and several other proteins with smaller molecular weight (e.g., 40, 43, and 55 kDa) were detected in livers of valproic acid–treated rats. The major protein adduct observed with sulindac (99) was the 110-kDa protein, with low levels found for the 140- and 200-kDa proteins. All the sulindac-modified protein adducts were shown to be concentrated in a subfraction derived from the bile canalicular region of the hepatocyte plasma membrane. Ibuprofen was the least toxic of carboxylic acids tested, and predominantly bound covalently to a 60-kDa protein with only relatively low levels of a 110-kDa adduct (99). Such selective modification of plasma membrane proteins by carboxylic acids, possibly containing new antigenic determinants, could become particularly important if the immune system were involved in the pathogenesis of carboxylic acid–induced liver injury (80).

VII. STEREOCHEMICAL ASPECTS OF ACYL GLUCURONIDES

Many of the carboxylic acid drugs belong to the class of 2-arylpropionic acid of profens, which have a chiral center at the carbon 2 of the propionic acid side chain. Only (*S*)-enantiomers have significant anti-inflammatory activity (107). Nevertheless, the clinically used profens are marketed as racemates with the notable exception of naproxen. A unique feature of the metabolism of this class of compounds is the inversion at the chiral center (carbon 2), generally referred to as chiral inversion, which is unidirectional in mammalian organisms. The pharmacologically inactive (*R*)-enantiomer is usually transformed to the active (*S*)-antipode, whereas the reverse reaction does not occur.

In general, the principal urinary metabolites of the profen drugs are their acyl glucuronides. Acyl glucuronidation of chiral carboxylic acids was reported to be enantioselective (112). Investigations of substrate enantioselectivity in the formation of acyl glucuronides have been performed in vitro with microsomes, solubilized microsomal protein, and immobilized protein obtained from animal and human liver as sources of UDP-glucuronosyltransferases. El Mouelhi et al. (46) have described species-dependent enantioselective formation of conjugates of naproxen, ibuprofen, and benoxaprofen. Similar results for benoxaprofen glucuronidation have been reported by Spahn et al. (43). Preferential glucuronidation of the (*R*)-enantiomer with rat liver microsomes was observed with various 2-arylpropionic acids, including 2-phenylpropionic acid (45), flunoxaprofen, flurbiprofen, indoprofen, pirprofen, benoxaprofen, and carprofen, with the exception of naproxen (108–110). In vitro glucuronidation studies of (*R*)- and (*S*)-ketoprofen in liver microsomes from a number of animal species demonstrated that the rate of glucuronidation of (*S*)-aglycone was 4.5-fold faster than that of (*R*)-enantiomer in dog liver microsomes, whereas no significant stereoselectivity was found in human, rat, or rabbit liver microsomes (49). With sheep liver microsome preparations, glucuronide yields were higher for (R)-flunoxaprofen (42,111) and (R)-fenoprofen (44) than for their respective (S)-glucuronides. Glucuronidation studies with enzyme-induced liver microsomes performed by Fournel-Gighleux et al. (45) with 2-phenylpropionic acid as the substrate clearly demonstrated that acyl glucuronide formation is significantly induced by phenobarbital, whereas other inducers (dexamethasone, 3-methylcholanthrene) lead to a minor increase of glucuronidation. The S/R ratio of acyl glucuronidation was not affected by any of the inducers. In each of those studies potential interference from stereoselective degradation of acyl glucuronides was minimized by rapid sample quenching, lowering the incubation pH to 5.5, or addition of specific esterase and β-glucuronidase inhibitors to prevent the enzymatic hydrolysis of acyl glucuronides (110,112).

In addition to stereoselective acyl glucuronidation, degradation of the diastereomeric acyl glucuronides (including hydrolysis and acyl migration) of various chiral carboxylic acids has also been shown to be stereoselective (112). In studies with benoxaprofen (43), flunoxaprofen (42), carprofen (75), naproxen (64), ketoprofen (49), and fenoprofen (62), the apparent first-order degradation half-lives of the (S)-acyl glucuronides were approximately twofold longer than those of their corresponding (R)-acyl glucuronides in a protein-free buffer system at pH 7.4, 37°C (Table 2). Stereoselective degradation of carprofen glucuronides under different conditions and the influence of HSA were characterized by our group (59). When (R)- and (S)-carprofen glucuronides were incubated at pH 7.0, 7.4, and 8.0 at 37°C in phosphate buffer, degradation was highly stereoselective at pH 7.0. Stereoselectivity decreased while degradation velocity increased with higher pH, as summarized in Table 3. At all pH values, the (R)-glucuronide conjugate of carprofen degraded more rapidly than the (S)-glucuronide. When HSA was added to the incubation medium, the stability of (S)-glucuronide was decreased, whereas the apparent half-life of (R)-glucuronide increased. Interestingly, the effect of fatty-acid-free HSA was much greater than

Table 3 Degradation Half-Lives of Carprofen β-1-O-Acyl Glucuronides: Influence of pH, Temperature, and Addition of Albumin on the Velocities of Degradation and Their Enantioselectivities

	Half-life (h)		
	(S)-glucuronide	(R)-glucuronide	S/R Ratio
1. pH effect at 37°C			
pH 7.0	6.42	2.60	2.43
pH 7.4	2.90	1.72	1.69
pH 8.0	0.85	0.60	1.41
2. Temperature dependence at pH 7.4			
4°C	>100	>100	1.0
25°C	11.8	7.80	1.51
37°C	2.90	1.72	1.69
3. Effect of HSA, pH 7.4, 37°C			
Without HSA	2.90	1.72	1.69
With 30 μM HSA (fatty-acid-free)	1.55	2.80	0.55
With 30 μM HSA (fraction V)	1.82	1.78	1.02

Source: Ref. 112.

that of fraction V HSA. This finding suggests that seemingly trivial differences in HSA purity could be important for the stability and chemical reactivity of acyl glucuronides (112). A similar stereoselective effect of HSA on the stability of diastereomeric glucuronides has been observed for naproxen glucuronides. The addition of HSA to the incubation medium not only increased the degradation rate of naproxen glucuronide, but also caused a change of the stereoselective stability where the (*R*)-naproxen glucuronide became more stable than the (*S*)-glucuronide (64).

In contrast to the well-documented stereoselective degradation studies of acyl glucuronides, relatively few studies have examined the potentially stereoselective nature of covalent binding of chiral carboxylic acids to protein via their acyl glucuronide conjugates. The covalent binding of carprofen to HSA after 1-h incubation was higher with (*S*)-carprofen glucuronide than (*R*)-glucuronide, whereas after 24 h, covalent binding was significantly higher for (*R*)-carprofen glucuronide incubations (75). In vitro covalent binding was also found to be higher for (*R*)-naproxen (64) than for (*S*)-naproxen when a 50-μM concentration of each epimeric glucuronide was incubated with HSA under physiological conditions (pH 7.4, 37°C). This stereoselective difference was observed with an HSA-containing medium as well as in rat and human plasma. No significant diastereoselective difference between the two beclobric acid enantiomers was detected with respect to the extent of in vitro covalent binding to HSA (27). Volland et al. (62) described significantly more covalent binding for the (*R*)-enantiomer of fenoprofen to human plasma protein in vitro; however, in vivo this stereoselectivity was reversed. This provides a clear example of competing enantioselective metabolism since (*R*)-fenoprofen is subjected to significant chiral inversion in humans, which will increase the exposure of (*S*)-fenoprofen and its glucuronide relative to its optical enantiomer in vivo.

Since acyl glucuronidation, stability under physiological conditions, and extent of covalent binding of diastereoisomeric acyl glucuronides to plasma proteins are stereoselective, one might consider toxicity of a racemic compound to be more extensively due to one enantiomer than to its antipode. However, at this stage, prediction of toxicity of carboxylic acids, including considerations concerning stereoselectivity, resulting from unstable acyl glucuronides are only speculative. Whether only (*S*)-enantiomers of the profen drugs should be marketed is still debatable.

VIII. PREDICTABILITY OF THE COVALENT BINDING OF ACIDIC DRUGS

The accumulated data from a number of studies suggest that the extent of covalent binding for carboxylic acid drugs in vitro may be predicted on the basis of the degradation rate constant (including hydrolysis and acyl migration) of the glucuronide conjugate. A synthesis of published data (59) on the covalent binding of several acyl glucuronides indicates that there is a good linear correlation between the apparent first-order disappearance rate constant for an acyl glucuronide in buffer, which is a measure of its chemical reactivity, and the maximum covalent binding observed when the glucuronide is incubated with HSA in vitro (Fig. 6). Acyl glucuronides of arylacetic acid (α-unsubstituted) such as tolmetin and zomepirac exhibit the highest covalent binding and lowest stability (highest degradation rate). The intermediate stable glucuronides of 2-arylpropionic acids (mono α-substituted), such as carprofen and fenoprofen, have lower covalent binding. Lowest covalent binding is observed for the most stable fully substituted carboxylic acids, such as beclobric acid and furosemide. Figure 6 summarizes data from our laboratories over a

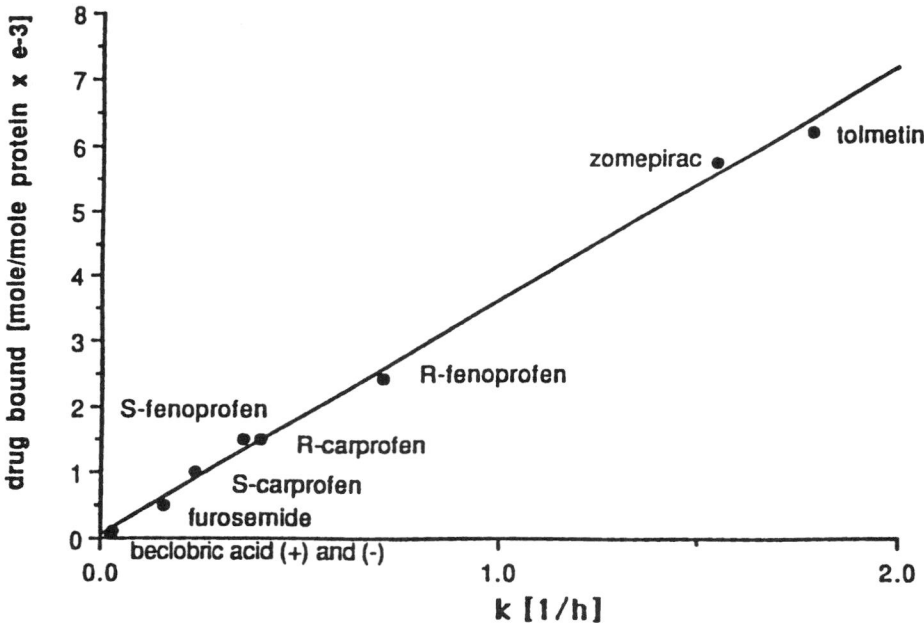

Figure 6 Plot of maximum epitope density (moles drug covalently bound per mole of protein × 10^3) versus degradation rate constant (h^{-1}) for the in vitro incubation of various acyl glucuronides (1 μM) in the presence of human serum albumin (0.5 mM). Degradation rates reflect both acyl migration and hydrolysis. Results are obtained from seven different studies over a 6-year period utilizing purified β-1-O-acyl glucuronides of zomepirac (72), tolmetin (25), carprofen (75), fenoprofen (62), furosemide (41,66), and beclobric acid (27). The data points for (+) and (−) enantiomers of beclobric acid are indistinguishable on the scale used. (From Ref. 59.)

6-year period with respect to in vitro degradation rates of the β-1-O-acyl glucuronides and the in vitro covalent binding for nine drug molecules, suggesting that the extent of in vitro covalent binding to albumin is predictable based on the chemical structure of the acid and depends on the degree of substitution at the alpha carbon to the carboxylic acid.

It may be expected that the relationship for in vivo covalent binding would be more complex than that of in vitro binding. However, the degree of covalent binding to plasma proteins should depend, at least, on the plasma concentrations of the acyl glucuronides and the degradation rate of each conjugate. The plasma concentrations of acyl glucuronides vary with the drug studied, and are dependent on the rate of formation, its degradation and elimination, as well as the administration dose. Acyl glucuronides of some carboxylic acids may reach significant concentrations in plasma of humans, as shown for zomepirac (95), tolmetin (113), diflunisal (76), beclobric acid (27), and etodolac (29), while no oxaprozin (16) and fenofibric acid (82) glucuronides have been detected in human plasma. In vivo studies (Table 4) with five carboxylic acid drugs, at their usual therapeutical doses, in five different sets of healthy volunteers, showed a 30-fold variation in AUCs for acyl glucuronides, whereas the maximum plasma protein binding showed a 25-fold variation. Since for each drug there is a direct relationship between the amount of covalent binding and the extent of exposure of acyl glucuronide (AUC), we normalize bound drug to AUC for comparison with in vitro glucuronide degradation rates, yielding a highly significant

Table 4 In Vivo Bound Drug, Area Under the Plasma Drug Glucuronide Concentration Time Curve (AUC), and In Vitro Acyl Glucuronide Degradation Rates[a]

Parent compound	Bound drug (mole/mole protein) $\times 10^4$	AUC glucuronide (mole $\times$ h/L) $\times 10^6$	Bound/AUC 10^{-2}	k hr^{-1}
Tolmetin	2.77 ± 1.54	3.72 ± 0.95	0.75	1.78
Zomepirac	2.33 ± 0.45	6.41 ± 2.14	0.36	1.54
(R)-fenoprofen	1.02 ± 0.32	6.31 ± 5.65	0.16	0.71
(S)-fenoprofen	3.23 ± 0.85	60.4 ± 24.7	0.054	0.36
Racemic carprofen	1.92 ± 1.28	40.9 ± 7.3	0.047	0.32
(+)-Beclobric acid	0.12 ± 0.03	8.16 ± 1.34	0.015	0.031
(−)-Beclobric acid	0.20 ± 0.11	8.31 ± 1.63	0.024	0.027

[a] Measurement of maximum amount of drug covalently bound to human serum albumin and area under the plasma concentration time curve (AUC) for the glucuronide conjugates measured in five different groups of healthy volunteers following oral dosing of either 400 mg of tolmetin (113), 100 mg of zomepirac (72), 600 mg of racemic fenoprofen (62), 50 mg of racemic carprofen (75), or 100 mg of racemic beclobric acid (27). When covalently bound drug is normalized to area under the curve for the respective glucuronide conjugates, an excellent correlation with the in vitro degradation rate constant (k) is obtained with an r^2 of 0.873.
Source: Ref. 59.

linear correlation ($r^2 = 0.873$). The findings presented in Table 4 suggest that the in vivo covalent binding of acidic drugs to albumin in humans is also predictable on the basis of the degradation rate constant of the glucuronide conjugate when the extent of covalent binding is corrected for the levels of the glucuronide present in plasma (AUC).

IX. POTENTIAL TOXICOLOGICAL SIGNIFICANCE OF THE REACTIVE ACYL GLUCURONIDES

It has been hypothesized that acyl glucuronides, owing to their reactive nature, may have a role in the observed toxicities associated with administration of a number of acidic compounds. It is striking that of 47 drugs withdrawn from U.S., British, and Spanish markets from 1964 through 1993 owing to severe toxicity (5,6), 10 are carboxylic acids. These drugs—alclofenac, bendazac, benoxaprofen, fenclofenac, ibufenac, indoprofen, pirprofen, suprofen, ticrynafen, and zomepirac—are primarily metabolized by humans to acyl glucuronides. For all these discontinued carboxylic acids, the most frequent types of adverse reaction leading to the decision to discontinue the products were idiosyncratic toxicities, such as liver damage, serious skin reactions, and renal toxicity, sometimes associated with fever, rash, and eosinophilia.

Covalent binding of carboxylic acids to proteins via their common reactive intermediates, acyl glucuronides, has been proposed to mediate such idiosyncratic toxicities associated with carboxylic acid–containing drugs (11,114). Both direct toxic effects and immune-mediated toxicity (hypersensitivity reactions) have been suggested as a possible mechanism of idiosyncratic liver injury (115). With direct toxicity, covalent protein binding via acyl glucuronides may disrupt the normal physiological function of a "critical" protein or some critical regulatory pathway, leading to cellular necrosis. Alternatively, the chemical reactive acyl glucuronides of carboxylic acids can act as a hapten and initiate an immune reaction that may be mediated via a specific humoral (antibody) response, a cellular response (T lymphocytes), or a combination of both (12,117). In most cases, the differentiation of these two forms of idiosyncratic toxicity is largely empirical as it is based on the clinical symptoms; for example, manifestations such as rash, fever, lymph-adenopathy, and eosinophilia all suggest drug hypersensitivity (immune-mediated toxic-ity). The lack of the clinical hallmarks of immunoallergic reactions, combined with the nature of the histological changes, may suggest a direct toxic reaction.

At present, the exact mechanisms responsible for the initiation and perpetuation of carboxylic acid–associated idiosyncratic organ (especially liver) toxicity and anaphylaxis remain poorly understood. Although it has not been ultimately proven that immune reac-tions are causally involved in such toxicities, a number of reports from the literature have provided evidence that immune-mediated toxicity plays an important role (1,116). Drug-specific antibodies have been detected in aspirin-hypersensitive patients (118) and in pa-tients receiving valproic acid therapy (35). Immunization with the mouse albumin conju-gate of tolmetin glucuronide has been demonstrated to stimulate an antibody response in mice (119). Antiadduct antibodies formed in mice following the administration of tol-metin-albumin adducts appeared to be specific for the aglycone and some cross-reactivity was observed for the structurally related carboxylic acids and their glucuronides. Recently, Kretz-Rommel and Boelsterli have characterized the selective covalent binding of diclo-fenac to rat and mice liver proteins in vivo, in cultured hepatocytes (105), and in subcellu-lar incubations (87). Since these selective protein adducts were shown not to exhibit a direct cytotoxic effect in short-term cultures of hepatocytes, the authors proposed that such selective covalent binding may be involved in the development of an immunogenic reaction in vivo (120). To confirm such a hypothesis, a murine ex vivo/in vitro mixed lymphocyte hepatocyte culture (MLHC) model was developed (120). Cultured hepatocytes from C57BL mice, preexposed to nontoxic concentrations of diclofenac, were cocultured with splenocytes derived from mice immunized with a synthetic diclofenac-protein adduct, that is, diclofenac covalently linked to the carrier protein, keyhole limpet hemocyanin (KLH). Splenocyte-mediated cytotoxicity was demonstrated by massively increased ala-nine aminotransferase release, an indicator of hepatocyte injury, apparent at 48 h in cocul-ture and present only in those cultures pretreated with diclofenac, not in the untreated controls or in the cocultures treated with KHL alone. These experiments imply a role for T cells in diclofenac-dependent cell killing and further support the possibility of immune-mediated toxicities (120).

In addition to drug hypersensitivity, direct disruption of function of critical proteins or important regulatory pathways by reactive acyl glucuronides may be involved in the idiosyncratic toxicities of carboxylic acids. For certain carboxylic acids, both mechanisms may be operative simultaneously.

The rare, but potentially lethal, idiosyncratic adverse reactions of carboxylic acids are highly host-dependent. The risk of the unpredictable hepatocytic injuries posed by carboxylic acids is small (121); nevertheless, fulminant hepatitis may develop in suscepti-ble patients, who may have abnormal metabolism or excretion of carboxylic acids, re-sulting in the overproduction and accumulation of reactive acyl glucuronides. Genetic and environmental variations in acyl glucuronidation, canalicular or sinusoidal secretion, and renal clearance of acyl glucuronides may all contribute to enhanced susceptibility, but these pathophysiological abnormalities have been poorly investigated. Specifically, interindividual variations in acyl glucuronidation in humans should be better characterized. Furthermore, the interindividual variations in canalicular excretion of acyl glucuronides may also need further characterization. Seitz et al. (122) have demonstrated that the reac-tive diclofenac glucuronide was selectively transported into rat bile via the canalicular conjugate export pump Mrp2 and that hepatobiliary transport is critical for diclofenac covalent binding to proteins in the biliary tree. By comparing the covalent binding pattern in normal Wistar rats with that in mutant Mrp2 transport-deficient (TR⁻) rats, the authors found that a major protein adduct of an apparent molecular mass of 118 kDa was selectively detected by immunoblotting in isolated canalicular, but not basolateral, membrane subfractions of wild-type rats, whereas no adducts could be identified in livers of TR⁻ rats (122). These results indicate the important role of transporters of acyl glucuronides in the selective covalent binding of carboxylic acids to proteins. Identification of potential genetic and environmental factors in the susceptible individuals will not only allow us to identify the vulnerable individuals, but also help us better understand the mechanism of toxicity.

ACKNOWLEDGMENT

Preparation of the manuscript and the studies from the authors' laboratory were supported by NIH Grant GM36633.

REFERENCES

1. Faed EM. Properties of acyl glucuronides: implications for studies of the pharmacokinetics and metabolism of acidic drugs. Drug Metab Rev 1984; 15:1213–1249.
2. Spahn-Langguth H, Benet LZ. Acyl glucuronides revisited: Is the glucuronidation process a toxification as well as detoxification mechanism? Drug Metab Rev 1992; 24:5–47.
3. Zimmerman HJ. Update of the hepatotoxicity due to classes of drugs in common clinical use: nonsteroidal drugs, anti-inflammatory drugs, antibiotics, antihypertensives, and cardiac and psychotropic agents. Semin Liver Dis 1990; 10:322–338.
4. Zimmerman HJ. Hepatic injury associated with nonsteroidal anti-inflammatory drugs. In: AJ Lewis, DE Furst, eds. Nonsteroidal Antiinflammatory Drugs: Mechanisms and Clinical Use. New York: Marcel Dekker, 1994:171–194.
5. Bakke OM, Wardell WM, Lasagna L. Drug discontinuations in the United Kingdom and the United States, 1964 to 1983: Issues of safety. Clin Pharmacol Ther 1984; 35:559–567.
6. Bakke OM, Manocchia M, de Abajo F, Kaitin KI, Lasagna L. Drug safety discontinuations in the United Kingdom, the United States and Spain from 1974 to 1993, a regulatory perspective. Clin Pharmacol Ther 1995; 58:108–117.
7. Stogniew M, Fenselau C. Electrophilic reactions of acyl-linked glucuronides, formation of clofibrate mercapturate in human. Drug Metab Dispos 1982; 10:609–613.
8. Shore LJ, Fenselau C, King AR, Dickinson RG. Characterization and formation of the glutathione conjugate of clofibric acid. Drug Metab Dispos 1995; 23:119–123.
9. Grillo MP, Benet LZ. In vitro studies of tolmetin metabolism in fresh isolated rat hepatocytes. Identification of a tolmetin-glycine amino acid conjugate. ISSX Proc 1995; 8:228.
10. van Breeman RB, Fenselau C. Reaction of 1-*O*-acyl glucuronides with 4-(*p*-nitrobenzyl)pyridine. Drug Metab Dispos 1986; 14:197–201.
11. Boelsterli UA, Zimmerman HJ, Kretz-Rommel A. Idiosyncratic liver toxicity of nonsteroidal antiinflammatory drugs: molecular mechanisms and pathology. Crit Rev Toxicol 1995; 25:207–235.
12. Park BK, Coleman JW, Kitteringham NR. Drug disposition and drug hypersensitivity. Biochem Pharmacol 1987; 36:581–590.
13. Burchell B, Brierley CH, Rance D. Specificity of human UDP-glucuronosyl transferases and xenobiotic glucuronidation. Life Sci 1995; 57:1819–1831.
14. Magdalou J, Chajes V, Lafaurie C, Siest G. Glucuronidation of 2-arylpropionic acids pirpro-

fen, flurbiprofen, and ibuprofen by liver microsomes. Drug Metab Dispos 1990; 18:692–697.

15. Panfil I, Lehman PA, Zimniak P, Ernst B, Franz T, Lester R, Radominska A. Biosynthesis and chemical synthesis of carboxyl-linked glucuronide of lithocholic acid. Biochim Biophys Acta 1992; 1126:221–228.

16. Ruelius RW, Kirkham SK, Young EM, Jassen FW. Reaction of oxaprozin-1-O-acyl glucuronide in solutions of human plasma and albumin. Adv Exp Med Biol 1986; 197:431–441.

17. Smith PC, Benet LZ, McDonagh AF. Covalent binding of zomepirac glucuronide to proteins: evidence for a Schiff base mechanism. Drug Metab Dispos 1990; 18:639–644.

18. Grubb N, Weil A, Caldwell J. Studies of the in vitro reactivity of clofibryl and fenofibryl glucuronides, evidence for protein binding via a schiff base mechanism. Biochem Pharmacol 1993; 46:357–364.

19. Parikh I, MacGlashan DW, Fenselau C. Immobilized glucuronosyltransferase for the synthesis of conjugates. J Med Chem 1976; 19:296–299.

20. Fenselau C, Pallante S, Parikh I. Solid-phase synthesis of drug glucuronides by immobilized glucuronosyltransferase. J Med Chem 1976; 19:679–683.

21. van Breemen RB, Fenselau C. Acylation of albumin by 1-O-acyl glucuronides. Drug Metab Dispos 1985; 13:316–320.

22. Bradow G, Kan L, Fenselau C. Studies of intramolecular rearrangements of acyl-linked glucuronides using salicylic acid, flufenamic acid, and (S)- and (R)-benoxaprofen and confirmation of isomerization in acyl-linked Δ^9-11-carboxyltetrahydrocannabinol glucuronide. Chem Res Toxicol 1989; 2:316–324.

23. Eggers NJ, Doust K. Isolation and identification of probenecid acyl glucuronide. J Pharm Pharmacol 1981; 33:123–124.

24. Hasegawa J, Smith PC, Benet LZ. Apparent intramolecular acyl migration of zomepirac glucuronide. Drug Metab Dispos 1982; 10:469–473.

25. Munafo A, McDonagh AF, Smith PC, Benet LZ. Irreversible binding of tolmetin glucuronic acid ester to albumin in vitro. Pharm Res 1990; 7:21–27.

26. Watt JA, King AR, Dickinson RG. Contrasting systemic stabilities of the acyl and phenolic glucuronides of diflunisal in the rat. Xenobiotica 1991; 21:403–415.

27. Mayer S, Mutschler E, Benet LZ, Spahn-Langguth H. In vitro and in vivo irreversible plasma protein binding of beclobric acid enantiomers. Chirality 1993; 5:120–125.

28. Iwakawa S, Suganuma T, Lee S, Spahn H, Benet LZ, Lin ET. Direct determination of diastereomeric carprofen glucuronides in human plasma and urine and preliminary measurements of stereoselective metabolic and renal elimination after oral administration of carprofen in man. Drug Metab Dispos 1989; 17:414–419.

29. Smith PC, Song WQ, Rodriguez RJ. Covalent binding of etodolac acyl glucuronide to albumin in vitro. Drug Metab Dispos 1992; 20:962–965.

30. Smith PC, Liu JH. Covalent binding of suprofen acyl glucuronide to albumin in vitro. Xenobiotica 1993; 23:337–348.

31. Castillo M, Smith PC. Disposition and reactivity of ibuprofen and ibufenac acyl glucuronides in vivo in the Rhesus monkey and in vitro with human serum albumin. Drug Metab Dispos 1995; 23:566–572.

32. Rachmel A, Hazelton GA, Yergey AL, Liberato DJ. Furosemide 1-O-acyl glucuronide, in vitro biosynthesis and pH-dependent isomerization to β-glucuronidase-resistant forms. Drug Metab Dispos 1985; 13:705–710.

33. McGurk KA, Remmel R, Hosagrahara VP, Tosh D, Burchell B. Reactivity of mefenamic acid 1-O-acyl glucuronide with proteins in vitro and ex vivo. Drug Metab Dispos 1996; 24:842–849.

34. Dickinson RG, Baker PV, King AR. Studies of the reactivity of acyl glucuronides. VII. Salicyl acyl glucuronide reactivity in vitro and covalent binding of salicylic acid to plasma protein of human taking aspirin. Biochem Pharmacol 1994; 47:469–476.

35. William AM, Worrall S, Jersey JD, Dickinson RG. Studies on the reactivity of acyl glucuronides. III. Glucuronide-derived adducts of valproic acid and plasma protein and anti-adduct antibody in humans. Biochem Pharmacol 1992; 43:745–755.

36. King AR, Dickinson RG. The utility of the bile-exteriorized rat as a source of reactive acyl glucuronides: studies with zomepirac. J Pharmacol Toxicol Method 1996; 36:131–136.

37. Sinclair KA, Caldwell J. The formation of β-glucuronidase resistant glucuronides by intramolecular rearrangement of glucuronic acid conjugates at mild alkaline pH. Biochem Pharmacol 1982; 31:953–957.

38. Hyneck ML, Smith PC, Unseld E, Benet LZ. High-performance liquid chromatographic determination of tolmetin glucuronide and its isomeric conjugates in plasma and urine. J Chromatogr 1987; 420:349–356.

39. Blanckaert N, Compernolle F, Leroy P, Van Hautte R, Fevery J, Heirwegh KPM. The fate of bilirubin-IX α glucuronide in cholestasis and during storage in vitro. Biochem J 1978; 171:203–214.

40. Hansen-Moller J, Cornett C, Dalgaard L, Hansen SH. Isolation and identification of the rearrangement products of diflunisal 1-O-acyl glucuronide. J Pharm Biomed Anal 1988; 6: 229–240.

41. Sekikawa H, Yagi N, Lin ET, Benet LZ. Apparent intramolecular acyl migration and hydrolysis of furosemide glucuronide in aqueous solution. Biol Pharm Bull 1995; 18:134–139.

42. Spahn H, Iwakawa S, Benet LZ. Stereoselective formation and degradation of flunoxaprofen glucuronides in microsomal incubations. Pharm Res 1988; 5(suppl):S200.

43. Spahn H, Iwakawa S, Lin ET, Benet LZ. Procedures to characterize in vitro and in vivo enantioselective glucuronidation properly: studies with benoxaprofen glucuronides. Pharm Res 1989; 6:125–132.

44. Volland C, Benet LZ. In vitro enantioselective glucuronidation of fenoprofen. Pharmacology 1991; 43:53–60.

45. Fournel-Gigleux S, Hammar-Hansen C, Motassim N, Atoine B, Mothe O, Decolin D, Caldwell J, Siest G. Substrate specific and enantioselectivity of arylcarboxylic acid glucuronidation. Drug Metab Dispos 1988; 16:627–634.

46. el Mouelhi M, Ruelius HW, Fenselau C, Dulik DM. Species-dependent enantioselective glucuronidation of three 2-arylpropionic acids, naproxen, ibuprofen, and benoxaprofen. Drug Metab Dispos 1987; 15:767–772.

47. Georges H, Persle N, Buronfosse T, Fournel-Gigleux S, Netter P, Magdalou J, Lapicque F. In vitro stereoselective degradation of carprofen glucuronide by human serum albumin: characterization of sites and reactive amino acids. Chirality 2000; 12:53–62.

48. Buszewski B, el Mouelhi M, Albert K, Bayer E. Influence of the structure of chemically bonded C18 phase on HPLC separation of naproxen glucuronide diastereomers. J Liq Chromatogr 1990; 13:505–524.

49. Chakir S, Maurice M, Magdalou J, Leroy P, Dubois N, Lapicque F, Abdelhamid Z, Nicolas A. High-performance liquid chromatographic enantioselective assay for the measurement of ketoprofen glucuronidation by liver microsomes. J Chromatogr B 1994; 654:61–68.

50. Heirwegh KP, Compernolle F. Micro-analytic detection and structure elucidation of ester-glycoside. Biochem Pharmacol 1979; 28:2109–2114.

51. Compernolle F, Blanckaert N, Heirweg KPM. The fate of bilirubin-IXα glucuronides in cholestatic bile: sequential migration of the 1-acylaglycone to 2-, 3-, and 4-positions of glucuronic acid. Biochem Soc Trans 1977; 5:317–319.

52. Smith PC, Benet LZ. Characterization of the isomeric esters of zomepirac glucuronide by proton NMR. Drug Metab Dispos 1986; 14:503–505.

53. Upton RA, Williams RL, Buskin JN, Jones RM. Effects of probenecid on ketoprofen kinetics. Clin Pharmacol Ther 1982; 31:705–712.

54. Haine AH. Relative reactivities of hydroxyl groups in carbohydrates. Adv Carbohydr Chem Biochem 1976; 33:101–109.

55. Illing HP, Wilson ID. pH dependent formation of β-glucuronidase resistant conjugates from the biosynthetic ester glucuronide of isoxepac. Biochem Pharmacol 1981; 30:3381–3384.

56. Dickinson RG, Hooper WD, Eadie MJ. pH-Dependent rearrangement of the biosynthetic ester glucuronide of valproic acid to β-glucuronidase-resistant forms. Drug Metab Dispos 1984; 12:247–252.

57. Yang DY, Benet LZ. Stability of diclofenac acyl glucuronide and irreversible binding to plasma proteins in vitro. Pharm Res 1995; 12:S-377.

58. Sallustio BC, Fairchild BA, Panall PR. Interaction of human serum albumin with the electrophilic metabolite 1-*O*-gemfibrozil-beta-D-glucuronide. Drug Metab Dispos 1997; 25:55–60.

59. Benet LZ, Spahn H, Iwakawa H, Volland C, Mizuma T, Mayer S, Mutschler E, Lin ET. Prediction of covalent binding of acidic drugs in man. Life Sci 1993; 53:PL141–146.

60. Smith PC, Hasegawa J, Langedijk PJ, Benet LZ. Stability of acyl glucuronides in blood, plasma, and urine: studies with zomepirac. Drug Metab Dispos 1985; 13:110–112.

61. Wells DS, Janssen FW. Interactions between oxaprozin glucuronide and human serum albumin. Xenobiotica 1987; 17:1437–1449.

62. Volland C, Sun H, Dammeyer J, Benet LZ. Stereoselective degradation of the fenoprofen acyl glucuronide enantiomers and irreversible binding to plasma protein. Drug Metab Dispos 1991; 19:1080–1086.

63. Hayball PJ, Nation RL, Bochner F. Stereoselective interactions of ketoprofen glucuronides with human plasma and serum albumin. Biochem Pharmacol 1992; 44:291–299.

64. Bischer A, Zia-Amirhosseini P, Iwaki M, McDonagh AF, Benet LZ. Stereoselective binding properties of naproxen glucuronide diastereomers to proteins. J Pharmacokinet Biopharm 1995; 23:379–395.

65. Watt J, Dickinson RG. Reactivity of diflunisal acyl glucuronide in human and rat plasma and albumin solutions. Biochem Pharmacol 1990; 39:1067–1075.

66. Mizuma T, Benet LZ, Lin ET. Interaction of human serum albumin with furosemide glucuronide: a role of albumin in isomerization, hydrolysis, reversible binding and irreversible binding of a 1-*O*-acyl glucuronide metabolite. Biopharm Drug Dispos 1999; 20:131–136.

67. Sudlow G, Birkett DJ, Wade DN. Further characterization of specific drug binding sites on human serum albumin. Mol Pharmacol 1976; 12:1052–1061.

68. Iwakawa S, Spahn H, Benet LZ, Lin ET. Stereoselective binding of the glucuronide conjugates of carprofen enantiomers to human serum albumin. Biochem Pharmacol 1990; 39:949–953.

69. Ojingwa JC, Spahn-Langguth H, Benet LZ. Reversible binding of tolmetin, zomepirac, and their glucuronide conjugates to human serum albumin and plasma. J Pharmacokin Biopharm 1994; 22:19–40.

70. Bischer A, Iwaki M, Zia-Amirhosseini P, Benet LZ. Stereoselective reversible binding properties of the glucuronide conjugates of fenoprofen enantiomers to human serum albumin. Drug Metab Dispos 1995; 23:900–903.

71. Kuenzle CC, Maier C, Ruttner JR. The nature of four bilirubin fractions from serum and of three bilirubin fractions from bile. J Lab Clin Med 1966; 67:294–306.

72. Smith PC, McDonagh AF, Benet LZ. Irreversible binding of zomepirac to plasma in vitro and in vivo. J Clin Invest 1986; 77:934–939.

73. Munafo A, Hyneck ML, Benet LZ. Pharmacokinetics and irreversible binding of tolmetin and its glucuronic acid esters in the elderly. Pharmacology 1993; 47:309–317.

74. Zia-Amirhosseini P, Ojingwa J, Spahn-Langguth H, McDonagh AF, Benet LZ. Enhanced covalent binding of tolmetin to proteins in humans after multiple dosing. Clin Pharmacol Ther 1994; 55:21–27.

75. Iwakawa S, Spahn H, Benet LZ, Lin ET. Carprofen glucuronide: stereoselective degradation and interaction with human serum albumin. Pharm Res 1988; 5(suppl):S-214.

76. McKinnon GE, Dickinson RG. Covalent binding of diflunisal and probenecid to plasma pro-

tein in humans: persistence of the adducts in the circulation. Res Commun Chem Pathol Pharmacol 1989; 3:1033–1039.

77. Sallustio BC, Knights KM, Roberts BJ, Zacest R. In vivo covalent binding of clofibric acid to human plasma proteins and rat liver proteins. Biochem Pharmacol 1991; 42:1421–1425.

78. Pohl LR, Branchflower RV. Covalent binding of electrophilic metabolites to macromolecules. Meth Enzymol 1981; 77:43–50.

79. Pumford NR, Halmes NC, Hinson JA. Covalent binding of xenobiotics to specific proteins in the liver. Drug Metab Rev 1997; 29:39–57.

80. Cohen SD, Pumford NR, Khairallah EA, Boekelheide K, Pohl LR, Amouzadeh HR, Hinson JA. Selective protein covalent binding and target organ toxicity. Toxicol Appl Pharmacol 1997; 143:1–12.

81. Pumford NR, Myers TG, Davila JC, Highet RJ, Pohl LR. Immunochemical detection of liver protein adducts of the nonsteroidal antiinflammatory drug diclofenac. Chem Res Toxicol 1993; 6:147–150.

82. Wel A, Guichard JP, Caldwell J. Interactions between fenofibryl glucuronides and human serum albumin or human plasma. In: G Siest, J Magdalou, B Burchell, eds. Cellular and Molecular Aspect of Glucuronidation. Colloque INSERM/John Libbey Eurotext Ltd. Montrouge, France, 1988; 173:233–236.

83. Dubois N, Lapicque F, Maurice M, Pritchard M, Fournel-Gigleux S, Magdalou J, Abiteboul M, Siest G, Netter P. In vitro irreversible binding of ketoprofen glucuronide to plasma proteins. Drug Metab Dispos 1993; 21:617–623.

84. Hansen-Moller J, Schmit U. Rapid high-performance liquid chromatographic assay for the simultaneous determination of probenecid and its glucuronide in urine. Irreversible binding of probenecid to serum albumin. J Pharm Biomed Anal 1991; 9:65–73.

85. Ojingwa JC, Spahn-Langguth H, Benet LZ. Irreversible binding of tolmetin to macromolecules via its glucuronide: binding to blood constituents, tissue homogenates and subcellular fractions in vitro. Xenobiotica 1994; 24:495–506.

86. Bailey MJ, Worrall S, de Jersey J, Dickinson RG. Zomepirac acyl glucuronide covalently modifies tubulin in vitro and in vivo and inhibits its assembly in an in vitro system. Chem Biol Intercations 1998; 115:153–166.

87. Kretz-Rommel A, Boelsterli UA. Mechanism of covalent adduct formation of diclofenac to rat hepatic microsome proteins, retention of the glucuronic acid moiety in the adduct. Drug Metab Dispos 1994; 22:956–961.

88. McDonagh AF, Palma LA, Lauff JJ, Wu T-W. Origin of mammalian biliprotein and rearrangement of bilirubin glucuronide in vivo in the rat. J Clin Invest 1984; 74:763–770.

89. van Breemen RB, Fenselau C, Mogilevsky W, Odell GB. Reaction of bilirubin glucuronides with serum albumin. J Chromatogr 1986; 383:287–392.

90. Garlick RL, Mazer JS. The principal site of non-enzymatic glycosylation of human serum albumin in vivo. J Biol Chem 1983; 258:6142–6146.

91. Dickinson RG, King AR. Studies on the reactivity of acyl glucuronides. II. Interaction of diflunisal acyl glucuronide and its isomers with human serum albumin in vitro. Biochem Pharmacol 1991; 42:2301–2306.

92. Ding A, Ojingwa JC, McDonagh AF, Burlingame AL, Benet LZ. Evidence for covalent binding of acyl glucuronides to serum albumin via an imine mechanism as revealed by tandem mass spectrometry. Proc Natl Acad Sci USA 1993; 90:3797–3801.

93. Ding A, Zia-Amirhosseini P, McDonagh AF, Burlingame AL, Benet LZ. Reactivity of tolmetin glucuronide with human serum albumin, identification of binding sites and mechanisms of reaction by tandem mass spectrometry. Drug Metab Dispos 1995; 23:369–375.

94. Qiu Y, Burlingame A, Benet LZ. Mechanisms for covalent binding of benoxaprofen glucuronide to human serum albumin, studies by tandem mass spectrometry. Drug Metab Dispos 1998; 26:246–256.

95. Smith PC, Langendijk PNJ, Bosso JA, Benet LZ. Effect of probenecid on the formation and

elimination of acyl glucuronides: studies with zomepirac. Clin Pharmacol Ther 1985; 38: 121–127.

96. King AR, Dickinson RG. Studies on the reactivity of acyl glucuronides. IV. Covalent binding of diflunisal to tissues of rat. Biochem Pharmacol 1993; 45:1043–1047.

97. Williams AM, Worrall S, Jersey JD, Dickinson RG. Studies on the reactivity of acyl glucuronides. VIII. Generation of an antiserum for the detection of diflunisal-modified proteins in diflunisal-dosed rats. Biochem Pharmacol 1995; 49:209–217.

98. Dickinson RG, King AR. Studies on the reactivity of acyl glucuronides. V. Glucuronide-derived covalent binding of diflunisal to bladder tissue of rats and its modulation by urine pH and β-glucuronidase. Biochem Pharmacol 1993; 46:1175–1182.

99. Wade LT, Kenna JG, Caldwell J. Immunochemical identification of mouse hepatic protein adducts derived from the nonsteroidal anti-inflammatory drugs diclofenac, sulindac, and ibuprofen. Chem Res Toxicol 1997; 10:546–555.

100. Bailey MJ, Dickinson RG. Chemical and immunochemical comparison of protein adduct formation of four carboxylate drugs in rat liver and plasma. Chem Res Toxicol 1996; 9:659–666.

101. Sallustio BC, Foster DJ. Reactivity of gemfibrozil 1-O-β-acylglucuronide, pharmacokinetics of covalently bound gemfibrozil-protein adducts in rats. Drug Metab Dispos 1995; 23:892–899.

102. Kitteringham NR, Maggs JL, Newby S, Park BK. Drug-protein conjugates. VIII. The metabolic fate of the dinitrophenyl hapten conjugated to albumin. Biochem Pharmacol 1995; 34: 1763–1771.

103. Dahms M, Spahn-Langguth H. Covalent binding of acidic drugs via reactive intermediates; detection of benoxaprofen and flunoxaprofen protein adducts in biological material. Pharmazie 1996; 51:874–881.

104. Hargus SJ, Amouzedeh HR, Pumford NR, Myers TG, McCoy SC, Pohl LR. Metabolic activation and immunochemical localization of liver protein adducts of the nonsteroidal anti-inflammatory drug diclofenac. Chem Res Toxicol 1994; 7:575–582.

105. Kretz-Rommel A, Boelsterli UA. Selective protein adducts to membrane proteins in cultured rat hepatocytes exposed to diclofenac: radiochemical and immunochemical analysis. Mol Pharmacol 1994; 45:237–244.

106. Gil ML, Ramirez MC, Terencio MC, Castell JV. Immunochemical detection of protein adducts in cultured human hepatocytes exposed to diclofenac. Biochim Biophys Acta 1995; 1272:140–146.

107. Shen TY. Nonsteroidal anti-inflammatory agents. In: ME Wolf, ed. Burger's Medicinal Chemistry, 4th ed., Part III. New York: Wiley Interscience, 1981:1205–1271.

108. Spahn H. Assay method for product formation in in vitro enzyme kinetic studies of uridine disposphate glucuronyltransferases: 2-arylpropionic acid enantiomers. J Chromatogr 1988; 430:368–375.

109. Spahn H, Benet LZ. Enantioselectivity of hepatic UDP-glucuronyltransferase in rat liver microsomes towards 2-arylpropionic acids: glucuronidation of naproxen enantiomers. Third European Congress on Biopharmaceutics and Pharmacokinetics Proceedings, Vol. II. In: JM Aiache, J Hirtz, eds. Experimental Pharmacokinetics. Freiburg, 1987:261–268.

110. Hayball P. Formation and reactivity of acyl glucuronides: the influence of chirality. Chirality 1995; 7:1–9.

111. Spahn H, Iwakawa S, Ojingwa J, Benet LZ. Glucuronidation of flunoxaprofen enantiomers by UDPGTs from different sources. International Conference on Pharmaceutical Sciences and Clinical Pharmacology, Jerusalem, May/June 1988.

112. Spahn-Langguth H, Benet LZ, Zia-Amirhosseini P, Iwakawa H, Langguth P. Kinetics of reactive phase II metabolites: stereochemical aspects of formation of epimeric acyl glucuronides and their reactivity. In: HY Aboul-Enein, IW Wainer, eds. The impact of stereochem-

istry on drug development and use. Chemical Analysis Series, Vol. 142. New York: Wiley, 1997:125–170.

113. Hyneck ML, Smith PC, Munafo A, McDonagh AF, Benet LZ. Disposition and irreversible plasma protein binding of tolmetin in humans. Clin Pharmacol Ther 1988; 44:107–114.

114. Pumford NR, Halmes NC. Protein targets of xenobiotic reactive intermediates. Annu Rev Pharmacol Toxicol 1997; 37:91–117.

115. Pirmohamed M, Madden S, Park BK. Idiosyncratic drug reactions metabolic bioactivation as a pathogenic mechanism. Clin Pharmacokinet 1996; 31:215–230.

116. Benet LZ, Spahn H. Acyl migration and covalent binding of drug glucuronides—potential toxicity mediators. In: G Siest, J Magdalou, B Burchell, eds. Cellular and Molecular Aspects of Glucuronidation. Colloque INSERM/John Libbey Eurotext Ltd. Montrouge, France. 1988; 173:261–269.

117. Pohl LR, Satoh H, Christ DD, Kenna JG. The immunological and metabolic basis of drug hypersensitivities. Annu Rev Pharmacol 1988; 28:367–387.

118. Amos HE, Wilson DV, Taussig MJ, Carlton SJ. Hypersensitivity reactions to acetylsalicylic acid. Clin Exp Immunol 1971; 8:563–572.

119. Zia-Amirhosseini P, Harris R, Brodsky FM, Benet LZ. Hypersensitivity to nonsteroidal anti-inflammatory drugs. Nature Med 1995; 1:2–4.

120. Kretz-Rommel A, Boelsterli UA. Cytotoxic toxicity of T cells and non-T cells from diclofenac-immunized mice against cultured syngeneic hepatocytes exposed to diclofenac. Hepatology 1995; 22:213–222.

121. Garcia Rodriguez LA, Williams R, Derby LE, Dean AD, Jick H. Acute liver injury associated with nonsteroidal anti-inflammatory drugs and the role of risk factor. Arch Intern Med 1994; 154:311–316.

122. Seitz S, Kretz-Rommel A, Elferink RPJO, Boelsterli UA. Selective protein adduct formation of diclofenac glucuronide is critically dependent on the rat canalicular conjugate export pump (Mrp2). Chem Res Toxicol 1998; 11:513–519.

123. Dickinson RG, King AR. Reactivity considerations in the analysis of glucuronide and sulfate conjugates of diflunisal. Ther Drug Monit 1989; 11:712–720.

124. Sallustio BC, Fairchild BA. Biosynthesis, characterization and direct high-performance liquid chromatographic analysis of gemfibrozil 1-O-β-acylglucuronide. J Chromatogr B 1995; 665: 345–353.

125. van Breemen RB, Fenselau CC, Dulik DM. Activated phase II metabolites: comparison of alkylation by 1-O-acyl glucuronides and acyl sulfates. Adv Exp Med Biol 1986; 197:423–429.

126. Akira K, Taira T, Hasegawa H, Sakuma C, Shinohara Y. Studies on the stereoselective internal acyl migration of ketoprofen glucuronide using ^{13}C labeling and nuclear magnetic resonance spectroscopy. Drug Metab Dispos 1998; 26:457–464.

127. Ruelius RW, Young EM, Kirkman SK, Schilings RT, Sisenwine SF, Jassen FW. Biological fate of acyl glucuronides in the rat: the role of rearrangement, intestinal enzyme and reabsorption. Biochem Pharmacol 1985; 34:451–452.

128. Sekikawa H, Yagi N, Oda K, Kenmotsu H, Takada M, Chen H, Lin ET, Benet LZ. Biliary excretion of furosemide glucuronide in rabbits. Biol Pharm Bull 1995; 18:447–453.

9

Nonparenchymal Cells, Inflammatory Macrophages, and Hepatotoxicity

DEBRA L. LASKIN and CAROL R. GARDNER

Rutgers University, Piscataway, New Jersey, U.S.A.

I. INTRODUCTION

Over the past several years considerable evidence has accumulated demonstrating that hepatotoxicity induced by a diverse group of drugs and chemicals is due not only to a direct effect of these compounds on the liver, but also indirectly to the actions of inflammatory mediators released by nonparenchymal cells, in particular macrophages, endothelial cells, and stellate cells, as well as infiltrating leukocytes. Following exposure of experimental animals to hepatotoxicants, these cells become "activated." This involves alterations in their functional and biochemical properties leading to the release of an array of proinflammatory and cytotoxic mediators that have the capacity to promote liver damage. These findings, together with the observation that hepatotoxicity can be modified by agents that modulate inflammatory cell and mediator activity, provide direct evidence that these cells contribute to tissue injury. The mediators involved in the cytotoxic process include reactive oxygen and reactive nitrogen intermediates, proinflammatory cytokines, proteolytic enzymes, eicosanoids, and/or bioactive lipids released at sites of injury. Whereas some of these mediators are directly cytotoxic (e.g., hydrogen peroxide, nitric oxide, peroxynitrite), others degrade the extracellular matrix (e.g., collagenase, elastase) and/or promote inflammatory cell adhesion and infiltration, and nonparenchymal cell proliferation and activation [e.g., interleukin-1 (IL-1), interleukin-6 (IL-6), tumor necrosis factor-α (TNFα), transforming growth factor-β, (TGFβ), platelet-activating factor (PAF), chemokines, and colony-stimulating factors]. There is also evidence that some of the mediators produced by activated nonparenchymal cells and inflammatory macrophages can modify hepatocyte protein and nucleic acid biosynthesis, as well as cytochrome P450–mediated xenobiotic metabolism, which may also contribute to hepatotoxicity. In this chapter experimental evidence implicating nonparenchymal cells and inflammatory macrophages and mediators produced by these cells in hepatotoxicity is reviewed.

II. HEPATIC NONPARENCHYMAL CELLS AND TISSUE INJURY

The liver is comprised of two main cell populations: parenchymal cells or hepatocytes and nonparenchymal cells, the majority of which reside within the hepatic sinusoids, positioned between the arterial vasculature and the parenchyma. Sinusoidal cells consist mainly of Kupffer cells, endothelial cells, and stellate cells. A small population (about 3%) of pit cells are also found within the hepatic sinusoids. These are the natural killer cells of the liver. Over the past several years evidence has accumulated demonstrating that in addition to their normal function within the tissue, each of these sinusoidal cell populations has the potential to contribute to xenobiotic-induced liver injury. Moreover, cross-talk between these cells may augment their toxicological potential.

A. Kupffer Cells and Inflammatory Macrophages

Kupffer cells constitute approximately 30% of the hepatic sinusoidal cells and represent the largest population (80–90%) of all the macrophages in the body. They are predominantly localized in periportal and central regions of the liver lobule and are anchored to the lumen of the endothelium by long cytoplasmic processes (1). Thus they are well positioned to remove particulate and foreign materials from the portal circulation, primarily through phagocytosis. Kupffer cells possess Fc and C3 receptors, as well as scavenger receptors, carbohydrate receptors, and cell adhesion molecules, which facilitate their ability to phagocytize opsonized and nonopsonized particles, apoptotic and damaged cells, neutrophils, and tumor cells (2–11). A major function of Kupffer cells is uptake and detoxification of gut-derived endotoxin (12,13). This is accomplished by binding of lipopolysaccharide (LPS), the toxic moiety in endotoxin to CD14, Toll 4-like receptors, scavenger receptors, and/or macrosialin (4,14–16). Kupffer cells are among the most active secretory cells in the body releasing hundreds of different products with inflammatory, growth-promoting, and regulatory activity. These include superoxide anion, hydrogen peroxide, nitric oxide, peroxynitrite, proteolytic enzymes, and eicosanoids that aid in antigen destruction (7,17–24). They also release a number of different cytokines with immunoregulatory and proinflammatory actions including TNFα, IL-1, IL-6, IL-8, IL-10, IL-18, PAF, TGFβ, and interferon (24–26). Kupffer cells also elaborate growth factors involved in regulating the proliferation of hepatocytes, endothelial cells, and inflammatory macrophages (22,24,27–30). Because of their continuous exposure to endotoxin in the portal circulation, Kupffer cells are in a constant state of activation and are therefore primed to respond to tissue injury. Thus after exposure to inflammatory stimuli, Kupffer cells exhibit markedly increased chemotactic and phagocytic activity and display significantly greater oxidant-dependent and oxidant-independent cytotoxicity (6–9,17–21,31–36). Moreover, release of cytotoxic and proinflammatory mediators by these cells is greatly increased. These findings, together with the observation that hepatic macrophages increase in number in response to tissue injury, suggest that these cells have the capacity to modulate both normal and pathological processes in the liver. Recent studies have demonstrated that Kupffer cells, like resident macrophages present in other tissues, express MHC class II antigens and act as antigen-presenting cells for the induction of specific T-lymphocyte responses (37–39). This indicates that Kupffer cells can also contribute to specific immune responses of the liver to antigens.

A growing body of literature has been generated over the past several years that has provided strong evidence implicating liver macrophages in hepatotoxicity induced by a diverse group of agents (Table 1). These include acetaminophen, endotoxin, carbon tetrachloride, galactosamine, 1,2-dichlorobenzene, allyl alcohol, cadmium, and ethanol. With each of these compounds, hepatotoxicity is abrogated or prevented by pretreatment of experimental animals with agents such as gadolinium chloride, which block macrophage activity. The fact that the mechanisms underlying tissue injury induced by these different toxins are distinct suggests that an involvement of macrophages may be a critical step in the pathogenic process leading to hepatotoxicity.

One of the first lines of evidence suggesting that macrophages contribute to hepatotoxicity was the observation that there are increased numbers of these cells in the liver following exposure of animals to hepatotoxicants (7,18,40–45). These cells are typically observed in the liver prior to histological evidence of frank necrosis. Moreover, their specific location within the liver lobule varies with the chemical agent and is directly

Table 1 Agents Whose Toxicity Is Associated with Macrophages and Inflammatory Mediators

Toxicant	Response of liver macrophages	Ref.
Acetaminophen	Increase number, chemotaxis, phagocytosis, cytotoxicity, ROI, RNI, IL-1, TNFα, HO-1, chemokines, eicosanoids	18,48,118,165,173,203,206,228, 301,302
Endotoxin	Increased number, chemotaxis, phagocytosis, ROI, RNI, IL-1, TNFα, IL-6, PAF, lipids, I-CAM	6–9,17,20–22,25,32,35,36,43,74, 168,233,266,267,270,286
Carbon tetrachloride	Increased number, ROI, RNI, IL-1, IL-10, TNFα, IL-6, TGFβ, MCP-1	42,46,47,55,73,89,170,186,190,194, 198,224,225,253,303
Ethanol	Increased I-CAM, ROI, RNI, IL-1, TNFα, MIP-2, CINC, TGFβ	52,54,70,166,167,187,195,199,201, 202,252
1,2-Dichlorobenzene	Increased ROI	67,227
Galactosamine	Increased number, increased ROI, TNFα	33,41,44,50,57,79,178,184
Cadmium	Increased phagocytosis, IL-1, TNFα, CINC	68,69,71,179
Allyl alcohol	Increased ROI, TNFα	45,185

ROI, reactive oxygen intermediates; RNI, reactive nitrogen intermediates; HO-1, heme oxygenase-1.

correlated with areas of the tissue that subsequently exhibit signs of injury. For example, after administration of acetaminophen or carbon tetrachloride, agents that induce centrilobular hepatic necrosis, macrophages are observed in these regions of the liver (18,46–48). In contrast, macrophages that localize in the liver following endotoxin, phenobarbital, *Corynebacterium parvum*, or galactosamine treatment of rats are scattered in clusters throughout the liver lobule, which is consistent with patterns of injury observed after exposure to these toxins (7,40,41,49,50).

Inflammatory cell accumulation in tissues is generally considered to be an early marker of tissue injury. It is likely that the cells accumulating in the liver after hepatotoxicant exposure consist of both resident Kupffer cells and mononuclear phagocytes that have infiltrated into the tissue in response to damage. Both of these cell populations are highly sensitive to early-response cytokines such as TNFα and IL-1, rapidly generated at sites of tissue injury, and become "activated." Under homeostatic conditions macrophage activation is carefully regulated. However, following exposure of experimental animals to hepatotoxicants, resident Kupffer cells and inflammatory macrophages may become "overactivated" or "hyperresponsive" and produce excessive quantities of cytotoxic mediators. In this regard, a number of studies have demonstrated that macrophages isolated from livers of hepatotoxicant-treated animals display morphological and functional properties of "activated" mononuclear phagocytes (Fig. 1). Thus these cells appear larger and more stellate than cells from untreated rats, are highly vacuolated, and display an increased cytoplasmic : nuclear ratio (7,17,18,40,51). In addition, macrophages from animals treated with hepatotoxicants such as phenobarbital, acetaminophen, or endotoxin adhere to and spread on culture dishes more rapidly than resident Kupffer cells (7,18,40). These properties are characteristic of morphologically "activated" macrophages. Liver macrophages from animals treated with hepatotoxicants also exhibit varying degrees of functional activation including increased expression of cell adhesion molecules, and enhanced phagocytic, chemotactic, cytotoxic, and metabolic activity, as well as increased release of superoxide anion, hydrogen peroxide, nitric oxide, peroxynitrite, proteolytic enzymes, eicosanoids, IL-1, IL-6, TNFα, and chemokines (7,9,17,18,25,31–36,40,49,52–57). Activated Kupffer cells and infiltrating macrophages are thought to promote hepatic damage through the release of these toxic secretory products (58).

A second line of evidence supporting a role for macrophages in hepatotoxicity is derived from experiments in which animals are pretreated with agents that either inhibit

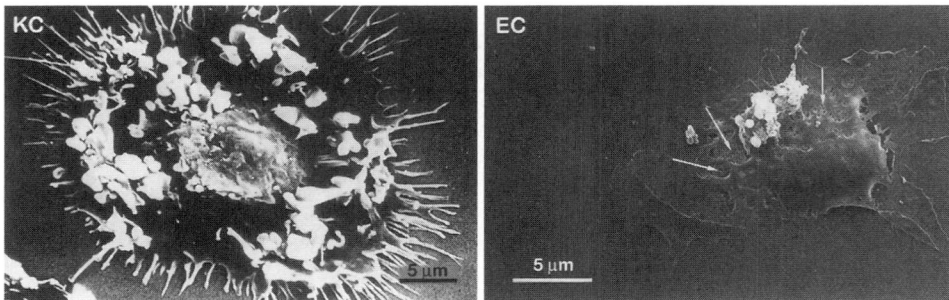

Figure 1   Scanning electron micrographs of an activated Kupffer cell (KC) and endothelial cell (EC) from an endotoxin-treated rat. Arrows indicate fenestrae in the endothelial cell. (Photo credit: Dr. Jay Wasserman, Bristol-Myers Squibb.)

or enhance macrophage activity and tissue injury is then assessed. Data from these studies clearly demonstrate that the degree of hepatic injury induced by a number of different chemicals is directly correlated with macrophage functioning. Thus, agents that depress macrophage functioning reduce toxicity, while compounds that augment macrophage activity enhance tissue injury. For example, drugs such as hydrocortisone, certain synthetic steroids, and natural substances that block inflammatory responses have been reported to protect against liver injury induced by carbon tetrachloride and acetaminophen (59,60). Similarly, the accumulation of macrophages in the liver and subsequent toxicity of acetaminophen, carbon tetrachloride, or endotoxin is prevented by pretreatment of animals with gadolinium chloride, carbon particles, dextran sulfate, or liposome-encapsulated dichloromethylene diphosphonate, compounds known to depress macrophage activity (61–64). Hepatoprotective effects of gadolinium chloride against 1,2-dichlorobenzene, diethyldicarbamate, galactosamine, ethanol, endotoxin, allyl alcohol, and cadmium-induced injury have also been described (45,65–72). Several studies have also demonstrated that activation of hepatic macrophages augments hepatic injury induced by toxic xenobiotics. Thus, pretreatment of rats with macrophage activators such as endotoxin, glucan, vitamin A, or latex beads aggravates liver injury induced by carbon tetrachloride, galactosamine, allyl alcohol, and C. parvum (20,32,49,55,72–80). Taken together, these observations support the hypothesis that macrophages contribute to hepatotoxicity. The specific mediators released by these cells that are involved in the pathogenic process appears to depend on the nature of the hepatotoxicant, as well as the levels of the mediator generated in the tissue and the extent to which other inflammatory signals are produced.

Recent studies have focused on analyzing mechanisms regulating macrophage activation following hepatotoxicant exposure. It has been suggested that this process involves inappropriate activation of biochemical signaling pathways in the cells leading to increased gene expression and inflammatory mediator production. For example, following acetaminophen administration to animals, a rapid increase in nuclear binding activity of the transcription factor, NF-κB has been observed in the liver (81). Similar effects have been described after treatment of animals with carbon tetrachloride, ethanol, endotoxin, or galactosamine (82–86). NF-κB is a ubiquitous transcription factor known to regulate the activity of numerous genes involved in inflammatory responses including inducible nitric oxide synthase (NOSII), cyclooxygenase-2 (COX-2), TNFα, and I-CAM-1 (87). Enhanced NF-κB expression induced by toxicants presumably modulates liver injury through an effect on the synthesis of these mediators (88). This idea is supported by the findings that mice lacking the p50 subunit of NF-κB do not generate TNFα and are protected from carbon tetrachloride–induced toxicity (89). Increased nuclear binding activity of the transcription factor AP-1 has also been described in the liver after treatment of animals with acetaminophen, carbon tetrachloride, or endotoxin (47,90,91). The fact that this activity is prevented by pretreatment of animals with gadolinium chloride demonstrates that Kupffer cells are crucial in the process. The proteins c-jun and c-fos constitute inducible transcription factors in signal transduction and regulate the activation of a battery of genes involved in cell growth. Recent studies have shown that c-fos and c-jun levels are also increased following administration of carbon tetrachloride or acetaminophen (85,92).

B. Sinusoidal Endothelial Cells in Hepatotoxicity

Endothelial cells form the walls of the hepatic sinusoids and represent the major fraction of hepatic sinusoidal cells (approximately 48%). Unlike endothelial cells in other vascular beds, hepatic sinusoidal endothelial cells are devoid of basement membrane (93). Moreover, they possess pores or fenestrae, which provides an opportunity for direct contact between plasma and hepatocytes. Thus sinusoidal endothelial cells function as a selective barrier between the blood and the liver parenchyma. Endothelial cells also possess unique "bristle-coated" membrane invaginations and vesicles, and lysosome-like vacuoles, and are thought to play a role in the clearance of macromolecules from the circulation. Through Fc, carbohydrate, and scavenger receptors, endothelial cells endocytose a variety of particles in the portal circulation including glycoproteins, lipoproteins, albumin, lactoferrin, and hyaluronic acid (2,4,5,10,94–101). It has been reported that endocytosis is upregulated in endothelial cells when Kupffer cell functioning is impaired (94,96,102–105). In response to inflammatory cytokines and bacterially derived lipopolysaccharide, hepatic endothelial cells, like Kupffer cells, can be "activated" to release mediators that regulate the function of parenchymal and nonparenchymal liver cells. These include chemokines, IL-1, IL-6, PAF, fibroblast growth factor, interferons, endothelin, eicosanoids, proteolytic enzymes, reactive oxygen, and nitrogen intermediates (17,22,25,106–112). Expression of cell adhesion molecules such as I-CAM and P-selectin, which facilitate inflammatory cell emigration into the liver, is also upregulated (6,113,114). These studies suggest that endothelial cells are important in inflammatory responses in the liver. The findings that endothelial cells also express CD40, CD80, CD86, and MHC class II molecules, which are markers of antigen-presenting cells, indicate that they may also play a role in immune surveillance and potentially in the development of tolerance in the liver (115,116).

A number of studies have demonstrated that endothelial cells also increase in number and become "activated" following exposure of experimental animals to hepatotoxicants such as acetaminophen, endotoxin, or ethanol (Fig. 1) (17,21,25,112,117,118). Like "activated" hepatic macrophages, these cells appear larger and more granular than cells from untreated rats, and produce increased amounts of reactive oxygen and nitrogen intermediates, eicosanoids, endothelin, IL-1, IL-6, TGFβ, fibroblast growth factor, and interferon (17,108,110,112,118). Moreover, expression of cell adhesion molecules, as well as receptors for TNFα and IL-6, are upregulated on these cells and their proliferative capacity increases (6,22,119–124). The ability of endothelial cells to produce and respond to these mediators may represent an important mechanism by which they participate in inflammatory and immune reactions associated with hepatotoxicity.

C. Stellate Cells in Hepatotoxicity and Fibrosis

Stellate cells, also referred to as Ito cells, fat-storing cells, perisinusoidal cells, and lipocytes, constitute approximately 20% of the hepatic sinusoidal cells. These cells normally reside in a quiescent, resting state within the space of Disse between endothelial cells and hepatocytes or between hepatocytes. Morphologically, stellate cells resemble fibroblasts in that they possess numerous extensions, as well as dilated rough endoplasmic reticulum. Stellate cells store vitamin A, which is localized in intracellular lipid droplets in the form of retinyl esters (125,126). Stellate cells also have the capacity to synthesize large quantities of extracellular matrix proteins, including types I, III, and IV collagen, as well as matrix metalloproteinases (MMP) and tissue inhibitors of metalloproteinase (TIMP), and there is evidence that they play a major role in collagen synthesis in both normal and fibrotic liver (127–131). It has been suggested that stellate cells can contribute to inflammatory responses in the liver. Following exposure of animals to toxicants such as ethanol or carbon tetrachloride, stellate cells undergo a process of activation (132–134).

This involves a loss of lipid droplets and vitamin A storage capacity, migration to sites of liver injury, and transformation into highly proliferative myofibroblast-like cells (133,135,136). Activated stellate cells also express increased quantities of the cell adhesion molecules, I-CAM-1, and V-CAM-1, as well as receptors for C5a, endothelin, eicosanoids, TNFα, IL-1, and platelet-derived growth factor (PDGF) (137–143). They are also primed to release cytotoxic and inflammatory mediators including IL-1, IL-6, IL-10, PAF, colony-stimulating factor-1, nitric oxide, hydrogen peroxide, superoxide anion, eicosanoids, gelatinase, fibronectin, TGFβ, endothelin, macrophage chemotactic protein-1, and CINC (129,144–151). Activation and transformation of stellate cells during the pathogenesis of tissue injury and fibrosis, as well as collagen deposition, appear to be mediated by cytokines and growth factors elaborated by parenchymal and nonparenchymal liver cells. These are largely divided into mitogenic mediators (TGFα, PDGF, IL-1, TNFα, and insulin-like growth factor) that stimulate proliferation and transformation of stellate cells and fibrogenic mediators including TGFβ and IL-6 that induce collagen gene expression (142).

Hepatic fibrosis represents the liver's wound healing response to injury and is characterized by excessive accumulation of interstitial matrix components within the tissue. A number of factors have been proposed to initiate and perpetuate the fibrogenic process in stellate cells including the accumulation of inflammatory cytokines and growth factors, alterations in the extracellular matrix, and oxidative stress (152). Xenobiotics such as alcohol or carbon tetrachloride can induce fibrogenesis by activating stellate cells. This can occur through the generation of lipid peroxides from damaged hepatocytes and/or oxidants and cytokines released from activated Kupffer cells and inflammatory macrophages (153). During the pathogenesis of fibrosis, stellate cells exhibit increased sensitivity to inflammatory mediators such as TNFα. This can enhance the production of chemotactic and fibrogenic mediators by liver cells and may contribute to the maintenance of an inflammatory infiltrate dominated by macrophages (154).

III. INFLAMMATORY MEDIATORS IMPLICATED IN HEPATOTOXICITY

Among the more prominent proinflammatory and cytotoxic mediators that have been implicated in hepatotoxicity are cytokines, reactive oxygen intermediates, reactive nitrogen intermediates, bioactive lipids, and hydrolytic enzymes. These mediators are likely to act in concert to promote hepatotoxicity.

A. Cytokines

Cytokines are cell-derived proteins that act in an autocrine and paracrine manner to regulate immune and inflammatory responses. Hepatic nonparenchymal cells and inflammatory macrophages are known to release a number of different cytokines that may play a role in the pathogenesis of tissue injury. Whereas some of these promote the inflammatory response (e.g., IL-1, IL-6, TNFα, interferon-γ, TGFβ, chemokines), others exert anti-inflammatory activity (e.g., IL-4, IL-10, IL-13). The overall outcome of the inflammatory response depends on the balance between levels of pro- and anti-inflammatory cytokines that are generated in the liver.

1. Proinflammatory Cytokines

IL-1 and TNFα are low-molecular-weight multifunctional proteins that induce a number of both distinct and overlapping functions (155–157). They are produced in large part by macrophages in response to inflammatory stimuli and are thought to play a prominent role in initiating the inflammatory response. Both IL-1 and TNFα stimulate the production of chemotactic factors and upregulate expression of cell adhesion molecules, thus promoting phagocyte margination and emigration to sites of injury. IL-1 also exerts mitogenic effects on macrophages and endothelial cells and induces the release of prostaglandins, metalloproteinases, and colony-stimulating factor (52,76,155–158). In the liver, IL-1 and TNFα activate Kupffer cells and infiltrating macrophages for cytotoxicity and stimulate the release of cytotoxic mediators including reactive nitrogen intermediates and reactive oxygen intermediates (24,155–159). They also induce the release of IL-1, IL-6, colony-stimulating factor, PAF, and eicosanoids from parenchymal and nonparenchymal liver cells (24,25). In conjunction with IL-6, IL-1 and TNFα regulate hepatocyte acute-phase protein and gene expression and cytochrome P450 activity (155–158,160,161). TNFα is unique among inflammatory cytokines in that it has the capacity to induce cytotoxicity directly. In hepatocytes, TNFα stimulates nitric oxide production and induces both necrosis and apoptosis (162–164). However, the biological effects of TNFα appear to be related to levels of this mediator generated. Thus at low concentrations, TNFα exerts homeostatic functions such as initiation of tissue repair, while at high concentrations it causes damage to endothelium, microthrombosis, and tissue injury (155–158).

Cytokines such as IL-1, IL-6, and TNFα, as well as interferon-γ, which are known to activate macrophages, have been directly implicated in hepatotoxicity in a number of experimental models. Following exposure of animals to ethanol, endotoxin, turpentine, carbon tetrachloride, cadmium, zymosan, galactosamine, dimethylnitrosamine, or acetaminophen, expression of these cytokines increases in the liver (25,46,165–173). Moreover, many of the observed clinical features of liver disease and injury including fever, inflammation, cirrhosis, and acute-phase protein production can be induced by administration of proinflammatory cytokines (155,174–176). Conversely, administration of neutralizing antibodies to IL-1, TNFα, IL-6, or interferon-γ, soluble cytokine receptors, or cytokine receptor antagonists reduces inflammatory cell accumulation, acute-phase protein production, and tissue injury induced by toxicants such as carbon tetrachloride, acetaminophen, endotoxin, ethanol, allyl alcohol, zymosan, and cadmium (160,165,177–185). Protection against toxicants by blocking antibodies is paralleled in many models by results obtained using transgenic animals. For example, recent studies have demonstrated that mice lacking the gene for the p55 TNFα receptor I or expressing only the membrane-bound form of the cytokine are protected from the toxic effects of carbon tetrachloride, ethanol, or the combination of endotoxin and galactosamine (89,184,186,187). Similarly, mice lacking the gene for IL-1 receptor or overexpressing IL-1 receptor antagonist exhibit an attenuated inflammatory response to turpentine (182), and IL-6 knockout mice are protected against the toxicity of zymosan (188). In contrast, mice lacking the p55 receptor of TNFα or the soluble form of TNFα have been reported to be more sensitive to the toxic effects of acetaminophen (189), and mice deficient in IL-6 exhibit a greater hepatotoxic response to carbon tetrachloride (190,191). These findings suggest that these cytokines can exert both protective and proinflammatory/cytotoxic activity, which depend on the toxicant, levels of cytokine produced, and the extent to which other inflammatory mediators are generated in the liver.

2. Transforming Growth Factor-β (TGFβ)

Studies with neutralizing antibodies and transgenic animal models have also provided evidence for a critical role of TGFβ in nonparenchymal cell activation and fibrosis. TGFβ is produced by activated liver macrophages in response to injury and infection. In addition to its autocrine actions, TGFβ acts on stellate cells to prolong their survival and induce collagen gene expression (192,193). Following exposure of animals to fibrogenic doses of toxicants such as carbon tetrachloride, vitamin A, or alcohol, production of TGFβ increases in the liver (150,194,195). These findings, together with the observation that carbon tetrachloride–induced increases in collagen deposition are reduced by 80% in transgenic mice with a targeted disruption of the TGFβ gene, or in mice treated with antibodies to TGFβ (196), provide strong support for an involvement of this cytokine in tissue injury and fibrosis.

3. Chemokines

Recent studies have focused on another class of proinflammatory cytokines that exhibit chemotactic activity. These belong to a superfamily of low-molecular-weight proteins that play a key role in orchestrating the inflammatory response. Chemotactic cytokines or chemokines are divided into two subfamilies: C-X-C proteins (e.g., IL-8 or CINC), which are mainly neutrophil chemoattractants, and C-C chemokines (e.g., MIP-1, MIP-2, MCP-1, MCP-2, MCP-3, RANTES), which induce migration and activation of macrophages/monocytes and lymphocytes (197). Continuous local release of chemokines at sites of injury is thought to mediate the ongoing migration of effector cells into lesions during inflammatory responses. Chemokines such as MIP-1α, MCP-1, RANTES, and CINC have been implicated in a variety of pathogenic processes in the liver including chemically induced toxicity (198,199). These chemokines, which are produced in large part by Kupffer cells and endothelial cells (54,200,201), are upregulated in the liver after administration of endotoxin, ethanol, cadmium, or acetaminophen to animals (68,198,199,201–204). However, the precise role of chemokines in the pathogenesis of toxicity is controversial. Whereas some studies have indicated that they contribute to injury (205), others suggest that they may in fact act to reduce hepatotoxicity (206), which is most likely related to the production of anti-inflammatory mediators by newly infiltrated phagocytes (207). Thus mice lacking the gene for CCR2, the receptor for MCP-1, were found to be more sensitive to the toxic effects of acetaminophen, a response that was correlated with increases in TNFα and interferon-γ in the liver (206). Similarly, administration of MCP-1 protected mice from endotoxin toxicity and decreased hepatic TNFα levels (208). These data support the concept that inflammatory cytokines can both prevent and augment hepatotoxicity (209).

Hepatocytes treated with toxicants like acetaminophen, galactosamine, or alcohol have also been reported to release phagocyte chemotactic and activating factors (41,210,211). Biochemical characterization studies have suggested that these factors are members of the chemokine family. Production of chemokines by hepatocytes is upregulated in response to Kupffer cell-derived TNFα and IL-1 (212,213). Thus, parenchymal cells apparently participate in inflammatory cell recruitment into the liver and activation during the pathogenesis of injury.

4. Anti-inflammatory Cytokines

Anti-inflammatory cytokines such as IL-4, IL-10, and IL-13 are also expressed in the liver following hepatotoxicant exposure (207,213–215). These cytokines facilitate the recovery of the liver from acute injury and inhibit the production of proinflammatory cytokines (214,216–218). They also enhance the production of IL-1 receptor antagonist (219). That these cytokines are important in toxicity is supported by the findings that administration of IL-13 protects mice from lethal endotoxemia and that anti-IL-13 antibodies significantly decrease survival rate (215). Similarly hepatic fibrosis is increased in IL-10 knockout mice after repeated carbon tetrachloride administration (214).

B.   Reactive Oxygen Intermediates

Reactive oxygen intermediates including superoxide anion, hydrogen peroxide, and hydroxyl radical are produced in significant quantities in cells by a variety of oxido-reductase reactions and during mitochondrial respiration. Although under physiological conditions these mediators destroy invading pathogens and particulates, when generated in excessive amounts, they can induce oxidative injury. This includes cell membrane, protein, and DNA damage, lipid peroxidation, and cytotoxicity (220–223). Peroxidation of membrane lipids by reactive oxygen intermediates can also induce the formation and release of other inflammatory mediators including prostaglandins, thromboxanes, and leukotrienes (see below). Macrophages, and in some models, endothelial cells and stellate cells isolated from the livers of hepatotoxicant-treated rats, have been reported to be "activated" to release increased quantities of reactive oxygen intermediates (7,17,18,20,40,67,70,224). Moreover, stimulation of hepatic macrophages to produce additional reactive oxygen intermediates by administration of agents such as retinol, glucan, or latex beads augments liver injury induced by agents such as *C. parvum*, carbon tetrachloride, 1,2-dichlorobenzene, and galactosamine. In contrast, administration of antioxidants like superoxide dismutase, catalase, allopurinol, *N*-acetylcysteine, methyl palmitate, endotoxin, or quinone derivatives is hepatoprotective (32,43,55,65,74,78,225–233). These studies support the hypothesis that oxygen-derived free radicals contribute to the pathogenesis of chemically induced hepatotoxicity.

Reactive oxygen intermediates also appear to play an important role in fibrosis. Both expression and synthesis of TGFβ are modulated via redox-sensitive reactions (151). Moreover, activation of stellate cells, as well as expression of metalloproteinases and their inhibitors, is dependent on reactive oxygen intermediates and lipid peroxidation products. The importance of oxidants in fibrosis is underscored by the finding that there is marked oxidative stress in the liver in most chronic disease processes affecting the tissue. It has been suggested that reactive oxidants contribute to both the onset and progression of fibrosis induced by alcohol, carbon tetrachloride, viruses, iron, copper overload, cholestasis, and hepatic blood congestion (118,134,151).

C.   Reactive Nitrogen Intermediates

Nitric oxide and its oxidation products have been implicated in altered hepatic functioning following xenobiotic exposure and in tissue injury (234–236). Nitric oxide is generated from 1-arginine by the NADPH-dependent enzyme, nitric oxide synthase. Three major isoforms of nitric oxide synthase have been identified: types I and III, which are produced in cells constitutively and are calcium and calmodulin-dependent, and type II nitric oxide synthase (NOSII), which is induced after activation of cells by bacterially derived pathogens or cytokines (237). Whereas the type I form is largely localized in neuronal tissue, the type III form is found in vascular endothelium. In contrast, type II nitric oxide synthase (NOSII) has been identified in both resident and inflammatory liver macrophages, as well as in hepatocytes, endothelial cells, stellate cells, smooth muscle cells, fibroblasts, and certain epithelial cells (21,24,25,48,144,145,162,209,234–239). Toxicity associated with excessive nitric oxide production is generally thought to be due to the actions of NOSII (209,240).

Nitric oxide is a small, relatively stable free radical gas that readily diffuses into cells and cell membranes where it reacts with molecular targets such as heme- and thiol-containing proteins and amines (237,240). This can result in decreased cellular proliferation and nucleic acid biosynthesis as well as altered enzyme activity, cytotoxicity, and apoptosis (234,238,240,241). Nitric oxide also binds to heme-containing proteins and this can result in either inhibition or activation of enzymes involved in hepatic drug metabolism. It has also been established that nitric oxide produced by macrophages is involved in the destruction of certain intracellular pathogens and tumor cells and in cytostasis (159,237,242,243). Nitric oxide is also known to react rapidly with superoxide anion–generating peroxynitrite, a relatively long-lived cytotoxic oxidant that has been implicated in stroke, heart disease, and immune complex–mediated pulmonary edema (244–247). Peroxynitrite can also induce lipid peroxidation and can react directly with sulfhydryl groups in cell membranes leading to cytotoxicity and/or apoptosis (248–250). Peroxynitrite can also react with metals or metalloproteinases such as superoxide dismutase to form nitronium ion, a potent and toxic nitrosylating species (251). After treatment of animals with hepatotoxicants such as acetaminophen, carbon tetrachloride, ethanol, or endotoxin, Kupffer cells, as well as inflammatory macrophages, sinusoidal endothelial cells, stellate cells, and/or hepatocytes have been reported to express NOSII and to produce excessive quantities of nitric oxide (23,48,73,143,144,239,252–255). This has been correlated with nitrotyrosine staining of the liver (256,257). However, the role of nitric oxide and peroxynitrite in hepatotoxicity is controversial. Thus, while some studies have suggested that their actions are toxic, in other models, reactive nitrogen intermediates appear to play a protective role. For example, in animals pretreated with inhibitors of NOSII, such as aminoguanidine, or in transgenic mice with a targeted disruption of NOSII, hepatotoxicity induced by acetaminophen, or endotoxin is significantly reduced (23,48,236,258–261). In contrast, hepatotoxicity is augmented in NOSII knockout mice treated with carbon tetrachloride (89). Similar increases in carbon tetrachloride- or endotoxin/*C. parvum*-induced hepatotoxicity have been described in animals pretreated with NOSII inhibitors (253,263–265), which is thought to be due to the ability of nitric oxide to reduce levels of cytotoxic oxidants (244–246,266). These data indicate that the relative pathological or protective roles of nitric oxide and peroxynitrite in toxicity depends on the nature of the toxicant and the extent to which tissue injury is mediated by reactive oxygen intermediates.

D. Bioactive Lipids

Bioactive lipids constitute a broad range of mediators with both pro- and anti-inflammatory activity. The largest group are eicosanoids, which are derived from membrane-bound arachidonic acid. Prostaglandins (PG) and thromboxanes (Tx) are generated from arachidonic acid via the enzyme cyclooxygenase (COX). Two isoforms of this enzyme have been identified: a constitutive form (COX-1), which is thought to provide cytoprotective function, and an inducible form (COX-2), which is involved in the generation of inflammatory PG. Metabolism of arachidonic acid via the enzyme lipoxygenase leads to the formation of leukotrienes (LT). Although activated liver macrophages, as well as endothelial cells, stellate cells, and hepatocytes have been reported to synthesize a large number of different eicosanoids including LTB_4, TxA_2, PGE_2, PGD_2, $PGF_{2\gamma}$, and PGI_2, their response to these mediators is distinct (24,106,145,267,268). This is most likely due to differential expression of eicosanoid receptors on these cells (140). The precise role of these eicosanoids in hepatotoxicity is unclear. Prostaglandins such as PGE_2 and PGD_2 are known to play a key role in regulating inflammatory and immune reactions and also have the capacity to modify hepatocyte carbohydrate metabolism, calcium homeostasis, as well as protein synthesis and phosphorylation (268–270). Enhanced release of prostaglandins has been described following exposure of animals to toxins such as acetaminophen, ethanol, and endotoxin (268,271–274). Moreover, administration of cyclooxygenase inhibitors to animals prevents tissue injury induced by these toxicants (60,79,268,270,274–277). Similarly, inhibition of TxB_2 synthase protects against endotoxic shock and liver injury (278,279). In contrast, recent studies have demonstrated some PG may be hepatoprotective, presumably because of their ability to block inflammatory mediator production. Thus PGE_2 pretreatment prevents endotoxin-induced liver injury by downregulating TNFα and IL-12 and upregulating the anti-inflammatory cytokine IL-10 (280). Similarly, protection against galactosamine-induced hepatotoxicity by administration of PGE_1 was correlated with decreased TNFα release (281).

A number of leukotrienes also exhibit proinflammatory activity and are thought to play a role in chemically induced tissue injury (44,268,281). For example, LTB_4 is known to be a potent polymorphonuclear leukocyte chemoattractant and to induce monocyte IL-1, TNFα, and hydrogen peroxide production (267,282–284). Thus, release of LTB_4 by macrophages in the liver following hepatotoxicant exposure may constitute a local control mechanism for the recruitment and activation of inflammatory cells. Kupffer cells and endothelial cells have been shown to express mRNA for 5-lipoxygenase, a major enzyme mediating the production of leukotrienes, while LTC_4 synthase mRNA has been identified mainly in hepatocytes and endothelial cells (285). Endotoxin administration increases the expression of LTC_4 synthase mRNA, and protein in hepatocytes, which may contribute to hepatocellular injury during inflammation (285). The finding that administration of lipoxygenase inhibitors or antagonists to mice protected against galactosamine-induced hepatitis suggests that leukotrienes have the capacity to contribute to inflammatory liver disease and injury (41,276).

PAF is a phospholipid mediator that has also been implicated in tissue injury. It is released by a variety of cell types including macrophages, neutrophils, and endothelial cells and is thought to act in an autocrine and paracrine manner to amplify and propagate early stages of the inflammatory response. Thus PAF released from inflammatory phagocytes stimulates macrophage and neutrophil chemotaxis and oxidative metabolism and nitric oxide generation (107,286–289). Following exposure of animals to endotoxin, liver macrophages and endothelial cells produce increased quantities of PAF (266,286,288). Interestingly, these cells also express increased numbers of functionally active receptors for PAF (290). Upregulation of PAF receptors may represent an important mechanism underlying macrophage and endothelial cell activation following hepatotoxicant exposure. In support of this possibility is the finding that administration of a PAF receptor antagonist reduces tissue injury induced by endotoxin (291).

E. Hydrolytic Enzymes

Macrophages and endothelial cells activated by inflammatory stimuli can also generate proteolytic and lysosomal enzymes. These include various proteases, lipases, matrix metalloproteinases, plasminogen activator, acid phosphatase, and cathepsin D (19,24,292–296). These can act directly on hepatocyte membranes to induce damage. Several of these enzymes have been shown to play a role in macrophage-mediated target cell destruction, as well as in altered hepatocyte functioning (19,24,297) and similar effects may occur in vivo after hepatotoxicant exposure. In contrast, the matrix metalloproteinases (e.g., collagenase, gelatinase, and stromelysin) may contribute to recovery from liver fibrosis and play a role in fibrolysis during cirrhosis (295,298–300).

IV. CONCLUSION

Evidence has accumulated over the past several years demonstrating that chemically induced toxicity is a multifactorial process involving direct tissue injury as well as a cascade of protein and lipid mediators generated by cells in the liver. These include not only resident cells (hepatocytes, Kupffer cells, stellate cells, and endothelial cells), but also infiltrating leukocytes. Cytokines and reactive mediators, including nitric oxide, peroxynitrite, superoxide anion, hydrogen peroxide, hydroxyl radicals, and eicosanoids, produced by "activated" nonparenchymal cells and/or infiltrating leukocytes may be cytotoxic, proinflammatory, and can compromise normal liver functioning (Fig. 2). Defining the precise role of each of these mediators in tissue injury is essential for our understanding of the mechanism of action of hepatotoxic chemicals and for devising steps to prevent or abrogate toxicity.

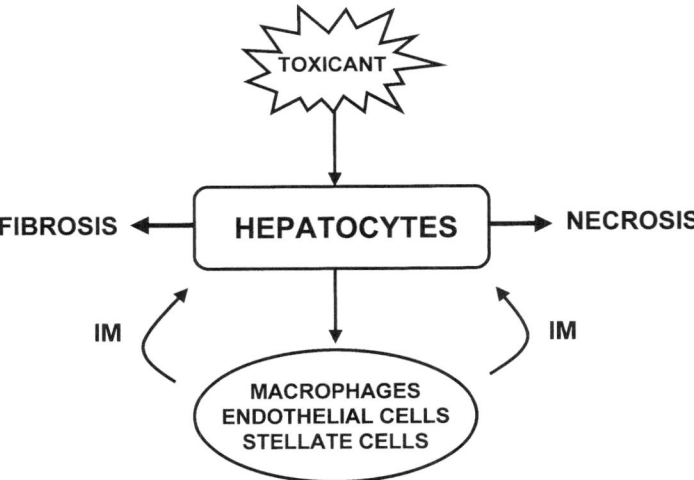

Figure 2 Model for the role of macrophages, endothelial cells, and stellate cells in hepatotoxicity. Toxicants such as acetaminophen and carbon tetrachloride cause injury to hepatocytes. This leads to the release of cytokines and/or growth factors that recruit and activate Kupffer cells, endothelial cells, stellate cells, and inflammatory macrophages to sites of injury. These cells become activated and release inflammatory mediators (IM) such as reactive oxygen intermediates, reactive nitrogen intermediates, TNFα, IL-1, bioactive lipids, hydrolytic enzymes, and/or growth factors that contribute to hepatic necrosis and fibrosis.

ACKNOWLEDGMENTS

Dr. Laskin is a Burroughs Wellcome Toxicology Scholar. This work was supported by an award from the Burroughs Wellcome Fund and by USPHS National Institutes of Health Grants GM34310, ES04738, ES06897, and ES05022.

REFERENCES

1. Bouwens L, Baekeland M, De Zanger R, Wisse E. Quantitation, tissue distribution and proliferation kinetics of Kupffer cells in normal rat liver. Hepatology 1986; 6:718–722.
2. Caperna TJ, Garvey JS. Antigen handling in aging. II. The role of Kupffer and endothelial cells in antigen processing in Fischer 344 rats. Mech Ageing Dev 1982; 20:205–221.
3. Terpstra V, van Berkel TJ. Scavenger receptors on liver Kupffer cells mediate the in vivo uptake of oxidatively damaged red blood cells in mice. Blood 2000; 95:2157–2163.
4. van Oosten M, van de Bilt E, van Berkel TJ, Kuiper J. New scavenger receptor-like receptors for the binding of lipopolysaccharide to liver endothelial and Kupffer cells. Infect Immun 1998; 66:5107–5112.
5. Sano A, Taylor ME, Leaning MS, Summerfield JA. Uptake and processing of glycoproteins by isolated rat hepatic endothelial and Kupffer cells. J Hepatol 1990; 10:211–216.
6. Ahmad N, Gardner CR, Yurkow EJ, Laskin DL. Inhibition of macrophages with gadolinium chloride alters intercellular adhesion molecule-1 expression in the liver during acute endotoxemia in rats. Hepatology 1999; 29:728–736.
7. Pilaro AM, Laskin DL. Accumulation of activated mononuclear phagocytes in the liver following lipopolysaccharide treatment of rats. J Leukoc Biol 1986; 40:29–41.
8. Gardner CR, Wasserman AJ, Laskin DL. Differential sensitivity of tumor targets to liver macrophage-mediated cytotoxicity. Cancer Res 1987; 47:6686–6691.
9. Gardner CR, Wasserman AJ, Laskin DL. Liver macrophage mediated cytotoxicity involves phagocytosis of tumor targets. Hepatology 1991; 14:318–324.
10. Løvdal T, Andersen E, Brech A, Berg T. Fc receptor mediated endocytosis of small soluble immunoglobulin G immune complexes in Kupffer cells and endothelial cells from rat liver. J Cell Sci 2000; 113:3255–3266.
11. Shi J, Fujieda H, Kokubo Y, Wake K. Apoptosis of neutrophils and their elimination by Kupffer cells in rat liver. Hepatology 1996; 24:1256–1263.
12. Mathison JC, Ulevitch RJ. The clearance, tissue distribution, and cellular localization of intravenously injected lipopolysaccharide in rabbits. J Immunol 1979; 123:2133–2143.
13. Nolan J. Endotoxin, reticuloendothelial function and liver injury. Hepatology 1981; 1:458–465.
14. Lukkari TA, Jarvelainen HA, Oinonen T, Kettunen E, Lindros KO. Short-term ethanol exposure increases the expression of Kupffer cell CD14 receptor and lipopolysaccharide binding protein in rat liver. Alcohol Alcohol 1999; 34:311–319.
15. Su GL, Klein RD, Aminlari A, Zhang HY, Steinstraesser L, Alarcon WH, Remick DG, Wang SC. Kupffer cell activation by lipopolysaccharide in rats: role for lipopolysaccharide binding protein and toll-like receptor 4. Hepatology 2000; 31:932–936.
16. Shnyra A, Lindberg AA. Scavenger receptor pathway for lipopolysaccharide binding to Kupffer and endothelial liver cells in vitro. Infect Immun 1995; 63:865–873.
17. McCloskey TW, Todaro JA, Laskin DL. Lipopolysaccharide treatment of rats alters antigen expression and oxidative metabolism in hepatic macrophages and endothelial cells. Hepatology 1992; 16:191–203.
18. Laskin DL, Pilaro AM. Potential role of activated macrophages in acetaminophen hepatotoxicity. I. Isolation and characterization of activated macrophages from rat liver. Toxicol Appl Pharmacol 1986; 86:204–215.

19. Tanner A, Keyhani A, Reiner R, Holdstock G, Wright R. Proteolytic enzymes released by liver macrophages may promote injury in a rat model of hepatic damage. Gastroenterology 1981; 80:647–654.

20. Liu P, McGuire GM, Fisher MA, Farhood A, Smith CW, Jaeschke H. Activation of Kupffer cells and neutrophils for reactive oxygen formation is responsible for endotoxin-enhanced liver injury after hepatic ischemia. Shock 1995; 3:56–62.

21. Laskin DL, Heck DE, Gardner CR, Feder LS, Laskin JD. Distinct patterns of nitric oxide production in hepatic macrophages and endothelial cells following acute exposure of rats to endotoxin. J Leukoc Biol 1994; 56:751–758.

22. Feder LS, Laskin DL. Regulation of hepatic endothelial cell and macrophage proliferation and nitric oxide production by GM-CSF, M-CSF and IL-1β following acute endotoxemia. J Leukoc Biol 1994; 55:507–513.

23. Laskin DL. Xenobiotic-induced inflammation and injury in the liver. In: RS McCuskey, DL Earnst, eds. Comprehensive Toxicology. Vol. 9. Hepatic and Gastrointestinal Toxicology. New York: Pergamon, 1997:151–164.

24. Decker K. Biologically active products of stimulated liver macrophages (Kupffer cells). Eur J Biochem 1990; 192:245–261.

25. Feder LS, Todaro JA, Laskin DL. Characterization of interleukin-1 and interleukin-6 production by hepatic endothelial cells and macrophages. J Leukoc Biol 1993; 53:126–132.

26. Tsutsui H, Matsui K, Okamura H, Nakanishi K. Pathophysiological roles of interleukin-18 in inflammatory liver diseases. Immunol Rev 2000; 174:192–209.

27. Noji S, Tashiro K, Koyama E, Nohno T, Ohyama K, Taniguchi S, Nakamura T. Expression of hepatocyte growth factor gene in endothelial and Kupffer cells of damaged rat livers, as revealed by in situ hybridization. Biochem Biophys Res Commun 1990; 173:42–47.

28. Boulton RA, Alison MR, Golding M, Selden C, Hodgson HJ. Augmentation of the early phase of liver regeneration after 70% partial hepatectomy in rats following selective Kupffer cell depletion. J Hepatol 1998; 29:271–280.

29. Takeishi T, Hirano K, Kobayashi T, Hasegawa G, Hatakeyama K, Naito M. The role of Kupffer cells in liver regeneration. Arch Histol Cytol 1999; 62:413–422.

30. Roth S, Gong W, Gressner AM. Expression of different isoforms of TGF-β and the latent TGF-β binding protein (LTBP) by rat Kupffer cells. J Hepatol 1998; 29:915–922.

31. Abril ER, Simm WE, Earnest DL. Kupffer cell secretion of cytotoxin cytokines is enhanced by hypervitaminosis A. In: E Wisse, DL Knook, K Decker, eds. Cells of the Hepatic Sinusoid. Vol. 2. Rijswijk: Kupffer Cell Foundation, 1989:73–75.

32. Arthur MJP, Bentley IS, Tanner A, Saunders PK, Millward-Sadler GH, Wright R. Oxygen-derived free radicals promote hepatic injury in the rat. Gastroenterology 1985; 89:1114–1122.

33. Shiratori Y, Takikawa H, Kawase T, Sugimoto T. Superoxide anion generating capacity and lysosomal enzyme activities of Kupffer cells in galactosamine-induced hepatitis. Gastroenterol Jpn 1986; 21:135–144.

34. Mochida S, Ogata I, Ohta Y, Yamada S, Fujiwara K. In situ evaluation of the stimulatory state of hepatic macrophages based on their ability to produce superoxide anions in rats. J Pathol 1989; 158:67–71.

35. Bautista AP, Meszaros K, Bojta J, Spitzer JJ. Superoxide anion generation in the liver during the early stages of endotoxemia in rats. J Leukoc Biol 1990; 48:123–128.

36. Bautista AP, Spitzer JJ. Superoxide anion generation by in situ perfused rat liver: effect of in vivo endotoxin. Am J Physiol 1990; 259:G907–G912.

37. Rogoff TM, Lipsky PE. Antigen presentation by isolated guinea pig Kupffer cells. J Immunol 1980; 124:1740–1744.

38. Itoh Y, Okanoue T, Morimoto M, Nagao Y, Mori T, Hori N, Kagawa K, Kashima K. Functional heterogeneity of rat liver macrophages: interleukin-1 secretion and Ia antigen expression in contrast with phagocytic activity. Liver 1992; 12:26–33.

39. Lohse AW, Knolle PA, Bilo K, Uhrig A, Waldmann C, Ibe M, Schmitt E, Gerken G, Meyer Zum Buschenfelde KH. Antigen-presenting function and B7 expression of murine sinusoidal endothelial cells and Kupffer cells. Gastroenterology 1996; 110:1175–1181.
40. Laskin DL, Robertson FM, Pilaro AM, Laskin JD. Activation of liver macrophages following phenobarbital treatment of rats. Hepatology 1988; 8:1051–1055.
41. Shiratori Y, Hai K, Takada H, Kiriyama H, Nagura T, Matsumoto K, Kamii K, Okano K, Tanaka M. Mechanism of accumulation of macrophages in galactosamine-induced liver injury: effect of lipoxygenase inhibitors on chemotaxis of spleen cells. Pathobiology 1992; 60: 316–321.
42. Thompson WD, Jack AS, Patrick RS. Possible role of macrophages in transient hepatic fibrogenesis induced by acute carbon tetrachloride injury. J Pathol 1980; 130:65–73.
43. Shiratori Y, Tanaka M, Hai K, Kawase T, Shirna S, Sugimoto T. Role of endotoxin-responsive macrophages in hepatic injury. Hepatology 1990; 11:183–192.
44. Jonker AM, Kijkhuis FW, Kroese FG, Hardonk MJ, Grond J. Immunopathology of acute galactosamine hepatitis in rats. Hepatology 1990; 11:622–627.
45. Przybocki JM, Reuhl KR, Thurman RG, Kauffman FC. Involvement of nonparenchymal cells in oxygen-dependent hepatic injury by allyl alcohol. Toxicol Appl Pharmacol 1992; 115:57–63.
46. Orfila C, Lepert JC, Alric L, Carrera G, Beraud M, Vinel JP, Pipy B. Expression of TNF-α and immunohistochemical distribution of hepatic macrophage surface markers in carbon tetrachloride-induced chronic liver injury in rats. Histochem J 1999; 31:677–685.
47. Camandola S, Aragno M, Cutrin JC, Tamagno E, Danni O, Chiarpotto E, Parola M, Leonarduzzi G, Biasi F, Poli G. Liver AP-1 activation due to carbon tetrachloride is potentiated by 1,2-dibromoethane but is inhibited by alpha-tocopherol or gadolinium chloride. Free Radic Biol Med 1999; 26:1108–1116.
48. Gardner CR, Heck DE, Yang CS, Thomas PE, Zhang X-J, DeGeorge GL, Laskin JD, Laskin DL. Role of nitric oxide in acetaminophen-induced hepatotoxicity in the rat. Hepatology 1998; 26:748–754.
49. Arthur MJP, Kowalski-Sanders P, Wright R. *Corynebacterium parvum*–elicited hepatic macrophages demonstrate enhanced respiratory burst activity compared with resident Kupffer cells in the rat. Gastroenterology 1986; 91:174–181.
50. MacDonald JR, Beckstead JH, Smuckler EA. An ultrastructural and histochemical study of the prominent inflammatory response in D(+)-galactosamine hepatotoxicity. Br J Exp Pathol 1987; 68:189–199.
51. Earnst DL, Brouwer A, Sim W, Horan MA, Hendriks HF, De Leeuw AM, Knook DL. Hypervitaminosis A activates Kupffer cells and lowers the threshold for endotoxin liver injury. In: A Kirn, DL Knook, E Wisse, eds. Cells of the Hepatic Sinusoid. Vol. 1. Rijswijk: Kupffer Cell Foundation, 1986:277–283.
52. Kamimura S, Tsukamoto H. Cytokine gene expression by Kupffer cells in experimental alcoholic liver disease. Hepatology 1995; 22:1304–1309.
53. Armendariz-Borunda J, Seyer JM, Postlethwaite AE, Kang AH. Kupffer cells from carbon tetrachloride-injured rat livers produce chemotactic factors for fibroblasts and monocytes: the role of tumor necrosis factor-alpha. Hepatology 1991; 14:895–900.
54. Bukara M, Bautista AP. Acute alcohol intoxication and gadolinium chloride attenuate endotoxin-induced release of CC chemokines in the rat. Alcohol 2000; 20:193–203.
55. elSisi AE, Earnest DL, Sipes IG. Vitamin A potentiation of carbon tetrachloride hepatotoxicity: role of liver macrophages and active oxygen species. Toxicol Appl Pharmacol 1993; 119:295–301.
56. Ferluga J, Allison AC. Role of mononuclear infiltrating cells in the pathogenesis of hepatitis. Lancet 1978; 2:610–611.
57. Freudenberg MA, Keppler D, Galanos C. Requirement for lipopolysaccharide-responsive

macrophages in galactosamine-induced sensitization to endotoxin. Infect Immun 1986; 51: 891–895.

58. Laskin DL, Pendino KJ. Macrophages and tissue injury. Annu Rev Pharmacol Toxicol 1995; 35:655–677.

59. Sudhir S, Budhiraja RD. Comparison of the protective effect of Withaferin-A and hydrocortisone against CCl$_4$ induced hepatotoxicity in rats. Indian J Physiol Pharmacol 1992; 36:127–129.

60. Ben-Zvi Z, Weissman-Teitellman B, Katz S, Dannon A. Acetaminophen hepatotoxicity: is there a role for prostaglandin synthesis? Arch Toxicol 1990; 64:299–304.

61. Edwards MJ, Keller BJ, Kauffman FC, Thurman RG. The involvement of Kupffer cells in carbon tetrachloride toxicity. Toxicol Appl Pharmacol 1993; 119:275–279.

62. Laskin DL, Gardner CR, Price VF, Jollow DJ. Modulation of macrophage functioning abrogates the acute hepatotoxicity of acetaminophen. Hepatology 1995; 21:1045–1050.

63. Stenger RJ, Petrelli M, McPath DCP, Segel A. Modification of carbon tetrachloride hepatoxicity by prior loading of the reticuloendothelial system with carbon particles. Am J Pathol 1969; 57:689–697.

64. Deaciuc IV, Bagby GJ, Niesman MR, Skrepnik N, Spitzer JJ. Modulation of hepatic sinusoidal endothelial cell function by Kupffer cells: an example of intercellular communication in the liver. Hepatology 1994; 19:464–470.

65. Ishiyama H, Ogino K, Hobara T. Kupffer cells in rat liver injury induced by diethyldithiocarbamate. Eur J Pharmacol 1995; 292:135–141.

66. Iimuro Y, Yamamoto M, Kohno H, Itakura J, Fujii H, Matsumoto Y. Blockade of liver macrophages by gadolinium chloride reduces lethality in endotoxemic rats—analysis of mechanisms of lethality in endotoxemia. J Leukoc Biol 1994; 55:723–728.

67. Hoglen NC, Younis HS, Hartley DP, Gunawardhana L, Lantz RC, Sipes IG. 1,2-dichlorobenzene-induced lipid peroxidation in male Fischer 344 rats is Kupffer cell dependent. Toxicol Sci 1998; 46:376–385.

68. Yamano T, DeCicco LA, Rikans LE. Attenuation of cadmium-induced liver injury in senescent male Fischer 344 rats: role of Kupffer cells and inflammatory cytokines. Toxicol Appl Pharmacol 2000; 162:68–75.

69. Sauer JM, Waalkes MP, Hooser SB, Kuester RK, McQueen CA, Sipes IG. Suppression of Kupffer cell function prevents cadmium induced hepatocellular necrosis in the male Sprague-Dawley rat. Toxicology 1997; 121:155–164.

70. Yokoyama H, Fukuda M, Okamura Y, Mizukami T, Ohgo H, Kamegaya Y, Kato S, Ishii H. Superoxide anion release into the hepatic sinusoid after an acute ethanol challenge and its attenuation by Kupffer cell depletion. Alcohol Clin Exp Res 1999; 23:71S–75S.

71. Rikans LE, Yamano T. Mechanisms of cadmium-mediated acute hepatotoxicity. J Biochem Mol Toxicol 2000; 14:110–117.

72. Al-Tuwaijri A, Akdamar K, Di Luzio NR. Modification of galactosamine-induced liver injury in rats by reticuloendothelial system stimulation or depression. Hepatology 1981; 1:107–113.

73. Chamulitrat W, Blazaka ME, Jordan SJ, Luster MI, Mason RP. Tumor necrosis factor-α and nitric oxide production in endotoxin-primed rats administered carbon tetrachloride. Life Sci 1995; 57:2273–2280.

74. Shiratori Y, Kawase T, Shiina S, Okano K, Sugimoto T, Teraoka H, Matano S, Matsumoto K, Kamii K. Modulation of hepatotoxicity by macrophages in the liver. Hepatology 1988; 8:815–821.

75. Chojkier M, Fierer J. D-Galactosamine hepatotoxicity is associated with endotoxin sensitivity and mediated by lymphoreticular cells in mice. Gastroenterology 1985; 88:115–121.

76. Galanos C, Freudenberg MA, Reuter W. Galactosamine-induced sensitization to the lethal effects of endotoxin. Proc Natl Acad Sci USA 1979; 76:5939–5943.

77. Nolan JP, Leibowitz AI. Endotoxin and the liver. III. Modification of acute carbon tetrachloride injury by polymyxin B—an antiendotoxin. Gastroenterology 1978; 75:445–449.

78. Sauer JM, Hooser SB, Badger DA, Baines A, Sipes IG. Alterations in chemically induced tissue injury related to all-*trans*-retinol pretreatment in rodents. Drug Metabol Rev 1995; 27: 299–323.

79. Tiegs G, Wolter M, Wendel A. Tumor necrosis factor is a terminal mediator in galactosamine/endotoxin-induced hepatitis in mice. Biochem Pharmacol 1989; 38:627–631.

80. Sauer JM, Sipes IG. Modulation of chemical-induced lung and liver toxicity by all-*trans*-retinol in the male Sprague-Dawley rat. Toxicology 1995; 105:237–249.

81. Blazka ME, Germolec DR, Simeonova P, Bruccoleri A, Pennypacker KR, Luster MI. Acetaminophen-induced hepatotoxicity is associated with early changes in NF-κB and NF-IL6 DNA binding activity. J Inflamm 1996; 47:138–150.

82. Ahmad N, Chen C, Martey CA, Ricketts SG, Laskin JD, Laskin DL. Acute endotoxemia is associated with increased STAT1 and NF-κB nuclear binding activity in hepatic macrophages and endothelial cells (abstr). Toxicol Sci 2000; 54:140.

83. Fox ES, Cantrell CH, Leingang KA. Inhibition of the Kupffer cell inflammatory response by acute ethanol: NF-κB activation and subsequent cytokine production. Biochem Biophys Res Commun 1996; 225:134–140.

84. Essani NA, McGuire GM, Manning AM, Jaeschke H. Endotoxin-induced activation of the nuclear transcription factor κB and expression of E-selectin messenger RNA in hepatocytes, Kupffer cells, and endothelial cells. J Immunol 1996; 156:2956–2963.

85. Gruebele A, Zawaski K, Kaplan D, Novak RF. Cytochrome P4502E1- and cytochrome P4502B1/2B2-catalyzed carbon tetrachloride metabolism: effects on signal transduction as demonstrated by altered immediate-early (*c*-Fos and *c*-Jun) gene expression and nuclear AP-1 and NF-κB transcription factor levels. Drug Metab Dispos 1996; 24:15–22.

86. Nanji AA, Jokelainen K, Rahemtulla A, Miao L, Fogt F, Matsumoto H, Tahan SR, Su GL. Activation of nuclear factor kappa B and cytokine imbalance in experimental alcoholic liver disease in the rat. Hepatology 1999; 30:934–943.

87. Miyamoto S, Verma IM. Rel/NF-κB/IκB story. Adv Cancer Res 1995; 66:255–292.

88. Liu SL, Degli Esposti S, Yao T, Diehl AM, Zern MA. Vitamin E therapy of acute CCl$_4$-induced hepatic injury in mice is associated with inhibition of nuclear factor kappa B binding. Hepatology 1995; 22:1474–1481.

89. Morio LA, Chiu H, Sprowles KA, Zhou P, Heck DE, Gordon MK, Laskin DL. Distinct roles of tumor necrosis factor-α and nitric oxide in acute liver injury induced by carbon tetrachloride in mice. Toxicol Appl Pharmacol 2001; 172:44–51.

90. Blazka ME, Bruccoleri A, Simeonova P, Germolec DR, Pennypacker KR, Luster MI. Acetaminophen-induced hepatotoxicity is associated with early changes in AP-1 DNA binding activity. Res Commun Mol Pathol Pharmacol 1996; 92:259–273.

91. Tran-Thi TA, Decker K, Baeuerle P. Differential activation of transcription factors NF-κB and AP-1 in rat liver macrophages. Hepatology 1995; 22:613–619.

92. Schiaffonati L, Tiberio L. Gene expression in liver after toxic injury: analysis of heat shock response and oxidative stress-inducible genes. Liver 1997; 17:183–191.

93. Hahn E, Wick G, Pencev D, Timpl R. Distribution of basement membrane protein in normal and fibrotic human liver: collagen type IV, laminin, and fibronectin. Gut 1980; 21:63–71.

94. Praaning-van Dalen DP, De Leeuw AM, Brower A, Knook DL. Rat liver endothelial cells have a greater capacity than Kupffer cells to endocytose *N*-acetylglucosamine- and mannose-terminated glycoproteins. Hepatology 1987; 7:672–679.

95. Dini L, Lentini A, Diez GD, Rocha M, Falasca L, Serafino L, Vidal-Vanaclocha F. Phagocytosis of apoptotic bodies by liver endothelial cells. J Cell Sci 1995; 108:967–973.

96. Kosugi I, Muro H, Shirasawa H, Ito I. Endocytosis of soluble IgG immune complex and its transport to lysosomes in hepatic sinusoidal endothelial cells. J Hepatol 1992; 16:106–114.

97. Smedsrod B, Pertoft H, Gustanson S, Laurent TC. Scavenger functions of the liver endothelial cell. Biochem J 1990; 266:313–327.

98. Oynebraten I, Hansen B, Smedsrod B, Uhlin-Hansen L. Serglycin secreted by leukocytes is

efficiently eliminated from the circulation by sinusoidal scavenger endothelial cells in the liver. J Leukoc Biol 2000; 67:183–188.

99. Zhou B, Oka JA, Singh A, Weigel PH. Purification and subunit characterization of the rat liver endocytic hyaluronan receptor. J Biol Chem 1999; 274:33831–33834.

100. Yoshioka T, Yamamoto K, Kobashi H, Tomita M, Tsuji T. Receptor-mediated endocytosis of chemically modified albumins by sinusoidal endothelial cells and Kupffer cells in rat and human liver. Liver 1994; 14:129–137.

101. Esbach S, Stins MF, Brouwer A, Roholl PJ, van Berkel TJ, Knook DL. Morphological characterization of scavenger receptor-mediated processing of modified lipoproteins by rat liver endothelial cells. Exp Cell Res 1994; 210:62–70.

102. Smedsrod B, Pertoft H, Gustanfson S, Laurent TC. Scavenger functions of the liver endothelial cell. Biochem J 1990; 266:313–327.

103. Steffan A-M, Gendrault J-L, McCuskey RS, McCuskey PA, Kirn A. Phagocytosis, an unrecognized property of murine endothelial liver cells. Hepatology 1986; 6:830–836.

104. Shiratori Y, Jin'nai H, Teraoka H, Matano S, Matsumoto K, Kamii K, Tanaka M, Okano K. Phagocytic properties of hepatic endothelial cells and splenic macrophages compensating for a decreased phagocytic function of Kupffer cells in the chronically ethanol-fed rats. Exp Cell Biol 1989; 57:300–309.

105. Bogers WMJM, Stad RK, Janssen DJ, Prins FA, Van Rooijen N, Van Es LA, Daha MR. Kupffer cell depletion in vivo results in clearance of large-sized IgA aggregates in rats by liver endothelial cells. Clin Exp Immunol 1991; 85:128–136.

106. Hashimoto N, Watanabe T, Shiratori Y, Ikeda Y, Kato H, Han K, Yamada H, Toda G, Kurokawa K. Prostanoid secretion by rat hepatic sinusoidal endothelial cells and its regulation by exogenous adenosine triphosphate. Hepatology 1995; 21:1713–1718.

107. Gardner CR, Laskin JD, Laskin DL. Platelet-activating factor-induced calcium mobilization and oxidative metabolism in hepatic macrophages and endothelial cells. J Leukoc Biol 1993; 53:190–196.

108. Spolarics Z. Endotoxin stimulates gene expression of ROS-eliminating pathways in rat hepatic endothelial and Kupffer cells. Am J Physiol 1996; 270:G660–G666.

109. Misquith S, Wattiaux-De Coninck S, Wattiaux R. Intracellular degradation by liver endothelial cells. Mol Cell Biochem 1989; 91:63–74.

110. Eakes AT, Olson MS. Regulation of endothelin synthesis in hepatic endothelial cells. Am J Physiol 1998; 274:G1068–G1076.

111. Mizoguchi Y, Ichikawa Y, Kioka K, Kawada N, Kobayashi K, Yamamoto S. Effects of arachidonic acid metabolites and interleukin-1 on platelet activating factor production by hepatic sinusoidal endothelial cells from mice. J Gastroenterol Hepatol 1991; 6:283–288.

112. Arii S, Imamura M. Physiological role of sinusoidal endothelial cells and Kupffer cells and their implications in the pathogenesis of liver injury. J Hepatobil Pancreat Surg 2000; 7:40–48.

113. Komatsu Y, Shiratori Y, Kawase T, Hashimoto N, Han K, Shiina S, Matsumura M, Niwa Y, Kato H, Tada M, et al. Role of polymorphonuclear leukocytes in galactosamine hepatitis: mechanism of adherence to hepatic endothelial cells. Hepatology 1994; 20:1548–1556.

114. Scoazec JY, Feldmann G. The cell adhesion molecules of hepatic sinusoidal endothelial cells. J Hepatol 1994; 20:296–300.

115. Knolle PA, Gerken G. Local control of the immune response in the liver. Immunol Rev 2000; 174:21–34.

116. Leifield L, Trautwein C, Dumoulin FL, Manns MP, Sauerbruch T, Spengler U. Enhanced expression of CD80 (B7-1), CD86 (B7-2), and CD40 and their ligands CD28 and CD154 in fulminant hepatic failure. Am J Pathol 1999; 154:1711–1720.

117. Sarphie G, D'Souza NB, Van Thiel DH, Hill D, McClain CJ, Deaciuc IV. Dose- and time-dependent effects of ethanol on functional and structural aspects of the liver sinusoid in the mouse. Alcohol Clin Exp Res 1997; 21:1128–1136.

118. Laskin DL. Nonparenchymal cells and hepatotoxicity. Semin Liver Dis 1990; 10:293–304.

119. Deaciuc IV, Alappat JM, D'Souza NB. Effect of acute and chronic alcohol administration to rats on the expression of interleukin-6 cell-surface receptors of hepatic parenchymal and nonparenchymal cells. Alcohol Clin Exp Res 1994; 18:1207–1214.

120. Deaciuc IV, D'Souza NB, Spitzer JJ. Tumor necrosis factor-alpha cell-surface receptors of liver parenchymal and nonparenchymal cells during acute and chronic alcohol administration to rats. Alcohol Clin Exp Res 1995; 19:332–338.

121. Nanji AA, Griniuviene B, Yacoub LK, Fogt F, Tahan SR. Intercellular adhesion molecule-1 expression in experimental alcoholic liver disease: relationship to endotoxemia and TNF alpha messenger RNA. Exp Mol Pathol 1995; 62:42–51.

122. Nanji AA, Tahan SR. Association between endothelial cell proliferation and pathologic changes in experimental alcoholic liver disease. Toxicol Appl Pharmacol 1996; 140:101–107.

123. Wisse E, Braet F, Luo D, De Zanger R, Jans D, Crabbe E, Vermoesen A. Structure and function of sinusoidal lining cells in the liver. Toxicol Pathol 1996; 24:100–111.

124. van Oosten M, van de Bilt E, de Vries HE, van Berkel TJ, Kunkel SL. Vascular adhesion molecule-1 and intercellular adhesion molecule-1 expression on rat liver cells after lipopolysaccharide administration in vivo. Hepatology 1995; 22:1538–1546.

125. Blomhoff R, Wake K. Perisinusoidal stellate cells of the liver: important roles in retinol metabolism and fibrosis. FASEB J 1991; 5:271–277.

126. Hendriks HF, Verhoofstad WA, Brouwer A, De Leeuw AM, Knook DL. Perisinusoidal fat-storing cells are the main vitamin A storage cells in rat liver. Exp Cell Res 1985; 160:138–149.

127. Ogata I, Mochida S, Tomiya T, Fujiwara W. Minor contribution of hepatocytes to collagen production in normal and early fibrotic rat livers. Hepatology 1991; 14:361–367.

128. Shiratori Y, Ichida T, Geerts A, Wisse E. Modulation of collagen synthesis by fat-storing cells, isolated from CCl_4- or vitamin A–treated rats. Dig Dis Sci 1987; 32:1281–1289.

129. Arthur MJ, Stanley A, Iredale JP, Rafferty JA, Hembry RM, Friedman SL. Secretion of 72 kDa type IV collagenase/gelatinase by cultured human lipocytes. Analysis of gene expression, protein synthesis and proteinase activity. Biochem J 1992; 287:701–707.

130. Friedman SL. Cellular sources of collagen and regulation of collagen production in liver. Semin Liver Dis 1990; 10:20–29.

131. Friedman SL, Roll FJ, Boyles JK, Bissell DM. Hepatic lipocytes: the principle collagen-producing cells of normal rat liver. Proc Natl Acad Sci USA 1985; 82:8681–8685.

132. French SW, Takahashi H, Wong K, Mendenhall CL. Ito cell activation induced by chronic ethanol feeding in the presence of different dietary fats. Alcohol Alcohol 1991; 1(suppl): 357–361.

133. Gressner AM. Transdifferentiation of hepatic stellate cells (Ito cells) to myofibroblasts: a key event in hepatic fibrogenesis. Kidney Int 1996; 54(suppl):S39–S45.

134. Kim KY, Choi I, Kim SS. Progression of hepatic stellate cell activation is associated with the level of oxidative stress rather than cytokines during CCl_4-induced fibrogenesis. Mol Cells 2000; 10:289–300.

135. Ikeda K, Wakahara T, Wang YQ, Kadoya H, Kawada N, Kaneda K. In vitro migratory potential of rat quiescent hepatic stellate cells and its augmentation by cell activation. Hepatology 1999; 29:1760–1767.

136. Friedman SL. Molecular mechanisms of hepatic fibrosis and principles of therapy. J Gastroenterol 1997; 32:424–430.

137. Knittel T, Dinter C, Kobold D, Neubauer K, Mehde M, Eichhorst S, Ramadori G. Expression and regulation of cell adhesion molecules by hepatic stellate cells (HSC) of rat liver: involvement of HSC in recruitment of inflammatory cells during hepatic tissue repair. Am J Pathol 1999; 154:153–167.

138. Hellerbrand C, Wang SC, Tsukamoto H, Brenner DA, Rippe RA. Expression of intracellular adhesion molecule 1 by activated hepatic stellate cells. Hepatology 1996; 24:670–676.

139. Schieferdecker HL, Schlaf G, Koleva M, Gotze O, Jungermann K. Induction of functional anaphylatoxin C5a receptors on hepatocytes by in vivo treatment of rats with IL-6. J Immunol 2000; 164:5453–5458.

140. Gandhi CR, Uemura T, Kuddus RH. Endotoxin causes up-regulation of endothelin receptors in cultured hepatic stellate cells via nitric oxide-dependent and -independent mechanisms. Br J Pharmacol 2000; 131:319–327.

141. Fennekohl A, Schieferdecker HL, Jungermann K, Püschel GP. Differential expression of prostanoid receptors in hepatocytes, Kupffer cells, sinusoidal endothelial cells and stellate cells of rat liver. J Hepatol 1999; 30:38–47.

142. Tsukamoto H. Cytokine regulation of hepatic stellate cells in liver fibrosis. Alcohol Clin Exp Res 1999; 23:911–916.

143. Wong L, Yamasaki G, Johnson RJ, Friedman SL. Induction of beta-platelet-derived growth factor receptor in rat hepatic lipocytes during cellular activation in vivo and in culture. J Clin Invest 1994; 94:1563–1569.

144. Helyar L, Bundschuh DS, Laskin JD, Laskin DL. Hepatic fat storing cells produce nitric oxide and hydrogen peroxide in response to bacterially-derived lipopolysaccharide. In: DL Knook, K Decker, eds. Cells of the Hepatic Sinusoid. Vol. 3. Amsterdam: Kupffer Cell Foundation, 1993:394–396.

145. Helyar L, Bundschuh DS, Laskin JD, Laskin DL. Induction of hepatic Ito cell nitric oxide production by acute endotoxemia. Hepatology 1994; 12:1509–1515.

146. Athari A, Hanecke K, Jungermann K. Prostaglandin F_2 alpha and D_2 release from primary Ito cell cultures after stimulation with noradrenaline and ATP but not adenosine. Hepatology 1994; 20:142–148.

147. Xu Y, Rojkind M, Czaja MJ. Regulation of monocyte chemoattractant protein 1 by cytokines and oxygen free radicals in rat hepatic fat-storing cells. Gastroenterology 1996; 110:1870–1877.

148. Knittel T, Janneck T, Muller L, Fellmer P, Ramadori G. Transforming growth factor beta 1–regulated gene expression of Ito cells. Hepatology 1996; 24:352–360.

149. Ramadori G, Knittel T, Odenthal M, Schwogler S, Neubauer K, Meyer zum Buschenfelde K. Synthesis of cellular fibronectin by rat liver fat-storing (Ito) cells: regulation by cytokines. Gastroenterology 1992; 103:1313–1321.

150. Davis BH, Kramer RT, Davidson NO. Retinoic acid modulates rat Ito cell proliferation, collagen, and transforming growth factor beta production. J Clin Invest 1990; 86:2062–2070.

151. Poli G. Pathogenesis of liver fibrosis: role of oxidative stress. Mol Aspects Med 2000; 21:49–98.

152. Britton RS, Bacon BR. Intracellular signaling pathways in stellate cell activation. Alcohol Clin Exp Res 1999; 23:922–925.

153. Friedman SL. Stellate cell activation in alcoholic fibrosis—an overview. Alcohol Clin Exp Res 1999; 23:904–910.

154. Sprenger H, Kaufmann A, Garn H, Lahme B, Gemsa D, Gressner AM. Differential expression of monocyte chemotactic protein-1 (MCP-1) in transforming rat hepatic stellate cells. J Hepatol 1999; 30:88–94.

155. Larrick JW, Kunkel SL. The role of tumor necrosis factor and interleukin 1 in the immunoinflammatory response. Pharmaceut Res 1988; 5:129–139.

156. Whicher JT, Evans SW. Cytokines in disease. Clin Chem 1990; 36/7:1269–1281.

157. Cerami A. Inflammatory cytokines. Clin Immunol Immunopathol 1992; 62:S3–S10.

158. Punjabi CJ, Laskin JD, Hwang S, MacEachern L, Laskin DL. Enhanced production of nitric oxide by bone marrow cells and increased sensitivity to macrophage colony-stimulating factor (CSF) and granulocyte-macrophage CSF after benzene treatment of mice. Blood 1994; 83:3255–3262.

159. Lavnikova N, Drapier J-C, Laskin DL. A single exogenous stimulus activates rat macrophages for nitric oxide production and cytotoxicity. J Leukoc Biol 1993; 54:322–328.

160. Sharma RJ, Macallan DC, Sedgwick P, Remick DG, Griffin GE. Kinetics of endotoxin-induced acute-phase protein gene expression and its modulation by TNF-α monoclonal antibody. Am J Physiol 1992; 262:R786–R793.

161. Sujita K, Okuno F, Tanaka Y, Hirano Y, Inamoto Y, Eto S, Arai M. Effect of interleukin 1 (IL-1) on the level of cytochrome P-450 involving IL-1 receptor on the isolated hepatocytes of rat. Biochem Biophys Res Commun 1990; 168:1217–1222.

162. Curran RD, Billiar TR, Stuehr DJ, Ochoa JB, Harbrecht BG, Flint SG, Simmons RL. Multiple cytokines are required to induce hepatocyte nitric oxide production and inhibit total protein synthesis. Ann Surg 1990; 212:462–469.

163. Wang JH, Redmond HP, Watson RW, Bouchier-Hayes D. Role of lipopolysaccharide and tumor necrosis factor-α in induction of hepatocyte necrosis. Am J Physiol 1995; 269:G297–G304.

164. Leist M, Gantner F, Bohlinger I, Germann PG, Tiegs G, Wendel A. Murine hepatocyte apoptosis induced in vitro and in vivo by TNF-α requires transcriptional arrest. J Immunol 1994; 153:1778–1788.

165. Blazka ME, Wilmer JL, Holladay SD, Wilson RE, Luster MI. Role of proinflammatory cytokines in acetaminophen hepatotoxicity. Toxicol Appl Pharmacol 1995; 133:43–52.

166. McClain CJ, Barve S, Deaciuc IV, Kugelmas M. Cytokines in alcoholic liver disease. Semin Liver Dis 1999; 19:205–219.

167. Fang C, Lindros KO, Badger TM, Ronis MJ, Ingelman-Sundberg M. Zonated expression of cytokines in rat liver: effect of chronic ethanol and the cytochrome P450 2E1 inhibitor, chlormethiazole. Hepatology 1998; 27:1304–1310.

168. Aono K, Isobe K, Kiuchi K, Fan ZH, Ito M, Takeuchi A, Miyachi M, Nakashima I, Nimura Y. In vitro and in vivo expression of inducible nitric oxide synthase during experimental endotoxemia: involvement of other cytokines. J Cell Biochem 1997; 65:349–358.

169. Scotte M, Hiron M, Masson S, Lyoumi S, Banine F, Teniere P, Lebreton JP, Daveau M. Differential expression of cytokine genes in monocytes, peritoneal macrophages and liver following endotoxin- or turpentine-induced inflammation in rat. Cytokine 1996; 8:115–120.

170. Horn TL, O'Brien TD, Schook LB, Rutherford MS. Acute hepatotoxicant exposure induces TNFR-mediated hepatic injury and cytokine/apoptotic gene expression. Toxicol Sci 2000; 54:262–273.

171. Wang J, Wendel A. Studies on the hepatotoxicity of galactosamine/endotoxin or galactosamine/TNF in the perfused mouse liver. Biochem Pharmacol 1990; 39:267–270.

172. Schook LB, Lockwood JF, Yang SD, Myers MJ. Dimethylnitrosamine (DMN)-induced IL-1 beta, TNF-alpha, and IL-6 inflammatory cytokine expression. Toxicol Appl Pharmacol 1992; 116:110–116.

173. Blazka ME, Elwellk MR, Holladay SD, Wilson RE, Luster MI. Histopathology of acetaminophen-induced liver changes: role of interleukin 1α and tumor necrosis factor α. Toxicol Pathol 1996; 24:181–189.

174. Shedlofsky SI, McClain CJ. Hepatic dysfunction due to cytokines. In: ES Kimball, ed. Cytokines and Inflammation. Boca Raton, FL: CRC Press, 1991:235–273.

175. Dinarello CA. Interleukin-1 and its biologically related cytokines. Adv Immunol 1989; 44:153–205.

176. Tracey KJ, Beutler B, Lowry SF, Merryweather J, Wolpe S, Milsark IW, Hariri RJ, Fahey TJ, Zentella A, Albert JD, et al. Shock and tissue injury induced by recombinant human cachectin. Science 1986; 234:470–474.

177. Fiedler VB, Loof I, Sander E, Voehringer V, Galanos C, Fournel MA. Monoclonal antibody to tumor necrosis factor-alpha prevents lethal endotoxin sepsis in adult rhesus monkeys. J Lab Clin Med 1992; 120:574–588.

178. Hishinuma I, Nagakawa J, Hirota K, Miyamoto K, Tsukidate K, Yamanaka T, Katayama

K, Yamatsu I. Involvement of tumor necrosis factor-α in development of hepatic injury in galactosamine-sensitized mice. Hepatology 1990; 12:1187–1191.

179. Kayama F, Yoshida T, Elwell MR, Luster MI. Role of tumor necrosis factor-alpha in cadmium-induced hepatotoxicity. Toxicol Appl Pharmacol 1995; 131:224–234.

180. Czaja MJ, Xu J, Alt E. Prevention of carbon tetrachloride-induced rat liver injury by soluble tumor necrosis factor receptor. Gastroenterology 1995; 108:1849–1854.

181. Dinarello CA. Interleukin-1 and interleukin-1 antagonism. Blood 1991; 77:1627–1652.

182. Josephs MD, Solorzano CC, Taylor M, Rosenberg JJ, Topping D, Abouhamze A, MacKay SL, Hirsch E, Hirsh D, Labow M, Moldawer LL. Modulation of the acute phase response by altered expression of the IL-1 type 1 receptor or IL-1ra. Am J Physiol 2000; 278:R824–R830.

183. Iimuro Y, Gallucci RM, Luster MI, Kono H, Thurman RG. Antibodies to tumor necrosis factor alfa attenuate hepatic necrosis and inflammation caused by chronic exposure to ethanol in the rat. Hepatology 1997; 26:1530–1537.

184. Nowak M, Gaines GG, Rosenberg J, Mintner R, Bahajat FR, Rectenwald J, MacKay SL, Edwards CK, Moldawer LL. LPS-induced liver injury in D-galactosamine-sensitized mice requires secreted TNF-alpha and the TNF-p55 receptor. Am J Physiol 2000; 278:R1202–R1209.

185. Sneed RA, Buchweitz JP, Jean PA, Ganey PE. Pentoxifylline attenuates bacterial lipopolysaccharide-induced enhancement of allyl alcohol hepatotoxicity. Toxicol Sci 2000; 56:203–210.

186. Yamada Y, Fausto N. Deficient liver regeneration after carbon tetrachloride injury in mice lacking type 1 but not type 2 tumor necrosis factor receptor. Am J Pathol 1998; 152:1577–1589.

187. Yin M, Wheeler MD, Kono H, Bradford BU, Gallucci RM, Luster MI, Thurman RG. Essential role of tumor necrosis factor alpha in alcohol-induced liver injury in mice. Gastroenterology 1999; 117:942–952.

188. Cuzzocrea S, de Sarro G, Costantino G, Mazzon E, Laura R, Ciriaco E, de Sarro A, Caputi AP. Role of interleukin-6 in a non-septic shock model induced by zymosan. Eur Cytokine Network 1999; 10:191–203.

189. Dambach DM, Gardner CR, Chiu H, Marion MW, Durham SK, Laskin DL. Increased sensitivity of tumor necrosis factor-α (TNF-α) knockout mice to acetaminophen (AA) is mediated by nitric oxide (abstr). Toxicologist 1999; 48:257.

190. Katz A, Chebath J, Friedman J, Revel M. Increased sensitivity of IL-6-deficient mice to carbon tetrachloride hepatotoxicity and protection with an IL-6 receptor-IL-6 chimera. Cytokines Cell Mol Ther 1998; 4:221–227.

191. Kovalovich K, DeAngelis PA, Li W, Furth EE, Ciliberto G, Taub R. Increased toxin-induced liver injury and fibrosis in interleukin-6-deficient mice. Hepatology 2000; 31:149–159.

192. Saile B, Matthes N, Knittel T, Ramadori G. Transforming growth factor-β and tumor necrosis factor-α inhibit both apoptosis and proliferation of activated rat hepatic stellate cells. Hepatology 1999; 30:196–202.

193. Dooley S, Delvoux B, Lahme B, Mangasser-Stephan K, Gressner AM. Modulation of transforming growth factor beta response and signaling during transdifferentiation of rat hepatic stellate cells to myofibroblasts. Hepatology 2000; 31:1094–1106.

194. Armendariz-Borunda J, Katai H, Jones CM, Seyer JM, Kang AH, Raghow R. Transforming growth factor-β gene expression is transiently enhanced at a critical stage during liver regeneration after CCl$_4$ treatment. Lab Invest 1993; 69:283–294.

195. Jarvelainen HA, Fang C, Ingelman-Sundberg M, Lindros KO. Effect of chronic coadministration of endotoxin and ethanol on rat liver pathology and proinflammatory and anti-inflammatory cytokines. Hepatology 1999; 29:1503–1510.

196. Hellerbrand C, Stefanovic B, Giordano F, Burchardt ER, Brenner DA. The role of TGFβ$_1$ in initiating hepatic stellate cell activation in vivo. J Hepatol 1999; 30:77–87.

197. Feng L. Role of chemokines in inflammation and immunoregulation. Immunol Res 2000; 21:203–210.

198. Czaja MJ, Geerts A, Xu J, Schmiedeberg P, Ju Y. Monocyte chemoattractant protein 1 (MCP-1) expression occurs in toxic liver injury. J Leukoc Biol 1994; 55:120–126.

199. Maher JJ. Rat hepatocytes and Kupffer cells interact to produce interleukin-8 (CINC) in the setting of ethanol. Am J Physiol 1995; 269:G518–G523.

200. Ohkubo K, Masumoto T, Horiike N, Onji M. Induction of CINC (interleukin-8) production in rat liver by non-parenchymal cells. J Gastroenterol Hepatol 1998; 13:696–702.

201. Bautista AP. Impact of alcohol on the ability of Kupffer cells to produce chemokines and its role in alcoholic liver disease. J Gastroenterol Hepatol 2000; 15:346–356.

202. Afford SC, Fisher NC, Neil DAH, Fear J, Brun P, Hubscher SG, Adams DH. Distinct patterns of chemokine expression are associated with leukocyte recruitment in alcoholic hepatitis and alcoholic cirrhosis. J Pathol 1998; 186:82–89.

203. Lawson JA, Farhood A, Hopper RD, Bajt ML, Jaeschke H. The hepatic inflammatory response after acetaminophen overdose: role of neutrophils. Toxicol Sci 2000; 54:509–516.

204. Kopydlowski KM, Salkowski CA, Cody MJ, Van Rooijen N, Major J, Hamilton TA, Vogel SN. Regulation of macrophage chemokine expression by lipopolysaccharide in vitro and in vivo. J Immunol 1999; 163:1537–1544.

205. Zhang P, Xie M, Zagorski J, Spitzer J, Spitzer JA. Attenuation of hepatic neutrophil sequestration by anti-CINC antibody in endotoxic rats. Shock 1995; 4:262–268.

206. Hoagboam CM, Bone-Larson CL, Steinhauser ML, Matsukawa A, Gosling J, Boring L, Charo IF, Simpson KJ, Lukacs NW, Kunkel SL. Exaggerated hepatic injury due to acetaminophen challenge in mice lacking C-C chemokine receptor 2. Am J Pathol 2000; 156:1245–1252.

207. Rai RM, Loffreda S, Karp CL, Yang S-Q, Lin H-Z, Diehl AM. Kupffer cell depletion abolishes induction of interleukin-10 and permits sustained overexpression of tumor necrosis factor alpha messenger RNA in the regenerating rat liver. Hepatology 1997; 25:889–895.

208. Zisman DA, Kunkel SL, Strieter RM, Tsai WC, Wilkowski J, Standiford TJ. MCP-1 protects mice in lethal endotoxemia. J Clin Invest 1997; 99:2832–2836.

209. Gardner CR, Laskin DL. Protective and pathologic roles of nitric oxide in tissue injury. In: JD Laskin, DL Laskin, eds. Cellular and Molecular Biology of Nitric Oxide. New York: Marcel Dekker, 1999:225–246.

210. Shiratori Y, Takada H, Hai K, Kiriyama H, Nagura T, Tanaka M, Matsumoto K, Kamii K. Generation of chemotactic factor by hepatocytes isolated from chronically ethanol-fed rats. Dig Dis Sci 1992; 37:650–658.

211. Laskin DL, Pilaro AM, Ji S. Potential role of macrophages in acetaminophen hepatotoxicity. II. Mechanisms of macrophage accumulation and activation. Toxicol Appl Pharmacol 1986; 86:216–226.

212. Mawet E, Shiratori Y, Hikiba Y, Takada H, Yoshida H, Okano K, Komatsu Y, Matsumura M, Niwa Y, Omata M. Cytokine-induced neutrophil chemoattractant release from hepatocytes is modulated by Kupffer cells. Hepatology 1996; 23:353–358.

213. Thornton AJ, Ham J, Kunkel SL. Kupffer cell-derived cytokines induce the synthesis of a leukocyte chemotactic peptide, interleukin-8, in human hepatoma and primary hepatocyte cultures. Hepatology 1991; 14:1112–1122.

214. Louis H, Van Laethem J-L, Wu W, Quertinmont E, Degraef C, Van den Berg K, Demols A, Goldman M, Le Moine O, Geerts A, Devière J. Interleukin-10 controls neutrophilic infiltration, hepatocyte proliferation, and liver fibrosis induced by carbon tetrachloride in mice. Hepatology 1998; 28:1607–1615.

215. Matsukawa A, Hoagboam CM, Lukacs NW, Lincoln PM, Evanoff HL, Strieter RM, Kunkel SL. Expression and contribution of endogenous IL-13 in an experimental model of sepsis. J Immunol 2000; 164:2738–2744.

216. Minty RR, Chalon P, Derocq J-M, Dumont X, Cuillemont J-C, Kaghad M, Labit C, Leplatois

P, Liauzun P, Milox B, Minty C, Casellas P, Loison G, Lupker J, Shire D, Ferrara P, Caput D. Interleukin-13 is a new human lymphokine regulating inflammatory and immune responses. Nature 1993; 362:248–250.

217. de Waal Malefyt R, Figdor CG, Huijbens RG, Mohan-Peterson S, Benett B, Culpepper J, Dang W, Zurawski G, de Vries JE. Effects of IL-13 on phenotype, cytokine production, and cytotoxic function of human monocytes: comparison with IL-4 and modulation by IFN-γ or IL-10. J Immunol 1993; 151:6370–6381.

218. Loyer P, Ilyin G, Abdel-Razzak Z, Banchereau J, Dezier JF, Campion JP, Guguen-Guillouzo C, Guillouzo A. Interleukin 4 inhibits the production of some acute-phase proteins by human hepatocytes in primary culture. FEBS Lett 1993; 336:215–220.

219. Gabay C, Porter B, Guenette D, Billir B, Arend WP. Interleukin-4 (IL-4) and IL-13 enhance the effect of IL-1 beta on production of IL-1 receptor antagonist by human primary hepatocytes and hepatoma HepG2 cells: differential effect on C-reactive protein production. Blood 1999; 93:1299–1307.

220. Babior BM. Oxidants from phagocytes: agents of defense and destruction. Blood 1984; 64: 959–966.

221. Halliwell B, Gutteridge JMC. Oxygen toxicity, oxygen radicals, transition metals and disease. Biochem J 1984; 219:1–14.

222. Rubin R, Farber JL. Mechanisms of the killing of cultured hepatocytes by hydrogen peroxide. Arch Biochem Biophys 1984; 228:450–459.

223. Sevanian A, Hochstein P. Mechanisms and consequences of lipid peroxidation in biological systems. Annu Rev Nutr 1985; 5:365–390.

224. Sipes IG, el Sisi AE, Sim WW, Mobley SA, Earnest DL. Reactive oxygen species in the progression of CCl_4-induced liver injury. Adv Exp Med Biol 1991; 283:489–497.

225. Towner RA, Reinke LA, Janzen EG, Yamashiro S. In vivo magnetic resonance imaging study of Kupffer cell involvement in CCl_4-induced hepatotoxicity in rats. Can J Physiol Pharmacol 1994; 72:441–446.

226. Arai M, Mochida S, Ohno A, Ogata I, Fujiwara K. Sinusoidal endothelial cell damage by activated macrophages in rat liver necrosis. Gastroenterology 1993; 104:466–471.

227. Guanawardhana L, Mobley SA, Sipes IG. Modulation of 1,2-dichlorobenzene hepatotoxicity in the Fischer-344 rat by a scavenger of superoxide anions and an inhibitor of Kupffer cells. Toxicol Appl Pharmacol 1993; 119:205–213.

228. Nakae D, Yamamoto K, Yoshiji H, Kinugasa T, Maruyama H, Farber JL, Konishi Y. Liposome-encapsulated superoxide dismutase prevents liver necrosis induced by acetaminophen. Am J Pathol 1990; 136:787–795.

229. Fujita S, Arai S, Monden K, Adachi Y, Funaki N, Higashitsuji H. Participation of hepatic macrophages and plasma factors in endotoxin-induced liver injury. J Surg Res 1995; 59: 263–270.

230. Amimoto T, Matsura T, Koyama SY, Nakanishi T, Yamada K, Kajiyama G. Acetaminophen-induced hepatic injury in mice: the role of lipid peroxidation and effects of pretreatment with coenzyme Q10 and alpha-tocopherol. Free Radic Biol Med 1995; 19:169–176.

231. Nagabubu E, Sesikeran B, Lakshmaiah L. The protective effects of eugeol on carbon tetra-chloride induced hepatotoxicity in rats. Free Radic Res 1995; 23:617–627.

232. Sugino K, Dohi K, Yamada K, Kawaski T. Changes in the levels of endogenous antioxidants in the liver of mice with experimental endotoxemia and the protective effects of antioxidants. Surgery 1989; 105:200–206.

233. Ghezzi P, Saccardo B, Bianchi M. Role of reactive oxygen intermediates in the hepatotoxicity of endotoxin. Immunopharmacology 1986; 12:241–244.

234. Nussler AK, Beger H-G, Liu ZZ, Billiar TR. Nitric oxide, hepatocytes and inflammation. Res Immunol 1995; 146:671–677.

235. Milbourne EA, Bygrave FL. Does nitric oxide play a role in liver function? Cell Signal 1995; 7:313–318.

236. Losser M-R, Payen D. Mechanisms of liver damage. Semin Liver Dis 1996; 16:357–367.

237. Moncada S, Palmer RM, Higgs EA. Nitric oxide: physiology, pathophysiology, and pharmacology. Pharmacol Rev 1991; 43:109–142.

238. Lavnikova N, Lakhotia A, Patel N, Prokhorova S, Laskin DL. Cytostasis is required for IL-1 induced nitric oxide production in transformed hamster fibroblasts. J Cell Physiol 1996; 169:532–537.

239. Laskin DL, Rodriguez del Valle M, Heck DE, Hwang S, Ohnishi ST, Durham S, Goller N, Laskin JD. Hepatic nitric oxide production following acute endotoxemia in rats is mediated by increased nitric oxide synthase gene expression. Hepatology 1995; 22:223–234.

240. Gross SS, Wolin MS. Nitric oxide: pathophysiological mechanisms. Annu Rev Physiol 1995; 57:737–769.

241. Hodgson PD, Renton KW. The role of nitric oxide generation in interferon-evoked cytochrome P450 down-regulation. Int J Immunopharmacol 1995; 17:995–1000.

242. MacMicking J, Xie QW, Nathan C. Nitric oxide and macrophage function. Annu Rev Immunol 1997; 15:323–350.

243. Lavnikova N, Burdelya L, Lakhotia A, Patel N, Prokhorova S, Laskin DL. Macrophage and interleukin-1 induced nitric oxide production and cytostasis in hamster tumor cells. J Leukoc Biol 1997; 61:452–458.

244. Beckman J. The double-edged role of nitric oxide in brain function and superoxide-mediated injury. J Dev Physiol 1991; 15:53–59.

245. Beckman JS, Crow JP. Pathological implications of nitric, superoxide and peroxynitrite formation. Biochem Soc Trans 1993; 21:330–334.

246. Freeman B. Free radical chemistry of nitric oxide: looking at the dark side. Chest 1994; 105:79S–84S.

247. Beckman JS, Koppenol WH. Nitric oxide, superoxide, and peroxynitrite: the good, the bad, and ugly. Am J Physiol 1996; 271:C1424–C1437.

248. Radi R, Beckman JS, Bush KM, Freeman B. Peroxynitrite oxidation of sulfhydryls: The cytotoxic potential of superoxide and nitric oxide. J Biol Chem 1991; 266:4244–4250.

249. Radi R, Beckman JS, Bush KM, Freeman B. Peroxynitrite-induced membrane lipid peroxidation: the cytotoxic potential of superoxide and nitric oxide. Arch Biochem Biophys 1991; 288:481–487.

250. Lin KT, Xue JY, Nomen M, Spur B, Wong PY. Peroxynitrite-induced apoptosis in HL-60 cells. J Biol Chem 1995; 270:16487–16490.

251. Ischiropoulos H, Zhu L, Chen J, Tsai M, Martin JC, Smith CD. Peroxynitrite-mediated tyrosine nitration catalyzed by superoxide dismutase. Arch Biochem Biophys 1992; 298:431–437.

252. Matsumoto H, Nishitani Y, Minowa Y, Fukui Y. Role of Kupffer cells in the release of nitric oxide and change of portal pressure after ethanol perfusion in the rat liver. Alcohol Alcohol 2000; 35:31–34.

253. Zhu W, Fung PC. The roles played by crucial free radicals like lipid free radicals, nitric oxide, and enzymes NOS and NADPH in CCl_4-induced acute liver injury of mice. Free Radic Biol Med 2000; 29:870–880.

254. Rockey DC, Chung JJ. Regulation of inducible nitric oxide synthase and nitric oxide during hepatic injury and fibrogenesis. Am J Physiol 1997; 273:G124–G130.

255. Spitzer JA, Spitzer JJ. Lipopolysaccharide tolerance and ethanol modulate hepatic nitric oxide production in a gender-dependent manner. Alcohol 2000; 21:27–35.

256. Hinson JA, Pike SL, Pumford NR, Mayeux PR. Nitrotyrosine-protein adducts in hepatic centrilobular areas following toxic doses of acetaminophen in mice. Chem Res Toxicol 1998; 11:604–607.

257. Gardner CR, Dambach DM, Durham SK, Cohen SD, Bruno MK, Salzman AL, Southan GJ, Laskin DL. Role of peroxynitrite (PN) in acetaminophen (AA)-induced hepatotoxicity (abstr). Toxicologist 2000; 54:41.

258. Wright CE, Rees DD, Moncada S. Protective and pathological roles of nitric oxide in endotoxin shock. Cardiovasc Res 1992; 26:48–57.
259. Ialenti A, Ianaro A, Moncada S, Di Rosa M. Modulation of acute inflammation by endogenous nitric oxide. Eur J Pharmacol 1992; 211:177–182.
260. Tanaka N, Tanaka K, Nagashima Y, Kondo M, Sekihara H. Nitric oxide increases hepatic arterial blood flow in rats with carbon tetrachloride-induced acute hepatic injury. Gastroenterology 1999; 117:173–180.
261. Al-Shabanah OA, Alam K, Nagi MN, Al-Rikabi AC, Al-Bekairi AM. Protective effect of aminoguanidine, a nitric oxide synthase inhibitor, against carbon tetrachloride induced hepatotoxicity in mice. Life Sci 2000; 66:265–270.
262. Billiar TR, Curran RD, Harbrecht BG, Stueher DJ, Demetris AJ, Simmons RL. Modulation of nitrogen oxide synthesis in vivo: N^G-monomethyl-L-arginine inhibits endotoxin-induced nitrite/nitrate biosynthesis while promoting hepatic damage. J Leukoc Biol 1990; 48:565–569.
263. Harbrecht BG, Billiar TR, Stadler J, Demetris AJ, Ochoa JB, Curran RD, Simmons RL. Inhibition of nitric oxide synthesis during endotoxemia promotes intrahepatic thrombosis and an oxygen radical-mediated hepatic injury. J Leukoc Biol 1992; 52:390–394.
264. Muriel P. Nitric oxide protection of rat liver from lipid peroxidation, collagen accumulation, and liver damage induced by carbon tetrachloride. Biochem Pharmacol 1998; 56:773–779.
265. Taylor BS, Alarcon LH, Billiar TR. Inducible nitric oxide synthase in the liver: regulation and function. Biochemistry (Mosc) 1998; 63:766–781.
266. Decker K. Eicosanoids, signal molecules of liver cells. Semin Liver Dis 1985; 5:175–190.
267. Keppler D, Hagmann W, Rapp S, Denzlinger C, Koch HK. The relation of leukotrienes to liver injury. Hepatology 1985; 5:883–891.
268. vom Dahl S, Hallbrucker C, Lang F, Haussinger D. Role of eicosanoids, inositol phosphates and extracellular Ca^{2+} in cell-volume regulation of rat liver. Eur J Biochem 1991; 198:73–83.
269. Ogle CK, Wu JZ, Alexander JW, Fischer JE, Ogle JD. The effects of in vivo administration of endotoxin on the functions and interaction of hepatocytes and Kupffer cells. Prostaglandins 1991; 41:169–183.
270. Rodriguez de Turco EB, Spitzer JA. Eicosanoid production in nonparenchymal liver cells isolated from rats infused with *E. coli* endotoxin. J Leukoc Biol 1990; 48:488–494.
271. Enomoto N, Ikejima K, Yamashina S, Enomoto A, Nishiura T, Nishimura T, Brenner DA, Schemmer P, Bradford BU, Rivera CA, Zhong Z, Thurman RG. Kupffer cell–derived prostaglandin E_2 is involved in alcohol-induced fat accumulation in rat liver. Am J Physiol Gastrointest Liver Physiol 2000; 279:G100–G106.
272. McClain CJ, Price S, Barve S, Devalarja R, Shedlofsky S. Acetaminophen hepatotoxicity: an update. Curr Gastroenterol Rep 1999; 1:42–49.
273. Horton AA, Wood JM. Effects of inhibitors of phospholipase A_2, cyclooxygenase and thromboxane synthase on paracetamol hepatotoxicity in the rat. Eicosanoids 1989; 2:123–129.
274. Mancuso G, Cusumano V, Cook JA, Smith E, Squadrito F, Blandino G, Teti G. Efficacy of tumor necrosis factor alpha and eicosanoid inhibitors in experimental models of neonatal sepsis. FEMS Immunol Med Microbiol 1994; 9:49–54.
275. Shiratori Y, Tanaka M, Umihara J, Kawase T, Shiina S, Sugimoto T. Leukotriene inhibitors modulate hepatic injury induced by lipopolysaccharide-activated macrophages. J Hepatol 1990; 10:51–61.
276. Tiegs G, Wendel A. Leukotriene-mediated liver injury. Biochem Pharmacol 1988; 37:2569–2573.
277. Casey LC, Fletcher JR, Zmudka MI, Ramwell PW. The role of thromboxane in primate endotoxin shock. J Surg Res 1985; 39:140–149.
278. Smith EF, Jugus M, Kinter LB. Effect of thromboxane receptor antagonist, BM 13.505, on the sequelae of endotoxemia in the conscious rat. Eicosanoids 1998; 1:27–33.

279. Takano M, Nishimura H, Kimura Y, Washizu J, Mokuno Y, Nimura Y, Yoshikai Y. Prostaglandin E_2 protects against liver injury after *Escherichia coli* infection but hampers the resolution of the infection in mice. J Immunol 1998; 161:3019–3025.

280. Muntané J, Rodriguez FJ, Segado O, Quintero A, Lozano JM, Siendones E, Pedraza CA, Delgado M, O'Valle F, Garcia R, Montero JL, De la Mata M, Miño G. TNF-α dependent production of inducible nitric oxide is involved in PGE_1 protection against acute liver injury. Gut 2000; 47:553–562.

281. Muntané J, Montero JL, Lozano JM, Miranda-Vizuete A, De la Mata M, Miño G. TNF-α but not IL-1α is correlated with PGE_1-dependent protection against acute D-galactosamine-induced liver injury. Can J Gastroenterol 2000; 14:175–180.

282. Hagmann W, Denzlinger C, Keppler D. Role of peptide leukotrienes and their hepatobilliary elimination in endotoxin action. Circ Shock 1984; 14:223–235.

283. Henderson WR. The role of leukotrienes in inflammation. Ann Intern Med 1994; 121:684–697.

284. Goetzl EJ, Pickett WC. Novel structural determinants of the human neutrophil chemotactic activity of leukotriene B. J Exp Med 1981; 153:482–487.

285. Shimada K, Navarro J, Goeger DE, Mustafa SB, Weigel PH, Weinman SA. Expression and regulation of leukotriene-synthesis enzymes in rat liver cells. Hepatology 1998; 28:1275–1281.

286. Mustafa SB, Flickinger BD, Olson MS. Suppression of lipopolysaccharide-induced nitric oxide synthase expression by platelet-activating factor receptor antagonists in the rat liver and cultured rat Kupffer cells. Hepatology 1999; 30:1206–1214.

287. Dieter P, Schulze-Specking A, Decker K. Differential inhibition of prostaglandin and superoxide production by dexamethasone in primary cultures of rat Kupffer cells. Eur J Biochem 1986; 159:451–457.

288. Sakaguchi T, Nakamura S, Suzuki S, Oda T, Ichiyama A, Baba S, Okamoto T. Participation of platelet-activating factor in the lipopolysaccharide-induced liver injury in partially hepatectomized rats. Hepatology 1999; 30:959–967.

289. Anderson BO, Bensard DD, Harken AH. The role of platelet activating factor and its antagonists in shock, sepsis and multiple organ failure. Surg Gynecol Obstet 1991; 172:415–424.

290. Gardner CR, Laskin JD, Laskin DL. Distinct biochemical responses of hepatic macrophages and endothelial cells to platelet-activating factor during endotoxemia. J Leukoc Biol 1995; 57:269–274.

291. Yue TL, Farhat M, Rabinovici R, Perera PY, Vogel SN, Feuerstein G. Protective effect of BN 50739, a new platelet-activating factor antagonist, in endotoxin-treated rabbits. J Pharmacol Exp Ther 1990; 254:976–981.

292. Tanner A, Keyhani A, Wright R. The influence of endotoxin in vitro on hepatic macrophage lysosomal enzyme release in different models of hepatic injury. Liver 1983; 3:151–160.

293. Magilavy DB, Zhan R, Black DD. Modulation of murine hepatic lipase activity by exogenous and endogenous Kupffer-cell activation. Biochem J 1993; 292:249–252.

294. Winwood PJ, Schuppan D, Iredale JP, Kawser CA, Docherty AJ, Arthur MJP. Kupffer cell–derived 95-kd type IV collagenase/gelatinase B: characterization and expression in cultured cells. Hepatology 1995; 22:304–315.

295. Peinado-Onsurbe J, Soler C, Galan X, Proveda B, Soley M, Llobera M, Ramirez I. Involvement of catecholamines in the effect of fasting on hepatic endothelial lipase activity in the rat. Endocrinology 1991; 129:2599–2606.

296. Hironaka K, Sakaida I, Matsumura Y, Kaino S, Miyamoto K, Okita K. Enhanced interstitial collagenase (matrix metalloproteinase-13) production of Kupffer cell by gadolinium chloride prevents pig serum–induced rat liver fibrosis. Biochem Biophys Res Commun 2000; 267:290–295.

297. Knittel T, Mehde M, Kobold D, Saile B, Dinter C, Ramadori G. Expression patterns of matrix

metalloproteinases and their inhibitors in parenchymal and non-parenchymal cells of rat liver: regulation by TNF-α and TGF-β1. J Hepatol 1999; 30:48–60.

298. Hamilton JA. Stimulation of macrophage prostaglandin and neutral protease production by phorbol esters as a model for the induction of vascular changes associated with tumor promotion. Cancer Res 1980; 40:2273–2280.

299. Arthur MJ. Degradation of matrix proteins in liver fibrosis. Pathol Res Pract 1994; 190:825–833.

300. Ueno T, Sujaku K, Tamaki S, Ogata R, Kin M, Nakamura T, Sakamoto M, Torimura T, Mitsuyama K, Sakisaka S, Sata M, Tanikawa K. OK-432 treatment increases matrix metalloproteinase-9 production and improves dimethylnitrosamine-induced liver cirrhosis in rats. Int J Mol Med 1999; 3:497–503.

301. Michael SL, Pumford NR, Mayeux PR, Niesman MR, Hinson JA. Pretreatment of mice with macrophage inactivators decreases acetaminophen hepatotoxicity and the formation of reactive oxygen and nitrogen species. Hepatology 1999; 30:186–195.

302. Chiu H, Laskin DL. Induction of heme oxygenase (HSP 32) in hepatic macrophages during acetaminophen hepatotoxicity (abstr). Toxicol Sci 2000; 54:42.

303. Thompson K, Maltby J, Fallowfield J, McAulay M, Millward-Sadler H, Sheron N. Interleukin-10 expression and function in experimental murine liver inflammation and fibrosis. Hepatology 1998; 28:1597–1606.

10

Roles of Cytokines and Growth Factors in Liver Regeneration, Repair, and Fibrosis after Liver Injury

REBECCA TAUB, MEENA BANSAL, and WEI LEI

University of Pennsylvania School of Medicine, Philadelphia, Pennsylvania, U.S.A.

I. INTRODUCTION

After liver injury or resection the liver has the capacity to regenerate, ultimately leading to repair and restoration of normal liver architecture. The great majority of liver cells are involved in this process including mature nonparenchymal cells and hepatocytes. The signals that initiate regeneration are mediated by paracrine pathways involving cytokines (TNFα and IL-6) and growth factors (e.g., HGF) acting in concert to regulate this complex process. During regeneration multiple growth factor, signal transduction, and transcriptional pathways are activated and large numbers of genes are upregulated. Interleukin-6 is a critical component for normal regeneration that occurs in the face of several types of liver injury and hepatic resection. In the face of repetitive liver injury in IL-6 knockout animals, reduction in the ability of the hepatocyte to undergo normal regeneration, progression through the cell cycle, and replication ultimately lead to prolonged stellate cell activation and increased liver fibrosis. Similarly, HGF deficiency exacerbates liver injury and fibrosis. Telomerase-deficient animals, which have a hepatocyte replicative defect, demonstrate increased liver fibrosis in response to repetitive liver injury. A major question that remains is whether reduced hepatocyte proliferation in the face of chronic liver injury is itself fibrogenic as is suggested in the telomerase-deficient model and supported partially by the IL-6−/− and HGF models. Alternatively or in addition, HGF and IL-6 may regulate a protein or gene expression program that directly block fibrosis by reducing the level of TGFβ or profibrogenic metalloproteinases produced by hepatic stellate cells.

II. LIVER REGENERATION AFTER PARTIAL HEPATECTOMY: COMPLEX PATHWAYS DISSECTED USING GENE EXPRESSION STUDIES

The liver has the capacity for self-renewal in which parenchymal cells normally in the G_0 phase of the cell cycle may be induced to proliferate following toxic damage, hepatitis, and surgical resection (1–4). The partial hepatectomy model of liver regeneration clearly demonstrates the liver's compensatory growth response that culminates in the rapid restoration of hepatic parenchyma. A number of growth factors and cytokines have been implicated as having a role in the regenerative response including HGF, EGF, TNF, and IL-6 (Fig. 1), and can be divided into cytokine-dependent and independent pathways. Cytokine-dependent pathways involve the activation of the TNFα/IL-6 axis in which these cytokines are released from Kupffer cells in response to changes in the level of portal lipopolysaccharide that occur after liver injury or partial hepatectomy. Other growth factors such as HGF are apparently released from other hepatic cells such as Ito cells. A number of other growth factors have been proposed as emanating from other organs and tissues and regulating proliferation of the hepatocyte.

Partial hepatectomy and toxic liver damage induce signals in the liver that result in rapid changes in the transcriptional milieu including activation of latent transcription factors such as NF-κB and STAT3, and induction of expression of early growth response genes during the G_0 to G_1 transition (3,4). In a multipathway cascade of intra- and intercellular signaling, hepatocytes and nonparenchymal liver cells progress through G_1 and enter S, G_2, and M phases in a synchronous fashion that ultimately leads to restoration of liver mass within a few days. Dissection of the early signals required to trigger liver regeneration has relied in part on gene expression analyses. More than 100 genes are known to be transcriptionally activated in the early phases of liver regeneration, and gene array studies will undoubtedly identify many others. The categories of genes that are induced during liver regeneration parallel those in many other growth-factor-activated systems including proto-oncogene transcription factors (AP-1, egr-1, myc), cell signaling molecules, growth factors, and apoptotic pathway proteins. However, induced genes include some liver-specific proteins as well, such as glucose-6-phosphatase and insulin-like-

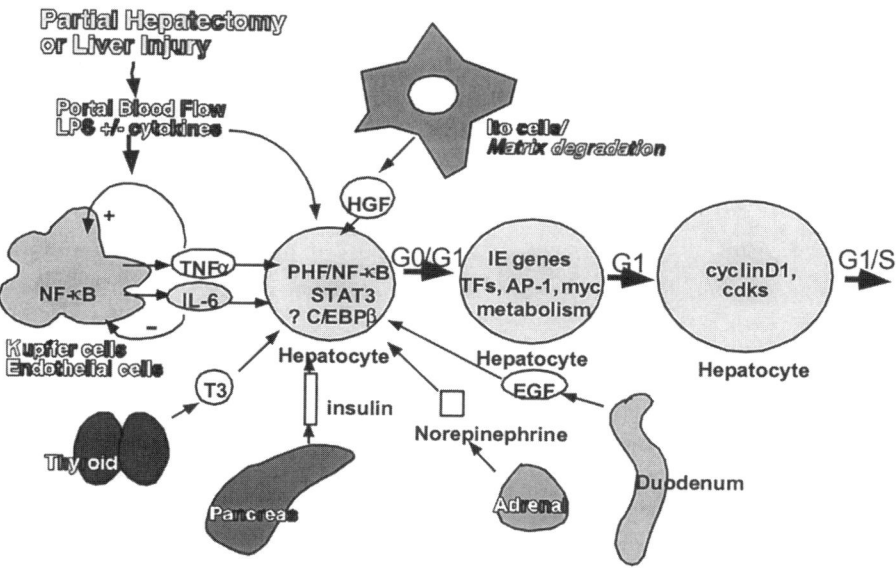

Figure 1 Model for growth factor pathways postulated to regulate liver regeneration after injury or partial hepatectomy.

growth factor binding protein-1 (5), that are important for the adaptive response of the liver to liver injury and allow for the maintenance of metabolic function during regeneration.

Studies identifying latent transcription factors that were rapidly activated in the remnant liver immediately posthepatectomy were originally helpful in identifying pathways that are involved in regeneration. For example, rapid changes in STAT3 and NF-κB transcription factor activity pointed to the importance of cytokine pathways including TNFα and IL-6 (6–8). The finding that genes such as IkBα that are activated by cytokines were rapidly induced during liver regeneration provided additional support for the role of IL-6 and TNFα in regulating hepatic regeneration. TNFα and IL-6 are presumably released from nonparenchymal liver cells within minutes of the hepatectomy. Based primarily on data from knockout mice (9–11), IL-6 and TNFα have been shown to be critical factors in the mitogenic response during liver regeneration. IL-6, which is downstream of TNFα signaling, is important both for cell cycle progression and protection from liver injury. However, neither IL-6 nor TNFα is a complete factor in that they are responsible for only a subset of the gene expression changes that occur posthepatectomy, and alone are insufficient to cause hepatic DNA synthesis. Likewise, knockout mouse studies indicate that C/EBPβ, a leucine zipper transcription factor that is also activated by cytokines, acts in an IL-6-independent fashion to induce a separate set of genes and proteins, and is also required for normal liver regeneration (2,12). Moreover, some early growth response genes are induced normally in the absence of C/EBPβ and IL-6 and highlight the role of other regulatory pathways in the early phases of liver regeneration. Thus, cytokine-dependent and independent pathways act cooperatively to control the complex series of events that result in liver regeneration. The requirement for multiple signals also protects the liver from undergoing hyperplasia in the absence of a compensatory need.

III. INSIGHT FROM REGENERATION STUDIES IN GENE KNOCKOUT MICE

Which of these genes rapidly induced during liver regeneration encode proteins that are essential for liver regeneration is largely unknown. However, regeneration studies performed in mice with gene knockouts have highlighted the importance of specific genes (Table 1) (13–18). Unfortunately, some of the genes of greatest interest to the field resulted in embryonic lethality after gene knockout. For example, HGF, *c*-Jun and NF-κB/p65 are all required for normal liver development, and therefore studies of regeneration in these models are not possible. Nonetheless, the finding of apoptosis in the developing liver in these gene knockouts provides evidence for the critical importance of these proteins in the liver. In the case of HGF this is particularly frustrating because HGF has long been felt to be a critical regulator of liver regeneration (1). However, it has been difficult to demonstrate that HGF is active during the initial phases of regeneration. Studies indicate that treatment with HGF promotes regeneration and hepatocyte proliferation, and reduces hepatic apoptosis and fibrosis, CCl_4-mediated injury (19,20). Antibodies to HGF at the time of CCl_4 injection blocked the regenerative response but the study did not assess the degree of injury (and therefore the requirement for regeneration) (21). Ultimately other models in which HGF or Met receptor are conditionally eliminated from the liver after birth will allow for an assessment of the requirement of HGF during regeneration.

Several of the gene knockout models showing impaired liver regeneration involve cytokine-dependent pathways. For example, it appears that TNF is required for induction of IL-6 after partial hepatectomy, and iNos, which helps prevent liver injury after hepatec-

Table 1 Mouse Genetics: Defining Molecular Pathways in Liver Development and Regeneration[a]

Defective liver development
  HGF
  p65/NF-κB
  c-Jun
  XBP-1
Defective liver regeneration
  IL-6
  TNF receptor I
  iNOS
  CREM
  C/EBPbeta
  Keratin 8
  Plasminogen
  Telomerase

[a] Gene deletions in mice that result either in abnormal liver development or defective liver regeneration.
HGF, hepatocyte growth factor; IL-6, interleukin-6; TNF, tumor necrosis factor; iNOS, inducible nitric oxide synthase; CREM, cAMP regulatory element; C/EBP, caat enhancer binding protein.

tomy, is a possible target gene of these cytokines (9,11,17). TNFα, IL-6, and normal iNos regulation are all required for normal liver regeneration. CEBPβ, a leucine zipper transcriptional factor, considered to be a cytokine-regulated factor, is also required for normal liver regeneration (12). How the activity of C/EBPβ is regulated by extracellular signals posthepatectomy is not known. There is some support for the hypothesis that the relative level of proproliferative forms of C/EBPβ is important in supporting liver growth, and balances antiproliferative forms and C/EBPα, an antiproliferative factor. Interestingly, C/EBPβ regulates a distinct set of genes posthepatectomy as compared to those regulated by IL-6 (2). Additional studies performed in TNF receptor I and IL-6 knockout animals suggest that NF-κB helps to protect the liver against TNF-mediated injury and allows for the proproliferative activity of TNF. As discussed below, IL-6 is important in reducing injury due to liver toxins and ischemia and reduces hepatic apoptosis and fibrosis.

IV. IL-6-INDUCED LIVER REGENERATION AFTER PARTIAL HEPATECTOMY AND TOXIC LIVER INJURY: REDUCED HEPATOCYTE PROLIFERATION AND PERSISTENT INJURY

IL-6−/− livers have been shown to respond abnormally to a variety of liver injury models including partial hepatectomy, CCl$_4$, ischemia reperfusion, and bile duct ligation (9,22–27). As such IL-6−/− mice provide an excellent model system to examine the relationship between liver regeneration, repair, and ultimately fibrogenesis. The operating hypothesis is that impaired hepatocyte replication leads to increased fibrogenesis due to protracted injury and therefore protracted stellate cell activation. However, it is also possible that IL-6 has a direct antifibrogenic effect through the modulation of fibrogenic proteins including metalloproteinases (MMPs).

Following partial hepatectomy, IL-6−/− livers have impaired liver regeneration characterized by liver necrosis and failure, a blunted DNA response in hepatocytes, and discrete G$_1$ phase abnormalities, including absence of STAT3 activation, and selective abnormalities in gene expression (9,25). Partial hepatectomy in IL-6−/− livers is not associated with increased hepatocyte apoptosis. Treatment of IL-6−/− mice with a single preoperative dose of IL-6 returns STAT3 binding, gene expression, and hepatocyte proliferation to near normal and prevents liver damage, establishing IL-6 as a critical component of the regenerative response following partial hepatectomy (9). Additional data support the critical role of IL-6 in liver regeneration and have defined TNFα as an upstream inducer of IL-6 expression during liver regeneration (11).

Several studies have examined the role of IL-6 in liver injury following ischemia reperfusion. In one study both hepatectomy and ischemia were simultaneously applied. It was found that hepatic ischemia in combination with hepatectomy significantly reduced the mitogenic response in mouse livers (24). Treatment with IL-6 improves the mitogenic response in the face of ischemic injury back to the normal level. In warm/ischemia reperfusion models, IL-6 is protective against ischemic injury and IL-6−/− livers show increased injury. In this model TNFα results in injury as antibodies to TNFα are able to reduce ischemic injury to a similar degree as administration of IL-6 (23). A program of gene expression, activation of STAT3, NF-κB, and a high degree of hepatocyte proliferation similar to that in the hepatectomy model have been observed in transplanted rodent livers subjected to prolonged warm ischemia (27), indicating that IL-6-dependent hepatic regeneration occurs following ischemic liver injury.

IL-6 also ameliorates acute toxic liver injury (22). CCl_4 is a hepatotoxin that causes direct hepatocyte injury by altering permeability of cellular, lysosomal, and mitochondrial membranes (28). Highly reactive free radicals are also formed from the metabolism of CCl_4 by cytochrome P450 Cyp2E1 of the hepatocyte causing centrizonal necrosis. CCl_4 causes not only primary liver necrosis but also hepatocyte apoptosis (29,30). CCl_4 liver injury is associated with increased cytokine levels including TNFα, which is felt to enhance CCl_4-mediated injury as CCl_4-induced liver necrosis can be significantly ameliorated by treatment with anti-TNFα antibodies (31). Tumor necrosis factor receptor I knockout (TNFRI−/−) livers subjected to CCl_4 have a reduced DNA synthetic response when compared to wild-type livers, but the effect on the amount of liver injury is not clear (32). TNFα is also an established inducer of hepatocyte apoptosis although TNFα-mediated activation of NF-κB provides some cellular protection against apoptosis (33–35).

Following acute carbon tetrachloride (CCl_4) treatment, IL-6−/− mice develop increased hepatocellular injury and defective regeneration with significant blunting of STAT3 and NF-κB activation and reduced hepatocyte DNA synthetic and mitotic responses (22). After CCl_4 treatment, unlike partial hepatectomy, increased hepatocyte apoptosis is noted in IL-6−/− livers. Pretreatment with IL-6 prior to CCl_4 reduces acute CCl_4 injury and apoptosis, and accelerates regeneration in both IL-6+/+ and −/− livers.

Two major defects are seen in IL-6−/− livers subjected to a single dose of CCl_4. First, despite having more extensive injury, IL-6−/− livers show reduced hepatocyte proliferation. Unlike the hepatectomy model in which additional IL-6 given to wild-type mice has little impact on the course of regeneration, treatment with IL-6 clearly accelerates the proliferative response in both IL-6+/+ and −/− livers. Peak entry into S phase occurs at 36 h rather than 48 h. This response further defines the role of IL-6 as a cell-cycle-progression factor. The second major finding in IL-6−/− livers is a dramatic increase in the degree of liver injury following CCl_4 toxicity (roughly two-thirds greater than wild type). IL-6−/− livers also have an increase in apoptotic hepatocytes following a single dose of CCl_4 that was not noted after partial hepatectomy. Treatment with IL-6 has a profound impact on both IL-6−/− and +/+ livers in reducing the amount of CCl_4-induced injury. IL-6 treatment also reduces the number of apoptotic hepatocytes in both IL-6−/− and +/+ livers.

CCl_4-induced liver injury is associated with high levels of TNFα. TNFα enhances CCl_4-mediated injury since this injury can be significantly ameliorated by treatment with anti-TNFα antibodies (31). In another model of liver injury associated with high levels of TNFα, the Con A T-cell activation liver model, antibodies to TNFα reduced injury as did injection of recombinant IL-6 (36). IL-6 may be functioning downstream of TNFα to ameliorate liver injury. However, further data are required to elucidate this mechanism.

Along with decreasing CCl_4-induced liver injury, IL-6 decreases hepatocyte apoptosis, a component of CCl_4-induced liver injury. In this model, it is not clear whether reduction in apoptosis is due to an overall reduction in injury or whether IL-6 exerts a primary antiapoptotic effect that serves to rescue hepatocytes. Increased levels of NF-κB and STAT3 two antiapoptotic transcription factors are found in IL-6+/+ as compared with −/− livers. As NF-κB is considered to be upstream, not downstream of IL-6, indirect effects could have led to its increase in IL-6+/+ livers (37). A number of in vitro studies have demonstrated an antiapoptotic effect of IL-6 and STAT3 in nonhepatic cell lines (38–42). Fas ligation, a purer model of hepatocyte apoptosis than CCl_4 toxicity, is likely to provide more insight into mechanisms by which IL-6 reduces hepatocyte apoptosis (Kovalovich, Li, and Taub, unpublished data). At least in the Fas model, neither STAT3 nor NF-κB appears to be mediating the decreased apoptosis observed in IL-6+/+ livers (Kovalovich and Taub, unpublished).

V. THE ROLE OF INTERLEUKIN-6 IN CHRONIC LIVER INJURY AND FIBROSIS

Given the increased level of injury in IL-6−/− livers following acute CCl$_4$ injury, it is important to consider the impact of IL-6 in chronic liver injury. Studies have demonstrated that mice chronically exposed to CCl$_4$ are resistant to cirrhosis (43–47). In mouse livers sparse amounts of localized fibrosis have been induced with CCl$_4$ after 8–12 weeks of exposure. There are a very limited number of mouse models of lobular fibrosis, which include: quartz-induced cirrhosis, which requires 12 weeks of therapy; fibrosis induced by intrahepatic injection of human pathogenic mycoplasma-like organisms, which is limited by availability and high animal mortality; low protein–low choline–high fat diet, which requires >12–24 weeks of treatment. A chronic CCl$_4$ injury model combining CCl$_4$ and phenobarbital in rats was adapted to mice and demonstrated a relatively rapid and reliable fibrotic response in wild-type livers with a low mortality level (22).

Repetitive doses of CCl$_4$ in the presence or absence of phenobarbital result in increased injury and fibrosis in IL-6−/− compared with +/+ livers. After acute and chronic injury, IL-6−/− livers demonstrate the protracted presence of α-smooth muscle actin associated with activated stellate cells suggesting a disturbed response in wound healing that progresses to fibrosis. These data support a role for IL-6 in reducing toxin-mediated acute and chronic liver injury and fibrosis.

A similar effect of IL-6 is found on the development of biliary cirrhosis, another model of chronic liver injury, again using the IL-6−/− mouse model (25). In this study, IL-6+/+ and −/− mice were subjected to bile duct ligation for 3 months. This results in protracted liver injury, and chronic biliary epithelial and hepatocyte proliferation. IL-6−/− mice develop more severe liver disease, reduced hepatocyte proliferation, reduced liver mass increase, more advanced biliary fibrosis, and a higher mortality rate. Treatment with recombinant IL-6 for several weeks improved several parameters including liver mass restitution. The authors concluded that IL-6 had the dual effect of contributing to biliary tree integrity and maintenance of hepatocyte mass during chronic injury. The absence of IL-6 led to increased fibrosis.

Normally, acute liver injury is followed by a wound-healing response that seeks to contain the injury, reconstitute lost liver cell mass, and restore the extracellular framework of the liver (48,49). Cytokines, which may be pro- or antifibrogenic, have been shown to play a major role in the wound-healing response to liver injury. Though the precise mechanisms remain unclear, we noted the IL-6−/− livers have persistent stellate cell activation following acute injury. Activation denotes a conversion from a resting, vitamin A–rich, perisinusoidal cell to one that is proliferative, fibrogenic, and contractile. Following resolution of injury, it is postulated that activated stellate cells may be eliminated by apoptosis although reversion back to a resting state has not been fully explored (50). Absence of IL-6 may cause a persistence of activated stellate cells that would otherwise be eliminated, leading to increased chronic liver injury and fibrosis.

Contradictory results were obtained using a chronic CCl$_4$ model in IL-6−/− mice incompletely backcrossed onto a Balb/c stain (51). In this model increased fibrosis was observed in IL-6+/+ (pure Balb/c) as compared to the IL-6−/− (six-generation Balb/c) livers. The degree of fibrosis was significantly lower than was observed by Kovalovich et al. (22). Conceivably, this difference could be due to different susceptibilities of various mouse strains.

The mechanisms underlying the protective effects of IL-6 in both chronic injury models remain to be elucidated. The critical question is whether IL-6 deficiency results in protracted injury and activated stellate cells due to increased injury and reduced hepatocyte proliferation, or whether IL-6 has a direct role in regulating the fibrogenic process. IL-6 has effects on many cells in the liver including stellate cells where it has been reported to be profibrogenic in culture. However, in vivo models as discussed above suggest an antifibrotic role. Stellate cells actively produce many proteinases that degrade normal basement membrane and type IV collagen. The action of stellate cells in physiological repair is important in restoring normal liver architecture. However, prolonged activation of stellate cells as in the IL-6−/− livers results in buildup of pathological collagens and ultimately cirrhosis. IL-6 may have a direct antifibrotic role. IL-6 has an important role in the stimulation of the acute-phase response proteins (52,53). Many of the acute-phase proteins expressed in hepatocytes and stellate cells in response to IL-6 have antiproteolytic activities (54). It is possible (as depicted in the model, Fig. 2) that IL-6 by controlling specific proteolytic activities in the liver regulates the level of MMPs that lead to the deposition of pathological collagens and persistent stellate cell activation.

Active matrix metalloproteinase-2 (MMP-2) has been shown to be elevated in both rat models of chronic liver injury and in human cirrhotic livers and thus, may have a profibrogenic role (55,56). An interplay between MMP-2 and IL-6 in modulating hepatic

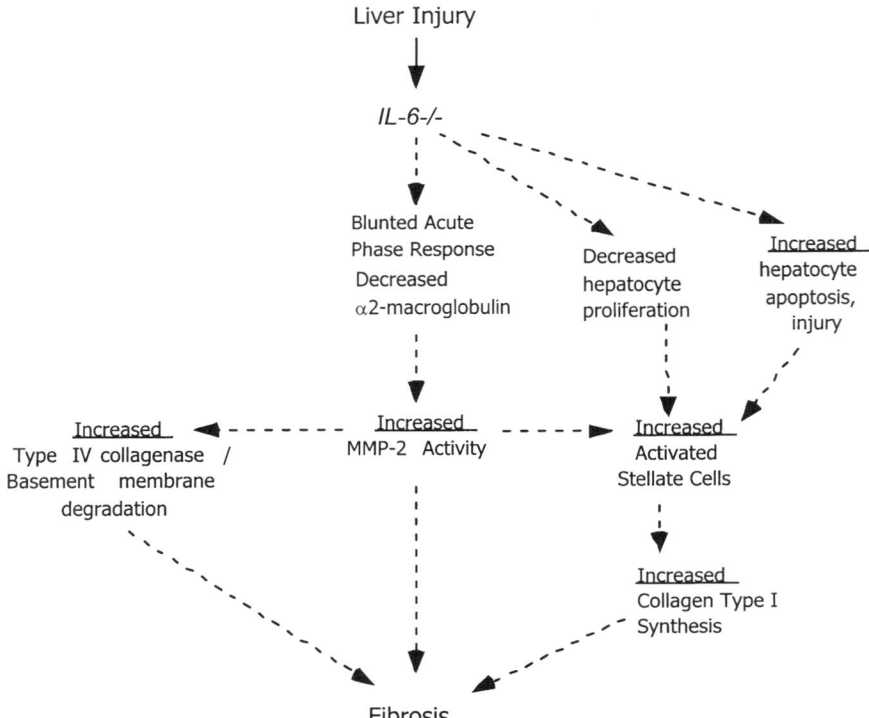

Figure 2   Hypothetical model showing how IL-6 may regulate liver fibrosis.

injury and fibrosis is a possible explanation for the fibrotic response to IL-6 deficiency. After acute and chronic CCl_4 treatment, increased MMP-2 is observed in areas of necrosis but staining is consistently higher in the IL-6$-/-$ livers (57). At 120 h after CCl_4, IL-6$+/+$ livers demonstrate evidence of wound healing and IL-6$-/-$ livers persistent injury as reflected by histological changes, increased α-SMA staining, and increased MMP-2 staining. A greater than 10-fold increase in active MMP-2 protein is found in IL-6$-/-$ livers beginning at 24 h, the time correlating with peak histological injury. In chronic CCl_4 injury, IL-6-deficient livers have increased MMP-2 staining and persistent α-SMA staining correlating with increased collagen type I staining. In addition, the peak in MMP-2 activation correlates with a decline in $α_2$-macroglobulin protein expression, an endogenous proteinase inhibitor. $α_2$-Macroglobulin, an IL-6-regulated gene, is secreted by hepatocytes as a feature of the acute-phase response and by activated stellate cells in culture. $α_2$-Macroglobulin has been shown to bind MMP-2 thereby resulting in sequestration and degradation of MMP-2 (58). These findings suggest that upregulation of MMP-2 in the IL-6-deficient livers may be important for mediating increased injury, delayed healing, and progression to fibrosis. In addition, downregulation of $α_2$-macroglobulin may contribute to increased proteolytic activity of MMP-2, further intensifying its potentially deleterious effects. Further studies will determine whether MMP-2 is directly regulated by IL-6 either transcriptionally or posttranscriptionally and whether MMP-2 is actually involved in the pathogenesis leading to liver fibrosis.

These results suggest that IL-6 functions in as-yet-unknown manner to stimulate rescue factors or reduce/inhibit proinjury factors that preserve hepatocyte viability and decreased liver injury. An accelerated hepatocyte proliferative response occurs following liver injury in mice with an intact endogenous IL-6 response. Further research into the mechanisms by which IL-6 ameliorates liver injury and fibrosis, and possibly hepatocyte apoptosis, has obvious therapeutic implications. Another possible therapeutic role for IL-6 involves situations of acute massive liver injury associated with a high risk of liver failure and death (e.g., drugs, toxins, acute viral hepatitis). Administration of IL-6 or targeting of factor(s) downstream of IL-6 may reduce injury and accelerate the restitution of functional liver mass.

VI. TELOMERASE-DEFICIENT MICE HAVE IMPAIRED HEPATOCYTE REGENERATION AND ARE PREDISPOSED TO FIBROSIS

Like the IL-6 knockout, the telomerase gene knockout provides a possible link between defective hepatocyte replication and persistent hepatic injury that ultimately leads to fibrosis (18). The results from three analyses strongly suggest that, even in the absence of pathologically activated proteases that provoke stellate cell activation, reduced or arrested hepatocyte proliferation may be a primary stimulus leading to stellate cell activation and ultimately fibrosis and cirrhosis.

Mice knocked out for the telomerase RNA (mTR) gene are normal. However, after six generations, telomerase dysfunction occurs and affects highly proliferative tissues such as bone marrow and gut. Liver development is normal in these mice. When crossed with the Alb-UPA transgene that causes increased hepatocyte turnover, late-generation mTR$-/-$ livers fail to provide sufficient replicative hepatocytes to overcome the high hepatocyte turnover. Increased hepatocyte apoptosis is also observed. After partial hepatectomy mTR$-/-$ livers demonstrate delayed regeneration and reduced progression through mitosis owing to the formation of aberrant mitotic spindles. After chronic CCl_4

treatment, mTR−/− livers showed increased fibrosis, which was reduced by treatment with an adenovirus containing the mTR gene. This was associated with increased hepatocyte proliferation thereby providing additional evidence for a strong correlation between hepatocyte proliferation and reduction in chronic injury and fibrosis.

However, one caveat of these studies is that few known proliferation-regulated signaling pathways have been examined in mTR−/− livers subjected to injury. Thus it is possible that in addition to defects in hepatocytes, defects in other cells such as Kupffer cells could result in reduced production of cytokines produced in mTR−/− livers. Against this possibility is the finding that transduction by adenovirus containing telomerase cures the regenerative defect. It is believed that adenovirus targets specifically to hepatocytes, not nonparenchymal liver cells. Thus any defect in nonparenchymal cells should have remained following the adenovirus transduction.

VII. HEPATOCYTE GROWTH FACTOR INDUCES LIVER REGENERATION AND BLOCKS FIBROSIS

Like IL-6, HGF regulates a variety of processes in the liver in addition to being a direct stimulant of hepatocyte proliferation. It was shown that infusion of HGF into rodents reduces the level of CCl_4-induced hepatic injury (19,20). However, the effect on specific signaling pathways leading to regeneration was not studied. In a rat model of liver cirrhosis produced by dimethylnitrosamine, HGF produced following gene transfections into skeletal muscles induced a high plasma level of human HGF resulting in activation of the c-Met/HGF receptor (19). The increase in transforming growth factor-beta1 (TGF-β1) normally associated with dimethylnitrosamine was reduced, but it was not clear whether this was a direct effect of HGF or resulted from the fact that there was less liver injury in the HGF-infused animals. HGF infusion inhibited fibrogenesis and hepatocyte apoptosis. It produced resolution of fibrosis in an already cirrhotic liver and improved survival rate of rats. Again, as in the case of IL-6, conclusions cannot be drawn as to whether the effect of HGF is limited to hepatocyte proliferation.

The effects of HGF on liver injury are very similar to those of IL-6, but thus far attempts to link these two cytokine/growth factors have failed. Although HGF may be directly upregulated by IL-6 treatment in vitro, in fact, there is no change in HGF signaling or HGF mRNA levels in IL-6−/− livers (9). Moreover, although abnormal regulation of plasminogen, which regulates HGF activity, is seen in IL-6−/− livers (59), no difference in HGF-mediated signaling has been detected. It remains to be seen whether the similar effects of IL-6 and HGF on hepatocyte apoptosis, injury, and regeneration are mutually exclusive yet overlapping.

VIII. CONCLUSIONS

Gene expression and gene knockout studies have yielded great advances in the understanding of signaling pathways that occur within the liver as it regenerates in response to a variety of insults or resection. The link between the ability of the liver to regenerate in response to chronic injury and the development of cirrhosis is disclosed here in the context of three required factors for normal liver regeneration: IL-6, telomerase, and HGF. Interestingly, all of these proteins either provided in excess (HGF, IL-6) or to correct a deficiency (IL-6, telomerase) are able not just to induce normal regeneration, but to reduce acute liver injury and the development of liver cirrhosis. Ultimately it will be important to determine whether HGF and IL-6 are directly antifibrogenic or instead simply reduce fibrosis by allowing regeneration and repair.

REFERENCES

1. Michalopoulos GK, DeFrances MC. Liver regeneration. Science 1997; 276:60–66.
2. Taub R, Greenbaum LE, Peng Y. Transcriptional regulation signals define cytokine-dependent and -independent pathways in liver regeneration. Semin Liver Dis 1999; 19(2):117–127.
3. Taub R. Liver regeneration in health and disease. Clin Lab Med 1996; 16:341–360.
4. Taub R. Liver regeneration 4: transcriptional control of liver regeneration. FASEB J 1996; 10:413–427.
5. Leu JI, Crissey MAS, Leu JP, Ciliberto G, Taub R. Interleukin-6-induced STAT3 and AP-1 amplify hepatocyte nuclear factor 1-mediated transactivation of hepatic genes, an adaptive response to liver injury. Mol Cell Biol 2001; 21(2):414–424.
6. Cressman DE, Greenbaum LE, Haber BA, Taub R. Rapid activation of posthepatectomy factor/nuclear factor-κB in hepatocytes, a primary response in the regenerating liver. J Biol Chem 1994; 269:30429–30435.
7. Cressman DE, Greenbaum LE, Haber BA, Taub R. Rapid activation of the STAT3 transcription complex in liver regeneration. Hepatology 1995; 21:1443–1449.
8. Taga T, Kishomoto T. GP130 and the interleukin-6 family of cytokines. Annu Rev Immunol 1997; 15:797–819.
9. Cressman DE, Greenbaum LE, DeAngelis RA, Ciliberto G, Furth EE, Poli V, Taub R. Liver failure and defective hepatocyte regeneration in interleukin-6-deficient mice. Science 1996; 274:1379–1383.
10. Akerman P, Cote P, Yang SQ, McClain C, Nelson S, Bagbt GJ, Diehl AM. Antibodies to tumor necrosis factor-alpha inhibit liver regeneration after partial hepatectomy. Am J Physiol 1992; 263:G579–G585.
11. Yamada Y, Kirillova I, Peschon JJ, Fausto N. Initiation of liver growth by tumor necrosis factor: defective liver regeneration in mice lacking type I tumor necrosis factor receptor. Proc Natl Acad Sci USA 1997; 94:1441–1446.
12. Greenbaum LE, Li W, Cressman DE, Ciliberto G, Poli V, Taub R. CCAAT enhancer-binding protein b is required for normal hepatocyte proliferation in mice after partial hepatectomy. J Clin Invest 1998; 102:996–1007.
13. Fausto N. Lessons from genetically engineered animal models. V. Knocking out genes to study liver regeneration: present and future. Am Physiol Soc 1999; 277:G917–G921.
14. Smith AJ, Elferink PJOE. Liver gene disruption: winners by KO? J Hepatol 1999; 31:752–759.
15. Loranger A, Duclos S, Grenier A, Price J, Wilson-Heiner M, Baribault H, Marceau N. Simple epithelium keratins are required for maintenance of hepatocyte integrity. Am J Pathol 1997; 151(6):1673–1683.
16. Reimold AM, Etkin A, Clauss I, Perkins A, Friend DS, Zhang J, Horton HF, Scott A, Orkin SH, Byrne MC, Grusby MJ, Glimcher LH. An essential role in liver development for transcription factor XBP-1. Genes Dev 2000; 14:152–157.
17. Rai RM, Lee FYJL, Rosen A, Yang SQ, Lin HZ, Koteish A, Liew FY, Zaragoza C, Lowenstein C, Diehl AM. Impaired liver regeneration in inducible nitric oxide synthase-deficient mice. Proc Natl Acad Sci USA 1998; 95:13829–13834.
18. Rudolph KL, Chang S, Millard M, Schreiber-Agus N, DePinho RA. Inhibition of experimental liver cirrhosis in mice by telomerase gene delivery. Science 2000; 287:1253–1258.
19. Ueki T, Kaneda Y, Tsutsui H, Nakanishi K, Sawa Y, Morishita R, Matsumoto K, Nakamura T, Takahashi H, Okamoto E, Fujimoto J. Hepatocyte growth factor gene therapy of liver cirrhosis in rats. Nature Med 1999; 5(2):226–230.

20. Matsuda Y, Matsumoto K, Yamada A, Ichida T, Asakura H, Komoriya Y, Nishiyama E, Nakamura T. Preventive and therapeutic effects in rats of hepatocyte growth factor infusion on liver fibrosis/cirrhosis. Hepatology 1997; 26(1):81–89.

21. Burr AW, Toole K, Chapman C, Hines JE, Burt AD. Anti-hepatocyte growth factor antibody inhibits hepatocyte proliferation during liver regeneration. J Pathol 1998; 185:298–302.

22. Kovalovich K, DeAngelis RA, Li W, Furth EE, Ciliberto G, Taub R. Increased toxin-induced liver injury and fibrosis in interleukin-6-deficient mice. Hepatology 2000; 31(1):149–159.

23. Camargo CA, Madden JF, Gao W, Selvan RS, Clavien P. Interleukin-6 protects liver against warm ischemia/reperfusion injury and promotes hepatocyte proliferation in the rodent. Hepatology 1997; 26(6):1513–1520.

24. Selzner M, Camargo CA, Clavien P-A. Ischemia impairs liver regeneration after major tissue loss in rodents: protective effects of interleukin-6. Hepatology 1999; 30(2):469–475.

25. Ezure T, Sakamoto T, Tsuji H, Lunz JG 3rd, Murase N, Fung JJ, Demetris AJ. The development and compensation of biliary cirrhosis in interleukin-6-deficient mice. Am J Pathol 2000; 156:1627–1639.

26. Sakamoto T, Liu Z, Murase N, Ezure T, Yokomuro S, Poli V, Demetris AJ. Mitosis and apoptosis in the liver of interleukin-6-deficient mice after partial hepatectomy. Hepatology 1999; 29(2):403–411.

27. Debonera F, Aldeguer X, Shen X, Gelman AE, Gao F, Que X, Greenbaum LE, Furth EE, Taub R, Olthoff KM. Activation of IL-6/STAT3 and liver regeneration following transplantation. J Surgical Res 2001; 96:289–295.

28. Berger ML, Bhatt H, Combes B, Estabrook R. CCl₄-induced toxicity in isolated hepatocytes: the importance of direct solvent injury. Hepatology 1966; 6:36–45.

29. Slater TF. Necrogenic action of carbon tetrachloride in the rat: a speculative mechanism based on activation. Nature 1966; 209:36–40.

30. Shi J, Aisaki K, Ikawa Y, Wake K. Evidence of hepatocyte apoptosis in rat liver after the administration of carbon tetrachloride. Am J Pathol 1998; 153:515–525.

31. Czaja MJ, Xu J, Alt E. Prevention of carbon tetrachloride-induced rat liver injury by soluble tumor necrosis factor receptor. Gastroenterology 1995; 108:1849–1854.

32. Yamada Y, Fausto N. Deficient liver regeneration after carbon tetrachloride injury in mice lacking type 1 but not type 2 tumor necrosis factor receptor. Am J Pathol 1998; 152:1577–1589.

33. Kondo T, Suda T, Fukuyama H, Adachi M, Nagata S. Essential roles of the Fas ligand in the development of hepatitis. Nature Med 1997; 3:409–413.

34. Beg AA, Baltimore D. An essential role for NF-kappaB in preventing TNF-alpha-induced cell death. Science 1996; 274:782–784.

35. Beg AA, Sha WC, Bronson RT, Ghosh S, Baltimore D. Embryonic lethality and liver degeneration in mice lacking the RelA component of NF-kappa B. Nature 1995; 376:167–170.

36. Mizuhara H, O'Neill E, Seki N, Ogawa T, Kusunoki C, Otsuka K, Satoh S, Niwa M, Senoh H, Fujiwara H. T cell activation-associated hepatic injury: mediation by tumor necrosis factors and protection by interleukin 6. J Exp Med 1994; 179:1529–1537.

37. Ravi R, Bedi A, Fuchs EJ, Bedi A. CD95 (Fas)-induced caspase-mediated proteolysis of NF-κB. Cancer Res 1998; 58:882–886.

38. Liu J, Li H, De Tribolet N, Jaufeerally R, Hamou MF, Van Meir EG. IL-6 stimulates growth and inhibits constitutive, protein synthesis-independent apoptosis of murine B-cell hybridoma 7TD1. Cell Immunol 1994; 155:428–435.

39. Smith MR, Xie T, Joshi I, Schilder RJ. Dexamethasone plus retinoids decrease IL-6/IL-6 receptor and induce apoptosis in myeloma cells. Br J Haematol 1998; 102:1090–1097.

40. Bellido T, O'Brien CA, Roberson PK, Manolagas SC. Transcriptional activation of the p21^{WAF1,CIP1,SDI1} gene by interleukin-6 type cytokines. J Biol Chem 1998; 273:21137–21144.

41. Schwarze MMK, Hawley RG. Prevention of myeloma cell apoptosis by ectopic bcl-2 expression or interleukin-6 mediated up-regulation of bcl-x₁. Cancer Res 1995; 55:2262–2265.

42. Fukada T, Hibi M, Yamanaka Y, Takahashi-Tezuka M, Fujitani Y, Yamaguchi T, Nakajima K, Hirano T. Two signals are necessary for cell proliferation induced by a cytokine receptor gp130: involvement of STAT3 in anti-apoptosis. Immunity 1996; 5:449–460.

43. Tsukamoto H, Matsuoka M, French SW. Experimental models of hepatic fibrosis: a review. Semin Liv Dis 1990; 10:56–65.

44. Brenner DA, Veloz L, Jaenisch R, Alcorn JM. Stimulation of the collagen alpha 1 (I) endogenous gene and transgene in carbon tetrachloride-induced hepatic fibrosis. Hepatology 1993; 17:287–292.

45. Ogawa M, Mori T, Mori Y, Ueda S, Azemoto R, Makino Y, Ohto M, Wakashin M, Yoshida H et al. Study on chronic renal injuries induced by carbon tetrachloride: selective inhibition of the nephrotoxicity by irradiation. Nephron 1992; 60:68–73.

46. Olufemi Williams S, Knapton AD. Hepatic silicosis, cirrhosis, and liver tumors in mice and hamsters: studies of transforming growth factor b expression. Hepatology 1996; 23:1268–1275.

47. Johnson LA, Wirostko E, Wirostko BM. Experimental murine chronic hepatitis: results following intrahepatic inoculation of human uveitis mycoplasma-like organisms. Int J Exp Pathol 1993; 74:325–331.

48. Friedman SL. Cytokines and fibrinogenesis. Semin Liver Dis 1999; 19(2):129–140.

49. Davis BH, Kresina TF. Hepatic fibrogenesis. Clin Lab Med 1996; 16:361–375.

50. Iredale JP, Benyon RC, Pickering J, et al. Mechanisms of spontaneous resolution of rat liver fibrosis: hepatic stellate cell apoptosis and reduced hepatic expression of metalloproteinase inhibitors. J Clin Invest 1998; 102:538–549.

51. Natsume M, Tsuji H, Harada A, Akiyama M, Yano T, Ishikura H, Nakanishi I, Matsushima K, Kaneko S, Mukaida N. Attenuated liver fibrosis and depressed serum albumin levels in carbon tetrachloride-treated IL-6-deficient mice. J Leukoc Biol 1999; 66:601–608.

52. Fattori E, Cappelletti M, Costa P, Sellitto C, Cantoni L, Carelli M, Fabbioni R, Fantuzzi G, Ghezzi P, Poli V. Defective inflammatory response in interleukin 6–deficient mice. J Exp Med 1994; 180:1243–1250.

53. Kopf M, Baumann H, Freer G, Freudenberg M, Lamers M, Kishimoto T, Zinkernagel R, Bluethmann H, Kohler G. Impaired immune and acute-phase responses in interleukin-6-deficient mice. Nature 1994; 368:339–342.

54. Gabay C, Kushner I. Acute-phase proteins and other systemic responses to inflammation. N Engl J Med 1999; 340(6):448–454.

55. Takahara T, Furui K, Tata Y, Jin B, Zhang LP, Nanbu S, Sato H, Seiki M, Watanabe A. Dual expression of matrix metalloproteinase in fibrotic human livers. Hepatology 1997; 26(6):1521–1529.

56. Nagase H. Matrix metalloproteinases. J Biol Chem 1999; 274:21491–21494.

57. Bansal MB, Kovalovich K, Li W, Taub R. The biologic interplay between IL-6 and MMP-2 in modulating hepatic injury and fibrosis. Hepatology 2000; 32(4):110A.

58. Nagase H, Itoh Y, Binner S. Interaction of alpha-2 macroglobulin with matrix metalloproteinases and its use for identification of their active fors. Ann NY Acad Sci 1994; 732:294–302.

59. Li W, Liang X, Lev J, Kovalovich K, Ciliberto G, Taub R. Global changes in interleukin-6 dependent gene expression patterns in mouse livers after partial hepatectomy. Hepatology 2001; 33:1377–1386.

11

Clinicopathological Patterns of Drug-Induced Liver Disease

WILLIS C. MADDREY

University of Texas Southwestern Medical Center, Dallas, Texas, U.S.A.

I. INTRODUCTION

The liver ranks high on the list of targets affected by adverse reactions to therapeutic or environmental agents (1–3). Therefore, detection of hepatic abnormalities receives considerable attention during testing and following release of new agents. Awareness of drug-induced reactions affecting the liver has become increasingly a matter of concern and searches have intensified for more effective ways to identify drugs that are likely to cause liver injury as well as subsets of patients who are at increased risk.

Hepatotoxicity has been one of the major reasons that otherwise effective therapeutic agents have failed during preapproval trials or have been withdrawn following release. In the absence of specific tests to establish a drug as the cause of a liver disease, it is often impossible to confidently establish a cause-effect relationship between the use of a drug and the appearance of an injury. There is hardly a drug in use that has not been proven, or at least suggested, to cause some type of adverse reaction affecting the liver. Clinical acceptance and success of a drug in the market depend on perceptions of efficacy and recognition of risks. Furthermore, concern regarding hepatotoxicity has limited the use of many drugs.

There are many reasons that the hepatotoxic potential of a drug might not be recognized until after a drug has been approved and is in widespread use. Even with several thousand patients receiving a drug during testing, rare events may be missed. Likewise, the population of patients studied before approval may not fully reflect the population who will take the drug after its release.

II. SPECTRUM OF DRUG-INDUCED LIVER DISORDERS

Hepatic manifestations of drug-induced liver injury can mimic almost the entire spectrum of liver diseases (1–3) (Table 1). Hepatocellular injury may be manifested as minimal biochemical abnormalities occurring in patients in whom there is no evidence of liver disease, or it may present as acute hepatitis, acute liver failure (fulminant hepatocellular failure), chronic hepatitis, and cirrhosis. In addition, cholestatic disorders ranging from those that are so mild as to be found only on routine biochemical testing to symptomatic cholestatic syndromes closely resembling primary biliary cirrhosis and primary sclerosing cholangitis are established manifestations of reactions to several drugs. Infiltration of fat into the liver, both microvesicular and macrovesicular, may result as an expected event because of the established mechanism of action of a drug, or as a clinically important untoward event occurring in a few individuals (4). There has been increased attention to the effects of drugs on mitochondrial respiration, which may lead to microvesicular fat, fatty acid accumulation, and decreased ATP levels (5,6). Furthermore, drugs are established causes of hepatic granulomatous inflammation indistinguishable from those found in a variety of infections and sarcoidosis (Table 2) (7–9).

In some situations hepatotoxicity is manifested as acquired phospholipidosis and as hepatic vein obstruction (Budd-Chiari syndrome). Tumors induced or promoted by therapeutic drugs range from benign hepatic adenomas, which have been associated with long-term use of oral contraceptives, to angiosarcomas, cholangiocarcinomas, and hepatocellular carcinomas.

III. IDENTIFICATION AND DIAGNOSIS OF DRUG-INDUCED LIVER INJURY

The difficulties in establishing a drug cause for a liver injury and in determining its importance reflect the protean manifestations of drug-induced hepatic injury and the absence of specific diagnostic features. Drug-induced liver disease is usually indistinguishable clinically from other types of injury and may only be detected through awareness, suspicion in a given situation, careful history, and inquisitive persistence by the clinician as to possible environmental or workplace exposure.

Table 1 Spectrum of Drug-Induced Liver Disorders

Type of injury	Features	Selected examples
Hepatocellular injury		
Elevated aminotransferase levels	Often asymptomatic	Almost all drugs
Acute hepatitis	Mimics acute viral hepatitis	Isoniazid
		Ketoconazole
		Troglitazone[a]
		Bromfenac[a]
		Diclofenac
		Methyldopa
Chronic hepatitis	May closely resemble auto-immune hepatitis	Nitrofurantoin
		Minocycline
		Methyldopa
		Oxyphenisatin[a]
Acute hepatic failure	Overwhelming liver failure	Halothane
		Isoniazid
Cholestatic reactions		
Cholestasis	Often prolonged course	Chlorpromazine
	Oral contraceptives may simulate bile duct obstruction	Benoxaprofen[a]
Simulate primary biliary cirrhosis	Antimitochondrial antibody negative	Chlorpromazine
Simulate primary sclerosing cholangitis		Floxuridine
Granulomas	Wide spectrum of diseases with and without evidence of hypersensitivity reaction	Phenylbutazone Carbamazepine (Table 2)
Simulate alcoholic hepatitis		Amiodarone
Steatohepatitis		Amiodarone
Phospholipidosis		Amiodarone
Vascular lesions		
Perisinusoidal fibrosis		Vitamin A
Peliosis hepatis	Hepatomegaly	Oral contraceptives
		Anabolic steroids
		Azathioprine
Hepatic vein obstruction	Congestive hepatopathy	Oral contraceptives
Veno-occlusive disease	Congestive hepatopathy	Oral contraceptives
Sinusoidal dilation	Hepatomegaly	Cytotoxics
		Oral contraceptives
Neoplasms		
Hepatic adenoma		Oral contraceptives
		Anabolic steroids
Cholangiocarcinoma		Anabolic steroids
		Thorotrast
Angiosarcoma		Vinyl chloride
		Anabolic steroids
		Thorotrast
Hepatocellular carcinoma		Danazol

[a] Drugs withdrawn after marketing.

Table 2 Hepatic Granulomas from
Therapeutic Drugs (62)

Allopurinol
Phenylbutazone
Sulfonamides
Carbamazepine
Quinidine
Hydralazine
Methyldopa
Phenytoin
Amoxicillin-clavulanic acid
Procainamide
d-Penicillamine

It is well recognized that many drugs cause minimal elevations in biochemical tests of the liver that are not accompanied by any signs or symptoms suggesting liver disease. These patients are identified only through random or preplanned blood testing. Many of the mild elevations (especially of aminotransferase levels) represent transient adaptation to the introduction of a new chemical compound, and with time, alternative pathways of disposition develop leading to resolution of the abnormal level. Alternatively, finding elevated levels of biochemical tests soon after introduction of a drug, and during a time when there are no symptoms or signs of liver injury, may indicate that the liver injury will progress and lead to clinically apparent liver disease. The unresolved dilemmas are in the identification of individuals who are susceptible and determination of effective ways to detect an adverse reaction that is likely to progress before serious liver injury develops.

The diagnosis of hepatic injury caused by a drug is usually based on circumstantial evidence, depending largely on suspicion by the clinician who recognizes that the time of onset and type of liver injury may be related to an adverse reaction to a therapeutic or environmental agent. Ingenuity and persistence are often required to determine whether a liver abnormality represents an adverse drug reaction and to establish whether a drug or environmental agent is actually the cause. For example, in a patient who develops an angiosarcoma of the liver, exposure to vinyl chloride may have occurred many years before. The development of reliable tests to detect hepatitis A–E has made the task of excluding viral hepatitis easier. The finding of a positive antimitochondrial antibody test in a patient who has jaundice and biochemical evidence of cholestasis may resolve concern as to whether the patient has primary biliary cirrhosis or a drug-induced syndrome that resembles the disorder.

Since the clinical and laboratory abnormalities of drug-induced injuries may be indistinguishable from liver disorders from other causes, the strongest supportive evidence implicating a drug may be resolution of manifestations of liver injury (deceleration) following withdrawal of the drug. In patients who have drug-induced hepatocellular injury, there is usually a marked decrease in elevated aminotransferase levels within 2 weeks of removing the drug. However, in patients who have predominantly cholestatic injury, there may be a delay of weeks or months before the elevated alkaline phosphatase and bilirubin levels fall to any major extent. Rechallenge with a suspected drug to establish a diagnosis is seldom necessary and in patients in whom acute hepatitis has occurred may be contraindicated. Even histological evaluation of the liver is rarely diagnostic, often allowing recognition of type and extent of injury present, rather than clearly incriminating a drug or environmental agent as the cause.

There are the additional difficulties in determining a drug-induced injury in a patient who has another known factor that could explain the liver injury. A well-known example includes the heightened toxicity of acetaminophen in patients who are chronic users of alcohol.

A. Acetaminophen

It has been well established that ingestion of excessive amounts of acetaminophen ($>$10–15 g), often in suicidal attempts, predictably leads to liver injury ranging from acute hepatitis to acute liver failure and death (10–12). In therapeutic doses ($\leq$4 g/day), acetaminophen is usually quite safe and well tolerated. However, patients who are regular users of alcohol appear to be especially likely to develop acetaminophen-induced liver injury (10–12). Hepatic injury from acetaminophen is caused by the effects of a reactive metabolic product, N-acetyl-benzoquinone-imide (NAPQI). Acetaminophen is predominantly metabolized by conjugation reactions to form sulfate and glucuronide metabolites, which are excreted in the urine. A lesser amount is metabolized by cytochrome P450 2E1 to form NAPQI, which is rapidly bound to intracellular glutathione and is excreted in the urine as mercapturic acid. When large doses of acetaminophen are ingested, the ability of the liver to form sulfate and glucuronide metabolites is overwhelmed and metabolism by cytochrome P450 2E1 becomes of much greater importance. In these situations, the capacity of glutathione to serve as an effective hepatoprotectant is negated, and the hepatocyte is vulnerable to an attack by highly reactive damaging intermediates.

Careful questioning to elicit factors that predispose patients to hepatic injury from acetaminophen in nonsuicidal situations is important. First and most important is the dose of acetaminophen. Patients may have underestimated or understated the amount ingested, especially since acetaminophen is present in many combination products. The intracellular concentration of NAPQI and dose of acetaminophen are clearly associated. Second is the concomitant use of alcohol. Cytochrome P450 2E1 is the P450 subspecies involved both in metabolism of ethanol and in the metabolism of acetaminophen. Prolonged regular use of ethanol induces P450 2E1 activity. In individuals who are regularly using alcohol, doses of acetaminophen near or within the suggested therapeutic range may lead to liver injury, especially if there is a coexistent decrease in intracellular glutathione. Cytochrome P450 2E1 is induced in patients regularly using alcohol, and therefore more acetaminophen is metabolized to yield NAPQI. In addition, the intracellular concentration of glutathione may be lowered in patients who regularly use alcohol. No clinical features specifically define these patients. Suspicion, careful history, and determination of blood acetaminophen levels should lead to the diagnosis.

IV. CLINICAL FEATURES OF DRUG-INDUCED LIVER DISEASE

A few broad generalizations may be drawn regarding clinical and laboratory manifestations of liver injury from therapeutic drugs and environmental agents, especially those causing hepatocellular necrosis. There may be few, if any, clinical signs suggesting liver injury, even in a patient who has biochemical and histological evidence of considerable damage. Early symptoms sometimes associated with these injuries are usually nonspecific and include loss of appetite, fatigue, lassitude, and occasionally a dull discomfort more prominent in the right upper quadrant of the abdomen. These are the same signs and symptoms found (or not found!) in patients who have chronic viral hepatitis or alcohol-induced liver disease. With a few drugs, there is the concomitant presence of fever, rash, or eosinophilia—the hallmarks of hypersensitivity reactions.

With many drugs, the appearance of clinical jaundice in a patient with hepatic injury is an indication of an adverse prognosis, with a fatal outcome occurring in approximately 10% (3). Therefore, jaundice appearing in a patient who has or might have a drug-induced liver disease is a cause for concern.

A. Isoniazid (INH)

A remarkable range of manifestations of hepatocellular injury can be caused by isoniazid (3,13–15). Approximately 1% of patients receiving INH develop clinically evident hepatic injury with an acute and occasionally overwhelming hepatitis. However, 10–20% of patients receiving INH have some increase in aminotransferase levels with onset within the first several days to weeks after beginning administration of the agent, and the vast majority of these patients are asymptomatic. In most, there is a return to or toward normal despite continued use of INH. Several important susceptibility factors affect the likelihood of developing severe hepatic injury. INH hepatitis is rare in patients below 20 years of age, whereas patients older than 35 years have an incidence of liver disease of at least 1.5% (3,15). Prodromal signs and symptoms are vague. If clinically apparent jaundice develops, there is an approximate 10% mortality.

There is general agreement that hepatotoxicity from INH results from the effects of an intermediary metabolite. The specific toxin has not been definitely established. Concomitant use of rifampicin increases the likelihood of an adverse reaction. Continued use of INH after the appearance of even nonspecific symptoms is associated with a likelihood of developing severe liver injury (13). Heightened awareness of the risk of isoniazid-induced liver injury and regular monitoring of aminotransferase levels in patients receiving isoniazid have proven effective in identifying evidence of hepatic injury that resolves following drug withdrawal.

V. NONSTEROIDAL ANTI-INFLAMMATORY DRUGS (NSAIDS)

Clinically significant adverse reactions affecting the liver are fortunately rare with all the NSAIDs presently in use (1–3,16). However, reactions of many types do occur and need to be recognized as drug-related. The spectrum of liver manifestations resulting from NSAIDs encompasses minimal abnormalities in biochemical tests in asymptomatic patients to acute hepatitis, cholestatic hepatitis, and, in rare instances, acute hepatic failure. Particular attention was directed to these drugs when benoxaprofen was removed from the market following recognition of a progressive downhill course and death from hepatic and renal failure in a number of patients (3,17). Elderly females were especially vulnerable to develop severe injury from benoxaprofen.

A. Sulindac

Occasionally patients receiving sulindac present with evidence of acute liver injury (18). Liver injury from sulindac appears within a few days to 6 weeks after therapy is initiated. Fever, rash, eosinophilia, and edema are frequently found in association with evidence of liver injury. Many of the patients have a predominantly cholestatic injury. There have been a few deaths. The mechanism of sulindac-related injury is uncertain but likely results from an immune reaction to a metabolic product.

B. Diclofenac

The NSAID that has received particular scrutiny as regards hepatotoxicity is diclofenac (19). Liver injury from this drug presents predominantly as hepatocellular injury with several instances of severe hepatocellular necrosis and death. Females appear to be at increased risk. Onset of liver abnormalities most often appears within 3 months of beginning therapy, although in a few patients, a much longer presymptomatic interval has been noted. The role of prospective monitoring of biochemical tests in identifying early injury, and thereby reducing the risk of developing severe injury, is uncertain.

C. Bromfenac

Bromfenac, a nonsteroidal drug approved for short term (10 days or less) use in the management of pain, was withdrawn from the marketplace in 1998 shortly after its release because of several instances of severe hepatocellular necrosis and acute liver failure requiring liver transplantation (20). Several deaths were attributed to the use of bromfenac (21–23). Patients in whom severe hepatic toxicity developed had often received the drug for longer than the approved 10-day course.

VI. SIGNALS OF HEPATOTOXICITY

Therapeutic drugs that are likely to damage the liver in many recipients at doses needed to elicit a response are usually identified during preapproval evaluation and discarded. The process of determining safety of a new agent extends over several years and observations are required in several thousands of patients before approval is granted. However, the rarer the event, the more likely a signal will be missed (Table 3).

During preapproval testing, clinical and laboratory manifestations indicating actual or potential hepatotoxicity are recorded and evaluated. There are several levels of concern (Table 3). Signals indicating hepatotoxicity that may be seen in prerelease approval include the appearance of any instances of overt hepatocellular failure leading to death or liver transplantation. Even one such patient brings the proposed drug under great scrutiny and consideration as to whether development should continue. One level less severe is the recognition of patients who have acute hepatitis with symptoms of malaise, anorexia, right-

Table 3 Signals Regarding Hepatotoxicity

Major	Development of acute liver failure
	Development of symptoms
	Onset of clinically apparent jaundice
	Appearance of ascites, encephalopathy, coagulopathy
Intermediate	ALT > 8× ULN
	ALT > 5× ULN
	ALT > 3× ULN
Minor	Any elevation ALT (<3× ULN) in asymptomatic patient

upper-quadrant abdominal pain, and especially jaundice. Most of these patients survive although, as noted previously, clinical jaundice carries an ominous prognosis. The most difficult signals to interpret are elevated aminotransferase or alkaline phosphatase levels in patients who are asymptomatic or in whom it is not possible to separate the drug-induced symptoms from those that may be from the underlying disease. As a general guideline, slight increases in ALT ($<3\times$ ULN) in asymptomatic patients who received a new agent, and in whom there were normal aminotransferase levels before beginning the drug, continue in the trials. Patients who have elevations to $>3\times$ ULN to $<8\times$ ULN (and with some agents $>3\times$ ULN to $<5\times$ ULN), even when asymptomatic, are evaluated more extensively including immediate redetermination to note whether further increases are occurring. Many drug evaluation protocols have mandatory drug withdrawal if the aminotransferase level is $>8\times$ ULN (and in some instances $>5\times$ ULN) even in asymptomatic patients.

There are several axioms regarding drug-induced liver disease that serve as general guides:

1. Clinical manifestations of drug-induced hepatotoxicity are usually indistinguishable from those of liver disease caused by other etiologies. Therefore, the diagnosis is often (almost always) made after exclusion of other possible etiologies.
2. In patients who develop hepatocellular injury from a drug, the appearance of clinically apparent liver disease, especially when associated with clinical jaundice, has a much less favorable prognosis than in patients who have acute viral hepatitis with an apparently similar degree of initial injury.
3. Any instance of acute hepatic failure leading to death, liver transplantation, or near death may lead to drug withdrawal or at least a requirement that the drug be intensely scrutinized. In these situations there is consideration of institution of a monitoring schedule in an effort to detect injury at a time that withdrawal is likely to be effective in avoiding severe liver disease.
4. Histological evidence of injury, especially in patients who have hepatocellular injury, is often more severe than is suggested by clinical signs or laboratory studies.
5. Even large and extensive testing programs in which several thousand patients are evaluated may not detect an idiosyncratic event that occurs in the range of 1 in 10,000 to 1 in 100,000 individuals. Therefore, compilation of data in the first 1 or 2 postrelease years, when many are exposed, may be necessary to identify toxicity.
6. A few drugs slip through the safety screens during preapproval evaluation and must be withdrawn based on unfavorable experience in the marketplace.
7. Hepatic injury from a drug may have a signature as regards time of onset, type of injury, and propensity to develop severe disease (e.g., hepatocellular or cholestatic manifestations).
8. In general, drugs that cause hepatocellular injury are more likely to produce serious, even life-threatening injury than are drugs that cause cholestatic injury.
9. Some drugs (e.g., phenylbutazone) lead to two patterns of injury. In those patients in whom granulomatous inflammation is found, liver disease tends to be less than in those in whom hepatocellular injury in the absence of granulomas is found (7).

VII. ASSESSMENT OF POSSIBLE DRUG-INDUCED HEPATOTOXICITY

It may be difficult or impossible to assess a drug's contribution to hepatic injury in a patient who has an underlying disease known also to produce liver injury. There may be masking of the effects of the drug on the liver because of abnormalities associated with the underlying disease. Examples would include overlooking drug-induced hepatic injury in patients who have HIV infection and acquired immune deficiency syndrome, a setting in which several other liver disorders are often found (24–27). Furthermore, there are difficulties in determining a drug-induced cause of liver injury in patients who are receiving many agents for treatment of a malignancy or disseminated infection. In addition, decisions regarding attribution of an injury to a drug are especially difficult in patients (often elderly) who are receiving many drugs (often from several physicians) (1–3). In these situations the clinician often must make a judgment call and withdraw the drug suspected of causing an injury, and then observe whether the liver abnormalities resolve.

In some patients considerable liver damage may occur and progress without any clinical signs or symptoms in the early stages. There are ample examples of liver injury progressing subclinically until there has been damage that is irreversible. Examples include progressive fibrosis and cirrhosis induced in some by prolonged use of methotrexate, and the hepatic failure that may develop in patients who have received amiodarone over prolonged intervals (3). In these situations clinical evidence of severe liver disease may be lacking.

A. Amiodarone

Amiodarone, a benzofuran derivative used in the treatment of ventricular and atrial tachyarrhythmias, is an established cause of hepatic injury and acquired phospholipidosis (3,28–30). There are many side effects from amiodarone including pulmonary, thyroid, corneal, renal, and neurological toxicities. Liver injury is overall the most important side effect. Amiodarone is a cationic amphiphilic compound that accumulates in lysosomes. The drug and its major metabolite desethylamiodarone are stored in lysosomes within hepatocytes and bile duct epithelium, thereby leading to phospholipidosis. Evidence of hepatic toxicity may appear within the first several months of beginning therapy with amiodarone or may become apparent after more than a year of treatment. Manifestations of liver injury may be subtle and include anorexia and fatigue. Hepatomegaly is often present.

Types of liver injury associated with amiodarone in addition to phospholipidosis include acute liver failure, cholestatic hepatitis, steatohepatitis, and cirrhosis (30). Elevations in aminotransferase levels are found in 15–50% of patients, usually in the range of 2–10 times the upper limit of normal. In most of these patients, elevations in aminotransferases occur in the absence of any signs or symptoms suggesting liver disease. Occasionally severe cholestasis occurs. Amiodarone-induced liver injury may closely simulate hepatic injury caused by alcohol with fibrosis, Mallory bodies, and active cirrhosis on liver biopsy. The relation of the phospholipidosis to the hepatocellular injury is uncertain and may be unrelated. The phospholipidosis likely results from a drug-induced inhibition of lysosomal phospholipases.

An unfortunate feature of amiodarone-induced injury is that even upon recognition of the relation of the drug to the liver injury and withdrawal of the drug, there may be continued damage for months caused by the release of active drug from lysosomal reservoirs (31). Some patients have died from decompensated liver disease. There are no reliable ways to predict when hepatic toxicity from amiodarone is near a dangerous level, no way to accelerate removal of the drug from the lysosomal stores, and unfortunately for many patients, no equally effective and less toxic therapy for the ventricular arrhythmias.

VIII. RISK-BENEFIT CONSIDERATIONS

With some drugs, the decision is made to accept the risk of hepatotoxicity to favorably treat a serious problem, especially if there are few, if any, effective alternatives. Such was the case with the drug tacrine used in the treatment of Alzheimer's disease (32). Even though half of all patients receiving tacrine exhibited increases in serum aminotransferases, the possible benefits of the drug led to the decision to approve it albeit with a stringent monitoring schedule. These issues are important to the clinician who must determine whether abnormalities in biochemical tests or clinically apparent liver injury have resulted from an adverse drug reaction or have been caused by an underlying medical problem. Sorting out the likely role of a drug in liver injury is often difficult and occasionally impossible.

A. Tacrine

Tacrine, a reversible cholinesterase inhibitor that is used in the treatment of Alzheimer's disease, is frequently associated with elevated aminotransferase levels (32). Approximately 50% of approximately 2500 patients who received the drug during clinical trials had elevations in serum aminotransferase levels. ALT levels greater than 3 times the upper limit of normal occurred in 25% and greater than 20 times the upper level of normal in 2%. Ninety percent of initial ALT elevations occur within 12 weeks of beginning therapy (32). Women were more likely to have elevations than were men. Elevations were noted after 12 weeks of therapy in only 10% of patients. Eosinophilia appeared to be associated with increased ALT levels, although fatigue, malaise, nausea, and vomiting did not occur more frequently in patients with elevated ALT levels compared to these manifestations in patients in the trials in whom ALT elevations did not occur. Through use of a frequent monitoring program, patients who have considerable elevations in aminotransferase levels are identified and the drug withdrawn. P450 1A2 has a major role in tacrine metabolism (33). It is of note that P450 1A2 is inhibited by cimetidine, metabolizes theophylline, and is increased by smoking. Fortunately, in most patients there is resolution of the abnormal elevations of aminotransferases within several weeks after drug withdrawal. However, at least one death has been suggested to have been the result of tacrine-induced liver injury (34).

Drugs that have established benefit yet show evidence of hepatic toxicity may remain on the market until either safer drugs that achieve the same benefit are developed, or the accumulation of evidence of severe hepatotoxicity leads to a decision to withdraw the agent. An example is troglitazone, which has been withdrawn because of hepatotoxicity and has been replaced by pioglitazone and rosiglitazone.

B. Troglitazone

Troglitazone, a thiazolidinedione agent that decreases hepatic glucose output and increases insulin-dependent glucose metabolism in skeletal muscle, has been withdrawn from clinical use because of hepatic toxicity (35). Several instances of acute liver failure leading to death or the need for liver transplantation occurred after the drug was approved in 1997 and was subsequently widely used. In the prerelease clinical trials of troglitazone, 2510 patients received the drug (35). Elevation in aminotransferase levels to >3× ULN was found in 1.9% of the patients as compared to an incidence of 0.6% in patients receiving placebo. Two treated patients became clinically jaundiced during the trial. No deaths or instances of acute liver failure occurred and biochemical abnormalities seen during the trial returned to normal following drug withdrawal with no evidence of any residual problems.

The hepatic injuries in patients who developed liver injury following release of troglitazone were predominantly hepatocellular. Several patients developed acute liver failure and died or required liver transplantation (36–41). No supportable mechanism to explain troglitazone-induced liver injury has been established. Because of the many favorable benefits of troglitazone for diabetics, the drug continued to be marketed with a mandated regular monitoring schedule. However, in 2000 it was decided to withdraw the drug from the market. Other drugs in the glitazone family (pioglitazone and rosiglitazone) have been approved and will be closely scrutinized to determine whether similar hepatic problems develop. One patient who presumably developed hepatic failure from rosiglitazone has been reported (42).

IX. DRUG-INDUCED CHRONIC HEPATITIS

Several drugs cause chronic hepatitis syndromes that are often indistinguishable from autoimmune hepatitis (43–45). It is most important to recognize the drug cause for the liver injury. Misdiagnosing those patients as having autoimmune hepatitis may lead to the institution of corticosteroid therapy and continuation of the drug, a situation in which the corticosteroids may blunt the manifestations of the injury while continued drug use leads to further damage. Generally drugs that cause chronic hepatitis are taken for prolonged intervals and the extent of the injury correlates to some extent with the duration of therapy. Issues include whether the chronic hepatitis results from continued ongoing acute injury from the drug administered over a prolonged interval or whether the drug unmasks an injury in a genetically susceptible patient.

With some drugs (e.g., nitrofurantoin, minocycline, and methyldopa), liver disease clinically and serologically closely mimics autoimmune hepatitis type I. Most of these patients are female, have increased serum globulin levels, and display the presence of autoantibodies, especially increased titers of serum antinuclear antibodies. The clinical onset of illness may be that of an apparent acute hepatitis in a patient in whom liver biopsy changes suggesting long-standing disease are found (an acute or chronic pattern). Or the illness may develop as insidious hepatic failure in a patient who has hepatosplenomegaly and evidence of portal hypertension or ascites. On liver biopsy chronic inflammation including many plasma cells is often found.

A. Nitrofurantoin

Several types of liver injury, including asymptomatic increases in serum aminotransferases, acute hepatitis, cholestatic hepatitis, and chronic hepatitis, have been attributed to adverse reactions to nitrofurantoin (3,46–49). Nitrofurantoin-induced chronic hepatitis has occurred almost exclusively in women who are middle-aged or older, and the most usual presentation is the insidious development of liver disease. Many of these patients have received nitrofurantoin for urinary antisepsis for longer than 6 months. Ascites, hypoalbuminemia, and hyperglobulinemia have been prominent features. In these patients, liver biopsy showed chronic hepatitis with bridging necrosis and occasionally cirrhosis. The hepatic manifestations of nitrofurantoin-induced injury closely simulate those of autoimmune hepatitis and observations of improvement following withdrawal of the drug may be required to make a confident diagnosis. Some patients have died of progressive liver failure even following drug withdrawal.

B. Minocycline

Minocycline, a second-generation tetracycline used in the long-term treatment of acne, has been reported to cause several types of liver damage including acute hepatitis, often with features of hypersensitivity and rarely acute liver failure. Occasional cholestatic features predominate (50–55). A chronic hepatitis syndrome with features simulating autoimmune hepatitis has been reported. Furthermore, minocycline has been implicated in causing a drug-induced lupus syndrome (50,54).

Although most patients who have minocycline-induced liver disease have been women, both sexes have been affected. Some patients have reported joint and muscle aches and pains as well as muscle stiffness. Hyperglobulinemia and the presence of ANA and anti-DNA antibodies have been reported.

C. Oxyphenisatin

The first drug recognized as causing drug-induced chronic hepatitis was oxyphenisatin, a former component of several laxatives, which led to chronic hepatitis, cirrhosis, and liver failure—especially in older women who had received prolonged exposure (56). The clinical resemblance of oxyphenisatin-induced liver injury to the progressive liver disease of autoimmune hepatitis was often so close that many of these patients were treated with corticosteroids while continuing the drug. Once the drug relationship was noted and the agent withdrawn, resolution of at least the acute ongoing component of the injury occurred, although some patients were left with considerable damage. A quite similar chronic hepatitis syndrome occurred in patients receiving long-term treatment with the once widely used antihypertensive medication methyldopa (57).

Two drugs, dihydralazine and tienilic acid, have been implicated as the cause of chronic hepatitis resembling autoimmune hepatitis, in which there is evidence of formation of antibodies against components of the cytochrome P450 system (45).

D. Tienilic Acid

Tienilic acid was on the market as a uricosuric diuretic and was withdrawn following recognition of hepatotoxicity (3,58). Laboratory and clinical manifestations of liver disease caused by this drug, as well as dihydralazine, are quite similar to those found in autoimmune hepatitis type I. Of additional interest is the observation that patients who developed liver injury from the uricosuric diuretic tienilic acid often had extensive hepatic injury in a setting in which there was development of anti-LKM2 antibodies. These antibodies were targeted against the cytochrome P450 (CYP 2C9) enzyme that catalyzes the hydroxylation of tienilic acid, therefore establishing that a drug can induce production of an autoantibody. Several of these patients had histological findings compatible with those found in classic chronic hepatitis. Tienilic acid was removed from the marketplace because of hepatotoxicity.

E. Dihydralazine

In dihydralazine-induced hepatitis, the predominant autoantibody is directed against CYP1A2, which is a liver microsomal protein (45).

X. MECHANISMS OF INJURY: EFFECTS ON CLINICAL AND PATHOLOGICAL MANIFESTATIONS

For some drugs there is evidence that genetically controlled pathways of metabolism play important roles in determining which individuals are likely to have an adverse reaction affecting the liver. Undoubtedly in the future, identification of genetic control of susceptibility factors will become even more important and useful. A well-studied example of genetic susceptibility to hepatic injury is in the oxidative polymorphism of debrisoquine-4-hydroxylase, an enzyme important in the metabolism of several drugs (1–3). Individuals who have genetically determined impairment of debrisoquine-4-hydroxylase (up to 10% of the population) are at increased risk of developing an adverse reaction due to increased blood levels if exposed to a group of drugs that are metabolized by the enzyme, such as propranolol, quinidine, and desipramine, and are at increased risk of hepatic injury from perhexiline maleate, due to increased accumulation of the parent drug.

A. Diphenylhydantoin

An additional interesting story with genetic implications is that of adverse hepatic reactions that occur in patients receiving diphenylhydantoin. The hepatic injury that occasionally develops in these patients may be severe, with intense liver necrosis often occurring as part of a syndrome that includes fever, exfoliative dermatitis, and eosinophilia (Stevens-Johnson syndrome) (59,60). The onset of evidence of an adverse reaction is usually within 4 weeks of beginning the drug. Up to half of the affected patients who develop the full syndrome died. Many features of diphenylhydantoin injury suggest important roles for immunological (hypersensitivity) reactions. However, it has been established that many of the patients have a genetically determined defect in detoxification (61), the nature of which is not certain.

REFERENCES

1. Farrell GC. Drug-Induced Liver Disease. New York: Churchill Livingstone, 1994.
2. Larrey D. Drug-induced liver diseases. J Hepatol 2000; 32(suppl 1):77–88.
3. Zimmerman HJ. Hepatotoxicity: The Adverse Effects of Drugs and Other Chemicals on the Liver. 2nd ed. Philadelphia: Lippincott Williams & Wilkins, 1999.
4. Bryant AE, Dreifuss FE. Valproic acid hepatic fatalities. III. U.S. experience since 1986. Neurology 1996; 46:465–468.
5. Berson A, De Beco V, Lettéron P, Robin MA, et al. Steatohepatitis-inducing drugs cause mitochondrial dysfunction and lipid peroxidation in rat hepatocytes. Gastroenterology 1998; 114:765–774.
6. Day CP, James OFW. Steatohepatitis: a tale of two "hits"? Gastroenterology 1998; 114:842–845.
7. Ishak KG, Kirchner JP, Dhar JK. Granulomas and cholestic-hepatocellular injury associated with phenylbutazone. Am J Dig Dis 1977; 22:611–617.
8. Mitchell MC, Boitnott JK, Arregui A, Maddrey WC. Granulomatous hepatitis associated with carbamazepine therapy. Am J Med 1981; 71:722–735.

9. Maddrey WC. Granulomas of the Liver. In: ER Schiff, MS Sorrell, WC Maddrey, eds. Schiff's Diseases of the Liver. 8th ed. Philadelphia: Lippincott-Raven. 1999:1571–1585.

10. Seeff LB, Cucherini BA, Zimmerman HJ, Adler E, et al. Acetaminophen hepatotoxicity in alcoholics: a therapeutic misadventure. Ann Intern Med 1986; 104:399–404.

11. Schenker S, Maddrey WC. Subliminal drug-drug interactions: users and their physicians take notice. Hepatology 1991; 13:995–998.

12. Zimmerman HJ, Maddrey WC. Acetaminophen hepatotoxicity in alcoholics. Hepatology 1995; 22:767–773.

13. Maddrey WC, Boitnott JK. Isoniazid hepatitis. Ann Intern Med 1973; 79:1–12.

14. Maddrey WC. Isoniazid-induced liver disease. Semin Liver Dis 1981; 1:77–84.

15. Black M, Mitchell JR, Zimmerman HJ, et al. Isoniazid-associated hepatitis in 114 patients. Gastroenterology 1975; 69:289.

16. Tolman KG. Hepatotoxicity of non-narcotic analgesics. Am J Med 1998; 105:13S–19S.

17. Taggart HM, Alderdice JM. Fatal cholestatic jaundice in elderly patients taking benoxaprofen. Br Med J 1982; 284:1372.

18. Tarazi EM, Harter JG, Zimmerman HJ, Ishak KG, et al. Sulindac-associated hepatic injury: analysis of 91 cases reported to the Food and Drug Administration. Gastroenterology 1993; 104:569–574.

19. Banks AT, Zimmerman HJ, Ishak KG, Harter JG. Diclofenac-associated hepatotoxicity: analysis of 180 cases reported to the Food and Drug Administration as adverse reactions. Hepatology 1995; 22:820–827.

20. Hunter EB, Johnston PE, Tanner G, Pinson CW, et al. Bromfenac (Duract)-associated hepatic failure requiring liver transplantation. Am J Gastroenterol 1999; 94:2299–2301.

21. Fontana RJ, McCashland TM, Benner KG, Appleman HD, et al. Acute liver failure associated with prolonged use of bromfenac leading to liver transplantation. Liver Transplant Surg 1999; 5:480–484.

22. Moses PL, Schroeder B, Alkhatib O, Ferrentino N, et al. Severe hepatotoxicity associated with bromfenac sodium. Am J Gastroenterol 1999; 94:1393–1396.

23. Rabkin JM, Smith MJ, Orloff SL, Corless CL, et al. Fatal fulminant hepatitis associated with bromfenac use. Ann Pharm 1999; 33:945–947.

24. Fortgang HS, Belitsos PC, Chaisson RE, Moore RD. Hepatomegaly and steatosis in HIV-infected patients receiving nucleoside analog antiretroviral therapy. Am J Gastroenterol 1995; 90:1433–1436.

25. Bräu N, Leaf HL, Wieczorek RL, Margolis DM. Severe hepatitis in three AIDS patients treated with indinavir. Lancet 1997; 349:924–926.

26. Vergis E, Paterson DL, Singh N. Indinavir-associated hepatitis in patients with advanced HIV infection. Int J STD AIDS 1998; 9:53.

27. Sulkowski MS, Thomas DL, Chaisson RE, Moore RD. Hepatotoxicity associated with antiretroviral therapy in adults infected with human immunodeficiency virus and the role of hepatitis C or B virus infection. JAMA 2000; 283:74–80.

28. Rigas B, Rosenfeld LE, Barwick KW, et al. Amiodarone hepatotoxicity: a clinicopathologic study of five patients. Ann Intern Med 1986; 104:348.

29. Rinder HM, Love JC, Wexler R. Amiodarone hepatotoxicity. N Engl J Med 1986; 324:318.

30. Snir Y, Pick N, Riesenberg K, Yanai-Inbar I, et al. Fatal hepatic failure due to prolonged amiodarone treatment. J Clin Gastroenterol 1995; 20:265–266.

31. Chang CC, Petrelli M, Tomashefski JF, McCullough AJ. Severe intrahepatic cholestasis caused by amiodarone toxicity after withdrawal of the drug. Arch Pathol Lab Med 1999; 123:251–256.

32. Watkins PB, Zimmerman HJ, Knapp MJ, Gracon SI, et al. Hepatotoxic effects of tacrine administered in patients with Alzheimer's disease. JAMA 1994; 271:992–998.

33. Becquemont L, Ragueneau I, Le Bot MA, Riche C, et al. Influence of the CYP1A inhibitor fluvoxamine on tacrine pharmacokinetics in humans. Clin Pharmacol Ther 1997; 61:619–627.

34. Blackard WG Jr, Sood GK, Crowe DR, Fallon MB. Tacrine: a cause of fatal hepatotoxicity? J Clin Gastroenterol 1998; 26:57–59.

35. Watkins PB, Whitcomb RW. Hepatic dysfunction associated with troglitazone. N Engl J Med 1998; 338:916–917.

36. Gitlin N, Julie NL, Spurr CL, Lim KN, et al. Two cases of severe clinical and histologic hepatotoxicity associated with troglitazone. Ann Intern Med 1998; 129:26–37.

37. Shibuya A, Watanabe M, Fijita Y, Saigenji K, et al. An autopsy case of troglitazone-induced fulminant hepatitis. Diabetes Care 1998; 21:2140–2143.

38. Neuschwander-Tetri BA, Isley WL, Oki JC, Ramrakhiani S, et al. Troglitazone-induced hepatic failure leading to liver transplantation. Ann Intern Med 1998; 129:38–41.

39. Fukano M, Amano S, Sato J, Yamamoto K, et al. Subacute hepatic failure associated with a new antidiabetic agent, troglitazone: a case report with autopsy examination. Hum Pathol 2000; 31:250–253.

40. Murphy EJ, Davern TJ, Shakil O, Shick L, et al. Troglitazone-induced fulminant hepatic failure. Dig Dis Sci 2000; 45:549–553.

41. Kohlroser J, Mathai J, Reichheld, Banner BF, et al. Hepatotoxicity due to troglitazone: Report of two cases and review of adverse events reported to the United States Food and Drug Administration. Am J Gastroenterol 2000; 95:272–276.

42. Forman LM, Simmons DA, Diamond RH. Hepatic failure in a patient taking rosiglitazone. Ann Intern Med 2000; 132:118–121.

43. Maddrey WC, Boitnott JK. Drug-induced chronic liver disease. Gastroenterology 1977; 72: 1348–1353.

44. Farrell GC. Drug-induced hepatic injury. J Gastroenterol Hepatol 1997; 12(suppl):S242–S250.

45. Czaja AJ. Autoimmune liver disease. Curr Opin Gastroenterol 2000; 16:262–270.

46. Black M, Rabin L, Schatz N. Nitrofurantoin-induced chronic active hepatitis. Ann Intern Med 1980; 92:62.

47. Sharp JR, Ishak KG, Zimmerman HJ. Chronic active hepatitis and severe hepatic necrosis associated with nitrofurantoin. Ann Intern Med 1980; 92:14.

48. Stricker BHCh, Blotz APR, Claas FHJ, et al. Hepatic injury associated with the use of nitrofurans: a clinicopathological study of 52 reported cases. Hepatology 1988; 8:599.

49. Schattner A, Von Der Walde J, Kozak N, Sokolovskaya N, et al. Nitrofurantoin-induced immune-mediated lung and liver disease. Am J Med Sci 1999; 317:336–340.

50. Golstein PE, Deviere J, Cremer M. Acute hepatitis and drug-related lupus induced by minocycline treatment. Am J Gastroenterol 1997; 92:143–146.

51. Tamm M, Sieber C, Schnyder F, Haefeli WE. Moxonidine-induced cholestatic hepatitis. Lancet 1997; 350:1822.

52. Bhat G, Jordan Jr. J, Sokalski S, Bajaj V, Marshall R, et al. Minocycline-induced hepatitis with autoimmune features and neutropenia. J Clin Gastroenterol 1998; 27:74–75.

53. Angulo JM, Sigal LH, Espinoza LR. Coexistent minocycline-induced systemic lupus erythematosus and autoimmune hepatitis. Semin Arthritis Rheum 1998; 28:187–92.

54. Schlienger RG, Bircher AJ, Meier CR. Minocycline-induced lupus: a systematic review. Dermatology 2000; 200:223–231.

55. Teitelbaum JE, Perez-Atayde AR, Cohen M, Bousvaros A, et al. Minocycline-related autoimmune hepatitis: case series and literature review. Arch Pediatr Adolesc Med 1998; 152:1132–1136.

56. Reynolds TB, Peters RL, Yamada S. Chronic active and lupoid hepatitis caused by a laxative, oxyphenisatin. N Engl J Med 1971; 280:813–820.

57. Maddrey WC, Boitnott JK. Severe hepatitis from methyldopa. Gastroenterology 1975; 68: 351–360.

58. Zimmerman HJ, Lewis JH, Ishak KG, Maddrey WC. Ticrynafen associated hepatic injury: analysis of 340 cases. Hepatology 1984; 4:3115–323.

59. Spielberg SP, Gordon GB, Blake DA, Goldstein DA, et al. Predisposition to phenytoin hepato-toxicity assessed in vitro. N Engl J Med 1981; 305:722–727.

60. Mullick FG, Ishak KG. Hepatic injury associated with diphenylhydantoin therapy: a clinico-pathological study of 20 cases. Am J Clin Pathol 1980; 74:442–452.

61. Gennis MA, Vemuri R, Burns EA, Hill JF, et al. Familial occurrence of hypersensitivity to phenytoin. Am J Med 1991; 91:631–634.

62. Maddrey, WC. Granulomas of the liver. In: ER Schiff, MF Sorrell, WC Maddrey, eds. Schiff's Diseases of the Liver. 8th ed. Vol. 2. Philadelphia: Lippincott-Raven. 1999:1571–1585.

12

Histopathology of Drug-Induced Liver Disease

GARY C. KANEL

University of Southern California, Los Angeles, California, U.S.A.

I. INTRODUCTION

As the liver is the major site for drug metabolism, it is not surprising that drug toxicity and adverse drug reactions would incite variable functional, histological, and ultrastructural hepatic abnormalities (1–9). Up to 10% of cases associated with abnormal liver tests are found to be drug- or toxin-induced, with the incidence rising to over 40% in patients over the age of 50 (10). Drug-induced liver injury is estimated to occur in from 2 to 5% of hospitalized patients with jaundice, and is responsible for up to 15–20% of cases of intrahepatic cholestasis, 15–30% of cases of fulminant hepatic failure, and 20–50% of cases of nonviral chronic hepatitis (11–17). The type of liver cell injury may be intrinsic

Table 1 Drug and Toxin-Induced Liver Cell Injury: Morphological Variants (11,19,57)

Morphology	Examples
Hepatocellular injury	
Lobular necrosis with minimal to absent inflammation	
Zonal: Perivenular (zone 3)	Alpha-methyldopa, acetaminophen, mushrooms
Midzonal (zone 2)	Beryllium, dioxane
Periportal (zone 1)	Allyl formate, phosphorus, ferrous salts
Diffuse (confluent)	Halogenated hydrocarbons, mushrooms
Lobular necrosis with inflammation	Isoniazid, phenytoin
Lobular confluent necrosis with inflammation	Niacin, troglitazone
Fatty change—macrovesicular	Ethanol, rifampin, corticosteroids
—microvesicular	Valproate, tetracycline, nucleosides
Granulomas	Diazepam, ranitidine, allopurinol
Mallory bodies	Amiodarone, griseofulvin
Cholestatic injury	
Cholestasis, simple	Oral contraceptives, methimazole, cyclosporin
Cholestasis with inflammation	Indomethacin, tamoxifen, carbamazapine, erythromycins, chlorpromazine, sulindac, amoxicillin + clavulanic acid
Bile duct injury	
Inflammation by neutrophils	Allopurinol, hydralazine
Inflammation by lymphocytes, ductopenia (duct loss)	Cimetidine, tolbutamide
Periductal fibrosis	Floxuridine
Vascular injury	
Sinusoids	
Peliosis	Arsenic, phalloidin
Dilatation	Oral contraceptives
Veno-occlusive disease	Pyrrolizidine alkaloids, cyclophosphamide
Thrombosis, fibrous obliteration	Ethanol, oral contraceptives
Vasculitis	Allopurinol, phenylbutazone
Portal fibrosis	
Progression to cirrhosis	Methotrexate, ethanol
Without progression to cirrhosis	Arsenic, vitamin A
Neoplasia	
Benign	Oral contraceptives, toxic (rapeseed) oil
Malignant	Aflatoxins, thorotrast
Miscellaneous	
Inclusions	
Hepatocytes	Procainamide, lead
Reticuloendothelial	Polyvinyl pyrrolidone, thorotrast
Pigments	
Lipochrome	Carbamazepine, nitrofurantoin
Hemosiderin	Ethanol, cimetidine
Radiopaque	Thorotrast
Anthracite	(Coal miners, city dwellers)
Gold	Gold sodium thiomalate

and dose-dependent (18); the mechanism may relate either to formation of free radicals or electrophilic intermediates, or to the production of reactive oxygen species, which, like free radicals, leads to lipid peroxidation (19–21). On the other hand, liver cell damage may be idiosyncratic and dose-independent, i.e., dependent on host susceptibility, and may be either immunologically or metabolically mediated (11,22). A wide variety of hepatic histological changes have been documented as secondary to drugs and toxins (Table 1); in addition, up to 1000 drugs and toxins have been implicated in causing these histological changes (23–25). Although the morphological features are usually reversible with stoppage of the medication and toxin exposure, unfortunately, in severe (fulminant) hepatitis and certain forms of chronic hepatitis, discontinuance of the drug does not alleviate the sometimes drastic outcomes. This chapter divides drugs and toxins into the various histological features seen on biopsy.

II. HEPATOCELLULAR INJURY

A. Lobular Necrosis with Minimal to Absent Inflammation

This type of liver cell injury is usually related to direct effects of the drug itself or its metabolites (19). Unlike drug-induced hypersensitivity reactions, the type of liver cell necrosis can be predicted, and is most often zonal in distribution. Usually the liver cell injury is coagulative in type, whereby the damaged liver cells become shrunken, with eosinophilic cytoplasm, and hyperchromatic nuclei with eventual nuclear pyknosis and karyorrhexis. Although an inflammatory reaction is not characteristic of this type of liver cell injury, a histological response to the necrotic hepatocytes may secondarily occur, with

Table 2 Lobular Necrosis with Minimal to Absent Inflammation

	Perivenular (zone 3)	
Alpha-methyldopa	Ethionamide	Propylthiouracil
Acetaminophen	Halogenated hydrocarbons	Pyrrolizidine alkaloids
Aflatoxin B1	Ketoconazole	Tannic acid
Carbon tetrachloride	Metoprolol	Tetrachlorethylene
Chloroform	Mithramycin	Tricrynafen
Copper	Mushrooms	Urethane
Dimethylnitrosamine	Phalloidin	Valproate

Midzonal (zone 2)	*Periportal (zone 1)*
Beryllium	Allyl formate
Dioxane	Endotoxin from *Proteus vulgaris*
	Ferrous sulfate
	Phosphorus

Perivenular or periportal	*Diffuse confluent*
Cocaine	Galactosamine
	Halogenated hydrocarbons
	Mushrooms
	2-Nitropropane
	Phenelzine
	Tetrachlorethane
	Trinitrotoluene

this type of inflammatory reaction predominantly neutrophilic. A zonal nature is often characteristic of specific drugs; most frequently the injury is perivenular (zone 3), but other zones may be specifically affected (Table 2, Figs. 1–5). In the more severe cases, bridging confluent necrosis may be seen involving two zones or the entire lobule, and is usually associated with high mortality. Often the borders of the areas of necrosis are sharply divided and distinct from the adjacent viable hepatocytes; the spared liver cells with time may show a ballooning change *not* representing liver cell injury but instead representing *regenerative* activity. Sometimes fatty change secondary to intrinsic damage may also occur. When there is impediment to bile flow, cholestasis may also be present.

B. Lobular Necrosis with Inflammation

As opposed to direct injury, drugs may induce a hypersensitivity reaction. Patients with this type of drug-induced injury may exhibit both clinical and histological features of *acute hepatitis* (Table 3, Figs. 6–12). The portal tracts show an inflammatory infiltrate that is most often lymphocytic, although coexisting eosinophils and sometimes neutrophils may also be seen. The parenchyma shows variable degrees of spotty necrosis either without a zonal distribution pattern, or slight accentuation in zone 3 (perivenular zone) in early-stage disease. The hepatocytes often show both hydropic ballooning changes as well as formation of individual cell necrosis ("acidophil" bodies), with an associated, usually mononuclear (lymphocytic), inflammatory infiltrate and Kupffer cell hyperplasia. Although cholestasis may also be seen, it usually is not pronounced except in cases of severe hepatitis when there is significant impediment to bile flow. Although the histology in many ways is similar to that seen in acute viral hepatitis, the degree of portal infiltrates in drug-induced injury is usually not as striking. In addition, a helpful clue to drug-induced injury

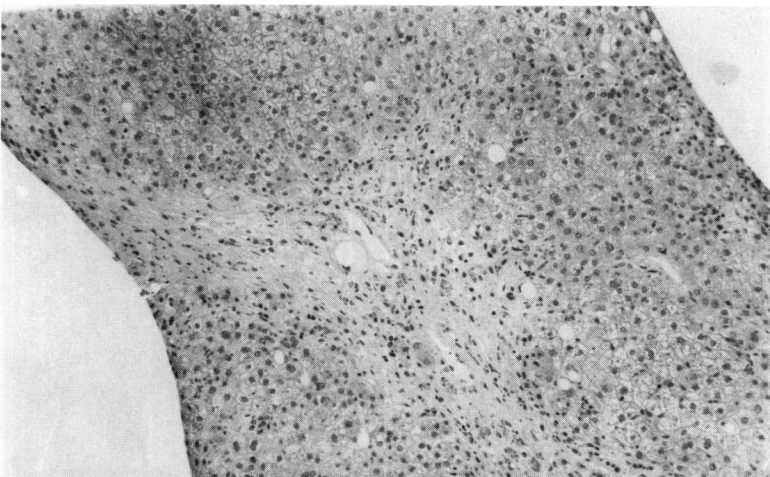

Figure 1 Acetaminophen. This low-power field shows prominent perivenular (zone 3) liver cell dropout with collapse of the reticulin framework in this patient who consumed approximately 10 g approximately 8 days prior to biopsy. Note that the adjacent viable parenchyma shows no inflammatory infiltrate.

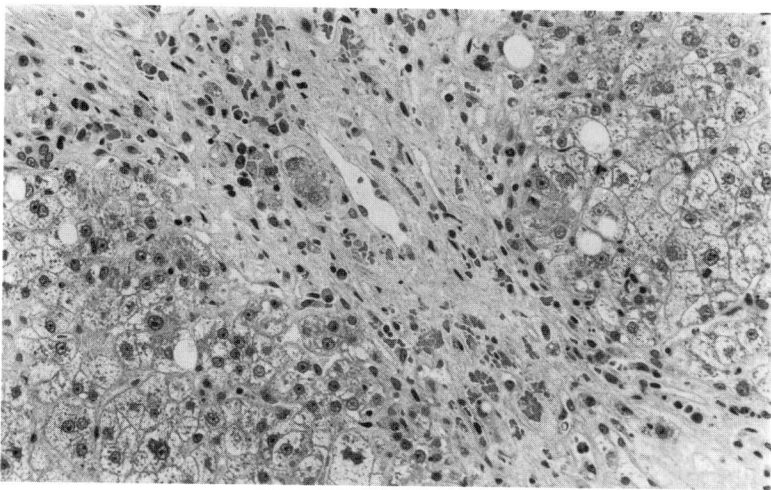

Figure 2 Acetaminophen. This high-power field from the same patient as in Fig. 1 exhibits lobular perivenular collapse with reactive histiocytic infiltrates. The coagulative-type necrosis seen in earlier-stage lesions is absent in the present biopsy owing to phagocytosis of the dead liver cells by histiocytes and Kupffer cells.

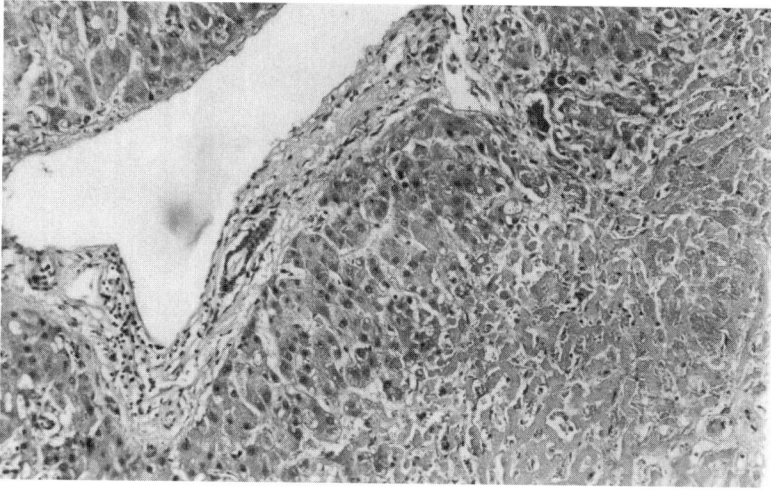

Figure 3 Cocaine. Cocaine hepatotoxicity may exhibit necrosis in various zones of the lobules. In this photomicrograph, the portal tract at the left of the field shows a mild lymphocytic infiltrate, with the hepatocytes in the periportal zone appearing viable, without an accompanying inflammatory infiltrate; however, the liver cells in the midzone and perivenular zone to the right of the field show extensive coagulative-type necrosis.

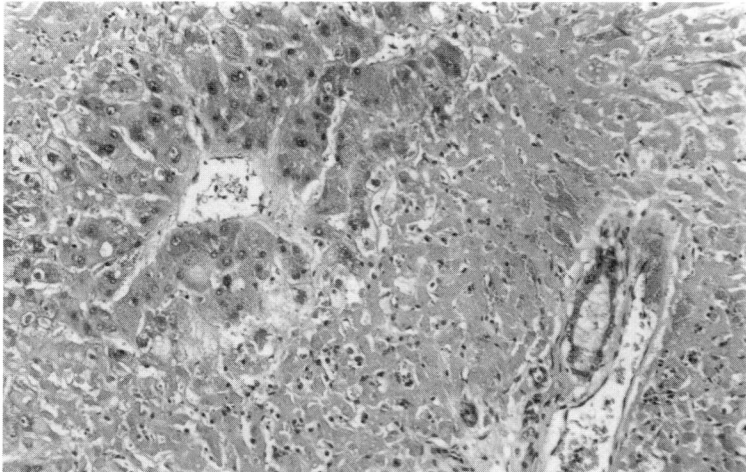

Figure 4 Cocaine. This example of cocaine hepatotoxicity shows extensive coagulative-type necrosis in the liver cells occupying the periportal zone, while the perivenular hepatocytes toward the left of the field are intact.

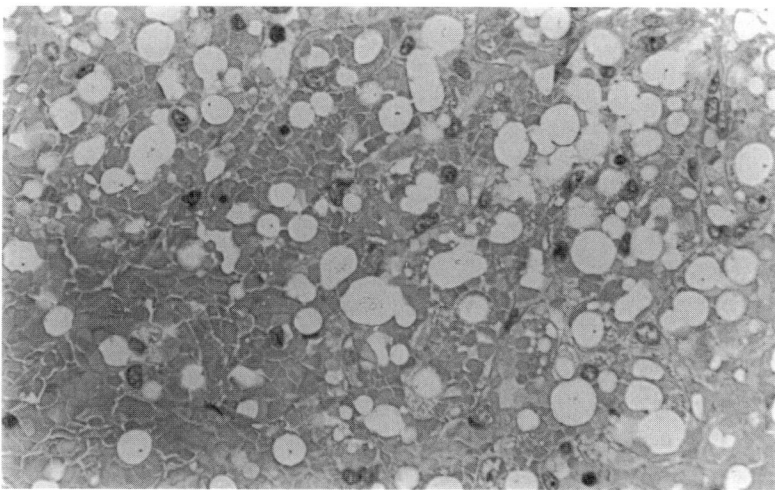

Figure 5 Mushrooms. Although mushroom hepatotoxicity may cause fatty change (as seen in this field and in Fig. 17), this high-power photomicrograph shows extensive necrosis of the hepatocytes containing the fat. No viable liver cell cytoplasm is seen, and only few nuclei are evident. Numerous red blood cells are seen within the sinusoids.

Table 3 Lobular Necrosis with Inflammation

Alpha-methyldopa	Glyburide	Pemoline
Aspirin	Halogenated hydrocarbons	Perhexilene maleate
Benzarone	Indomethacin	Phenylbutazone
Bupropion	Isoniazid	Phenytoin
Chlorpromazine	Ketoconazole	Pirprofen
Clarithromycin	Lisinopril	Propylthiouracil
Clometacin	Methotrexate	Rifampin
Dantrolene	Minocycline	Sulfadoxine
Dapsone	Naproxen	Sulfasalazine
Diclofenac	Niacin	Suloctidil
Dihydralazine	Nitrofurantoin	Sulfonamides
Disulfiram	Oxacillin	Toxic oil (rapeseed)
Ethanol	Oxaprozin	Trazodone
Etretinate	Oxyphenisatin	Tricrynafen
Fenofibrate	Papaverine	Troglitazone
Germander	Para-aminosalicylic acid	

is a prominent portal eosinophilic infiltrate, which unfortunately is seen in only a minority of cases of drug-induced liver cell injury.

In instances of ongoing necroinflammatory change, a *chronic hepatitis* may also ensue, with persistently abnormal aminotransferase elevations. The histological features may show progression with time, with variable degrees of periportal inflammatory activity (periportal or interface hepatitis, "piecemeal" necrosis), portal fibrosis, and bridging fibrosis if the drug is not discontinued (see below for drugs that may cause a chronic hepatitis with fibrosis); although cirrhosis may eventually occur, this feature nowadays is quite uncommon.

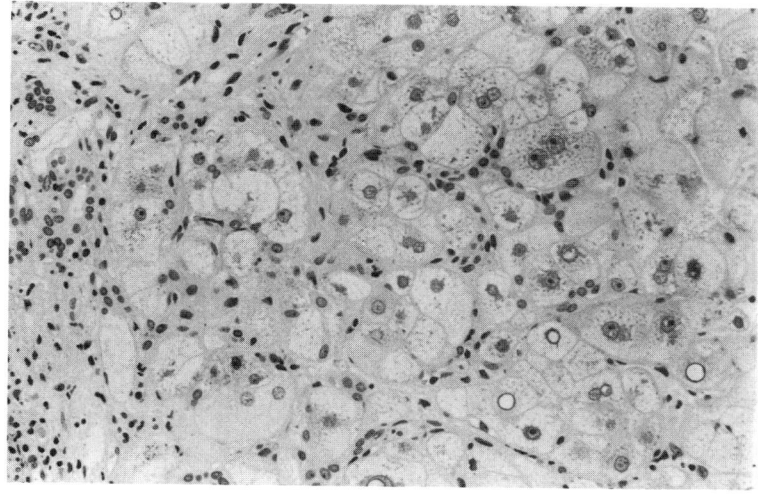

Figure 6 Methotrexate. Diffuse lymphocytic infiltrates are seen within the lobule. Scattered glycogenated nuclei are also present toward the right of the field.

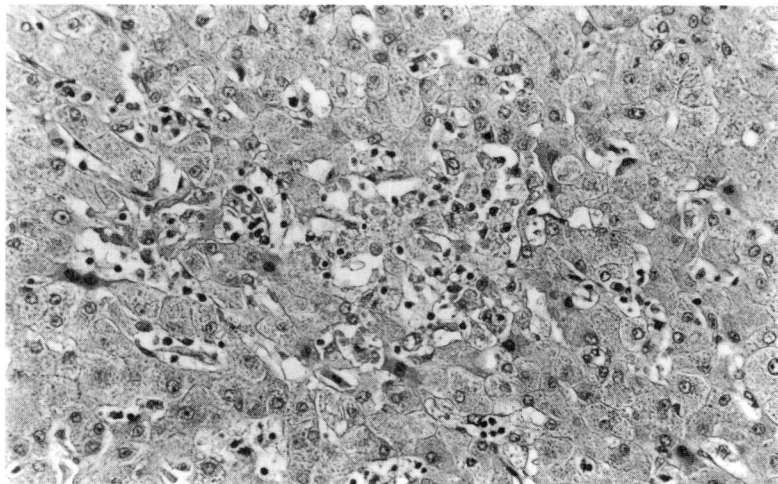

Figure 7 Troglitazone. The liver cells show variable hydropic change with focal lymphocytic infiltrates. Hypertrophic Kupffer cells and macrophages are seen within the sinusoids in areas of necrosis owing to phagocytosis of the damaged liver cells.

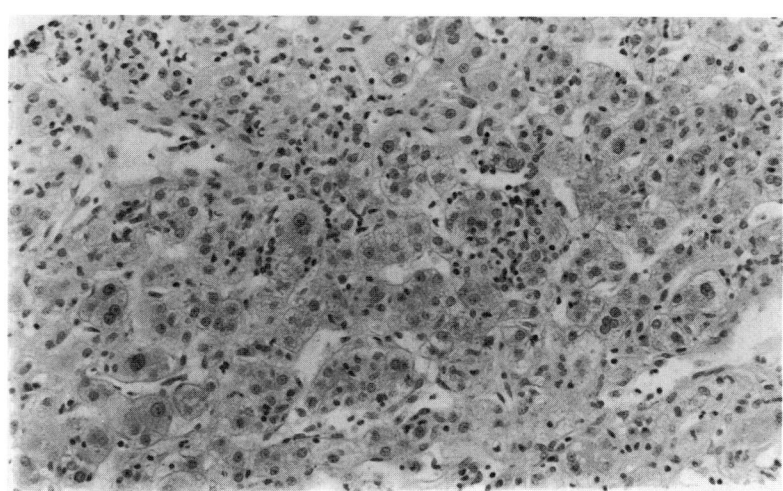

Figure 8 Isoniazid. The inflammatory infiltrate seen in this field is diffuse and chiefly lymphocytic. Mild hydropic change of the hepatocytes is also seen.

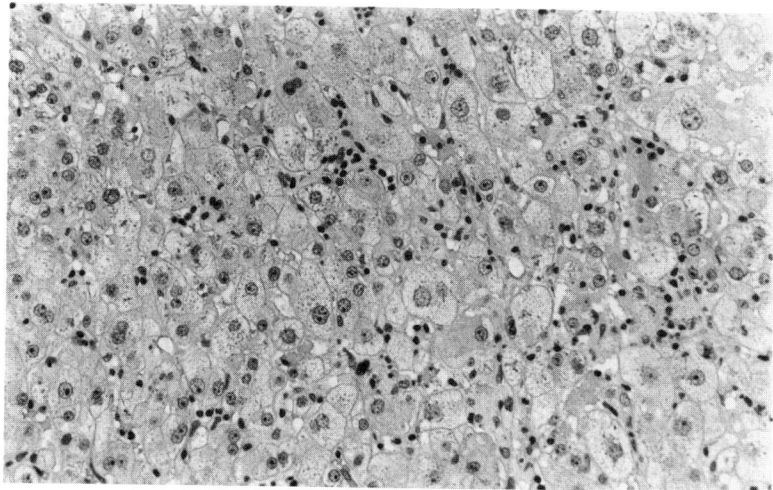

Figure 9 Phenytoin. The inflammatory component is lymphocytic. Note also that increased numbers of lymphocytes are also apparent within the sinusoids, histologically resembling that seen in cytomegalovirus and Epstein-Barr virus infection in immunocompetent patients ("mononucleosis-type" changes).

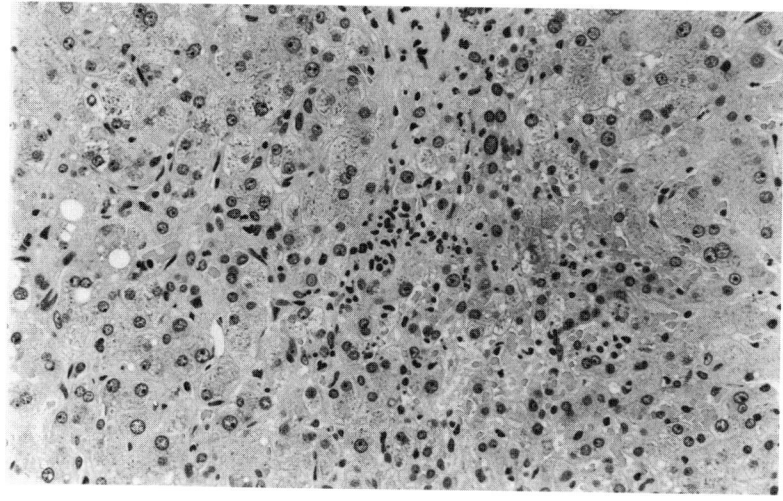

Figure 10 Rifampin. The lobular inflammatory infiltrate is chiefly lymphocytic, with mild hydropic change of the liver cells.

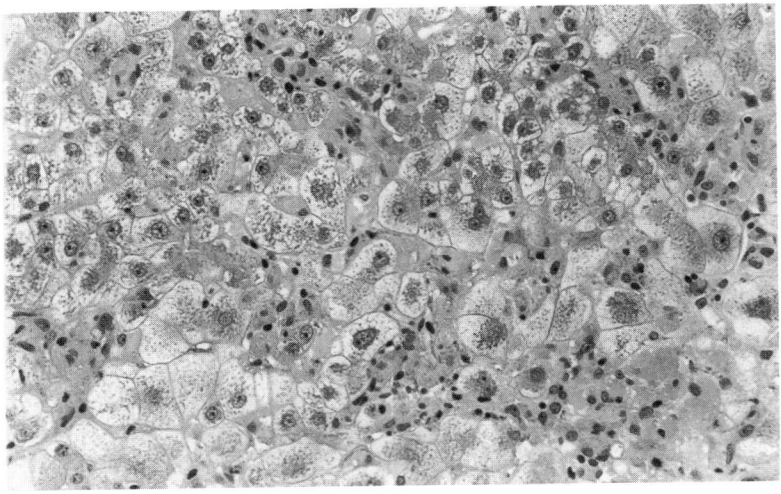

Figure 11   Alpha-methyldopa. The liver cells are quite hydropic, with associated lymphocytic infiltrates and hypertrophic Kupffer cells in areas of necrosis.

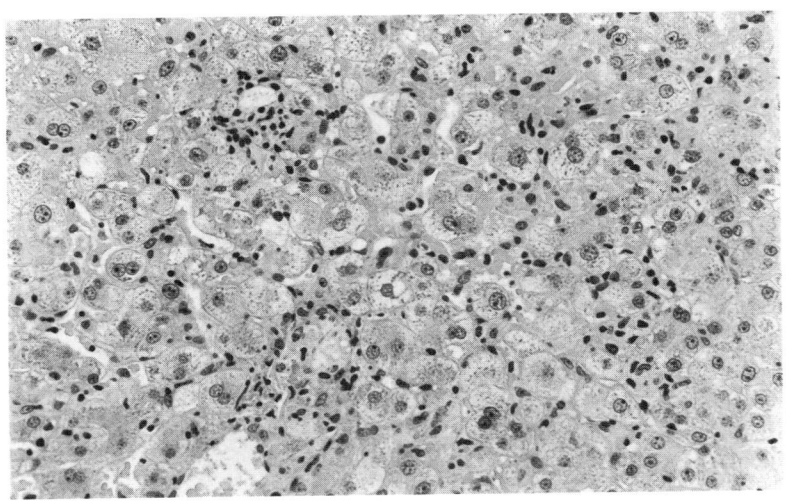

Figure 12   Bupropion. The lymphocytic inflammatory infiltrate is diffuse, with mild hydropic change of the liver cells.

Table 4 Lobular Confluent Necrosis with Inflammation

Alpha-methyldopa	Gold sodium thiomalate	Phenelzine sulfate
Allopurinol	Halogenated hydrocarbons	Phenylbutazone
Bromofenac	Hydralazine	Phenytoin
Captopril	Indomethacin	Piroxicam
Carbamazepine	Iprocloziden	Probenecid
Chlordiazepoxide	Isoniazid	Prochlorperazine
Clarithromycin	Ketoconazole	Propylthiouracil
Cimetidine	Mithramycin	Sulfamethoxazole
Dacarbazine	Mitomycin	Sulfasalazine
Dideoxyinosine	Niacin	Sulfonamides
Erythromycin	Nicotinic acid	Ticrynafen
Ethacrynic acid	Nitrofurantoin	Troglitazone
Ethionamide	Pemoline	Valproic acid

C. Lobular Confluent Necrosis with Inflammation

The more severe forms of acute hepatitis are associated with significant liver cell necrosis with prominent liver cell dropout and associated collapse of the reticulin framework (*confluent* or *submassive* necrosis), and may clinically present as a fulminant hepatitis (Table 4, Figs. 13–16). The necrosis usually involves an entire zonal population of cells, most often the perivenular zone (zone 3); however, more than one zone is frequently involved. When all three zones are affected, a *panacinar* (*massive*) necrosis is present, associated with an ominous prognosis. A portal and lobular inflammatory component is

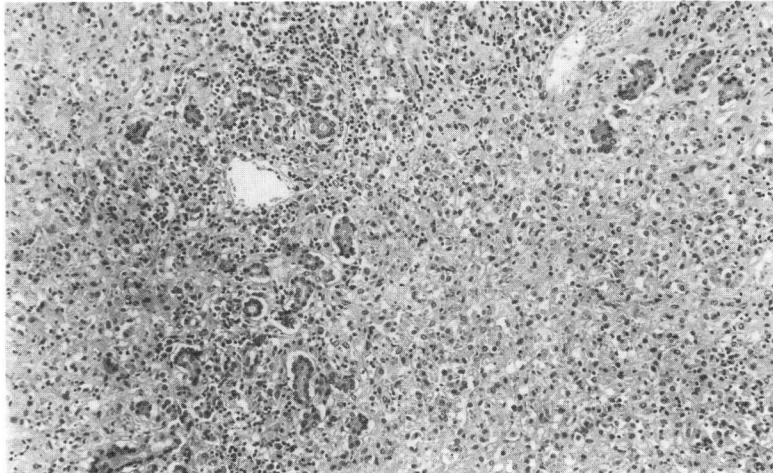

Figure 13 Isoniazid. Although isoniazid hepatotoxicity shows an acute hepatitis-like reaction (refer to Fig. 8), that change is reversible if the drug is discontinued in time; however, this photomicrograph shows extensive liver cell dropout with a prominent portal and lobular lymphocytic infiltrate in this patient, who unfortunately developed fulminant hepatitis and died.

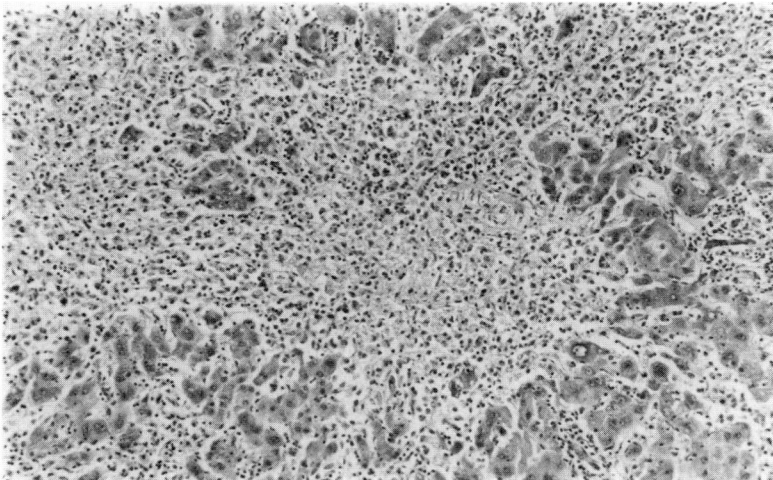

Figure 14 Halothane. The perivenular zone and midzone show extensive liver cell necrosis and dropout with a prominent lymphocytic infiltrate. The inflammatory component also involves the periportal zone as well.

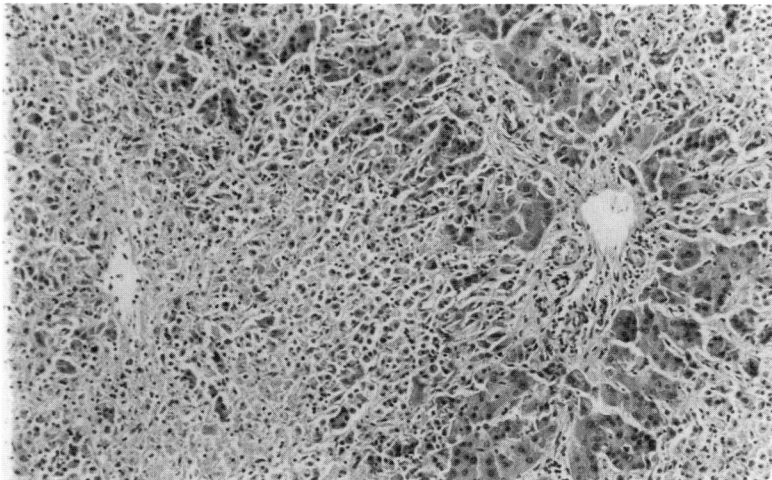

Figure 15 Halothane. The perivenular and midzonal liver cells again demonstrate prominent liver cell necrosis with a lymphocytic inflammatory infiltrate. The portal tract at the right of the field also shows a mild lymphocytic infiltrate.

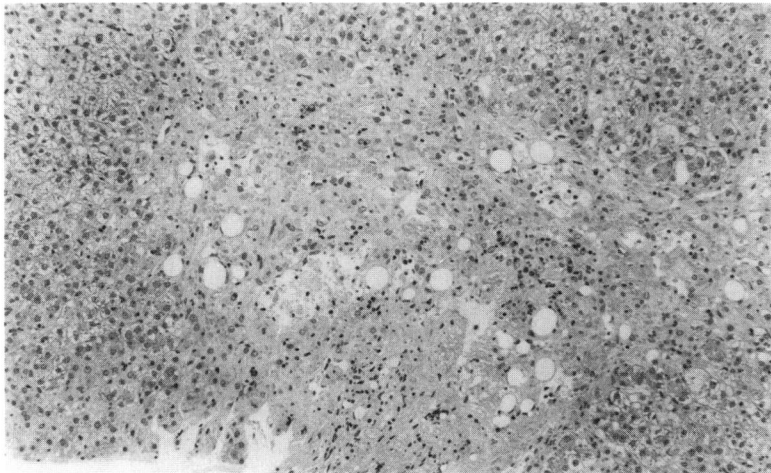

Figure 16 Niacin. Prominent perivenular and midzonal dropout of liver cells is apparent, with an accompanying predominantly lymphocytic infiltrate. Residual fatty change is seen, which represents the fat originally present within the damaged liver cells that were phagocytized by the Kupffer cells and reactive macrophages.

present and is predominantly lymphocytic, with a prominent lobular Kupffer cell reaction. The hepatocytes that are viable show variable and often prominent ballooning degeneration with an accompanying mononuclear inflammatory infiltrate. Regenerative activity may also be seen, although the incidence of recovery is meager. In this type of hepatitis, cholestasis in the surviving lobules may be pronounced when associated with impaired regeneration (26).

D. Fatty Change

Fatty change may be due to a number of factors, including [1] inability of the liver cell to excrete synthesized fat owing to defective or deficient assembly of the lipid transport moiety apoprotein VLDL, [2] increased mobilization of lipids from peripheral stores, [3] increased synthesis but decreased oxidation of fatty acids, and [4] mitochondrial dysfunction (19,21,27–29). The type of fat may be either *macrovesicular* (equal to or larger than the liver cell nucleus) or *microvesicular* (smaller than the nucleus) (Table 5, Figs. 17–25). A "mixed" pattern may also be seen. In addition, sometimes the microvesicles may be extremely small (*foamy change*) and difficult to identify on routine histological sections unless the cut sections are thin (1–2 microns). Although sometimes a zonal distribution pattern is seen, often the feature is spotty or diffuse. The fatty change may be the only histological feature present, without accompanying liver cell necrosis, whereby the change is more incidental. At other times, liver cell necrosis may also be present, either without an accompanying inflammatory reaction (e.g., mushroom hepatotoxicity) or with a mononuclear and/or neutrophilic infiltrate (e.g., amiodarone hepatotoxicity). The latter condition is also termed "steatohepatitis" and is sometimes associated with Mallory body

Table 5 Fatty Change

Macrovesicular

Acetaminophen	Ethanol	Microcycline
Acetylsalicylic acid	Ethionine	Minocycline
Alpha-methyldopa	Ethyl chloride	Mitomycin
Amanitin	Ethyl bromide	Mushrooms
Asparaginase	Etretinate	Nitrofurantoin
Azidothymidine (AZT)	Fialuridine	Organic solvents
Bleomycin	Floxuridine	Orotic acid
Borates	Flurazepam	Perhexilene maleate
Cadmium	Gold sodium thiomalate	Phosphorus
Carbon tetrachloride	Halogenated hydrocarbons	Rifampin
Chloroform	Hydrazine	Sulfasalazine
Chromate	Ibuprofen	Sulindac
Cisplatin	Indomethacin	Tamoxifen
Clometacin	Isoniazid	Tannic acid
Cocaine	L-Asparaginase	Tetrachloroethane
Corticosteroids	Methimazole	Tetrachloroethylene
Cyanamide	Methotrexate	Total parenteral nutrition
Dantrolene	Methyl chloride	Trichlorethylene
Dichloroethylene	Methyl bromide	Uranium compounds
Dimethylformamide	Methyldichloride	Warfarin

Microvesicular

Acetylsalicylic acid	Dideoxyinosine	Phalloidin
Aflatoxin	Dimethylformamide	Phosphorus
Amineptine	Ethanol	Piroxicam
Amiodarone	Ethionine	Pirprofen
Antiemetics	Fialuridine	Pyrrolizidine alkaloids
Aspirin	Hypoglycin A	Rolitetracycline
Boric acid	Ibuprofen	Tetracycline
Calcium hopantenate	Ketoprofen	Thallium compounds
Camphor	Margosa oil	Tolmetin
Chlortetracycline	Methyl salicylate	Valproic acid
Cocaine	Mushrooms	Vitamin A[a]
Demeclocycline	Oxytetracycline	Warfarin
Desferrioxamine	Pennyroyal oil	
Didanosine	Pentenoic acid	

Fatty change + inflammation (steatohepatitis)

Amiodarone	Perhexiline maleate
Methotrexate	Sulfasalazine
Naproxen	Spironolactone

Phospholipidosis

Amiodarone	Gentamycin
Amitriptyline	Ketaconazole
Chloramphenicol	Perhexilene maleate
Chloroquine	Promethazine
Chlorpheniramine	Sulfamethoxazole-trimethoprim
Chlorpromazine	Thioridazine
Coralgil	

[a] Fat within sinusoidal stellate cells.

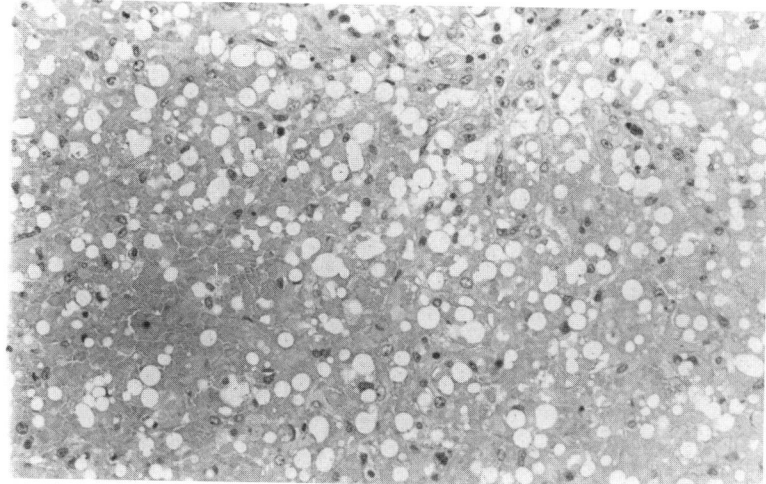

Figure 17 Mushrooms. Diffuse macrovesicular fatty change is seen within all zones. The liver cells also have undergone extensive necrosis, which is also a feature that may be seen in mushroom hepatotoxicity (refer to Fig. 5).

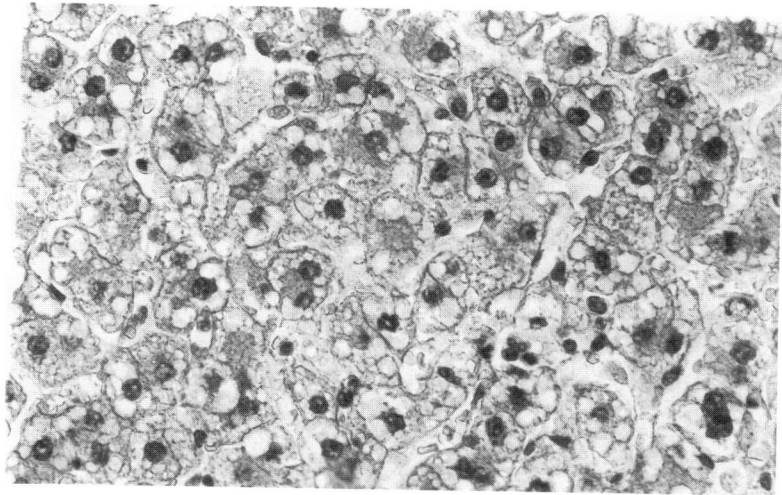

Figure 18 Tetracycline. Microvesicular fatty change (the fat globules smaller than the size of the nucleus) is seen involving all the liver cells. The fat in this field shows readily distinct globules that are equal in size or smaller than the nucleus. Depending on the time of biopsy, sometimes macrovesicular fat can also be seen (recovery phase).

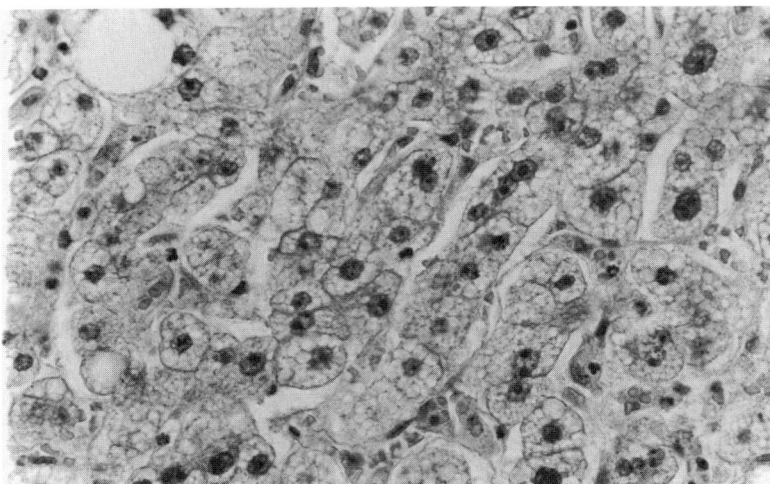

Figure 19 Tetracycline. In some instances, microvesicular fat is difficult to appreciate on typical hematoxylin-eosin stain owing to the extremely small size of the microvesicles ("foamy" change), as evident in this biopsy specimen; in these instances, frozen section on fresh or formalin-fixed tissue will confirm the presence of fat by strong uptake on Oil Red O stain.

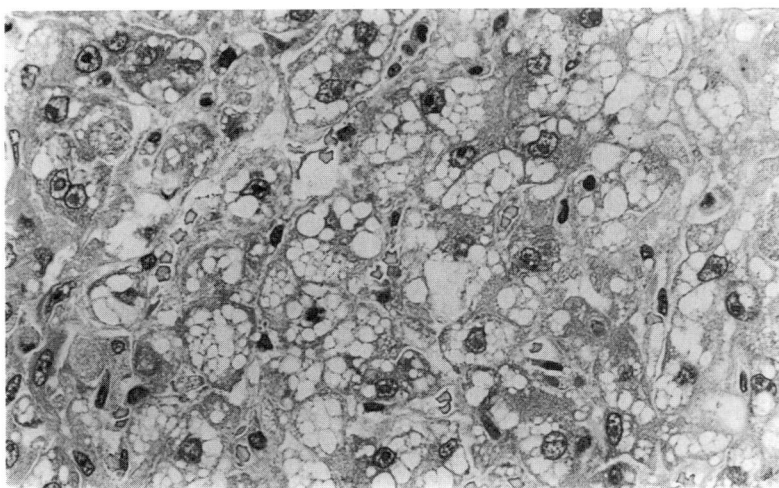

Figure 20 Cocaine. Both macrovesicular and microvesicular fatty change can sometimes be seen in cocaine-induced hepatotoxicity in the viable hepatocytes adjacent to areas of coagulative-type necrosis (the latter demonstrated in Figs. 3 and 4).

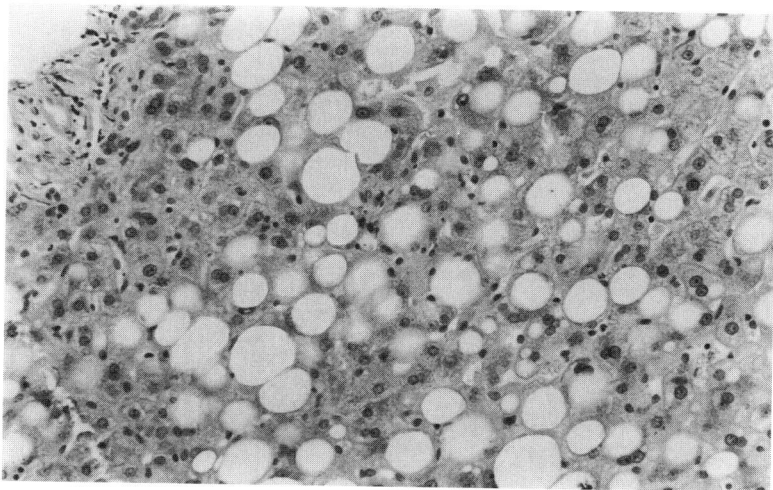

Figure 21 Sulfasalazine. Macrovesicular fatty change is present diffusely within the parenchyma, the fat chiefly macrovesicular.

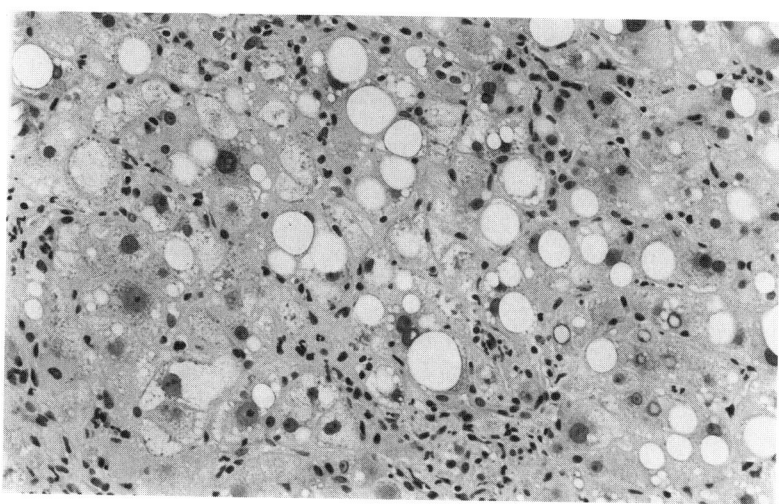

Figure 22 Methotrexate. Both fatty change and inflammation ("steatohepatitis") are present in this example. The inflammatory component is usually lymphocytic, although neutrophils can also occasionally be present. Portal fibrosis and intrasinusoidal collagen deposition may also be seen; if the medication is not then discontinued, a micronodular cirrhosis can eventually occur (refer to Fig. 47).

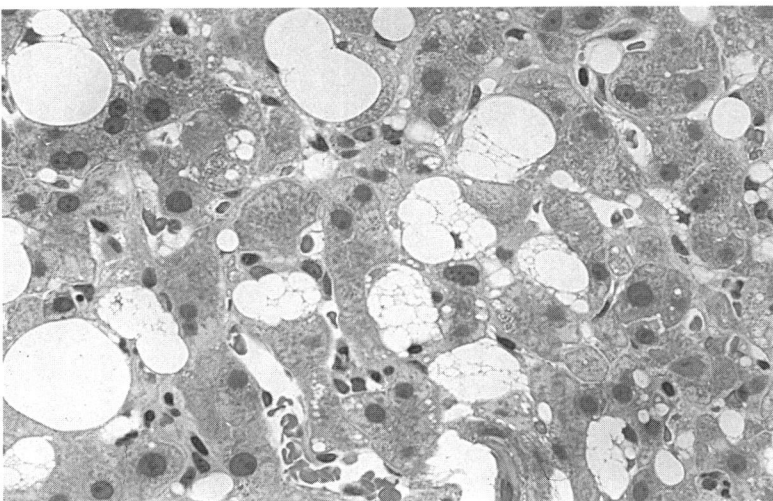

Figure 23 Hypervitaminosis A. The fat globules are present within stellate (Ito or "fat-storing") cells, and are seen as both large and small droplets. These stellate cells contain abundant vitamin A, which can be demonstrated by autofluorescence on frozen sections of fresh or formalin-fixed material.

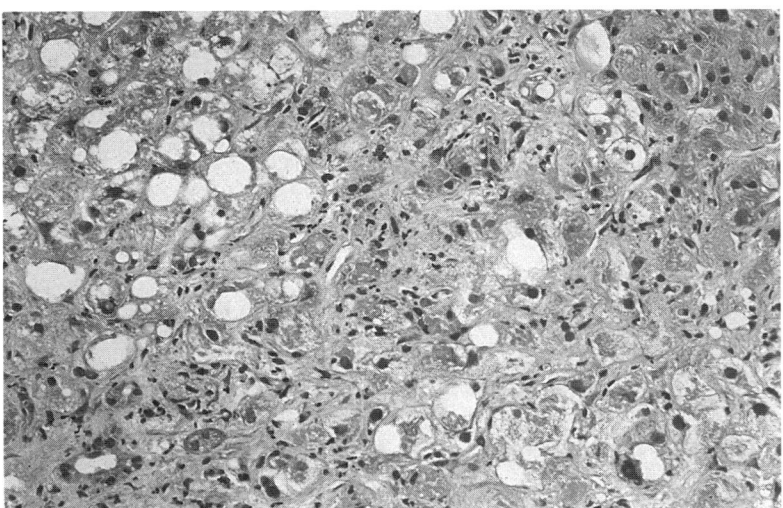

Figure 24 Amiodarone. This photomicrograph shows not only fatty change, but also a prominent inflammatory component consisting of both lymphocytes and scattered neutrophils ("steatohepatitis"). In addition, occasional Mallory bodies are also seen. These combined histological features mimic those seen in acute alcoholic hepatitis.

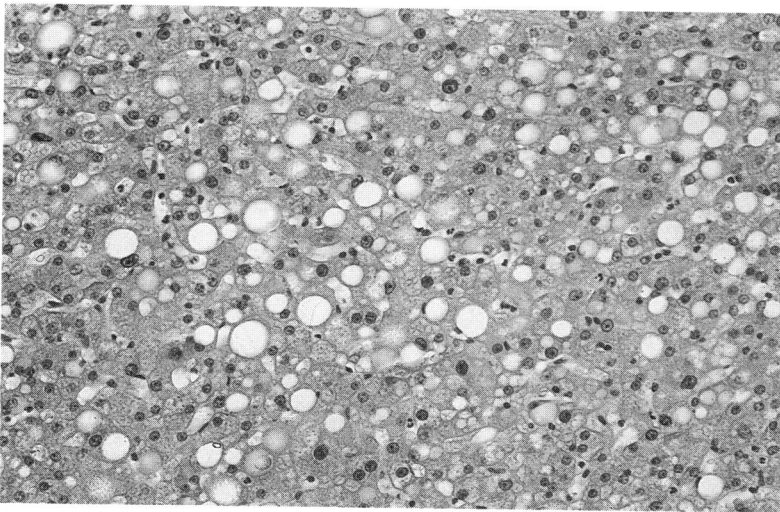

Figure 25 Methotrexate. Fatty change without an accompanying inflammatory component is seen diffusely within the lobule, with the fat chiefly macrovesicular.

deposition. The histological features then may mimic those seen in acute alcoholic hepatitis ("acute sclerosing hyaline necrosis"), necessitating careful history with appropriate laboratory interpretation. For example, in drug-induced steatohepatitis, the AST and ALT activities are usually equally elevated or the ALT is greater than the AST (30), in contrast to the increased AST:ALT ratio in alcoholic liver disease.

A variant of fatty change involves foamy lipid deposition within hepatocytes (*phospholipidosis*) (19,31,32). These phospholipids accumulate within the lysosomes due to inhibition of phospholipase A from lipid hydrolysis. Many of the drugs that are associated with this morphological feature also may be responsible for Mallory body deposition.

E. Granulomas

Hepatic granulomas are loosely defined as distinct clusters of inflammatory cells, and may be seen more frequently within the lobules, although portal tracts may also be involved (Table 6, Figs. 26–30). Granulomas are the result of a cellular immune reaction by the hepatic reticuloendothelial system to a drug or toxin (33). The granulomas may be small, poorly circumscribed, and may contain a mixed inflammatory infiltrate consisting of lymphocytes, histiocytes, neutrophils, and eosinophils (*inflammatory* type). These granulomas may infrequently contain multinucleated giant cells. Granulomas may also be sharply circumscribed, and composed chiefly of lymphocytes and activated macrophages that have clear large nuclei and abundant eosinophilic cytoplasm (*epithelioid* type), often with multinucleated giant cells. Central necrosis is seldom seen in drug-induced granulomatous necrosis, and coalescence of granulomas, a feature sometimes seen in sarcoidosis or tuberculosis, is uncommon. However, more often than not the histological changes in drug-induced granulomatous hepatitis are indistinguishable from other causes of hepatic granulomas. The diagnosis then rests on exclusion (34).

Table 6 Granulomas

Acitretin	Glyburide	Phenytoin
Allopurinol	Gold sodium thiomalate	Polyvinyl pyrrolidone
Alpha-methyldopa	Green-lipped mussel (Seatone)	Prajmalium
Amiodarone	Halogenated hydrocarbons	Procainamide
Amoxicillin-clavulanic acid	Hydralazine	Procarbazine
Aprindine	Interferon	Pronestyl
Aspirin	Isoniazid	Quinidine
Azapropazone	Mestranol	Quinine
Barium	Metahydrin	Ranitidine
Bacille Calmette-Guerin (BCG)	Metalazone	Salicylazosulfapyridine
therapy or vaccination	Methimazole	Silica
Beryllium	Methotrexate	Succinylsulfathiazole
Carbamazepine	Metolazone	Sulfasuxidine
Carbutamide	Mineral oil	Sulfadiazine
Cephalexin	Nitrofurantoin	Sulfadimethoxine
Chlorpromazine	Nomifensine	Sulfadoxine-pyrimethamine
Chlorpropamide	Norethindrone	Sulfamethoxazole-trimethoprim
Copper	Norethynodrel	Sulfanilamide
Dapsone	Norgestrel	Sulfasalazine
Detajmium tartrate	Oral contraceptives	Sulfathiazole
Diazepam	Oxacillin	Sulfonamide
Dideoxyinosine	Oxyphenbutazone	Sulfonylurea agents
Diltiazem	Oxyphenisatin	Tacrine
Dimethicone	Papaverine	Thorotrast
Disopyramide	Penicillin	Tocainide
Feprazone	Phenazone	Tolbutamide
Glibenclamide	Phenprocoumon	Trichlormethiazide
	Phenylbutazone	Verapamil

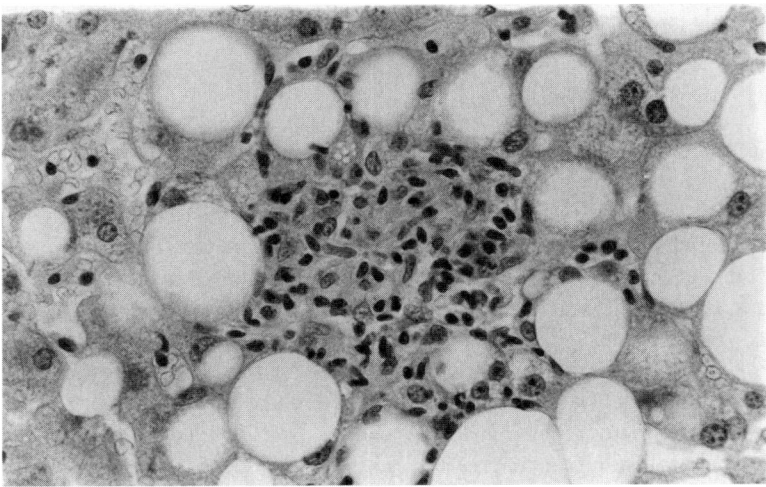

Figure 26 Sulfasalazine. The granuloma is composed of a mixture of lymphocytes and histiocytes without multinucleated glant cells.

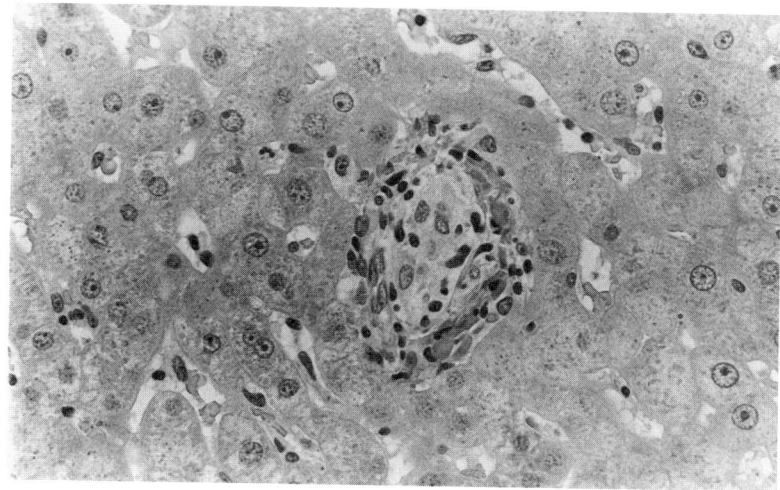

Figure 27 Chlorpromazine. This "microgranuloma" contains a small cluster of epithelioid cells surrounded by lymphocytes.

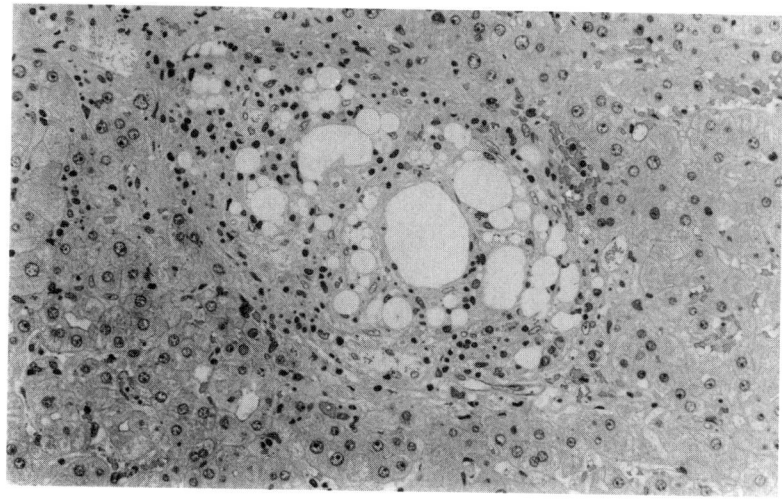

Figure 28 Mineral oil. The mineral oil itself is contained in variably sized foamy macrophages admixed with scattered lymphocytes ("lipogranuloma"); these granulomas can appear not only within portal tracts but also in close proximity to the terminal hepatic venules.

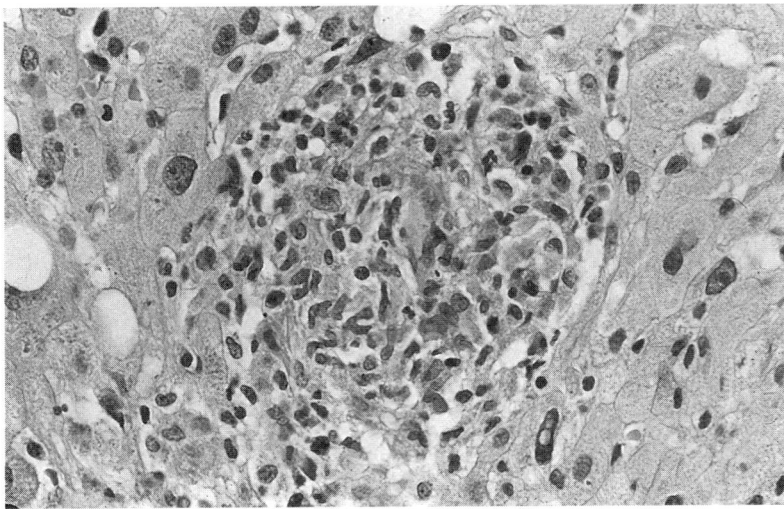

Figure 29   Sulfomadies. A granuloma is present within the parenchyma, and is composed of lymphocytes, histiocytes, neutrophils, and eosinophils.

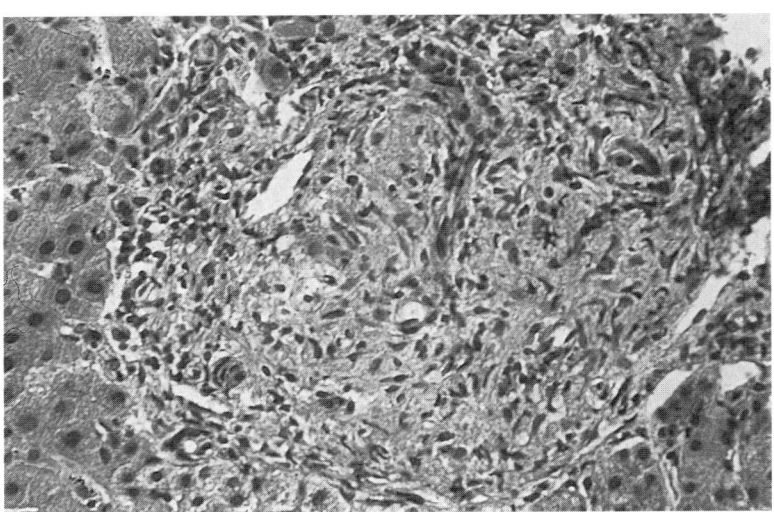

Figure 30   Phenylbutazone. A granuloma is present within this portal tract and is composed chiefly of epithelioid cells with scattered lymphocytes. No multinucleated giant cells are seen in this example.

Table 7 Mallory Bodies

Amiodarone	Griseofulvin
Collidine	Methotrexate
Coralgil	Nicardipine
4,4′-Diethylaminoethoxyhexestrol	Nifedipine
Diethylstilbestrol	Perhexiline maleate
Diltiazem	Tamoxifen
Estrogens	Tetracycline
Ethanol	Valproic acid
Glucocorticoids	Vitamin A

F. Mallory Bodies

Mallory bodies represent eosinophilic ropy cytoplasmic inclusions within hepatocytes. These are most characteristic of both acute and chronic alcoholic liver injury, although a variety of nonalcoholic liver diseases (such as nonalcoholic steatohepatitis, primary biliary cirrhosis, Wilson's disease) as well as various drugs and toxins may also be associated with Mallory body deposition (19,35–38) (Table 7, Figs. 31,32). The Mallory bodies in part represent proliferation and derangement of *intermediate filaments*, which constitute the cytoskeleton of the hepatocyte (35,36). The Mallory bodies located within the liver cell cytoplasm may appear alone or be associated with an inflammatory component that is usually but not always neutrophilic. The cells containing the Mallory bodies have a tendency to be located within the perivenular zone (zone 3), although exceptions do occur. When induced by alcohol, associated sinusoidal collagen deposition and fatty change are characteristic, although some drugs such as amiodarone may also demonstrate histological features quite similar to alcoholic liver disease.

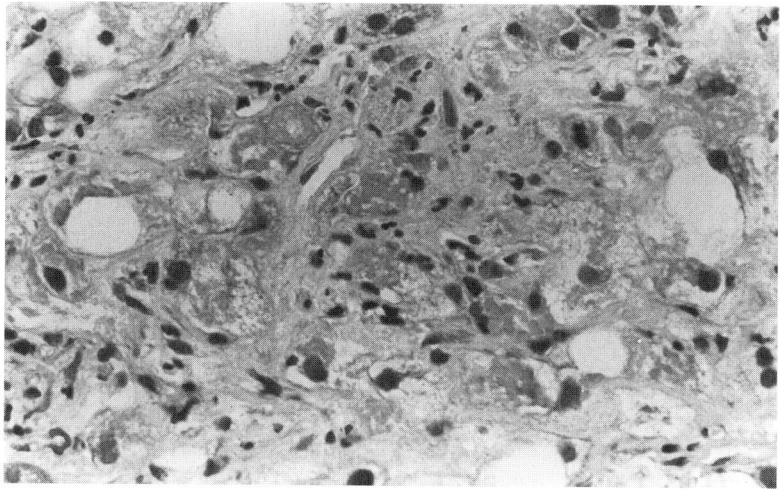

Figure 31 Amiodarone. Mallory bodies are seen here surrounded by neutrophils ("satellitosis"). Variable fatty change and intrasinusoidal collagen deposition are also present.

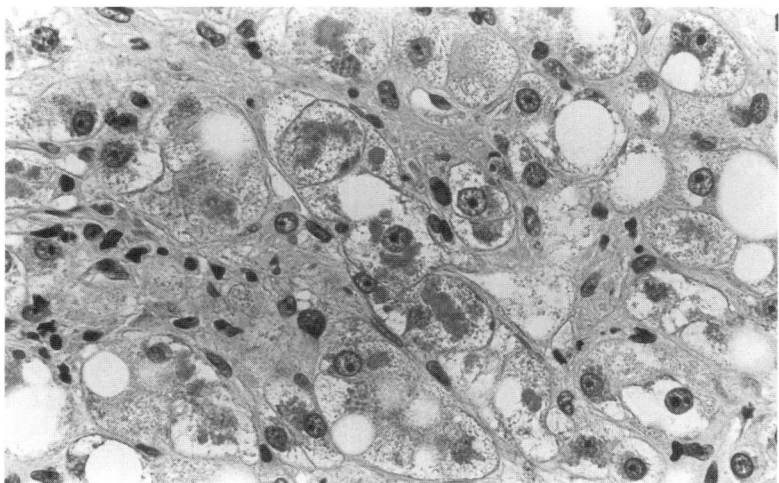

Figure 32 Ethanol. Active alcoholic liver disease characteristically exhibits Mallory bodies, which are accentuated in the perivenular zones.

III. CHOLESTATIC INJURY

A. Cholestasis, Simple

This form of cholestatic liver cell injury is limited to impaired transport and secretion of bile *without* an accompanying inflammatory infiltrate or injury to bile ducts (11,12,39). The drugs most often associated with this form of hepatic dysfunction are listed in Table 8 (Figs. 33–35). The bile plugs are most often conspicuous in the perivenular zone (zone 3), and are histologically manifested by both an intracytoplasmic and intracanalicular component. In some instances the midzone and periportal zone may also be involved, although much less frequently. In the latter instance, proliferation of cholangioles containing bile concretions may be seen, often associated with a mild neutrophilic infiltrate. The interlobular bile ducts are spared. The hepatocytes are histologically uninvolved. Portal inflammatory changes are minimal to absent. What is most important in histological diagnosis is assessment of the interlobular bile ducts, as one of the most common causes of cholestasis is extrahepatic biliary tract obstruction. The interlobular bile ducts in obstruction are characteristically increased in number, often ectatic, and may show periductal edema, periductal fibrosis, and/or acute cholangitis. In drug-induced cholestatic liver cell injury, the interlobular bile ducts are usually normal, exceptions being the rare examples of direct bile duct damage caused by certain drugs; however, in very early stages of bile

Table 8 Cholestasis, Simple

Anabolic steroids (oxymetholone)	Methandrostenolone	Oral contraceptives
Cyclosporin A	Methimazole	Piroxicam
Ethchlorvynol	Methyltestosterone	Prochlorperazine
Fluoxymesterone	Norethindrone	Warfarin
Gold sodium thiomalate	Norethynodrel	
Mestranol	Norgestrel	

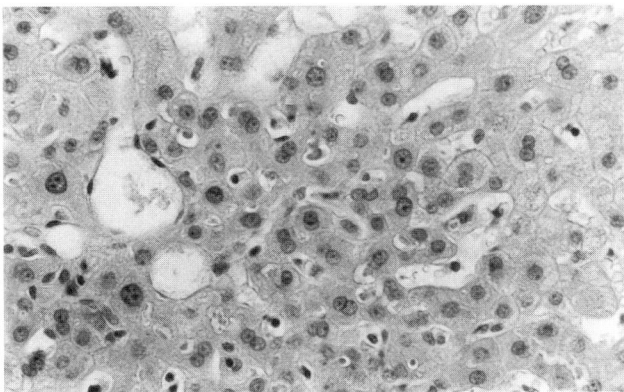

Figure 33 Methyltestosterone. Bile plugs can be seen within dilated canaliculi within the perivenular zone and midzones. There is no necrosis or inflammation in this example of simple cholestasis.

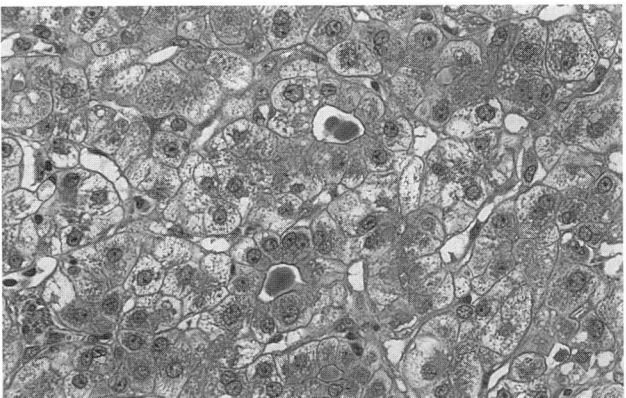

Figure 34 Oral contraceptives. Bile plugs can be seen within dilated canaliculi. The adjacent hepatocytes show mild hydropic change without an accompanying inflammatory infiltrate.

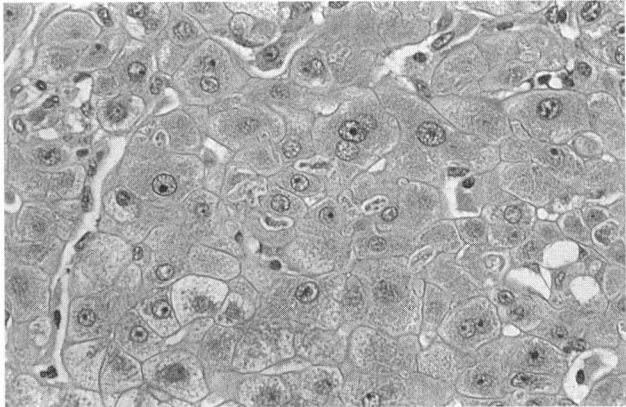

Figure 35 Methimazole. Bile plugs are conspicuous within dilated canaliculi. The adjacent parenchyma is devoid of inflammatory cells.

Table 9 Cholestasis with Inflammation

Alpha-methyldopa	Erythromycin	Phenylbutazone
Acetaminophen	Ethchlorvynol	Phenytoin
Acetohexamide	Ethionamide	Piperazine
Allopurinol	Flucloxacillin	Piroxicam
Aminoglutethimide	Fluoxymesterone	Pizotyline
Aminosalicylic acid	Fluphenazine	Polythiazide
Amitriptyline	Flurazepam hydrochloride	Prajmalium bitartrate
Amoxicillin-clavulanic acid	Flutamide	Prochlorperazine
Aprindine	Glibenclamide	Propoxyphene hydrochloride
Atenolol	Gold sodium thiomalate	Quinethazone
Azathioprine	Griseofulvin	Ranitidine
Benoxaprophen	Halogenated hydrocarbons	Rifampin
Captopril	Haloperidol	Sulfasalazine
Carbamazepine	Imipramine	Sulfonamides
Carbarsone	Indomethacin	Sulindac
Carbimazole	Iodipamide meglumine	Tamoxifen
Carisoprodol	Isocarboxazid	Thiabendazole
Cefadroxil monohydrate	Isoniazid	Thiopental sodium
Cefazolin sodium	Ketoconazole	Thioridazine
Chlorambucil	Meprobamate	Ticlopidine
Chlordiazepoxide	6-Mercaptopurine	Tocainide
Chlorothiazide	Naproxen	Tolazamide
Chlorpromazine	Nicotinic acid	Tolbutamide
Chlorpropamide	Niacin	Total parenteral nutrition
Chlortetracycline	Nifedipine	Toxic oil (rapeseed)
Chlorthalidone	Nitrofurantoin	Tranylcypromine sulfate
Cimetidine	Nomifensine	Triazolam
Cisplatin	Oxacillin	Trifluoperazine hydrochloride
Clarithromycin	Oxaprozin	Trimethobenzamide hydrochloride
Clorazepate dipotassium	Oxyphenisatin	Trimethoprim-sulfamethoxazole
Cyclosporine	Papaverine hydrochloride	Tripelennamine
Dacarbazine	Para-aminosalicylic acid	Troleandomycin
Dantrolene sodium	Penicillamine	Valproic acid
Diazepam	Penicillin	Verapamil
Diclofenac	Perphenazine	Zimelidine
Disopyramide phosphate	Phenobarbital	
Enalapril		

duct obstruction, the portal duct changes may be subtle, and other parameters such as imaging studies may be most important in identifying the cause.

B. Cholestasis with Inflammation

Cholestatic drug-induced liver cell injury may also be associated with a lobular inflammatory infiltrate (39) (Table 9, Figs. 36–38). The inflammation is usually mild with the cholestatic component more striking. The inflammation is usually composed of mononuclear cells. Cholestasis with inflammation is often enhanced in the perivenular zone (zone 3), although in severe cases the features may be diffuse. In contrast to simple cholestasis,

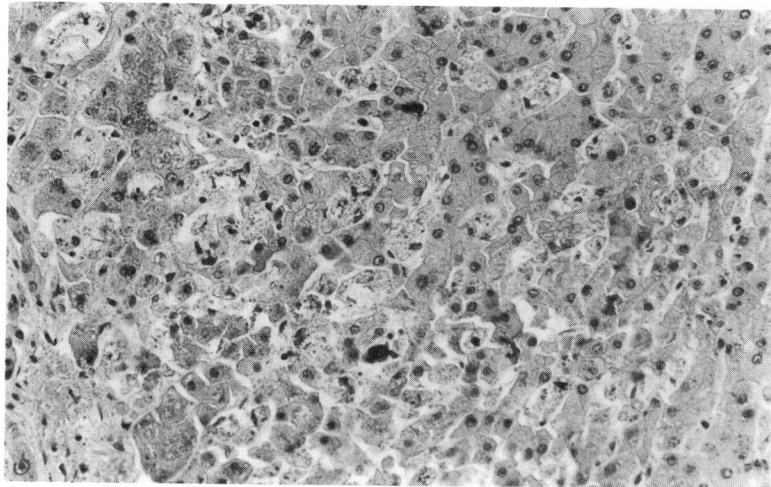

Figure 36 Ketoconazole. Bile plugs can be seen with an associated inflammatory infiltrate, the latter most evident in this biopsy specimen by numerous clusters of macrophages and Kupffer cells in areas of necrosis.

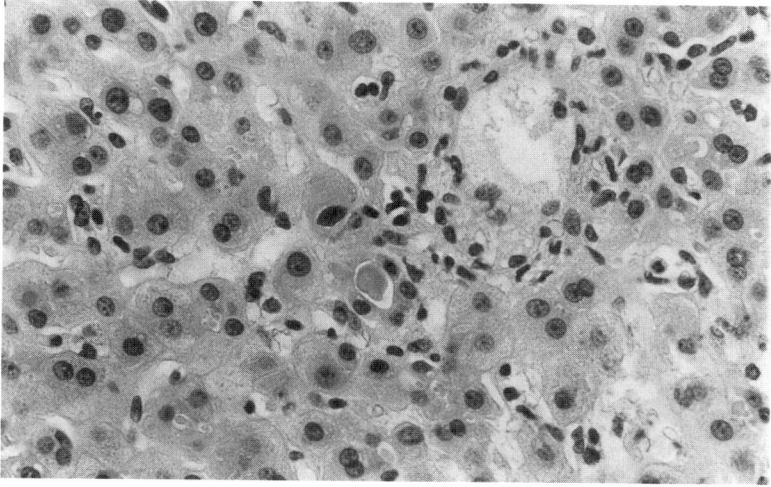

Figure 37 Niacin. A bile plug within a dilated canaliculus is seen in the perivenular zone (center of this field). Smaller bile plugs are also present. There is a mild coexisting lymphocytic infiltrate as well.

cholestasis with inflammation is associated with a portal inflammatory component, which may be predominantly lymphocytic but also may include eosinophils and neutrophils. Bile ducts do not show signs of obstruction (e.g., ectasia, periductal edema, or periductal fibrosis); however, drug-induced bile duct injury has nonetheless been described, with the inflammatory infiltrate neutrophilic or lymphocytic.

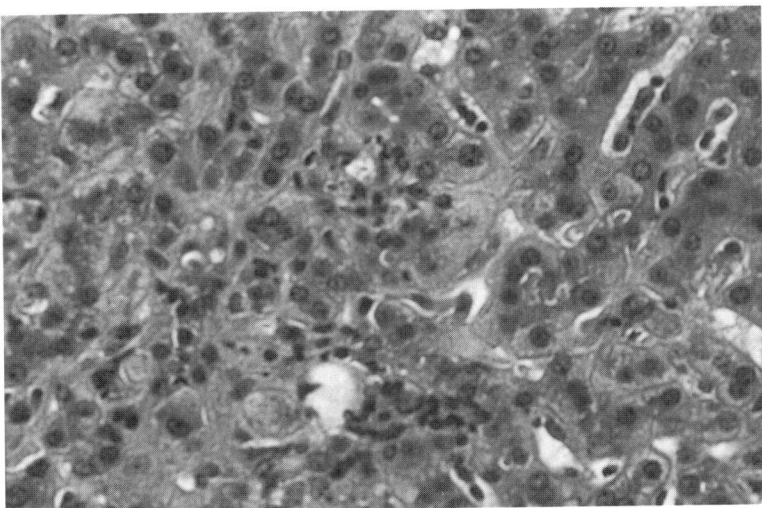

Figure 38 Chlorpromazine. Dilated canaliculi containing bile plugs are present in the perivenular zone, with bile also noticed within the cytoplasm of the liver cells. A moderate accompanying lymphocytic infiltrate is also apparent.

Table 10 Bile Ducts: Inflammation and Injury

Inflammation by neutrophils

Allopurinol	Flucloxacillin
Chlorpromazine	Hydralazine
Chlorpropamide	Sulindac (clinoril)
Chlorthiazide	

Inflammation by lymphocytes, ductopenia

Acetaminophen	Chlorthiazide	Piroxicam
Ajmaline (alkaloid isolated from	Cimetidine	Prochlorperazine
Rauwolfia serpentina)	Cromolyn	Sporidesmin
Allopurinol	Cyproheptadine	Sulfonurea agents
Amineptine	Diazepam	Tetracycline
Amitriptyline	Dicloxacillin	Thiabendazole
Amoxicillin-clavulanate	Erythromycin	Tiopronin
Ampicillin	Flucloxacillin	Tolazemide
Arsenicals	Haloperidol	Tolbutamide
Azathioprine	Imipramine	Toxic oil (rapeseed)
Carbamazepine	Methylenediame	Trifluoperazine
Carbutamide	Methyltestosterone	Troleandomycin
Chlorpromazine	Phenylbutazone	Xenelamine
Chlorpropamide	Phenytoin	

Periductal fibrosis
Floxuridine

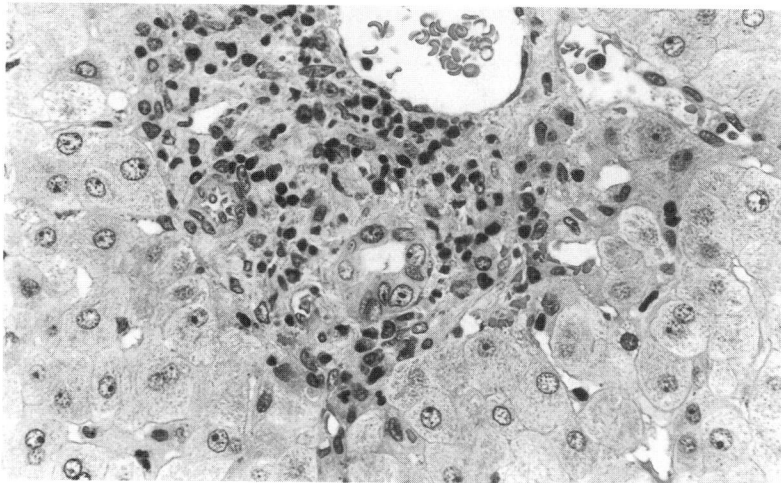

Figure 39 Chlorpropamide. Both this photomicrograph and Fig. 40 are from the same patient, and exhibit prominent cytological duct atypia. This field shows prominent duct distortion, with overlapping nuclei, prominent nucleoli, and irregular nuclear outlines. No inflammatory cells are seen directly infiltrating into this duct, although the duct is surrounded by a prominent inflammatory infiltrate.

IV. BILE DUCT INJURY

Interlobular bile ducts may show histological damage, evident by variable hydropic change of the cytoplasm, nuclear irregularity with pyknosis, and individual cell necrosis. There is most often an accompanying inflammatory reaction oriented to the bile ducts (Table 10, Figs. 39–42), and may be neutrophilic (*acute cholangitis*) or lymphocytic (*nonsuppurative*

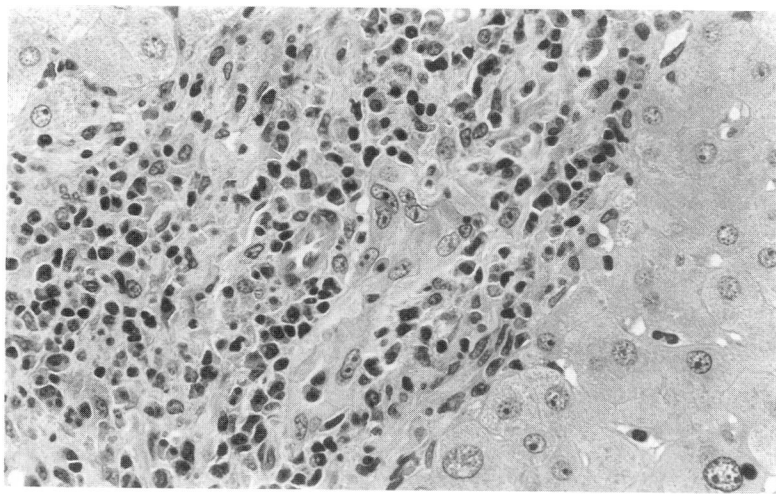

Figure 40 Chlorpropamide. This field shows similar cytological duct distortion, with lymphocytes infiltrating through the duct wall and into the lumen.

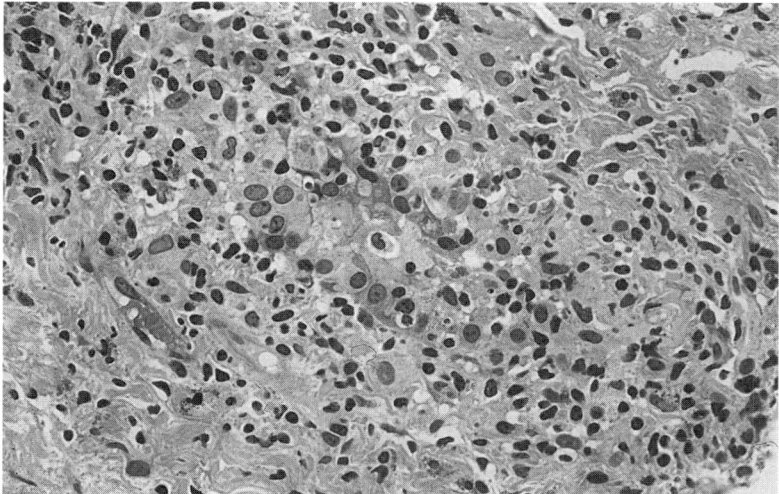

Figure 41 Chlorpromazine. An interlobular bile duct in the center of the field is surrounded and infiltrated by lymphocytes, with considerable cytological atypia of the duct epithelium. Lymphocytes and eosinophils can also be seen in the portal tract as well.

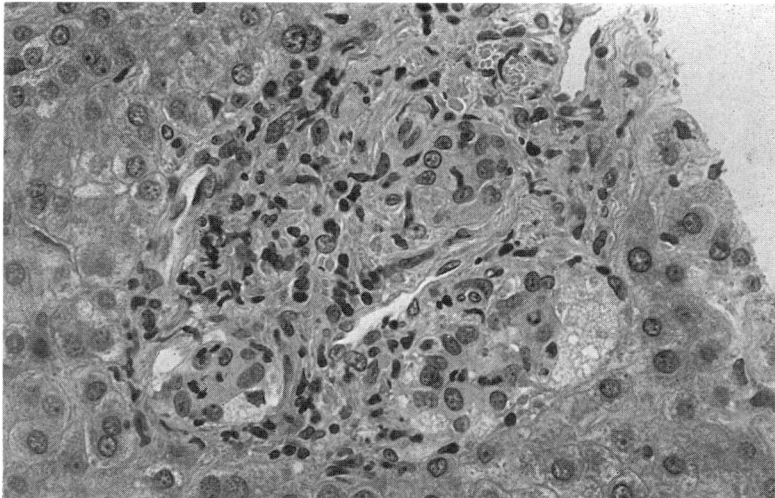

Figure 42 Chlorthiazide. The interlobular bile ducts are surrounded and infiltrated by a mixed inflammatory infiltrate consisting predominantly of neutrophils with occasional lymphocytes. It is important in instances such as this to rule out more common causes of acute cholangitis such as bile duct obstruction.

cholangitis). Persistence of duct inflammation and damage may eventually lead to duct loss (ductopenia) (12,40). When ductopenia occurs, other etiologies for duct loss, such as primary biliary cirrhosis, primary sclerosing cholangitis, and autoimmune hepatitis (*autoimmune cholangiopathy*), must be considered. An uncommon bile duct change induced by floxuridine in treatment of hepatic tumors (41,42) is periductal fibrosis (*biliary sclerosis*), which histologically mimics bile duct obstruction and primary sclerosing cholangitis.

Table 11   Hepatic Lesions

Sinusoids: peliotic lesions

Androgenic/anabolic steroids (oxymetholone)	Glucocorticoids	Steroids, endogenous production (adrenal tumor)
Arsenic	Hydroxyprogesterone	Tamoxifen
Azathioprine	Hydroxyurea	Testosterone
Busulfan	Medroxyprogesterone	6-Thioguanine
Danazol	6-Mercaptopurine	Thorotrast
Diethylstilbestrol	Methandrostenolone	Vinyl chloride
Estrone sulfate	Methotrexate	Vitamin A
Fluoxymesterone	Methyltestosterone	
	Phalloidin	

Sinusoids: dilatation
Oral contraceptives
Metoclopramide

Veno-occlusive disease

Actinomycin D	Cytosine arabinoside	Indicine
Adriamycin	Dacarbazine	Mate tea
Aflatoxins	Dactinomycin	Mechlorethamine
Arsenicals	Danazol	6-Mercaptopurine
Azathioprine	Daunorubicin	Mitomycin C
Busulfan	Decarbazine	Pyrrolizidine alkaloids
Carboplatin	Dimethylbusulfan	Tamoxifen
Carmustine (BCNU)	Dimethylnitrosamine	6-Thioguanine
Cisplatin	Doxorubicin	Urethane
Cyclophosphamide	Estramustine	Vinblastine
Cysteamine	Floxuridine	Vincristine
Cytarabine		

Hepatic vein thrombosis/fibrous obliteration
Ethanol
Oral contraceptives

Vasculitis

Allopurinol	Phenylbutazone
Chlorothiazide	Phenytoin
Chlorpropamide	Sulfonamides
Penicillin	

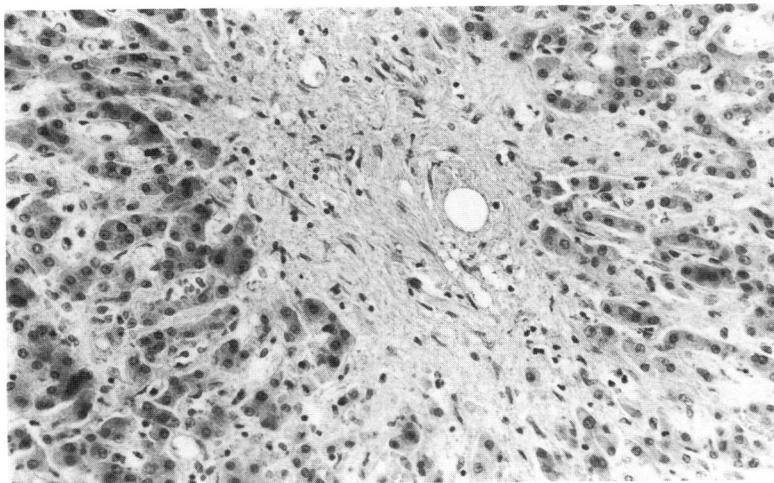

Figure 43 Ethanol. The terminal hepatic venule shows total intraluminal fibrous obliteration. Perivenular sinusoidal collagen deposition is also present.

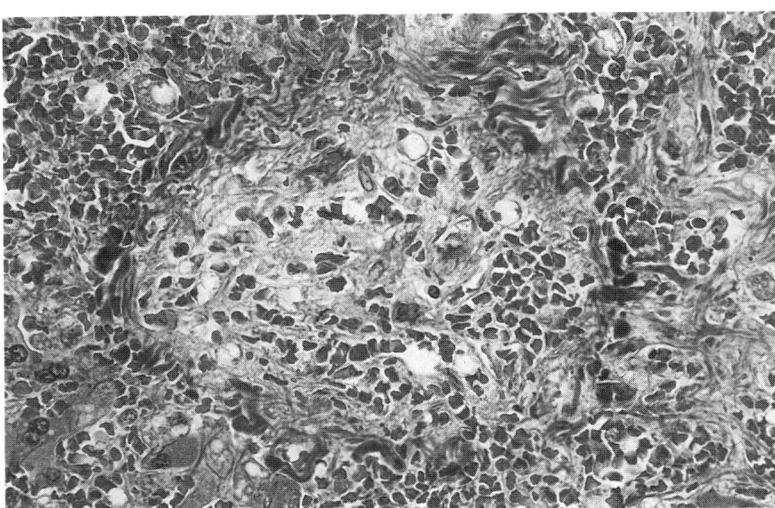

Figure 44 Conditioning regimen for bone marrow transplant. This liver biopsy is from a 46-year-old man with multiple myeloma who died with veno-occlusive disease 31 days posttransplant. The conditioning regimen consisted of busulfan followed by cyclophosphamide. The terminal hepatic venule on trichrome stain shows intraluminal fibrosis and hemorrhage. Endothelial cells are damaged and depleted (Courtesy Dr. Howard Shulman, Fred Hutchison Cancer Research Center, Seattle, WA.)

V. VASCULAR INJURY

A number of different vascular hepatic lesions may be seen in drug-induced injury (Table 11, Figs. 43,44) (43). Weakening and damage to the lobular reticulin network can cause microcystic lobular changes that fill with red blood cells, these small cysts usually but not always devoid of an endothelial lining (*peliosis hepatis*) (40,44–46). Sometimes these lesions may be large enough to be visualized on imaging; rarely the lesions may rupture with intra-abdominal hemorrhage. *Sinusoidal dilatation* may be induced in livers that also demonstrate peliosis, but also may be seen in the periportal zone (zone 1) secondary to oral contraceptive usage (40,47,48). *Veno-occlusive disease* is associated with endothelial damage of the terminal hepatic venules, with endothelial loss, sinusoidal fibrosis, and variable intraluminal occlusion (49). It is seen in conjunction with exposure to pyrrolizidine alkaloids, but also is seen in patients after bone marrow transplant on various conditioning regimens (49–52). *Hepatic vein thrombosis* has been reported in patients on oral contraceptives (53). Chronic alcoholic liver disease shows characteristic *fibrous obliteration* of the terminal hepatic venules and sublobular veins due to activation of stellate cells (54–56). *Arteritis* seldom directly involves the arterioles, and usually the small arteries are also spared. Medium-sized vessels are most often affected; hence the morphological features can be missed on biopsy unless a larger portal tract is present for evaluation (57).

VI. PORTAL FIBROSIS

Both toxin exposure and long-term usage of certain drugs may cause a chronic liver disease with portal fibrosis that in some instances may with time progress to cirrhosis (Table 12, Figs. 45–47). Hepatic stellate cells play a central role in extracellular fibrogenesis with these drugs and toxins; following injury, the stellate cells undergo morphological and

Table 12 Portal Fibrosis

Cirrhosis, or portal fibrosis with progression to cirrhosis on serial biopsies		
Alpha-methyldopa	Etretinate	Oxyphenisatin
Acetaminophen	Fenofibrate	Papaverine
Acetohexamide	Ferrous fumarate	Perhexilene maleate
Amiodarone	Isoniazid	Phenylbutazone
Chlorpromazine	Lisinopril	Propylthiouracil
Chlorthiazide	Mercaptopurine	Pyrrolizidine alkaloids[a]
Coralgil	Methotrexate	Tamoxifen
Dantrolene	Methyltestosterone	Thiabendazole
Diclofenac	Nitrofurantoin	Total parenteral nutrition
Ethanol	Oral contraceptives[a]	Valproic acid

Portal fibrosis without progression to cirrhosis (noncirrhotic portal fibrosis)	
Anabolic steroids	Toxic oil syndrome
Arsenicals	Vinyl chloride
Thorotrast	Vitamin A

[a]Cardiac cirrhosis.

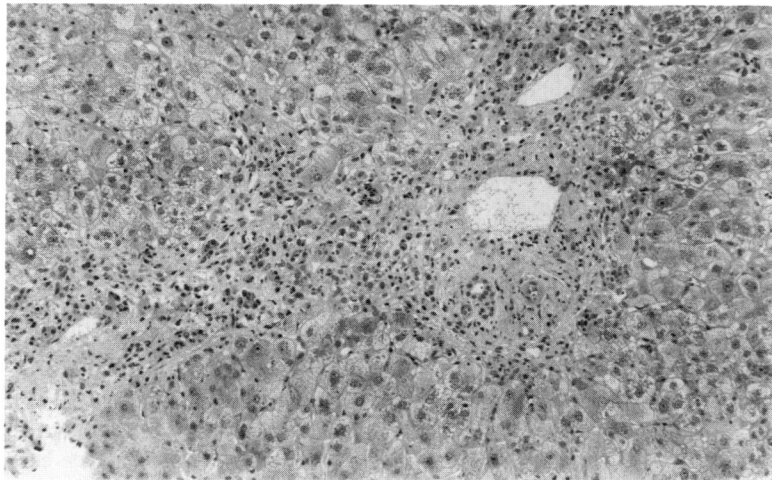

Figure 45 Alpha-methyldopa. Portal fibrosis with portal-to-portal bridging fibrosis is seen. The portal tracts exhibit a moderate lymphocytic infiltrate, with mild periportal inflammatory activity ("piecemeal" necrosis).

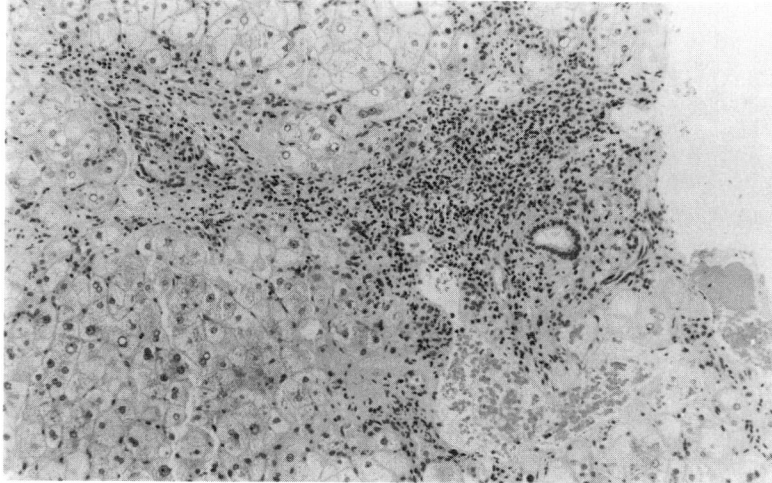

Figure 46 Methotrexate. Portal-to-portal bridging fibrosis is seen, the portal tracts exhibiting a moderate lymphocytic infiltrate. Mild periportal activity ("piecemeal" necrosis) is also present. The adjacent liver cells are rather large and hydropic, with scattered glycogenated nuclei of hepatocytes.

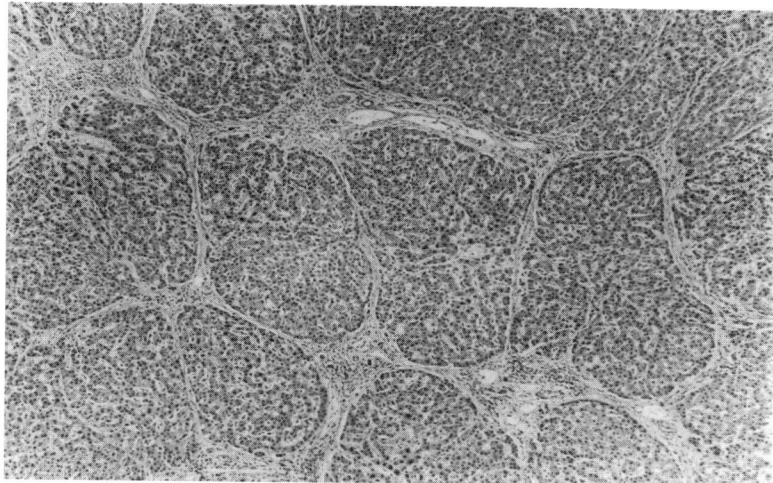

Figure 47 Methotrexate. Fibrous septa with regenerative nodule formation are seen; the nodules are small ("micronodular" cirrhosis). The degree of liver cell dysplasia often seen in methotrexate hepatotoxicity is not present in this specimen, as methotrexate therapy for psoriasis had been discontinued 1 year earlier.

phenotypic alterations resulting in their activation and eventual extracellular matrix deposition (58–60). Knowledge of these drugs with appropriate screening on biopsy has virtually eliminated development of advanced liver disease, an excellent example being methotrexate in treatment of rheumatoid arthritis. When cirrhosis develops, the subtype may be *macronodular* (regenerative nodules > 3mm in diameter) or *micronodular* (regenerative nodules ≤ 3 mm in diameter). A *biliary* pattern ("geographic" appearance of the nodules) has also been described in instances where the primary liver injury is directed to bile ducts, with eventual duct depletion (ductopenia). Sometimes portal fibrosis will occur with clinical manifestations of portal hypertension, *without* eventual progression of the liver disease to the cirrhotic stage ("noncirrhotic portal fibrosis"). When secondary to thorotrast, polyvinyl chloride, or arsenic exposure, this hepatic disorder is also associated with the development of malignant primary tumors (most often angiosarcoma and cholangiocarcinoma) (57,61,62).

VII. NEOPLASIA

Certain drugs and toxins may with time induce formation of both benign and malignant neoplastic lesions (Table 13, Figs. 48–50) (11,57), which may be single or multiple. Oral contraceptive usage and liver cell adenomas is a well-known example (63). These adenomas may disappear when the drug is discontinued, although more often the mass lesions persist. Liver cell adenomas have also been reported to progress to hepatocellular carcinoma (64), although the aggressiveness of this malignant lesion is questionable, with no known cases having metastasized. Hepatocellular carcinoma and cholangiocarcinoma are both associated with long-term drug or toxin exposure. Angiosarcoma, which is a very rare primary liver cell neoplasm, has a remarkably high incidence in patients with exposure

Table 13   Neoplasia

Benign		
Liver cell adenoma	Focal nodular hyperplasia	Nodular regenerative hyperplasia
Anabolic steroids (oxymetholone)	Estrogens	Anabolic steroids
Oral contraceptives		Copper
Toxic oil (rapeseed)		Corticosteroids
		Ethanol
		Oral contraceptives
		Thorotrast
		Toxic oil (rapeseed)
		Vinyl chloride

Malignant		
Hepatocellular carcinoma	Angiosarcoma	Cholangiocarcinoma
Aflatoxin	Anabolic steroids	Alpha-methyldopa
Anabolic steroids	Arsenic	Anabolic steroids
Arsenic	Copper	Isoniazid
Ethanol	Diethylstilbestrol	Oral contraceptives
Methotrexate	Oral contraceptives	Thorotrast
Oral contraceptives	Phenelzine	
Thorotrast	Thorotrast	
Vinyl chloride	Vinyl chloride	

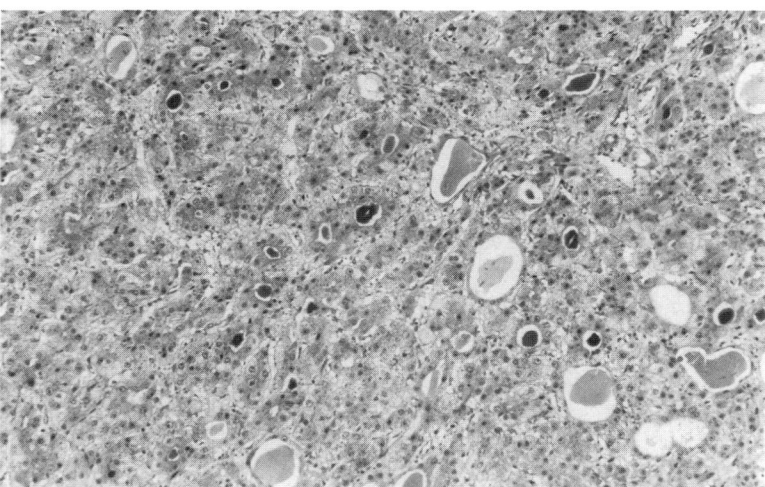

Figure 48   Oxymethalone. The tumor is composed of cytologically benign hepatocytes forming normal-sized cords (*liver cell adenoma*). Numerous dilated canaliculi forming acinar structures are seen, these structures filled with bile plugs.

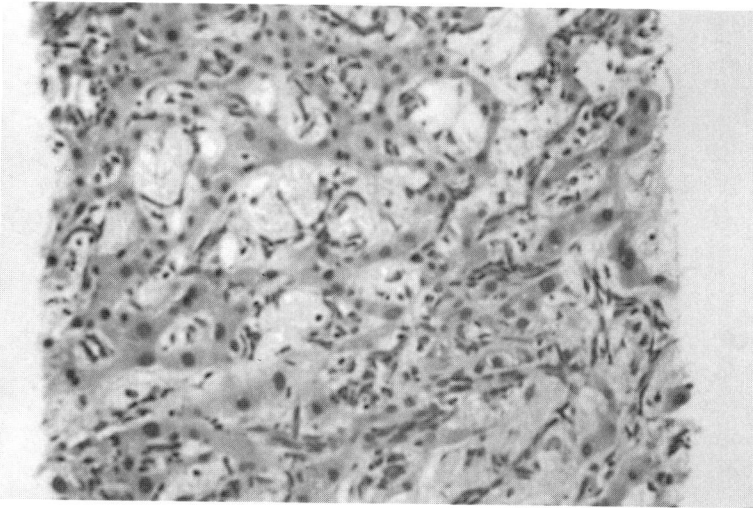

Figure 49 Thorotrast. The same case as in Figure 52 also demonstrates an adjacent angiosarcoma, characterized by numerous plump hyperchromatic, closely packed endothelial cells lining dilated hepatic sinusoids.

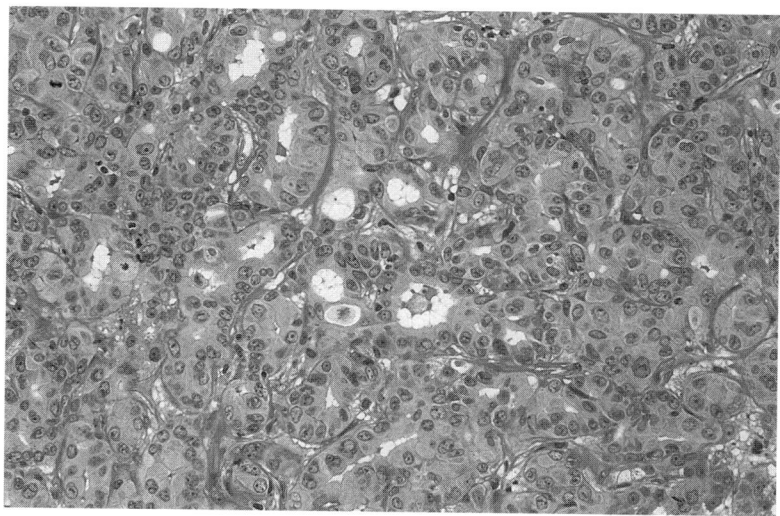

Figure 50 Thorotrast. Adjacent to the portal tract shown in Figure 53 is a cholangiocarcinoma, with moderately differentiated gland formation.

Table 14 Inclusions

Hepatocytes		
Cytoplasmic	Nuclear	Ground glass-like hepatocytes
Procainamide	Lead	Azathioprine
		Chlorpromazine
		Cyanamide (periportal)
		Phenytoin
		Glucocorticoids
		Phenobarbital
Kupffer cells, portal macrophages		
Polyvinyl pyrrolidone		
Silicone rubber (damaged cardiac prosthetic valves)		
Talc, particulate material		
Thorotrast		

to thorotrast (thorium dioxide, an alpha, beta, gamma emitter used from 1930 to 1953 as an arteriographic agent), arsenic, copper, or polyvinyl chloride (61).

VIII. MISCELLANEOUS

A. Inclusions

Inclusion bodies secondary to drugs and toxins can be seen within liver cell cytoplasm, liver cell nuclei, and Kupffer cells (Table 14, Fig. 51). The inclusions may be distinct and well circumscribed (e.g., procainamide usage); however, sometimes the liver cell cyto-

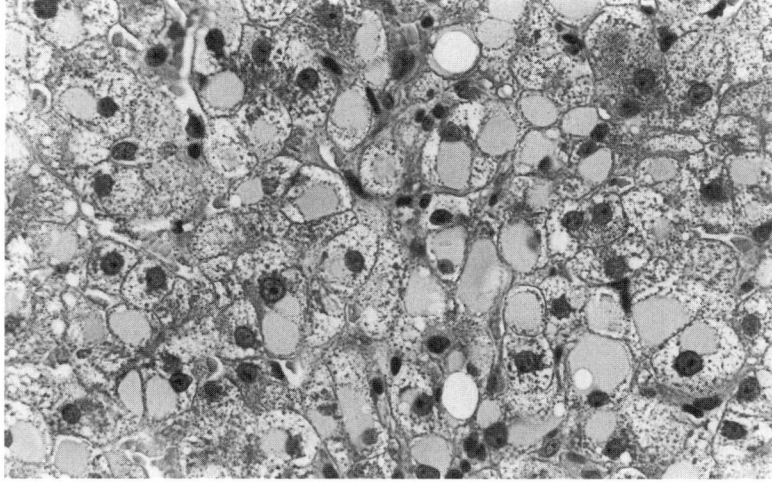

Figure 51 Procainamide. The liver cells exhibit numerous well-demarcated compact eosinophilic cytoplasmic globules.

Table 15 Pigments

Lipochrome (hepatocytes)	*Hemosiderin (hepatocytes, Kupffer cells, portal macrophages)*	*Radiopaque (Kupffer cells, portal macrophages)*
Acetylsalicylic acid	Cimetidine	Thorotrast
Aminopyrine	Ethanol	
Carbamazepine	Hexachlorobenzene	
Cascara sagrada	Iron (oral/parenteral)	
Chenodeoxycholic acid		
Chlordecone (kepone)		
Chlorinated biphenyls		
Chlorpromazine		
Halothane		
Insecticides		
Nitrofurantoin		
Phenacetin		
Phenothiazines		
Rifampin		

Black pigments
(Kupffer cells, portal macrophages)
Anthracite
Gold sodium thiomalate
Titanium

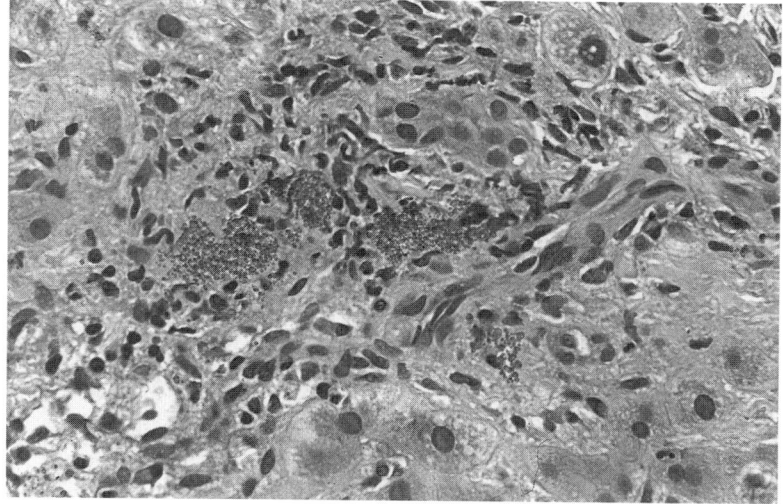

Figure 52 Thorotrast. The granular gray-green thorotrast pigment in this first case example is present within portal macrophages, with an associated portal lymphocytic infiltrate.

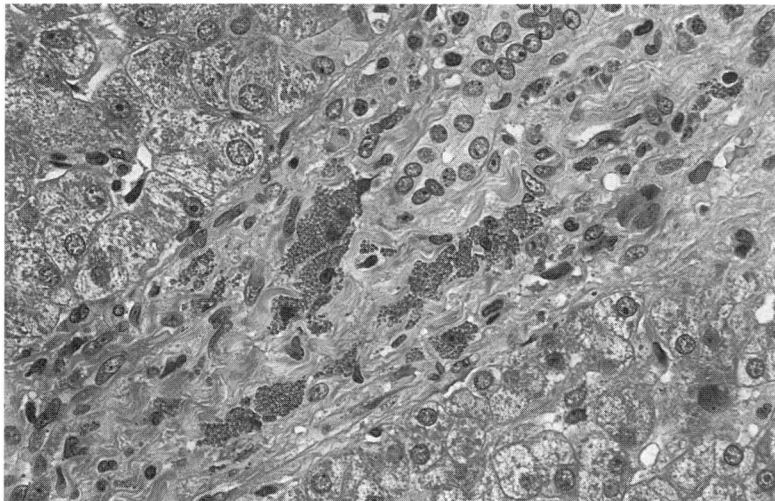

Figure 53 Thorotrast. The thorotrast pigment in this second case example is present within portal macrophages.

plasm has a diffuse "ground-glass" appearance, with or without distinct inclusions, as seen with phenobarbital usage and cyanamide exposure. The inclusions are in part secondary to hypertrophy of the smooth endoplasmic reticulum (65). Particulate material showing positive birefringence under polarized light may be identified within portal tracts and occasionally within Kupffer cells in long-term intravenous drug users, and represents the injectant used.

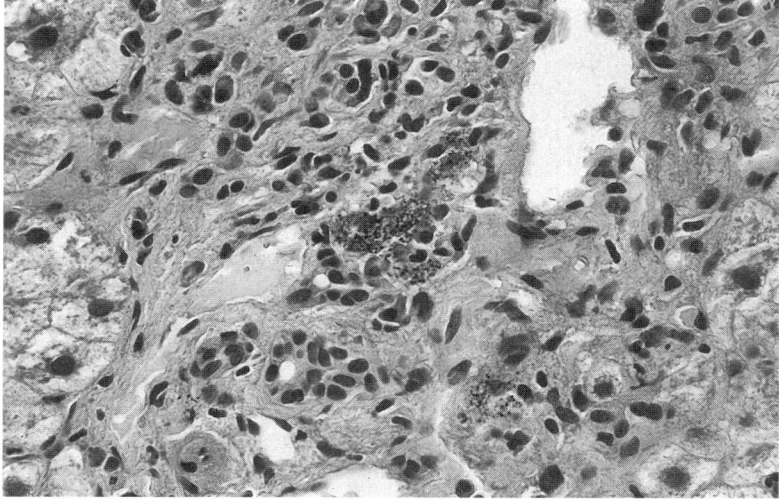

Figure 54 Anthracite. This dark black granular pigment is present within portal macrophages, and is most frequently seen in city dwellers or coal mine workers.

B. Pigments

Various pigments secondary to drugs and toxins (Table 15, Figs. 52–54) may also be identified, and can be confirmed with special stains (Ziehl-Neelsen acid-fast stain to highlight some examples of lipochrome, Perls' iron stain for hemosiderin). Although lipochrome generally is most prominent in the elderly population, in some instances this pigment deposition can be enhanced in individuals on certain medications such as phenacetin (11). Certain pigments may have a tinctorial quality that is unique, such as the gray-green thorotrast pigment, or the dark black granular anthracotic pigment sometimes seen in city dwellers and coal miners. The pigment is most often seen in portal macrophages and Kupffer cells, although sometimes the pigment appears extracellular.

IX. SUMMARY

The histological changes seen in the liver in drug-induced and toxic hepatic injury are complex. A whole spectrum of morphological changes are observed, and unfortunately, with rare exceptions (e.g., demonstration of thorotrast pigment), no histological features are diagnostic. The distinction in the vast majority of cases rests upon eliminating other causes of liver disease, as no reliable approach outside of discontinuing the medication and observing improvement of liver tests is feasible. Usually the degree of active liver disease manifested by monitoring of hepatic function will resolve within 1–2 weeks, although in some instances the abnormal liver tests may persist for considerable time periods (66). In instances of hypersensitivity reactions, rechallenging the patient will demonstrate conclusively the diagnosis, but should be approached cautiously to avoid serious liver cell injury.

REFERENCES

1. Larrey D. Drug-induced liver diseases. J Hepatol 2000; 32(suppl):77–88.
2. Amacher DE. Serum transaminase elevations as indicators of hepatic injury following the administration of drugs. Regul Toxicol Pharmacol 1998; 27:119–130.
3. Rubin E. Iatrogenic hepatic injury. Hum Pathol 1980; 11:312–331.
4. Kaplowitz N, Aw TY, Simon FR, Stolz A. Drug-induced hepatotoxicity. Ann Intern Med 1986; 104:826–839.
5. Lee WM. Drug-induced hepatotoxicity. N Engl J Med 1995; 333:1118–1127.
6. Ishak KG, Zimmerman HJ. Morphologic spectrums of drug-induced liver disease. Gastroenterol Clin North Am 1995; 24:759–786.
7. Phillips MJ, Poucell S, Patterson J, Valencia P. The Liver. An Atlas and Text of Ultrastructural Pathology. New York: Raven Press, 1987.
8. Hall P de la M. Histopathology of drug-induced liver disease. In: GC Farrell, ed. Drug-Induced Liver Diseases. Edinburgh: Churchill Livingstone, 1994:115–151.
9. Black M. Drug-induced liver disease. Clin Liver Dis 1998; 2:457–647.
10. Benhamos JP. Drug-induced hepatitis: clinical aspects. In: JP Fillastre, ed. Hepatotoxicity of Drugs. Rouen: Université de Rouen, 1985:22–30.
11. Zimmerman HJ. Hepatotoxicity: The Adverse Effects of Drugs and Other Chemicals on the Liver. Philadelphia: Lippincott Williams & Wilkins, 1999.
12. Zimmerman HJ, Lewis JH. Drug-induced cholestasis. Med Toxicol 1987; 2:112–160.
13. Matzen P, Malchow-Moller A, Hilden J, et al. Computer icterus group: differential diagnosis of jaundice: a pocket diagnostic chart. Liver 1984; 4:360–371.

14. Dossing M, Sonne J. Drug-induced hepatic disorders. Incidence, management and avoidance. Drug Safety 1993; 9:441–449.

15. Devictor D, Desplanques L, Debray D, Ozier Y, Dubousset AM, Valayer J, Houssin D, Bernard O, Huault G. Emergency liver transplantation for fulminant liver failure in infants and children. Hepatology 1992; 16:1156–1162.

16. Hoofnagle JH, Carithers RL Jr, Shapiro C, Ascher N. Fulminant hepatic failure: summary of a workshop. Hepatology 1995; 21:240–252.

17. Lewis JH, Zimmerman HJ. Drug-induced liver disease. Med Clin North Am 1989; 73:775–792.

18. Zimmerman HJ, Ishak KG. Hepatic injury due to drugs and toxins. In: RB MacSween, P Anthony, P Scheuer, AD Burt, BC Portmann, eds. Pathology of the Liver. 3rd ed. Edinburgh: Churchill Livingstone, 1994:563–633.

19. Zimmerman HJ. Drug-induced liver disease. In: ER Schiff, MF Sorrell, WC Maddrey, eds. Schiff's Diseases of the Liver. 8th ed. Philadelphia: Lippincott-Raven, 1999:973–1064.

20. DeLeve LD, Kaplowitz N. Mechanism of drug-induced liver disease. Gastroenterol Clin North Am 1995; 24:787–810.

21. Pessayre D. Role of reactive metabolites in drug-induced hepatitis. J Hepatol 1995; 23(suppl 1):16–24.

22. Neuberger J. Immune mechanisms in drug hepatotoxicity. Clin Liver Dis 1998; 2:471–482.

23. Farrell GC. Drug-induced chronic active hepatitis. In: GC Farrell, ed. Drug-Induced Liver Disease. Edinburgh: Churchill-Livingstone, 1994:413–430.

24. Stricker BH, Blok AP, Class FH, Van Parys GE, Desmet VJ. Hepatic injury associated with the use of nitrofurans: a clinicopathological study of 52 reported cases. Hepatology 1988; 8:599–606.

25. Zimmerman HJ. Update of hepatotoxicity due to classes of drugs in common clinical use: non-steroidal drugs, anti-inflammatory drugs, antibiotics, antihypertensives, and cardiac and psychotropic agents. Semin Liver Dis 1990; 10:322–338.

26. Peters RL. Viral inflammatory disease. In: RL Peters, JR Craig, eds. Liver Pathology. New York: Churchill Livingstone, 1986:73–123.

27. Dianzani MU. Toxic liver injury by protein synthesis inhibitors. Prog Liver Dis 1976; 5:232–245.

28. Stein O, Bar-On H, Stein Y. Lipoproteins and the liver. Prog Liver Dis 1972; 4:45–62.

29. Pessayre D, Mansouri A, Haouzi D, Fromenty B. Hepatotoxicity due to mitochondrial dysfunction. Cell Biol Toxicol 1999; 15:367–373.

30. Lewis JH, Ranard RC, Caruso A, Jackson LK, Mullick F, Ishak KG, Seeff LB, Zimmerman HJ. Amiodarone hepatotoxicity: prevalence and clinicopathologic correlations among 104 patients. Hepatology 1989; 9:679–685.

31. Poucell S, Ireton J, ValenciaMayoral P, et al. Amiodarone associated phospholipidosis and fibrosis of the liver: light, immunohistochemical and electron microscopic studies. Gastroenterology 1984; 86:926–936.

32. Lullman H, Lullman-Rauch R. Drug induced lysosomal storage disease of the liver. In: W Fillastre, ed. Hepatotoxicity of Drugs. Rouen: Université de Rouen, 1986:127–137.

33. Kanel GC, Reynolds TB. Hepatic granulomas. In: N Kaplowitz, ed. Liver and Biliary Diseases. 2nd ed. Baltimore: Williams & Wilkins, 1996:455–462.

34. Ishak KG, Zimmerman HJ. Drug-induced and toxic granulomatous hepatitis. Baillieres Clin Gastroenterol 1988; 2:463–480.

35. French SW. The Mallory body: structure, composition and pathogenesis. Hepatology 1981; 1:76–83.

36. Phillips MJ, Poucell S, Patterson J, Valencia P. The Liver: An Atlas and Text of Ultrastructural Pathology. New York: Raven Press, 1987:393–446.

37. Kanel GC. Hepatic lesions resembling alcoholic liver disease. In: LD Ferrell, ed. Diagnostic Problems in Liver Pathology. Philadelphia: Hanley & Belfus, 1994:77–104.

38. Zetterman RK. Nonalcoholic steatohepatitis. In: ER Schiff, MF Sorrell, WC Maddrey, eds. Schiff's Diseases of the Liver. 8th ed. Philadelphia: Lippincott-Raven, 1999:1179–1183.

39. Simon FR. Drug-induced cholestasis: pathobiology and clinical features. Clin Liver Dis 1998; 2:483–499.

40. Ishak KG. The liver. In: RH Riddell, ed. Pathology of Drug-Induced and Toxic Diseases. New York: Churchill Livingstone, 1982:457–513.

41. Ludwig J, Kim CH, Wiesner GH, Krom RA. Floxuridine-induced sclerosing cholangitis: an ischemic cholangiopathy. Hepatology 1989; 9:215–218.

42. Kemeny MM, Battifora H, Blayney DW, Cecchi G, Goldberg DA, Leong LA, Margolin KA, Terz JJ. Sclerosing cholangitis after continuous hepatic artery infusion of FUDR. Ann Surg 1985; 202:176–181.

43. Gitlin N. Drug-induced hepatic vascular abnormalities. Clin Liver Dis 1998; 2:591–606.

44. Zafrani ES, Pinaudeau Y, Dhumeaux D. Drug-induced vascular lesions of the liver. Arch Intern Med 1983; 143:495–502.

45. Bagheri SA, Boyer JL. Peliosis hepatis associated with androgenic-anabolic steroid therapy: a severe form of hepatic injury. Ann Intern Med 1974; 81:610–618.

46. Yanoff M, Rawson AJ. Peliosis hepatis: an anatomic study with demonstration of two varieties. Arch Pathol 1964; 77:159–165.

47. Altmann H-W. Drug-induced liver reactions: a morphological approach. Curr Top Pathol 1980; 69:69–142.

48. Winkler K, Poulsen H. Liver disease with periportal sinusoidal dilatation: a possible complication to contraceptive steroids. Scand J Gastroenterol. 1975; 10:699–704.

49. DeLeve LD, McCuskey RS, Wang X, Hu L, McCuskey MK, Epstein RB, Kanel GC. Characterization of a reproducible rat model of hepatic veno-occlusive disease. Hepatology 1999; 29:1779–1791.

50. Shulman HM, Fisher LB, Schoch HG, Henne KW, McDonald GB. Venoocclusive disease of the liver after marrow transplantation: histological correlates of clinical signs and symptoms. Hepatology 1994; 19:1171–1180.

51. Lee JL, Gooley T, Bensinger W, Schiffman K, McDonald GB. Veno-occlusive disease of the liver after busulfan, melphalan, and thiotepa conditioning therapy: incidence, risk factors, and outcome. Biol Blood Marrow Transplant 1999; 5:306–315.

52. Schiano TD. Liver injury from herbs and other botanicals. Clin Liver Dis 1998; 2:607–630.

53. Maddrey WC. Hepatic vein thrombosis (Budd-Chiari syndrome): possible association with the use of oral contraceptives. Semin Liver Dis 1987; 7:32–39.

54. French SW, Nash J, Shitabata P, Kachi K, Hara C, Chedid A, Mendenhall CL, VA Cooperative Study Group 119. Pathology of alcoholic liver disease. Semin Liver Dis 1993; 13:154–169.

55. Nakano M, Worner TM, Lieber CS. Perivenular fibrosis in alcoholic liver injury: ultrastructural and histologic progression. Gastroenterology 1982; 83:777–785.

56. Goodman ZD, Ishak KG. Occlusive venous lesions in alcoholic liver disease: a study of 200 cases. Gastroenterology 1982; 83:786–796.

57. Kanel GC, Korula J. Liver Biopsy Evaluation: Histologic Diagnosis and Clinical Correlations. Philadelphia: W.B. Saunders, 2000.

58. Patel T. Apoptosis in hepatic pathophysiology. Clin Liver Dis 2000; 4:295–317.

59. Rockey DC. The cell and molecular biology of hepatic fibrogenesis: clinical and therapeutic implications. Clin Liver Dis 2000; 4:319–355.

60. Li D, Friedman SL. Liver fibrogenesis and the role of hepatic stellate cells: new insights and prospects for therapy. J Gastroenterol Hepatol 1999; 14:618–633.

61. Popper H, Thomas LB, Telles NC, et al. Development of hepatic angiosarcoma in man induced by vinyl chloride, thorotrast, and arsenic: comparison with cases of unknown etiology. Am J Pathol 1978; 92:349–376.

62. Almoudarres M, Vega KJ, Trotman BW. Noncirrhotic portal hypertension in the adult: case report and review of the literature. J Assoc Acad Minor Phys 1998; 9:53–55.

63. Edmondson HA, Henderson B, Benton B. Liver-cell adenomas associated with use of oral contraceptives. N Engl J Med 1976; 294:470–472.
64. Korula J, Yellin A, Kanel G, Nichols P. Hepatocellular carcinoma coexisting with hepatic adenoma: incidental discovery after long-term oral contraceptive use. West J Med 1991; 155: 416–418.
65. Pamperl H, Gradner W, Frittlich H, et al. Influence of long-term anti-convulsant treatment on liver ultrastructure in man. Liver 1984; 4:294–300.
66. Kaplowitz N. Drug metabolism and hepatotoxicity. In: N Kaplowitz, ed. Liver and Biliary Diseases. 2nd ed. Baltimore: Williams & Wilkins, 1996:103–120.

13

Mechanisms of Acetaminophen-Induced Liver Disease

SIDNEY D. NELSON and SAM A. BRUSCHI

University of Washington School of Pharmacy, Seattle, Washington, U.S.A.

I. INTRODUCTION

Acetaminophen is the generic name in the United States for 4′-hydroxyacetanilide, the *N*-acetylated derivative of *p*-aminophenol (paracetamol is the generic name used in Great Britain and several other countries). This nonnarcotic analgesic/antipyretic, available over the counter in the United States since 1960, is one of the most widely used drugs in the world, and is available alone and in combination with many other drugs (1). In recommended doses, acetaminophen is considered to be efficacious and safe, and is not associated with the high incidence of gastrointestinal bleeding caused by aspirin and nonsteroidal antiinflammatory drugs, or with the development of Reye's syndrome.

Although many different kinds of toxic effects have been attributed to acetaminophen use and abuse, except for hepatotoxicity and nephrotoxicity, their incidence is very low and in many cases considered insignificant (for reviews see refs. 1 and 2). Even the incidence of nephrotoxicity is low, with an estimated occurrence of acute tubular necrosis of less than 2% of all acetaminophen poisonings (3), and there is an insignificant association between acetaminophen use and chronic renal injury, such as nephropathy (4,5).

Thus, the major toxicity caused by acetaminophen is hepatotoxicity characterized by acute hepatocellular damage primarily in zone 3, the centrilobular region of the liver. It is not the intent of this chapter to describe the clinical and morphological characteristics of acetaminophen hepatotoxicity; readers are referred to several excellent reviews on acetaminophen for further information in this area (1,6,7). Suffice it to say that acetaminophen is a major cause of acute liver failure in the United States, United Kingdom, and Australia (8–10), and accounts for a high percentage of inquiries to poison centers ($>$100,000 cases/ year) and deaths from poisonings (11,12). In the United States, initial results from a multicenter study suggest that a little over one-third of cases of acute liver failure are caused by acetaminophen, with approximately 40% of those cases due to intentional overdose, and 60% classified as accidental or therapeutic misadventures where high therapeutic doses are taken by individuals who are alcoholics, have other severe illness, and/or are malnourished (13). The percentages are reversed in the United Kingdom, with more individuals taking intentional overdoses (9). Interestingly, reports have recently appeared that restricting the availability of acetaminophen in the United Kingdom in 1998 by requiring blister packs of only 32 tablets has apparently decreased the incidence of severe acetaminophen poisoning (14,15). Longer-term follow-up will be required to substantiate this claim.

The remainder of this chapter will focus on mechanisms of acetaminophen hepatotoxicity with discussion of events involved in initiation or early stages of hepatotoxicity followed by discussion of events involved in progression of the injury to hepatic necrosis. Some limited discussion of factors (e.g., age, diet, other drugs) that may influence the metabolism and disposition of acetaminophen will be included as they relate to the mechanisms proposed.

II. EARLY EVENTS IN ACETAMINOPHEN-INDUCED HEPATOTOXICITY

A. Pathways of Acetaminophen Metabolism

1. Introduction and General Scheme

After hepatotoxicity caused by acetaminophen was reported in animals (16,17) and humans (18,19) in the mid-1960s, several investigations commenced on the mechanism. In 1973, Mitchell and colleagues published a series of classic papers (20–22) that outlined a scheme for the metabolic activation of acetaminophen to an electrophilic quinone imine, N-acetyl-p-benzoquinone imine (NAPQI), that covalently bound to hepatic proteins, mostly in centrilobular liver cells that became necrotic. The role of glutathione (GSH) in protecting liver cells from injury also was elucidated (23), and this led to the development of N-acetylcysteine as an effective antidote that is still widely successful today in the management of acetaminophen toxicity (24–26).

A scheme for the metabolism of acetaminophen is shown in Fig. 1 (27). Work from several laboratories has contributed to the development of this and related metabolic schemes as reviewed in more detail elsewhere (1,2,6,7,28), and pathways and enzymes primarily related to metabolism in humans will be highlighted in the following discussion.

2. Major Non-P450 Pathways

The two major pathways of acetaminophen metabolism in all species are glucuronidation and sulfation of the phenolic group. After therapeutic doses of acetaminophen, humans

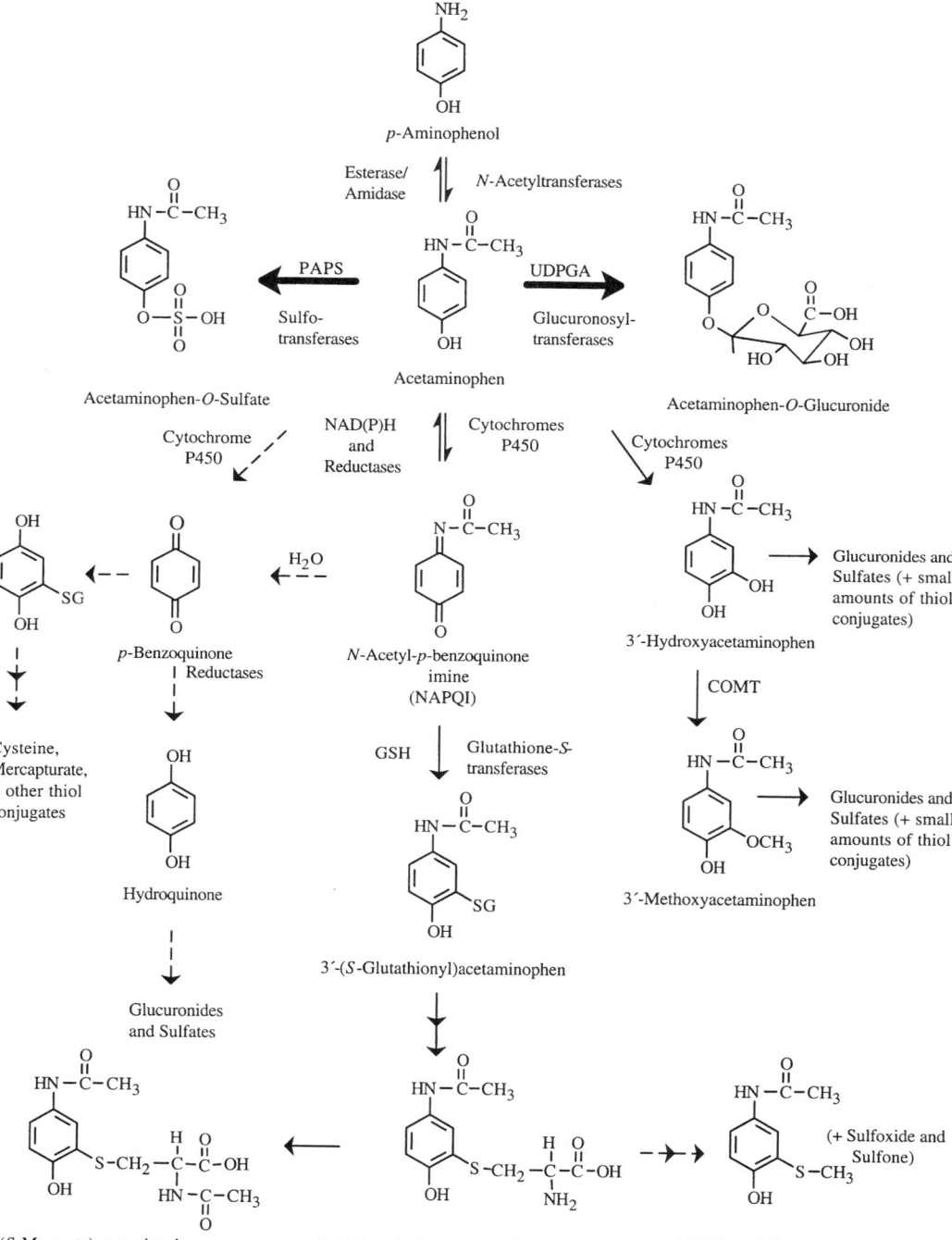

Figure 1 Metabolic pathways of acetaminophen. Bold arrows indicate major pathways, normal arrows indicate intermediate pathways, and broken arrows indicate minor pathways. Benzoquinone metabolites have been detected only in mice, whereas all other pathways have been detected in several species, including humans.

excrete approximately 50% of the dose as the phenolic O-glucuronide and approximately 30% as the O-sulfate. These nontoxic metabolites are selectively formed by UGT1*6, a human isoform of the uridine diphosphate (UDP)-glucuronosyltransferase family of enzymes (29), and members of the SULT1 family of phenol sulfotransferases (30). Decreased elimination of acetaminophen as its glucuronide in congenic rats with a hereditary deficiency in UDP-glucuronosyltransferase activity (31) or in cats with a similar deficiency (32) makes these animals significantly more susceptible to acetaminophen-induced hepatotoxicity, and in humans, increased susceptibility to acetaminophen-induced hepatotoxicity may occur in Gilbert's disease (33,34). However, except for one case report of a possible Zidovudine interaction (35), there is no evidence that patients who receive drugs that competitively inhibit the glucuronidation of acetaminophen are at increased risk of acetaminophen-induced hepatotoxicity (1,27). Moreover, there have been no reports of effects on the sulfation pathway where increased toxicity to acetaminophen has been observed. It appears that if glucuronidation of acetaminophen is decreased, there is a compensatory increase in sulfation, and conversely, decreased sulfation is offset by increases in glucuronidation.

Carboxylesterases of the CES1 family and N-acetyltransferases (both NAT1 and NAT2) likely contribute to the hydrolysis of approximately 10% of a dose of acetaminophen to p-aminophenol and its reacetylation back to acetaminophen, a "futile cycling" that has been documented in rats (36). The extent to which this occurs in humans is unknown, but may be more related to the risk of nephrotoxicity from acetaminophen than hepatotoxicity, since p-aminophenol is a known nephrotoxicant that has been implicated in nephrotoxicity caused by acetaminophen in rats (37,38). With regard to drug interactions, it has been found that therapeutic doses of acetaminophen in humans can inhibit the polymorphic NAT2 (39).

3. Cytochrome P450 Oxidation Pathways

Cytochrome P450 (CYP)-catalyzed oxidation of acetaminophen to NAPQI is the major metabolic pathway leading to hepatotoxicity (22,40). Originally, N-hydroxyacetaminophen was proposed as a precursor to NAPQI (24), but kinetic (41) and carrier-trapping (42) experiments both showed that if this metabolite is formed, it decomposes before it leaves the CYP active site. NAPQI has been synthesized (43,44), and has the chemical, biochemical, and toxicological properties consistent with its role as the major ultimate toxic metabolite of acetaminophen (43–48). Because of its short half-life in biological systems [~0.7 s (45)], NAPQI is usually detected as thioether conjugates (49,50), but it has also been detected directly in incubations of acetaminophen with purified rat CYP 1A1 (51). Also, because of its reactivity, NAPQI causes necrosis of cells in the periportal region of the livers of rats infused with NAPQI through the portal vein (Fig. 2), rather than in the centrilobular region as occurs when acetaminophen is administered (see ref. 1 for a review and photomicrographs).

Thiol ether metabolites of acetaminophen are excreted into urine as an indicator of NAPQI formation (Fig. 1), and represent 5–10% of normal therapeutic doses in humans (1,52). However, this is probably an underestimation of the extent of oxidation of acetaminophen to NAPQI because this highly reactive quinone imine can be reduced back to acetaminophen by several reductases and their reducing cofactors including NADPH-cytochrome P450 reductase and NADPH (40,53,54), and via *ipso* adduct decomposition reactions (55,56).

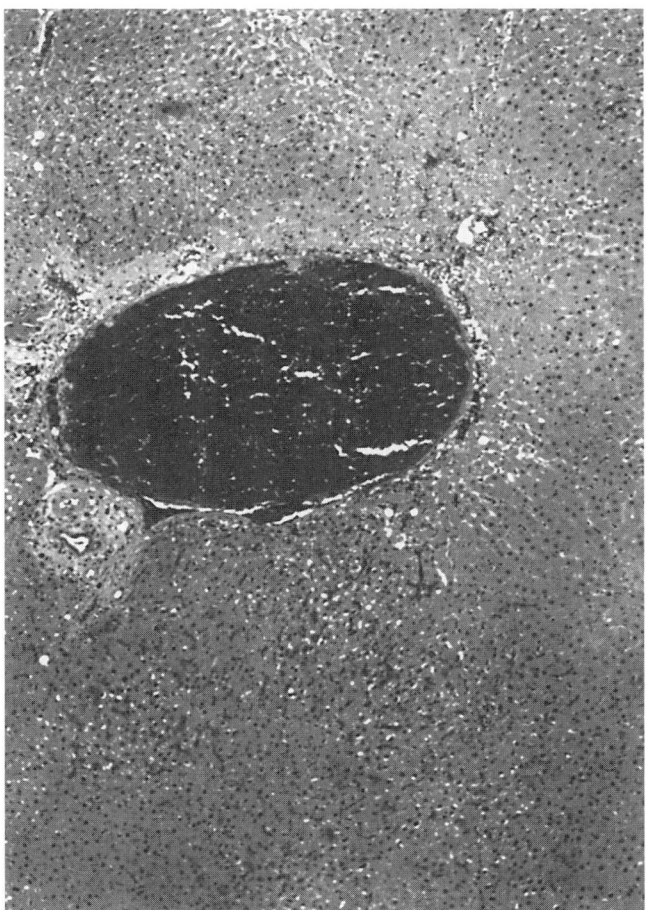

Figure 2 Section of rat liver obtained 5 h after intraportal infusion of a 20 mg/kg dose of NAPQI in FC-43 emulsion (Oxypherol). Hematoxylin-and-eosin-stained micrograph shows necrosis of cells proximal to the periportal vein and portal triad. The FC-43 vehicle does not cause cellular damage.

A catechol metabolite of acetaminophen, 3-hydroxyacetaminophen (Fig. 1), is apparently formed in a classical CYP monooxygenase reaction, inasmuch as the hydroxyl group oxygen is derived from molecular oxygen (57). This catechol is nontoxic based on studies in mice (58), though small amounts of thioether metabolites of the catechol and its 3-O-methylated metabolite are formed ($<0.5\%$) indicating their further oxidation to electrophilic quinones and quinone imines. Overall, the catechol and catechol-derived metabolites account for 4–8% of therapeutic doses of acetaminophen in humans (1,52).

There are several reports concerning the specific CYP isoforms that are involved in the oxidation of acetaminophen to NAPQI in laboratory animals and humans, and the reader is referred to refs. 1 and 2 for reviews. The following discussion will focus on relative efficiencies of expressed and, in some cases, purified human CYP isoforms with a comparison to information obtained with human liver microsomes and in vivo studies in humans.

Table 1 Kinetic Parameters for Purified Human CYP Isoforms Involved in Acetaminophen
Oxidation to Its Toxic Metabolite, NAPQI, Measured as Its Glutathione Conjugate, 3′-
(Glutathion-S-yl) Acetaminophen (GS-APAP), and the Nontoxic Catechol Metabolite, 3′-
Hydroxyacetaminophen (3-OH-APAP)

Purified human isoform	GS-APAP			3-OH-APAP		
	K_m (mM)	V_{max} (nmol/min/nmolP450)	V/K	K_m (mM)	V_{max} (nmol/min/nmolP450)	V/K
CYP 1A2	1.4	14.4	10.3	ND	0.1	ND[a]
CYP 2A6	4.6	7.9	1.7	2.2	14.2	6.5
CYP 2C8	1.0	0.2	0.2	ND	0.1	ND[a]
CYP 2C9	1.1	0.1	0.1	ND	ND	ND[b]
CYP 2D6	1.8	3.0	1.7	ND	ND	ND[b]
CYP 2E1	1.3	6.9	5.2	4.0	2.5	0.6
CYP 3A4	0.14	1.5	10.5	ND	0.1	ND[b]

[a] Although CYP 1A2, CYP 2C8, and CYP 3A4 did form measurable amounts of the catechol metabolite (V_{max} ≈ 0.1 nmol/min/nmol P450), limits of detection of the HPLC/EC assay were not sufficient to accurately determine K_m values.
[b] CYP 2C9 and CYP 2D6 did not form detectable amounts of the catechol metabolite.

The data in Table 1 compare data obtained in our laboratory with human liver CYP
isoforms purified to homogeneity from baculovirus expression systems (59–63). Other
human CYP isoforms (1B1, 2B6, 2C19) were obtained as Supersomes (Gentest Corp.)
and showed no detectable formation of either NAPQI or the catechol metabolite, whereas
human CYP 1A1 was nearly as active as CYP 1A2. However, CYP 1A1 is not normally
expressed in human liver, and is therefore unlikely to play a role in bioactivation of acetaminophen to its proximal reactive intermediate in hepatocytes.

In assessing the data in Table 1, one should consider the following. First, as discussed previously, the kinetic parameters are apparent only for NAPQI formation since
GS-APAP is the product of a very reactive metabolite that can undergo other undetectable
reactions. Second, the values obtained with the purified enzymes are not the same as
those obtained by others using partially purified preparations and transfected cells (64,65).
However, the relative importance of these human isoforms in forming the major hepatotoxicant from acetaminophen is fairly consistent among the various studies with the possible
exception of CYP 1A2. The possible significance of each major isoform is discussed
below.

CYP 1A2. Although purified CYP 1A2 is one of the most efficient catalysts of NAPQI
formation, its importance in acetaminophen metabolism and toxicity is unclear. Induction
of this isoform in humans (e.g., charcoal-broiled meat, cigarette smoking, omeprazole)
does not increase the formation of NAPQI based on amounts of thioether metabolites
formed (66–69). Furthermore, *Cyp 1a2* null mice are not significantly more susceptible
to acetaminophen-mediated hepatotoxicity than wild-type mice (70). However, CYP 1A2
is involved in acetaminophen oxidation to NAPQI in human liver microsomes (64), and
when mice have deletions of both the *Cyp 2e1* and *Cyp 1a2* genes, they are less susceptible
to acetaminophen hepatotoxicity than just *Cyp 2e1* null mice (71,72). These results suggest
that some CYPs may function differently in intact cells, or even in their membrane-bound

states, which is consistent with much higher K_m (3–4 mM) and lower V_{max} (0.3–3 nmol/min/nmol P450) values for CYP 1A2 in these preparations (61,64,65). Whether it is altered reductase interactions or other factors that modulate CYP 1A2 activity in membranes is unknown.

CYP 2A6. CYP 2A6 appears to be the major human CYP isoform that catalyzes the oxidation of acetaminophen to its catechol metabolite (Table 1) (60). It also forms NAPQI, but the relatively high K_m for this reaction suggests that this would be important only at relatively high hepatotoxic doses of acetaminophen. There is one report that methoxsalen, a relatively specific inhibitor of CYP 2A6, decreases the formation of NAPQI from acetaminophen in humans (73). Methoxsalen does decrease hepatotoxicity caused by acetaminophen in mice (74).

CYP 2D6. Overall CYP 2D6 plays a minor role in the oxidation of acetaminophen to NAPQI (ranging from 4.5% to 22% of total thioether conjugates formed in a panel of human liver microsomes) as would be expected based on kinetic parameters (Table 1) (62). However, CYP 2D6 is polymorphically expressed in humans, and it could contribute significantly in CYP 2D6 ultrarapid and extensive metabolizers (75), and put some populations at greater risk of acetaminophen hepatotoxicity (76).

CYP 2E1. Although CYP 2E1 only accounts for about 5–10% of total P450 in most human livers (77), this isoform appears to be the major isoform that catalyzes the oxidation of acetaminophen to NAPQI in humans (60,64,65,78). It also forms significant amounts of the catechol metabolite (Table 1) (60). CYP 2E1 will be discussed further below.

CYP 3A4. CYP 3A4 is the most efficient P450 in the oxidation of acetaminophen to NAPQI (Table 1) (63,65). Its high abundance in human liver (about 30% of total hepatic P450) (77) and relatively low K_m would suggest that CYP 3A4 should be the most important contributor to NAPQI formation from acetaminophen given at therapeutic doses in humans. However, studies in vitro in human liver microsomes using troleandomycin as an inhibitor of CYP 3A4 (63), and in vivo in humans using rifampin to induce CYP 3A4 (78), indicate that CYP 3A isoforms only contribute to about 10% of the oxidation of acetaminophen to NAPQI. Because of its low K_m and low V_{max}, it is unlikely that CYP 3A4 is a major contributor at concentrations of acetaminophen (≥ 1 mM) that are normally achieved in cases of hepatotoxicity (79).

B. Factors that Influence Acetaminophen Metabolism and Hepatotoxicity

This section will be limited to a discussion of those cases where there is substantial evidence for modulating the hepatotoxicity caused by acetaminophen in humans. A much more detailed discussion is provided in ref. 1.

1. Age

One of the few factors that has been reasonably well documented in humans that affects the incidence of hepatotoxicity is age, and only in the sense that young children appear to be less susceptible to hepatotoxicity caused by acetaminophen than adults (80). This has been attributed to increased rates of sulfation of acetaminophen in children (81), and to increased rates of glutathione resynthesis when the liver is challenged based on studies in rats (82). When used properly in children, acetaminophen appears to be a very safe drug (83), but unintentional multiple overdoses of acetaminophen in children have led to several cases of hepatotoxicity (84–89). A recommendation is that 60–90 mg/kg/day is a reasonable therapeutic dose, but that repeated supratherapeutic dosing of greater than 90 mg/kg/day is inappropriate (90).

2. Drug-Drug Interactions

Although several chemicals, including many drugs, can induce CYPs that oxidize acetaminophen to NAPQI (27) (Table 14.1 in ref. 1), in only a few cases in humans on anticonvulsant drugs has the induction apparently led to hepatotoxicity caused by acetaminophen (91–93). It may be that some drugs such as rifampin (94) also induce enzymes involved in clearance of acetaminophen through nontoxic pathways, such as glucuronidation. Propoxyphene is an analgesic often used in combination with acetaminophen that can cause deaths in humans (95). This has been attributed to respiratory depression caused by propoxyphene although some cases may involve induction of acetaminophen metabolism and hepatotoxicity (95). In contrast, propoxyphene forms a tight-binding metabolite inhibitory complex with P450 heme (96) that may have protected against hepatotoxicity after ingestion of a normally hepatotoxic dose of acetaminophen by an individual (97).

Other drugs known to inhibit and induce CYP isoforms involved in acetaminophen oxidation in humans are isoniazid (98,99) and ethanol (100,101). A model of time-dependent induction of CYP 2E1 by ligand stabilization, such that inhibition is observed while the inducer is present and enhancement of activity occurs with removal of the inducer, has been proposed (102) and was very predictive of the ethanol-acetaminophen interaction in humans (101). Also, isoniazid was found to inhibit the oxidation of acetaminophen to NAPQI in humans for nearly 24 h after coadministration (98,103), but between 24 and 48 h after administration, significant increases in its formation were observed that may have contributed to hepatotoxicity and nephrotoxicity in some patients who received acetaminophen after taking isoniazid (104–106).

Although it seems clear that chronic ingestion of alcohol puts humans at greater risk of acetaminophen-mediated hepatotoxicity (for reviews see refs. 1,107–109), the majority of cases appear to involve accidental overdoses of acetaminophen in chronic alcohol abusers (110,111). Also, as previously discussed (100,101), induction of CYP 2E1 by ethanol stabilization of this isoform is likely to increase NAPQI formation only 2–3-fold, and additional factors such as other mechanisms of CYP 2E1 induction (112), alterations in hepatic GSH status (113,114), and poor nutritional status (115–117) are likely to be important contributors to hepatotoxicity. Furthermore, induction of other CYP isoforms (such as CYP 3A isoforms) by ethanol and other alcohols present in alcoholic beverages may play a role in increased risk of hepatotoxicity caused by chronic alcohol ingestion based on studies in animals (118,119), although induction of CYP 3A isoforms in humans does not appear to significantly increase acetaminophen oxidation to NAPQI (78).

Acetaminophen has been safely used for many years as the analgesic/antipyretic of choice in patients taking the narrow therapeutic index anticoagulant warfarin, with only a few case reports of enhanced anticoagulant effect (120–123). However, a retrospective study (124) has suggested that acetaminophen is an underrecognized cause of excessive anticoagulation in elderly patients. Results of a more recent case-controlled study did not reveal any pharmacokinetic or pharmacodynamic alterations of warfarin caused by acetaminophen (125), and acetaminophen does not significantly inhibit CYP 2C9 hydroxylation of S-warfarin (126). However, unrecognized genetic and/or nongenetic factors may put some individuals at risk of hypocoagulation as a result of acetaminophen therapy with warfarin.

C. Mechanisms of Reactive Metabolite Formation

Mechanisms of the oxidation of acetaminophen by cytochrome P450s to NAPQI, 3-hydroxyacetaminophen, and *p*-benzoquinone have been reviewed elsewhere (2,127). Briefly, differential CYP isoform selectivity in the formation of NAPQI and the catechol metabolite strongly implies that acetaminophen orients differently in the active sites of different CYP isoforms, such that hydrogen atom removal by a high valency heme iron-oxo complex, usually depicted as FeO^{3+} or $Fe^v = O$, occurs to generate either an amide nitrogen radical that rebounds to form a ternary enzyme-oxy-acetaminophen complex that essentially dehydrates to yield NAPQI, or a phenoxy radical that rebounds via generation of a stabilized semiquinone aryl radical to form the catechol metabolite.

Although there is no direct evidence to support these reactions, indirect evidence from NMR paramagnetic-relaxation studies has demonstrated that acetaminophen binds to the resting, ferric form of different rat CYPs consistent with the selective formation of NAPQI by CYP 1A1 and 3-hydroxyacetaminophen by CYP 2B1 (128). Recently, we have shown similar results with two purified human CYPs (61). The results show that acetaminophen preferentially orients in CYP 2E1, which selectively forms NAPQI (60), with the amide group significantly closer to the heme iron than the phenolic group (Fig. 3A), whereas the reverse is true with CYP 2A6 (Fig. 3B), which selectively forms the catechol metabolite (60). It should be emphasized that these results do not confirm mechanism, since it is known from time-resolved crystallographic studies of CYP 101 that changes in its active site structure occur at every step of the reaction (129), and structural changes upon reduction and oxygenation occur with other CYP active sites as well (130,131). Nonetheless, based on the distances from the heme iron obtained for acetaminophen in the NMR paramagnetic relaxation studies and a CYP 2E1 homology model, a possible mode of interaction of acetaminophen in the active site of human CYP 2E1 has been described (132), and awaits testing and refining.

D. Reactive Metabolite Disposition

The discussion in this section will focus on the reactions of the major reactive and toxic metabolite of acetaminophen, NAPQI. Although small amounts of quinones and quinoneimines of the catechol and its methylated metabolite are formed in mice (Fig. 1), they are formed in larger amounts from a nonhepatotoxic regioisomer of acetaminophen, 3'-hydroxyacetanilide (133–135), and therefore, are unlikely to contribute significantly to hepatotoxicity. Since NAPQI is a quinone imine that is both a strong oxidant and electrophile, it can react in more than one way leading to both covalent and noncovalent modifications of cellular constituents (1,2,6,7,28,56,127,136–138). A major unresolved question is how important each of these modifications is in the pathogenesis of liver cell injury.

1. Covalent Binding to Hepatocellular Proteins

At the organ level, covalent binding of acetaminophen to the liver of mice occurs in hepatocytes in the centrilobular region, and this binding precedes cellular necrosis of those hepatocytes (21,139,140). One study (140) showed colocalization of CYP 2E1 in necrotic

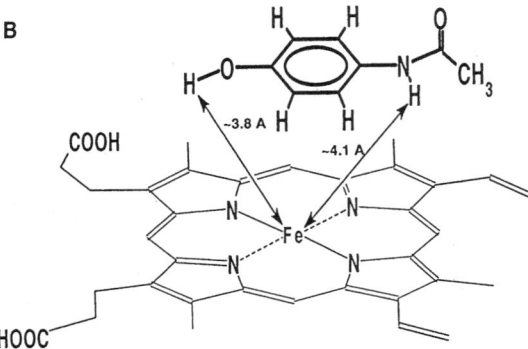

Figure 3 (A) The favored orientation of acetaminophen in relation to the heme iron at the active site of CYP 2E1 based on ^{1}H-NMR relaxation studies. (B) The favored orientation of acetaminophen in relation to heme iron at the active site of CYP 2A6 based on ^{1}H-NMR relaxation studies.

cells in the liver and other necrotic tissues in mice that contained protein-bound acetaminophen. Studies of postmortem human livers from acetaminophen overdose cases have shown acetaminophen adducts to proteins in the necrotic centrilobular regions (141), and a strong correlation between plasma ALT and 3-(cysteinyl-S-yl) acetaminophen protein adducts has also been observed in human acetaminophen overdose cases (142).

NAPQI is a soft electrophile that appears to form covalent adducts primarily, though not exclusively, with cysteine residues on proteins (56,143–146). One study has provided evidence that oxidation of acetaminophen by mouse liver microsomes yields lysine amino adducts with some proteins (147), and minor amounts of noncysteinyl adducts of acetaminophen have been detected in mouse liver (148).

Acetaminophen has been found to bind covalently in a stable enough form to several hepatic proteins in the mouse that has allowed for the identification of the proteins (for reviews, see refs. 1,2,149–151). For many of the proteins, investigations have not been carried out to determine whether their function has been altered as a result of adduction by NAPQI, but for a few, decreased catalytic activity or changes in function have been measured (Table 2).

Table 2 Modifications to Proteins in Mouse Liver After In Vivo Administration of Hepatotoxic Doses of Acetaminophen (see individual references for doses used and when livers were obtained for measurements)

Protein and subcellular localization	Adduct (ref.)	Activity (ref.)[a]	Protein level[b]
Cytoplasm			
Selenium-binding proteins	Yes (151–153)		↓↓
N-10-Formyl tetrahydrofolate dehydrogenase	Yes (158)	↓↓ (158)	↓
Glyceraldehyde-3-phosphate dehydrogenase	Yes (146)	↓↓ (146)	
Albumin			↑↑
Glutathione peroxidases	Yes (151)	↓↓ (136,159)	↓
Thioether S-methyltransferase	Yes (151)		↓
Aryl sulfotransferase	Yes (151)		
Inorganic pyrophosphatase	Yes (151)		↓
Proteasome subunit C8	Yes (151)		
Methionine adenosyl transferase (synthetases)	Yes (151)		↓↓
Aldehyde dehydrogenases	Yes (151)		↓
Osteoblast-specific factor 3	Yes (151)		
Glutathione S-transferase Pi	Yes (151)		↓
Glutathione S-transferase Alpha			↓↓
Carbonic anhydrase III	Yes (151)		↑[c]
Sorbitol dehydrogenase (fragment)	Yes (151)		↓↓[d]
Glycine N-methyl transferase	Yes (151)		
3-Hydroxyanthranilate 3,4-dioxygenase	Yes (151)		↓
Adenosine kinase			↓
Phosphoenolpyruvate carboxykinase			↓↓[e]
Superoxide dismutase [Cu-Zn]			↓↓
Thioredoxin peroxidase 1			↓[d]
Endoplasmic Reticulum			
Glutamine synthetase	Yes (160)	↓↓ (160,161)	
Calreticulin precursor (crp 55, erp 60)	In vitro only (147)		↑
A probable protein disulfide isomerase (er-60)	In vitro only (147)		↓↓[d]
Mitochondria			
Aldehyde dehydrogenase	Yes (151,162)	↓↓ (162)	↓[d]
Glutamate dehydrogenase	Yes (163)	↓↓ (163)	↓[d]
Carbamyl phosphate synthetase-I	Indirect evidence only (161)	↓↓ (161)	↓
ATP synthetase α subunit	Yes (151)		
Housekeeping protein	Yes (151)		
Matrix protein P1 (hsp-60, GroEl protein)			↓↓
Mitochondrial stress-70 protein precursor (grp 75)			↓↓
Thioredoxin-dependent peroxide reductase 2			↓↓

Table 2   Continued

Protein and subcellular localization	Adduct (ref.)	Activity (ref.)[a]	Protein level[b]
Nucleus			
Lamin A	Yes (156)		
Cytoskeleton			
Tropomyosin 5	Yes (151)		↓[d]
Actin			↓[d]
Peroxisomes			
Likely 2,4-dienoyl-CoA reductase	Yes (151)		
Urate oxidase	Yes (151)		↓
Catalase			↓[d]
Other			
Tumor necrosis factor, type 1 receptor associated protein			↓↓
Senescence marker protein-30 (smp-30)			↓↓

[a] Double arrows indicate significant decreases in enzyme activity were observed. Note: The relatively nonhepatotoxic regioisomer 3′-hydroxyacetanilide caused significantly less decrease in the activity of glyceraldehyde-3-phosphate dehydrogenase (146) and glutathione peroxidase (136). The effects of this isomer on other enzyme activities have not yet been determined.

[b] See ref. 154 for more information. A double arrow indicates significant decreases (↓↓) or increases (↑↑) in levels of proteins 8 h after doses of 300 mg/kg in mice. A single arrow indicates a trend toward a decrease (↓) or increase (↑). Note: The relatively nonhepatotoxic regioisomer 3′-hydroxyacetanilide did not significantly change protein expression levels except as indicated below.

[c] The relatively nonhepatotoxic regioisomer 3′-hydroxyacetanilide caused a small increase in protein expression level.

[d] The relatively nonhepatotoxic regioisomer 3′-hydroxyacetanilide caused a small decrease in protein expression level.

[e] The relatively nonhepatotoxic regioisomer 3′-hydroxyacetanilide caused a significant decrease in protein expression level.

The first protein, or group of proteins, that were well characterized as forming adducts with reactive metabolites of acetaminophen were 55–58-kDa cytosolic proteins that are very similar to cytosolic selenium-binding proteins whose function is not well understood (2,152,153). These proteins have also been found to decrease in concentration in mouse liver after acetaminophen treatment, but not after treatment with the nonhepatotoxic regioisomer 3′-hydroxyacetanilide (154) (Table 2). This regioisomer does form reactive metabolites that covalently bind to the same set of selenium-binding proteins, but the adducts seem to be less stable (155). Preliminary evidence has been presented that the acetaminophen-adducted protein translates to the nucleus as a possible signal of electrophile damage (156). A recent report also implicates a 56-kDa selenium-binding protein in intra-Golgi protein transport (157), and it will be of interest to determine whether acetaminophen affects this function.

From Table 2 it can be seen that several cellular dehydrogenases form adducts with acetaminophen reactive metabolites, and where measured, their activities are significantly decreased. Such reactions would favor an oxidant state in cells, and ATP synthesis could be impaired. It is interesting that *ipso* adduct forms of NAPQI (see discussion below) resemble the NADH and NADPH products of cofactor reduction, which may explain in part the selectivity of NAPQI for these enzymes. Moreover, a mitochondrial housekeeping protein that is a precursor to thioredoxin reductase, a selenoprotein requiring NADPH for its activity (164–166), is also adducted (Table 2) (151).

In general, mitochrondria appear to be an important target for the pathogenesis of acetaminophen hepatotoxicity. This organelle sustains high levels of protein adduct formation after hepatotoxic doses of acetaminophen in mice. In comparison, there is little binding to mitochrondrial proteins with doses of the relatively nonhepatotoxic analog 3′-hydroxyacetanilide, despite similar amounts of overall cellular adduct formation (134, 135,167). However, when mitochrondrial GSH is depleted in mice, 3′-hydroxyacetanilide does bind to hepatic mitochrondrial proteins, alters mitochrondrial function, and hepatotoxicity ensues (168). Mitochrondria are also one of the earliest organelles to undergo both morphological (169,170) and functional (134,136,171–177) changes in hepatocytes after hepatotoxic doses of acetaminophen. Significant decreases in rates of ATP synthesis (177) and ATP concentrations (136,175,177–179) occur, and mitochrondrial ATP synthetase appears to be a target of acetaminophen-mediated damage (151,180).

Several other enzymes, and a few receptor and structural proteins, form covalent adducts with reactive metabolites of acetaminophen (Table 2) but it is not yet known if their activities or functions are affected. Furthermore, the time courses of adduct formation, repair, and/or degradation, and of activity and function are unknown for most of the proteins identified (see below). Finally, the effects of acetaminophen on human liver proteins and their activities have not been investigated. The use of human liver tissue, liver slices, and hepatocytes, and functional proteomics approaches should yield substantial new information in all of these areas.

2. "Noncovalent" Interactions with Cellular Proteins

As evident from Table 2, there are some hepatic proteins whose basal levels are decreased after acetaminophen administration to mice, yet no protein adducts have been identified. Additionally, it is known that hepatotoxic doses of acetaminophen affect some hepatocyte enzyme activities early in the pathogenesis of toxicity without detectable adduct formation. For example, there is evidence that acetaminophen, through its reactive metabolite NAPQI, inhibits calcium-dependent ATPases (134,136,181–185), but no adducts to these ATPases have been identified. Hepatocyte plasma membrane Na^+/K^+-ATPase activity is also significantly inhibited after hepatoxic doses of acetaminophen in rats (186), and despite attempts to detect adducts, none have been detected to this ATPase (150). Xanthine dehydrogenase in mouse liver is converted to its oxidase form after administration of hepatotoxic doses of acetaminophen (136,179) and may represent another indicator and mediator of oxidant stress. Finally, protein phosphatase activity is decreased prior to evidence of cytotoxicity in mouse hepatocytes after exposure to toxic concentrations of acetaminophen, with no evidence of acetaminophen binding to the phosphatase enzymes (187).

Although there are several possible explanations for these observations, including activation of proteases and/or signal transduction pathways, another possibility is that protein *ipso* adducts of NAPQI may form that react with cellular thiols to form *S*-thiolated proteins with modified activities. Glutathionyl and cysteinyl *ipso* adducts of NAPQI have been characterized, and evidence for protein *ipso* adducts of NAPQI with inhibition of protein activity has been presented (55,56,185). It is unlikely that these *ipso* adducts are stable enough to be detected as protein adducts under the conditions of gel electrophoresis that have been used to separate adducted proteins prior to their identification by either mass spectral or immunochemical methods. However, there is evidence that *S*-glutathionylated

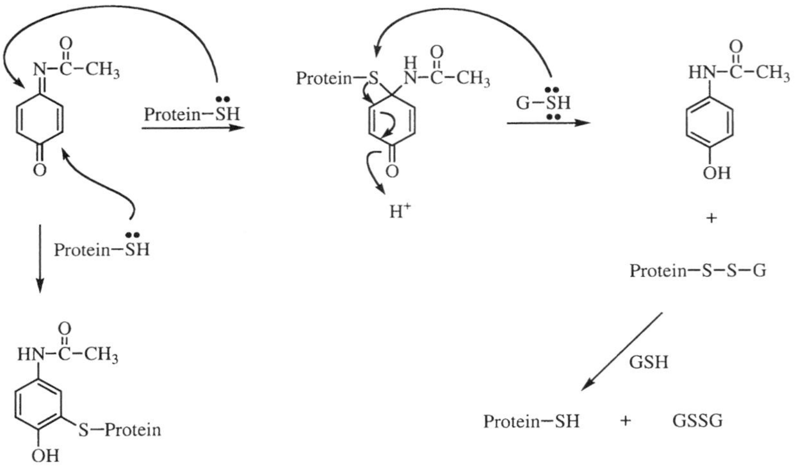

Figure 4 Possible reactions of NAPQI with protein thiols to generate a stable 3′-protein thiol adduct and unstable *ipso* protein thiol adduct that can form *S*-glutathionylated proteins that can further react with GSH to regenerate the free protein thiol and oxidized glutathione (GSSG).

proteins formed from these *ipso* adducts contribute to hepatocellular damage. First, both hepatic nonprotein and protein thiols are oxidized in mice within the first few hours after administration of hepatotoxic doses of acetaminophen (136,179). Second, some thiol compounds protect against hepatocellular injury caused by acetaminophen and NAPQI without significantly decreasing the levels of acetaminophen protein adducts (188–191). Third, 3′-hydroxyacetaminophen covalently binds to proteins but causes very little protein thiol oxidation and is relatively nonhepatotoxic (136,188). Finally, the time course of increases in GSSG concentrations in hepatic tissue in the pathogenesis of acetaminophen toxicity is consistent with the resynthesis of GSH a few hours after its initial rapid depletion by both covalent interaction with NAPQI and formation of protein *ipso* adducts of NAPQI (Fig. 4), and is consistent with reaction of the newly synthesized GSH with the *ipso* adducts to form GSSG and *S*-glutathionylated proteins (56,134,188). Alternatively, increases in GSSG in hepatocytes, observed particularly in mitochondria, does occur in the 4–6-h time period after acetaminophen administration when hepatocytes begin to show overt signs of pathophysiological damage, and may simply be a result of tissue injury (138,192–194).

3. Lipid Peroxidation and Related Oxidative Events

Although some products of lipid peroxidation have been observed in mice and rats after hepatotoxic doses of acetaminophen (195–197), the products generally appear after hepatic damage has commenced, whereas they occur in the initiation stages of liver injury caused by such agents as carbon tetrachloride (198–201). In humans, F_2-isoprostanes were measured as a sensitive marker of lipid peroxidation and were significantly (~9-fold) elevated in the plasma of 10 patients with acute liver and renal failure associated with acetaminophen overdose (202), but this was most likely late in the course after severe injury since serum F_2-isoprostanes are not elevated in the first 6 h after hepatotoxic doses of acetaminophen in rats (201).

Other products of oxidative stress potentially caused by acetaminophen radicals and their secondary oxyradical products include protein carbonyls. However, these products were not increased in rats administered hepatotoxic doses of acetaminophen, though they were increased with the hepatotoxic redox cycling compound diquat (203). Protein carbonyls were modestly elevated in livers of mice administered hepatotoxic doses of acetaminophen, but only when the mice were pretreated with ferrous sulfate (204). It is also noteworthy that agents that protect against radical-mediated oxidant stress, such as the iron chelator deferoxamine, can delay the development, but not decrease the extent, of hepatotoxicity caused by acetaminophen (205–207). Again, the data suggest that oxyradical-mediated oxidant events are not initiating events in the course of acetaminophen hepatotoxicity, but rather occur later, likely as a result of Kupffer cell activation (208,209), and protection afforded against acetaminophen hepatotoxicity by such agents as liposome-encapsulated superoxide dismutase in vivo in rats (210) is most likely related to scavenging of superoxide generated by phagocytic cells.

One mechanism for radical-mediated oxidation would be redox cycling of NAPQI. Although the semiquinone imine radical of NAPQI can be formed either by one-electron oxidation of acetaminophen by cyclooxygenases (211,212) and peroxidases (213,214), or by one-electron reduction of NAPQI (215,216), the semiquinone imine radical has a relatively high redox potential that would not favor direct reduction of oxygen to the superoxide radical anion (217). However, superoxide anion may be generated in coupled reactions of the semiquinone imine with glutathione or NAD(P)H (218,219) or the ferrous-oxy form of cytochrome P450 (220). Thus, we cannot rule out the possibility that, under some conditions, radical-mediated oxidant stress may play a role in the initiating events leading to hepatocellular injury, and new functional genomic and proteomic approaches may help resolve this issue.

III. LATE EVENTS IN ACETAMINOPHEN-INDUCED HEPATOTOXICITY

A. Introduction

According to the "covalent binding hypothesis," the events that follow bioactivation and covalent modification of cellular macromolecules by reactive metabolite(s) result in subsequent chemically induced cell death and organ damage. In the case of liver injury produced by acetaminophen, an unequivocal causal relationship between the loss of function of a protein "target" and eventual cell death has not yet been demonstrated. Nonetheless, the molecular mechanisms of acetaminophen-induced hepatotoxicity represent an active area of research with considerable relevance to other drug- and chemically induced injuries. In this section more recent studies will be reviewed, in particular those utilizing transgenic or knockout approaches. Where possible, these will be placed into perspective with the considerable body of work available on acetaminophen-mediated hepatotoxicity.

For ease of study, the organ damage produced by acetaminophen can be subdivided into two components, namely an initial (or *intrinsic*) cell death phase followed by a delayed (or *extrinsic*) phase. These correlate approximately with the stage 1 and stage 2 classifications of Bessems and Vermeulen (2). The intrinsic phase is widely believed to result from the loss of a critical cellular function(s) after covalent modification of an important target protein or proteins. Although many biochemical parameters associated with the typical centrilobular hepatocyte death observed after acetaminophen overdose have been studied, especially in animal systems, the consequences of such alterations to cellular homeostasis are still mostly unknown. As will be discussed further below, the pathological sequelae of acetaminophen-induced hepatotoxicity are likely to be considerably more complex than outlined by Prescott in 1996; i.e., "Overall, the probable mechanism was depletion of cellular glutathione by *N*-acetyl-*p*-benzoquinone imine followed by covalent binding to, and oxidative depletion of, protein thiol groups causing disturbances of intermediary metabolism and calcium homeostasis" (1, p. 330).

The extrinsic phase of acetaminophen-induced liver injury is equated with the recruitment of immune surveillance and represents the response to loss of cellular integrity during the intrinsic phase. Consequently, this phase of acetaminophen-induced hepatotoxicity adds to the complexity of the initial intrinsic damage with the addition of cytokine/chemokine mediators and further nonparenchymal and nonhepatic cell types. With such increased complexity the probability for simple therapeutic interventions may be appropriately decreased, although recent animal studies have shown promise in protecting against hepatotoxicity by inhibiting aspects of the extrinsic inflammatory response. At present the only clinical strategy of choice for the treatment of acetaminophen-induced hepatotoxicity remains *N*-acetylcysteine (221). The benefit of *N*-acetylcysteine is maximal early after poisoning, most likely either by increasing intracellular GSH levels or by acting as an antioxidant during the intrinsic phase, but can be useful for late presenters (10–24 h). The prospect remains that more effective clinical strategies to treat acetaminophen-induced hepatotoxicity, or other drug-induced hepatotoxicities, will result from the interest now evident in the mechanistic aspects of intrinsic cell death and modifications to the extrinsic pathway of damage to the liver.

B. The Intrinsic Cell Death Pathway

Historically, the mechanisms of acetaminophen-induced cell death have focused on the broad classifications of protein modification by arylation or indices of cellular oxidative stress (e.g., lipid peroxidation; see above) (137,150,204). The hepatotoxicity produced from an excessive acetaminophen dose is distinctive in that both protein covalent modification events *and* oxidative stress appear to be important in the final development of (cyto)toxicity. Nonetheless, as indicated earlier, the relative contribution of protein modification in comparison to cellular redox alterations has not been well defined for acetaminophen-induced cytotoxicity.

In short, although an excellent correlation has generally been observed between the extent of damage and the magnitude and location of covalent binding, some studies have dissociated the two phenomena (222–224). There are no examples, however, where cell death or liver injury caused by acetaminophen has been shown in the absence of covalent binding of the reactive intermediate(s). This has led to a paradigm shift favoring the existence of critical protein targets in the ultimate expression of acetaminophen-induced cell death. As detailed earlier and in Table 2, proteomic and more traditional protein identification methods have identified a complete complement of cellular proteins modified by NAPQI. Their identities provide support for the perturbation of cellular homeostasis by redox and nonredox mechanisms (refer, for example, to arylation of the proteasome C8 subunit, ATP synthetase α subunit, thioredoxin reductase, and GSH peroxidase) (151). Significantly, some of the most prominently modified proteins either have no known biological function (i.e., selenium- or acetaminophen-binding protein) or have many functions (glyceraldehyde-3-phosphate dehydrogenase) (225). Moreover, many in vitro studies, using modifying agents such as antioxidants or metal ion chelators (226), have indicated that cellular oxidative stress plays a significant factor in acetaminophen-induced acute cytotoxicity (227,228). These studies also invariably indicate that injury progression can be delayed but not totally inhibited. In comparison, there have been relatively few in vivo studies that address the role of reactive oxygen species (ROS) in acetaminophen-mediated cell death. Furthermore, although methodological considerations frequently limit direct comparison, many studies appear in conflict (136,161,229–231). As a specific example, Gupta and colleagues (161) have recently confirmed their earlier work indicating no protein sulfhydryl (PSH) loss after acetaminophen treatment yet Birge and co-workers (231)—using essentially identical procedures of monobromobimane fluorescence and gel electrophoresis—found clear PSH losses. A further limitation is that the extent of inhibition of damage by antioxidant or chelator treatment in vivo is usually far less than that observed with "comparable" in vitro studies (207,232).

There are, however, carefully designed in vivo studies that are strongly suggestive of a ROS contribution and these provide a basis for ultimately resolving this intriguing issue (210,233,234). These are discussed further in the following section and are noteworthy as an illustration of the extent of protection, or exacerbation, of damage possible in various transgenic lines modulating responses to ROS production.

1. Glutathione and Other Detoxification Pathways in Acetaminophen-Induced Hepatotoxicity

Transgenic and knockout animal studies have offered the promise of resolving these questions and also providing new avenues for the study of acetaminophen-induced hepatotoxicity. The findings to date, however, have only added to the enigma that is acetaminophen-induced cell death and liver injury. Nowhere is the conflict between traditional biochemical toxicology and more recent genetically based animal studies more apparent than with the role of nucleophilic tripeptide glutathione (GSH) in detoxification. Conjugative (phase 2) metabolism of acetaminophen with GSH has generally been considered straightforward—if not trivial. Consequently, enzymatic or nonenzymatic nucleophilic addition of GSH with NAPQI is thought to provide the terminal metabolic step in the liver. Several new studies, from diverse sources, now challenge this simplistic view and provide renewed interest in the field.

Henderson et al. (233) have examined the absence of glutathione S-transferase isozymes Pi1 and Pi2 on acetaminophen-induced hepatotoxicity. Contrary to expectations the homozygously deficient $GstP1/P2$ $(-/-)$ animals were protected from the hepatotoxic effects of acetaminophen. Protection in the nulled animals could not be attributed to alterations in bioactivation of acetaminophen to NAPQI as acetaminophen metabolism and binding were unaffected. Moreover, in keeping with the extent of liver damage, resistant $GstP1/P2$ $(-/-)$ animals showed a good recovery of hepatic glutathione to near-normal levels after an initial decline whereas no recovery was evident in $GstP1/P2$ $(+/+)$ animals. The rebound in free hepatic GSH in the $GstP1/P2$ $(-/-)$ group after acetaminophen administration is consistent with an upregulation of novel compensatory processes to prevent cellular redox status changes and may even be compatible with the recently proposed function for selenium/acetaminophen-binding proteins as redox stress sensors (2). Alternatively, upregulation of either γ-glutamylcysteine synthetase or glutathione synthetase may be occurring. The authors, however, report no change in the content of either of these GSH synthetic enzymes and enzymatic activities were not determined. Given the poor correlation between γ-glutamylcysteine synthetase protein levels and activity (235) it will be of interest to determine γ-glutamylcysteine synthetase activities in *GstP1/P2* (−/−) mice in the future.

These findings also hint at additional, as yet uncharacterized, functions for GST Pi within the hepatocyte. This possibility is raised with the observation that GST Pi activity inhibits Jun *N*-terminal kinase (JNK). Consequently, removal of GST Pi activity may constitutively activate JNK, a condition associated with the induction of cell death by apoptosis (236). On a more speculative note, GST Pi may be involved in glutathiolation pathways thereby inhibiting signal-transducing activities such as protein tyrosine phosphatase 1B (237)—an activity also inhibited with excessive acetaminophen concentrations (187). Potential transport of NAPQI from its site of generation in the endoplasmic reticulum to mitochondria and other target organelles may be made possible via transient *ipso* adduct formation (see above) with GST. Consequently, the removal of the GST protein target could decrease intracellular transport of the reactive intermediate, thereby limiting damage within the hepatocyte.

Finally, it should be emphasized that GST Pi is itself arylated by acetaminophen (151) (Table 2). As will be discussed below, this is likely to impact on the cellular homeostasis of GST Pi deficient transgenic animals following acetaminophen overdose.

The intriguing observations of Henderson et al. (233) are supported by the complementary findings of Rzucidlo et al. (238), who examined acetaminophen hepatotoxicity in animals with elevated GSH levels via transgenic overexpression of glutathione synthetase. Again, contrary to expectation, elevated hepatic GSH levels failed to protect against acetaminophen-induced damage. Both biochemical and histopathological criteria indicated increased hepatic injury in the transgenic animals with ≥200% elevation of serum ALT levels and increased severity and extent of centrilobular necrosis. Moreover, the level of hepatotoxicity was further increased by injection of the GSH synthetase substrate γ-glutamylcysteine ethyl ester (γ-GCE), which resulted in additional liver GSH levels. Although evidence for nephrotoxicity was minimal in nontransgenic animals, it was clearly evident in acetaminophen-treated GSH-overproducing transgenics presumably via downstream mercapturate pathway processing of systemically elevated acetaminophen-GSH conjugate.

A comprehensive study of the effects of transgenic overexpression of three enzymes important in protection against ROS, namely glutathione peroxidase extracellular form (GPe), glutathione peroxidase intracellular form (GPi), and Cu/Zn-SOD (SOD1), was undertaken by Mirochnitchenko et al. (234). The results indicated that overexpression of either GPe or SOD1 resulted in near-total protection from acetaminophen-induced hepatotoxicity and morbidity indicating that circulating levels of ROS contribute significantly to the ultimate expression of injury. Moreover, Mirochnitchenko et al. (234) observed that intravenously injected glutathione peroxidase protected against subsequent acetaminophen challenge, thereby elegantly confirming from two perspectives the earlier work of Nakae et al. (210). As further confirmation of many previous reports, the authors also observed a lack of correlation between hepatotoxicity and animal survival with the level of lipid peroxidation.

However, in a surprising finding that parallels the observations of Henderson et al. (233) and Rzucidlo et al. (238), transgenic overexpression of GPi produced considerably more hepatotoxicity and decreased survival (234). One possible interpretation of these data is that GPi overexpression results in an alteration of the cellular redox setpoint toward reductive stress, thereby increasing intrinsic injury. The complexity of this issue is illustrated by the growing body of evidence indicating that there is a fine line between cellular protection and cellular toxicity with regard to ROS production. For example, using knock-out transgenic animal models, the importance of Mn-SOD (SOD2) and Cu/Zn-SOD (SOD1) in protecting against ROS-mediated damage has been shown (239–242). However, enzymes that metabolize reactive oxygen species can also have prooxidant effects depending on the level of expression and the balance with other enzymes. As with the present case of GPi overexpression in acetaminophen-mediated injury, there are examples of SOD overexpression resulting in increased ROS production and cell death (243,244). We note here again that the increased toxicity associated with GPi overexpression is in a protein previously identified as a target for the reactive metabolite of acetaminophen (151) (Table 2). The potential significance of this is discussed later.

In contrast to traditional biochemical toxicology studies (e.g., 245–247) the unexpected findings from these transgenic and knockout experiments require an examination of the role of GSH conjugation in acetaminophen metabolism and toxicity. The acetaminophen-GSH conjugate itself may have cytotoxic potential possibly from further metabolism within the hepatocyte and warrants further investigation.

The data of Mirochnitchenko et al. (234) indicating a sizable oxidative stress component to acetaminophen-induced liver damage are supported by the findings of Enomoto et al. (247). Substantial, but not complete, protection from acetaminophen-induced liver damage was evident using very young mice deficient in the antioxidant-responsive element (ARE)-directed transcription factor NRF2 (247). As several important detoxification enzymes (notably catalase, SOD1, γ-glutamylcysteine synthetase, and UDP-GTs) are under ARE control, these findings suggest the important contribution of these components in the detoxification pathways of acetaminophen metabolism. However, the authors did not confirm the contribution of oxidative stress more specifically by assessing catalase and/or SOD1 activities in $nfr2$ $(-/-)$ animals, inasmuch as upregulation of γ-glutamylcysteine synthetase and UDP-GTs can protect by mechanisms unrelated to oxidative stress.

General agreement exists for a protective role for metallothionein during acetaminophen-induced hepatotoxicity. Both Rofe et al. (248) and Liu et al. (249) have observed an exacerbation of injury in mice nulled in both the metallothionein-I and metallothionein-II genes [MT $(-/-)$]. Rofe et al. (248) observed large increases in biochemical indices of hepatotoxicity, and commensurate alterations to plasma and tissue zinc levels, with MT $(-/-)$ mice after acetaminophen dosing. Of relevance to the mechanism of injury was the observation that toxicity was not found when glycolytic capacity, and presumably hepatic ATP, were maintained (see below). Essentially identical findings were observed by Liu and colleagues (249) with only minor discrepancies likely attributable to variations in the genetic background of the animals (i.e., mice were less sensitive to acetaminophen). Both studies attribute the protective effects of metallothionein I and II to the antioxidant properties of metallothionein although other mechanisms were not considered. For example, the contribution of changes in cellular zinc levels on apoptotic processes should not be underestimated. Liu and colleagues (249) further proposed, by association, an early lipid peroxidation component to injury. As a corollary, the possibility remains that the protective effects observed with $nrf2$ $(-/-)$ mice (247) are mediated in part via metallothionein I, since metallothionein I is regulated by the ARE (250).

2. Cell Biology of Acetaminophen-Induced Cytotoxicity

The downstream cellular responses to acetaminophen-initiated damage are clearly multifaceted and complex. These pleiotypic effects include the well-studied examples of GSH depletion, cellular redox imbalances, oxidation of protein thiols, and alterations to calcium homeostasis with associated DNA fragmentations (reviewed in refs. 1,2,6,127,150,204). Other cell biological changes are only now being addressed. These include, but may not be limited to:

Arylation-mediated disruption of protein structure and induction of stress proteins
Organellar/cellular effects of ATP/NAD(P)H declines following inhibition of intermediary metabolism (e.g., autophagy and/or mitochondrial proliferation)
Perturbations of cellular regulatory and housekeeping pathways (e.g. proteolysis)
Pathological changes to signal transduction pathways

How these areas integrate with the mechanism of cell death and the identities of proteins modified by reactive intermediate(s) of acetaminophen is not known, but exciting glimpses of future directions are becoming evident. For example, stress proteins are induced during acetaminophen-induced injury as might be expected from the protein-denaturing capacity of acetaminophen-reactive intermediate(s) (251). In particular, the inducible form of cytosolic stress protein 70 kDa (HSP70i) and HSP25 are elevated following acetaminophen exposure within, or proximal to, the area of damage. In comparison, HSP70i or HSP25 were not induced following treatment with the relatively nonhepatotoxic isomer 3′-hydroxyacetanilide, despite equivalent levels of reactive intermediate binding. The authors attribute these differences to the specific targets adducted by acetaminophen in comparison to 3′-hydroxyacetanilide. This is supported by the published and preliminary findings that acetaminophen hepatotoxicity is distinguished by covalent modification of mitochondrial proteins (134,155,252).

The data of Salminen and colleagues (251) are given additional significance with recent reports indicating that HSP70i can bind to, and inhibit, APAF1 (cytosolic apoptotic protease activating factor 1). When fully active, APAF1 is a large complex consisting of cytochrome c, procaspase 9, and dATP/ATP that is of central importance to apoptotic cell death (253,254).

Considerable debate and confusion surround the mechanism of acetaminophen-induced intrinsic cell death (i.e., prior to immune system involvement). Acetaminophen-induced cell death and hepatotoxicity have been traditionally viewed as necrotic, although some recent studies have proposed an apoptotic component (232,255). In keeping with HSP70i induction and inhibition of APAF1 (251,253,254), two recent studies have failed to find evidence of caspase activation after hepatotoxic doses of acetaminophen (246,256). As the caspase family of proteases represents the primary proteolytic component of the better-studied examples of apoptosis, these studies would appear to negate an apoptotic involvement in acetaminophen-mediated cell death. Our own data support the relative absence of caspase activation with marginal, and most likely biologically insignificant, increases in caspase-3-like (DEVDase), caspase-9 and caspase-6 levels during acetaminophen treatment in vivo (257) or in vitro (258). Nonetheless, we have observed alterations to hepatic subcellular processing and localization of the proapoptotic BCL-2 family member, BAX, very early after acetaminophen administration (257). Moreover, acetaminophen-induced cytotoxicity can be efficiently prevented by overexpression of BCL-X$_L$, the predominant antiapoptotic BCL-2 family member found in the liver (259,260).

Consequently, given these conflicting signals occurring early in the intrinsic cell death process, it may not be appropriate to classify acetaminophen-induced cell death as either apoptotic or necrotic. The question that should be addressed then is "What are the defining attributes of acetaminophen-induced cell death?" instead of "Is acetaminophen-mediated cell death apoptotic or necrotic?" Moreover, increasing evidence now points not

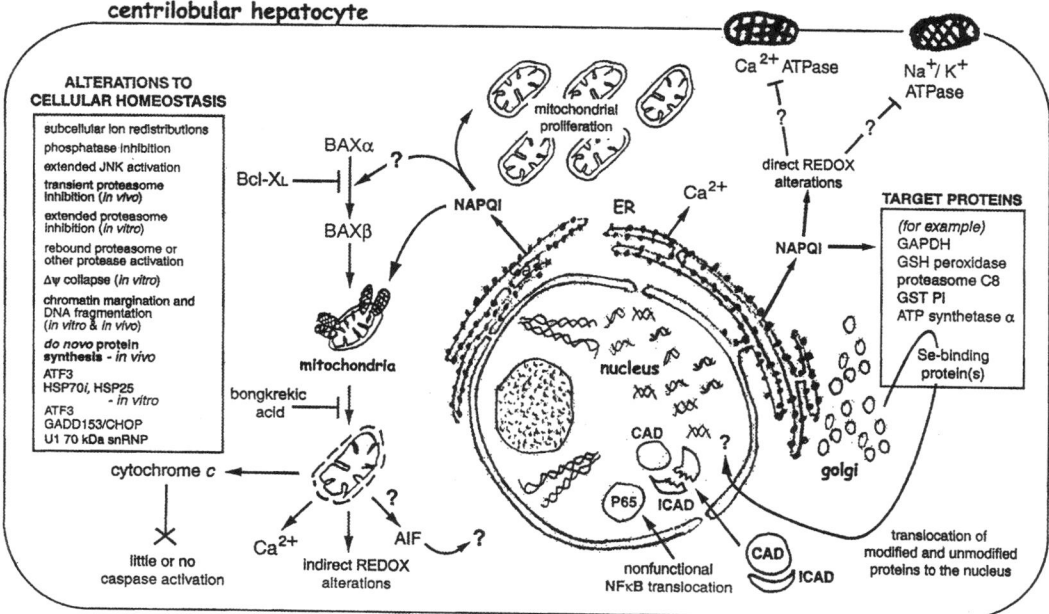

Figure 5 Depiction of several cellular organelles and biochemical pathways that appear to be affected in the hepatocyte as a result of NAPQI formation from acetaminophen and that appear to be involved in the pathogenesis of hepatocellular injury. The scheme does not include events and pathways extrinsic to the hepatocyte (see text for discussion).

to a bipolar pattern of physiological or pathological cell death. Instead, a spectrum of characteristics define cell death with apoptosis and necrosis occupying the extreme ends of the classification (261). From this viewpoint differing aspects of the cell death routine may be initiated depending on various factors, including ATP depletion (262) and/or the concentration of the toxicant (263). As discussed previously, excessive acetaminophen concentrations will result in the arylation of the ATP synthetase α subunit (151), and large depletions of cellular adenine pools (in particular ATP) are an early functional consequence of this modification (136,175,177–179). Such depletions of ATP (approximately 60% of total hepatic content, and probably near-complete depletion within the area of centrilobular damage) must clearly impact on a considerable number of cellular processes. Therefore, it is perhaps not surprising that changes in cell death phenotype are observed with modulations of cellular ATP content (264).

The multifaceted nature of the cellular events occurring in response to acetaminophen exposure is represented in Fig. 5 and is by necessity incomplete. A challenge for the future will be to determine the critical pathways ultimately determining cell death susceptibility amid this considerable complexity.

3. A Model for Future Genetic Studies Examining the Cell Biology of Acetaminophen-Induced Cytotoxicity

Aside from the well-studied examples of acetaminophen-induced lipid peroxidation and sulfhydryl/redox status, many of the cellular alterations occurring within the hepatocyte are mostly unexplored and represent nascent areas for investigation (Fig. 5). An important area that has received little attention to date is the impact of acetaminophen on the removal of abnormally folded proteins prior to aggregation. The unexpected results of Henderson et al. (233) and Mirochnitchenko et. al. (234) provide support for this as they share a common attribute, namely, the genetic modification of acetaminophen target proteins previously identified from proteomic studies. Since *both* GST Pi class and GPi are arylated (151), the extent of cell death may be particularly prone to either overexpression (234) or ablation (233) of the target protein. Consequently, overexpression of an acetaminophen target protein, irrespective of its biological function, may be expected to increase cell death and hepatotoxicity by providing a "sink" for generated reactive intermediates (NAPQI) (234). Under conditions of sizable ATP depletion the consequences of this would be overloading of the proteolytic quality control and removal systems of the hepatocyte (Fig. 6). The opposite would be true for ablation of an acetaminophen target, as indeed found by Henderson et al. (233), with protection of damage after removal of this important detoxification enzyme.

One would predict that, with cellular ATP depletion, the overexpression of any identified acetaminophen target protein would increase hepatotoxicity, whereas the null genotype would correspondingly prevent liver damage after acetaminophen dosing. Fortunately, there are many alternatives available from the list of identified acetaminophen target proteins to test this hypothesis (146,150,151). Finally, as has been observed throughout the literature, increased glycolysis and elevated cellular ATP levels can be hepatoprotective (248,265). Under conditions of surplus ATP, cellular proteolytic capacity is maintained and the elimination of acetaminophen-modified target proteins is not compromised (Fig. 6).

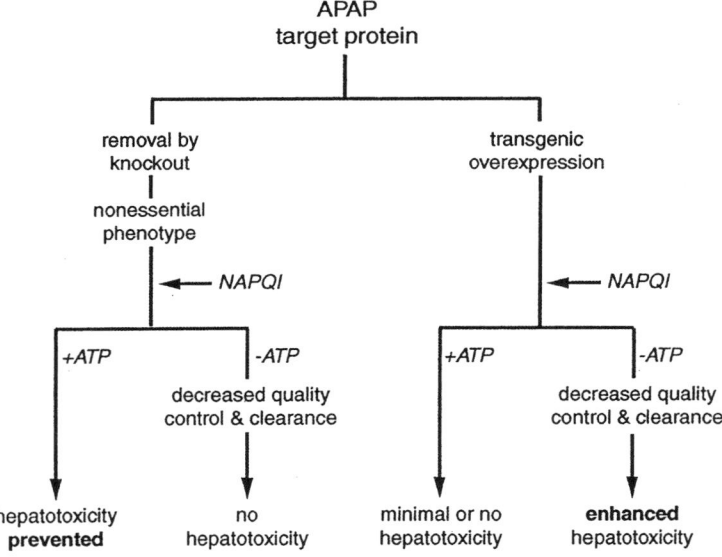

Figure 6   Hypothetical scheme for how the removal or overexpression of target proteins may affect hepatotoxic response to acetaminophen.

Determining the significant cell biological effects of acetaminophen-induced organ damage and its relationship to early adduction events appears to be the key to defining the mechanism of intrinsic cell death. How the hepatocyte responds to acetaminophen-mediated postadduction events will also likely reveal fundamental principles of the cellular response(s) to other hepatotoxicants.

C. The Extrinsic Cell Death Pathway

1. Role of Cytokine Mediators During Acetaminophen-Induced Liver Injury

The liver is an organ capable of mounting a major inflammatory response. Up to 35% of all liver cells are nonparenchymal (constituting the sinusoidal endothelium, Kupffer cells, and Ito cells). These cell types, in addition to infiltrating cells such as macrophages, are implicated in both the protective and the pathological (i.e., necrosis/fibrosis) responses of immune activation (266–268).

Although many cytokines/chemokines have been proposed to participate in the responses to acetaminophen exposure, the proinflammatory mediators have come under the most scrutiny. The role of inflammation in acetaminophen-mediated liver injury is complex with many proinflammatory mediators being implicated (e.g., TNF, Fas, IL-6/8, MIP-2, MCP-1). With the influx of activated cells such as macrophages, neutrophils, and monocytes comes the involvement of nitric oxide, superoxide anions, and other ROS. The release of proteases from degranulation events further adds to the complexity. Nonetheless, good evidence points to the potential for increased injury after hepatotoxicant exposure as a result of such proinflammatory processes (269). As a consequence, the possibility exists for the prevention of injury with treatments designed to inhibit extrinsic injury. As mentioned earlier, Mirochnitchenko et al. (234) have observed substantial success in preventing mortality after acetaminophen treatment in a transgenic mouse line overexpressing serum GPe enzyme. These data ultimately hold promise for a clinical alternative to N-acetylcysteine since GPe would act at the level of inhibiting circulating ROS and peroxides during the extrinsic (delayed) phase of injury progression.

Other strategies have also been employed to block inflammation and inhibit the severity of extrinsic hepatitis after acetaminophen overdose. In a novel study, effective protection against acetaminophen-induced hepatotoxicity was observed in mice treated with an antisense oligonucleotide (ISIS 22023) specifically directed to inhibit Fas/CD95 expression as confirmed by a sensitive ribonuclease protection assay (270). These promising findings are in agreement with other studies that indicate a role for TNF in the delayed progression of acetaminophen-mediated liver injury (271,272). However, an important caveat is provided. The authors note that ISIS 22023 was not effective at higher doses of acetaminophen, which "suggests that a reduction of Fas expression can reduce the severity of liver damage caused by low dose, but cannot completely block the effects of high doses of (acetaminophen)." Furthermore, the relative effectiveness of Fas-directed antisense treatments with a more clinically relevant protocol was not examined. It would have been of particular interest to determine the relative effectiveness of ISIS 22023 given at increasing intervals after acetaminophen exposure. Under these more clinically realistic scenarios, any reductions to the severity of hepatotoxicity (e.g., >12 h after acetaminophen) would constitute an improvement on current N-acetylcysteine strategies (221).

The redundancy in function of proinflammatory mediators is illustrated by the well-conducted TNF/lymphotoxin-α knockout studies of Boess et al. (273) and by analysis of

TNF genotype in patients presenting with severe acetaminophen-induced hepatotoxicity (274). Both studies concluded that TNF, or more widely sepsis, was unlikely to be a primary factor in this form of hepatotoxicity. The complex interrelationship between acetaminophen and the extrinsic immune response is also highlighted by an observation that acetaminophen itself can inhibit Fas/CD95 activation at the level of downstream caspase-3 activation thereby blocking resultant apoptosis (256).

Taken collectively, the failure of ISIS 22023 and TNF receptor knockouts to prevent hepatotoxicity at higher doses of acetaminophen argues for the importance of other mediators in the acetaminophen-generated extrinsic pathway. Indeed, TNF ligands and receptors have many members and are accorded superfamily status (275). The apoptotic actions of several proinflammatory agents, e.g., TNF and IL-1β, are considered to be mediated by nitric oxide (NO). During inflammation an excessive production of reactive nitrogen and oxygen species is typical, and the term "nitrosative stress" has been proposed as the nitrosative counterpart of oxidative stress (276). However, NO is also associated with antiapoptotic actions and recent work indicates that these apparent discrepancies can be rationalized based on the concentration of NO and duration of release (277). The prevailing opinion is that of a continuum with nitosative events, mediated through NO, serving signaling functions whereas more irreversible oxidative modifications are associated with toxicity (278). In this manner protein nitrosylation can be envisaged to either provide transient cellular protection against damage or initiate cell death programs in the longer term.

Protein nitrotyrosine formation has been detected after acetaminophen administration and, in addition, the subsequent acetaminophen-induced liver damage can be mostly prevented with inhibitors of macrophage activation (e.g., gadolinium chloride or dextran sulfate) without observable inhibition of the extent of acetaminophen bioactivation (279–283). Nonetheless, these animal studies have all required prior treatment with inhibitors of macrophage/Kupffer cell activation. The relative effectiveness of more clinically realistic treatment regimes, i.e., administration at increasing intervals after acetaminophen dosing, is important and not known at present.

As with other areas in NO research, many issues that impact on the role of nitrosative stress during acetaminophen-mediated injury have not yet been adequately defined. S-Nitrosylation, particularly of cysteine thiols, is a major component of the biological effects of NO (278) and has not yet been detected in acetaminophen-mediated hepatotoxicity. Furthermore, the identification of nitrotyrosylated proteins in the area of centrilobular damage is correlative only. Despite this good correlation, further studies will be needed to identify nitrosylated proteins and relate protein identity to cell death in mechanistic terms. For example, a speculation raised recently is that phosphatidylinositol 3-kinase may be a nitrosylated species during acetaminophen-induced hepatotoxicity (280). If confirmed, this would still fall short of a causal relationship between phosphatidylinositol 3-kinase and acetaminophen-induced cell death.

IV. CONCLUSIONS

Recent work has raised the possibilities of novel and more effective strategies to treat accidental or intentional acetaminophen-induced hepatotoxicity. For example, confirmation of a central role for BAX in the early cellular response to acetaminophen, as has been shown for the CNS toxicant 1-methyl-4-phenyl-1,2,3,6-tetrahydropyridine (284), may allow for the therapeutic use of low-molecular-weight inhibitors of BAX oligomerization to prevent early events in acetaminophen-induced hepatotoxicity.

The possibility of effective, yet safe, inhibitors of the extrinsic response will allow for treatment beyond the current time window available with N-acetylcysteine. However, the lack of therapeutic strategies that stem from research in the secondary, extrinsic pathway argues for a degree of immune complexity that may preclude effective clinical strategies. Given this multifactorial complexity of the inflammatory response to acetaminophen-mediated intrinsic injury, it may not be surprising if treatments designed to specifically modulate only one chemokine/cytokine will turn out to be of limited clinical applicability. Nonetheless, recent work with animal models holds considerable promise for future developments in this area.

In conclusion, determining the significant cell biological aspects of acetaminophen-induced hepatotoxicity remains a formidable problem. How the hepatocyte responds to the initiation of damage via protein adduction will undoubtedly reveal fundamental aspects of hepatocyte biology and its response to external stress. In addition, the elucidation of functions for the protein targets of NAPQI will provide information with respect to basic processes in cell biology (e.g., protein processing, transport, and compartmentation). Acetaminophen-induced hepatotoxicity, now considered an excellent model for chemically induced cell death, is still an enigma and remains a challenge despite over 20 years of intensive study.

REFERENCES

1. Prescott LF. Paracetamol (Acetaminophen): A Critical Bibliographic Review. London: Taylor & Francis, 1996.
2. Bessems JGM, Vermeulen, NPE. Paracetamol (acetaminophen)-induced toxicity: molecular and biochemical mechanisms, analogues and protective approaches. Crit Rev Toxicol 2001; 31:55–138.
3. Blakely P, McDonald BR. Acute renal failure due to acetaminophen ingestion: a case report and review of the literature. J Am Soc Nephrol 1995; 6:48–53.
4. De Broe ME, Elseviers MM. Analgesic nephropathy. N Engl J Med 1998; 338:446–452.
5. Feinstein AR, Heinemann LAJ, Curham GC, Delzell E, DeSchepper PJ, Fox JM, Graf H, Luft FC, Michielsen P, Mihatsch MJ Suissa S, van der Woude F, Willich S. Relationship between nonphenacetin combined analgesics and nephropathy: a review. Kidney Int 2000; 58:2259–2264.
6. Hinson JA. Biochemical toxicology of acetaminophen. Rev Biochem Toxicol 1980; 2:103–130.
7. Black M. Acetaminophen hepatotoxicity. Annu Rev Med 1984; 35:577–593.
8. Schiødt FV, Rochling FA, Casey DL, Lee WM. Acetaminophen toxicity in an urban county hospital. N Engl J Med 1997; 337:1112–1117.
9. Makin AJ, Wendon J, Williams R. A 7-year experience of severe acetaminophen-induced hepatotoxicity (1987–1993). Gastroenterology 1995; 109:1907–1916.
10. Gow PJ, Smallwood RA, Angus PW. Paracetamol overdose in a liver transplantation centre: an 8-year experience. J Gastroenterol Hepatatol 1999; 14:817–821.
11. Litovitz TL, Klein-Schwartz W, Dyer KS, Shannon M, Lee S, Powers M. Annual report of the American Association of Poison Control Centers toxic exposure surveillance system. Am J Emerg Med 1998; 16:443–497.
12. Vale JA, Proudfoot AT. Paracetamol (acetaminophen) poisoning. Lancet 1995; 346:547–552.
13. Lee WM, personal communication, 2000.
14. Price MI, Thomas SHL, James OFW, Hudson M. Reduction in incidence of severe paracetamol poisoning. Lancet 2000; 355:2047–2048.

15. Turvill JL, Burroughs AK, Moore KP. Changes in occurrence of paracetamol overdose in UK after introduction of blister packs. Lancet 2000; 355:2048–2049.

16. Eder H. Chronic toxicity studies on phenacetin, *N*-acetyl-*p*-aminophenol (NAPA) and acetyl-salicylic acid on cats. Acta Pharmacol Toxicol 1964;21:197–204.

17. Boyd EM, Bereczky GM. Liver necrosis from paracetamol. Br J Pharmacol 1966; 26:606–614.

18. Davidson DGD, Eastham WN. Acute liver necrosis following overdose of paracetamol. Br Med J 1966; 2:497–499.

19. Thomson JS, Prescott LF. Liver damage and impaired glucose tolerance after paracetamol overdosage. Br Med J 1966; 2:506–507.

20. Mitchell JR, Jollow DJ, Potter WZ, Davis DC, Gillette JR, Brodie BB. Acetaminophen-induced hepatic necrosis. I. Role of drug metabolism. J Pharmacol Exp Ther 1973; 187:185–194.

21. Jollow DJ, Mitchell JR, Potter WZ, Davis DC, Gillette JR, Brodie BB. Acetaminophen-induced hepatic necrosis. II. Role of covalent binding in vivo. J Pharmacol Exp Ther 1973; 187:195–202.

22. Potter WZ, Davis DC, Mitchell JR, Jollow DJ, Gillette JR, Brodie BB. Acetaminophen-induced hepatic necrosis. III. Cytochrome P-450–mediated covalent binding in vitro. J Pharmacol Exp Ther 1973; 187:203–210.

23. Mitchell JR, Jollow DJ, Potter WZ, Gillette JR, Brodie BB. Acetaminophen-induced hepatic necrosis. IV. Protective role of glutathione. J Pharmacol Exp Ther 1973; 187:211–217.

24. Mitchell JR, Thorgeirsson SS, Potter WZ, Jollow DJ, Keiser H. Acetaminophen-induced hepatic injury: protective role of glutathione in man and rationale for therapy. Clin Pharmacol Ther 1974; 16:676–684.

25. Smilkstein MJ, Knapp GL, Kulig KW, Rumack BH. Efficacy of oral *N*-acetylcysteine in the treatment of acetaminophen overdose: analysis of the National Multicenter Study (1975 to 1985). N Engl J Med 1988; 319:1557–1562.

26. Routledge P, Vale JA, Bateman DN, Johnston GD, Jones A, Judd A, Thomas S, Volans G, Prescott LF, Proudfoot A. Paracetamol (acetaminophen) poisoning: no need to change current guidelines to accident departments. Br Med J 1998; 317:1609–1611.

27. Nelson SD. Analgesic-antipyretics. In: RH Levy, KE Thummel, WF Trager, PD Hansten, ME Eichelbaum, eds. Metabolic Drug Interactions. Philadelphia: Lippincott Williams & Wilkins, 2000:447–455.

28. Nelson SD. Molecular mechanisms of the hepatotoxicity caused by acetaminophen. Semin Liver Dis 1990; 10:267–278.

29. Burchell B, Brierley CH, Rance D. Specificity of human UDP-glucuronosyltransferases and xenobiotic glucuronidation. Life Sci 1995; 57:1819–1831.

30. Duffel MW. Sulfotransferases. In: FP Guengerich, ed. Comprehensive Toxicology. Vol. 3. Biotransformation. Oxford: Elsevier, 1997:365–383.

31. deMorais SMF, Chow SYM, Wells PG. Biotransformation and toxicity of acetaminophen in congenic RHA rats with or without a hereditary deficiency in bilirubin UDP-glucuronosyl-transferase. Toxicol Appl Pharmacol 1992; 117:81–87.

32. Court MH, Greenblatt DJ. Molecular basis for deficient acetaminophen glucuronidation in cats. Biochem Pharmacol 1997; 53:1041–1047.

33. deMorais SMF, Uetrecht JP, Wells PG. Decreased glucuronidation and increased bioactivation of acetaminophen in Gilbert's syndrome. Gastroenterology 1992; 102:577–586.

34. Esteban A, Perez-Mateo M. Gilbert's disease: a risk factor for paracetamol overdosage? J Hepatol 1993; 18:247–258.

35. Richman DD, Fischl MA, Grieco MH, Gottlieb MS, Volberding PA, Laskin OL, Leedom JM, Groopman JE, Mildvan D, Hirsch MS, Jackson GG, Durack DT, Nusinoff-Lehrman S. AZT Collaborative Working Group: the toxicity of azidothymine (AZT) in the treatment of patients with AIDS and AIDS-related complex. N Engl J Med 1987; 317:192–197.

36. Nicholls AW, Caddick S, Wilson ID, Farrant RD, Lindon JC, Nicholson JK. High resolution NMR spectroscopic studies on the metabolism and futile deacetylation of 4-hydroxyacetanilide (paracetamol) in the rat. Biochem Pharmacol 1995; 49:1155–1164.

37. Newton JF, Kuo CH, DeShone GM, Hoeffle DF, Berstein J, Hook JB. The role of *p*-aminophenol in acetaminophen-induced nephrotoxicity: effect of bis(*p*-nitrophenyl) phosphate on acetaminophen and *p*-aminophenol nephrotoxicity and metabolism in Fischer 344 rats. Toxicol Appl Pharmacol 1985; 81:416–430.

38. Mugford CA, Tarloff JB. The contribution of oxidation and deacetylation to acetaminophen nephrotoxicity in female Sprague-Dawley rats. Toxicol Lett 1997; 93:15–22.

39. Rothen JP, Haefeli WE, Meyer UA, Todesco L, Wenk M. Acetaminophen is an inhibitor of hepatic *N*-acetyltransferase 2 in vitro and in vivo. Pharmacogenetics 1998; 8:553–559.

40. Dahlin DC, Miwa GT, Lu AYH, Nelson SD. *N*-Acetyl-*p*-benzoquinone imine: a cytochrome P-450-mediated oxidation product of acetaminophen. Proc Natl Acad Sci USA 1984; 81:1327–1331.

41. Hinson JA, Pohl LR, Gillette JR. *N*-Hydroxyacetaminophen: a microsomal metabolite of *N*-hydroxyphenacetin but apparently not acetaminophen. Life Sci 1979; 24:2133–2138.

42. Nelson SD, Forte AJ, Dahlin DC. Lack of evidence for *N*-hydroxyacetaminophen as a reactive metabolite of acetaminophen in vitro. Biochem Pharmacol 1980; 29:1617–1620.

43. Blair IA, Boobis AR, Davies DJ, Cresp TM. Paracetamol oxidation: synthesis and reactivity of *N*-acetyl-*p*-benzoquinone imine. Tetrahedron Lett 1980; 21:4947–4950.

44. Dahlin DC, Nelson SD. Synthesis, decomposition kinetics and preliminary toxicological studies on pure *N*-acetyl-*p*-benzoquinone imine, a proposed toxic metabolite of acetaminophen. J Med Chem 1982; 25:885–886.

45. Miner DJ, Kissinger PT. Evidence for the involvement of *N*-acetyl-*p*-benzoquinone imine in acetaminophen metabolism. Biochem Pharmacol 1979; 28:3285–3290.

46. Corcoran GB, Mitchell JR, Vaishnav YN, Horning EC. Evidence that acetaminophen and N-hydroxyacetaminophen form a common arylating intermediate, *N*-acetyl-*p*-benzoquinone imine. Mol Pharmacol 1980; 18:536–542.

47. Holme JA, Dahlin DC, Nelson SD, Dybing E. Cytotoxic effects of *N*-acetyl-*p*-benzoquinone imine, a common arylating intermediate of paracetamol and *N*-hydroxyparacetamol. Biochem Pharmacol 1984; 33:401–406.

48. Albano E, Rundgren M, Harvison PJ, Nelson SD, Moldéus P. Mechanisms of *N*-acetyl-*p*-benzoquinone imine cytotoxicity. Mol Pharmacol 1985; 280:306–311.

49. Nelson SD, Vaishnav Y, Kambara H, Baillie TA. Comparative EI, CD and FD mass spectra of some thioether metabolites of acetaminophen. Biomed Mass Spectrom 1981; 8:244–251.

50. Hinson JA, Monks TJ, Hong M, Highet RJ, Pohl LR. 3-(Gluthathione-*S*-yl) acetaminophen: a biliary metabolite of acetaminophen. Drug Metab Dispos 1982; 10:47–50.

51. Harvison PJ, Guengerich FP, Rashed MS, Nelson SD. Cytochrome P450 isozyme selectivity in the oxidation of acetaminophen. Chem Res Toxicol 1988; 1:47–52.

52. Slattery JTS, Wilson JM, Kalhorn TF, Nelson SD. Dose-dependent pharmacokinetics of acetaminophen: evidence of glutathione depletion in humans. Clin Pharmacol Ther 1987; 41:413–418.

53. Powis G, Svingen BA, Dahlin DC, Nelson SD. Enzymatic and nonenzymatic reduction of *N*-acetyl-*p*-benzoquinone imine. Biochem Pharmacol 1984; 33:2367–2370.

54. Powis G, See KL, Santone KS, Melder DC, Hodnett EM. Quinone imines as substrates for quinone reductase (NAD(P)H: (quinone-acceptor) oxido reductase) and the effect of dicoumarol on their cytotoxicity. Biochem Pharmacol 1987; 36:2473–2479.

55. Coles B, Wilson I, Wardman P, Hinson JA, Nelson SD, Ketterer B. The spontaneous and enzymatic reduction of *N*-acetyl-*p*-benzoquinone imine with glutathione: a stopped-flow kinetic study. Arch Biochem Biophys 1988; 264:253–260.

56. Chen W, Shockor JP, Tonge R, Hunter A, Gartner C, Nelson SD. Protein and nonprotein

cysteinyl thiol modification by *N*-acetyl-*p*-benzoquinone imine via a novel *ipso* adduct. Biochemistry 1999; 38:8159–8166.

57.   Hinson JA, Pohl LR, Monks TJ, Gillette JR, Guengerich FP. 3-Hydroxyacetaminophen: a microsomal metabolite of acetaminophen. Drug Metab Dispos 1980; 8:289–294.

58.   Forte AJ, Wilson JM, Slattery JT, Nelson SD. The formation and toxicity of catechol metabolites of acetaminophen in mice. Drug Metab Dispos 1984; 12:484–491.

59.   Regal KM. Caffeine as an active site probe of cytochrome P4501A2. Ph.D. dissertation, University of Washington, Seattle, 1998.

60.   Chen W, Koenigs LL, Thompson SJ, Peter RM, Rettie AE, Trager WF, Nelson, SD. Oxidation of acetaminophen to its toxicity quinone imine and nontoxic catechol metabolites by baculovirus-expressed and purified human cytochromes P450 2E1 and 2A6. Chem Res Toxicol 1998; 11:295–301.

61.   Chen W. Mechanistic studies on the formation of oxidative metabolites of acetaminophen. Ph.D. dissertation, University of Washington, Seattle, 1998.

62.   Dong H, Haining RL, Thummel KE, Rettie AE, Nelson SD. Involvement of human cytochrome P450 2D6 in the bioactivation of acetaminophen. Drug Metab Dispos 2000; 28: 1397–1400.

63.   Thummel KE, Lee CA, Kunze KL, Nelson SD, Slattery JT. Oxidation of acetaminophen to *N*-acetyl-*p*-benzoquinone imine by human CYP3A4. Biochem Pharmacol 1993; 45:1563–1569.

64.   Raucy JL, Lasker JM, Lieber CS, Black M. Acetaminophen activation by human liver cytochromes P450IIE1 and P450IA2. Arch Biochem Biophys 1989; 271:270–283.

65.   Pattern CJ, Thomas PE, Guy RL, Lee M, Gonzalez FJ, Guengerich FP, Yang CS. Cytochrome P450 enzymes involved in acetaminophen activation by rat and human liver microsomes and their kinetics. Chem Res Toxicol 1993; 6:511–518.

66.   Anderson KE, Schneider J, Pantuck EJ, Pantuck CB, Mudge GH, Welch RM, Conney AH, Kappas A. Acetaminophen metabolism in subjects fed charcoal-broiled beef. Clin Pharmacol Ther 1983; 34:369–374.

67.   Miners JO, Attwood J, Birkett DJ. Determinants of acetaminophen metabolism: effects of inducers and inhibitors of drug metabolism on acetaminophen's metabolic pathways. Clin Pharmacol Ther 1984; 35:480–486.

68.   Bock KW, Wiltfang J, Blume R, Ullrich D, Bircher J. Paracetamol as a test drug to determine glucuronide formation in man: effects of inducers and of smoking. Eur J Clin Pharmacol 1987; 32:677–683.

69.   Sarich T, Kalhorn T, Magee S, Al-Sayegh F, Adam S, Slattery J, Goldstein J, Nelson S, Wright J. The effect of omeprazole pretreatment on acetaminophen metabolism in rapid and slow metabolizers of *S*-mephenytoin. Clin Pharmacol Ther 1997; 62:21–28.

70.   Tonge RP, Kelly EJ, Bruschi SA, Kalhorn T, Eaton DL, Nebert DW, Nelson SD. Role of CYP1A2 in the hepatotoxicity of acetaminophen: investigations using *Cyp1a2* null mice. Toxicol Appl Pharmacol 1998; 153:102–108.

71.   Zaher H, Buters JTM, Ward JM, Bruno MK, Lucas AM, Stern ST, Cohen SD, Gonzalez FJ. Protection against acetaminophen toxicity in CYP1A2 and CYP2E1 double-null mice. Toxicol Appl Pharmacol 1998; 152:193–199.

72.   Lee SST, Buters JTM, Pineau T, Fernandez-Salguero P, Gonzalez FJ. Role of CYP2E1 in the hepatotoxicity of acetaminophen. J Biol Chem 1996; 271:12063–12067.

73.   Amouyal G, Larrey D, Letteron P, Genéve J, Labbe G, Belghiti J, Pessayre D. Effects of methoxsalen on the metabolism of acetaminophen in humans. Biochem Pharmacol 1987; 36: 2349–2352.

74.   Letteron P, Descatoire V, Larrey D, Degott C, Tinel M, Genéve J, Pessayre D. Pre- or post-treatment with methoxsalen prevents the hepatotoxicity of acetaminophen in mice. J Pharmacol Exp Ther 1986; 239:559–567.

75.   Johansson I, Lundquist E, Bertilsson L, Dahl ML, Sjoquist F, Ingelman-Sundberg M. Inher-

ited amplification of an active gene in the cytochrome P450 CYP2D locus as a cause of ultrarapid metabolism of debrisoquine. Proc Natl Acad Sci USA 1993; 90:P11825–11829.

76. Aklillu E, Persson I, Bertilsson L, Johansson I, Rodriguez F, Ingelman-Sundberg M. Frequent distribution of ultrarapid metabolizers of debrisoquine in an Ethiopian population carrying duplicated and multiduplicated functional CYP2D6 alleles. J Pharmacol Exp Ther 1996; 278: 441–446.

77. Shimada T, Yamazaki H, Mimura M, Inui Y, Guengerich FP. Interindividual variations in human liver cytochrome P-450 enzymes involved in the oxidation of drugs, carcinogens and toxic chemicals: studies with liver microsomes of 30 Japanese and 30 Caucasians. J Pharmacol Exp Ther 1994; 270:414–423.

78. Manyike PT, Kharasch ED, Kalhorn TF, Slattery JT. Contribution of CYP2E1 and CYP3A to acetaminophen reactive metabolite formation. Clin Pharmacol Ther 2000; 67:275–282.

79. Prescott LF, Howie D, Darrien I, Adriaenssens P. Paracetamol hepatotoxicity in man. In: H Bundgaard, P Juul, H Kofod, eds. Drug Design and Adverse Reactions. Cophenhagen: Munksgaard, 1977:99–108.

80. Rumack BH. Acetaminophen overdose in young children. Am J Dis Child 1984; 138:428–433.

81. Miller RP, Roberts RJ, Fischer LJ. Acetaminophen elimination kinetics in neonates, children, and adults. Clin Pharmacol Ther 1976; 19:284–294.

82. Lauterberg BH, Vaishnav Y, Stillwell B, Mitchell JR. The effects of age and glutathione depletion on hepatic glutathione turnover in vivo determined by acetaminophen probe analysis. J Pharmacol Exp Ther 1980; 213:54–58.

83. Lesko SM, Mitchell AA. The safety of acetaminophen and ibuprofen among children younger than two years old. Pediatrics 1999; 104:1–5.

84. Alonso EM, Sokol RJ, Hart J, Tyson RW, Narkewicz MR, Whitington PF. Fulminant hepatitis association with centrilobular hepatic necrosis in young children. J Pediatr 1995; 127: 888–894.

85. Rivera-Penera T, Gugig R, Davis J, McDiarmid S, Vargas J, Rosenthal P, Berquist W, Hegman MB, Ament ME. Outcome of acetaminophen overdose in pediatric patients and factors contributing to hepatotoxicity. J Pediatr 1997; 130:300–304.

86. Heubi JE, Barbacci MB, Zimmerman HJ. Therapeutic misadventures with acetaminophen: hepatotoxicity after multiple doses in children. J Pediatr 1998; 132:22–27.

87. Miles FK, Kamath R, Dorrey SFA, Gaskin KJ, O'Loughlin EV. Accidental paracetamol overdosing and fulminant hepatic failure in children. Med J Aust 1999; 171:472–475.

88. Hynson JL, South M. Childhood hepatotoxicity with paracetamol doses less than 150 mg/ kg per day. Med J Aust 1999; 171:497.

89. Caravati EM. Unintentional acetaminophen ingestion in children and the potential for hepatotoxicity. Clin Toxicol 2000; 38:291–296.

90. Daly FFS, Dart RC, Prescott LF. Accidental paracetamol overdosing and fulminant hepatic failure in children. Med J Aust 2000; 173:558–559.

91. Wright JN, Prescott LF. Potentiation by previous drug therapy of hepatotoxicity following paracetamol overdosage. Scott Med J 1973; 18:56–58.

92. Wilson JT, Kasantikul V, Harbison R, Martin D. Death in an adolescent following an overdose of acetaminophen and phenobarbital. Am J Dis Child 1978; 132:466–473.

93. Minton NA, Henry JA, Frankel RJ. Fatal paracetamol poisoning in an epileptic. Hum Toxicol 1988; 7:33–34.

94. Prescott LF, Critchley JAJH, Balali-Mood M, Pentland B. Effects of microsomal enzyme induction on paracetamol metabolism in man. Br J Clin Pharmacol 1981; 12:149–153.

95. Robinson AE, Sattar H, McDowell RD, Holder AT, Powell R. Forensic toxicology of some deaths associated with the combined use of propoxyphene and acetaminophen (paracetamol). J Forens Sci 1977; 22:708–717.

96. Peterson GR, Hostetler RM, Lehman T, Covault HP. Acute inhibition of oxidative drug metabolism by propoxyphene. Biochem Pharmacol 1979; 28:1783–1789.

97. Pond SM, Tong TG, Kaysen GA, Menke DJ, Galinsky RE, Roberts SM, Levy G. Massive intoxication with acetaminophen and propoxyphene: unexplained survival and unusual pharmacokinetics of acetaminophen. J Toxicol Clin Toxicol 1982; 19:1–16.

98. Zand R, Nelson SD, Slattery JT, Thummel KE, Kalhorn TF, Adams SP, Wright JM. Inhibition and induction of cytochrome P4502E1-catalyzed oxidation by isoniazid in humans. Clin Pharmacol Ther 1993; 54:142–149.

99. Chien JY, Peter RM, Nolan CM, Wartell C, Slattery JT, Nelson SD, Carithers Jr. RL, Thummel KE. Influence of polymorphic N-acetyltransferase phenotype on the inhibition and induction of acetaminophen bioactivation with long-term isoniazid. Clin Pharmacol Ther 1997; 61:24–34.

100. Slattery JT, Nelson SD, Thummel KE. The complex interaction between ethanol and acetaminophen. Clin Pharmacol Ther 1996; 60:241–246.

101. Thummel KE, Slattery JT, Ro H, Chien JY, Nelson SD, Lown LE, Watkins PB. Ethanol and production of the hepatotoxic metabolite of acetaminophen in healthy adults. Clin Pharmacol Ther 2000; 67:591–599.

102. Chien JY, Thummel KE, Slattery JT. Pharmacokinetic consequences of induction of CYP2E1 by ligand stabilization. Drug Metab Dispos 1997; 25:1165–1174.

103. Epstein MM, Nelson SD, Slattery JT, Kalhorn TF, Wall RA, Wright JM. Inhibition of the metabolism of paracetamol by isoniazid. Br J Clin Pharmacol 1991; 31:139–142.

104. Murphy R, Scartz R, Watkins PB. Severe acetaminophen toxicity in a patient receiving isoniazid. Ann Intern Med 1990; 113:799–800.

105. Moulding TS, Redeker AG, Kanel GC. Acetaminophen, isoniazid, and hepatic toxicity. Ann Intern Med 1991; 114:431.

106. Nolan CM, Sandblom RE, Thummel KE, Slattery JT, Nelson SD. Hepatotoxicity associated with acetaminophen use in patients receiving multiple drug therapy for tuberculosis. Chest 1994; 105:408–411.

107. McClain CJ, Kromhaut JP, Peterson FJ, Holtzman JL. Potentiation of acetaminophen hepatotoxicity by alcohol. JAMA 1980; 244:251–253.

108. Benjamin SB. Acetaminophen toxicity in the alcoholic: a therapeutic misadventure. Ann Intern Med 1986; 104:399–404.

109. Zimmerman HJ, Maddrey WC. Acetaminophen (paracetamol) hepatotoxicity with regular intake of alcohol: analysis of instances of therapeutic misadventure. Hepatology 1995; 22:767–773.

110. Prescott LF. Paracetamol, alcohol and the liver. Br J Clin Pharmacol 2000; 49:291–301.

111. Makin A, Williams R. Paracetamol hepatotoxicity and alcohol consumption in deliberate and accidental overdose. Q J Med 2000; 93:341–349.

112. Takahashi T, Lasker J, Rosman A, Lieber C. Induction of cytochrome P-4502E1 in the human liver is caused by corresponding increase in encoding messenger RNA. Hepatology 1993; 17:236–245.

113. Hirano T, Kaplowitz N, Tsukamoto H, Kamimura S, Fernandez-Checa J. Hepatic mitochondrial glutathione depletion and progression of experimental alcoholic liver disease in rats. Hepatology 1992; 16:1423–1427.

114. Garcia-Ruiz C, Morales A, Ballesta A, Rodes J, Kaplowitz N, Fernandez-Checa J. Effect of chronic ethanol feeding on glutathione and functional integrity of mitochondria in periportal and perivenous rat hepatocytes. J Clin Invest 1994; 94:193–201.

115. Lauterburg BH, Velez ME. Glutathione deficiency in alcoholics: risk factor for paracetamol hepatotoxicity. Gut 1988; 29:1153–1157.

116. Whitcomb DC, Block GD. Association of acetaminophen hepatotoxicity with fasting and ethanol use. JAMA 1994; 272:1845–1850.

117. Hu Y, Ingelman-Sandberg M, Lindros KO. Induction mechanisms of cytochrome P450 2E1

in liver: interplay between ethanol treatment and starvation. Biochem Pharmacol 1995; 50: 155–161.

118. Sinclair JF, Szakacs JG, Wood SG, Kotrubsky VE, Jeffrey EH, Wrighton SA, Bement WJ, Wright D, Sinclair PR. Acetaminophen hepatotoxicity precipitated by short-term treatment of rats with ethanol and isopentanol. Biochem Pharmacol 2000; 59:445–454.

119. Sinclair JF, Szakacs JG, Wood SG, Walton HS, Bement JL, Gonzalez FJ, Jeffery EH, Wrighton SA, Bement WJ, Sinclair PR. Short-term treatment with alcohols causes hepatic steatosis and enhances acetaminophen hepatotoxicity in *Cyp2e1 (−/−)* mice. Toxicol Appl Pharmacol 2000; 168:114–122.

120. Autlitz AM, Mead JA, Tolentino MA. Potentiation of oral anticoagulant therapy by acetaminophen. Curr Ther Res 1968; 10:501–507.

121. Boejings JJ, Boerstra EE, Ris P. Interaction between paracetamol and coumarin anticoagulants. Lancet 1982; 1:506.

122. Rubin RN, Mentzner RL, Budzynski AZ. Potentiation of anticoagulant effect of warfarin by acetaminophen: Tylenol. Clin Res 1984; 32:698a.

123. Bartle WR, Blakely JA. Potentiation of warfarin anticoagulation by acetaminophen. JAMA 1991; 265:1260.

124. Hylek EM, Heiman H, Skates SJ, Sheehan MA, Singer DE. Acetaminophen and other risk factors for excessive warfarin anticoagulation. JAMA 1998; 279:657–662.

125. Kwan D, Bartle WR, Walker SE. The effects of acetaminophen on pharmacokinetics and pharmacodynamics of warfarin. J Clin Pharmacol 1999; 39:68–75.

126. Takigawa T, Tainaka H, Mihara K, Ogata H. Inhibition of S-warfarin metabolism by nonsteroidal antiinflammatory drugs in human liver microsomes in vitro. Biol Pharmacol Bull 1998; 21:541–543.

127. Nelson SD. Mechanisms of the formation and disposition of reactive metabolites that can cause acute liver injury. Drug Metab Rev 1995; 27:147–177.

128. Myers TG, Thummel KE, Kalhorn TF, Nelson SD. Preferred orientations in the binding of 4′-hydroxyacetanilide (acetaminophen) to cytochrome P450 1A1 and 2B1 isoforms as determined by ^{13}C- and ^{15}N-NMR relaxation studies. J Med Chem 1994; 37:860–867.

129. Schlichting I, Berendzen J, Chu K, Stock AM, Maves SA, Benson DE, Sweet BM, Ringe D, Petsko GA, Sligar SG. The catalytic pathway of cytochrome P450cam at atomic resolution. Science 2000; 287:1615–1622.

130. Hasemann CA, Kurumbail RG, Boddupalli SS, Peterson JA, Deisenhofer J. Structure and function of cytochrome P450: a comparative analysis of three crystal structures. Structure 1995; 2:41–62.

131. Modi S, Primrose WU, Boyle JMB, Gibson CF, Lian YF, Roberts GCK. NMR studies of substrate binding to cytochrome P450 BM3: comparison to cytochrome P450cam. Biochemistry 1995; 34:8982–8988.

132. Lewis DFV, Bird MG, Dickins M, Lake BG, Eddershaw PJ, Tarbit MH, Goldfarb PS. Molecular modelling of human CYP2E1 by homology with the CYP102 haemoprotein domain: investigation of the interactions of substrates and inhibitors within the putative active site of the human CYP2E1 isoform. Xenobiotica 2000; 30:1–25.

133. Rashed MS, Myers TG, Nelson SD. Hepatic protein arylation, glutathione depletion, and metabolite profiles of acetaminophen and a non-hepatotoxic regioisomer, 3′-hydroxyacetanilide, in the mouse. Drug Metab Dispos 1990; 18:765–770.

134. Tirmenstein MA and Nelson SD. Subcellular binding effects on calcium homeostasis produced by acetaminophen and a non-hepatotoxic regioisomer, 3′-hydroxyacetanilide. J Biol Chem 1989; 264:9814–9819.

135. Roberts SA, Price VF, Jollow DJ. Acetaminophen structure-toxicity studies: in vivo covalent binding of a non-hepatotoxic analog, 3′-hydroxyacetanilide. Toxicol Appl Pharmacol 1990; 105:195–208.

136. Tirmenstein MA, Nelson SD. Acetaminophen-induced oxidation of protein thiols: contribu-

tion of impaired thiol metabolizing enzymes and the breakdown of adenine nucleotides. J Biol Chem 1990; 265:3059–3065.

137.   Nelson SD, Pearson PG. Covalent and noncovalent interactions in acute lethal cell injury caused by chemicals. Annu Rev Pharmacol Toxicol 1990; 30:169–195.

138.   Rogers LK, Valentine CJ, Szczpyka M, Smith CV. Effects of hepatotoxic doses of acetaminophen and furosemide on tissue concentrations of CoASH and CoASSG in vivo. Chem Res Toxicol 2000; 13:873–882.

139.   Roberts DW, Bucci TJ, Benson RW, Warbritton AR, McRae TA, Pumford NR, Hinson JA. Immunohistochemical localization and quantification of the 3-(cystein-S-yl)-acetaminophen protein adduct in acetaminophen hepatotoxicity. Am J Pathol 1991; 138:359–371.

140.   Hart SGE, Cartun RW, Wyand DS, Khairallah EA, Cohen SD. Immunohistochemical localization of acetaminophen in target tissues of the CD-1 mouse: correspondence of covalent binding with toxicity. Fund Appl Toxicol 1995; 24:260–274.

141.   Bartalone JB, Beierschmitt WP, Birge RB, Hart SGE, Wyand DS, Cohen SD, Khairallah EA. Selective acetaminophen metabolite binding to hepatic and extrahepatic proteins: an in vivo and in vitro analysis. Toxicol Appl Pharmacol 1989; 99:240–249.

142.   Hinson JA, Roberts DW, Benson RW, Dalhoff K, Loft S, Poulsen HE. Mechanism of paracetamol toxicity. Lancet 1990; 335:732.

143.   Streeter AJ, Dahlin DC, Nelson SD, Baillie, TA. The covalent binding of acetaminophen to protein: evidence for cysteine residues as major sites of arylation in vitro. Chem-Biol Interact 1984; 48:349–366.

144.   Hoffman K-J, Streeter AJ, Axworthy DB, Baillie TA. Identification of the major covalent adduct formed in vitro and in vivo between acetaminophen and mouse liver proteins. Mol Pharmacol 1985; 27:566–573.

145.   Potter DW, Pumford NR, Hinson JA, Benson RW, Roberts DW. Epitope characterization of acetaminophen bound to protein and nonprotein sulfhydryl groups by an enzyme-linked immunosorbent assay. J Pharmacol Exp Ther 1989; 248:182–189.

146.   Dietze EC, Schäfer A, Omichinski JG, Nelson SD. Inactivation of glyceraldehyde-3-phosphate dehydrogenase by a reactive metabolite of acetaminophen and mass spectral characterization of an arylated active site peptide. Chem Res Toxicol 1997; 10:1097–1103.

147.   Zhou L, McKenzie BA, Eccleston Jr ED, Srivasta SP, Chen N, Erickson RR, Holtzman JL. The covalent binding of [^{14}C] acetaminophen to mouse hepatic microsomal proteins: the specific binding to calreticulin and the two forms of the thiol: protein disulfide oxidoreductases. Chem Res Toxicol 1996; 9:1176–1182.

148.   Matthews AM, Roberts DW, Hinson JA, Pumford NR. Acetaminophen-induced hepatotoxicity. Analysis of total covalent binding vs. specific binding to cysteine. Drug Metab Dispos 1996; 24:1192–1196.

149.   Cohen SD, Khairallah EA. Selective protein arylation and acetaminophen-induced hepatotoxicity. Drug Metab Rev 1997; 29:59–77.

150.   Pumford NR, Halmes NC. Protein targets of xenobiotic reactive metabolites. Annu Rev Pharmacol Toxicol 1997; 37:91–117.

151.   Qiu Y, Benet LZ, Burlingame AL. Identification of the hepatic protein targets of reactive metabolites of acetaminophen in vivo in mice using two-dimensional gel electrophoresis and mass spectrometry. J Biol Chem 1998; 273:17940–17953.

152.   Bartolone JB, Birge RB, Bulera SJ, Bruno MK, Nishanian EV, Cohen SD, Khairallah EA. Purification, antibody production, and partial amino acid sequence of the 58-kDa acetaminophen-binding liver proteins. Toxicol Appl Pharmacol 1992; 113:19–29.

153.   Pumford NR, Martin BM, Hinson JA. A metabolite of acetaminophen covalently binds to the 56 kDa selenium binding protein. Biochem Biophys Res Commun 1992; 182:1348–1355.

154.   Fountoulakis M, Berndt P, Boelsterli UA, Crameri F, Winter M, Albertini S, Suter L. Two-dimensional database of mouse liver proteins: changes in hepatic protein levels following

treatment with acetaminophen or its nontoxic regioisomer 3-acetamidophenol. Electrophoresis 2000; 21:2148–2161.

155. Myers TG, Dietz EC, Anderson NL, Khairallah EA, Cohen SD, Nelson SD. A comparative study of mouse liver proteins arylated by reactive metabolites of acetaminophen and its non-hepatotoxic regioisomer, 3'-hydroxyacetanilide. Chem Res Toxicol 1995; 8:403–413.

156. Khairallah EA, Bruno MK, Hong M, Cohen SD. Cellular consequences of protein adduct formation. Toxicologist 1995; 15:86 (abstr).

157. Porat A, Sagiu Y, Elazar Z. A 56-kDa selenium-binding protein participates in intra-Golgi protein transport. J Biol Chem 2000; 275:14457–14465.

158. Pumford NR, Halmes NC, Martin BM, Cook RJ, Wagner C, Hinson JA. Covalent binding of acetaminophen to N-10-formyl-tetrahydrofolate dehydrogenase in mice. J Pharmacol Exp Ther 1997; 280:501–505.

159. Arnaiz SL, Llesuy S, Cutrín JC, Boveris A. Oxidative stress by acute acetaminophen administration in mouse liver. Free Radic Biol Med 1995; 19:303–310.

160. Bulera SJ, Birge RB, Cohen SD, Khairallah EA. Identification of the mouse liver 44-kDa acetaminophen-binding protein as a subunit of glutamine synthetase. Toxicol Appl Pharmacol 1995; 134:313–320.

161. Gupta S, Rogers LK, Taylor SK, Smith CV. Inhibition of carbamyl phosphate synthetase-I and glutamine synthetase by hepatotoxic doses of acetaminophen in mice. Toxicol Appl Pharmacol 1997; 146:317–327.

162. Landin JS, Cohen SD, Khairallah EA. Identification of a 54-kDa mitochondrial acetaminophen-binding protein as aldehyde dehydrogenase. Toxicol Appl Pharmacol 1996; 141:299–307.

163. Halmes NC, Hinson JA, Martin BA, Pumford NR. Glutamate dehydrogenase covalently binds to a reactive metabolite of acetaminophen. Chem Res Toxicol 1996; 9:541–546.

164. Luthman M, Holmgren A. Rat liver thioredoxin and thioredoxin reductase: purification and characterization. Biochem 1982; 21:6628–6633.

165. Gadaska PY, Gadaska JR, Cochran S, Powis, G. Cloning and sequencing of human thioredoxin reductase. FEBS Lett 1995; 373:5–9.

166. Gladyshev VN, Jeang K, Stadtman TC. Selenocysteine, identified as the penultimate C-terminal residue in human T-cell thioredoxin reductase, corresponds to TGA in the human placental gene. Proc Natl Acad Sci USA 1996; 93:6146–6174.

167. Matthews AM, Hinson JA, Roberts DW, Pumford NR. Comparison of covalent binding of acetaminophen and the regioisomer 3'-hydroxyacetanilide to mouse liver protein. Toxicol Lett 1997; 90:77–82.

168. Tirmenstein MA, Nelson SD. Hepatotoxicity after 3'-hydroxyacetanilide administration to buthionine sulfoximine pretreated mice. Chem Res Toxicol 1991; 4:214–217.

169. Dixon MF, Dixon B, Aparici SR, Lowey DP. Experimental paracetamol-induced hepatic necrosis: a light- and electron-microscope and histochemical study. J Pathol 1975; 116:17–29.

170. Walker RM, Racz WJ, McElligott TF. Acetaminophen-induced hepatotoxicity in mice. Lab Invest 1980; 42:181–189.

171. Meyers LL, Beierschmitt WP, Khairallah EA, Cohen SD. Acetaminophen-induced inhibition of hepatic mitochrondrial respiration in mice. Toxicol Appl Pharmacol 1988; 93:378–387.

172. Katyare SS, Satav JG. Impaired mitochondrial oxidative energy metabolism following paracetamol-induced hepatotoxicity in the rat. Br J Pharmacol 1989; 96:51–58.

173. Ramsay RR, Rashed MS, Nelson SD. In vitro effects of acetaminophen metabolites and analogs on the respiration of mouse liver mitochrondria. Arch Biochem Biophys 1989; 273:449–457.

174. Burcham PC, Harman AW. Acetaminophen toxicity results in site-specific mitochrondrial damage in isolated mouse hepatocytes. J Biol Chem 1991; 266:5049–5054.

175. Strubelt O, Younes M. The toxicological relevance of paracetamol-induced inhibition of hepatic respiration and ATP depletion. Biochem Pharmacol 1992; 44:163–170.

176. Donnelly PJ, Walker RM, Racz WJ. Inhibition of mitochrondrial respiration in vivo is an early event in acetaminophen hepatotoxicity. Arch Toxicol 1994; 68:110–118.

177. Vendemiale G, Grattagliano I, Altomare E, Turturro N, Guerrieri F. Effect of acetaminophen administration on hepatic glutathione compartmentation and mitochrondrial energy metabolism in the rat. Biochem Pharmacol 1996; 52:1147–1154.

178. Martin, FL, McLean AEM. Adenosine triphosphate (ATP) levels in paracetamol-induced cell injury in the rat in vivo and in vitro. Toxicology 1995; 104:91–97.

179. Jaeschke H. Glutathione disulfide formation and oxidant stress during acetaminophen-induced hepatotoxicity in mice in vivo: the protective effect of allpurinol. J Pharmacol Exp Ther 1990; 255:935–941.

180. Parmer DV, Ahmed G, Khandkar MA, Katyare SS. Mitochondrial ATPase: a target for paracetamol-induced hepatotoxicity. Eur J Pharmacol 1995; 293:225–229.

181. Moore M, Thor H, Moore G, Nelson S, Moldéus P, Orrenius S. The toxicity of acetaminophen and N-acetyl-p-benzoquinone imine in isolated hepatocytes is associated with thiol depletion and increased cytosolic Ca^{2+}. J Biol Chem 1985; 260:13035–13040.

182. Tsokos-Kuhn JO, Todd EL, McMillin-Wood JB, Mitchell JR. ATP-dependent calcium uptake by rat liver plasma membrane vesicles: effect of alkylating hepatotoxins in vivo. Mol Pharmacol 1985; 28:56–61.

183. Lauterburg BH. Early disturbance of calcium translocation across the plasma membrane in toxic liver injury. Hepatology 1987; 7:1179–1183.

184. Burcham PC, Harman AW. Effect of acetaminophen hepatotoxicity on hepatic mitochondrial and microsomal calcium contents in mice. Toxicol Lett 1988; 44:91–99.

185. Nicotera P, Rundgren M, Porubek DJ, Cotgreave I, Moldéus P, Orrenius S, Nelson SD. On the role of Ca^{2+} in the toxicity of alkylating and oxidizing quinone imines in isolated hepatocytes. Chem Res Toxicol 1989; 2:46–50.

186. Corcoran GB, Chung SJ, Salazar DE. Early inhibition of the Na^+/K^+-ATPase ion pump during acetaminophen-induced hepatotoxicity in rat. Biochem Biophys Res Commun 1987; 149:203–207.

187. Bruno MK, Khairallah EA, Cohen SD. Inhibition of protein phosphatase activity and changes in protein phosphorylation following acetaminophen exposure in cultured mouse hepatocytes. Toxicol Appl Pharmacol 1998; 153:119–132.

188. Nelson, SD, Tirmenstein MA, Rashed MS, Myers TG. Acetaminophen and protein thiol oxidation. In: CM Witmer, RR Snyder, DJ Jollow, GF Kalf, JJ Kocsis, IG Sipes, eds. Biological Reactive Intermediates IV. New York: Plenum, 1991:579–588.

189. Labadorios D, David M, Portmann B, Williams R. Paracetamol-induced hepatic necrosis in the mouse: relationship between covalent binding, hepatic glutathione depletion and the protective effect of alpha-mercaptopropionyl glycine. Biochem Pharmacol 1977; 26:31–35.

190. Albano E, Rundgren M, Harvison PJ, Nelson SD, Moldéus P. Mechanisms of N-acetyl-p-benzoquinone imine cytotoxicity. Mol Pharmacol 1985; 280:306–311.

191. Tee LBG, Boobis AR, Hugett AC, Davies DS. Reversal of acetaminophen toxicity in isolated hamster hepatocytes by dithiothreitol. Toxicol Appl Pharmacol 1986; 83:294–314.

192. Lauterburg BH, Smith CV, Hughs H, Mitchell JR. Biliary excretion of glutathione and glutathione disulfide in the rat: regulation and response to oxidative stress. J Clin Invest 1984; 73:124–133.

193. Smith CV, Mitchell JR. Acetaminophen hepatotoxicity in vivo. Free Radic Biol Med 1991; 10:217–224.

194. Smith CV. Correlations and apparent contradictions in assessment of oxidant stress status in vivo. Free Radic Biol Med 1991; 10:217–224.

195. Wendel A, Feuerstein S, Konz K-H. Acute paracetamol intoxication of starved mice leads to lipid peroxidation in vivo. Biochem Pharmacol 1979; 28:2051–2055.

196. Fairhurst S, Barber DJ, Clark B, Horton AA. Studies on paracetamol-induced lipid peroxidation. Toxicology 1982; 23:249–259.

197. Amimoto T, Matsura T, Koyama S-Y, Nakanishi T, Yamada K, Kajiyama G. Acetaminophen-induced hepatic injury in mice: the role of lipid peroxidation and effects of pretreatment with coenzyme Q_{10} and α-tocopherol. Free Radic Biol Med 1995; 19:169–176.

198. Burk RF, Lane JM. Ethane production and liver necrosis in rats after administration of drugs and other chemicals. Toxicol Appl Pharmacol 1979; 50:467–478.

199. Walker RM, Massey TE, McElligott TF, Racz WJ. Acetaminophen toxicity in fed and fasted mice. Can J Physiol Pharmacol 1982; 60:399–404.

200. Kamiyama T, Sato C, Liu J, Tajin K, Miyaka H, Marumo F. Role of lipid peroxidation in acetaminophen-induced hepatotoxicity: comparison with carbon tetrachloride. Toxicol Lett 1993; 66:7–12.

201. Morrow JD, Awad JA, Kato T, Takahashi K, Badr KF, Roberts LJ, Burk RF. Formation of novel non-cyclooxygenase-derived prostanoids (F_2-isoprostanes) in carbon tetrachloride hepatotoxicity. J Clin Invest 1992; 90:2502–2507.

202. Morrow JD, Chen Y, Brame CJ, Yang J, Sanchez SC, Xu J, Zackert WE, Awad JA, Roberts LJ. The isoprostanes: unique prostaglandin-like products of free radical-initiated lipid peroxidation. Drug Metab Rev 1999; 31:117–139.

203. Gupta S, Rogers LK, Smith CV. Biliary excretion of lysosomal enzymes, iron, and oxidized protein in Fischer-344 and Sprague-Dawley rats and the effects of diquat and acetaminophen. Toxicol Appl Pharmacol 1994; 125:42–50.

204. Gibson JD, Pumford NR, Samokyszyn VM, Hinson JA. Mechanism of acetaminophen-induced hepatotoxicity: covalent binding versus oxidative stress. Chem Res Toxicol 1996; 9:580–585.

205. Younes M, Siegers C-P. The role of iron in the paracetamol-and CCl_4-induced lipid peroxidation and hepatotoxicity. Chem-Biol Interact 1985; 55:327–334.

206. Younes M, Sause C, Siegers C-P, Lemoine R. Effect of deferrioxamine and diethyldithiocarbamate on paracetamol-induced hepato- and nephrotoxicity: the role of lipid peroxidation. J Appl Toxicol 1988; 8:261–265.

207. Schnellmann JG, Pumford NR, Kusewitt DF, Bucci TJ, Hinson JA. Deferoxamine delays the development of the hepatotoxicity of acetaminophen in mice. Toxicol Lett 1999; 106:79–88.

208. Laskin DL, Pilaro AM. Potential role of activated macrophages in acetaminophen hepatotoxicity. Toxicol Appl Pharmacol 1986; 86:204–215.

209. Elisi AED, Hall P, Sim W-L, Earnest DL, Sipes IG. Characterization of vitamin A potentiation of carbon tetrachloride-induced liver injury. Toxicol Appl Pharmacol 1993; 9:280–288.

210. Nakae D, Yamamoto K, Yoshijitt, Kinugasa T, Maruyama H, Farber JL, Konishi Y. Liposome-encapsulated superoxide dismutase prevents liver necrosis induced by acetaminophen. Am J Pathol 1990; 136:787–795.

211. Potter DW, Hinson JA. The 1- and 2-electron oxidation of acetaminophen catalyzed by prostaglandin H synthase. J Biol Chem 1987; 262:974–980.

212. Harvison PJ, Egan RW, Gale PH, Christian GD, Hill BS, Nelson SD. Acetaminophen and analogs as cosubstrates and inhibitors of prostaglandin H synthase. Chem-Biol Interact 1988; 64:251–266.

213. West PR, Harman LS, Josephy PD, Mason RP. Acetaminophen: enzymatic formation of a transient phenoxy free radical. Biochem Pharmacol 1984; 33:2933–2936.

214. Potter DW, Miller DW, Hinson JA. Identification of acetaminophen polymerization products catalyzed by horseradish peroxidase. J Biol Chem 1985; 260:12174–12180.

215. Powis G, Svingen BA, Dahlin DC, Nelson SD. Enzymatic and non-enzymatic reduction of N-acetyl-p-benzoquinone imine and some properties of the N-acetyl-p-benzoquinone imine radical. Biochem Pharmacol 1984; 33:2367–2370.

216. Fischer V, West PR, Nelson SD, Harvison PJ, Mason RP. Formation of 4-aminophenoxyl

free radical from the acetaminophen metabolite *N*-acetyl-*p*-benzoquinone imine. J Biol Chem 1985; 260:11446–11450.

217. Bisby RH, Tabassum N. Properties of the radicals formed by one-electron oxidation of acetaminophen—a pulse radiolysis study. Biochem Pharmacol 1988; 37:2731–2738.

218. Ross D, Albano E, Nilsson U, Moldéus P. Thiyl radicals—formation during peroxidase-catalyzed metabolism of acetaminophen in the presence of thiols. Biochem Biophys Res Commun 1984; 125:109–115.

219. Keller RJ, Hinson JA. Mechanism of acetaminophen-stimulated NADPH oxidation catalyzed by the peroxidase-H_2O_2 system. Drug Metab Dispos 1991; 19:184–187.

220. Van de Straat R, de Vries J, Vermeulen NPE. Role of hepatic microsomal and purified cytochrome P-450 in one-electron reduction of two quinone imines and concomitant reduction of molecular oxygen. Biochem Pharmacol 1987; 36:613–619.

221. Chitturi S, Farrell GC. Drug-induced liver disease. Curr Treat Options Gastroenterol 2000; 3:457–462.

222. Streeter AJ, Bjorge SM, Axworthy DB, Nelson SD, Baillie TA. The microsomal metabolism and site of covalent binding to protein of 3′-hydroxyacetanilide, a nonhepatotoxic positional isomer of acetaminophen. Drug Metab Dispos 1984; 12:565–576.

223. Devalia JL, McLean AE. Covalent binding and the mechanism of paracetamol toxicity. Biochem Pharmacol 1983; 32:2602–2603.

224. Devalia JL, Ogilvie RC, McLean AE. Dissociation of cell death from covalent binding of paracetamol by flavones in a hepatocyte system. Biochem Pharmacol 1982; 31:3745–3749.

225. Sirover MA. New insights into an old protein: the functional diversity of mammalian glyceraldehyde-3-phosphate dehydrogenase. Biochim Biophys Acta 1999; 1432:159–184.

226. Shen W, Kamendulis LM, Ray SD, Corcoran GB. Acetaminophen-induced cytotoxicity in cultured mouse hepatocytes: effects of $Ca^{(2+)}$-endonuclease, DNA repair, and glutathione depletion inhibitors on DNA fragmentation and cell death. Toxicol Appl Pharmacol 1992; 112:32–40.

227. Kyle ME, Miccadei S, Nakae D, Farber JL. Superoxide dismutase and catalase protect cultured hepatocytes from the cytotoxicity of acetaminophen. Biochem Biophys Res Commun 1987; 149:889–896.

228. Gerson RJ, Casini A, Gilfor D, Serroni A, Farber JL. Oxygen-mediated cell injury in the killing of cultured hepatocytes by acetaminophen. Biochem Biophys Res Commun 1985; 126:1129–1137.

229. Smith CV, Mitchell JR. Acetaminophen hepatotoxicity in vivo is not accompanied by oxidant stress. Biochem Biophys Res Commun 1985; 133:329–336.

230. Kyle ME, Sakaida I, Serroni A, Farber JL. Metabolism of acetaminophen by cultured rat hepatocytes. Depletion of protein thiol groups without any loss of viability. Biochem Pharmacol 1990; 40:1211–1218.

231. Birge RB, Bartolone JB, Nishanian EV, Bruno MK, Mangold JB, Cohen SD, Khairallah EA. Dissociation of covalent binding from the oxidative effects of acetaminophen. Studies using dimethylated acetaminophen derivatives. Biochem Pharmacol 1988; 37:3383–3393.

232. Ray SD, Mumaw VR, Raje RR, Fariss MW. Protection of acetaminophen-induced hepatocellular apoptosis and necrosis by cholesteryl hemisuccinate pretreatment. J Pharmacol Exp Ther 1996; 279:1470–1483.

233. Henderson CJ, Wolf CR, Kitteringham N, Powell H, Otto D, Park BK. Increased resistance to acetaminophen hepatotoxicity in mice lacking glutathione *S*-transferase Pi. Proc Natl Acad Sci USA 2000; 97:12741–12745.

234. Mirochnitchenko O, Weisbrot-Lefkowitz M, Reuhl K, Chen L, Yang C, Inouye M. Acetaminophen toxicity: opposite effects of two forms of glutathione peroxidase. J Biol Chem 1999; 274:10349–10355.

235. Kitteringham NR, Powell H, Clement YN, Dodd CC, Tettey JN, Pirmohamed M, Smith DA, McLellan LI, Kevin Park B. Hepatocellular response to chemical stress in CD-1 mice: induc-

tion of early genes and gamma-glutamylcysteine synthetase. Hepatology 2000; 32:321–333.

236. Chen YR, Wang X, Templeton D, Davis RJ, Tan TH. The role of c-Jun N-terminal kinase (JNK) in apoptosis induced by ultraviolet C and gamma radiation: duration of JNK activation may determine cell death and proliferation. J Biol Chem 1996; 271:31929–31936.

237. Barrett WC, DeGnore JP, Konig S, Fales HM, Keng YF, Zhang ZY, Yim MB, Chock PB. Regulation of PTP1B via glutathionylation of the active site cysteine 215. Biochemistry 1999; 38:6699–6705.

238. Rzucidlo SJ, Bounous DI, Jones DP, Brackett BG. Acute acetaminophen toxicity in transgenic mice with elevated hepatic glutathione. Vet Hum Toxicol 2000; 42:146–150.

239. Williams MD, Van Remmen H, Conrad CC, Huang TT, Epstein CJ, Richardson A. Increased oxidative damage is correlated to altered mitochondrial function in heterozygous manganese superoxide dismutase knockout mice. J Biol Chem 1998; 273:28510–28515.

240. Tsan MF, White JE, Caska B, Epstein CJ, Lee CY. Susceptibility of heterozygous MnSOD gene-knockout mice to oxygen toxicity. Am J Respir Cell Mol Biol 1998; 19:114–120.

241. Warner B, Papes R, Heile M, Spitz D, Wispe J. Expression of human Mn SOD in Chinese hamster ovary cells confers protection from oxidant injury. Am J Physiol 1993; 264:L598–605.

242. Majima HJ, Oberley TD, Furukawa K, Mattson MP, Yen HC, Szweda LI, St Clair DK. Prevention of mitochondrial injury by manganese superoxide dismutase reveals a primary mechanism for alkaline-induced cell death. J Biol Chem 1998; 273:8217–8224.

243. Fullerton HJ, Ditelberg JS, Chen SF, Sarco DP, Chan PH, Epstein CJ, Ferriero DM. Copper/zinc superoxide dismutase transgenic brain accumulates hydrogen peroxide after perinatal hypoxia ischemia. Ann Neurol 1998; 44:357–364.

244. Amstad P, Moret R, Cerutti P. Glutathione peroxidase compensates for the hypersensitivity of Cu,Zn- superoxide dismutase overproducers to oxidant stress. J Biol Chem 1994; 269: 1606–1609.

245. Seo KW, Kim JG, Park M, Kim TW, Kim HJ. Effects of phenethylisothiocyanate on the expression of glutathione S-transferases and hepatotoxicity induced by acetaminophen. Xenobiotica 2000; 30:535–545.

246. Hentze H, Gantner F, Kolb SA, Wendel A. Depletion of hepatic glutathione prevents death receptor-dependent apoptotic and necrotic liver injury in mice. Am J Pathol 2000; 156:2045–2056.

247. Enomoto A, Itoh K, Nagayoshi E, Haruta J, Kimura T, O'Connor T, Harada T, Yamamoto M. High sensitivity of Nrf2 knockout mice to acetaminophen hepatotoxicity associated with decreased expression of ARE-regulated drug metabolizing enzymes and antioxidant genes. Toxicol Sci 2001; 59:169–177.

248. Rofe AM, Barry EF, Shelton TL, Philcox JC, Coyle P. Paracetamol hepatotoxicity in metallothionein-null mice. Toxicology 1998; 125:131–40.

249. Liu J, Liu Y, Hartley D, Klaassen CD, Shehin-Johnson SE, Lucas A, Cohen SD. Metallothionein-I/II knockout mice are sensitive to acetaminophen-induced hepatotoxicity. J Pharmacol Exp Ther 1999; 289:580–586.

250. Dalton T, Palmiter RD, Andrews GK. Transcriptional induction of the mouse metallothionein-I gene in hydrogen peroxide-treated Hepa cells involves a composite major late transcription factor/antioxidant response element and metal response promoter elements. Nucleic Acids Res 1994; 22:5016–5023.

251. Salminen WF, Voellmy R, Roberts SM. Differential heat shock protein induction by acetaminophen and a nonhepatotoxic regioisomer, 3′-hydroxyacetanilide, in mouse liver. J Pharmacol Exp Ther 1997; 282:1533–1540.

252. Qiu Y, Benet LZ, Burlingame AL. Identification of mouse liver protein targets for reactive intermediates of nonhepatotoxic acetaminophen regioisomer, 3′-hydroxyacetanilide. 46th

ASMS Conference on Mass Spectrometry and Allied Topics, Orlando, FL, May 31–June 4, 1998, p. 1136.

253. Saleh A, Srinivasula SM, Balkir L, Robbins PD, Alnemri ES. Negative regulation of the Apaf-1 apoptosome by Hsp70. Nat Cell Biol 2000; 2:476–483.

254. Beere HM, Wolf BB, Cain K, Mosser DD, Mahboubi A, Kuwana T, Tailor P, Morimoto RI, Cohen GM, Green DR. Heat-shock protein 70 inhibits apoptosis by preventing recruitment of procaspase-9 to the Apaf-1 apoptosome. Nat Cell Biol 2000; 2:469–475.

255. Wiger R, Finstad HS, Hongslo JK, Haug K, Holme JA. Paracetamol inhibits cell cycling and induces apoptosis in HL-60 cells. Pharmacol Toxicol 1997; 81:285–293.

256. Lawson JA, Fisher MA, Simmons CA, Farhood A, Jaeschke H. Inhibition of Fas receptor (CD95)-induced hepatic caspase activation and apoptosis by acetaminophen in mice. Toxicol Appl Pharmacol 1999; 156:179–186.

257. Adams ML, Pierce RH, Vail ME, Tonge RP, Fausto N, Nelson SD, Bruschi SA. Enhanced acetaminophen hepatotoxicity in transgenic mice overexpressing BCL-2. Mol Pharmacol 2001; 60:907–915.

258. Pierce RH, Tonge RP, Chen W, Fausto N, Nelson SD, Bruschi SA. Acetaminophen, and its nonhepatotoxic regioisomer, induce cell death by anomalous apoptosis in vitro and in vivo. Toxicologist 1999; 48:1457 (abstr).

259. Bruschi SA, Pritchard L, Poot M, Pierce RH, Fausto N, Nelson SD, Campbell JS. Early ATF3-mediated stress responses accompany mitochondrial alterations and precede cell death by necrosis or mixed apoptosis/necrosis. Toxicologist 2001; 60:182 (abstr).

260. Tzung SP, Fausto N, Hockenbery DM. Expression of Bcl-2 family during liver regeneration and identification of Bcl-x as a delayed early response gene. Am J Pathol 1997; 150:1985–1995.

261. Nicotera P, Leist M, Ferrando-May E. Intracellular ATP, a switch in the decision between apoptosis and necrosis. Toxicol Lett 1998; 102–103:139–142.

262. Leist M, Single B, Castoldi AF, Kuhnle S, Nicotera P. Intracellular adenosine triphosphate (ATP) concentration: a switch in the decision between apoptosis and necrosis. J Exp Med 1997; 185:1481–1486.

263. Bonfoco E, Krainc D, Ankarcrona M, Nicotera P, Lipton SA. Apoptosis and necrosis: two distinct events induced, respectively, by mild and intense insults with N-methyl-D-aspartate or nitric oxide/superoxide in cortical cell cultures. Proc Natl Acad Sci USA 1995; 92:7162–7166.

264. Single B, Leist M, Nicotera P. Differential effects of bcl-2 on cell death triggered under ATP-depleting conditions. Exp Cell Res 2001; 262:8–16.

265. Mourelle M, Beales D, McLean AE. Prevention of paracetamol-induced liver injury by fructose. Biochem Pharmacol 1991; 41:1831–1837.

266. Laskin DL, Pendino KJ. Macrophages and inflammatory mediators in tissue injury. Ann Rev Pharmacol Toxicol 1995; 35:655–677.

267. Blazka ME, Germolec DR, Simeonova P, Bruccoleri A, Pennypacker KR, Luster MI. Acetaminophen-induced hepatotoxicity is associated with early changes in NF-kB and NF-IL6 binding activity. J Inflamm 1995–1996; 47:138–150.

268. DeLeve LD, Wang X, Kaplowitz N, Shulman HM, Bart JA, van der Hoek A. Sinusoidal endothelial cells as a target for acetaminophen toxicity. Biochem Pharmacol 1997; 53:1339–1345.

269. Blazka ME, Wilmer JL, Holladay SD, Wilson RE, Luster MI. Role of proinflammatory cytokines in acetaminophen hepatotoxicity. Toxicol Appl Pharmacol 1995; 133:43–52.

270. Zhang H, Cook J, Nickel J, Yu R, Stecker K, Myers K, Dean NM. Reduction of liver Fas expression by an antisense oligonucleotide protects mice from fulminant hepatitis. Nat Biotechnol 2000; 18:862–867.

271. Blazka ME, Elwell MR, Holladay SD, Wilson RE, Luster MI. Histopathology of acetaminophen-induced liver changes: role of interleukin 1 alpha and tumor necrosis factor alpha. Toxicol Pathol 1996; 24:181–189.

272. Hogaboam CM, Bone-Larson CL, Steinhauser ML, Matsukawa A, Gosling J, Boring L, Charo IF, Simpson KJ, Lukacs NW, Kunkel SL. Exaggerated hepatic injury due to acetaminophen challenge in mice lacking C-C chemokine receptor 2. Am J Pathol 2000; 156:1245–1252.

273. Boess F, Bopst M, Althaus R, Polsky S, Cohen SD, Eugster HP, Boelsterli UA. Acetaminophen hepatotoxicity in tumor necrosis factor/lymphotoxin-alpha gene knockout mice. Hepatology 1998; 27:1021–1029.

274. Bernal W, Donaldson P, Underhill J, Wendon J, Williams R. Tumor necrosis factor genomic polymorphism and outcome of acetaminophen (paracetamol)-induced acute liver failure. J Hepatol 1998; 29:53–59.

275. Locksley RM, Killeen N, Lenardo MJ. The TNF and TNF receptor superfamilies: Integrating mammalian biology. Cell 2001; 104:487–501.

276. Hausladen A, Stamler JS. Nitrosative stress. Methods Enzymol 1999; 300:389–395.

277. Beltran B, Mathur A, Duchen MR, Erusalimsky JD, Moncada S. The effect of nitric oxide on cell respiration: A key to understanding its role in cell survival or death. Proc Natl Acad Sci USA 2000; 97:14602–14607.

278. Stamler JS, Hausladen A. Oxidative modifications in nitrosative stress. Nat Struct Biol 1998; 5:247–249.

279. Hinson LA, Pike SL, Pumford NR, Mayeux PR. Nitrotyrosine-protein adducts in hepatic centrilobular areas following toxic doses of acetaminophen in mice. Chem Res Toxicol 1998; 11:604–607.

280. Hinson JA, Michael SL, Ault SG, Pumford NR. Western blot analysis for nitrotyrosine protein adducts in livers of saline-treated and acetaminophen-treated mice. Toxicol Sci 2000; 53:467–473.

281. Michael SL, Pumford NR, Mayeux PR, Niesman MR, Hinson JA. Pretreatment of mice with macrophage inactivators decreases acetaminophen hepatotoxicity and the formation of reactive oxygen and nitrogen species. Hepatology 1999; 30:186–195.

282. Gardner CR, Heck DE, Yang CS, Thomas PE, Zhang XJ, DeGeorge GL, Laskin JD, Laskin DL. Role of nitric oxide in acetaminophen-induced hepatotoxicity in the rat. Hepatology 1998; 27:748–754.

283. Goldin RD, Ratnayaka ID, Breach CS, Brown IN, Wickramasinghe SN. Role of macrophages in acetaminophen (paracetamol)-induced hepatotoxicity. J Pathol 1996; 179:432–435.

284. Vila M, Jackson-Lewis V, Vukosavic S, Djaldetti R, Liberatore G, Offen D, Korsmeyer SJ, Przedborski S. Bax ablation prevents dopaminergic neurodegeneration in the 1-methyl-4-phenyl-1,2,3,6-tetrahydropyridine mouse model of Parkinson's disease. Proc Natl Acad Sci USA 2001; 98:2837–2842.

14

Acetaminophen: Pathology and Clinical Presentation of Hepatotoxicity

WILLIAM M. LEE and GEORGE OSTAPOWICZ

University of Texas Southwestern Medical Center, Dallas, Texas, U.S.A.

I. INTRODUCTION

Acetaminophen (called paracetamol outside the United States) is a popular and widely used analgesic and antipyretic agent. First synthesized in 1893, it was introduced for prescription use in the United States in 1955 and approved for over-the-counter use in 1960 (1). It is frequently combined with codeine or other analgesic agents, decongestants, and antihistamines. Over 300 different preparations are now available in the United States with more than one billion pills sold annually. Acetaminophen's popularity has in part arisen from its apparent lack of side effects. Unlike aspirin and other nonsteroidal anti-inflammatory drugs (NSAIDs) it does not cause gastric irritation or erosions. Although it is remarkably safe when used at usual therapeutic doses, it has a relatively narrow therapeutic window.

Reports of fatal and nonfatal hepatic necrosis following suicide attempts first began to appear in the mid-1960s (2,3) in Great Britain and in the mid-1970s in the United States (4). Acetaminophen self-poisoning, in fact, has now became one of the most popular means of attempting suicide in Great Britain (5,6). Significant hepatic necrosis related to acetaminophen is also being seen more frequently in the United States (7,8). More recently it has also become evident that even therapeutic doses can be hepatotoxic in some individuals, especially in the presence of chronic alcohol consumption and fasting (therapeutic misadventure) (7,9–11). An important problem in this scenario is the public's perception of acetaminophen as a safe drug and the lack of awareness of the potential dangers of its ingestion in just above therapeutic doses. Acetaminophen is now the single most important cause of acute liver failure in both the United States (12) and United Kingdom (13). Unlike most other causes of acute liver failure, however, timely use of the antidote *N*-acetylcysteine will prevent its development, or at least lessen the severity of hepatic damage. The liver damage results from the metabolism of acetaminophen by the cytochrome P450 system and the production of the highly reactive metabolite *N*-acetyl-benzoquinone-imine (NAPQI). This is discussed in detail in another chapter.

II. TOXIC DOSES

The recommended maximum "safe" dose of acetaminophen that can be ingested over 24 h is 4 g in adults and 60 mg/kg in children. While acetaminophen is the classical example of a dose-dependent hepatotoxic drug, there is no definite threshold dose for hepatic injury. The amount of acetaminophen ingested as a single dose required to produce injury is relatively variable. Single doses of acetaminophen exceeding 7–10 g in adults or 150 mg/kg body weight in children are enough to cause significant hepatocellular necrosis; however, this is not inevitable. Severe liver injury, defined as ALT or AST greater than 1000 IU/L, or fatal cases usually involve doses of at least 15–25 g (14). Ingested doses have exceeded 15 g (>200 mg/kg) in 80% of serious and fatal cases (15). As acetaminophen metabolism and susceptibility to toxicity differ between individuals, survival is possible even after ingestion of massive doses as large as 75 g. Among subjects with significant acetaminophen overdose who did not undergo treatment, severe liver injury was reported in only 20%, and among those with severe liver injury, the mortality was 20% (14). On the other hand, daily doses as low as 2–6 g have been associated with fatal hepatotoxicity in heavy drinkers (11,16).

It must be remembered, however, that calculation of an accurate ingested dose has often been made difficult by the failure of patients to provide exact information, either because of intoxication or drowsiness caused by coingested substances, or through lack of cooperation. Early vomiting has also interfered with the calculation of the real amount ingested.

III. RISK FACTORS FOR ACETAMINOPHEN-INDUCED HEPATOTOXICITY

While dose of acetaminophen ingested is clearly important in the development of hepatotoxicity, as discussed above, a number of other risk factors can predispose to liver damage. It has been suggested that children are relatively resistant to acetaminophen hepatotoxicity (17). It is unclear whether this is related to vomiting part of the ingested dose, or to biological resistance, or both. Children have a different relative importance of the metabolic pathways involved, with a lower ratio of glucuronidation to sulfation, which may protect them against liver damage (18).

A number of studies have now established that chronic alcohol use increases the individual's susceptibility to acetaminophen-induced hepatotoxicity (9–11,19–23). The mechanisms appear to include both the induction of the cytochrome P450 (CYP450) system and glutathione depletion. Results suggesting enhanced acetaminophen metabolism have been reported. In this study, the disappearance of acetaminophen after ingestion of 1 g was faster in chronic alcoholics than in normal individuals (24). The alcohol consumption threshold that predisposes to hepatic injury is uncertain, but may be relatively low. A retrospective analysis of patients with severe acetaminophen-induced liver injury found a higher mortality in men consuming more than 24 g alcohol/day and women consuming more than 16 g/day compared to those who drank less (25). Hepatic injury may occur even at therapeutic doses of acetaminophen in alcoholics. A recent study assessing therapeutic misadventures in a group of individuals, most of whom drank more than 60 g alcohol per day, found that 60% had ingested less than 6 g/day and 40% less than 4 g/day (11). Of these patients, 95% developed transaminase elevations greater than 1000 IU/L and 18% died. Other studies have reported similar findings with daily acetaminophen doses ranging from 2.6 to 16.5 g/day (10,20). The association between chronic alcohol ingestion and enhanced acetaminophen hepatotoxicity has recently been questioned however (26). In a review of acetaminophen and alcohol interactions, and clinical reports of toxicity, the author states that the evidence is largely anecdotal and inconclusive. Nevertheless, he concludes that such an association is possible and alcoholics must be considered at increased risk of hepatotoxicity.

Conversely, acute intoxication without chronic alcohol use does not predispose to acetaminophen hepatotoxicity (27). In fact, it may have some protective effect, presumably due to competition of alcohol and acetaminophen resulting in less formation of NAPQI.

Fasting or malnourished patients have an increased susceptibility to acetaminophen hepatotoxicity presumed due to depressed levels of hepatic glutathione and induction of CYP2E1. While the chronically malnourished alcoholic is a classic example of this scenario, the average individual may become at risk after a subacute systemic illness that causes nausea and vomiting with a resulting decrease in food intake. Chronic cardiopulmonary insufficiency has also been reported to predispose to liver damage after short-term ingestion of therapeutic doses of acetaminophen (<9 g over 3 days) (28). Consequent drug metabolism studies indicated that this patient had decreased rates of hepatic metabolism of acetaminophen to its primary nontoxic metabolites. It was speculated that limited hepatic blood flow and nutrient supply, resulting in reduced glutathione levels, may have played a role.

Concurrent use of other medications such as phenobarbital (29), phenytoin (30,31), isoniazid (32,33), and zidovudine (34) is also a risk factor for hepatotoxicity. These agents induce CYP450 or compete with glucuronidation pathways resulting in the increased production of NAPQI. The presence of underlying chronic liver disease or cirrhosis does not predispose to acetaminophen hepatotoxicity. The clinical presentation may be more severe, however, in persons with underlying liver damage because of limited hepatic reserve.

IV. SUICIDAL POISONING

Historically, the majority of cases of acetaminophen-induced hepatic damage have occurred as a result of a single large ingestion taken by an individual attempting suicide, or as a parasuicidal gesture—"a cry for help." Ingestion of moderate to large amounts of alcohol around the time of the overdose is common. Such persons often take the drug on impulse and many do not want to actually die. They later regret their actions when they present to the emergency room to receive appropriate treatment.

V. ACCIDENTAL POISONING (THERAPEUTIC MISADVENTURE)

Significant hepatic injury and death have also been reported in persons taking acetaminophen with therapeutic intent (7,9–11,20,35). These accidental poisonings have been termed "therapeutic misadventures." In contrast to suicidal poisoning, these individuals ingest smaller amounts of acetaminophen for periods ranging from a few days to, less frequently, a few weeks. This is most likely to occur in the setting of an acute or subacute painful illness or condition, including febrile illness with severe myalgias, dental or traumatic pain, headache, acute exacerbation of chronic back pain, pancreatitis, and even hangover. The typical presentation involves the use of higher-than-recommended doses with ingestions of 10–20 g over 2–3 days. Up to 40% of patients claimed to have taken less than 4 g/day (11). While most ingestions occur over less than 7 days, up to one-third of patients have reported using acetaminophen preparations for at least 30 days (11,36). As outlined above, this scenario occurs most frequently in chronic alcohol users or in the presence of illness-related fasting or underlying malnutrition. A summary of the clinical characteristics of accidental and suicidal poisonings is given in Table 1.

Table 1 Characteristics of Accidental and Suicidal Acetaminophen Ingestions

Feature	Accidental	Suicidal
Presentation	Late	Early
Dose ingested	Small	Large
Association with alcohol abuse	Frequent	Present but less frequent
Blood acetaminophen levels	Seldom elevated	Usually elevated
Key to diagnosis	High aminotransferases, history	History, toxic blood levels
N-Acetylcysteine effective	Usually of value	Definitely effective
Severity	>60% severe	Occasionally (20%) severe
Mortality	High	Low
Typical hospital stay	Long	Short

Source: Adapted from Schiødt et al. (7).

Multiple preparations under different trade names as well as the various acetaminophen and narcotic combinations result in some persons taking a few different trade name tablets each containing acetaminophen, without realizing their combined toxic potential. In addition, such individuals often present late, at the stage of symptomatic hepatic injury, with a consequent increase in their mortality. Patients who develop jaundice on the background of significant alcohol use may be misdiagnosed as having alcoholic hepatitis (37). The key to diagnosis is the extreme transaminase elevation, which is never seen with alcohol alone, and levels greater than 5000 IU/L are rarely seen in viral hepatitis. A high index of suspicion is required as these patients may benefit from treatment with N-acetylcysteine.

Accidental poisoning has recently also been reported in children ranging in age from 5 weeks to over 12 years (17,38–44). The typical setting is the administration of frequent doses over a few days by parents or on occasion by hospital staff, to children who have a febrile acute or subacute illness. As in the adult cases, supratherapeutic doses (greater than 150 mg/kg/24 h) are often used, although smaller doses have frequently been reported. Doses used have ranged from 20 to over 600 mg/kg/24 h taken over periods of 1 day–6 weeks (40,42). The association of a febrile illness with or without vomiting, resulting in a decreased oral intake, is likely to have made the children acutely malnourished and predisposed them to acetaminophen hepatotoxicity at lower-than-expected doses. In children with significant acetaminophen hepatotoxicity, progression to acute liver failure has been reported in over 20% of cases with a significant mortality rate (39,40).

Dosing errors most frequently made by parents result from a variety of mistakes, including: adult preparations used instead of infant or children's preparations; dosing instructions misread or misunderstood; or extra doses given when symptoms persist despite recommended dosing (40). Failure to recognize the potential danger and the resulting delays in presentation and management further predispose to hepatotoxicity. It remains worrisome that some children appear to develop significant hepatic injury after receiving what are thought to be safe, though repetitive, doses of acetaminophen. Dose undercalculation cannot be discounted in at least some of these cases. The associated underlying febrile illness in addition to causing acute malnutrition also raises the possibility of viral cofactors playing a role in the hepatic damage. The typical course and outcome of this scenario is, however, more in keeping with acetaminophen-induced hepatotoxicity rather than fulminant viral or indeterminate hepatitis (45).

In summary, significant hepatocellular injury from acetaminophen in children is relatively uncommon, occurring in less than 10% of cases in which potentially toxic doses of drug had been ingested (17,44). Accidental acetaminophen poisoning is, however, a major cause of overdose in children 10 years of age or younger and can lead to acute liver failure and death (39). Repetitive doses of acetaminophen, even when in the therapeutic range, need to be given with caution to children suffering from a febrile illness associated with nausea and anorexia.

VI. CHRONIC TOXICITY

Possible chronic hepatotoxicity has been reported in a person who had ingested therapeutic or near-therapeutic doses (2–6 g/day) over a prolonged period. Bonkowsky and colleagues (46) have described significant histological damage, including fibrosis, in a male who had ingested 4 g acetaminophen per day for 1 year. On stopping the drug, the elevated transaminases returned to near normal. Rechallenge with a dose of 1325 mg was associated with a rise in transaminases within 18 h. This scenario is similar to the classic therapeutic misadventure, although the duration of ingestion was significantly longer. While some persons may be predisposed to developing liver damage, it remains unclear why the damage did not occur earlier or whether other drugs, toxins, or intercurrent illnesses may have made the liver more susceptible to acetaminophen-induced hepatotoxicity or, indeed, were responsible for some of the injury. Chronic acetaminophen hepatotoxicity remains unproven.

In contrast, some individuals ingest otherwise toxic amounts of acetaminophen over prolonged periods without developing any obvious signs of liver injury. Doses ranging from 3 g to 65 g/day have been reported (47–49). A recent study demonstrated that repeat exposure to incremental acetaminophen doses provides protection in an animal model, as a possible explanation for this scenario (49).

VII. EPIDEMIOLOGY OF ACETAMINOPHEN POISONING

Acetaminophen poisoning is predominantly a Western phenomenon, although even here the incidence varies between different countries. Intentional overdose with acetaminophen is one of the most popular means of attempting suicide in the United Kingdom (50). It is of further concern that acetaminophen overdoses and toxicity appear to be on the increase in the United States (8,12). Over 110,000 cases of acetaminophen poisoning are reported per year in the United States (51) and an estimated 70,000 cases in the United Kingdom (52). Some 150–200 deaths from acetaminophen occur annually in the United Kingdom compared to approximately 100 in the United States. Case fatality rates have been estimated to be 0.4% in the United Kingdom (53), and 0.1% in the United States (51) and France (53). Accidental overdoses or therapeutic misadventures have been reported predominantly from the United States and may comprise 30–50% of cases of severe hepatic injury (7,36).

While a number of social and psychological factors interact in predisposing individuals to take overdoses, there is a clear correlation between acetaminophen availability and sales, and the incidence of overdose (53,54). Countries such as Australia that limit the number of acetaminophen tablets available per packet and encourage the use of blister packaging have a significantly lower incidence of severe hepatic injury. Some evidence is now becoming available that severe acetaminophen hepatotoxicity may be decreasing in the United Kingdom since availability has been limited (55,56). Widespread public education campaigns warning of the dangers of acetaminophen and chronic alcohol use are also needed, in addition to specific medication label warnings, to decrease the prevalence of therapeutic misadventures.

VIII. CLINICAL FEATURES

The clinical characteristics of acetaminophen hepatotoxicity can be divided into four stages (57). Stage 1 occurs within a few hours of ingestion. It consists of acute gastrointestinal symptoms, including anorexia, abdominal pain, nausea, and vomiting as well as general malaise, diaphoresis, and occasional vascular collapse. Drowsiness is more likely to occur with concomitant ingestion of narcotics or sedatives. Some patients may experience little or no symptoms. Stage 2 is seen 24–48 h after ingestion. During this period the patients are relatively well and may, in fact, be totally asymptomatic.

Stage 3 is seen only in those patients who develop significant liver injury. Clinical signs of liver injury are usually present 2–5 days after ingestion. In addition to the gastrointestinal symptoms outlined above, patients develop lethargy, dark urine, jaundice, and hepatic tenderness. In more severe cases overt acute liver failure is seen with the development of hepatic encephalopathy. While this generally occurs 3–4 days after poisoning, occasionally it may be delayed for up to 6 days. Acute liver failure may be accompanied by renal failure, multiple organ failure, sepsis, and cerebral edema, which may lead to death. Stage 4, the recovery phase, is usually seen 5–10 days after ingestion in those who survive the hepatic insult. As full recovery takes place, all symptoms gradually resolve. In those with more severe hepatic injury, jaundice and renal failure may be more prolonged. Permanent liver damage is seen very infrequently after acetaminophen overdose (58) and liver function returns to normal in those without underlying liver disease.

IX. BIOCHEMICAL AND OTHER LABORATORY FEATURES

A summary of laboratory values seen in acetaminophen hepatotoxicity is given in Table 2. Patients who are treated with *N*-acetylcysteine within 8–12 h of ingestion will often display few or no laboratory abnormalities, even in the presence of a "high risk" serum acetaminophen level. Those treated later, or not at all, develop a number of typical biochemical and hematological abnormalities. These laboratory features in themselves are, however, not diagnostic of acetaminophen hepatotoxicity. Serum levels of alanine aminotransferase (ALT) and aspartate aminotransferase (AST), which are markers of hepatocellular injury, can become markedly elevated, occasionally reaching over 10,000 IU/L (11). Transaminase levels generally increase approximately 24 h after admission, occasionally as early as 8 h, and peak at day 2 or 3 (60). Levels usually return to normal, or near normal, within 7–10 days of the insult. Transaminase levels of the magnitude seen in acetaminophen hepatotoxicity are rarely seen in other causes of hepatic injury with the

Table 2 Biochemical Characteristics of Acetaminophen Toxicity

Laboratory value	Minor to moderate toxicity	Severe toxicity
AST/ALT	Normal to mildly elevated (up to 1000 IU/L)	Often very elevated; >3000 IU/L; typically peak at day 2–3 after ingestion
Bilirubin	Normal to moderately elevated (up to 100 μmol/L or 5.9 mg/dL)	Continues to increase, even after transaminases improve
INR	Normal to moderately prolonged up to 2	Very prolonged; may be >10 elevation out of proportion to level of encephalopathy
Creatinine	Usually normal	Acute renal failure occurs frequently in patients with ALF
Acid-base balance	Respiratory alkalosis, pH usually <7.60	Metabolic acidosis; admission arterial pH <7.30 is a poor sign
Platelets	Usually normal	Thrombocytopenia (<100 × 10⁹) common in patients with ALF
Blood glucose	Usually normal or slightly decreased	Severe hypoglycemia may be seen in ALF

Source: Adapted from Schiødt and Lee (59).

exception of ischemic hepatitis or heat stroke and rare cases of viral hepatitis. Serum bilirubin elevation occurs in more severe cases. Typically bilirubin levels peak later than transaminases and may continue to increase after ALT/AST levels have begun to improve. Maximum bilirubin elevations are lower than seen in viral hepatitis or idiosyncratic drug reactions. Very high bilirubin levels may be seen in the presence of acute renal failure. Hepatic production of clotting factors becomes reduced with a resulting prolongation in the prothrombin time (and INR) (61). In severe cases the INR may be greater than 10. The INR prolongation is often out of proportion to the level of encephalopathy seen in acute liver failure.

Serum creatinine may be elevated in cases of severe poisoning, resulting from direct acetaminophen nephrotoxicity (62). As with hepatotoxicity, chronic alcohol ingestion has been reported to predispose to the development of renal damage and failure (63,64). Acute renal failure occurs in approximately 50% of patients with acute liver failure with grade III or IV encephalopathy as part of the multisystem failure syndrome (65). Acid-base disturbances are frequently seen (66). While respiratory alkalosis secondary to hyperventilation occurs in the milder cases, lactic acidosis is a poor prognostic sign in hepatic encephalopathy (67). Severe hypoglycemia requiring concentrated glucose infusions may be seen in acute liver failure. Moderate thrombocytopenia can also occur in hepatic failure.

X. PATHOLOGICAL FEATURES

The characteristic histological changes seen with acetaminophen poisoning are centrilobular (zone III) hepatic necrosis and sinusoidal congestion (58,68). In severe cases, submassive (bridging) or panacinar (massive) necrosis is seen. This pattern of necrosis reflects the role of CYP2E1, which is located in this part of the hepatic acinus, and glutathione levels that are lower. Inflammation is not a significant feature. On recovery, complete resolution without fibrosis occurs. In the kidney, necrosis of the proximal and distal tubules is the most prominent finding. Myocardial necrosis and pancreatitis have also been reported (69,70).

XI. ACETAMINOPHEN-INDUCED ACUTE LIVER FAILURE

Hepatic injury, defined as a transaminase level greater than 1000 IU/L, is seen relatively frequently in acetaminophen poisoning if treated late or untreated. The percentage of patients who develop acute liver failure (ALF) is, however, actually quite small (7,71). In a series of 71 hospitalized patients from a county hospital in the United States, 14% developed ALF and 7% died (7); all but one patient was in the accidental poisoning group. Series from Australia have reported even lower morbidity and mortality. Acute liver failure was seen in 7% of 306 hospitalized patients, with no deaths (72). Two more recent studies found ALF in 9% of 151 patients with one death (0.6%) (73), and only two deaths (0.2%) among 981 patients (74). Factors associated with more severe liver injury and the development of ALF included late presentation and treatment, ingestion of large amounts of acetaminophen, chronic alcohol ingestion, and accidental overdose.

The epidemiology of acetaminophen-induced ALF varies widely in countries around the world (Table 3). It is the most common cause of ALF in both the United Kingdom and United States, being responsible for 60% (13,76) and up to 35% (12) of all cases, respectively. On the other hand, it plays a less important role in other European countries and is not seen at all in Eastern countries such as India (77–79). The clinical features

Table 3 Etiology of ALF in Different Countries

	HAV (%)	HBV (%)	Drug reactions (%)	Acetaminophen (%)	Other[a] (%)
UK: 1993–1994 (n = 342)	2	2	2	73	21
France: 1972–1990 (n = 502)	4	32	17	2	45
India: 1987–1993 (n = 423)	2	31	5	0	62
Denmark: 1973–1990 (n = 160)	1	7	10	45	37
USA: 1994–1996 (n = 295)	7	10	12	20	51

[a] Includes NANB, HEV, and miscellaneous.
Source: Adapted from Lee and Schiødt (75).

of acetaminophen-caused ALF are different from those of other etiologies. The onset of symptoms is typically very rapid (hyperacute), extremely high transaminases are frequently seen, and the INR is often elevated out of proportion to the encephalopathy grade. The time course of clinical and laboratory abnormalities is quite rigid for suicidal ingestions.

XII. DIAGNOSIS

The diagnosis is straightforward in those who present with a clear history of ingestion including the amount and time taken. Such a history is not always available, however. Individuals may have a depressed level of consciousness due to alcohol intoxication or coingestion of sedatives or other drugs. Others may be simply uncooperative. A high index of suspicion is required in all potential suicidal overdose cases. Acetaminophen poisoning must also be suspected in all persons with elevated transaminases, especially if the levels are greater than 1000 IU/L. It must be remembered that transaminases will be normal soon after ingestion. In those with accidental poisoning, careful questioning regarding all medications taken is imperative, as these persons will not be aware of the potential implications of their analgesic use. The reported dose may be inaccurate owing to either underreporting or partial vomiting, so this cannot be relied on completely. Paracetamol serum levels checked at 4 h after ingestion or presentation (if later than 4 h) can be very useful in assessing the potential for significant hepatotoxicity, but have their limitations especially when the time interval between ingestion and measurement is uncertain. In some cases repeating the measurement in another 4 h, if this is within 8 h of ingestion, and calculation of the acetaminophen half-life may be of help. Those who have a half-life of less than 4 h are unlikely to develop significant hepatotoxicity. Acetaminophen levels may be normal in accidental poisoning because of both later presentations and smaller individual doses. Transaminase levels may be of more help in this setting.

Matthew-Rumack nomogram (see Fig. 1) (80), often used to decide on the need for *N*-acetylcysteine treatment, was developed after assessment of a group of untreated patients for hepatotoxicity, defined as ALT or AST above 1000 IU/L. Plasma acetaminophen level is plotted on the Y axis and time from ingestion on the X axis. When plotted above

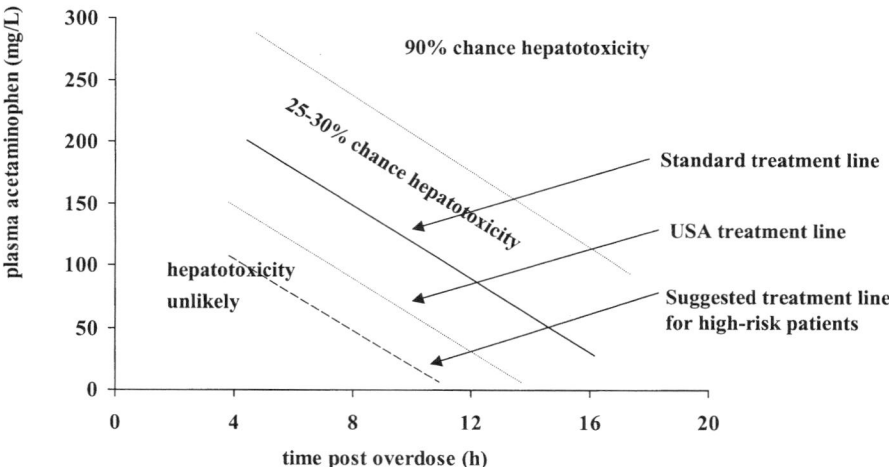

Figure 1   Matthew-Rumack nomogram for plasma acetaminophen after a single acetaminophen ingestion. Plots in the area between the standard treatment line (solid) and the slashed line represent a 25–30% risk of hepatotoxicity, while those above the slashed line represent a 90% risk of hepatotoxicity. Treatment with NAC is instituted when a result is above either the standard treatment line or the U.S. treatment line. It has been recommended that treatment be started at lower plasma levels for those predisposed to acetaminophen hepatotoxicity, hence the treatment line for high-risk patients.

the line starting at a plasma level of 300 mg/L at 4 h, there is a 90% chance of developing hepatotoxicity. Treatment is usually instituted when values fall above the standard treatment line starting at a plasma level of 200 mg/L at 4 h. The nomogram is, however, of limited use in predicting hepatotoxicity under several circumstances. It is only of benefit in a single point ingestion, not in repeated doses as occurs in accidental poisoning. Also, the absorption of extended-release acetaminophen preparations may be more prolonged and thus the original "safe" values may be misleading (81). The nomogram cannot be safely applied in patients at high risk for acetaminophen hepatotoxicity. Consequently, a treatment line starting at a plasma level of 100 mg/L at 4 h has been suggested for high-risk patients (82). Finally, the interval since ingestion may be uncertain or unknown. In any case, when doubt exists about the potential toxicity of the ingestion, treatment must be instituted.

XIII. TREATMENT

The principles of treatment of acetaminophen poisoning are interruption of drug absorption, use of a specific antidote—*N*-acetylcysteine—and supportive care. Prompt treatment with *N*-acetylcysteine is, however, central to the successful management of acetaminophen toxicity.

An effort to decrease acetaminophen absorption should be made unless it is clear that ingestion occurred more than 24 h earlier. Gastric lavage can be useful in patients who present within 4 h of ingestion; many, however, present later. Oral activated charcoal has been shown to reduce acetaminophen absorption by binding to it in the lumen of the stomach. It appears to be superior to both gastric lavage and ipecac (83). Charcoal is unlikely to interfere with the efficacy of oral N-acetylcysteine (84).

N-Acetylcysteine (NAC) is the established antidote for acetaminophen poisoning. It is the N-acetylated derivative of the sulfhydryl amino acid L-cysteine and its sulfhydryl group is thought to be essential for its early antidote effects. Its most important action is the replenishment of glutathione stores, which inhibits the damaging effects of the breakdown product NAPQI (85,86). Other actions of NAC include vasodilatation, increased tissue oxygen uptake, antioxidant effects, and suppression of TNFα (87–90). These actions may in part explain the continued benefit of NAC once hepatic injury and even acute liver failure have developed.

A number of different NAC regimens exist in clinical practice. Oral NAC is used in the United States as the intravenous form has not been approved by the Food and Drug Administration. The oral regimen involves a loading dose of 140 mg/kg and is followed by maintenance doses of 70 mg/kg, every 4 h for 72 h (91). Total NAC dose given is 1330 mg/kg. Many patients have significant nausea with or without vomiting after acetaminophen poisoning, and the oral preparation of NAC with its strong unpleasant odor is difficult to ingest. As a result, some units in the United States have been using intravenous preparations (of the oral form) without any apparent problems (92,93). The standard intravenous protocol is given as an infusion in 5% dextrose over 20 h (94). This includes a loading dose of 150 mg/kg given over 15 min–1 h, followed by 50 mg/kg over 4 h, then 100 mg/kg over 16 h. Total NAC dose given is 300 mg/kg and volume of dextrose required about 1800 mL. This protocol may be extended in patients presenting late with significant hepatotoxicity. Infusions of 150 mg/kg over 24 h can be given for a further 24–48 h. Another intravenous regimen involves the intermittent doses based on the oral version (95). Each dose is given over 1 h, every 4 h, for 48 h. Total NAC dose given is 980 mg/kg. Oral versus intravenous regimens have never been compared directly. A recent meta-analysis of seven studies reported that prevention of hepatotoxicity was similar in both groups (74). The authors concluded that intravenous NAC may be preferable because of a shorter hospital stay, patient convenience, and concerns over the bioavailability of oral NAC in the presence of nausea and vomiting.

While none of the original NAC studies were of optimal design, lacking randomization and using only historical controls, the use of NAC within 10 h of ingestion is associated with a definite protective effect. Less than 10% of patients developed hepatic damage if given NAC within 10 h, and almost complete protection is seen within 8 h (91). In patients who received NAC 10–24 h after ingestion, 26–63% developed hepatic damage with a mortality of 2–7% (94). This contrasts with the development of hepatic injury in more than 80% of historical controls. Some benefit is seen even in individuals given NAC 72 h after overdose with less frequent progression to grade III or IV encephalopathy and a lower mortality (96,97). Furthermore, a randomized controlled trial in patients with acetaminophen-induced ALF found that those given NAC were less likely to develop hypotension and cerebral edema, and had a higher rate of survival (96).

N-Acetylcysteine is a safe treatment. Adverse effects have been reported in about 5–14% of patients (92,98). They occur more frequently with intravenous infusions than oral regimens. Most represent a mild anaphylactoid reaction and include pruritus, mild urticaria, flushing, or wheezing. Rare serious adverse reactions including arrhythmias, angioedema, hypotension, and death have been reported. It is very likely that factors other than NAC played important roles in the development of these events. Treatment includes slowing or stopping the infusion and/or antihistamine or, rarely, corticosteriod injection. Invariably the infusion is continued without further adverse effects. Most reactions occur early in the front-loaded infusion and giving the first dose over 60 min, instead of 15 min, decreases the incidence of reactions (74).

In the patients who develop ALF, supportive treatment in an intensive care unit is of paramount importance (99). Supportive care includes the close monitoring and correction of blood glucose levels and electrolyte abnormalities. Any signs of sepsis are treated aggressively with broad-spectrum antibiotics until results of cultures are known. Some units use prophylactic antibiotics. Sedation or analgesics are generally contraindicated. Dialysis may be required in patients with acute renal failure who develop serious electrolyte disturbances or fluid overload. Signs of increased intracranial pressure are treated immediately with intravenous mannitol. Patients with grade III or IV encephalopathy are usually intubated and ventilated. Transfer to a specialist liver unit must be considered to allow for urgent liver transplantation in deteriorating individuals before irreversible cerebral edema or multisystem failure occurs. Unfortunately, many of these patients are not transplant candidates because of underlying psychiatric histories or substance abuse.

XIV. OUTCOME

The outcome of acetaminophen poisoning is largely related to the absolute amount of drug taken and the time interval between ingestion and administration of the antidote. While the overall estimated case fatality rates are very small, ranging from 0.1 to 0.4%, this figure does not fully represent the morbidity and overall impact on both individuals and Western societies of acetaminophen poisoning. In those persons who develop ALF the spontaneous survival of 65% is significantly better than in ALF from other etiologies (25%) (12). Only a small percentage undergo liver transplantation (<10%); however, significant numbers still die (28%) either on the transplant list or after exclusion from transplantation for psychosocial reasons. Those who undergo transplantation are faced with lifelong immunosuppression for what was potentially a reversible condition.

A number of clinical features on presentation have been found to be associated with a poor outcome. These include acidosis, severe coagulopathy, low plasma coagulation factors V and VIII, high creatinine and bilirubin, and the presence of grade III or IV encephalopathy. Accurate prognostic criteria are important to predict who is likely to require a liver transplant or, conversely, survive without the need for transplantation. The King's College criteria from London (Table 4) are among the most commonly used (67).

Table 4   Indications for Liver Transplantation in Acetaminophen-Induced ALF Patients Developed at King's College Hospital, London

King's College Hospital Criteria
pH < 7.3 (irrespective of encephalopathy grade)
or
Prothrombin time > 100 s (INR > 7.0) and serum creatinine >300 µmol/L (> 3.4 mg/dL) in patients with grade III or IV encephalopathy

Fulfillment of the criteria was originally associated with an 80% probability to require liver transplantation. As these criteria were developed some years ago, they may not be totally applicable currently in units in other countries. A recent report concluded that fulfillment of King's criteria usually predicts a poor outcome (good positive predictive value) but lack of fulfillment of the criteria does not predict survival (low negative predictive value) (100). Analysis of the U.S. Acute Liver Failure Study Group data (79 cases of acetaminophen toxicity), on the other hand, revealed a poor positive predictive value (54%) and moderate negative predictive value (73%) (unpublished data). Other scoring systems such as the APACHE II (101) and III (102) have also been investigated and may be better predictors; however, the advantage appears relatively small. Clearly, a need exists for the development of better prognostic criteria.

XV. CONCLUSION

Acetaminophen is one of the most readily available and widely used analgesics. Although side-effect-free and relatively safe at recommended doses, it has a narrow therapeutic window. Both suicidal overdose and the more recently recognized accidental poisoning or therapeutic misadventure are major causes of hepatotoxicity in Western countries. Acetaminophen hepatotoxicity is the most common cause of acute liver failure in both the United States and United Kingdom and is associated with a significant number of deaths. The timely use of N-acetylcysteine prevents significant hepatotoxicity in the majority of cases. More importantly, measures should to be undertaken to prevent the large number of poisonings that continue to occur in the developed world. Limiting the availability of acetaminophen in countries such as the United States is central to these measures. Alerting the public to the potential dangers of acetaminophen use, especially with chronic alcohol ingestion, without emphasizing its suicidal potential, is another challenge.

REFERENCES

1. Black M. Acetaminophen hepatotoxicity. Annu Rev Med 1984; 35:577–593.
2. Davidson DG, Eastham WN. Acute liver necrosis following overdose of paracetamol. Br Med J 1966; 2:497–499.
3. Thompson JS, Prescott LF. Liver damage and impaired glucose tolerance after paracetamol overdose. 1966; 2:506–507.
4. McJunkin B, Barwick KW, Little WC, Winfield JB. Fatal massive hepatic necrosis following acetaminophen overdose. JAMA 1976; 236:1874–1875.
5. Clark R, Borirakchanyavat V, Davidson AR, Thompson RP, Widdop B, Goulding R, Williams R. Hepatic damage and death from overdose of paracetamol. Lancet 1973; 1:66–70.
6. Hamlyn AN, Douglas AP, James O. The spectrum of paracetamol (acetaminophen) overdose: clinical and epidemiological studies. Postgrad Med J 1978; 54:400–404.
7. Schiødt FV, Rochling FA, Casey DL, Lee WM. Acetaminophen toxicity in an urban county hospital. N Engl J Med 1997; 337:1112–1117.
8. Schiødt FV, Atillasoy E, Shakil AO, Schiff ER, Caldwell C, Kowdley KV, Stribling R, Crippin JS, Flamm S, Somberg KA, Rosen H, McCashland TM, Hay JE, Lee WM, Acute Liver Failure Study Group. Etiology and outcome for 295 patients with acute liver failure in the United States. Liver Transplant Surg 1999; 5:29–34.
9. Maddrey WC. Hepatic effects of acetaminophen: enhanced toxicity in alcoholics. J Clin Gastroenterol 1987; 9:180–185.

10. Whitcomb DC, Block GD. Association of acetaminophen hepatotoxicity with fasting and alcohol use. JAMA 1994; 272:1845–1850.

11. Zimmermann HJ, Maddrey WC. Acetaminophen (paracetamol) hepatotoxicity with regular intake of alcohol: analysis of instances of therapeutic misadventure. Hepatology 1995; 22: 767–773.

12. Ostapowicz G, Fontana R, Larson AM, Davern T, Lee WM, ALF Study Group. Etiology and outcome of acute liver failure in the USA: preliminary results of a prospective multi-center study. Hepatology 1999; 30(suppl):221A.

13. Tibbs C, Williams R. Viral causes and management of acute liver failure. J Hepatol 1995; 22(1 suppl):68–73.

14. Prescott LF, Critchley JA. The treatment of acetaminophen poisoning. Annu Rev Pharmacol Toxicol 1983; 23:87–101.

15. Hamlyn AN, Douglas AP, James O. The spectrum of paracetamol (acetaminophen) overdose: clinical and epidemiological studies. Postgrad Med J 1978; 54:400–404.

16. Denison H, Kaczynski J, Wallerstedt S. Paracetamol medication and alcohol abuse: a danger-ous combination for the liver and the kidney. Scand J Gastroenterol 1987; 22:701–704.

17. Rumack BH. Acetaminophen overdose in young children. Am J Dis Child 1984; 138:428–433.

18. Miller RP, Roberts RJ, Fischer LJ. Acetaminophen elimination kinetics in neonates, children, and adults. Clin Pharmacol Ther 1976; 19:284–294.

19. McClain CJ, Kromhout JP, Peterson FJ, Holtzman JL. Potentiation of acetaminophen hepato-toxicity by alcohol. JAMA 1980; 244:251–253.

20. Seeff LB, Cuccherini BA, Zimmerman HJ, Adler E, Benjamin SB. Acetaminophen hepato-toxicity in alcoholics: a therapeutic misadventure. Ann Intern Med 1986; 104:399–404.

21. Lesser PB, Vietti MM, Clark WD. Lethal enhancement of therapeutic doses of acetamino-phen by alcohol. Dig Dis Sci 1986; 3:103–105.

22. Wootton FT, Lee WM. Acetaminophen hepatotoxicity in the alcoholic. South Med J 1990; 83:1047–1049.

23. Johnston SC, Pelletier LL. Enhanced hepatotoxicity of acetaminophen in the alcoholic pa-tient: two case reports and a review of the literature. Medicine 1997; 76:185–191.

24. Girre C, Hispard E, Palombo S, N'Guyen C, Dally S. Increased metabolism of acetaminophen in chronically alcoholic patients. Alcohol Clin Exp Res 1993; 17:170–173.

25. Bray GP, Mowat C, Muir DF, Tredger JM, Williams R. The effect of chronic alcohol intake on prognosis and outcome in paracetamol overdose. Hum Exp Toxicol 1991; 10:435–438.

26. Prescott LF. Paracetamol, alcohol and the liver. Br J Clin Pharmacol 2000; 49:291–301.

27. Banda PW, Quart BD. The effect of mild alcohol consumption on the metabolism of acet-aminophen in man. Res Commun Chem Pathol Pharamacol 1982; 38:57–70.

28. Bonkovsky HL, Kane RE, Jones DP, Galinsky RE, Banner B. Acute hepatic and renal toxicity from low doses of acetaminophen in the absence of alcohol abuse or malnutrition: evidence for increased susceptibility to drug toxicity due to cardiopulmonary and renal insufficiency. Hepatology 1994; 19:1141–1148.

29. Pirotte JH. Apparent potentiation of hepatotoxicity from small doses of acetaminophen by phenobarbital. Ann Intern Med 1984; 101:403.

30. McClements BM, Hyland M, Callender ME, Blair TL. Management of paracetamol poison-ing complicated by enzyme induction due to alcohol or drugs. Lancet 1990; 335:1526.

31. Bray GP, Harrison PM, O'Grady JG, Tredger JM, Williams R. Long-term anticonvulsant therapy worsens outcome in paracetamol-induced fulminant hepatic failure. Hum Exp Tox-icol 1992; 11:265–270.

32. Murphy R, Swartz R, Watkins PB. Severe acetaminophen toxicity in a patient receiving isoniazid. Ann Intern Med 1990; 113:799–800.

33. Crippin JS. Acetaminophen hepatotoxicity: potentiation by isoniazid. Am J Gastroenterol 1993; 88:590–592.

34. Shriner K, Goetz MB. Severe hepatotoxicity in a patient receiving both acetaminophen and zidovudine. Am J Med 1992; 93:94–96.

35. Eriksson LS, Broome U, Kalin M, Lindholm M. Hepatotoxicity due to repeated intake of low doses of paracetamol. J Intern Med 1992; 231:567–570.

36. Larson AM, Ostapowicz G, Fontana R, Shakil AO, Lee WM, ALF Study Group. Outcome of acetaminophen-induced liver failure in the USA in suicidal vs accidental overdose: preliminary results of a prospective multi-center trial. Hepatology 2000; 32(suppl):396A.

37. Kumar S, Rex DK. Failure of physicians to recognize acetaminophen hepatotoxicity in chronic alcoholics. Arch Intern Med 1991; 151:1189–1191.

38. Rumack BH, Peterson RG. Acetaminophen overdose: incidence, diagnosis and management in 416 patients. Pediatrics 1978; 62:898–903.

39. Rivera-Penera T, Gugig R, Davis J, McDiarmid S, Vargas J, Rosenthal P, Berquist W, Heyman MB, Ament ME. Outcome of acetaminophen overdose in pediatric patients and factors contributing to hepatotoxicity. J Pediatr 1997; 130:300–304.

40. Heubi JE, Barbacci MB, Zimmerman HJ. Therapeutic misadventures with acetaminophen: hepatotoxicity after multiple doses in children. J Pediatr 1998; 132:22–27.

41. Hynson JL, South M. Childhood hepatotoxicity with paracetamol doses less than 150 mg/kg per day. Med J Aust 1999; 171:497.

42. Miles FK, Kamath R, Dorney SF, Gaskin KJ, O'Loughlin EV. Accidental paracetamol overdosing and fulminant hepatic failure in children. Med J Aust 1999; 171:472–475.

43. Pershad J, Nichols M, King W. "The silent killer": chronic acetaminophen toxicity in a toddler. Pediatr Emerg Care 1999; 15:43–46.

44. Alander SW, Dowd MD, Bratton SL, Kearns GL. Pediatric acetaminophen overdose: risk factors associated with hepatocellular injury. Arch Pediatr Adolesc Med 2000; 154:346–350.

45. Alonso EM, Sokol RJ, Hart J, Tyson RW, Narkewicz MR, Whitington PF. Fulminant hepatitis associated with centrilobular hepatic necrosis in young children. J Pediatr 1995; 127:888–894.

46. Bonkowsky HL, Mudge GH, McMurtry RJ. Chronic hepatic inflammation and fibrosis due to low doses of paracetamol. Lancet 1978; 1:1016–1018.

47. McBride AJ, Meredith-Smith P. Compound opioid/paracetamol analgesics: misuse and dependence. Br J Clin Pract 1995; 49:268–269.

48. Tredger JM, Thuluvath P, Williams R, Murray-Lyon IM. Metabolic basis for high paracetamol dosage without hepatic injury: a case study. Hum Exp Toxicol 1995; 14:8–12.

49. Shayiq RM, Roberts DW, Rothstein K, Snawder JE, Benson W, Ma X, Black M. Repeat exposure to incremental doses of acetaminophen provides protection against acetaminophen-induced lethality in mice: an explanation for high acetaminophen dosage in humans without hepatic injury. Hepatology 1999; 29:451–463.

50. Hawton K, Fagg J. Trends in deliberate self poisoning and self injury in Oxford, 1976–90. Br Med J 1992; 304:1409–1411.

51. Litovitz TL, Klein-Schwartz W, White S, Cobaugh DJ, Youniss J, Drab A, Benson BE. 1999 Annual report of the American Association of Poison Control Centers Toxic Exposure Surveillance System. Am J Emerg Med 2000; 18:517–574.

52. Fagan E, Wannan G. Reducing paracetamol overdoses. Br Med J 1996; 313:1417–1418.

53. Gunnell D, Hawton K, Murray V, Garnier R, Bismuth C, Fagg J, Simkin S. Use of paracetamol for suicide and non-fatal poisoning in the UK and France: are restrictions on availability justified? J Epidemiol Commun Health 1997; 51:175–179.

54. Gilbertson RJ, Harris E, Pandey SK, Kelly P, Myers W. Paracetamol use, availability, and knowledge of toxicity among British and American adolescents. Arch Dis Child 1996; 75:194–198.

55. Prince MI, Thomas SH, James OF, Hudson M. Reduction in incidence of severe paracetamol poisoning. Lancet 2000; 355:2047–2048.

56. Turvill JL, Burroughs AK, Moore KP. Change in occurrence of paracetamol overdose in UK after introduction of blister packs. Lancet 2000; 355:2048–2049.

57. Rumack BH. Acetaminophen overdose. Am J Med 1983; 75:104–112.

58. Portmann B, Talbot IC, Day DW, Davidson AR, Murray-Lyon IM, Williams R. Histopathological changes in the liver following a paracetamol overdose: correlation with clinical and biochemical parameters. J Pathol 1975; 117:169–181.

59. Schiødt FV, Lee WM. Management of acetaminophen toxicity. In: EL Krawitt, ed. Medical Management of Liver Disease. New York: Marcel Dekker, 1999:325–337.

60. Singer AJ, Carracio TR, Mofenson HC. The temporal profile of increased transaminase levels in patients with acetaminophen-induced liver dysfunction. Ann Emerg Med 1995; 25:49–53.

61. Harrison PM, O'Grady JG, Keays RT, Alexander GJ, Williams R. Serial prothrombin time as prognostic indicator in paracetamol induced fulminant hepatic failure. Br Med J 1990; 301:964–966.

62. Cobden I, Record CO, Ward MK, Kerr DN. Paracetamol-induced acute renal failure in the absence of fulminant liver damage. Br Med J 1982; 284:21–22.

63. Kaysen GA, Pond SM, Roper MH, Menke DJ, Marrama MA. Combined hepatic and renal injury in alcoholics during therapeutic use of acetaminophen. Arch Intern Med 1985; 145:2019–2023.

64. Blakely P, McDonald BR. Acute renal failure due to acetaminophen ingestion: a case report and review of the literature. J Am Soc Nephrol 1995; 6:48–53.

65. Wendon JA, Ellis AJ. Circulatory derangements, monitoring and management: heart, kidney and brain. In: WM Lee, R Williams, eds. Acute Liver Failure. Cambridge: Cambridge University Press, 1997:132–143.

66. Gray TA, Buckley BM, Vale JA. Hyperlactataemia and metabolic acidosis following paracetamol overdose. QJ Med 1987; 65:811–821.

67. O'Grady J, Alexander GJM, Hayallar KM, Williams R. Early indicators of prognosis in fulminant hepatic failure. Gastroenterology 1989; 97:439–445.

68. Clark R, Borirakchanyavat V, Davidson AR, Thompson RP, Widdop B, Goulding R, Williams R. Hepatic damage and death from overdose of paracetamol. Lancet 1973; 1:66–70.

69. Will EJ, Tomkins AM. Acute myocardial necrosis in paracetamol poisoning. Br Med J 1971; 4:430–431.

70. Hamlyn AN, Douglas AP, James O. The spectrum of paracetamol (acetaminophen) overdose: clinical and epidemiological studies. Postgrad Med J 1978; 54:400–404.

71. Broughan TA, Soloway RD. Acetaminophen hepatotoxicity. Dig Dis Sci 2000; 45:1553–1558.

72. Brotodihardjo AE, Batey RG, Farrell GC, Byth K. Hepatotoxicity from paracetamol self-poisoning in western Sydney: a continuing challenge. Med J Aust 1992; 157:382–385.

73. Gow PJ, Smallwood RA, Angus PW. Paracetamol overdose in a liver transplant centre: an 8-year experience. J Gastroenterol Hepatol 1999; 14:817–821.

74. Buckley NA, Whyte IM, O'Connell DL, Dawson AH. Oral or intravenous N-acetylcysteine: which is the treatment of choice for acetaminophen (paracetamol) poisoning? Clin Toxicol 1999; 37:759–767.

75. Lee WM, Schiødt FV. Fulminant hepatic failure. In: ER Schiff, MF Sorrell, WC Maddrey, eds. Schiff's Textbook of Liver Diseases. New York: Lippincott-Raven, 1999:879–898.

76. Makin AJ, Wendon J, Williams R. A 7-year experience of sever acetaminophen induced hepatotoxicity (1987–1993). Gastroenterology 1995; 109:1907–1916.

77. Acharya SK, Dasarathy S, Kumer TL, Sushma S, Prasanna KS, Tandon A, Sreenivas V, Nijhawan S, Panda SK, Nanda SK, Irshad M, Joshi YK, Duttagupta S, Tandon RK, Tandon BN. Fulminant hepatitis in a tropical population: clinical course, cause, and early predictors of outcome. Hepatology 1996; 23:1448–1445.

78. Khuroo MS. Acute liver failure in India. Hepatology 1997; 26:244–246.

79. Acharya SK, Panda SK, Saxena A, Gupta SD. Acute liver failure in India: a perspective from the East. J Gastroenterol Hepatol 2000; 15:473–479.

80. Rumack BH, Matthew H. Acetaminophen poisoning and toxicity. Pediatrics 1975; 55:871–876.

81. Bizovi KE, Aks SE, Paloucek F, Gross R, Keys N, Rivas J. Late increase in acetaminophen concentration after overdose of Tylenol Extended Relief. Ann Emerg Med 1996; 28:549–551.

82. Bridger S, Henderson K, Glucksman E, Ellis AJ, Henry JA, Williams R. Deaths from low dose paracetamol poisoning. Br Med J 1998; 316:1724–1725.

83. Underhill TJ, Greene MK, Dove AF. A comparison of the efficacy of gastric lavage, ipecacuanha and activated charcoal in the emergency management of paracetamol overdose. Arch Emerg Med 1990; 7:148–154.

84. Spiller HA, Krenzelok EP, Grande GA, Safir EF, Diamond JJ. A prospective evaluation of the effect of activated charcoal before oral N-acetylcysteine in acetaminophen overdose. Ann Emerg Med 1994; 23:519–523.

85. Lauterburg BH, Corcoran GB, Mitchell JR. Mechanism of action of N-acetylcysteine in the protection against the hepatotoxicity of acetaminophen in rats in vivo. J Clin Invest 1983; 71:980–991.

86. Huggett A, Blair IA. The mechanism of paracetamol-induced hepatotoxicity: implications for therapy. Hum Toxicol 1983; 2:399–405.

87. Harrison PM, Wendon JA, Gimson AE, Alexander GJ, Williams R. Improvement by acetylcysteine of hemodynamics and oxygen transport in fulminant hepatic failure. N Engl J Med 1991; 324:1852–1857.

88. Peristeris P, Clark BD, Gatti S, Faggioni R, Mantovani A, Mengozzi M, Orencole SF, Sironi M, Ghezzi P. N-Acetylcysteine and glutathione as inhibitors of tumor necrosis factor production. Cell Immunol 1992; 140:390–399.

89. Henderson A, Hayes P. Acetylcysteine as a cytoprotective antioxidant in patients with severe sepsis: potential new use for an old drug. Ann Pharmacother 1994; 28:1086–1098.

90. Harrison P, Wendon J, Williams R. Evidence of increased guanylate cyclase activation by acetylcysteine in fulminant hepatic failure. Hepatology 1996; 23:1067–1072.

91. Smilkstein MJ, Knapp GL, Kulig KW, Rumack BH. Efficacy of oral N-acetylcysteine in the treatment of acetaminophen overdose: analysis of the national multicenter study (1976 to 1985). N Engl J Med 1988; 319:1557–1562.

92. Yip L, Dart RC, Hurlbut KM. Intravenous administration of oral N-acetylcysteine. Crit Care Med 1998; 26:40–43.

93. Falk JL. Oral N-acetylcysteine given intravenously for acetaminophen overdose: we shouldn't have to, but we must. Crit Care Med 1998; 26:7.

94. Prescott LF, Illingworth RN, Critchley JA, Stewart MJ, Adam RD, Proudfoot AT. Intravenous N-acetylcysteine: the treatment of choice for paracetamol poisoning. Br Med J 1979; 2:1097–1100.

95. Smilkstein MJ, Bronstein AC, Linden C, Augenstein WL, Kulig KW, Rumack BH. Acetaminophen overdose: a 48-hour intravenous N-acetylcysteine treatment protocol. Ann Emerg Med 1991; 20:1058–1063.

96. Harrison PM, Keays R, Bray GP, Alexander GJ, Williams R. Improved outcome of paracetamol-induced fulminant hepatic failure by late administration of acetylcysteine. Lancet 1990; 335:1572–1573.

97. Keays R, Harrison PM, Wendon JA, Forbes A, Gove C, Alexander GJ, Williams R. Intravenous acetylcysteine in paracetamol induced fulminant hepatic failure: a prospective controlled trial. Br Med J 1991; 303:1026–1029.

98. Dawson AH, Henry DA, McEwen J. Adverse reactions to N-acetylcysteine during treatment for paracetamol poisoning. Med J Aust 1989; 150:329–331.

99. Lee WM. Medical management of acute liver failure. In: WM Lee, R Williams, eds. Acute Liver Failure. Cambridge: Cambridge University Press, 1997:115–131.

100. Shakil AO, Kramer D, Mazariegos GV, Fung JJ, Rakela J. Acute liver failure: clinical features, outcome analysis, and applicability of prognostic criteria. Liver Transplant 2000; 6: 163–169.

101. Mitchell I, Bihari D, Chang R, Wendon J, Williams R. Earlier identification of patients at risk from acetaminophen-induced acute liver failure. Crit Care Med 1998; 26:279–284.

102. Bernal W, Wendon J, Rela M, Heaton N, Williams R. Use and outcome of liver transplantation in acetaminophen-induced acute liver failure. Hepatology 1998; 27:1050–1055.

15

Mechanisms Underlying the Hepatotoxicity of Nonsteroidal Anti-Inflammatory Drugs

URS A. BOELSTERLI

HepaTox Consulting and University of Basel, Basel, Switzerland

I. HEPATIC TOXICITY OF NSAIDs—A "CLASS EFFECT"?

Nonsteroidal anti-inflammatory drugs (NSAIDs) belong to a group of therapeutic agents that are frequently prescribed because of their analgesic and antipyretic properties. Many NSAIDs are even available without a prescription and are generally considered safe. However, because a large population of patients is exposed to these drugs, it is not surprising that a relatively large number of adverse effects have been reported. The extremely wide use worldwide has led to an extensive literature on the incidence and types of major and minor adverse effects. Although the most frequent adverse effects associated with the use of NSAIDs clearly occur in the gastrointestinal tract, other target organs, including the liver, have been identified. Comprehensive reviews are available that summarize the risk and the clinical manifestations of NSAID-related hepatic disorders (1–16).

Although new NSAIDs have been designed and are becoming increasingly important (e.g., NO-releasing compounds; highly selective COX-2 inhibitors), many of the "classical" NSAIDs, including oxicams, are still extensively used (5). In spite of the fact that in the last few decades further clinical development of a significant number of NSAIDs had to be stopped, or drugs even withdrawn from the market because of hepatic toxicity (16), new cases of hepatic toxicity are being increasingly reported (4,17). Therefore, the question arises whether this class of drugs has some common feature that would make them particularly prone to hepatic liability through the action of similar mechanisms. However, if one analyzes the relative incidence of acute or subacute liver injury caused by NSAIDs, it becomes apparent that the incidence is low, and not higher than that observed for other drugs (18). An exception may be sulindac: the unusually high incidence of approximately 150 cases of liver injury per 100,000 sulindac users suggests that there is a causal link between the use of this NSAID and an increased risk of hepatotoxicity (14,15). For other NSAIDs, the incidence is clearly lower. For example, it is intermediate for mefenamic acid (2.5 per 100,000), diclofenac (3.6), or naproxen (3.8), and lowest for ibuprofen (1.6) and other NSAIDs (14,15,18).

In general, the clinical manifestations of NSAID toxicity in the liver can present as two distinct forms. On the one hand, mild hepatic changes, evident as minor increases in liver enzymes in the plasma, are relatively frequent and have been estimated to range between 1 and 15% (13). They are usually observed in phase III clinical trials, prior to marketing. In contrast, and of greater concern, are the clinically more significant hepatic injuries, which become evident from case reports in the literature, and which sometimes can have a fatal outcome (8,16). These latter cases are very rare, but, in view of the great number of patients treated worldwide, the absolute numbers may be high. For example, in Denmark between 1978 and 1987, about 9% of all hepatic drug reactions could be attributed to NSAIDs (19). Whether the mild and severe forms of liver injury are causally linked to each other is currently not known.

Awareness of severe hepatic adverse effects of NSAIDs became more widespread when benoxaprofen was introduced into clinical use. Almost immediately after its introduction in 1982, the drug was withdrawn from the market because of hepatic toxicity. Subsequently, the FDA Arthritis Advisory Committee issued the statement that hepatotoxicity is a *class characteristic* of NSAIDs (20). NSAIDs are, however, chemically heterogeneous, comprising several distinct classes (e.g., aspirin and other salicylates, phenylacetic acid derivatives, propionic acid derivatives, indol acetic acid derivatives, pyrazolone derivatives, oxicams, anthranilic acid derivatives, and the more recently introduced coxibs). Meanwhile it has been recognized that this statement is an oversimplification for a number of reasons (21). For example, rates and types of injury vary within and between chemical classes. In addition, there is no consistent mechanism underlying all NSAID-induced liver injuries. A likely reason why hepatotoxicity has been attributed to the entire therapeutic class may simply be that these drugs are among the most widely used medications in the world and that, therefore, hepatic adverse effects seem common.

Nevertheless, most of those NSAIDs that have been associated with liver injury share some common structural features and follow similar pathways of hepatic metabolism and disposition. For example, they are weak acids (pK_a ~3.5–5.5), share a carboxylic acid moiety, and many of them feature lipophilic ring structures. They are often metabolized to acyl glucuronides, excreted, at least in part, via bile, and undergo enterohepatic circulation.

Although these features may be general and shared by many other drugs, they are high-lighted for a better understanding of some of the molecular mechanisms underlying the hepatobiliary toxicity of these drugs.

Only few reviews exist that describe the possible *mechanisms* underlying the hepatic toxicity of NSAIDs (21,22). Apart from in vitro data, the paucity of mechanistic data may reflect the fact that for most NSAIDs, mechanisms responsible for hepatic toxicity in vivo have remained largely enigmatic and speculative. In search of keys to unravel these mechanisms, the observed hepatic adverse effects of NSAIDs have often been grouped into two categories (often referred to as "mechanisms," which they are not). In some cases, hepatic injury seems to be driven by a clear dose-dependent intrinsic toxicity of the compound (e.g., aspirin-induced hepatotoxicity). In most other cases, however, the hepatic reaction is idiosyncratic; that is, the toxicity largely depends on a host-dependent component and occurs in selected individuals only who feature a genetic and/or acquired predisposition. Because it is difficult at present to analyze all the individual susceptibility factors leading to idiosyncratic toxicity, efforts have concentrated on identifying the toxic risk of a compound. This risk is not only determined by the drug's inherent toxic potential on the cellular or molecular level, but also driven by factors governing its disposition and metabolism.

II. DISPOSITION AND METABOLISM OF NSAIDs—IMPLICATIONS FOR HEPATIC ADVERSE EFFECTS

A. Plasma Protein Binding

An important feature of NSAIDs is their high degree of reversible plasma protein binding, which usually is higher than 99% (23). Although the overall bound fraction is high, individual NSAIDs can exhibit marked differences in their unbound fractions (23). This becomes important for risk assessment in humans or for a critical extrapolation from in vitro studies in microsomes, isolated mitochondria, or cellular systems. Often the incubation media do not contain exogenous albumin or other plasma proteins and results from in vitro assays can therefore be easily overestimated.

It is not only the parent compounds, but also the metabolites (including the glucuronoconjugates), that are highly protein-bound. For the glucuronides, the fraction of the free (nonbound) metabolite can even be considerably higher than that of the free parent compound. For example, although more than 90% of naproxen acyl glucuronide is bound to plasma proteins (24), the concentration of the free acyl glucuronide was approximately 10-fold higher than that of the free parent compound. Furthermore, the *iso*-glucuronides (spontaneously formed positional isomers of the acyl glucuronide) can exhibit an even lower degree of protein binding (e.g., 66% for naproxen) (24). As glucuronides play a putative role as pivotal mediators of NSAID hepatotoxicity, the sharp increase in concentration of the free circulating conjugates can become important.

B. Bioactivation to Reactive Metabolites

Some NSAIDs (e.g., diclofenac, piroxicam, ketoprofen) have been shown to form reactive metabolites (25), causing acute lethal cell injury in cultured rat hepatocytes. Unfortunately, there is no clear-cut correlation between the potential to form such reactive metabolites in vitro and the relative incidence of liver injury in patients. Acute cell killing triggered by high drug concentrations in cell culture systems (26) cannot be directly translated into

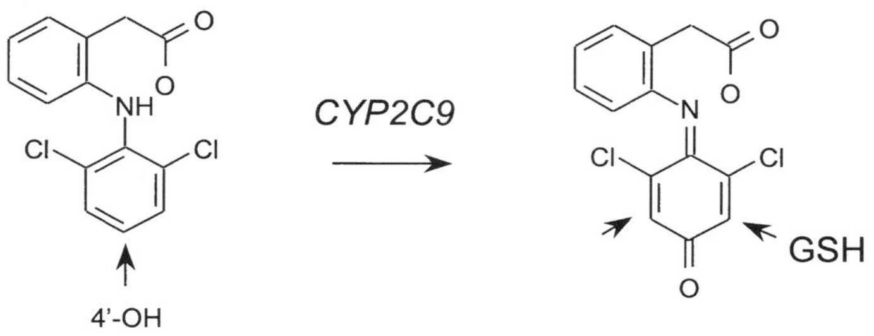

Figure 1 P450-mediated ring hydroxylation of diclofenac can result in the formation of quinone imines. For example, CYP2C9-catalyzed 4′-hydroxylation leads to the 1′4′-quinone imine, which exhibits electrophilic centers (arrows) that can react with glutathione or nucleophilic residues of proteins.

the human situation. However, such data may provide qualitative evidence for the generation of a reactive metabolite in the liver and can help to explain certain interactions of these intermediates with cellular macromolecules.

1. Cytochrome P450-Mediated Bioactivation

Some NSAIDs are ring-hydroxylated by selective P450 forms, which can lead to the formation of reactive intermediates. For example, diclofenac has been shown to form distinct *p*-benzoquinone imines (27), which are electrophilic species. In rats, these intermediates are readily conjugated with glutathione and excreted in bile as *S*-glutathionyl adducts (Fig. 1). Interestingly, the same adducts were detected in human hepatocytes (28,29). If glutathione levels are depleted or if a metabolite is highly reactive, one can surmise that the electrophilic intermediate will also arylate cellular proteins. Indeed, in rats one of the metabolites of diclofenac generated by CYP2C11-catalyzed reactions is so reactive that it forms a covalent adduct with P450 itself at the site of its generation (30). The toxicological implications of these reactions, however, are not clear.

2. Activation by Coenzyme A to Acyl-CoA Thioesters

Carboxylic acid–containing NSAIDs can be activated by acyl-coenzyme A synthetase (ACS1) to form acyl-CoA thioesters (31) (Fig. 2). The 2-arylpropionic acids (profens) are particularly prone to undergoing this reaction. The liver is quantitatively the most important site of activation of profens to CoA thioesters (32).

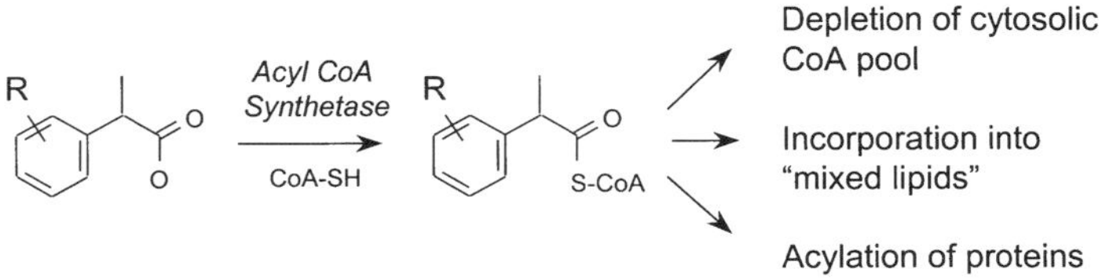

Figure 2 Some carboxylic acid–containing NSAIDs (e.g., 2-arylpropionic acids) can be biotransformed by acyl CoA synthetase to acyl-CoA thioesters. This bioactivation step can entail a number of toxicological consequences.

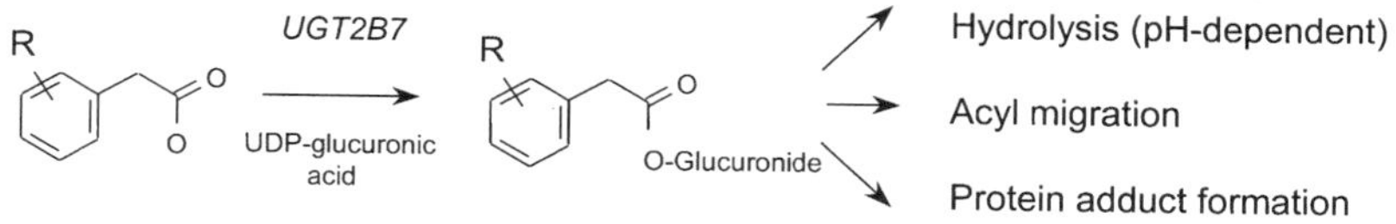

Figure 3 Carboxylic acid–containing NSAIDs can be bioactivated by glucuronosyltransferases (UGT) to β-1-*O*-glucuronides. These acyl (ester) glucuronides are reactive metabolites that can engage in a number of reactions with potential toxicological consequences.

If large amounts of a drug are converted to CoA thioesters, this conjugation reaction in hepatocytes can have several consequences. First, it can lead to a depletion of the cytosolic CoA pool. Furthermore, similar to activated fatty acids, these NSAID-CoA thioesters can enter the pathways of lipid biochemistry. For example, they can be conjugated with cholesterol, bile acids, carnitine, or other amino acids (33) or, alternatively, incorporated into glycerolipids or phospholipids (34,35). Finally, acyl-CoA-thioesters are protein-reactive intermediates that can directly acylate proteins (36). Thus, bioactivation by CoA is an important step in NSAID metabolism with possible toxicological implications.

Interestingly, activation of profens, which exhibit a chiral carbon atom at the α-carboxy position, to their thioesters is stereoselective. Because there is a great variability in the nature and extent of this stereoselectivity, both across species and across different NSAIDs (37), one can expect that the extent of interference of profens with lipid metabolism and their protein reactivity is subject to considerable variability.

3. Activation by UDP-Glucuronosyltransferase to Reactive Acyl Glucuronides and *iso*-Glucuronides

Many carboxylic acid-containing NSAIDs are glucuronidated by members of the UDP-glucuronosyltransferase (UGT) superfamily (reviewed in ref. 38) to their corresponding acyl (or ester) glucuronides. In particular, UGT2B7 has been implicated in catalyzing the glucuronidation of NSAIDs in humans (39,40) (Fig. 3). Because both acyl glucuronides and their positional isomers, generated after spontaneous acyl migration (Fig. 10), are protein-reactive metabolites, the glucuronoconjugation cannot be considered a mere detoxication step but must also be considered a bioactivating pathway.

UGT expression can vary interindividually, due to both environmental and genetic factors. On the one hand, UGTs can be selectively induced by a number of drugs and other chemicals (41). On the other hand, there exist genetic polymorphisms in the genes coding for UGT (42,43). It is likely that additional genetic variations in the human population will be detected that could perhaps help to explain the variability in the plasma or urine concentrations of NSAID glucuronides in the human population (43).

Although acyl glucuronidation is a common pathway, not all carboxylic acid–containing NSAIDs form these conjugates. For example, bromfenac metabolism by human microsomes does not produce an acyl glucuronide. Furthermore, rats administered bromfenac unexpectedly produced an acid-labile *N*-glucoside conjugate (44). It is not known whether this unusual conjugation step with glucose is related to the hepatic toxicity associated with bromfenac, which was recently withdrawn from the market (45–47).

C. Hydrolysis and Systemic Cycling

Acyl glucuronides are readily hydrolyzed, particularly in vivo (48). Serum albumin, to which most NSAIDs bind, can increase this process by interaction of the aglycone moiety

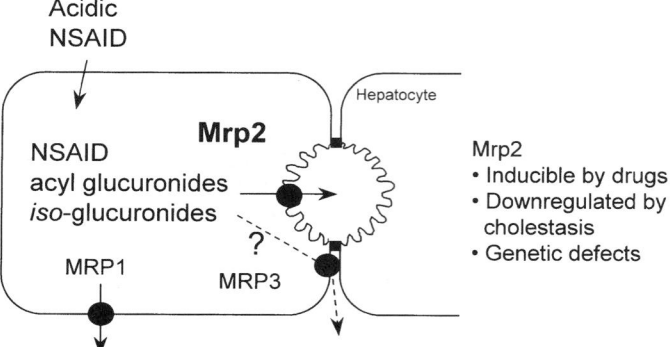

Figure 4 Acyl glucuronides or their positional isomers are transported across the canalicular plasma membrane by the canalicular isoform of the multidrug resistance–associated protein (Mrp2) into bile. Other Mrp isoforms can export the glucuronides across the basolateral membrane into blood. The expression of Mrp is highly regulated, and genetic variations exist.

with basic amino acids (49). Thus, the reversal of glucuronidation, coupled with reglucuronidation, can lead to a systemic cycling, resulting in increased exposure and reduced renal elimination (50).

D. Biliary Excretion

Biliary excretion is an important pathway of NSAID clearance. In particular, the glucuronoconjugates and glutathione S-conjugates are eliminated across the canalicular membrane into the biliary tree. In those cases where NSAIDs contain a chiral center (e.g., the 2-arylpropionic acids), the hepatocanalicular export can be stereoselective. For example, the S-diastereomer of naproxen glucuronide has a higher export rate than the R-diastereomer (51).

NSAID acyl glucuronides are selectively exported into bile by the canalicular isoform of the multidrug resistance–associated protein, Mrp2 (52) (Fig. 4). The hepatic expression of Mrp2 is inducible by a number of drugs (53). This may represent an adaptive response aimed at enhancing biliary elimination of the inducing drug and/or its metabolites. In contrast, under conditions of cholestasis, Mrp2 may disappear from the canalicular membrane, or be relocalized to other subcellular compartments (54). Genetic defects in the gene coding for the canalicular form of Mrp2, such as in the Dubin-Johnson syndrome in humans or in a number of transport-deficient rat models, have been described (55). These altered expression patterns of the canalicular conjugate export pump may have severe toxicokinetic and toxicodynamic consequences.

When biliary elimination is impaired by drugs or by obstruction of the bile duct, other pathways may be activated. For example, while under normal conditions acyl glucuronides and its isomers are excreted into bile (in the rat) and only a minor amount is excreted into the urine, experimental bile duct ligation caused the acyl glucuronide of zomepirac to be shunted into blood (56). These altered pathways can cause increased systemic exposure to the drug.

E. Enterohepatic Circulation

NSAID glucuronides that are excreted via the biliary tree into the gut can be deconjugated by several mechanisms. First, the slightly alkaline pH in bile and in the gastrointestinal

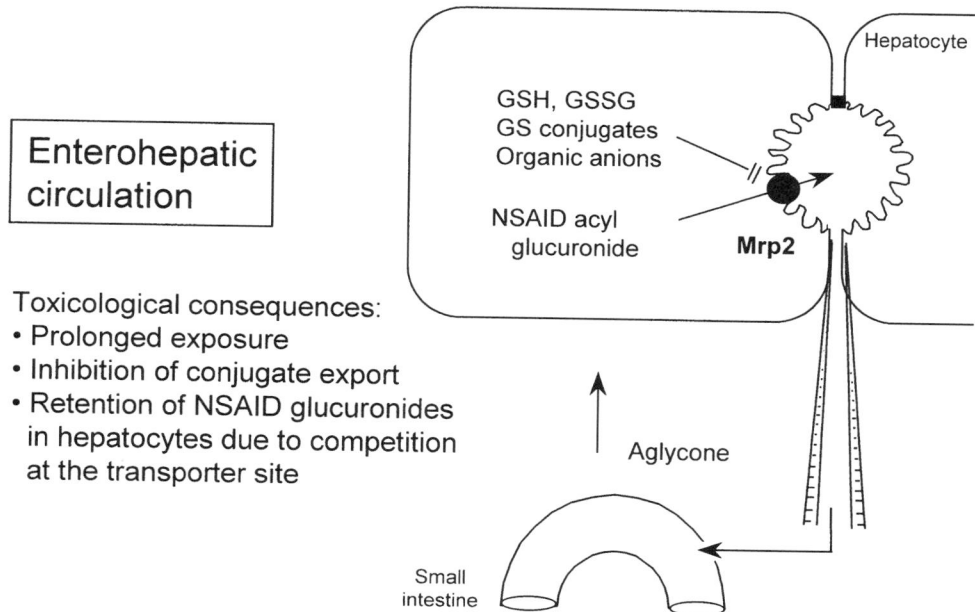

Figure 5   Biliary excretion of the glucuronides, hydrolysis in the biliary tree and/or small intestine, and reabsorption of the aglycone lead to extensive enterohepatic circulation of a number of acidic NSAIDs. This condition can have toxicological consequences, as indicated.

tract can favor hydrolysis of the alkali-labile acyl glucuronide. In addition, acyl glucuronides, but not the *iso*-glucuronides, can be cleaved by bacterial β-glucuronidase and nonspecific esterases. This leads to a rapid reuptake of the free parent drug and to enterohepatic circulation (57–60) (Fig. 5). Possible consequences of this repeated cycling are increased hepatic exposure and sustained interaction with hepatocanalicular transport, which is the rate-limiting site in drug elimination.

That enterohepatic circulation of NSAIDs is an important factor that determines their hepatic toxic potential can be illustrated by therapeutic studies in dogs. NSAIDs undergo extensive enterohepatic circulation in dogs and are therefore eliminated slowly. Carprofen administration has caused hepatopathy, manifested by increases in aminotransferase activity, cholestasis, hepatocellular degeneration, and necrosis (61,62). Similarly, dogs that received naproxen at therapeutic doses developed toxic side effects including increases in hepatic enzyme markers (63).

F.   Cholehepatic Circulation

Following excretion into the biliary tree, some NSAIDs can be readily reabsorbed. For example, it has long been suspected that sulindac (the aglycone, not the conjugated form) can undergo such cholehepatic circulation in humans (64). This has been confirmed in rats: following its canalicular secretion via the bile salt–exporting protein (cBsep), sulindac is reabsorbed across the bile duct epithelium. This results in decreased overall biliary excretion and higher blood levels during long-term administration of this drug (65). The possible consequences of cholehepatic circulation include increased exposure and possible compet-

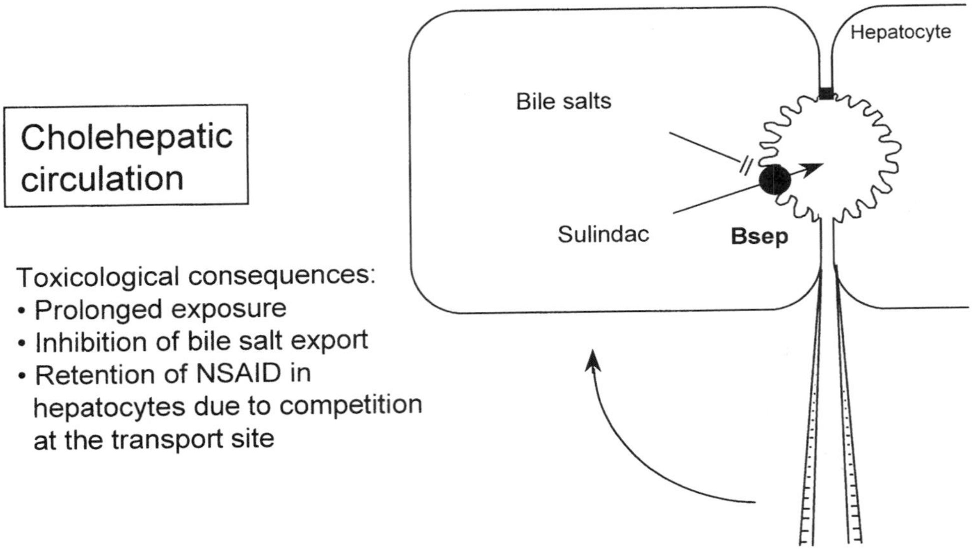

Figure 6   Hepatobiliary excretion of sulindac (parent compound) across the canalicular membrane via the bile salt–exporting protein (cBsep) and subsequent reabsorption in bile ducts leads to extensive cholehepatic circulation of this compound. This condition can have toxicological consequences, as indicated.

itive interaction at the hepatocanalicular transport site of bile salts and other substrates of the cBsep (Fig. 6).

G.   Renal Excretion

If the renal elimination of NSAID metabolites, e.g., acyl glucuronides, is impaired, this can lead to higher levels of circulating conjugates and hence to increased exposure to these potentially reactive metabolites. This was illustrated by experimental inhibition by probenecid of the renal elimination of zomepirac, which caused increased formation of drug adducts to plasma proteins (66).

III.   CELLULAR AND MOLECULAR MECHANISMS OF NSAID-INDUCED HEPATOTOXICITY

The "mechanisms" of NSAID hepatotoxicity are often classified as either intrinsic or idiosyncratic (4,12,16). However, this distinction is merely a phenotypical classification and reflects our lack of a clear understanding of the underlying mechanisms on a molecular and cellular basis.

For overt dose-dependent drug toxicity, the risk of toxicity can be more readily identified and taken into account for risk assessment. In contrast, for idiosyncratic drug toxicity, where the toxic manifestation is cryptic or latent and clearly host-dependent, the risk is much less easily determined because it does not manifest itself in most individuals. Both types of drug toxicity, however, harbor an intrinsic component, and some of the underlying cellular and molecular mechanisms may be similar.

In search of these mechanisms, a number of key pathways have been emerging. Apart from possible effects related to the pharmacological targets, three molecular mechanisms implicated in NSAID hepatotoxicity have been identified. These mechanisms are: (1) mitochondrial toxicity and interference with energy homeostasis, (2) protein binding of a reactive metabolite and subsequent hapten formation, and (3) interference of NSAIDs with hepatobiliary transport of cholephilic compounds, leading to intracellular accumulation of endogenous and/or exogenous compounds.

A. Pharmacological Targets—Are They Related to Hepatotoxic Side Effects?

The effectiveness of NSAIDs has been mostly attributed to cyclooxygenase (COX) inhibition, but other receptors, including the peroxisome proliferator-activated receptors (PPARs) have recently gained attention. Evidence relating NSAID hepatotoxicity to these pharmacological targets is scanty.

1. Cyclooxygenase (COX) Inhibition

NSAIDs are selective inhibitors of COX. This enzyme subfamily catalyzes the metabolic conversion of arachidonic acid to prostaglandins. Two isoforms of COX have been identified in mammalian cells. They are encoded from two different genes and exhibit tissue-specific expression. COX-1 is constitutively expressed and is a house-keeping enzyme, whereas COX-2 is an inducible form that is normally expressed at very low levels in many tissues but is upregulated by inflammatory mediators (67).

It is possible that inhibition of the degradation of arachidonic acid via the COX pathway by NSAIDs will in turn stimulate the alternative pathway of arachidonic acid metabolism, that is, activation of the lipoxygenase pathway. This would increase the formation of leukotrienes and could therefore alter microsomal membranes (68) via generation of hydroperoxy derivatives (69) and inflammatory responses (70,71). However, there is no experimental evidence that this pathway may be related to the hepatic liability associated with NSAIDs.

Recent efforts have aimed at developing selective COX-2 inhibitors that spare COX-1. Although these new drugs (e.g., celecoxib, rofecoxib) have not been associated with adverse effects in the liver, one cannot conclude from this safety profile that liver injury from traditional nonselective COX inhibitors is linked to COX-1 inhibition (72).

2. Peroxisome Proliferator-Activated Receptors (PPARs)

NSAIDs can bind to and activate PPARs, which are ligand-activated nuclear receptors that are involved in the regulation of lipid homeostasis. Among the several isoforms of PPAR, PPARα is abundant in liver and plays a key role in peroxisomal fatty acid β-oxidation and peroxisome proliferation. In fact, earlier observations had revealed that certain NSAIDs (e.g., ibuprofen and flurbiprofen) are inducers of peroxisomal β-oxidation (73). Although these compounds are structurally similar to clofibric acid, a powerful inducer of peroxisomal β-oxidation, NSAIDs are not as potent inducers as clofibric acid.

In contrast to PPARα, PPARγ is normally expressed at low levels in the liver. However, obesity and nutrition can upregulate PPARγ expression in the liver (74,75). PPARγ plays a key role in decreasing mitochondrial β-oxidation and in increasing fatty acid incorporation into storage lipid. In cell cultures, indomethacin, fenoprofen, ibuprofen, and flufenamic acid all have been shown to bind and activate PPARγ and to induce lipogenesis

(76). Interestingly, at low (nanomolar) concentrations, indomethacin blocked only COX activity, thus inhibiting the formation of prostaglandin derivatives that are activators of PPARγ, without directly binding to PPARγ. At higher (micromolar) concentrations, however, indomethacin not only inhibited COX activity but also activated PPARγ. Thus depending on the concentration, NSAIDs may function as either inhibitors or activators of PPARγ-mediated processes (76).

One of these PPARγ-mediated processes is apoptosis. NSAIDs have been shown to induce apoptosis in cell lines by a COX-independent pathway (77). This has been causally linked with the compounds' well-known chemopreventive activity against intestinal tumorigenesis (78–81).

In spite of these well-known interactions of NSAIDs with PPARs, the relevance of these findings for the liver has remained unclear.

B. Disruption of Mitochondrial Energy Production

Mitochondrial bioenergetics have been implicated as a potential target of the toxic action of NSAIDs in the liver. The underlying mechanisms of mitochondrial damage include uncoupling of oxidative phosphorylation, opening of the mitochondrial permeability transition pore, and inhibition of mitochondrial β-oxidation.

1. Uncoupling of Oxidative Phosphorylation

Mitochondrial uncoupling of oxidative phosphorylation is one of the most widely discussed mechanisms underlying the toxicity of NSAIDs (82–86). This effect can be explained by the chemical structure; many NSAIDs are monocarboxylic acids with one or more aromatic rings and most of them are lipophilic. These features are typical for uncoupling agents.

Uncoupling compounds short-circuit the proton gradient that is normally built up in the intermembraneous space during electron transport, by reversing the proton flux from the intermembraneous space back into the matrix (Fig. 7). The resulting dissipation of the proton gradient precludes the oxidative phosphorylation of ADP by the ATP synthetase. This ultimately leads to release of Ca^{2+} and to an energy crisis and cell demise (87–90).

At least three major mechanisms have been identified that form the basis of this

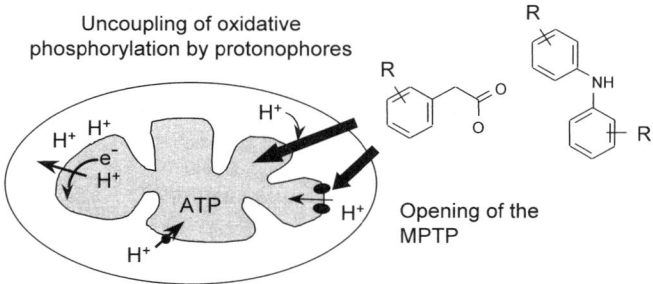

Figure 7 Acidic NSAIDs dissipate the mitochondrial membrane potential by facilitating proton reflux across the inner mitochondrial membrane. This can occur both by the protonophore activity of the carboxylic acid moiety or the diphenylamine structure of an NSAID, causing uncoupling of electron transport from ATP synthesis, and effects on the mitochondrial permeability transition pore (MPTP), which opens and allows rapid influx of protons.

uncoupling effect. First, the protonophoric activity of acidic NSAIDs shuttles the protons back into the matrix. Evidence indicates that the diphenylamine structure may also contribute to this effect (89,91). Second, NSAIDs can directly cause opening of the mitochondrial permeability transition pore, which allows rapid influx of protons into the matrix. Finally, there is evidence that the hydrophobic NSAIDs accumulate nonspecifically in the mitochondrial membranes and cause membrane disordering, which also could contribute to the uncoupling effects (85).

Most of the experiments demonstrating an uncoupling effect of NSAIDs were carried out either in isolated mitochondria (85) or in isolated or cultured hepatocytes. The concentrations needed to induce such mitochondrial changes ranged from low micromolar (for, e.g., mefenamic acid, flufenamic acid, diflunisal) (82), to high micromolar (100–250 µM for, e.g., diclofenac), to the millimolar range (e.g., for aspirin). Some NSAIDs did not inhibit hepatic mitochondrial ATP synthesis at all (e.g., indomethacin or sulindac), even at concentrations exceeding 5 mM (82). A comparison among NSAIDs of the IC_{50} values for inhibition of ATP synthesis and the relative incidence of inducing liver dysfunction in humans readily reveals that there is no positive correlation between the in vitro data and the hepatotoxic potential in humans. For example, sulindac, which is more frequently associated with hepatotoxicity than all other NSAIDs (92), was not cytotoxic and did not deplete hepatocellular ATP in rat hepatocyte cultures (89). In contrast, nimesulide and meloxicam have few hepatic side effects, yet are among the most potent uncouplers (86). Thus, uncoupling is not a general property of all NSAIDs and this effect is unlikely to contribute to the toxicity in vivo. In addition, most of the effects observed with isolated mitochondria or cell cultures were caused by high drug concentrations only. Because most NSAIDs are highly bound to plasma proteins in vivo (23), the concentration of "free" (unbound) drug is approximately three orders of magnitude smaller than the concentrations used in vitro.

2. Induction of the Membrane Permeability Transition in Mitochondria

In recent years, the mitochondrial membrane permeability transition (MPT) pore, a tightly regulated megachannel associated with Ca^{2+}-dependent increases in the permeability of ions and solutes with molecular masses ≤ 1500 D, has gained much attention. The MPT has been implicated in mitochondrial uncoupling and induction of apoptosis. A recent report indicates that induction of the MPT is a general response to short-chain carboxylic acids having a pK_a of 4–5 (93).

NSAIDs are able to differentially induce the mitochondrial MPT, leading to a collapse of the proton gradient and an energy crisis (91,94,95) (Fig. 7). While some NSAIDs (e.g., piroxicam, aspirin) exert this effect only at relatively high concentrations (500 µM), others (e.g., diclofenac, mefenamic acid) cause opening of the MPT pore at concentrations as low as 2 µM. The mechanism of MPT induction caused by NSAIDs is not well understood, but it has been suggested that oxidation of pyridine nucleotides or protein thiols may play a role.

3. Inhibition of Mitochondrial β-Oxidation

Inhibition of mitochondrial β-oxidation has been discussed as one of the mechanisms involved in NSAID hepatotoxicity, in particular that associated with 2-arylpropionic acid derivatives (96–101) (Fig. 8). Mitochondrial β-oxidation is the process by which nonesterified fatty acids (NEFAs) are oxidized and shortened into acetyl-CoA fragments, which in turn are either condensed to ketone bodies or further metabolized by entry into the

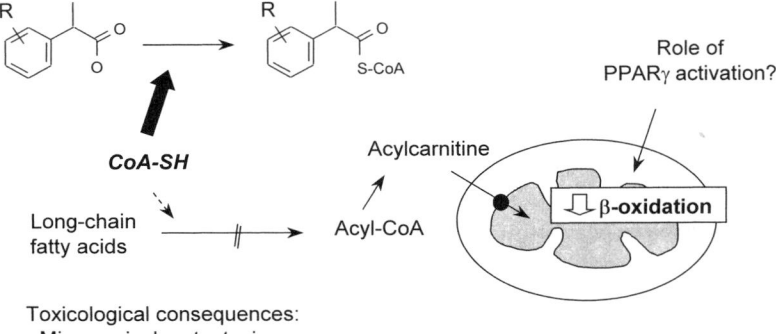

Figure 8   Inhibition by 2-arylpropionic acids of long-chain fatty acyl β-oxidation in mitochondria. CoA is sequestered by the acidic NSAIDs and is less available to activate long-chain fatty acids prior to their carnitine-mediated transport across the inner mitochondrial membrane. The ensuing accumulation of fatty acids in hepatocytes may lead to microvesicular steatosis.

citrate cycle. In contrast to short- and medium-chain NEFAs, which can readily penetrate into mitochondria, long-chain NEFAs have to be activated to an acyl-CoA intermediate prior to being transported across the inner mitochondrial membrane by the carnitine shuttle system. Inhibition of β-oxidation, which is an important sink for NEFAs in the liver, leads not only to decreased ATP production but also to an accumulation of fatty acids. Ultimately, this can develop into microvesicular steatosis.

The mechanism underlying NSAID-induced inhibition of β-oxidation has both a stereoselective and a nonstereoselective basis (97). The first mechanism can be explained by the stereoselective formation of 2-arylpropionic acid-CoA thioester formation, which can lead to extramitochondrial CoA sequestration. As a consequence, activation of long-chain NEFAs is inhibited and, hence, β-oxidation is decreased (100,102). Second, for those 2-arylpropionic acids that do not form CoA intermediates (e.g., flurbiprofen), a nonstereoselective, CoA-independent β-oxidation pathway has been described (83). The exact mechanism is not known but, because these drugs are also uncouplers, it has been suggested that the NSAID may enter mitochondria and directly inhibit β-oxidation (83). Finally, as many NSAIDs are activators of PPARγ, which is associated with downregulation of the mitochondrial β-oxidation pathway and accumulation of NEFAs, it is possible that the observed microvesicular steatosis in hepatic parenchymal cells could be attributed, at least in part, to activation of upregulated PPARγ in the liver.

The concentrations required to achieve a significant inhibition of β-oxidation in vitro are usually much higher than the therapeutic plasma concentrations, considering again that the nonbound ("free") drug is less than 1% of the total. Therefore, it is not likely that these effects will become important in the vast majority of patients. However, the data can explain a mechanism that may become relevant in compromised cells, in genetically altered mitochondrial β-oxidation (103), or at exceedingly high intracellular NSAID concentrations.

Indeed, microvesicular steatosis has been described in patients who received pirprofen (104), naproxen (105), ibuprofen (106), or ketoprofen (107). However, because microvesicular steatosis can be nonspecific and because it is more prevalent than previously

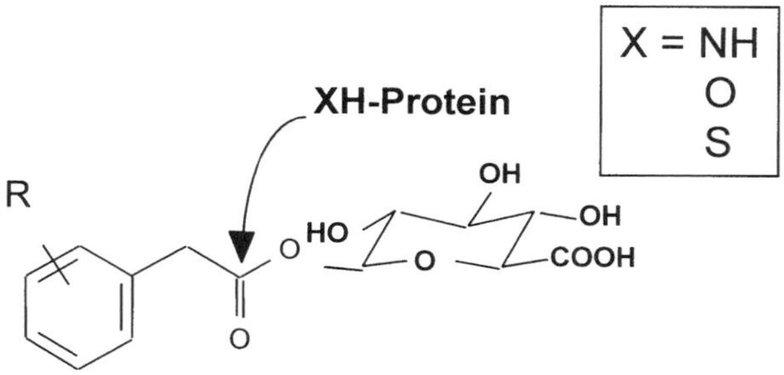

Figure 9 Covalent adduct formation of a NSAID acyl glucuronide (unsubstituted at the α-carbon atom) to a nucleophilic amino acid residue of a target protein by the transacylation mechanism.

suspected, a causal link with NSAIDs is often difficult to establish. A causal link can only be made with the use of aspirin (108).

C. Protein Adduct Formation and Immune-Mediated Toxicity

1. Mechanisms and Molecular Targets of NSAID Acyl Glucuronides and *iso*-Glucuronides

Carboxylic acid–containing NSAIDs are biotransformed both in the liver and extrahepatically to reactive metabolites. Among these, acyl glucuronides have gained special attention because they are quantitatively important and because they are protein-reactive. As a consequence of their moderate reactivity, they often do not react with target molecules in their immediate vicinity, but leave the site of their formation and reach the blood or biliary compartment. In the vascular system, acyl glucuronides can react with plasma proteins (109–112). Protein binding to, e.g., albumin, has also been demonstrated in vitro (113–120) and has been used to investigate the molecular mechanisms of binding.

For human serum albumin, the most prominent binding site for covalent interactions with NSAIDs has been determined. Following exposure to tolmetin acyl glucuronide, the intramolecular target has been identified as Lys-199 (117,121). This is particularly interesting, as Lys-199 is a lysine ε-amino group located in a hydrophobic region of the protein that is a target for covalent binding of penicillin derivatives, well-known immunogenic drugs (122).

One mechanism of covalent binding of an NSAID acyl glucuronide to protein is nucleophilic displacement or transacylation, whereby the NSAID acylates a nucleophilic amino acid residue of a target protein and the glucuronic acid moiety is released (Fig. 9). A second mechanism of binding is protein glycation, by which the glucuronic acid moiety is retained in the adduct. This reaction is made possible after intracellular rearrangement (acyl migration), where the acyl group migrates from the 1-*O*-position to the 2-, 3-, or 4-position of the sugar ring, exposing a new electrophilic center in the resulting *iso*-glucuronide (Fig. 10). Protein glycation by this mechanism is quite common, in particular by 2-arylpropionic acids (51,123). Protein adducts with *iso*-glucuronides may be quantitatively as important as those derived from the original acyl glucuronide (124). They may even become more relevant in toxicology as they are more persistent than the less stable adducts formed from the 1-*O*-acyl glucuronide.

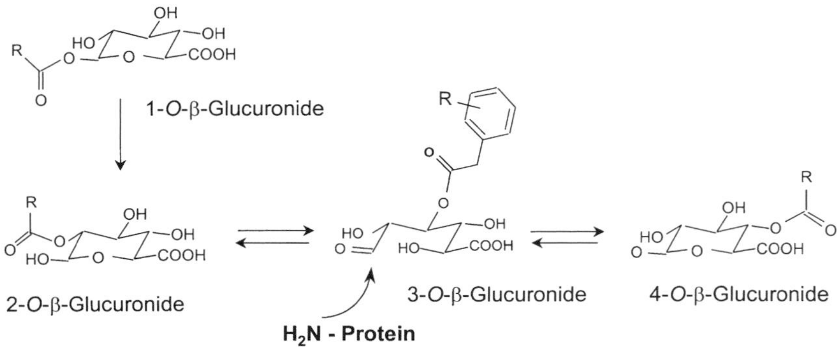

Figure 10 Covalent adduct formation of a NSAID *iso*-glucuronide to a target protein by the glycation mechanism. Following intracellular rearrangement (acyl migration of the aglycone along the sugar ring), positional isomers can be formed. These *iso*-glucuronides (in this example, the 3-*O*-glucuronide of an NSAID) can exist transiently in the open ring form, where the exposed aldehyde group is attacked by a nucleophilic amino acid residue.

There is a clear correlation between the stability of a formed acyl glucuronide and its reactivity (covalent binding) (125). For a number of acyl glucuronides, the apparent first-order disappearance rate constant in buffer correlated in a linear fashion with maximum irreversible binding to albumin in vitro. The degree of substitution at the α-carboxy atom is crucial in determining the stability; unsubstituted acetic acid derivatives are relatively unstable and exhibit high covalent binding. More stable glucuronides are mono-α-substituted acetic acids, which exhibit intermediate covalent binding. Finally, stable acids fully substituted at the α-carbon exhibit only little covalent binding (125). It has therefore been suggested that steric factors hindering the reaction may play a role in this differential reactivity. However, the predictability of covalent binding becomes less accurate for the in vivo situation: besides the degradation rate constant of a given glucuronide, many other factors can modify the site and extent of binding considerably, including differential bioactivation pathways and pharmacokinetic variables.

Stability and, hence, protein adduct formation of acyl glucuronides are pH-dependent. Acyl glucuronides are unstable at pH > 8, a pH that may occur in the biliary tree and the lower intestine. Therefore, covalent binding in the biliary tree will occur more extensively than under conditions of lower pH, as is found in blood.

In the liver, targeting of covalent protein binding does not occur at random, but is directed against selective proteins. A number of experimental studies have characterized or identified proteins that are preferentially alkylated or acylated by reactive NSAID metabolites (30,52,126–131). Which proteins are detected in Western blots or by fluorography depends on a number of factors, including the duration of drug administration and the time that has elapsed between the dose and the sacrificing of the animal. In most studies, persistent adducts were found to be associated with plasma membrane proteins (52,128,130–132) (Fig. 11).

Subcellular fractionation studies and immunohistochemical analysis have revealed that one (or one group of) particularly abundant adduct(s) is associated with proteins of the canalicular plasma membrane domain. Evidence suggests that the proteins targeted by a number of NSAIDs including diclofenac (52,128,131), sulindac (131), or benoxaprofen (133) may be identical. Specifically, they all are in the molecular mass range of 110–

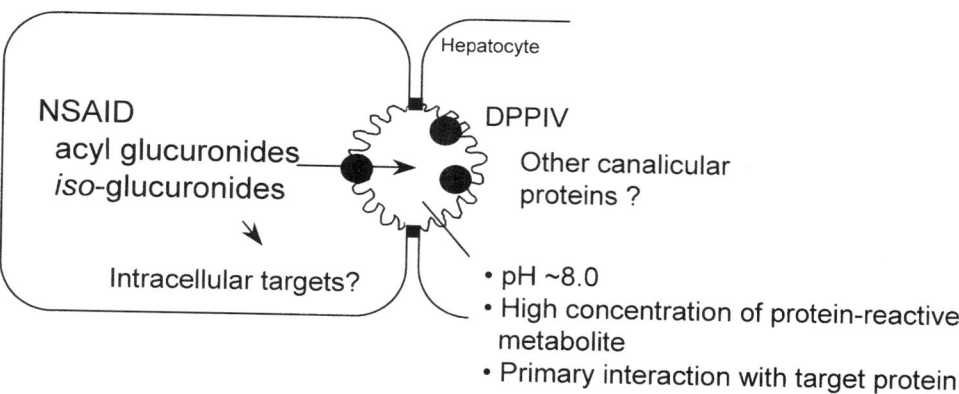

Figure 11 NSAID metabolites covalently bind to one or several 110–118-kDa plasma membrane proteins exposed to the canalicular lumen. One identified common target is dipeptidyl peptidase IV (DPPIV).

126 kDa, and one common target that has been identified is dipeptidyl peptidase IV (DPPIV) (130,134,135).

Adducts to canalicular membrane proteins are only generated when the protein-reactive metabolite (the acyl glucuronide or isomers) is transported from the hepatocyte across the canalicular membrane into the bile canalicular lumen (52). This was inferred from the observation that in mutant transport-deficient (TR⁻) rats, which do not express a functional export pump for the glucuronides (canalicular Mrp2), no membrane protein adducts were detectable after treatment with diclofenac. The reason for this compartment-selective reaction is severalfold. First, the reactive metabolite that is exported from the cell by an ATP-dependent transporter is upconcentrated in the canalicular lumen and reaches high concentrations. Second, the reactivity of the acyl glucuronides is increased in a slightly alkaline compartment, such as the biliary tree (136,137). Finally, the nature of the target protein(s) may favor a primary interaction with the glucuronide metabolite.

The role of covalent protein binding in NSAID hepatotoxicity is not clear. However, theoretically, adduct formation can have toxicological consequences, including inactivation of a critical target protein or hapten formation and an immunogenic response against the drug-altered protein.

2. Inactivation of Critical Protein Function

For some proteins covalently modified by NSAID metabolites, a clear functional impairment has been demonstrated. For example, the activity of DPPIV, which is an abundant ectoenzyme residing in the canalicular plasma membrane and a major target, was reduced by 22% in rats treated with diclofenac (130). The biological significance of this functional alteration has remained unclear, as there is no obvious relationship between the decrease in DPPIV activity and hepatotoxicity. In fact, NSAIDs that produce focal necrosis and apoptosis in rat liver (diclofenac and sulindac), as well as an NSAID that produces much less overt injury (ibuprofen), caused equal inhibition of DPPIV expression and activity (134).

The function of a number of other proteins covalently modified by NSAIDs was shown to be similarly compromised. For example, acute administration of diclofenac to rats resulted in covalent binding to CYP2C11 and a 72% decrease in the catalytic activity of this P450 (30). Furthermore, incubation of suprofen acyl glucuronide with human serum albumin or superoxide dismutase significantly inhibited both the binding capacity of albumin for other drugs and the catalytic activity of superoxide dismutase (138). Finally, the reactive acyl glucuronide of zomepirac covalently modified tubulin and inhibited its assembly into microtubules (139).

The relevance of these findings for NSAID hepatotoxicity is not clear. Acute damage of a protein and rapid replacement may not be so critical. Thus, for proteins featuring a relatively short half-life, such as albumin, binding may be less relevant than for proteins featuring a much slower turnover rate (e.g., collagen), where accumulating adducts may be more severe (138).

3. Hapten Formation and Immune-Mediated Hepatic Injury

Covalent binding of a reactive NSAID metabolite to hepatocellular proteins may lead to the formation of a hapten that could play a role in a possible immune response against the drug-altered self-protein (140). The hapten itself, or conformational changes of the target protein, could then result in the formation of structural and conformational epitopes, respectively. Direct evidence for the involvement of such a mechanism is, however, scanty.

Several requirements have to be fulfilled for an adduct to become immunogenic. First, the adduct density (mol adduct bound per mol protein) is an important determinant. Chronic treatment will increase the adduct density; indeed, multiple dosing, as opposed to single administration of an NSAID, can lead to accumulation of the protein adducts (112,141). Second, the half-life (stability) of the adduct itself may also determine its potential immunogenicity. The stability of an adduct is partially determined by the mechanism of covalent binding: for many drugs, adducts arising from the reactive *iso*-glucuronides are more stable than those arising from the acyl glucuronide. Often the adducts actually persist in plasma far beyond the period when concentrations of the parent compound and/or its glucuronides are measurable (112,141). For example, in human volunteers (6-day oral study), the terminal half-life of covalently bound diflunisal to plasma proteins was calculated to be 10 days (142). Long-lived adducts may lead to enhanced uptake by macrophages, resulting in greater processing and presentation of antigenic peptides compared with unaltered albumin (143).

Adduct formation alone, however, is not sufficient to trigger an immune response. In fact, most, if not all, recipients receiving NSAIDs form adducts and the formation of drug-altered peptides induces tolerance rather than an immune response. To stimulate B cells or T cells, peptides require presentation by MHC molecules. This process is limited in the liver: hepatocytes express MHC class I molecules at a very low level, and class II molecules are not expressed under normal conditions (144). MHC class I molecules can, however, be upregulated under pathophysiological conditions, including viral hepatitis, autoimmune liver disease, or cholestasis (145–147). Similarly, MHC II antigen can become expressed in hepatocytes following stimulation by cytokines or under pathophysiological conditions such as hepatitis (144,148–150). By implication, one can speculate that alkylated hepatic proteins ("nonself" peptides) are released during cell turnover or after toxic injury, phagocytosed by Kupffer cells, degraded, and presented in conjunction with MHC II, thus activating a particular Th cell clone bearing an appropriate T-cell receptor. The activated T-cell clone may begin to express IL-2 receptors and to secrete various immune modulators including IL-2 and IL-4, which will activate other immune cells, including B cells and cytotoxic T cells (Fig. 12).

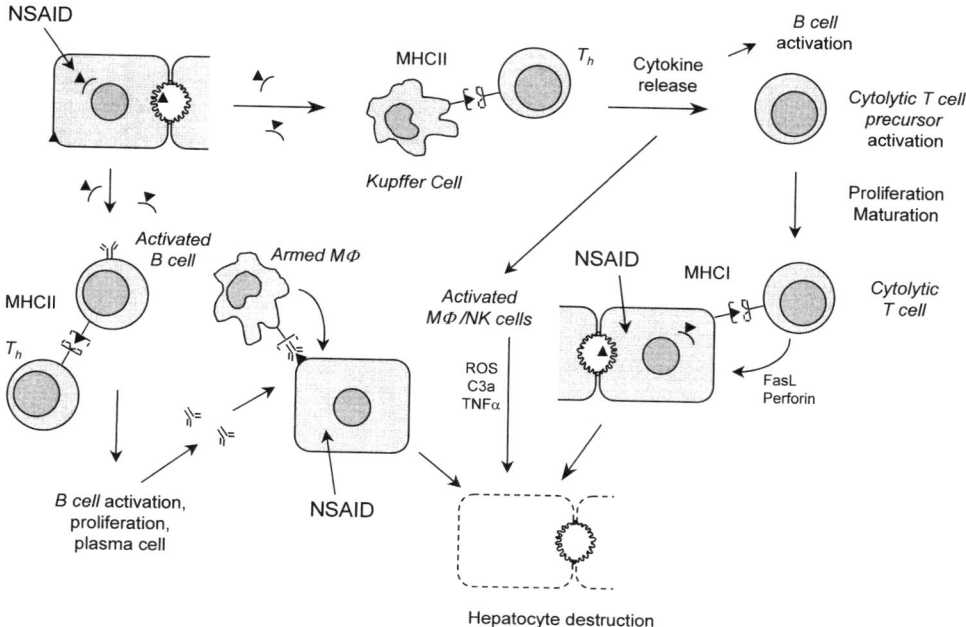

NSAID

MHCII

T_h Cytokine release

B cell activation

Cytolytic T cell precursor activation

Kupffer Cell

Proliferation Maturation

Activated B cell   Armed MΦ

NSAID   MHCI

Cytolytic T cell

MHCII

T_h

Activated MΦ/NK cells

ROS C3a TNFα

FasL Perforin

B cell activation, proliferation, plasma cell   NSAID

Hepatocyte destruction

Figure 12   Putative pathways of immune-mediated hepatocyte injury induced by NSAIDs. Covalent adducts of reactive metabolites of NSAIDs will be accessible to cells of the immune system following degradation of hepatocytes. Adducts are primarily formed in the endoplasmic reticulum and at the canalicular plasma membrane. Internalization of NSAID-modified proteins by antigen-presenting cells (e.g., Kupffer cells) is followed by processing and presentation of the peptides in conjunction with MHC class II. The hapten or conformational epitope of the peptides is recognized by the T-cell receptor of T helper cells. Cytokine release and subsequent activation of B cells and cytolytic T-cell precursors results in clonal expansion and maturation to cytolytic T cells. These T cells recognize the antigen presented in conjunction with MHCI on the hepatocytes and destroy the target cell. Activated macrophages or natural killer cells may also lyse target cells by various mediators. Alternatively, NSAID-altered proteins may interact with a B-cell receptor, followed by internalization, processing, and presentation by MHCII, which leads to activation and clonal expansion of B cells, maturation to plasma cells, and secretion of antibodies. These antibodies may bind to epitopes on the plasma membrane of hepatocytes (exposed protein adducts). This may result in nonspecific recognition and binding via the Fc receptor of killer cells and macrophages and killing of the target hepatocytes.

Immune-mediated liver injury could be mediated by a number of effector mechanisms. First, antibodies may bind to alkylated membrane proteins on the cell surface and induce cell lysis through complement or killer cells. Although, in some cases, such antibodies against NSAID-altered peptides have indeed been found, the pathophysiological significance of antibodies is not clear. In particular, it is not clear whether they are causally involved in the killing of target cells or merely markers for antigenicity. For example, two independent experiments have shown that immunization with a syngeneic serum albumin conjugate of a NSAID (diflunisal and tolmetin) acyl glucuronide stimulated an antibody response in rodents (151,152). These studies show that self-proteins covalently modified by incubation with a reactive NSAID glucuronide can be immunogenic. They do not, however, provide evidence that these antibodies are indeed causally involved in an aberrant immune response in the liver.

It is only in few cases that there is evidence that these antibodies may play a causative role in cell-mediated toxicity. For example, the addition of sera from patients with clometacine hepatitis to cultured human hepatocytes that had been exposed to clometacine resulted in hepatocellular injury when autologous lymphoid cells were added (153). The antiserum from such patients did not, however, recognize drug-modified proteins, but only native proteins. Therefore, it is likely that clometacine, and possibly other NSAIDs, can in rare cases induce autoimmune-type hepatitis. This has been inferred from the presence of accompanying high titers of anti-DNA or anti–smooth muscle antibodies, typical for autoimmune hepatitis (154). It is possible that the role of the drug, being one of the factors that add to the risk of developing autoimmune hepatitis, would be in revealing a latent autoimmune disease (155). One hypothesis involves autoreactive B cells that are normally quiescent but would present both the drug-altered protein and native peptides, triggering a Th response against the native protein (156). Recent evidence also indicates that drugs can disrupt the process of positive selection of immature T cells in the thymus that occurs throughout life, breaking the tolerance to self, and that this process can lead to autoimmune disease (157).

The second effector mechanism involves cytolytic T cells, following appropriate stimulation by Th cells. Cytolytic T cells would recognize the drug-modified peptides presented in conjunction with MHC I and destroy the target cells by Fas- or perforin-mediated mechanisms. Such a mechanism has not been proven in vivo, and to date there is no animal model available with which one could study these pathways. Limited evidence stems from a mouse study that has shown that in vivo activated T cells derived from diclofenac-immunized mice are able to kill hepatocytes that had been exposed in vitro to diclofenac (158) (Fig. 13).

In this ex vivo/in vitro model, C57BL/6 mice were immunized with diclofenac coupled to the carrier protein, keyhole limpet hemocyanin (KLH). To explore the role of a T-cell-mediated response directed against diclofenac-modified peptides, splenocytes from KLH-diclofenac (and KLH only) immunized mice were harvested and either used as a crude splenocyte fraction (containing T cells, B cells, NK cells, and macrophages) or

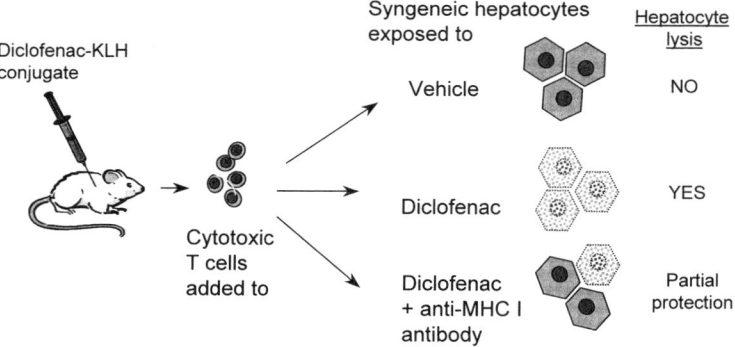

Figure 13 Cytotoxic T cells from diclofenac-immunized mice kill hepatocytes previously exposed to diclofenac in vitro. Immunization alone or exposure to diclofenac alone did not cause hepatocyte injury.

further purified to a T-cell-enriched fraction. These splenocytes were then combined with isolated and precultured syngeneic hepatocytes and kept in coculture for several days. Prior to being combined with splenocytes, the hepatocytes were exposed to high but nontoxic concentrations (100 μM) of diclofenac, which was biotransformed to a reactive metabolite and subsequently formed covalent adducts to hepatocellular proteins. Upon contact with these diclofenac-modified hepatocytes, the primed lymphocytes responded with a proliferative burst and an upregulation of interleukin-2 receptor expression, both specific markers of T-cell activation. Furthermore, the activated T cells were able to kill the diclofenac-pretreated hepatocytes as demonstrated by a delayed increase in ALT release from injured hepatocytes. Prior incubation of diclofenac-exposed hepatocytes with an anti-MHC I antibody afforded partial protection against T-cell-mediated cell killing. This indicates that hepatocyte injury was, at least in part, dependent on the T-cell receptor that recognized MHC class I–associated diclofenac-modified peptides, rather than being a nonspecific effect. A number of other observations also suggest that in this model cytolytic T cells were primarily involved as effectors of hepatocyte injury. For example, the highest degree of hepatocyte lysis was achieved when a T-cell-enriched fraction was used, as opposed to a crude splenocyte fraction. Furthermore, the supernatant from an activated lymphocyte culture, containing cytokines and other soluble mediators, alone had no damaging effect on hepatocytes unless effector cells were added. Importantly, control experiments revealed that immunization with diclofenac alone or exposure of hepatocytes to diclofenac alone was not sufficient to induce hepatocyte injury. However, because high effector cell/target cell ratios were required to elicit the cytotoxic effects, and because both the extent and molecular identity of the diclofenac adducts (or other forms of intracellular stress) generated by high concentrations of diclofenac in vitro are not directly comparable with those following in vivo exposure to diclofenac, caution has to be exerted in interpreting the data as a general mechanism.

Finally, another possible effector mechanism of NSAID-induced immune-mediated liver injury could involve lymphokine release by activated Th cells, which would recruit and activate macrophages, and which would result in tissue damage and inflammation.

Collectively, the evidence for immune-mediated reactions that are involved in NSAID-induced liver toxicity stems primarily from clinical criteria (delayed onset of disease, appearance of rash, fever, eosinophilia, rapid onset of symptoms after rechallenge with drug). When these criteria are employed, a number of NSAIDs, including clometacine, phenylbutazone, diclofenac, naproxen, piroxicam, and tolmetin, all exhibit, at least to some degree, signs of hypersensitivity. The molecular pathways that can trigger such an immune response and, even more important, the mechanisms underlying breaking of immune tolerance, are, however, poorly understood.

D. Impairment of Canalicular Transmembrane Transport of Endogenous Compounds and Retention of Toxic Bile Acids

Some NSAIDs can interfere directly with the hepatobiliary transport of endogenous or exogenous cholephilic compounds, such as bile salts (Fig. 6). For example, sulindac at high doses not only inhibits the basolateral uptake of bile salts, but also inhibits the ATP-dependent canalicular export of conjugated bile acids (65). In rats, this drug can induce cholestasis, leading to retention of bile salts in the hepatocytes. If toxic (hydrophobic) bile salts accumulate, they can pose an oxidative stress (159) and/or induce apoptosis and necrosis (160) by Fas-mediated pathways (161).

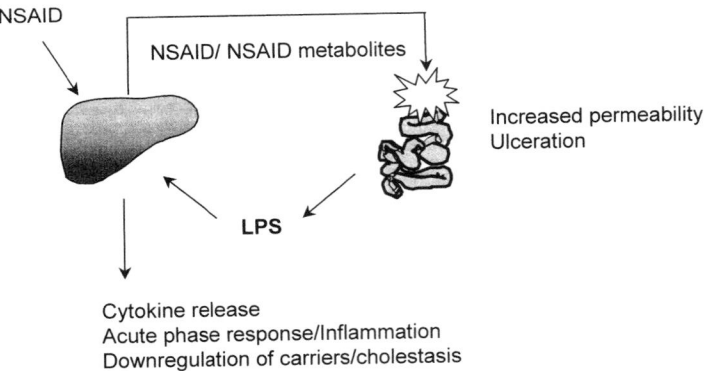

Figure 14   NSAID-associated enteropathy can lead to increased release of bacterial lipopolysaccharide and trigger secondary hepatic effects including downregulation of hepatobiliary transporters.

Alternatively, NSAIDs may impair the excretion of cholephilic compounds by pathways other than direct inhibition of the bile salt transporter, including secondary hepatic effects due to gastrointestinal injury. Because most NSAIDs affect the gastrointestinal epithelium and cause bleeding and ulceration in sensitive species even at low doses (60,162), intestinal injury could entail increases in the permeability of the small intestine. Increased release of bacterial endotoxin can not only cause cholestasis and impairment of liver function but also downregulate some hepatobiliary carriers including the conjugate export pump, Mrp2 (163,164). This condition may lead to an accumulation of the drug or drug conjugate in the hepatocyte (Fig. 14).

E.   Other Mechanisms

1.   Formation of Mixed Lipids

Because some carboxylic acids can be activated to acyl-CoA thioesters, they can enter the pathways of lipid biosynthesis, similar to endogenous fatty acids activated by CoA. For example, a number of 2-arylpropionic acids that are substrates for acyl CoA ligase thus become incorporated into "hybrid" triacylglycerol (165,166) (Fig. 15). This incorporation and accumulation of NSAIDs in endogenous lipid is stereoselective; only the *R*-enantiomer is activated and incorporated into lipids (35,167,168). Because hybrid triacylglycerides have the potential to form long-lasting residues in adipose tissues and to be incorporated into biomembranes, where they may disturb membrane function, their forma-

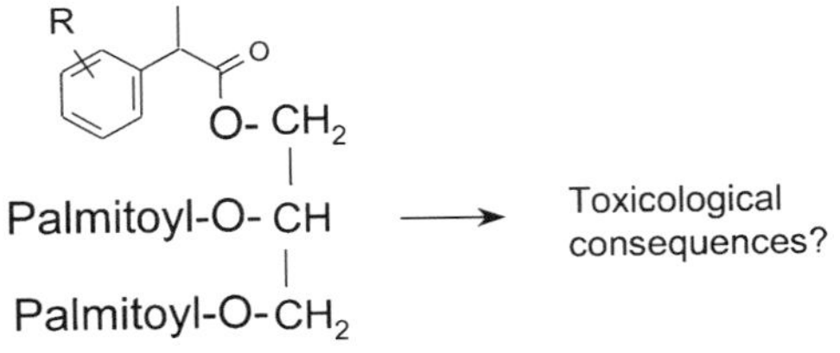

Figure 15   Steroselective activation by CoA and incorporation of 2-arylpropionic acids into "hybrid" triacylglycerols.

tion has been considered a potential pathway for toxicity (33,169,170). However, no clear mechanistic link to the hepatic toxicity of NSAIDs has been established.

2. Predisposition by Hepatic Changes Caused by Rheumatic Diseases for Which the NSAIDs Are Prescribed

In search of mechanisms of toxicity, it is often overlooked that the treated individuals are patients whose liver function may already be altered due to the disease and prior to the intake of the drug. For example, in patients with acute rheumatic fever, NSAID disposition can be altered: it has been shown that the unbound fraction of the drug in plasma was higher than that in healthy persons. This condition was not only inversely related to the serum albumin concentration, but also showed a positive correlation with increased aminotransferases (171). In fact, liver tests in rheumatoid arthritis patients or in systemic lupus erythematosus (SLE) patients are often abnormal, featuring increased serum activities of alkaline phosphatase and other liver-selective enzymes (13,172–174).

IV. IDIOSYNCRATIC LIVER TOXICITY CAUSED BY NSAIDs

The frequently used (and often misused) term "idiosyncratic" liver injury implies that toxicity occurs in a very small population subset and that the etiology is unknown. More importantly, it also implies that host-dependent factors govern whether the drug is well tolerated or whether liver injury will ensue. Traditionally, NSAID-associated idiosyncratic reactions have been considered largely dose-independent and have been subdivided into metabolic idiosyncrasy and hypersensitivity reactions (4,12,16).

More recent concepts have, however, slightly altered the view about the mechanisms underlying these rare toxicities (175). In particular, there is growing evidence that idiosyncratic liver toxicities are dose-dependent, too. Because "idiosyncrasy" does not refer to a mechanism, it is proposed here not to use this term any more in the context of mechanistic explanations of drug effects. Most NSAIDs that rarely cause liver injury are intrinsically toxic. In the vast majority of individuals, however, the risk is small and toxicity does not manifest itself because of a powerful system that mediates tolerance and/or secures cellular defense and repair, or simply because the exposure is too small. It is only a small subset of patients who exhibit a specific genetically determined abnormality or an acquired proclivity for altered toxicokinetics or toxicodynamics or for abnormal immune responses. If, in these patients, unusually large amounts of reactive metabolites are generated, combined with low levels of detoxifying pathways, or if factors causing intracellular accumulation or impaired transport prevail, then NSAIDs will eventually precipitate hepatic toxicity by the mechanisms discussed above (Fig. 16).

V. CONCLUSIONS

NSAID-induced hepatotoxicity has become a paradigm for studying drug-induced liver injury. The reason for this is not necessarily that these drugs are more toxic, but that they are more frequently used than other drugs, and that, therefore, the number of reported hepatic adverse effects has become significant.

It has become clear that multiple mechanisms are involved in NSAID toxicity to the liver and that not a single mechanism can be advocated for the adverse effects. Although mitochondrial injury, immune-mediated toxicity, and impaired hepatobiliary transport have all been discussed as potential mechanisms contributing to the toxicity, the evidence

Genetic Factors   **Environmental Factors**

Drug-metabolizing enzymes   Underlying disease
Hepatobiliary transporters   Infections
Cellular defense systems   Age
Immune system   Co-medication
Mitochondrial abnormalities   Acquired cholestasis
                                               Regulation of gene expression

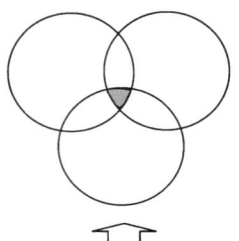

NSAID-induced "Danger Signal"

High dose
Cellular stress
Mitochondrial toxicity
High adduct levels
Cytotoxicity

Figure 16 NSAID-induced idiosyncratic reactions are multifactorial and become manifested when several critical risk factors (both genetically determined and acquired) are simultaneously expressed in an individual (overlapping area). The intrinsic toxicity of NSAIDs does not normally become apparent, owing to immune tolerance and/or cellular defense and repair systems.

has remained circumstantial. On this basis, a toxic hazard has been recognized for many NSAIDs.

Nevertheless, although the tools for both detecting mechanisms and calculating drug exposure have been improved, risk assessment and a reliable prediction of hepatic effects caused by NSAIDs in humans have remained difficult for a number of reasons. First, in spite of vigorous efforts, no animal model is available to study the hepatic toxicity of NSAIDs, in particular immune-mediated mechanisms (176). Furthermore, there is no clear correlation between the in vitro toxicity (e.g., mitochondrial toxicity) and the reported incidence of hepatic toxicity in patients. Finally, and importantly, it is impossible to date to define and detect the individual risk factors in the patient population.

Prediction of NSAID hepatotoxicity can be made at two different levels: at the drug level and at the patient level. Prediction for a chemical can only be made on the basis of a number of factors. These include the formation of acyl glucuronides and *iso*-glucuronides with a relatively high protein reactivity (137), the formation of canalicular membrane protein adducts in the molecular mass range of 110–120 kDa, and a high degree of entero-hepatic circulation. Prediction at the patient level is much more difficult. However, the advent of genomics, technologies that will allow us to detect specific genetic abnormalities, as well as novel techniques to detect the regulation of certain key genes, will hopefully lead to a better understanding of how and why NSAIDs can precipitate liver injury in some susceptible patients.

REFERENCES

1. O'Brien WM, Bagby GF. Rare adverse reactions to nonsteroidal antiinflammatory drugs. J Rheumatol 1985; 12:562–567.

2. Doube A. Hepatitis and non-steroidal anti-inflammatory drugs. Ann Rheum Dis 1990; 49: 489–490.

3. Tolman KG. Hepatotoxicity of antirheumatic drugs. J Rheumatol 1990; 17(suppl 22):6–11.

4. Zimmerman HJ. Update of hepatotoxicity due to classes of drugs in common clinical use: non-steroidal drugs, anti-inflammatory drugs, antibiotics, antihypertensives, and cardiac and psychotropic agents. Semin Liver Dis 1990; 10:322–338.

5. Garcia Rodriguez LA, Gutthann SP, Walker AM, Lueck L. The role of nonsteroidal anti-inflammatory drugs in acute liver injury. Br Med J 1992; 305:865–868.

6. Rabinovitz M, VanThiel DH. Hepatotoxicity of nonsteroidal anti-inflammatory drugs. Am J Gastroenterol 1992; 87:1696–1704.

7. Carson JL, Strom BL, Duff A, Gupta A, Das K. Safety of nonsteroidal anti-inflammatory drugs with respect to acute liver disease. Arch Intern Med 1993; 153:1331–1336.

8. Farrell GC. Liver disease produced by non-steroidal anti-inflammatory drugs. In: GC Farrell, ed. Drug-induced Liver Disease. Edinbourgh: Churchill Livingstone, 1994:371–388.

9. Garcia Rodriguez LA, Williams R, Derby LE, Dean AD, Jick H. Acute liver injury associated with nonsteroidal anti-inflammatory drugs and the role of risk factors. Arch Intern Med 1994; 154:311–316.

10. Johnson AG, Seidemann P, Day RO. NSAID-related adverse drug interactions with clinical relevance—an update. Int J Clin Pharm Thera 1994; 32:509–532.

11. Singh G, Ramey DR, Morfeld D, Fries JF. Comparative toxicity of non-steroidal anti-inflammatory agents. Pharmacol Ther 1994; 62:175–191.

12. Zimmerman HJ. Hepatic injury associated with nonsteroidal anti-inflammatory drugs. In: AJ Lewis, DE Furst, eds. Nonsteroidal Anti-inflammatory Drugs. New York: Marcel Dekker, 1994:171–194.

13. Fry SW, Seeff LB. Hepatotoxicity of analgesics and anti-inflammatory agents. Gastroenterol Clin North Am 1995; 24:875–905.

14. Manoukian AV, Carson JL. Nonsteroidal anti-inflammatory drug-induced hepatic disorders. Drug Safety 1996; 15:64–71.

15. Walker AM. Quantitative studies of the risk of serious hepatic injury in persons using nonsteroidal antiinflammatory drugs. Arthritis Rheum 1997; 40:201–208.

16. Zimmerman HJ. Hepatotoxicity. Philadelphia: Lippincott Williams & Wilkins, 1999.

17. Katsinelos P, Katsos I, Patsiaoura K, Xiarchos P, Goulis I, Eugenidis N. Tenoxicam-associated hepatic injury: a case report and review. Eur J Gastroenterol Hepatol 1997; 9:403–406.

18. Krähenbühl S, Reichen J. Drug hepatotoxicity. In: BR Bacon, AM DiBisceglie, eds. Liver Disease: Diagnosis and Management. New York: Churchill Livingston, 2000:294–309.

19. Friis H, Andreasen PB. Drug-induced hepatic injury—an analysis of 1100 cases reported to the Danish Committee on Adverse Drug Reactions between 1978 and 1987. J Intern Med 1992; 232:133–138.

20. Paulus HE. FDA Arthritis Advisory Committee meeting. Arthritis Rheum 1982; 25:1124–1125.

21. Tolman KG. Hepatotoxicity of non-narcotic analgesics. Am J Med 1998; 105:13S–19S.

22. Boelsterli UA, Zimmerman HJ, Kretz-Rommel A. Idiosyncratic liver toxicity of nonsteroidal antiinflammatory drugs: molecular mechanisms and pathology. Crit Rev Toxicol 1995; 25: 207–235.

23. Borga O, Borga B. Serum protein binding of nonsteroidal antiinflammatory drugs: a comparative study. J Pharmacokinet Biopharm 1997; 25:63–77.

24. Vree TB, Van den Biggelaar-Martea M, Verwey-Van Wissen CPWGM, Vree ML, Guelen PJM. The pharmacokinetics of naproxen, its metabolite O-desmethylnaproxen, and their acyl-glucuronides in humans: effect of cimetidine. Br J Clin Pharmacol 1993; 35:467–472.

25. Jurima-Romet M, Crawford K, Huang HS. Comparative cytotoxicity of nonsteroidal antiinflammatory drugs in primary cultures of rat hepatocytes. Toxicol In Vitro 1994; 8:55–66.

26. Sorensen EMB, Acosta D. Relative toxicities of several nonsteroidal antiinflammatory compounds in primary cultures of rat hepatocytes. J Toxicol Environ Health 1985; 16:425–440.

27. Shen S, Marchick MR, Davis MR, Doss GA, Pohl LR. Metabolic activation of diclofenac by human cytochrome P450 3A4: role of 5-hydroxydiclofenac. Chem Res Toxicol 1999; 12: 214–222.

28. Tang W, Stearns RA, Bandiera SM, Zhang Y, Raab C, Braun MP, Dean DC, Pang J, Leung KH, Doss GA, Strauss JR, Kwei GY, Rushmore TH, Chiu SHL, Baillie TA. Studies on cytochrome P-450-mediated bioactivation of diclofenac in rats and in human hepatocytes: Identification of glutathione conjugated metabolites. Drug Metab Dispos 1999; 27:365–372.

29. Tang W, Stearns RA, Wang RW, Chiu SHL, Baillie TA. Roles of human hepatic cytochrome P450s 2C9 and 3A4 in the metabolic activation of diclofenac. Chem Res Toxicol 1999; 12: 192–199.

30. Shen SJ, Hargus SJ, Martin BM, Pohl LR. Cytochrome P4502C11 is a target of diclofenac covalent binding in rats. Chem Res Toxicol 1997; 10:420–423.

31. Sevoz C, Benoit E, Buronfosse T. Thioesterification of 2-arylpropionic acids by recombinant acyl-coenzyme A synthetases (ACS1 and ACS2). Drug Metab Dispos 2000; 28:398–402.

32. Hall SD, Qian XT. The role of coenzyme a in the biotransformation of 2-arylpropionic acids. Chem Biol Interact 1994; 90:235–251.

33. Mayer JM, Testa B, Roy-de Vos M, Audergon C, Etter JC. Interactions between the in vitro metabolism of xenobiotics and fatty acids: the case of ibuprofen and other chiral profens. Arch Toxicol 1995; suppl 17:499–513.

34. Caldwell J, Marsh MV. Interrelationships between xenobiotic metabolism and lipid biosynthesis. Biochem Pharmacol 1983; 32:1667–1672.

35. Mayer JM, Roy de Vos M, Audergon C, Testa B, Etter JC. Interactions of anti-inflammatory 2-arylpropionates (profens) with the metabolism of fatty acids: in vitro studies. Int J Tissue React 1994; 16:59–72.

36. Sallustio BC, Nunthasomboon S, Drogemuller CJ, Knights KM. In vitro covalent binding of nafenopin-CoA to human liver proteins. Toxicol Appl Pharmacol 2000; 163:176–182.

37. Hayball PJ. Chirality and nonsteroidal anti-inflammatory drugs. Drugs 1996; 52:47–58.

38. Mackenzie PI, Owens IS, Burchell B, Bock KW, Bairoch A, Bélanger A, Fournel-Gigleux S, Green M, Hum DW, Iyanagi T, Lancet D, Louisot P, Magdalou J, Chowdhury JR, Ritter JK, Schachter H, Tephly TR, Tipton KF, Nebert DW. The UDP glycosyltransferase gene superfamily: recommended nomenclature update based on evolutionary divergence. Pharmacogenetics 1997; 7:255–269.

39. Jin C, Miners JO, Lillywhite KJ, Mackenzie PI. Complementary deoxyribonucleic acid cloning and expression of a human liver uridine diphosphate-glucuronosyltransferase glucuronidating carboxylic acid-containing drugs. J Pharmacol Exp Ther 1993; 264:475–479.

40. Burchell B, McGurk K, Brierley CH, Clarke DJ. UDP-glucuronosyltransferases. In: IG Sipes, CA McQueen, AJ Gandolfi, eds. Comprehensive Toxicology. New York: Elsevier, 1997: 401–435.

41. Le HT, Franklin MR. Selective induction of phase II drug metabolizing enzyme activities by quinolines and isoquinolines. Chem Biol Interact 1997; 103:167–178.

42. Patel M, Tang BK, Grant DM, Kalow W. Interindividual variability in the glucuronidation of (S) oxazepam contrasted with that of (R) oxazepam. Pharmacogenetics 1995; 5:287–297.

43. Coffman BL, King CD, Rios GR, Tephly TR. The glucuronidation of opioids, other xenobiotics, and androgens by human UGT2B7Y(268) and UGT2B7(268). Drug Metab Dispos 1998; 26:73–77.

44. Kirkman SK, Zhang MY, Horwatt PM, Scatina J. Isolation and identification of bromfenac glucoside from rat bile. Drug Metab Dispos 1998; 26:720–723.

45. Fontana RJ, McCashland TM, Brenner KG, Appelman HD, Gunartanam NT, Wisecarver JL, Rabkin JM, Lee WM. Acute liver failure associated with prolonged use of bromfenac leading to liver transplantation. Liver Transplant Surg 1999; 5:480–484.

46. Moses PL, Schroeder B, Alkhatib O, Ferrentino N, Suppan T, Lidofsky SD. Severe hepatotoxicity associated with bromfenac sodium. Am J Gastroenterol 1999; 94:1393–1396.

47. Skjodt NM, Davies NM. Clinical pharmacokinetics and pharmacodynamics of bromfenac. Clin Pharmacokinet 1999; 36:399–408.

48. Watt JA, King AR, Dickinson RG. Contrasting systemic stabilities of the acyl and phenolic glucuronides of diflunisal in the rat. Xenobiotica 1991; 21:403–415.

49. Georges H, Presle N, Buronfosse T, Fournel-Gigleux S, Netter P, Magdalou J, Lapique F. In vitro stereoselective degradation of carprofen glucuronide by human serum albumin. Characterization of sites and reactive amino acids. Chirality 2000; 12:53–62.

50. Hayball PJ. Formation and reactivity of acyl glucuronides: the influence of chirality. Chirality 1995; 7:1–9.

51. Iwaki M, Bischer A, Nguyen AC, Mcdonagh AF, Benet LZ. Stereoselective disposition of naproxen glucuronide in the rat. Drug Metab Dispos 1995; 23:1099–1103.

52. Seitz S, Kretz-Rommel A, Oude Elferink RPJ, Boelsterli UA. Selective protein adduct formation of diclofenac glucuronide is critically dependent on the rat canalicular conjugate export pump (Mrp2). Chem Res Toxicol 1998; 11:513–519.

53. Kauffmann HM, Keppler D, Gant TW, Schrenk D. Induction of hepatic *mrp2 (cmrp/cmoat)* gene expression in nonhuman primates treated with rifampicin or tamoxifen. Arch Toxicol 1998; 72:763–768.

54. Rost D, Kartenbeck J, Keppler D. Changes in the localization of the rat canalicular conjugate export pump Mrp2 in phalloidin-induced cholestasis. Hepatology 1999; 29:814–821.

55. Paulusma CC, Bosma PJ, Zaman GJR, Bakker CTM, Otter M, Scheffer GL, Scheper RJ, Borst P, Oude Elferink RPJ. Congenital jaundice in rats with a mutation in a multidrug resistance-associated protein gene. Science 1996; 271:1126–1128.

56. Wang M, Dickinson RG. Effect of cholestasis on adduct formation and disposition of zomepirac in rats. Life Sci 2000; 68:525–537.

57. Yesair DW, Callahan M, Remington L, Kensler CJ. Role of the entero-hepatic cycle of indomethacin on its metabolism, distribution in tissues and its excretion by rats, dogs and monkeys. Biochem Pharmacol 1970; 19:1579–1590.

58. Brune K. Is there a rational basis for the different spectra of adverse effects of nonsteroidal anti-inflammatory drugs (NSAIDs)? Drugs 1990; 40(suppl 5):12–15.

59. Reuter BK, Davies NM, Wallace JL. Nonsteroidal anti-inflammatory drug enteropathy in rats: role of permeability, bacteria, and enterohepatic circulation. Gastroenterology 1997; 112:109–117.

60. Seitz S, Boelsterli UA. Diclofenac acyl glucuronide, a major biliary metabolite, is directly involved in small intestinal injury in rats. Gastroenterology 1998; 115:1476–1482.

61. MacPhail CM, Lappin MR, Meyer DJ, Smith SG, Webster CRL, Armstrong PJ. Hepatocellular toxicosis associated with administration of carprofen in 21 dogs. J Am Vet Med Assoc 1998; 212:1895–1901.

62. Priymenko N, Garnier F, Ferre JP, Delatour P, Toutain PL. Enantioselectivity of the enterohepatic recycling of carprofen in the dog. Drug Metab Dispos 1998; 26:170–6.

63. Khan SA, Khan MA, Albretsen JC, Gwaltney SM. Naproxen toxicosis in dogs: A review of fifty-seven cases (abstr). Toxicol Sci 1999; 48(suppl):32.

64. Dobrinska MR, Furst DE, Spiegel T, Vincek WC, Tompkins R, Duggan DE, Davies RO, Paulus HE. Biliary secretion of sulindac and metabolites in man. Biopharm Drug Dispos 1983; 4:347–358.

65. Bolder U, Trang NV, Hagey LR, Schteingart CD, Ton-Nu HT, Cerrè C, Oude Elferink RPJ, Hofmann AF. Sulindac is excreted into bile by a canalicular bile salt pump and undergoes a cholehepatic circulation in rats. Gastroenterology 1999; 117:962–971.

66. Smith PC, McDonagh AF, Benet LZ. Irreversible binding of zomepirac to plasma protein in vitro and in vivo. J Clin Invest 1986; 77:934–939.

67. Needleman P, Isakson PC. The discovery and function of COX-2. J Rheumatol 1997; 24:6–8.

68. Pessayre D, Mazel P, Descatoire V, Rogier E, Feldmann G, Benhamou JP. Inhibition of hepatic drug-metabolizing enzymes by arachidonic acid. Xenobiotica 1979; 9:301–310.

69. Gasperini R, Leone R, Velo GP, Fracasso ME. The inhibition of hepatic microsomal drug metabolism in rats by non-steroidal anti-inflammatory drugs. Pharmacol Res 1990; 22(suppl 3):115–116.

70. Hagmann W, Kirn A, Keppler D. Role of leukotrienes in acute inflammatory liver disease. In: W. Reutter, P.C. Heinrich, H. Popper, D. Keppler, I.M. Arias and L. Landmann, eds. Modulation of Liver Cell Expression. Lancaster: MTP Press, 1987:423–433.

71. Trudell JR, Gut J, Costa AK. Leukotrienes in hepatocyte injury. In: W Reutter, PC Heinrich, H Popper, D Keppler, IM Arias, L Landmann, eds. Modulation of Liver Cell Expression. Lancaster: MTP Press, 1987:411–421.

72. Kaplan-Machlis B, Klostermeyer BS. The cyclooxygenase-2 inhibitors: safety and effectiveness. Ann Pharmacother 1999; 33:979–988.

73. Foxworthy PS, Perry DN, Eacho PI. Induction of peroxisomal β-oxidation by nonsteroidal anti-inflammatory drugs. Toxicol Appl Pharmacol 1993; 118:271–274.

74. Vidal-Puig AJ, Considine RV, Jimenez-Liñan M, Werman A, Pories WJ, Caro JF, Flier JS. Peroxisome proliferator-activated receptor gene expression in human tissues: effects of obesity, weight loss, and regulation by insulin and glucocorticoids. J Clin Invest 1997; 99:2416–2422.

75. Bedoucha M, Atzpodien E, Boelsterli UA. Diabetic KKA^y mice exhibit increased hepatic PPARγ1 gene expression and develop hepatic steatosis upon chronic treatment with antidiabetic thiazolidinediones. Hepatol 2001; 17:17–23.

76. Lehmann JM, Lenhard JM, Oliver BB, Ringold GM, Kliewer SA. Peroxisome proliferator-activated receptors α and γ are activated by indomethacin and other non-steroidal anti-inflammatory drugs. J Biol Chem 1997; 272:3406–3410.

77. Rahman MA, Dhar DK, Masunaga R, Yamanoi A, Kohno H, Nagasue N. Sulindac and exisulind exhibit a significant antiproliferative effect and induce apoptosis in human hepatocellular carcinoma cell lines. Cancer Res 2000; 60:2085–2089.

78. Shiff SJ, Qiao L, Tsai L, Rigas B. Sulindac sulfide, an aspirin-like compound, inhibits proliferation, causes cell cycle quiescence, and induces apoptosis in HT-29 colon adenocarcinoma cells. J Clin Invest 1995; 96:491–503.

79. Hanif R, Pittas A, Feng Y, Koutsos MI, Qiao L, Staianocoico L, Shiff SI, Rigas B. Effects of nonsteroidal anti-inflammatory drugs on proliferation and on induction of apoptosis in colon cancer cells by a prostaglandin-independent pathway. Biochem Pharmacol 1996; 52:237–245.

80. Shiff SJ, Koutsos MI, Qiao L, Rigas B. Nonsteroidal anti-inflammatory drugs inhibit the proliferation of colon adenocarcinoma cells: effects on cell cycle and apoptosis. Exp Cell Res 1996; 222:179–188.

81. Zhu GH, Wong BCY, Ching CK, Lai KC, Lam SK. Differential apoptosis by indomethacin in gastric epithelial cells through the constitutive expression of wild-type p53 and/or upregulation of c-myc. Biochem Pharmacol 1999; 58:193–200.

82. McDougall P, Markham A, Cameron I, Sweetman AJ. The mechanism of inhibition of mitochondrial oxidative phosphorylation by the non-steroidal anti-inflammatory agent diflunisal. Biochem Pharmacol 1983; 32:2595–2598.

83. Browne GS, Nelson C, Nguyen T, Ellis BA, Day RO, Williams KM. Stereoselective and substrate-dependent inhibition of hepatic mitochondrial β-oxidation and oxidative phosphorylation by the non-steroidal anti-inflammatory drugs ibuprofen, flurbiprofen, and ketorolac. Biochem Pharmacol 1999; 57:837–844.

84. Mahmud T, Scott DL, Bjarnason I. A unifying hypothesis for the mechanism of NSAID related gastrointestinal toxicity. Ann Rheum Dis 1996; 55:211–213.

85. Petrescu I, Tarba C. Uncoupling effects of diclofenac and aspirin in the perfused liver and isolated hepatic mitochondria of rat. Biochim Biophys Acta (Bioenergetics) 1997; 1318:385–394.

86. Moreno-Sanchez R, Bravo C, Vasquez C, Ayala G, Silveira LH, Martinez-Lavin M. Inhibi-

tion and uncoupling of oxidative phosphorylation by nonsteroidal anti-inflammatory drugs. Biochem Pharmacol 1999; 57:743–752.

87. Tokomitsu Y, Lee S, Ui M. In vitro effects of nonsteroidal anti-inflammatory drugs on oxidative phosphorylation in rat liver mitochondria. Biochem Pharmacol 1977; 26:2101–2106.

88. Knights KM, Drew R. The effects of ibuprofen enantiomers on hepatocyte intermediary metabolism and mitochondrial respiration. Biochem Pharmacol 1992; 44:1291–1296.

89. Masubuchi Y, Saito H, Horie T. Structural requirements for the hepatotoxicity of nonsteroidal anti-inflammatory drugs in isolated rat hepatocytes. J Pharmacol Exp Ther 1998; 287:208–213.

90. Ponsoda X, Bort R, Jover R, Gomezlechon MJ, Castell JV. Molecular mechanism of diclofenac hepatotoxicity: association of cell injury with oxidative metabolism and decrease in ATP levels. Toxicol In Vitro 1995; 9:439–444.

91. Masubuchi Y, Yamada S, Horie T. Possible mechanism of hepatocyte injury induced by diphenylamine and its structurally related nonsteroidal anti-inflammatory drugs. J Pharmacol Exp Ther 2000; 292:982–987.

92. Bjorkman D. Nonsteroidal anti-inflammatory drug-associated toxicity of the liver, lower gastrointestinal tract, and esophagus. Am J Med 1998; 105:17S–21S.

93. Wallace KB, Frederick CB. Induction of the mitochondrial permeability transition in vitro by carboxylic acids (abstr). Toxicol Sci 2000; 54(suppl):163.

94. Uyemura SA, Santos AC, Mingatto FE, Jordani MC, Curti C. Diclofenac sodium and mefenamic acid: potent inducers of the membrane permeability transition in renal cortex mitochondria. Arch Biochem Biophys 1997; 342:231–235.

95. Al-Nasser IA. Ibuprofen-induced liver mitochondrial permeability transition Toxicol Lett 2000; 111:213–218.

96. Geneve J, Hayat-Bonan B, Labbe G, Degott C, Lettéron C, Fréneaux E, LeDinh T, Larrey D, Pessayre D. Inhibition of mitochondrial β-oxidation of fatty acids by pirprofen. Role in microvesicular steatosis due to this nonsteroidal anti-inflammatory drug. J Pharmacol Exp Ther 1987; 242:1133–1137.

97. Freneaux E, Fromenty B, Berson A, Labbe G, Degott C, Lettéron P, Larrey D, Pessayre D. Stereoselective and nonstereoselective effects of ibuprofen enantiomers on mitochondrial β-oxidation of fatty acids. J Pharmacol Exp Ther 1990; 255:529–535.

98. Zhao B, Geisslinger G, Hall I, Day RO, Williams KM. The effect of the enantiomers of ibuprofen and flurbiprofen on the β-oxidation of palmitate in the rat. Chirality 1992; 4:137–141.

99. Fraser JL, Antonioli DA, Chopra S, Wang HH. Prevalence and nonspecificity of fatty change in the liver. Mod Pathol 1995; 8:65–70.

100. Fromenty B, Pessayre D. Inhibition of mitochondrial beta-oxidation as a mechanism of hepatotoxicity. Pharmacol Ther 1995; 67:101–154.

101. Fromenty B, Pessayre D. Impaired mitochondrial function in microvesicular steatosis. J Hepatol 1997; 26:43–53.

102. Deschamps D, Fisch C, Fromenty B, Berson A, Degott C, Pessayre D. Inhibition by salicylic acid of the activation and thus oxidation of long-chain fatty acids. Possible role in the development of Reye's syndrome. J Pharmacol Exp Ther 1991; 259:894–904.

103. Vianey-Liaud C, Divry N, Gregersen N, Mathieu M. The inborn errors of mitochondrial fatty acid oxidation. J Inher Metab Dis 1987; 10(suppl 1):159–198.

104. Danan G, Trunet P, Bernuau J, Degott C, Babany G, Pessayre D, Ruoff B, Benhamou JP. Pirprofen-induced fulminant hepatitis. Gastroenterology 1985; 89:210–213.

105. Victorino RMM, Silveria JCB, Baptista A, De Moura MC. Jaundice associated with naproxen. Postgrad Med J 1980; 56:368.

106. Bravo JF, Jacobson MP, Mertens BF. Fatty liver and pleural effusion with ibuprofen therapy. Ann Intern Med 1977; 87:200–201.

107. Dutertre JP, Bastides F, Jonville AP, DeMuret a, Sonneville A, Larrey D, Autret E. Microvesicular steatosis after ketoprofen administration. Eur J Gastroenterol Hepatol 1991; 3:953–954.

108. Fraser JL, Antonioli DA, Chopra S, Wang HH. Prevalence and nonspecificity of microvesicular fatty change in the liver. Mod Pathol 1995; 8:65–70.

109. Hyneck ML, Smith PC, Munafo A, McDonagh AF, Benet LZ. Disposition and irreversible plasma protein binding of tolmetin in humans. Clin Pharmacol Ther 1988; 44:107–114.

110. Smith PC, Benet LZ, McDonagh AF. Covalent binding of zomepirac glucuronide to proteins: evidence for a Schiff base mechanism. Drug Metab Disp 1990; 18:639–644.

111. King AR, Dickinson RG. Studies on the reactivity of acyl glucuronides. IV. Covalent binding of diflunisal to tissues of the rat. Biochem Pharmacol 1993; 45:1043–1047.

112. Zia-Amirhosseini P, Ojingwa JC, Spahn-Langguth H, McDonagh AF, Benet LZ. Enhanced covalent binding of tolmetin to proteins in humans after multiple dosing. Clin Pharmacol Ther 1994; 55:21–27.

113. Van Breemen RB, Fenselau C. Acylation of albumin by 1-*O*-acyl glucuronides. Drug Metab Dispos 1985; 13:318–320.

114. Iwakawa S, Spahn H, Benet LZ, Lin ET. Carprofen acyl glucuronides: stereoselective degradation and interaction with human serum albumin. Pharm Res 1988; 5(Suppl.):S-214.

115. Dickinson RG, King AR. Studies on the reactivity of acyl glucuronides—II. Interaction of diflunisal acyl glucuronide and its isomers with human serum albumin in vitro. Biochem Pharmacol 1991; 42:2301–2306.

116. Smith PC, Song WQ, Rodriguez RJ. Covalent binding of etodolac acyl glucuronide to albumin invitro. Drug Metab Dispos 1992; 20:962–965.

117. Ding A, Ojingwa JC, McDonagh AF, Burlingame AL, Benet LZ. Evidence for covalent binding of acyl glucuronides to serum albumin via an imine mechanism as revealed by tandem mass spectrometry. Proc Natl Acad Sci USA 1993; 90:3797–3801.

118. Dubois N, Lapicque F, Maurice MH, Pritchard M, Fournelgigleux S, Magdalou J, Abiteboul M, Siest G, Netter P. In vitro irreversible binding of ketoprofen glucuronide to plasma proteins. Drug Metab Dispos 1993; 21:617–623.

119. Smith PC, Liu JH. Covalent binding of suprofen acyl glucuronide to albumin in vitro. Xenobiotica 1993; 23:337–348.

120. Smith PC, Liu JH. Covalent binding of suprofen to renal tissue of rat correlates with excretion of its acyl glucuronide. Xenobiotica 1995; 25:531–540.

121. Ding A, Zia-Amirhosseini P, Mcdonagh AF, Burlingame AL, Benet LZ. Reactivity of tolmetin glucuronide with human serum albumin—identification of binding sites and mechanisms of reaction by tandem mass spectrometry. Drug Metab Dispos 1995; 23:369–376.

122. Yvon M, Wal JM. Identification of lysine residue 199 of human serum albumin as a binding site for benzylpenicilloyl groups. FEBS Lett 1988; 239:237–240.

123. Akira K, Hasegawa H, Shinohara Y, Imachi M, Hashimoto T. Stereoselective internal acyl migration of 1β-O-acyl glucuronides of enantiomeric 2-phenylpropionic acids. Biol Pharm Bull 2000; 23:506–510.

124. Iwaki M, Ogiso T, Inagawa S, Kakehi K. In vitro regioselective stability of β-1-O and 2-O-acyl glucuronides of naproxen and their covalent binding to human serum albumin. J Pharm Sci 1999; 88:52–57.

125. Benet LZ, Spahn-Langguth H, Iwakawa S, Volland C, Mizuma T, Mayer S, Mutschler E, Lin ET. Predictability of the covalent binding of acidic drugs in man. Life Sci 1993; 53:PL141–PL146.

126. Spahn H, Näthke I, Mohri K, Zia-Amirrhosseini P, Benet LZ. Preliminary characterization of proteins to which benoxaprofen glucuronide binds irreversibly. Pharm Res 1990; 7(suppl):S-257.

127. Pumford NR, Myers TG, Davila JC, Highet RJ, Pohl LR. Immunochemical detection of liver protein adducts of the nonsteroidal antiinflammatory drug diclofenac. Chem Res Toxicol 1993; 6:147–150.

128. Hargus SJ, Amouzedeh HR, Pumford NR, Myers TG, McCoy SC, Pohl LR. Metabolic activation and immunochemical localization of liver protein adducts of the nonsteroidal anti-inflammatory drug diclofenac. Chem Res Toxicol 1994; 7:575–582.

129. Kretz-Rommel A, Boelsterli UA. Selective protein adducts to membrane proteins in cultured rat hepatocytes exposed to diclofenac: radiochemical and immunochemical analysis. Mol Pharmacol 1994; 45:237–244.

130. Hargus SJ, Martin BM, George JW, Pohl LR. Covalent modification of rat liver dipeptidyl peptidase IV (CD26) by the nonsteroidal anti-inflammatory drug diclofenac. Chem Res Toxicol 1995; 8:993–996.

131. Wade LT, Kenna JG, Caldwell J. Immunochemical identification of mouse hepatic protein adducts derived from the nonsteroidal anti-inflammatory drugs diclofenac, sulindac, and ibuprofen. Chem Res Toxicol 1997; 10:546–555.

132. Myers TG, Pumford NR, Davila JC, Pohl LR. Covalent binding of diclofenac to plasma membrane proteins of the bile canaliculi in the mouse. Toxicologist 1992; 12:253.

133. Caldwell J, Fakurakzi S, Ramsay LA, Somchit N, Goldin RD. Benoxaprofen forms protein adducts in the bile canaliculi of female CD1 mice (abstr). Toxicol Sci Suppl 2000; 54:46.

134. Caldwell J, Somchit N, Ramsay LA, Kenna JG. Inhibition of canalicular plasma membrane dipeptidyl peptidase IV (DPP IV) is not associated with NSAID-induced hepatotoxicity in rat. Meeting Abstract, 5th International ISSX Meeting, Cairns, Australia, 1998, 13:151.

135. Wang M, Gorrell MD, McCaughan GW, Dickinson RG. Dipeptidyl peptidase IV is a target for covalent adduct formation with the acyl glucuronide metabolite of the anti-inflammatory drug zomepirac. Life Sci 2001; 68:785–797.

136. Boelsterli UA. Reactive acyl glucuronides: Possible role in small intestinal toxicity induced by nonsteroidal anti-inflammatory drugs. Toxic Subst Mech 1999; 18:83–100.

137. Boelsterli UA. Acyl glucuronides in idiosyncratic toxicity. In: V. Subrahmanyan, ed. Mechanisms, Models and Predictions of Idiosyncratic Drug Toxicity. Brentwood, MO: ISE Press, 2002. In press.

138. Chiou YJ, Tomer KB, Smith PC. Effect of nonenzymatic glycation of albumin and superoxide dismutase by glucuronic acid and suprofen acyl glucuronide on their functions in vitro. Chem-Biol Interact 1999; 121:141–159.

139. Bailey MJ, Worrall S, de Jersey J, Dickinson RG. Zomepirac acyl glucuronide covalently modifies tubulin in vitro and in vivo and inhibits its assembly in an in vitro system. Chem-Biol Interact 1998; 115:153–166.

140. De Weck AL. Immunopathological mechanisms and clinical aspects of allergic reactions to drugs. In: AL De Weck, H Bungaard, eds. Allergic Reactions to Drugs. Berlin: Springer Verlag, 1983:75–133.

141. Munafo A, Hyneck ML, Benet LZ. Pharmacokinetics and irreversible binding of tolmetin and its glucuronic acid esters in the elderly. Pharmacology 1993; 47:309–317.

142. McKinnon GE, Dickinson RG. Covalent binding of diflunisal and probenecid to plasma protein in humans: Persistence of the adducts in the circulation. Res Commun Chem Pathol Pharmacol 1989; 66:339–354.

143. Dohlman JG, Pillion DJ, Rokeach LA, Ramprasad MP. Identification of macrophage cell-surface binding sites for cationized bovine serum albumin. Biochem Biophys Res Comm 1991; 181:787–796.

144. Franco A, Barnaba V, Natali P, Balsano C, Musca A, Balsano F. Expression of class I and class II major histocompatibility complex antigens on human hepatocytes. Hepatology 1988; 8:449–454.

145. Harris HW, Gill TJ. Expression of class I transplantation antigens. Transplantation 1986; 42:109–116.

146. Calmus Y, Arvieux C, Gane P, Boucher E, Nordlinger B, Rouger P, Poupon R. Cholestasis induces major histocompatibility complex class-I expression in hepatocytes. Gastroenterology 1992; 102:1371–1377.

147. Arvieux C, Calmus Y, Gane P, Legendre C, Mariani P, Delelo R, Poupon R, Nordlinger B. Immunogenicity of rat hepatocytes in vivo—effect of cholestasis-induced changes in major histocompatibility complex expression. J Hepatol 1993; 18:335–341.

148. Lobo-Yeo A, Senaldi G, Portmann B, Mowat AP, Mieli-Vergani G, Vergani D. Class I and class II major histocompatibility complex antigen expression on hepatocyes: a study in children with liver disease. Hepatology 1990; 12:224–32.

149. Volpes R, Vandenoord JJ, Desmet VJ. Can hepatocytes serve as activated immunomodulating cells in the immune response. J Hepatol 1992; 16:228–240.

150. Chedid A, Mendenhall CL, Moritz TE, French SW, Chen TS, Morgan TR, Roselle GA, Nemchausky BA, Tamburro CH, Schiff ER, Mcclain CJ, Marsano LS, Allen JI, Samanta A, Weesner RE, Henderson WG. Cell-mediated hepatic injury in alcoholic liver disease. Gastroenterology 1993; 105:254–266.

151. Worrall S, Dickinson RG. Rat serum albumin modified by diflunisal acyl glucuronide is immunogenic in rats. Life Sci 1995; 56:1921–1930.

152. Zia-Amirhosseini P, Harris RZ, Brodsky FM, Benet LZ. Hypersensitivity to nonsteroidal anti-inflammatory drugs. Nature Med 1995; 1:2–4.

153. Sidrouphis L, Beaugrand, M., Malledant, Y., Brissot, P., Guguen-Guillouzo, C., Guillouzo, A. Use of adult human hepatocytes in primary culture of the study of clometacin-induced immunoallergic hepatitis. Toxic In Vitro 1991; 5:529–534.

154. Toh BH. Anti-cytoskeletal autoantibodies: diagnostic significance for liver diseases, infections and systemic autoimmune diseases. Autoimmunity 1991; 11:119–125.

155. Hillon P, Bedenne L, Piard F, Regis P. Clometacine-induced hepatitis. Dig Dis Sci 1988; 33:1045–1053.

156. Pessayre D. Physiopathologie des hépatopathies médicamenteuses. Gastroentérol Clin Biol 1993; 17:H3–H17.

157. Kretz-Rommel A, Rubin RL. Disruption of positive selection of thymocytes causes autoimmunity. Nature Med 2000; 6:298–305.

158. Kretz-Rommel A, Boelsterli UA. Cytotoxic activity of T cells and non-T cells from diclofenac-immunized mice against cultured syngeneic hepatocytes exposed to diclofenac. Hepatology 1995; 22:213–222.

159. Sokol RJ, Devereaux M, Khandwala R, Obrien K. Evidence for involvement of oxygen free radicals in bile acid toxicity to isolated rat hepatocytes. Hepatology 1993; 17:869–881.

160. Spivey JR, Bronk SF, Gores GJ. Glycochenodeoxycholate-induced lethal hepatocellular injury in rat hepatocytes. Role of ATP depletion and cytosolic free calcium. J Clin Invest 1993; 92:17–24.

161. Miyoshi H, Rust C, Roberts PJ, Burgart LJ, Gores GJ. Hepatocyte apoptosis after bile duct ligation in the mouse involves Fas. Gastroenterology 1999; 117:669–677.

162. Atchison CR, Hargus SJ, Daiker D, Aronson J, West B, M.T. M. Histopathology and diclofenac protein adducts in rat liver and intestine (abstr). Fund Appl Toxicol 1997; 36(suppl): 211.

163. Trauner M, Arrese M, Soroka CJ, Ananthanarayanan M, Koeppel TA, Schlosser SF, Suchy FJ, Keppler D, Boyer JL. The rat canalicular conjugate export pump (Mrp2) is downregulated in intrahepatic and obstructive cholestasis. Gastroenterology 1997; 113:255–264.

164. Paulusma CC, Kothe MJC, Bakker CTM, Bosma PJ, Van Bokhoven I, Van Marle J, Bolder U, Tytgat GNJ, Oude Elferink RPJ. Zonal down-regulation and redistribution of the multidrug resistance protein 2 during bile duct ligation in rat liver. Hepatology 2000; 31:684–693.

165. Fears R, Baggaley KH, Alexander R, Morgan B, Hindles RM. The participation of ethyl 4-benzoyloxybenzoate (BRL 10894) and other aryl-substituted acids in glycerolipid metabolism. J Lipid Res 1978; 19:3–11.

166. Mayer JM. Ibuprofen enantiomers and lipid metabolism. J Clin Pharmacol 1996; 36:27S–32S.

167. Williams K, Day R, Knihinicki R, Duffield A. The stereoselective uptake of ibuprofen enanti-omers into adipose tissue. Biochem Pharmacol 1986; 35:3403–3405.

168. Mayer JM. Stereoselective metabolism of anti-inflammatory 2-arylpropionates. Acta Pharm Nord 1990; 2:197–216.

169. Sherrat HSA. Acyl-CoA esters of xenobiotic carboxylic acids as biochemically active inter-mediates. Biochem Soc Trans 1985; 13:856–858.

170. Dodds PF. Incorporation of xenobiotic carboxylic acids into lipids. Life Sci 1991; 49:629–649.

171. Gitlin N. Salicylate hepatotoxicity: The potential role of hypoalbuminemia. J Clin Gastro-enterol 1980; 2:281.

172. Runyon BA, LaBrecque DR, Anuras S. The spectrum of liver disease in systemic lupus erythematosus: report of 33 histologically-proved cases and review of the literature. Am J Med 1980; 69:187–194.

173. Mills PR, Sturrock RD. Clinical associations between arthritis and liver disease. Ann Rheum Dis 1982; 41:295–307.

174. Weinblatt ME, Tesser J, Gilliam JH. The liver in rheumatic disease. Semin Arthritis Rheum 1982; 11:399–405.

175. Uetrecht JP. New concepts in immunology relevant to idiosyncratic drug reactions: The "Danger Hypothesis" and innate immune system. Chem Res Toxicol 1999; 12:387–395.

176. Furst SM, Gandolfi AJ. Immunologic mediation of chemical-induced hepatotoxicity. In: GL Plaa, WR Hewitt, eds. Toxicology of the Liver. 2nd ed. Washington: Taylor & Francis, 1998: 259–295.

16

Nonsteroidal Anti-Inflammatory Drugs: Pathology and Clinical Presentation of Hepatotoxicity

JAMES H. LEWIS

Georgetown University Medical Center, Washington, D.C., U.S.A.

I. INTRODUCTION

Nonsteroidal anti-inflammatory drugs (NSAIDs) as a class are an important cause of drug-induced toxic injury to several organ systems, including well-known injury to the gastrointestinal tract and kidneys. While perhaps less well appreciated, NSAIDs are a leading cause of drug-induced hepatotoxicity. For instance, in Denmark, NSAIDs accounted for approximately 9% (97 of 1100) of all drug-related liver injury reports between 1978 and 1987 (1) and they continue to be reported at a rate that often exceeds other drug classes (2).

The early history of NSAID-induced hepatic injury dates back more than 60 years (3). Cinchophen was one of the earliest agents to be associated with hepatotoxicity, with a case-fatality rate of nearly 50% that forced its withdrawal from clinical use (4,5). Over the ensuing decades, several other NSAIDs have been developed or introduced into practice only to be abandoned during pre- or postmarket evaluation owing to serious liver injury (3,6) (Table 1). Early examples included glafenine (7), an NSAID similar to cinchophen; ibufenac (8), a precursor of ibuprofen; fenclozic acid, an early acetic acid derivative NSAID (9); and fluproquazone, the precursor compound of quinazolone derivatives (3). However, it was not until the withdrawal of benoxaprofen (Oraflex) in 1982 owing to reports of fatal jaundice in the United Kingdom (10) that attention was intensively focused on the hepatotoxicity of NSAIDs as a group (3,6,11). At that time, the Arthritis Advisory Committee of the Food and Drug Administration concluded that hepatic injury should be considered a class characteristic of NSAIDs (12). However, this uniform characterization of hepatic injury obscures the many individual differences and potential for hepatic injury found within and among the different NSAID classes (13). Newer NSAIDs continue to include agents associated with instances of fulminant hepatic failure (FHF) that have forced their withdrawal, as most recently occurred with bromfenac (14). For others, such as diclofenac, liver enzyme monitoring to detect hepatoxicity is recommended to help prevent FHF (11). Several other agents, including sulindac, piroxicam, and mefenamic acid, also should be monitored closely for clinical signs of liver injury (11).

This chapter will review the clinical presentation and pathological features of the acute hepatic injury associated with the currently available NSAIDs. For many agents, liver injury has been well characterized; for several others, however, only limited data are available and clinical summaries are necessarily less complete.

Table 1 Examples of NSAIDs of Various Classes Withdrawn or Abandoned Due to Hepatotoxicity

Anthranilic acid derivatives
Cinchophen
Glafenine
Acetic acid derivatives
Amphenac
Fenclozic acid
Isoxepac
Bromfenac
Propionic acid derivatives
Benoxaprofen
Ibufenac
Pirprofen
Suprofen
Fenbufen
Pyrazolone derivatives
Phenylbutazone
Oxyphenbutazone
Oxicams
Isoxicam
Sudoxicam
Quinazonlone derivatives
Fluproquazone

II. INCIDENCE OF NSAID-INDUCED HEPATIC INJURY

It has been suggested that the occurrence of serious overt hepatic injury due to NSAIDs as a group is well under 0.1% (15), although figures to determine the true incidence of NSAID-induced hepatic damage are generally lacking. However, with upward of tens of millions of patients in the United States taking NSAIDs on a regular basis, even this very low incidence of injury may translate into a substantial number of affected individuals. For example, using Medicaid billing data from hospital admissions for acute liver disease in Michigan and Florida, Carson and colleagues (16) reported an annual incidence of acute hepatitis due to NSAIDs leading to hospitalization of 2.2 per 100,000 persons. However, when NSAID cases were compared with controls, none of the individual NSAIDs was associated with a statistically significant increased risk. In contrast, a large retrospective Canadian study involving nearly 230,000 patients and 650,000 person-years of NSAID exposure showed a risk of NSAID-associated hospitalization for acute (mostly cholestatic) liver injury of 1.7, based on an excess risk of injury of 5 per 100,000 person years (17). A similar estimate of the relative risk of NSAID-associated liver injury was also reported in Denmark for sulindac and fenbufen, which were reported more often than other NSAIDs (1). Incidence rates for individual agents have been reliably estimated for only a few drugs,

Table 2 Effects of Some Rheumatological Diseases on the Liver

	Disease	Hepatic abnormalities	Pathology
I.	Rheumatoid arthritis	Elevated alkaline phosphatase, GGT in 25–50%	Steatosis
			Nonspecific changes
		Hepatomegaly 10%	Mild portal inflammation
II.	Systemic lupus erythematosus	Elevated LAEs 20–50%	Steatosis
		Autoimmune (lupoid) hepatitis	Cholestasis
			CAH
		Hepatomegaly 20–25%	Granulomas
		Jaundice 4%	Cirrhosis
		Ascites 10%	
III.	Fetty's syndrome (RA, splenomegaly, neutropenia)	Elevated LAEs 33%	Nodular regenerative hyperplasia (up to 70%)
		Hepatomegaly 33–66%	Portal fibrosis
			Portal hypertension
IV.	Sjögren's syndrome	Elevated LAEs 5%	CAH
		Jaundice 2%	May be part of PBC
V.	Essential mixed cryoglobulinemia	Chronic hepatitis C in 40%	
VI.	Polyarteritis nodosa	Hepatitis B	HBs Ag-associated immune complexes; changes of vasculitis
		Hepatomegaly	
		Elevated LAEs	
		Acalculous cholecystitis	
VII.	Psoriatic arthritis	Elevated LAEs	Steatosis, inflammation, hepatic necrosis, fibrosis cirrhosis (<1%)

Source: After Refs. 20–23.
LAE, liver-associated enzymes (usually ALT, AST); CAH, chronic active hepatitis; PBC, primary biliary cirrhosis.

Table 3 Clincopathological Features of Hepatotoxicity due to NSAIDs

Class agent	Type of injury	Proposed mechanism	Susceptibility factors
Salicylates			
Aspirin	Acute H-cell, CAH?, Reye's syndrome	Intrinsic toxicity	JRA, SLE, RF
Sodium, choline salicylates	H-cell (minor)	Hypersensitivity	
Diflunisal (Dolobid)	Cholestatic, mixed	Hyposensitivity?	
Benorilate	Zone 3 necrosis	Intrinsic	
Salsalate (Disalcid)	H-cell (minor)	[a]	
Acetic acid derivatives			
Diclofenac (Voltaren)	Acute H-cell necrosis, autoimmune CAH-like	Metabolic idiosyncrasy	Elderly females with OA, cross-sensitivity with ibuprofen?
Etodolac (Lodine)	H-cell necrosis	Metabolic idiosyncrasy?	
Ketorolac (Toradol)	Not reported	—	
Bromfenac (Duract)	Massive necrosis	Metabolic idiosyncrasy	Prolonged use
Indomethacin (Indocin)	H-cell necrosis, microvesicular steatosis, cholestasis (less often)	Metabolic idiosyncrasy	Children
Sulindac (Clinoril)	Cholestasis or mixed, H-cell in 25%	Hypersensitivity	JRA, SLE
Tolmetin (Tolectin)	Jaundice, steatosis	Metabolic idiosyncrasy?	
Nabumetone (Relafen)	Cholestatic Jaundice	Metabolic idiosyncrasy?	
Clometacin	Autoimmune CAH, granulomas, cholestasis	Hypersensitivity	Elderly females

	Type of lesion	Mechanism	Risk factors	Cross-sensitivity
Propionic acid derivatives				
Ibuprofen (Motrin et al)	H-cell or mixed (rare), steatosis	Hypersensitivity?		Cross-sensitivity with diclofenac
Naproxen (Naprosyn et al)	H-cell jaundice, cholestasis	Hypersensitivity?		Cross-sensitivity with naproxen
Fenoprofen (Nalfon)	Cholestatic jaundice (rare)	Hypersensitivity?		
Flurbiprofen (Ansaid)	H-cell jaundice (rare)	Hypersensitivity?		
Oxaprozine (Daypro)	H-cell	Metabolic idiosyncrasy?		
Ketoprofen (Orudis)	H-cell jaundice (rare)	Metabolic idiosyncrasy?		
Benoxaprofen (Oraflex)	Cholestatic jaundice	Metabolic idiosyncrasy	Elderly females	
Oxicams				
Piroxicam (Feldene)	H-cell necrosis, cholestasis	Hypersensitivity		
Droxicam	Cholestasis	Hypersensitivity?	Elderly	
Pyrazolone derivatives				
Phenylbutazone	H-cell necrosis, steatosis or cholestasis, granulomas	Hypersensitivity (intrinsic toxicity in high doses)?	Adults, women	
Oxyphenbutazone	H-cell necrosis, granulomas	Hypersensitivity		
Fenamates				
Mefenamic acid (Ponstel)	H-cell necrosis (rare)	a		
Meclofenamic acid (Meclomen)	H-cell (minor)	a		
Cyclooxygenase-2 Inhibitors				
Nimesulide	H-cell necrosis, cholestasis less often	Metabolic idiosyncrasy (? hypersensitivity)		
Celecoxib	H-cell (rare)	?		
Rofecoxib	a	a		

CAH, chronic active hepatitis; H-cell, hepatocellular; JRA, juvenile rheumatoid arthritis; SLE, systemic lupus erythematosus; RF, rheumatic fever; LFT, liver function tests.
[a] Unknown, too little information available.

as will be presented. In general, spontaneous reports do not reliably reflect the results of large epidemiological studies (18,19).

III. EFFECT OF RHEUMATIC DISEASES ON THE LIVER

Any discussion of NSAID-induced hepatic injury must take into account the underlying rheumatic disease being treated that may also adversely affect the liver. Many rheumatic diseases may have hepatic-associated enzyme elevations that may mimic drug injury. For example, rheumatoid arthritis is associated with elevations of alkaline phosphatase levels in 25–50% of individuals not receiving drug treatment (20–23). Hepatic involvement in systemic lupus erythematosus (SLE) is present in as many as 20% of individuals with a twofold elevation in hepatic-associated enzymes (23,24). Hepatic abnormalities in biochemical testing as well as hepatic histology have also been observed in patients with Felty's syndrome, Sjögren's syndrome, progressive systemic sclerosis, polyarteritis nodosa, essential mixed cryoglobulinemia (which may be associated with underlying chronic hepatitis C infection), polymyalgia rheumatica, Reiter's syndrome, and occasionally even osteoarthritis (22,23) (Table 2). Data observed with agents such as diclofenac suggest that patients, of either gender, with osteoarthritis are more susceptible to minor drug-induced hepatic injury compared to those with rheumatoid arthritis, and that susceptibility to clinically significant injury is enhanced even further in women (3,13).

IV. CLINICAL AND BIOCHEMICAL SPECTRUM OF NSAID-INDUCED HEPATIC INJURY

While most NSAIDs that can produce overt hepatic injury (with jaundice) do so rarely, many agents are associated with mild abnormalities of hepatic enzymes such as aspartate aminotransferase (AST) and alanine aminotransferase (ALT). Elevations in AST and ALT values occur in 5–15% of patients taking NSAIDs as a class (15). Most of these levels remain less than three times the upper limits of normal (ULN), and in some cases may resolve despite continuation of the NSAID. In general, however, the higher the incidence of even mildly elevated aminotransferase levels (especially ALT), the more likely the risk of overt hepatic disease (12).

The histological lesions produced by NSAIDs depend on the agent involved and on the mechanism of injury. Table 3 lists the predominant types of injury for the currently available NSAIDs. Acute hepatocellular injury involves hepatic degeneration or cell necrosis, while cholestatic injury is characterized mainly by the agents that arrest bile flow. Mixed injury refers to hepatocellular (cytotoxic) injury and cholestasis. Intrinsic hepatotoxins cause injury that is mainly cytotoxic with necrosis, degeneration, and/or steatosis, although a few can cause cholestasis. In contrast, idiosyncratic injury results in cholestatic or hepatocellular injury (3,11).

The biochemical changes seen with NSAID-associated liver injury reflect the histological pattern of damage. Hepatocellular injury with necrosis resembles acute viral hepatitis with AST and ALT levels increased 10–100-fold or more and bilirubin levels that are variably increased. Serum alkaline phosphatase values are generally normal or only mildly elevated. Toxic microvesicular steatosis may resemble acute fatty liver of pregnancy or Reye's syndrome with aminotransferase values 5–20 times normal and up to threefold elevations in alkaline phosphatase and bilirubin (25).

Clinically, hepatocellular injury may cause anorexia, fatigue, nausea, malaise, and jaundice. Massive necrosis leading to fulminant hepatitis may result in hepatic coma, coagulopathy, ascites, and death. Drug-induced jaundice associated with hepatocellular injury must by regarded as a serious lesion since case fatality rates are 10% or more, depending on the agent. The prognosis of complete recovery is usually good for patients who survive the acute phase of injury (3).

Cholestatic injury is characterized by elevated alkaline phosphatase levels (3–10 times normal) with parallel increases in gamma glutamyl transpeptidase or 5′-nucleotidase and variable increases in serum bilirubin, with AST and ALT remaining normal or only modestly elevated. The predominant features of cholestatic injury are jaundice and pruritus. Some patients complain of abdominal pain that may mimic acute extrahepatic biliary obstruction. Rarely does intrahepatic cholestatic injury cause a fatal outcome, although prolonged jaundice may sometimes be seen (26).

V. HEPATIC INJURY DUE TO INDIVIDUAL NSAIDs

A. Salicylates

1. Aspirin (Acetylsalicylic Acid)

Several hundred of cases of aspirin-related hepatic injury have been reported since the 1970s (27). However, this represented a delay of more than 75 years before the hepatotoxic potential of aspirin was truly appreciated. In part this may have been due to the fact that the injury is often mild and anicteric and was overlooked in the era prior to routine enzymatic testing (3,27). Alternatively, the injury may have been attributed to the underlying rheumatic disease (21). In contrast, NSAIDs developed in the past two decades often have had hepatic injury observed during clinical trials or soon after initial marketing because of the routine use of biochemical testing (13).

Aspirin injury is primarily hepatocellular, but in general is clinically mild and reversible with ALT/AST levels <10-fold elevated. Bilirubin levels usually remain normal or are minimally elevated with jaundice seen in fewer than 5% of cases (27). Liver biopsy characteristically shows areas of focal necrosis with a mild inflammatory response in the portal areas. In addition, cellular unrest, ballooning, and eosinophilic degeneration have been described (27). Ultrastructural changes include increased numbers of lysosomes, peroxisomes, and mitochondria with dilation of the smooth and the rough endoplasmic reticulum (28).

Aspirin injury is both dose- and blood concentration–dependent consistent with intrinsic toxicity (27) as seen in both animals and cell culture experiments (29,30). The major metabolites of aspirin are salicyluric and salicylphenolic glucuronide. It has been suggested that these metabolic pathways are readily saturated in children as well as adults leading to the accumulation of an otherwise minor nontoxic metabolite that may become responsible for hepatic injury (31). The exact mechanism of the cellular injury is unclear, although several possible modes of action have been postulated. These include lipid peroxidation, mitochondrial damage, hydroxyl radical scavenging, and injury to hepatocyte membranes (30,32).

Hepatic damage as indicated by elevated AST and ALT levels is seen in up to 50% of patients taking sufficient aspirin to produce serum blood levels above 15 mg/dL, although hepatic injury has been noted with levels as low as 10 mg/dL (27). This appears to be a property of the salicylate molecule, since sodium and choline salicylate also lead to elevated aminotransferase values (6,33). Susceptibility to aspirin injury is reported to be greater in patients with juvenile rheumatoid arthritis, SLE, and rheumatic fever, perhaps because of the relatively higher doses taken for these disorders (21,27,33–37). The incidence of abnormal hepatic-associated enzymes detected in these patients ranges from 20 to 70% with children under age 12 having a higher incidence compared to adults (27,36). No gender differences in susceptibility have been observed, although a possible genetic predisposition for hepatotoxicity was reported for children with juvenile rheumatoid arthritis (JRA) who have the A2BW40 haplotype (37). Hypoalbuminemia has been reported to increase the risk from decreased protein binding (38), as has chronic liver disease in general, where more salicylate is free to distribute to the tissues and injure the liver (39).

Aspirin-associated injury, in general, has not been serious and resolves promptly when the drug is stopped. Severe injury occurs in less than 3% of patients and no convincing cases of fatal necrosis have been reported (3,27), although a few instances of fatal illness associated with encephalopathy and coagulopathy in patients with JRA and SLE receiving high doses were reported prior to 1980 (27,40), and possibly may have represented early examples of Reye's syndrome (RS), as will be discussed. Several reports have suggested that chronic active hepatitis may develop as a result of acute injury (41), although these cases antedated the availability of hepatitis C testing (12). Reports of aspirin-related chronic hepatitis are lacking in the hepatitis C era.

Epidemiological studies in the 1980s demonstrated a strong association between aspirin and RS in children with influenza or varicella (chickenpox) (42–44). Adults were also affected as evidenced by several reports of older individuals developing RS after taking aspirin for a presumed viral infection (45–47). Convincing evidence for the association also comes from the striking decline in the incidence of RS in the United States that paralleled the decreased use of aspirin (48,49). In work by Pinsky and colleagues (50), an increased risk of RS was associated with an increased dose of aspirin, although doses as low as 15 mg/kg/day (the equivalent of two 325-mg tablets in a 40-kg child) were associated with a substantially increased risk. As a result, the use of aspirin continues to be strongly discouraged in acute febrile illnesses, especially in children.

The mechanism by which aspirin acts with the viral illness to produce RS is unclear. Salicylate toxicity leads to mitochondrial injury resembling that of RS both in vivo and in vitro (51), although other antipyretics, including acetaminophen (not thought to be related to RS), have the potential in animal models to exacerbate the lethal effects of a viral infection by decreasing interferon-induced antiviral responses (52). Recently, the association between aspirin and RS in children has been challenged as more likely being the result of one of several inborn errors in ammonia metabolism that were first diagnosed in the 1980s. According to Orlowski (53), 69% of patients who survived a bout of RS in Australia were subsequently diagnosed as having medium-chain aryl–coenzyme A dehydrogenase deficiency or other now well-described metabolic disorders; none of their 49 original RS patients would be diagnosed as having definite RS by today's criteria.

2. Other Salicylates

Nonacetylated salicylates also appear able to produce hepatic injury with *sodium* and *choline salicylate* resulting in elevated aminotransferase levels and jaundice in some instances (6). A rather severe but reversible hypersensitivity reaction with markedly elevated AST and ALT values accompanied the injury reported in a 66-year-old woman who took *choline magnesium trisalicylate* after just 3 days (54). *Diflunisal* (Dolobid), a difluorophenol derivative of salicylic acid, has been incriminated in cholestatic and mixed chole-static hepatocellular jaundice in a few reports (55,56). Diflunisal does not undergo metabo-lism to salicylate, which may explain the relative absence of clinical hepatic injury (57), although experimentally, diflunisal causes cytotoxicity (58). Hypersensitivity has been suggested as the mechanism (52). *Benorilate* is an acetaminophen ester of acetylsalicylic acid cited as producing hepatic injury resembling that caused by acetaminophen (paraceta-mol) toxicity, namely zone 3 (centrilobular) necrosis, rather than degeneration and mi-crovesicular steatosis more typical of aspirin-related injury (59). *Salsalate* also has been reported to cause elevated aminotransferase values, but serious injury appears unlikely (13).

B. Acetic Acid Derivatives

1. Diclofenac

Diclofenac (Voltaren, Cataflam), a benzene–acetic acid derivative, is one of the most widely prescribed NSAIDs worldwide, having been introduced in the United States more than a decade ago. There are two formulations, a delayed-released enteric-coated diclo-fenac sodium and an immediate-release potassium formulation, which will be considered together for purposes of hepatic injury. The drug has been implicated as the cause of approximately 250 cases of hepatocellular damage in published reports, with a case-fatality rate of approximately 10% (60–63). Abnormal aminotransferase values develop in 15–20% of patients taking the drug that may not progress (62). It has been estimated that there are approximately one to two cases per million prescriptions of hepatic injury due to delayed-released diclofenac (63,64), although Food and Drug Administration (FDA) data suggest an incidence that may be two to three times higher (60). Diclofenac is more likely to produce hepatic injury than are most other NSAIDs, exceeded only by sulindac (60,65), although not all cohorts have demonstrated an increased risk (66).

Diclofenac injury is predominantly hepatocellular, resembling acute viral hepatitis. In the series by Banks and colleagues (60), 79% of affected individuals were women, most of whom were aged 60 or above, and two-thirds had underlying osteoarthritis. A majority of cases (67%) were initially detected on the basis of hepatic symptoms with the remainder identified by abnormal liver-associated enzymes. Latency periods were ob-served to be 1 month in 24% of cases, with cumulative rates of injury being 63% by 3 months and 85% by 6 months. Twelve percent of individuals had taken diclofenac for 6–12 months, and only 3% for more than 12 months, prior to the onset of hepatic injury.

Hepatocellular injury was apparent in 97 of the 180 patients studied (54%), of whom 60% were jaundiced. Mixed injury was seen in 12%, indeterminate injury in 26%, and intrahepatic cholestasis in 8%. When the alkaline phosphatase was elevated greater than three times the upper limits of normal, the injury was invariably mixed or cholestatic. However, published reports of acute cholestatic hepatitis with diclofenac are less common outside of this series (67). Most patients present with jaundice, fatigue, anorexia, nausea, and vomiting. Fever, rash, and eosinophilia are uncommonly seen (60). Aminotransferase levels range from 10 to 100 times the ULN, and jaundice may be prominent. Based on the biopsy or autopsy material available for review in 21 of the FDA series cases (60), the main lesion was acute hepatic necrosis (predominantly zone 3), the severity of which often matched the marked elevations of aminotransferase levels. Other histological find-ings included granulomas in one of 21 patients and changes of chronic hepatitis in six individuals. About 50% of the 180 cases reported to the FDA and analyzed by Banks and colleagues were anicteric with only modestly elevated aminotransferase values, and occurred in mostly asymptomatic individuals with elevated enzymes found during routine biochemical testing (60). Females and patients with osteoarthritis (OA) appear to have a significantly higher risk of hepatic injury than do males or rheumatoid arthritis patients. The average age of affected individuals has been 60 years, reflecting their underlying OA (60).

Autoimmune chronic active hepatitis has been suspected in several patients reported and summarized by Scully et al. (68) and by Sallie (69) based on the presence of antinuclear or anti–smooth muscle antibodies. Histological findings in these cases ranged from periportal inflammation with mild fibrosis to panlobular hepatitis (68).

The delayed onset of injury after taking diclofenac (up to 12 months) and a late response to rechallenge (as long as 5 weeks after readministration) suggest metabolic idiosyncrasy as the likely mechanism (60). While six of 21 patients in the collected series reported by Scully et al. had features of a hypersensitivity reaction, including peripheral eosinophilia and rash, the other 15 patients had injury in keeping with a metabolic abnormality (68). None of the patients in the larger FDA series had hypersensitivity features (60). Several investigators have identified reactive metabolites of diclofenac that are concentrated in bile canaliculi, decrease cellular ATP, and are presumably responsible for experimental liver toxicity (70–74) as well as that seen in humans (75).

Recovery is usually prompt after diclofenac is withdrawn, although as with other drug-induced hepatocellular injury, massive necrosis with fulminant hepatic failure and death is a feared complication that occurred in about 8% of icteric cases in the FDA series (60). A report from Japan cites the beneficial effects of an intravenous prostaglandin E infusion in combination with intravenous prednisolone that contributed to the recovery of a 56-year-old man who developed fulminant hepatitis from diclofenac (76). A few patients have received corticosteroids for presumed diclofenac-associated autoimmune hepatitis (68), although its value is unclear in this setting.

2. Etodolac (Lodine)

This pyranocarboxylic acid derivative rarely caused hepatic injury in clinical trials. A rise in aminotransferase levels or bilirubin values greater than 1.5 times ULN was seen in only 10 of 3302 patients in doses from 50 to 600 mg daily for 6 weeks to as long as 88 months (77). However, a recent report of fatal hepatitis underscores the possibility of serious hepatic injury (78). That case involved an obese 67-year-old woman who had taken etodolac 300 mg twice daily for about 4 months before developing a 1-week prodrome of nausea, vomiting, weakness, anorexia, jaundice, and confusion, followed by liver failure. At autopsy, the liver revealed submassive bridging necrosis, early fibrosis, and microvesicular steatosis. The mechanism of the hepatocellular injury, similar to other members of this class, was presumably metabolic idiosyncrasy. Etodolac undergoes extensive enterohepatic circulation and its elimination is markedly inhibited in rats with either hepatic or renal failure producing high plasma levels (79). A false-positive test for urinary bilirubin may occur due to its phenolic metabolite (80).

3. Ketorolac (Toradol)

I am not aware of any published report of hepatic injury with this agent although the manufacturer notes that patients with impaired hepatic function or other causes of hypoalbuminemia may be at risk for hepatic toxicity, including liver failure (81). Elevated AST and ALT values may be seen in patients with preexisting liver disease and the drug should be used with caution in this setting.

4. Bromfenac

This acetic acid derivative was introduced in 1997 as a nonnarcotic analgesic of the phenyl acetate class for short-term pain relief, but was removed from the market in 1998 owing to several instances of fulminant hepatic failure leading to death or transplant that occurred after prolonged administration (14,82–84). While the drug did not appear to be hepatotoxic during limited short-term use (less than 10 days), reports of severe hepatotoxicity began to appear in patients who were treated for periods exceeding 30–90 days. In a case-series reported by Fontana and colleagues (14) a prodrome of malaise and fatigue heralded severe hepatocellular injury progressing to fulminant hepatic failure. The histological findings included massive or submassive centrizonal necrosis accompanied by a lymphocytic infiltrate. Two patients with a protracted clinical course developed nodular regeneration. Resolution of fulminant hepatic failure within 3 months using supportive measures was seen in a patient reported by Moses and colleagues (78). Others have required liver transplantation (14,83), and deaths were reported (84).

No evidence of a hypersensitivity reaction was apparent in any of the reported cases. The drug binds to plasma albumin and is extensively metabolized (85). As a result, the mechanism of injury was thought to be metabolic idiosyncrasy. The inability to identify individuals at risk from prolonged use forced its withdrawal soon after initial fulminant hepatic failure cases were reported (14).

5. Fenclozic Acid

This early derivative of the arylakanoic acid group produced mixed or cholestatic jaundice in 10% of recipients and was withdrawn in 1970 (9,86).

6. Indomethacin (Indocin)

This indole acetic acid derivative has been available in the United States since 1963. Despite its use being limited by side effects that appear in up to 50% of patients, only a few instances of jaundice have been reported (6). An analysis of adverse reactions to NSAIDs during a 9-year period in the United Kingdom showed indomethacin to be responsible for more than 1260 total reactions, of which 114 were fatal. However, only approximately 3% of all reactions and about 6% of fatalities involved the liver in that series (8).

Indomethacin has produced mainly hepatocellular necrosis (massive or central), sometimes accompanied by microvesicular steatosis and striking cholestasis (87). A high case-fatality rate (approximately 15%) was estimated by Cuthbert in 1974 (8). Although there are few reports documenting indomethacin as the cause of fatal hepatic disease, children appear more vulnerable and the drug is not recommended in the pediatric age group based on several deaths involving hepatocellular necrosis in children with JRA (88–90).

Indomethacin is converted to active metabolites, and since none appear to be intrinsically hepatotoxic, metabolic idiosyncrasy seems the most likely mechanism (15). Experimentally, indomethacin has completely prevented the mortality and hemorrhagic hepatic necrosis caused by the mushroom toxin phallidin (91) and also protects against carbon tetrachloride–mediated injury, possibly increasing mitochondrial respiration (92). Nevertheless, it is suggested that individuals with underlying liver disease avoid this agent given the high case-fatality rate (3).

7. Sulindac (Clinoril)

This indene derivative, which bears a structural similarity to indomethacin, was approved for use in the United States in 1978 after several years of study in Europe. The overall incidence of adverse side effects has been 25%, and toxicity requiring withdrawal of the drug was seen in 5–7% of patients (93–95). It is considered one of the most likely NSAIDs to produce hepatic injury (96,97). More than two dozen published case reports or case series of sulindac-associated jaundice have been published (6). Among 338 cases of suspected sulindac hepatic injury reported to the FDA, and analyzed by Tarazi and colleagues (98), 91 were considered probably or definitely related. This relatively high case number is consistent with an incidence of sulindac-associated hepatic injury that exceeds that for most other NSAIDs and is comparable to that of diclofenac (1).

In the series by Tarazi and colleagues (98), the onset of illness usually occurred within 8 weeks of starting the drug and in many cases (48%) developed in less than 4 weeks. Histological material was available for review in 15 of these 91 cases, and revealed that most were cholestatic or had mixed jaundice. However, one-quarter of cases were hepatocellular, and another 20% were indeterminate (98). Women outnumbered men by 3.5 to 1 and 69% were over age 50 with only 6% of individuals being under age 20. The biochemical features of injury mimicked the histological picture; those with cholestatic injury had an alkaline phosphatase elevated $>2\times$ ULN ranging up to 3500 mU/mL with a mean bilirubin elevation of 7 mg/dL (ranging up to 35 mg/dL). AST and ALT values were raised $3–4\times$ ULN in this group. Among those with hepatocellular injury, mean elevations in AST and ALT were $20–25\times$ ULN ranging to more than 100-fold; mean bilirubin was 5.4 mg/dL and alkaline phosphatase was normal. Since sulindac has also led to pancreatitis (99), ductal obstruction due to pancreatitis may have contributed to some of the jaundiced cases.

Hypersensitivity features were present in most patients, with fever in 55%, rash in 48%, pruritus in 40%, and eosinophilia in 35% in the series reported by Tarazi et al. (98). These percentages are nearly identical to those reported in the literature and were uniformly distributed across the histological groups, except for eosinophilia, which was absent in patients whose ALT/AST values were elevated more than eightfold (98). Rechallenge with the drug after recovery has led to recurrence of hepatic injury within several days, as was seen in nearly one-quarter of cases overall, and supports drug allergy (immunological idiosyncrasy) as the mechanism of injury (98). Further support is found in cases of Stevens-Johnson syndrome reported with sulindac (100,100a).

Most patients recover within 1–2 months after stopping the drug (98), but recovery may be delayed for as long as 7 months (101). Case fatality rates are about 5%, and deaths appear to be due to severe generalized hypersensitivity, including toxic epidermal necrolysis and renal failure, rather than to hepatic disease alone, since the most common pattern is cholestatic injury. However, there have been a few cases of fatal hepatic necrosis (98). As with aspirin, children with rheumatoid arthritis and patients with SLE may be at increased risk of sulindac injury (102,103), although in general, factors associated with increased susceptibility include older age and female gender. While the use of NSAIDs (including sulindac) is not advised in patients with cirrhosis owing to the risk of renal toxicity and hepatorenal syndrome, sulindac is a less potent inhibitor of renal eicosanoids compared to other NSAIDs, such as ibuprofen, and is reported to have renal-sparing effects (104).

8. Tolmetin (Tolectin)

This pyrrole acetic acid derivative has been in use in the United States for about a decade. A few reports have been submitted to the FDA including cases of jaundice, although the rate of hepatic injury appears to be somewhat less than for other NSAIDs (3). One published case report involved microvesicular steatosis as part of widespread multisystem organ failure in a 15-year-old girl who died having a markedly elevated tolmetin blood level (105). It has been reported that about 5% of individuals receiving tolmetin develop minor elevations in aminotransferase levels that do not progress (106).

9. Nabumetone (Relafen)

This naphthyl acetic acid derivative includes mention of mild elevations in aminotransferases in the class labeling in the package insert based on <1% risk among 1677 patients in premarketing studies. Worldwide safety experience in nearly 38,000 patients does not include any reports of liver necrosis (107).

10. Clometacin

This agent is an isomer of indomethacin and is used primarily in France. It is not available in the United States. Clometacin has been associated with a form of autoimmune hepatitis that is seen in women after a latent period of 6 months to several years (2,3,108). In a series of 30 cases reported by Islam and colleagues (109), a female predominance of 29 to 1 was seen, with an age range of 32–84 years. Acute hepatitis with centrilubular necrosis was present in 17 of 25 patients undergoing liver biopsy, and eight showed chronic active hepatitis. Anti–smooth muscle (anti-actin) and antinuclear antibodies were found in 66% and 52%, respectively, in titers ranging to 1/2560. Seventy-three percent of these patients had hypergammaglobulinemia. The syndrome seen with clometacin was noted to be similar to that produced by the laxative oxyphenisatin (110). Renal injury, rash, and eosinophilia may accompany the hepatic disease (3). In addition to acute and chronic autoimmune hepatitis, other histological forms of injury seen with clometacin include granulomatous injury, multinuclear giant cell hepatitis, cholestatic hepatitis, and cirrhosis (3,110). The acute syndrome with fulminant hepatitis has been fatal in some instances (110,111). Immunological idiosyncrasy is the presumed mechanism of injury, although intrinsic toxicity has also been suspected as the basis of injury seen in overdose settings (3).

C. Propionic Acid Derivatives

1. Ibuprofen (Motrin, Advil, and Others)

This derivative of ibufenac [a drug withdrawn from use in the 1960s because of fatal hepatocellular injury (8)] has proven to be far less hepatotoxic (3,15). In fact, the relatively few reports of hepatic injury in early United Kingdom and FDA series suggest that ibuprofen is among the least likely of the commonly used NSAIDs to produce hepatic injury (15). Figures from the 1970s also indicated that adverse reactions to ibuprofen (4% overall) rarely involved the liver (8). More recent studies suggest that ibuprofen is safer compared to aspirin and oxaprozin in arthritis patients undergoing AST monitoring (112), consistent with its safety profile amassed over a 15-year period (113).

Occasional reports of acute hepatocellular or mixed cholestatic injury have appeared with ibuprofen (114–116), including a case of overlapping susceptibility with diclofenac (60). Fever and generalized hypersensitivity accompanied the injury and supported immunological idiosyncrasy as the mechanism. The occurrence of fatal steatosis in one patient (116) indicates that the injury may be metabolically mediated (15). Indeed, reactive metabolites have been demonstrated (70). A report of acute hepatocellular injury in a patient taking a large overdose (20 g) implies some intrinsic toxicity is also possible (117) and is supported by experimental studies of the relative hepatotoxicity of ibuprofen and related agents given in high doses (118). In vitro, ibuprofen alters mitochondrial membrane permeability (119) and induces hepatocellular hypertrophy and hyperplasia through an effect on peroxisomes (120).

While most ibuprofen-associated liver toxicity has been transient in nature, a report by Alam and colleagues (121) suggests that this agent should be added to the growing list of drugs causing prolonged cholestasis as part of the vanishing bile duct syndrome (26). They describe a 29-year-old man who presented with acute right-upper-quadrant pain, nausea, vomiting, hepatosplenomegaly, and jaundice 3 weeks after taking ibuprofen daily for body aches and headaches during hyposensitization treatment for common allergens. He had no prior exposure to ibuprofen. Values for liver-associated enzymes included a peak bilirubin of 24 mg/dL, an alkaline phosphatase of nearly 4000 IU/L, and an ALT of 488 IU/L. These abnormalities persisted over the next year, with serial liver biopsies that evolved from a marked portal inflammatory process with bile duct proliferation by neutrophils and eosinophils, to one of increased cholestasis, obliteration, and eventual paucity of bile ducts. Progressive xanthomatosis and hypercholesterolemia also developed, and the syndrome defied treatment, as well as any other explanation. When the report was published, the current status of the patient was unknown.

Riley and Smith (122) recently reported a provocative case series of possible increased susceptibility to ibuprofen-induced hepatotoxicity among three patients with chronic hepatitis C infection. Sudden rises in ALT and AST values to greater than 1000 IU/L were recorded after the brief use (up to 1 week) of ibuprofen for pain. These rises were reproducible in one of these patients on rechallenge. The transaminases slowly returned to baseline 2–3 months after ibuprofen was discontinued. I am currently unaware of any other reports that corroborate this observation, although caution and hepatic enzyme monitoring have been advised in this setting.

2. Naproxen (Naprosyn, Anaprox, and Others)

Only a few cases of hepatic injury have been reported (8) for this arylacetic acid derivative, including hepatocellular jaundice, cholestatic jaundice, a case of indeterminate jaundice, and a case with fulminant hepatic failure (123–125). Cuthbert (8) reported that 4% of 179 adverse reactions involved the liver in the United Kingdom in the 1970s. The onset of overt injury has been within 1–12 weeks of starting the drug and mild elevations in serum aminotransferases have regressed during continued therapy in some instances (6). Fever in one patient and hepatic eosinophilia in another indicated possible hypersensitivity (125). While there have been too few cases to precisely identify the mechanism, no evidence of intrinsic toxicity, following accidental overdose or experimental studies, has been seen (126,127).

3. Fenoprofen (Nalfon)

This drug resembles ibuprofen in its structure and metabolism, and also rarely results in hepatic injury (128), having been incriminated in only two instances (129,130). One patient developed cholestatic jaundice while initially taking a form of naproxen (125). After it was discontinued and recovery from jaundice was complete, rechallenge with fenoprofen led to recurrence of the abnormality, implying cross-sensitivity. In the other case, jaundice occurred after 7 weeks of therapy and resolved on discontinuation (130). Injury in animals has not been observed (128). A related agent, *fenbufen*, has produced AST/ALT elevations in 25% of recipients, possibly by a hypersensitivity and/or intrinsic mechanism (131). It is not available in the United States.

4. Flurbiprofen (Ansaid)

There has been only one published report of jaundice to my knowledge, in which the injury was apparently hepatocellular, and was accompanied by symptoms of hypersensitivity (132). The onset in that case, however, was unusually delayed for hypersensitivity, occurring 3 months after the drug was started.

5. Oxaprozin (Daypro)

This agent elevates aminotransferase levels in about 15% of patients, but only 1% had values exceeding a threefold elevation. In two-thirds of patients with abnormal ALT, the values decreased or remained essentially unchanged, despite continuation of the drug (133). Overt hepatitis appears to be rare, although at least two cases of symptomatic liver injury have been reported. In one, massive necrosis was fatal (134), and in the other, recovery from acute hepatocellular jaundice occurred (135). The mechanism is unknown, but is presumed to be a toxic metabolite.

6. Ketoprofen (Orudis)

A few instances of jaundice have been reported to the manufacturer (136), but the overall incidence of injury appears quite low and I am unaware of any published reports. In contrast, *pirprofen*, an earlier phenyl propionic acid derivative, was withdrawn from use after fatal liver toxicity was reported (137). Most of the cases of severe necrosis occurred in older women who had taken the drug for 1.5–9 months. An hepatotoxic metabolite was suspected from clinical and experimental data (93,137).

7. Benoxaprofen (Oraflex)

Benoxaprofen was approved in the United States in April 1982, only to be withdrawn 4 months later after several elderly patients in the United Kingdom had died with hepatic and renal disease (3,16,138). In Britain, about 500,000 patients took the drug, and the Committee on the Safety of Medicines received about 3500 reports of adverse reactions, most involving photosensitization of the skin (139,140). Other toxicity included gastrointestinal upset, a few cases of Stevens-Johnson-type reactions, and several instances of hepatic injury (6,10,139–141). Many of the fatalities had hepatic and renal involvement. While there were no published U.S. case reports, several hundred instances of hepatic disease were submitted to the Adverse Reaction Registry of the FDA (3). Although the validity of these reports has not been firmly established, the sheer number suggests hepatic injury occurred, and its historical importance warrants the inclusion of benoxaprofen in any discussion on NSAID-induced hepatotoxicity.

Hepatic injury appeared after the drug had been taken for 1–12 months in a daily dose of 600 mg. (10,141). The first prominent symptom was jaundice, although this was sometimes preceded by anorexia, nausea, and vomiting. Several patients had abdominal pain and hematemesis. Even after the drug had been stopped, some individuals continued to deteriorate with deepening jaundice, renal failure, and coagulopathy progressing to death.

Peak bilirubin levels ranged up to 17 mg/dL, although most were below 8 mg/dL. Aminotransferase levels were modestly elevated, exceeding eight times ULN in only a few individuals. Alkaline phosphatase levels were elevated threefold or more in about half of the patients. The histological features consisted of marked cholestasis and slight to moderate necrosis. Cholestasis was particularly evident in zone 3, and both cholangioles and canaliculi showed characteristic inspissated bile casts (6,26).

The lack of hypersensitivity hallmarks and the prolonged exposure to the drug prior to the injury suggest metabolic idiosyncrasy was responsible. About 50% of the drug is converted to a glucuronide, and concentrations of the drug found in bile canaliculi may have been composed of this or other poorly soluble metabolites. Precipitation of the drug in the small bile ducts apparently led to jaundice (26).

All but one of the published fatal cases involved women, most of whom were over the age of 70. Elderly individuals metabolize the drug much more slowly than younger people, the half-life of the drug being almost four times greater in elderly patients than in those 40 years and younger (142). Prolonged metabolism may have led to higher blood levels and, ultimately, biliary excretion of larger amounts of higher concentrations of a poorly soluble product that precipitated in the bile canaliculi.

In experimental studies using isolated rat hepatocytes, marked toxicity was seen independent of the P450-mediated metabolism of benoxaprofen (143). Injury, however, did correlate with both concentration and duration of exposure in this model. Injury was also demonstrated in a cultured rat hepatocyte model, where, again, dose-related injury was seen (144). More recent investigations have found that benoxaprofen has a molecular structure similar to clofibrate and may be a substrate for CYP4 resulting in hepatic peroxisomal proliferation. The structural similarity of benoxaprofen with psoralen explains its association to phototoxicity (145,146).

The cause of death in the patients who developed benoxaprofen jaundice remains unclear. Drug-induced cholestasis is rarely associated with case fatalities (26), yet 11 of the 14 individuals with benoxaprofen-induced cholestasis died (10). The biochemical data and histological features suggested that the parenchymal liver injury was not severe enough in most of these individuals to have led to death. It has been proposed that the slower metabolism in these older individuals led to higher benoxaprofen blood and tissue levels and that it was a combination of cholestasis and, perhaps more importantly, renal failure that led to their demise. As a result, death seemed more likely due to a generalized drug toxicity and renal failure than to hepatic injury alone (12).

D. Oxicams

The first member of this class of benzothiazine derivatives to be studied, *sudoxicam*, was implicated in several cases of hepatocellular jaundice, including fatal hepatic necrosis, and was withdrawn from further clinical trials in 1977 (3).

Piroxicam (Feldene) is a carboxamide derivative used as a once-a-day treatment for rheumatoid arthritis and osteoarthritis. It has been available since 1982 and a number of instances of severe hepatic necrosis and cholestatic jaundice have been reported (15,147–150). While most of these cases have occurred in patients over age 60, a report of transient hepatic dysfunction in a 2-year-old child who ingested an inadvertent overdose has been published (151). Some of the cases were fatal from massive or submassive necrosis, and several other individuals have had prolonged cholestatic jaundice (>4 months). Hypersensitivity is suspected given the short latency period (as early as 3 days) as well as the clinical features.

In the perfused rat liver, piroxicam has an effect on energy metabolism via its action to decrease mitochondrial ATP generation (152,153). Piroxicam has a possible protective effect on ethanol-induced glutathione depletion in rats that deserves further study (154).

Meloxicam (Mobic) is an enolic acid derivative that in clinical trials has not been associated with any hepatic abnormalities to date (155).

Droxicam and *tenoxicam* are oxicams available outside of the United States that are both associated with hepatic injury, mostly cholestatic (156). Eosinophilia in some cases suggests an immunoallergic mechanism of injury similar to piroxicam. In the case of *isoxicam*, reports of toxic epidermal necrolysis in association with cholestatic injury forced its withdrawal from clinical use (157).

E. Pyrazolone Derivatives

Phenylbutazone (PBZ, Butazolidin) was introduced in 1949 in the United States for the treatment of rheumatoid arthritis and related disorders. At present, it is no longer being manufactured for human use but is still used in veterinary medicine (158). Side effects were recorded in up to 45% of recipients and serious reactions in 10–15% of patients forced its withdrawal from the market several years ago (8,12). More than 100 cases of hepatic injury were described with an incidence of overt hepatotoxicity of 1–5%, depending on the series (15,159). Most patients who developed PBZ hepatotoxicity were adults who had taken the drug for 1–6 weeks. Men and women appeared to be affected equally; most were over age 30, and one-third were older than age 60. Nearly half had hypersensitivity hallmarks such as fever, rash, and eosinophilia. Hepatocellular injury predominated in two-thirds with cholestasis in one-third of cases. Hepatic granulomas were found in 30% of those who underwent liver biopsy (159). The relatively short, fixed latent period, a prompt response to rechallenge, and the high incidence of allergic manifestations and granulomatous hepatitis suggested an immunological mechanism, although intrinsic toxicity most likely explained the injury that was seen in children receiving an overdose, as well as in some experimental models (159). The prognosis from PBZ hepatotoxicity depended on the morphological form of injury. Those with cholestatic features or granulomas usually recovered within a few weeks or months, although one case evolved into chronic cholestasis. A case-fatality rate of 25% was recorded for those with severe hepatic necrosis (15,159). In mice, hepatic and renal cell tumors developed in long-term carcinogenicity studies (160).

Oxyphenbutazone is the hydroxylated derivative of *phenylbutazone* and one of its active metabolites. It shares a similar toxicity profile with the parent compound (8,161) and is not currently marketed.

Other pyrazolone derivatives that have been developed and were chemically related to phenylbutazone, include *azapropazone* and *feprazone*. They have side effect profiles similar to the parent compound and are not currently available (6,8). *Proquazone*, a quinazolone compound designed to replace fluproquazone, a parent compound that proved too hepatotoxic for clinical use (3), is not in use in the United States, although it produced a low incidence of elevated hepatic enzyme in initial clinical trials(162).

F. Fenamates (Anthranilic Acids)

Mefenamic acid (Ponstel) has been incriminated in at least one instance of severe but nonfatal necrosis (163). A related agent, *meclofenamic acid (Meclomen)*, leads to minor

Table 4 Current Monitoring Recommendations to Prevent NSAID Hepatotoxicity Among Agents Available in the United States

Class/agent	Manufacturer's product information	Manufacturer's monitoring recommendations
Salicylates		
Aspirin	Transient elevation LAEs, hepatitis	Reye's syndrome warning (for plain, enteric coated) Increased toxicity at high doses during pediatric use.
Diflunisal (Dolobid)	CL	Potentially life-threatening hypersensitivity involving the liver
Sodium, choline salicylate	—	—
Salsalate (Disalcid, salflex)	CL	Reye's syndrome warning, periodically monitor blood levels
Acetic acid derivatives		
Diclofenac (voltaren)	CL; FFH, OLT mentioned LAEs <3× ULN in 15% >3× in 4% >8× in 1%	No change in metabolism or elimination in cirrhosis; measure AST and ALT in first 4 weeks, and periodically to 24 weeks Inform patient of warning signs of hepatotoxicity
Indomethacin	CL; FFH mentioned	D/C for signs or symptoms of liver disease
Sulindac	CL; FFH mentioned Hypersensitivity including severe skin reactions	Hypersensitivity reactions and cholestatic hepatitis may occur, monitor closely in patients with poor liver function; LFTs checked whenever a patient develops hypersensitivity features and D/C drug
Tolmetin	CL; Anaphylaxis, FFH mentioned	Discontinue for signs of livery injury, hypersensitivity.
Nabumetone	CL; FFH mentioned	Use caution in patients with severe liver impairment as metabolism may be reduced
Etodolac	CL; FFH mentioned	No change in compensated cirrhosis but decrease dose in severe hepatic failure; false-positive urine test for bilirubin due to phenolic metabolites
Ketorolac	Modified CL Hepatitis, liver failure mentioned	Clearance not affected by low albumin in cirrhosis but preexisting liver dysfunction may lead to more severe hepatic reaction; D/C if abnormal LAEs occur

Drug		Recommendation
Propionic acid derivatives		
Ibuprofen	CL; FFH mentioned	Evaluate for evidence of more severe hepatic reaction if liver injury occurs; discontinue for signs of allergy
Naproxen	CL; FFH mentioned	Use caution in cirrhosis and in patients with renal impairment. D/C if LFTs worsen
Fenoprofen	CL; FFH mentioned	Use under strict observation in patients with impaired liver function; monitor LFTs periodically during long-term therapy
Flurbiprofen	—	—
Oxaprozin	CL; may be risk of fatal hepatitis	No dose adjustment necessary in compensated liver disease; use caution in severe liver disease; D/C if abnormal LFTs worsen
Ketoprofen	CL; serious hepatic reactions, jaundice reported	No change in drug disposition in cirrhosis but carefully monitor and keep dose at a minimum since unbound biologically active fraction is doubled in hypoalbuminemia; use lower doses in patients with albumin <3.5 g/dL or hepatic impairment
Oxicams		
Piroxicam	CL; FFH mentioned	Discontinue if signs of liver injury or allergy develop
Fenamates		
Mefenamic acid	CL; FFH mentioned	Reduce dose in liver dysfunction; discontinue if signs of liver injury persist or worsen
Meclofenamic acid	—	—
Cyclooxygenase-2 inhibitors		
Celecoxib	CL	Reduced dose for moderate hepatic impairment; not recommended for use in severe hepatic disease; monitor carefully if abnormal LFTs occur
Rofecoxib	CL	Limited data in patients with hepatic impairment; monitor carefully if abnormal LFTs occur

CL, class labeling (see text); FFH, fatal fulminant hepatitis; OLT, liver transplantation; D/C, discontinue elevation of aminotransferases in fewer than 5% of recipients who regress in many instances despite continued use of the drug (164).

G. Cyclooxygenase-2-Selective Inhibitors

1. Nimesulide

This sulfonamide derivative is currently available outside of the United States as one of the new selective COX-2 inhibitors that have fewer gastrointestinal side effects. In clinical trials, nimesulide rarely produced elevations in AST or ALT values (1.6% of patients treated for greater than 3 months), as reported by McCormick and colleagues (165). However, several recent reports of acute liver injury with this agent have subsequently appeared (165–171). Van Steenbergen and colleagues (166) from Belgium described four women with centrilobular or panlobular necrosis and two men with bland intrahepatic cholestasis, where jaundice was the presenting symptom in five of six. Two individuals (one man and one woman) had eosinophilia, suggesting drug allergy, but none of the others had any hypersensitivity signs or symptoms. All abnormal values returned to normal after the drug was discontinued, but this took between 6 and 17 months. One of their patients was diagnosed with pancreatic cancer and succumbed to that illness, which was considered unrelated to the drug. Other reports of acute cholestatic hepatitis from nimesulide have appeared (171), but are less common than hepatocellular injury.

Several reports of fulminant hepatic necrosis, some fatal, have been described with nimesulide. McCormick and colleagues (165) described a middle-aged woman who developed fulminant and hepatic failure after restarting nimesulide for back pain. She developed mild to moderate increases in aminotransferase values from a normal baseline, and subsequently developed jaundice and markedly elevated aminotransferases (AST 2014, ALT 2857) at which time the drug was discontinued. Despite undergoing an emergency liver transplant, she died of primary graft nonfunction. The explanted liver revealed massive necrosis.

Weiss and colleagues (167) reported six individuals (five of whom were women) with acute hepatitis that resolved when the drug was discontinued. Most had associated fatigue, nausea, and vomiting, with median ALT values elevated 15 times the upper limits of normal. These returned to normal within 2–4 months after the drug was stopped. One patient, however, continued the drug for 2 weeks after becoming symptomatic and developed a fatal subfulminant hepatic failure including hepatorenal syndrome and died 6 weeks later. These authors recommended liver enzyme monitoring with this agent and caution to discontinue it immediately if any biochemical or clinical symptoms of hepatitis develop.

Celecoxib and *rofecoxib*, are the two newest COX-2 selective inhibitors to be approved for use in the United States. Celecoxib is a nonarylamine benzene sulfonamide derivative that has been associated with hepatic injury in only a few reports (172). Rofecoxib does not contain a sulfonamide moiety and has not been associated with liver toxicity in any published reports as of yet (173).

VI. MONITORING FOR NSAID-INDUCED HEPATIC INJURY

Although the FDA considers hepatic injury to be a class effect of NSAIDs, the agency stopped short of recommending mandatory enzyme monitoring during NSAID therapy (12). However, in the case of diclofenac, monitoring has been recommended by other authorities (174). Table 4 includes the information from monitoring statements included in manufacturers' current package inserts. While class labeling varies somewhat, it generally mentions that for any given agent, liver abnormalities are possible and may progress, may remain unchanged, or may be transient with continued therapy.

For many compounds, the labeling adds that cases of severe hepatic injury, including jaundice and even fatal fulminant hepatitis, have been reported. For these particular agents, physicians should be aware of the potential toxicity and remain alert for abnormal hepatic enzymes that persist or worsen, to clinical signs and symptoms of liver disease, or systemic manifestations such as eosinophilia, rash, or fever. For a few agents, mention is made that they should be used cautiously in individuals with underlying chronic liver disease. NSAIDs, in general, are usually best avoided in cirrhosis because of a risk of renal toxicity leading to hepatorenal syndrome, the possible exceptions being sulindac and the newer COX-2-selective agents. More intensive monitoring in patients with chronic hepatitis or cirrhosis seems prudent for NSAIDs as well as other agents, but uniform recommendations await additional study.

It is recognized that liver enzyme monitoring is controversial from a clinical, as well as a cost, standpoint. For drugs whose incidence of injury is extremely low, routine monitoring is not warranted and, if prescribed, would probably not be followed. For injury due to hypersensitivity, a rational case for no biochemical monitoring also could be made, since the drug toxicity announces itself when the hypersensitivity reaction develops. It is unlikely that monitoring would serve as a harbinger of impending hepatic injury in this setting (3).

In contrast, drugs capable of causing severe hepatic injury and that act through metabolic idiosyncrasy should be monitored on a periodic basis (6,13,175). For those agents where a greater than threefold rise in ALT from a normal baseline is seen, the specter of hepatotoxicity is raised and the monitoring frequency should be increased. If the abnormality does not subside or if it progresses, the drug should probably be stopped. In the event that clinical signs of symptoms of liver disease develop (i.e., nausea, fatigue, lethargy, pruritus, abdominal discomfort, in addition to jaundice), the drug should be discontinued immediately. If the biochemical abnormality resolves despite continuation of therapy, the NSAID can be continued.

While the performance of biochemical testing and periodic symptoms assessment and physical examinations does not guarantee the detection or prevention of NSAID- or any drug-induced hepatic injury, it is the expectation of any reasonably designed monitoring program that abnormalities detected early will prevent progression to more serious or irreversible toxicity.

REFERENCES

1. Friis H, Andreasen PB. Drug-induced hepatic injury: an analysis of 1,100 cases reported to the Danish Committee on Adverse Drug Reactions between 1978 and 1987. J Intern Med 1992; 232:133–138.
2. Koff RS. Liver disease induced by nonsteroidal anti-inflammatory drugs. In: JT Borda, RS Koff, eds. NSAIDS: A Profile of Adverse Effects. St. Louis: Mosby-Year Book, 1992:133–145.
3. Zimmerman HJ. Hepatotoxicity: The Adverse Effects of Drugs and Other Chemicals on the Liver. 2nd ed. Philadelphia: Lippincott, William & Wilkins, 1999.
4. Palmer WL, Woodall PS, Wang KC. Cinchophen and toxic necrosis of the liver, a survey of the problem. Trans Assoc Am Physicians 1936; 51:381–393.

5. Heuper WE. Cinchophen (Atophan): a critical review. Medicine 1948; 27:43.

6. Lewis JH. Hepatic toxicity of nonsteroidal anti-inflammatory drugs. Clin Pharm 1984; 3: 128–138.

7. Stricker BHC, Blok AP, Bronkhorst FB. Glafenine-associated hepatic injury: analysis of 38 cases and review of the literature. Liver 1986; 6:63–72.

8. Cuthbert MF. Adverse reactions to nonsteroidal anti-inflammatory drugs. Curr Med Res Opin 1974; 2:600–610.

9. Hart FD, Bain LS, Huskisson EC, et al. Hepatic effects of fenclozic acid. Ann Rheum Dis 1970; 29:684.

10. Taggart HM, Alderdice JM. Fatal cholestatic jaundice in elderly patients taking benoxaprofen. Br Med J (Clin Res Ed) 1982; 284:1372.

11. Lewis JH. NSAID-induced hepatotoxicity. Clin Liver Dis 1998; 2:543–561.

12. Paulus HE. FDA Arthritis Advisory Committee meeting. Arthritis Rheum 1981; 25:1124–1125.

13. Lewis JH, Zimmerman HJ. NSAID hepatotoxicity. IM Intern Med 1996; 17:45–67.

14. Fontana RJ, McCashland TM, Benner KG, et al. Acute liver failure associated with prolonged use of bromfenac leading to liver transplantation: the acute liver failure study group. Liver Transpl Surg 1999; 5:480–484.

15. Zimmerman, HJ. Update of hepatotoxicity due to classes of drugs in common clinical use: Nonsteroidal anti-inflammatory drugs, antibiotics, antihypertensives, and cardiac and psychotropic agents. Semin Liver Dis 1990; 10:322–328.

16. Carson JL, Strom BL, Duff A, et al. Safety of nonsteroidal anti-inflammatory drugs with respect to acute liver disease. Arch Intern Med 1993; 153:1331–1336.

17. Garcia Rodriguez LA, Williams R, Derby LE, et al. Acute liver injury associated with nonsteroidal anti-inflammatory drugs and the role of risk factors. Arch Intern Med 1994; 154:311–316.

18. Singh G, Ramey DR, Morfeld D, et al. Comparative toxicity of non-steroidal anti-inflammatory agents. Pharmacol Ther 1994; 62:175–191.

19. Miwa LJ, Jones JK, Pathiyal A, et al. Value of epidemiologic studies in determining the true incidence of adverse events: the nonsteroidal anti-inflammatory drug story. Arch Intern Med 1997; 157:2129–2136.

20. Mills PR, Sturrock RD. Clinical associations between arthritis and liver disease. Ann Rheum Dis 1982; 41:295–307.

21. Seaman WE, Plotz PH. Effect of aspirin on liver tests in patients with RA and SLE and in normal volunteers. Arthritis Rheum 1976; 19:155–160.

22. Weinblatt ME, Tesser JR, Gilliam JH, et al. The liver in rheumatic disease. Semin Arthritis Rheum 1982; 11:399–405.

23. Bailey M, Chapin W, Licht H, et al. The effects of vasculitis on the gastrointestinal tract and liver. Gastroenterol Clin North Am 1998; 98:747–782.

24. Runyon BA, LaBrecque DR, Anuras S. The spectrum of liver disease in systemic lupus erythematosus: Report of 33 histologically proved cases and review of the literature. Am J Med 1980; 69:187–194.

25. Lewis JH. Drug-induced liver disease. Med Clin North Am 2000; 84:1275–1311.

26. Lewis JH, Zimmerman JH. Drug- and chemical-induced cholestasis. Clin Liver Dis 1999; 3:433–464.

27. Zimmerman HJ. Effects of aspirin and acetaminophen on the liver. Arch Intern Med 1981; 141:333–342.

28. Tomoda T, Kurashige T, Hayashi Y, et al. Primary changes in liver damage by aspirin in rats. Acta Paediatr Jpn 1998; 40:593–596.

29. Janota J, Wincey CW, Sandiford M, et al. Effect of salicylate on the activity of plasma enzymes in the rabbit. Nature 1960; 185:935–936.

30. Tolman KG, Peterson P, Gray P, et al. Hepatotoxicity of salicylates in monolayer cell cultures. Gastroenterology 1978; 74:205–208.

31. Levy G, Yaffe SJ. Clinical implications of salicylate-induced liver damage. Am J Dis Child 1975; 129:1385.

32. Ingleman-Sundberg M, Kaur H, Terelius Y, et al. Hydroxylation of salicylate by microsomal fractions and cytochrome P-450: lack of production of 2,3-dihydroxybenzoate unless hydroxyl radical formation is permitted. Biochem J 1991; 276:753–757.

33. O'Gorman T, Koff RS. Salicylate hepatitis. Gastroenterology 1977; 72:726–728.

34. Athreya BH, Moser G, Cecil HS, et al. Aspirin-induced hepatotoxicity in juvenile rheumatoid arthritis: a prospective study. Arthritis Rheum 1975; 18:347–352.

35. Rich RR, Johnson JJ. Salicylate hepatotoxicity in patients with juvenile rheumatoid arthritis. Arthritis Rheum 1973; 16:1–9.

36. Bernstein BH, Singsen GH, King KK, et al. Aspirin-induced hepatotoxicity and its effect on juvenile rheumatoid arthritis. Am J Dis Child 1977; 131:659–663.

37. Bell CL, Schur PH. Juvenile rheumatoid arthritis and salicylate related liver chemistry abnormalities: clinical and genetic considerations (abstr). Arthritis Rheum 1980; 22:592.

38. Gitlin N. Salicylate hepatotoxicity: The potential role of hypoalbuminemia. J Clin Gastroenterol 1980; 2:281.

39. Okamura H, Ichikawa T., Obayashi K, et al. Studies on aspirin-induced hepatic injury. Recent Adv Gastroenterol 1967; 3:223.

40. Koff RS, Galdabini JJ. Fever, myalgias and hepatic failure in a 17 year old girl. N Engl J Med 1977; 296:1337–1346.

41. Zimmerman HJ. Drug-induced chronic liver disease. Med Clin North Am 1979; 63:567–582.

42. Soller RW, Stander H. Association between salicylates and Reye's syndrome. JAMA 1983; 249:883.

43. Starko KM, Ray CG, Dominques LB, et al. Reye's syndrome and salicylate use. Pediatrics 1980; 66:859–864.

44. Arrowsmith JB, et al. National patterns of aspirin use and Reye syndrome reporting, United States, 1980–1985. Pediatrics 1987; 79:858–863.

45. Peters LJ, Wiener GJ, Gilliam J, et al: Reye's syndrome in adults: a case report and review of the literature. Arch Intern Med 1986; 146:2401.

46. Meythaler JM, Varma RR. Reye's syndrome in adults: diagnostic considerations. Arch Intern Med 1987; 147:61–64.

47. Forsyth BW, Horwithz RI, Acampora D, et al. New epidemiologic evidence confirming that bias does not explain the aspirin/Reye's syndrome association. JAMA 1989; 261:2517–2524.

48. Remington PL, Rawley D, McGee H, et al. Decreasing trend in Reye's syndrome and aspirin use in Michigan. 1979 to 1984. 1986; 77:93–98.

49. Belay ED, Bresee JS, Holman RC, et al. Reye's syndrome in the United States from 1981 through 1997. N Engl J Med 1999; 340:1377–1382.

50. Pinsky PF, Hurwitz ES, Schonberger LB, et al. Reye's syndrome and aspirin: evidence for a dose-response effect. JAMA 1988; 260:657–661.

51. Martens ME, Change CH, Lee CP. Reye's syndrome: mitochondrial swelling and calcium release induced by Reye's plasma, allantoin, and salicylate. Arch Biochem Biophys 1986; 244:773–786.

52. Crocker JF, Digout SC, Lee SH, et al. Effects of antipyretics on mortality due to influenza B virus in a mouse model of Reye's syndrome. Clin Invest Med 1998 21:192–202.

53. Orlowski JP. Whatever happened to Reye's syndrome? Did it ever really exist? Crit Care Med 1999; 27:1582–1587.

54. Nadkarni MM, Peller CA, Retig JR. Eosinophilic hepatitis after ingestion of choline magnesium trisalicylate. Am J Gastroenterol 1992; 87:151.

55. Cook DJ, Achong MR, Murphy FR. Three cases of diflunisal hypersensitivity. Can Med Assoc J 1988; 138:1029–1030.

56. Warren NS. Diflunisal-induced cholestatic jaundice. Br Med J 1978; 2:736–737.

57. Brogden RN, Heel RC, Pakes GE, et al. Diflunisal: a review of its pharmacological properties and therapeutic use in pain and musculoskeletal strains and sprains and pain in osteoarthritis. Drugs 1980; 19:84–106.

58. Masubuchi Y, Saito H, Horie T. Structural requirements for the hepatotoxicity of nonsteroidal anti-inflammatory drugs in isolated rat hepatocytes. J Pharmacol Exp Ther 1998; 287:208–213.

59. Symon DN, Gray ES, Hanmer OJ, et al. Fatal paracetamol poisoning from benorylate therapy in child with cystic fibrosis. Lancet 1982; 2:1151–1152.

60. Banks AT, Zimmerman HJ, Ishak KG, et al. Diclofenac-associated hepatotoxicity: analysis of 180 cases reported to the Food and Drug Administration. Hepatology 1995; 22:820–827.

61. Breen EG, McNicholl J, Cosgrove E, et al. Fatal hepatitis associated with diclofenac. Gut 1986; 27:1390–1393.

62. Helfgott SM, Sanberg-Cook J, Zakim D, et al. Diclofenac-associated hepatotoxicity. JAMA 1990; 264:2660–2662.

63. Purcell P, Henry D, Melville G. Diclofenac hepatitis. Gut 1991; 32:1381–1385.

64. Ciucci AG. A review of spontaneously reported adverse drug reactions with diclofenac sodium (Voltarol). Rheumatol Rehabil 1979; 2(suppl):116–121.

65. Fry SW, Seeff LB. Hepatotoxicity of analgesics and anti-inflammatory agents. Gastroenterol Clin North Am 1995; 24:875–905.

66. Perez-Gutthann S, Garcia-Rodriguez LA, Duque-Oliart A, et al. Low-dose diclofenac, naproxen, and ibuprofen cohort study. Pharmacotherapy 1999; 19:854–859.

67. Hackstein H, Mohl W, Puschel W, et al. Diclofenac-associated acute cholestatis hepatitis. Z Gastroenterol 1998; 36:385–389.

68. Scully W, Clarke D, Barr RJ. Diclofenac induced hepatitis: three cases with features of autoimmune chronic hepatitis. Dig Dis Sci 1993; 38:744–751.

69. Sallie R. Diclofenac hepatitis (letter). J Hepatol 1990; 11:281.

70. Wade LT, Kenna JG, Caldwell J. Immunochemical identification of mouse hepatic protein adducts derived from the nonsteroidal anti-inflammatory drugs diclofenac, sulindac, and ibuprofen. Chem Res Toxicol 1997; 10:546–555.

71. Masubuchi Y, Yamada S, Horie T. Possible mechanism of hepatocyte injury induced by diphenylamine and its structurally related nonsteroidal anti-inflammatory drugs. J Pharmacol Exp Ther 2000; 292:982–987.

72. Bort R, Ponsoda X, Jover R, et al. Diclofenac toxicity to hepatocytes: a role for drug metabolism in cell toxicity. J Pharmacol Exp Ther 1999; 288:65–72.

73. Seitz S, Kretz-Rommel A, Oude Elferink RP, et al. Selective protein adduct formation of diclofenac glucuronide is critically dependent on the rat canalicular conjugate export pump (Mrp2). Chem Res Toxicol 1998; 11:513–519.

74. Miyamoto G, Zahid N, Uetrecht JP. Oxidation of diclofenac to reactive intermediates by neutrophils, myeloperoxidase, and hypochlorous acid. Chem Res Toxicol 1997; 10:414–419.

75. Bort R, Mace K, Boobis A, et al. Hepatic metabolism of diclofenac: role of human CYP in the minor oxidative pathways. Biochem Pharmacol 1999; 58:787–796.

76. Ohana M, Hajiro K, Takakuwa H, et al. Recovery from diclofenac-induced hypersensitive fulminant hepatitis and prostaglandins. Dig Dis Sci 1997; 42:2031–2032.

77. Schattenkirchner M. An updated safety profile of etodolac in several thousand patients. Eur J Rheumatol Inflamm 1990; 10:56.

78. Mabee CL, Mabee SW, Baker PB, et al. Fulminant hepatic failure associated with etodolac use. Am J Gastroenterol 1995; 90:659.

79. Ogiso T, Kitagawa T, Iwaki M, et al. Pharmacokinetic analysis of enterohepatic circulation

of etodolac and effect of hepatic and renal injury on the pharmacokinetics. Biol Pharm Bull 1997; 20:405–410.

80. Etodolac product information. Physicians' Desk Reference. 54th ed. Montvale, NJ: Medical Economics Company, 2000.

81. Ketorolac product information. Physicians' Desk Reference. 54th ed. Montvale, NJ: Medical Economics Company, 2000.

82. Moses PL, Schroeder B, Alkhatib O, et al. Severe hepatotoxicity associated with bromfenac sodium. Am J Gastroenterol 1999; 94:1393–1396.

83. Hunter EB, Johnson PE, Tanner G, et al. Bromfenac (Duract)-associated hepatic failure requiring liver transplantation. Am J Gastroenterol 1999; 94:2299–2301.

84. Rabkin JM, Smith MJ, Orloff SL, et al. Fatal fulminant hepatitis associated with bromfenac use. Ann Pharmacother 1999; 33:945–947.

85. Skjodt NM, Davies NM. Clinical pharmacokinetics and pharmacodynamics of bromfenac. Clin Pharmacokinet 1999; 36:399–408.

87. Fenech FF, Bannister WH, Grech JL. Hepatitis with biliberdinaemia in association with indomethacin therapy. Br Med J 1967; 3:155–156.

88. Jacobs JS. Sudden death in arthritic children receiving large doses of indomethacin. JAMA 1967; 199:93.

89. Kelsey WM, Scharyi M. Fatal hepatitis probably due to indomethacin. JAMA 1967; 199: 154–155.

90. Boardman PL, Hart FD. Side-effects of indomethacin. Ann Rheum Dis 1967; 26:127–132.

91. Barriault C, Audet M, Yousef IM, et al. Protection of indomethacin against the lethality and hepatotoxicity of phalloidin in mice. Toxicol Lett 1994; 71:257–269.

92. Makogon NV, Lushnikova IV, Korneitchuk AN, et al. Effects of noridhydroguaiaretic acid and indomethacin on the viability and functional activities of normal and carbon tetrachloride-injured rat hepatocytes cultured alone and with Kupffer cells. Acta Physiol Pharmacol Bulg 1998; 23:33–38.

93. Smith FE, Lindberg PJ. Life-threatening hypersensitivity to sulindac. JAMA 1980; 244: 269.

94. Brogden RN, Heel RC, Speight TM, et al. Sulindac: a review of its pharmacological properties and therapeutic efficacy in rheumatic diseases. Drugs 1978; 16:97–114.

95. Park GD, Spector R, Headstream T, et al. Serious adverse reactions associated with sulindac. Arch Intern Med 1982; 142:1292–1294.

96. Garcia Rodriguez LA, Perez-Gutthann S, Walker AM, et al. The role of nonsteroidal antiinflammatory drugs in acute liver injury. Br Med J 1992; 305:865–868.

97. Kromann-Anderson H, Pedersen A. Reported adverse reactions and consumption of nonsteroidal anti-inflammatory drugs in Denmark over a 17-year period. Danish Med Bull 1988; 35:187–192.

98. Tarazi EM, Harter JG, Zimmerman HJ, et al. Sulindac-associated hepatic injury: Analysis of 91 cases reported to the Food and Drug Administration. Gastroenterology 1992; 104:569–574.

99. Lerche A, Vyberg M, Kirkegaard E. Acute cholangitis and pancreatitis associated with sulindac (Clinoril). Histopathology 1987; 11:647.

100. Levitt L, Pearson RW. Sulindac-induced Stevens-Johnson toxic epidermal neurolysis syndrome. JAMA 1980; 243:1262.

100a. Maquire FW. Stevens-Johnson syndrome due to sulindac: a case report and review of the literature. Del Med 1981; 53:193–197.

101. Whittaker SJ, Amar JN, Wanless IR, et al. Sulindac hepatotoxicity. Gut 1982; 23:875–877.

102. Calabro J, Marchesano J, Partirdge R, et al. Sulindac in juvenile rheumatoid arthritis. Clin Pharmacol Ther 1979; 25:216.

103. Park GD, Spector R, Headstream T, et al. Serious adverse reactions associated with sulindac. Arch Intern Med 1982; 142:1292–1294.

104. Laffi G, Daskalopoulos G, Kronborg I, et al. Effects of sulindac and ibuprofen in patients with cirrhosis and ascites: an explanation for the renal-sparing effect of sulindac. Gastroenterology 1986; 90:182–187.

105. Shaw GR, Anderson WR. Multisystem failure and hepatic microvesicular fatty metamorphosis associated with tolmetin ingestion. Arch Pathol Lab Med 1991; 115:818–821.

106. O'Brien WM. Long-term efficacy and safety of tolmetin sodium in treatment of geriatric patients with rheumatoid arthritis and osteoarthritis: a retrospective study. J Clin Pharmacol 1983; 23:309–323.

107. Bernhard GC. Worldwide safety experience with nabumetone. J Rheumatol 1992; 19(suppl): 48–57.

108. Pessayre D, Degos F, Feldmann G, et al. Chronic active hepatitis and giant multinucleated hepatocytes in adults treated with clometacin. Digestion 1982; 22:66–72.

109. Islam S, Mekhloufi F, Paul JM, et al. Characteristics of clometacin-induced hepatitis with special reference to the presence of anti-actin cable antibodies. Autoimmunity 1989; 2:213–221.

110. Tordjmann T, Grimbert S, Genestie C, et al. Adult multi-nuclear cell hepatitis: a study of 17 patients. Gastroenterol Clin Biol 1998; 22:305–310.

111. Poitrine A, Poynard T, Naveau S, et al. A new fatal case of hepatitis caused by clometacin. Gastroenterol Clin Biol 1983;7:99.

112. Freeland GR, Northington RS, Hedrich DA, et al. Hepatic safety of two analgesics used over the counter: ibuprofen and aspirin. Clin Pharmacol Ther 1988; 43:473–479.

113. Royer GL, Seckman CE, Welshman IR. Safety profile: fifteen years of clinical experience with ibuprofen. Am J Med 1984; 77:25–34.

114. Sternlieb P, Robinson RM. Stevens-Johnson syndrome plus toxic hepatitis due to ibuprofen. NY State J Med 1978; 78:1239–1243.

115. Stempel DA, Miller JJ III. Lymphopenia and hepatic toxicity with ibuprofen. J Pediatr 1977; 90:657–658.

116. Bravo JF, Jacobson MP, Mertens BF. Fatty liver and pleural effusion with ibuprofen therapy. Ann Intern Med 1977; 87:200–201.

117. Lee CY, Finkler A. Acute intoxication due to ibuprofen overdose. Arch Pathol Lab Med 1986; 110:747–749.

118. Castell JV, Larrauri A, Gomez-Lechon MJ. A study of the relative hepatotoxicity in vitro of the non-steroid anti-inflammatory drugs ibuprofen, flurbiprofen and butibufen. Xenobiotica 1988; 18:737–745.

119. Al-Nasser IA. Ibuprofen-induced liver mitochondrial permeability. Toxicol Lett 2000; 111: 213–218.

120. Bendele AM, Hulman JF, White S, et al. Hepatocellular proliferation in ibuprofen-treated mice. Toxicol Pathol 1993; 21:15–20.

121. Alam I, Ferrell LD, Bass NM. Vanishing bile duct syndrome temporally associated with ibuprofen use. Am J Gastroenterol 1996; 91:1626–1630.

122. Riley TR III, Smith JP. Ibuprofen-induced hepatotoxicity in patients with chronic hepatitis C: a case series. Am J Gastroenterol 1998; 93:1563–1565.

123. Bass BG. Jaundice associated with naproxen (letter). Lancet 1974; 1:998.

124. Giarelli L, Falconieri G, Delender M. Fulminant hepatitis following naproxen administration. Hum Pathol 1986; 17:1079.

125. Law JP, Knight H. Jaundice associated with naproxen. N Engl J Med 1976; 295:1201.

126. Fredell EW, Strand LJ. Naproxen overdose (letter). JAMA 1997; 238:938.

127. Brogden RN, Heel RC, Speight TM, et al. Naproxen up to date: a review of its pharmacological properties and therapeutic efficacy and use in rheumatic diseases and pain states. Drugs 1979; 18:241–277.

128. Brogden RN, Pinder RM, Speight TM, et al. Fenoprofen: a review of its pharmacological properties and therapeutic efficacy in rheumatic diseases. Drugs 1977; 13:241–265.

129. Andrejak M, Davion T, Gineston JL, et al. Cross hepatotoxicity between nonsteroidal anti-inflammatory drugs. Br Med J 1987; 295:180.

130. Stennett DJ, Simonson W, Hall CA. Fenoprofen-induced hepatotoxicity (letter). Am J Hosp Pharm 1978; 35:901.

131. Brogden RN, Heel RC, Speight TM, et al. Fenbufen: A review of its pharmacological properties and therapeutic use rheumatic disease and acute pain. Drugs 1981; 21:1–22.

132. Kotowski KE, Grayson MF. Side effects of non-steroidal anti-inflammatory drugs. Br Med J 1982; 285:377.

133. Zimmerman HJ. Hepatic effects of oxaprozin. Semin Arthritis Rheum 1986; 15:35–42.

134. Purdum PE, Shelden SL, Boyd JW, et al. Oxaprozin-induced fulminant hepatitis. Ann Pharmacother 1994; 28:1159.

135. Kethu SR, Rukkannagari S, Lansford CL. Oxaprozin-induced symptomatic hepatotoxicity. Ann Pharmacother 1999; 33:942–944.

136. Ketoprofen product information. Physicians' Desk Reference, 54th ed. Montvale, NJ: Medical Economics Company, 2000.

137. Depla ACTM, Vermeersch PHMJ, Gorp LHM, et al. Fatal acute liver failure associated with pirprofen. Report of a case and a review of the literature. Neth J Med 1990; 37:32.

138. Anonymous. Arthritis drug withdrawn. FDA Consum Bull 1982; 16:4.

139. Halsey J, Cardoe N. Benoxaprofen: Side effect profile in 300 patients. Br Med J (Clin Res Ed) 1982; 284:1385–1388.

140. Prescott LE, Leslie PJ, Padfield P. Side effects of benoxaprofen. Br Med J 1982; 284:1782.

141. Goudie BM, Birnie GF, Watkinson G, et al. Jaundice associated with the use of benoxaprofen. Lancet 1982; 1:959.

142. Hamdy RC, Murnang B, Pereran, et al. The pharmacokinetics of benoxaprofen in elderly subjects. Eur J Rheumatol Inflamm 1982; 5:69.

143. Knights KM, Cassidy MR, Drew R. Benoxaprofen induced toxicity in isolated rat hepatocytes. Toxicology 1986; 40:327–339.

144. Sorensen EM. Morphometric analysis of cultured hepatocytes exposed to benoxaprofen. Toxicol Lett 1986; 34:277–286.

145. Lewis DF, Ioannides C, Parke DV. A retrospective study of the molecular toxicology of benoxaprofen. Toxicology 1990; 65:33–47.

146. Ayrton AD, Ioannides C, Parke DV. Induction of the cytochrome P450 I and IV families and peroxisomal proliferation in the liver of rats treated with benoxaprofen. Possible implication in its hepatotoxicity. Biochem Pharmacol 1991; 42:109–115.

147. Lee SM, O'Brien CJ, Williams R., et al. Subacute hepatic necrosis induced by piroxicam. Br Med J 1986; 293:540–541.

148. Paterson D, Kerlin P, Walker N, et al. Piroxicam induced submassive necrosis of the liver. Gut 1992; 33:1436–1438.

149. Planas R, De Leon R, Quer JC, et al. Fatal submassive necrosis of the liver associated with piroxicam. Am J Gastroenterol 1990; 85:468–470.

150. Hepps KS, Maliha GM, Estrada R, et al. Severe cholestatic jaundice associated with piroxicam. Gastroenterology 1991; 101:1737–1740.

151. MacDougall LG, Taylor-Smith A, Rothberg AD, et al. Piroxicam poisoning in a 2-year-old child: a case report. S Afr Med J 1984; 66:31–33.

152. Salgueiro-Pagadigorria CL, Kelmer-Bracht AM, et al. Effects of nonsteroidal anti-inflammatory drug piroxicam on rat liver mitochondria. Comp Biochem Physiol C Pharmacol Toxicol Endocrinol 1996; 113:85–91.

153. Salgueiro-Pagadigorria CL, Constantin J, Bracht A, et al. Effects of nonsteroidal anti-inflammatory drug piroxicam on energy metabolism in the perfused rat liver. Comp Biochem Physiol C Pharmacol Toxicol Endocrinol 1996; 113:93–98.

154. Zentella de Pina M, Corona S, Rocha-Hernandez AE, et al. Restoration by prioxicam of liver glutathione levels decreased by acute ethanol intoxication. Life Sci 1994; 54:1433–1439.

155. Yocum D, Fleishmann R, Dalgin P, et al. Safety and efficacy of meloxicam in the treatment of osteoarthritis. Arch Intern Med 2000; 160:2947–2954.

156. Garcia Gonzalez M, Sanroman AL, Herrero C, et al. Hepatitis por droxicam. Descripcion de tres neuvos casos y revision de la leteratura. Rev. Clinca Espan 1994:170.

157. Ollagnon HO, Perpoint B, Decousus H, et al. Hepatitis induced by isoxicam. Hepatogastroenterology 1986; 33:109.

158. Carpenter SL, McDonnell WM. Misuse of veterinary phenylbutazone. Arch Intern Med 1995; 155:1229.

159. Benjamin SB, Ishak KG, Zimmerman HJ, et al. Phenylbutazone liver injury: A clinical pathologic survey of 23 cases and review of the literature. Hepatology 1981; 1:255–263.

160. Kari F, Bucher J, Haseman J, et al. Long-term exposure to the anti-inflammatory agent phenylbutazone induces kidney tumors in rats and liver tumors in mice. Jpn J Cancer Res 1995; 86:252–263.

161. Popper H, Rubin E, Gardio D, et al. Drug-induced liver disease: a penalty for progress. Arch Intern Med 1965; 115:128–136.

162. Gubler HU, Baggiolini M. Pharmacological properties of proquazone. Scand J Rheumatol 1978; 21(suppl):8–11.

163. Imoto S, Matzumoto H, Fujii M. Drug-related hepatitis (letter). Ann Intern Med 1979; 91: 129.

164. Preston SN. Safety of sodium meclofenamate (meclomen). Curr Ther Res 1978; 23(suppl): 5107–5112.

165. McCormick PA, Kennedy F, Curry M, et al. COX 2 inhibitor and fulminant hepatic failure. Lancet 1999; 353:40–41.

166. Van Steenbergen W, Peeters P, De Bondt J, et al. Nimesulide-induced acute hepatitis: evidence from six cases. J Hepatol 1998; 29:135–141.

167. Weiss P, Mouallem M, Bruck R, et al. Nimesulide-induced hepatitis and acute liver failure. Isr Med Assoc J 1999; 1:89–91.

168. Villa G. NSAIDs and hepatic reactions (letter). Lancet 1999; 353:846.

169. Rainsford KD. An analysis from clinico-epidemiological data of the principal adverse events from the COX-2 selective NSAID, nimesulide, with particular reference to hepatic injury. Inflammopharmacology 1998; 6:203–221.

170. Andrade RJ, Lucena MI, Fernandez MC, et al. Fatal hepatitis associated with nimesulide. J Jepatol 2000; 32:174.

171. Romero-Gomez M, Nevado Santos M, Otero Fernandez MA, et al. Acute cholestatic hepatitis by nimesulide. Liver 1999; 19:164–165.

172. Carrillo-Jimenez R, Nurnberger M. Celecoxib-induced acute pancreatitis and hepatitis: a case report. Arch Intern Med 2000; 160:553–554.

173. Fung HB, Kirschenbaum HL. Selective cyclooxygenase-2 inhibitors for the treatment of arthritis. Clin Ther 1999; 21:1131–1157.

174. Simon LS. Toxicity of the nonsteroidal anti-inflammatory drugs. Curr Opin Rheumatol 1991; 3:341.

175. Schiff ER. Can we prevent nonsteroidal anti-inflammatory drug-induced hepatic failure? Gastrointest Dis Today 1994; 3:768–770.

17

Mechanism, Pathology, and Clinical Presentation of Hepatotoxicity of Anesthetic Agents

J. GERALD KENNA

AstraZeneca Safety Assessment, Cheshire, England

I. INTRODUCTION

The advent of modern anesthesia occurred in the 1840s, when the clinical value of ether and chloroform was first described. These were the most popular anesthetic agents throughout the remainder of the nineteenth century and the first part of the twentieth century, even though they had significant practical disadvantages (1). Ether is highly combustible, irritates the respiratory tract, and has appreciable solubility in blood, which results in a slow onset of action and slow recovery. Chloroform is a cardiorespiratory depressant, has arrhythmogenic effects, and is both nephrotoxic and hepatotoxic. The organ toxicity of chloroform has been ascribed to bioactivation in liver and kidneys to reactive species that interact with macromolecules and cause cellular necrosis (2).

To circumvent these and other adverse effects, a range of alternative volatile agents were developed throughout the twentieth century. Halothane was introduced in the late 1950s and was shown to be potent, relatively fast-acting, nonirritant, and easy to use. However, cases of severe postoperative liver injury in patients exposed to halo-thane soon appeared in the medical literature and it is now well established that a small, but significant, proportion of the population (including certain medical personnel who undergo occupational exposure) are susceptible to "halothane hepatitis." Usage of halothane has declined markedly since the 1970s and a series of alternative agents (enflurane then isoflurane, followed more recently by sevoflurane and desflurane) have been introduced that have markedly reduced hepatotoxic potential. The purpose of this chapter is to review the clinical features of liver damage caused by halothane and the recent generation of volatile anesthetics, to evaluate the data obtained to date on un-derlying biochemical and cellular mechanisms, and to discuss individual susceptibility factors.

II. CLINICAL FEATURES OF VOLATILE ANESTHETIC-INDUCED HEPATOTOXICITY

A. Halothane

The clinical features and pathology of liver injury caused by halothane are now well documented and have been reviewed extensively (1,3–5). Typically, patients have no his-tory of preexisting liver disease, do not abuse alcohol, and have no concurrent intake of drugs with known hepatotoxic potential. The incidence of this adverse reaction is not known precisely but is low (between 1 in several thousand and 1 in 30,000 patients). This led to considerable debate over many years concerning whether halothane was the true causative agent, or patients with liver injury due to other causes (e.g., acute viral infection) were being misdiagnosed. Attempts to resolve the controversy by undertaking large retro-spective and prospective studies were inconclusive (6) and the matter was only resolved when diagnostic antibody tests were described (see below).

A substantial proportion of patients who sustain halothane hepatitis are frequently female and of late middle age, and obesity is common. Nevertheless, many cases of halo-thane hepatitis in nonobese males have been described (1,3–5), as have several well-documented cases in young children (7). Liver damage that can be attributed to occupa-tional halothane exposure has also been reported in medical personnel (8). The first symptoms displayed by patients frequently include malaise, anorexia, and nonspecific gastrointestinal symptoms (nausea and upper-abdominal discomfort). The majority of patients exhibit delayed-onset pyrexia, while some develop nonspecific rash and/or arthral-gia (3,9,10). These symptoms are followed by large elevations in serum transaminases and then by jaundice. The time to onset of jaundice is very variable, and may be greater than 28 days (11). In some patients the liver damage is severe and fulminant hepatic failure develops, which may require liver transplantation. However, many patients with halothane hepatitis do not sustain liver failure (11). Nonfatal cases have been reported to resolve progressively and uneventfully and not to be associated with development of chronic liver disease, provided further exposure to halothane (and to structurally related compounds, as discussed below) is avoided.

Investigations of liver pathology have shown that centrilobular hepatic necrosis is a common histological feature (1,9,12). A spectrum of severity ranging from panlob-ular and multifocal necrosis to massive necrosis has been observed, as has ballooning degeneration of hepatocytes, inflammatory infiltration, and fibrosis. Fatty infiltration has been reported in many patients, and in some cases granulomatous aggregates have also been observed (12). Mitochondrial membrane abnormalities have been identified by electron microscopy in some instances (9,13), but not in others (14). Overall, the pathological features of halothane hepatitis are not diagnostic and are similar to those described in cases of acute hepatitis due to acute viral infection and to various other drugs.

The vast majority of patients who develop halothane hepatitis have been anesthetized with halothane on multiple occasions. Halothane hepatitis has been described in cases where the interval between anesthetic exposure has been many years (11,15). However, retrospective analyses have indicated that the severity of liver injury and the interval from final anesthesia to onset of jaundice tend to be inversely related to the interval between anesthetics (3,11). A significant proportion of patients who sustain halothane hepatitis have exhibited adverse reactions (delayed-onset pyrexia or jaundice) following previous halothane exposure (3,11,16,17). Consequently it is important to take a careful clinical history before exposing patients to halothane. Halothane hepatitis is characterized by a high incidence of peripheral eosinophilia, circulating autoantibodies to tissue antigens, and cellular and humoral immune sensitization to reactive metabolite-modified liver neo-antigens (3–5,17). In view of this, it has been proposed that the disease process has a major immune component, which is discussed in detail below.

A much milder, and clinically unimportant, form of halothane-induced liver injury in humans has also been described. This was identified in prospective studies, which revealed that up to 30% of patients who underwent surgical anesthesia with halothane developed mild liver injury that resolved asymptomatically (18,19). Serological investigations revealed no evidence of immune activation in these patients, including no detectable antibodies to metabolite-modified liver neoantigens (20,21). It has been concluded that this mild form of liver injury does not have an immune component.

B. Other Volatile Agents (Enflurane, Isoflurane, Desflurane, and Sevoflurane)

A retrospective review of 24 cases of otherwise-unexplained liver damage in patients anesthetized with enflurane has indicated that, in common with halothane, this agent can cause severe liver damage in humans (22). The incidence of enflurane-induced liver injury is very low, and of the order of 1 in 800,000 exposed patients (23). The clinical, biochemical, and pathological features of patients with enflurane hepatitis are similar to those described for halothane hepatitis, including a delayed interval between anesthesia and onset of jaundice, frequently a previous history of exposure to enflurane of halothane, and a significant incidence of mortality due to liver failure (22). In addition, an association between prior exposure of certain patients to halothane and subsequent liver injury following anesthesia with enflurane has been reported (22,24,25). This can be attributed to immune cross-sensitization between the anesthetics (see below).

Numerous cases of liver injury that may be attributable to anesthesia with isoflurane have also been described (26–29), although the number reported to date is small when one considers the widespread worldwide use of this agent since its introduction in 1984. It is reasonable to conclude that the incidence of hepatitis due to isoflurane is far lower than the incidence of halothane hepatitis. Although causality has been difficult to establish, at least some cases of possible isoflurane hepatitis exhibit clinical and pathological features that are consistent with a "halothane hepatitis–like" mechanism. These are an association with multiple exposures to volatile anesthetics, a preponderance of females, obesity, and severe centrilobular hepatocellular injury (30). Detection of antibodies to metabolite-modified protein neoantigens has been described in two cases (31,32), which is consistent with an immune pathogenesis.

A single case of postoperative liver injury in a patient exposed to desflurane has been described (33). Antibodies that recognized metabolite-modified liver neoantigens were detected in the patient's serum and it was noted that the patient had a prior history of anesthesia with halothane (albeit 12 and 18 years previously). By analogy with halothane hepatitis, the proposed mechanism of liver injury was immunological.

Sevoflurane was introduced into anesthetic practice relatively recently in the Western world (in 1995), but prior to this was used widely as a surgical anesthetic for over 10 years in Japan. Cases of liver injury in patients anesthetized with sevoflurane have been described in the Japanese literature (34–36). However, it is unclear whether these can be attributed to the anesthetic agent (see below).

III. METABOLISM OF VOLATILE ANESTHETICS

A. Halothane

About 20% of an inhaled dose of halothane is metabolized in humans (37). This process is catalyzed by isozymes of hepatic cytochrome P450 and proceeds via distinct oxidative and reductive pathways that have been reviewed elsewhere (38) and are summarized in simplified form in Fig. 1. The reductive pathway is favored at reduced oxygen tensions but occurs only to a limited extent at normal oxygen tensions (i.e., during surgical anesthesia in humans) (39). The initial step in this pathway is insertion of a single electron to form the trifluorochlorobromoethyl radical, which undergoes a well-defined further series of chemical reactions and biotransformations to other chemically reactive species. These initiate lipid peroxidation, bind covalently to cellular macromolecules (both lipids and proteins), and/or are excreted as urinary and volatile metabolites. Oxidative metabolism is the major pathway of metabolism in humans (39). This proceeds via insertion of oxygen, which is followed by spontaneous debromination to produce a reactive species (trifluoroacetyl chloride) that reacts with water to form the major urinary metabolite trifluoroacetate (39). In addition, a small fraction of trifluoroacetyl chloride binds covalently to ε-amino groups of cellular phospholipids (i.e., phosphatidylethanolamine) and proteins (40–42), thereby generating trifluoroacetylated lipid and protein adducts (Fig. 1).

Several different cytochrome P450 isozymes have been shown to catalyze reductive and oxidative metabolism of halothane (43). However, oxidative metabolism is catalyzed preferentially by CYP 2E1 and this is the major isozyme responsible for bioactivation of halothane in humans (44,45).

B. Other Volatile Agents

In common with halothane, enflurane and isoflurane are metabolized by hepatic CYP 2E1 via oxidative dehalogenation (46,47). However, these compounds do not undergo reductive metabolism. The extent of metabolism in humans is 2–4% for enflurane (48) and about 0.2% for isoflurane (49), which is markedly lower than the extent of metabolism

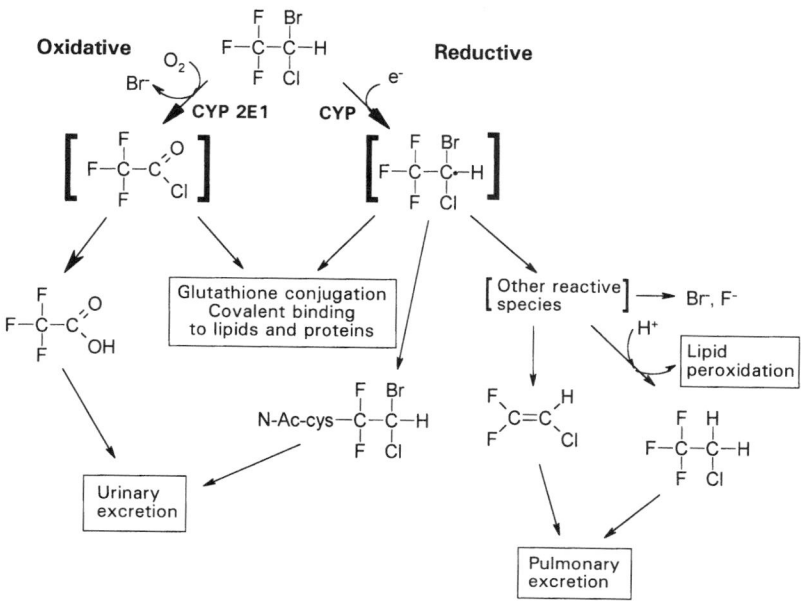

Figure 1   Metabolism of halothane. CYP, cytochrome P450; UGT.

of halothane (50). Metabolism of enflurane proceeds via a reactive intermediate that either reacts with water to form an acid that is excreted in urine as a glucuronide conjugate (51) or binds covalently to liver proteins to form protein adducts (52) (see Fig. 2). CYP 2E1-mediated oxidation of isoflurane results in renal excretion of inorganic fluoride and trifluoroacetic acid (53) and proceeds via reactive intermediates (believed to include trifluoroacetyl chloride) that covalently modify liver proteins and form protein adducts (52) (Fig. 2).

Desflurane is extremely resistant to biodegradation and the extent of metabolism in humans is no more than 10% of that described for isoflurane (i.e., less than 0.02%) (54). Trifluoroacetic acid has been identified as a urinary metabolite (54), which implies that metabolism of desflurane proceeds via pathways similar to those proposed for isoflurane and involves formation of protein adducts (33) (Fig. 2).

The rate of metabolism of sevoflurane by hepatic cytochromes P450 is markedly greater in vitro when compared with the other anesthetics described above (including halothane) (55) but is limited in vivo owing to its low blood and tissue solubility. Consequently, about 2–5% of an anesthetic dose of sevoflurane is metabolized in humans (56,57). In common with halothane, enflurane, isoflurane, and desflurane, the process is catalyzed in vivo by CYP 2E1 (57). The first step is oxidation of the fluoromethyl group (Fig. 3), which may involve generation of formyl fluoride. Since formyl fluoride is a highly reactive species, this is a possible mechanism of generation of novel liver protein adducts derived from sevoflurane. However, whether such adducts are actually produced in livers

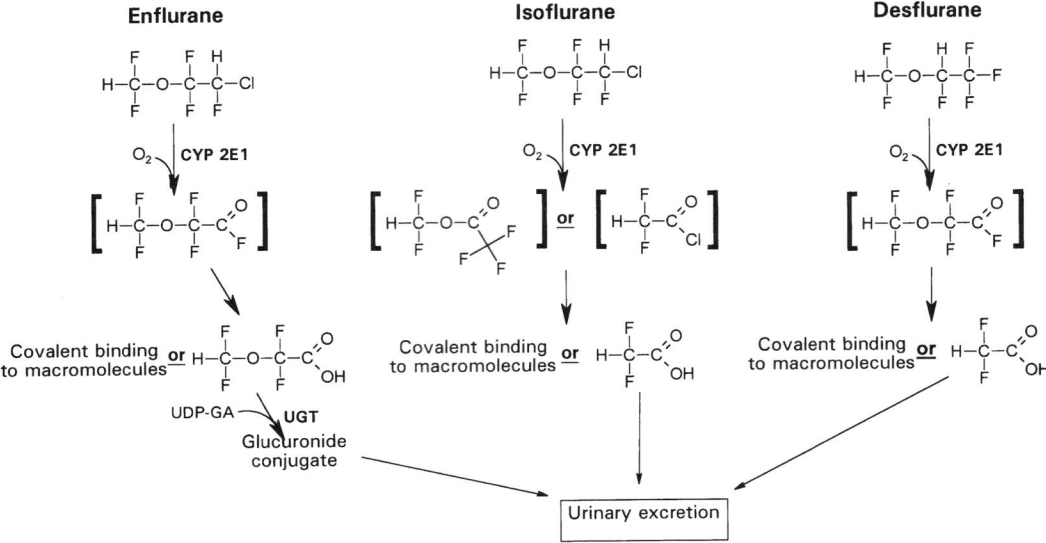

Figure 2 Metabolic bioactivation of enflurane, isoflurane, and desflurane (UGT = UDP-glucuronyltransferase).

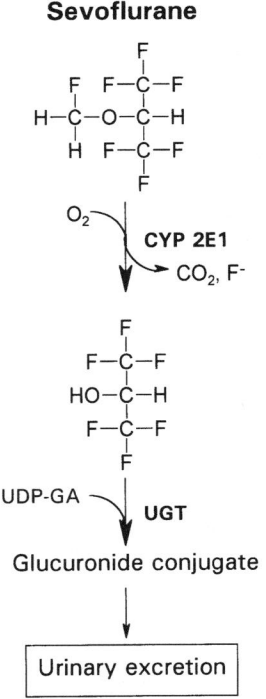

Figure 3 Metabolism of sevoflurane.

of sevoflurane-exposed animals or humans is unknown. Metabolism of sevoflurane results in liberation of inorganic fluoride and carbon dioxide and in formation of hexafluoroiso-propanol, which is excreted in urine as a glucuronide conjugate (57) (Fig. 3).

IV. ANIMAL MODELS OF ANESTHETIC-INDUCED LIVER INJURY

A. Halothane

Reproducible and dose-dependent hepatotoxicity has been produced by pretreatment of rats with polychlorinated biphenyls or with phenobarbitone to induce cytochromes P450, then exposure of the animals to halothane at reduced oxygen tensions to promote reductive metabolism (58–60). The liver injury produced in these models has been attributed to a combination of direct toxic effects of reductive reactive metabolites (which promote lipid peroxidation and bind covalently to hepatocellular lipids and proteins) plus ischemic injury caused by tissue hypoxia (61,62).

Liver toxicity that has been attributed to hypoxia alone has been observed in rats exposed to halothane at normal oxygen tensions, following pretreatment with triiodothyro-nine (63). In addition, two animal models have been described that involve hepatotoxicity mediated via oxidative metabolites of halothane. In the first of these models Fischer 344 rats were exposed to halothane at normal oxygen tensions following pretreatment with isoniazid, which is a potent CYP 2E1 inducer that increased oxidative metabolism of the anesthetic (64). In the second model, hepatotoxicity was produced in guinea pigs by expo-sure to halothane at normal oxygen tensions (65,66). Marked strain- and sex-dependent differences in susceptibility to halothane-induced liver injury were observed in the guinea pig model. These were not attributable to differences in oxidative metabolism of halothane, but could be a consequence of variable effects of halothane on hepatic blood flow (67) and/or due to variability in hepatic thiol status (which will affect capacity to detoxify electrophilic reactive intermediates, as illustrated in Fig. 1) (68).

Although the various animal model studies have demonstrated that both oxidative and reductive pathways of metabolism of halothane may mediate hepatotoxicity, the mechanisms underlying tissue injury remain largely undefined. Alteration in hepatic lipid peroxidation has been observed in the reductive rat models (69) and altered calcium homeostasis has been proposed to play a role in liver toxicity in the rat (70) and the guinea pig (71). It is notable that none of the models require multiple exposures to halothane, all are reproducible and dose-dependent, and none are characterized by the selective immune stimulation that is characteristic of halothane hepatitis in humans. Consequently, it is con-sidered that these models are not directly relevant to halothane hepatitis in humans. One or more of the models could explain why up to 30% of halothane-exposed patients sustain very mild and transient liver injury, however (38,62).

B. Other Volatile Agents

Hepatocellular liver injury has been produced by pretreatment of rats with triiodothyro-nine, then anesthesia with enflurane, isoflurane, or halothane (63). In addition, exposure of phenobarbitone-pretreated rats to halothane, enflurane, or isoflurane under markedly hypoxic conditions has been reported to result in liver damage (72–74). The toxicity ob-served in these studies has been attributed to ischemic liver damage caused by tissue hypoxia and not to specific toxic effects of the anesthetics themselves. This is because similar extents of liver injury were observed when rats that had been pretreated with phenobarbital were anesthetized intravenously with thiopental or fentanyl under hypoxic conditions, in place of the volatile agent (74). When rats were pretreated with phenobarbital and then anesthetized with halothane, enflurane, or isoflurane under mildly hypoxic conditions, liver injury was observed only in the group of rats that had received halothane (73). It was concluded that enflurane and isoflurane have minimal intrinsic hepatotoxic potential when compared with halothane. Hepatotoxicity has not been observed in the animal investigations undertaken to date with desflurane or sevoflurane.

V. THE IMMUNE HYPOTHESIS OF ANESTHETIC-INDUCED LIVER INJURY

A. Halothane

Immune responses to halothane metabolite–modified liver neoantigens in patients with halothane hepatitis was described initially by Vergani and co-workers. Specific cellular sensitization to such antigens in patients with halothane hepatitis, but not control individuals, was observed using the technique of in vitro leukocyte migration (75). In addition, antibody-dependent cytotoxic killing of hepatocytes from halothane-treated rabbits was demonstrated following incubation of the hepatocytes with sera from patients with halothane hepatitis (which had been adsorbed to deplete antibodies to normal liver antigens) and normal human leukocytes (76). The hepatocyte toxicity was not observed when experiments were undertaken using control hepatocytes, or hepatocytes from rabbits that had been anesthetized with ether, or when hepatocytes from halothane-treated rabbits were incubated with sera from various groups of control individuals (including anesthetists, patients exposed to halothane who did not sustain liver injury, patients with various other types of liver disease, and normal controls) (76,77). It was concluded that the cytotoxicity was mediated by antibodies in sera from patients with halothane hepatitis, that the antibody response to the antigens was specific to the patients, and that the target antigens were halothane-modified macromolecules expressed on the surface of hepatocytes (76).

Subsequent investigations, which have used a variety of other methods to detect the antibodies (including enzyme-linked immunosorbent assay and immunoblotting), have confirmed these findings and have shown that antibodies to halothane-induced neoantigens are predominantly of IgG class (78,79). The specificity of the immune response indicates that it is not simply a secondary consequence of halothane exposure and/or liver damage, while the finding of IgG-class antibodies implies that patients' immune responses have been sensitized to halothane-induced antigens following previous halothane exposures. This is consistent with the known association of halothane hepatitis with multiple exposures to the anesthetic.

The nature of the halothane-induced neoantigens has been explored by SDS–polyacrylamide gel electrophoresis (SDS-PAGE) and immunoblotting (which involves substantial protein denaturation due to exposure to the detergent SDS), and also using two nondenaturing approaches (ELISA and immunoprecipitation). The immunoblotting studies have identified a range of different liver microsomal polypeptide neoantigens expressed in halothane-exposed rabbits, humans, and rats, but not in livers from control animals or humans (79,80). The neoantigens were shown to be generated via oxidative cytochrome P450–mediated metabolism of halothane (81). As described previously, this proceeds via trifluoroacetyl chloride, which is a highly reactive intermediate that binds covalently to liver macromolecules (see Fig. 1). The neoantigens contain covalently bound trifluoroacetyl groups (which are bound to ε-amino groups on lysine residues of the carrier proteins) and comprise the major trifluoroacetylated proteins expressed in livers of halothane-exposed animals (81–84). Antibodies from patients with halothane hepatitis bind to epitopes that include the trifluoroacetyl group and also individual structural features (presumably amino acid residues adjacent to the covalently modified lysine residues) that are unique to each of the individual target proteins (81).

The ELISA and immunoprecipitation studies revealed the existence of an additional group of halothane-induced neoantigens that were recognized by antibodies from patients with halothane hepatitis, but were not detected by SDS-PAGE/immunoblotting (85,86). Generation of these neoantigens was also found to require oxidative metabolism of halothane, and the immunoprecipitation studies have established that the target proteins are trifluoroacetylated integral membrane proteins (85,86). In contrast, the neoantigens detected by immunoblotting are predominantly peripheral membrane proteins (87).

Many of the trifluoroacetylated liver target proteins have been characterized by amino acid sequence analysis and/or cDNA cloning (Table 1) (86,88–98). The majority are highly abundant and relatively long-lived peripheral membrane proteins that reside in the lumen of the endoplasmic reticulum (87). The trifluoroacetylated forms of these proteins accumulate progressively in the liver over a period of about 24 h and they persist for many days once formed (82). Presumably they become covalently modified in a relatively nonselective manner. Since the active site of CYP 2E1 (the enzyme responsible for neoantigen formation) is located on the cytosolic face of the endoplasmic reticulum, yet these target proteins are lumenal, it has been proposed that their generation requires diffusion of trifluoroacetyl chloride across the lipid bilayer (87), as illustrated in Fig. 4. The normal cellular functions of these proteins include calcium storage, carboxylesterase activity, shuffling of disulfide bonds on nascent polypeptide chains during folding of newly synthesized proteins, and mediation of protein folding via chaperone interactions, and are unrelated to metabolism of halothane or other xenobiotics.

The major conformation-dependent neoantigen detectable by immunoprecipitation comprises a trifluoroacetylated form of microsomal epoxide hydrolase (86), which is a

Table 1 Trifluoroacetylated Liver Neoantigens Derived from Halothane

Molecular mass (kDa) determined by SDS-PAGE	Identity of protein	Method initially used to detect neoantigen	Recognition by antibodies from patients with halothane hepatitis	Ref.
29	Cytosolic glutathione-S-transferase	Protein purification	Not demonstrated	88
50	Microsomal epoxide hydrolase	Immunoprecipitation	Yes	86
52	CYP 2E1	Immunoprecipitation	Yes (autoantibodies)	89,90
57	Protein disulfide isomerase	Immunoblotting	Yes	92
58	Unknown function	Immunoblotting	Yes	91
59	Microsomal carboxylesterase	Immunoblotting	Yes	93
63	Calreticulin	Immunoblotting	Yes	94
80	Erp72	Immunoblotting	Yes	95
82	BiP/GRP78	Immunoblotting	Yes	96
100	Endoplasmin/Erp99/GRP94	Immunoblotting	Yes	97
170	UDP-glucose:glycoprotein glucosyltransferase	Immunoprecipitation	Not demonstrated	98

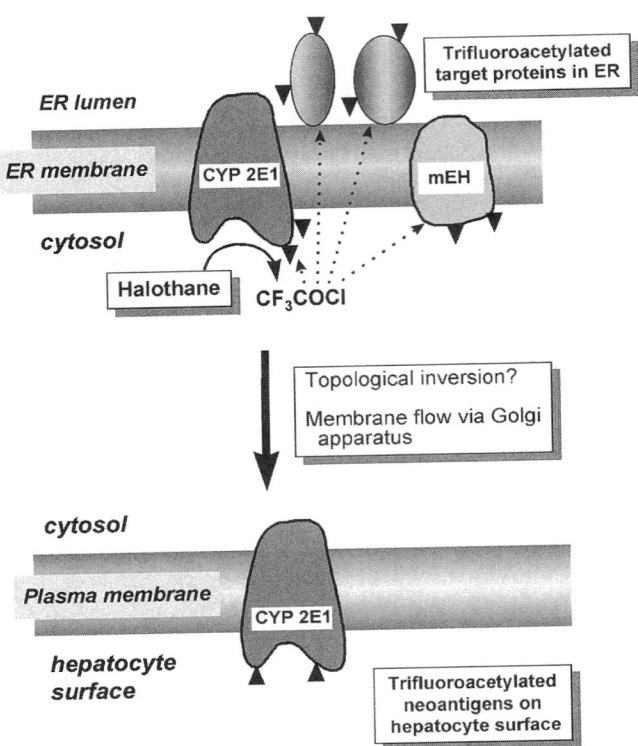

Figure 4 Proposed mechanism of generation of trifluoroacetylated protein neoantigens derived from halothane, and of cell surface expression of trifluoroacetylated CYP 2E1. ER, endoplasmic reticulum.

highly abundant integral membrane protein. In addition, a trifluoroacetylated form of CYP 2E1 has been detected in livers of halothane-treated rats by immunoprecipitation (89), and a high incidence of autoantibodies to a nontrifluoroacetylated form of CYP 2E1 has been demonstrated in sera from patients with halothane hepatitis (89,90). It has been proposed that these CYP 2E1 autoantibodies are generated because trifluoroacetylation of CYP 2E1 leads to a selective breakdown in immune tolerance (89,90). Similar processes may explain the presence of autoantibodies to unmodified forms of other trifluoroacetylated neoantigens in the patients' sera (91,92,95,99,100).

Expression of a low, but significant, fraction of total trifluoroacetylated CYP 2E1 on the hepatocyte plasma membrane has also been demonstrated (89). This is likely to occur via membrane flow through the Golgi apparatus, as has been described for other CYP isozymes (101), and could involve inversion of the normal topology of the protein in the endoplasmic reticulum (102) (see Fig. 4). Cell surface expression of other trifluoroacetylated neoantigens [particularly microsomal epoxide hydrolase (103)] is also likely, but has not yet been demonstrated directly.

The available data indicate that exposure of susceptible individuals to halothane "primes" immune effector mechanisms directed against trifluoroacetylated liver protein

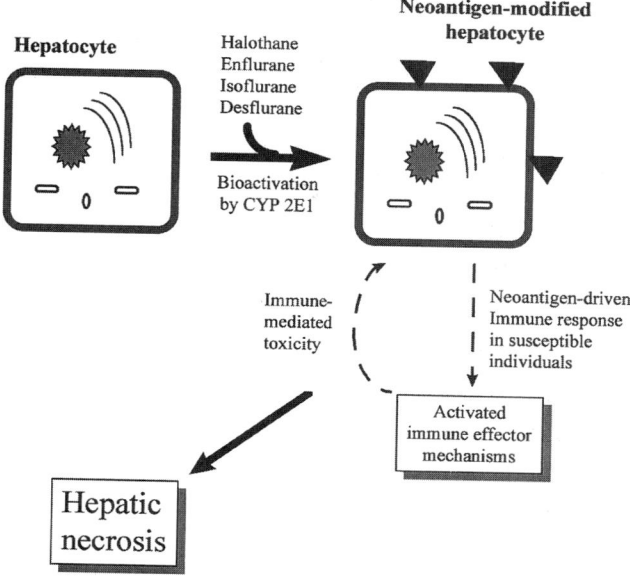

Figure 5 Proposed mechanism of immune-mediated hepatotoxicity of volatile anesthetics.

neoantigens, which mediate liver injury when the patients are rechallenged with halothane. This is illustrated schematically in Fig. 5.

B. Enflurane, Isoflurane, Desflurane, and Sevoflurane

Analysis of livers from rats treated with enflurane or isoflurane by immunoblotting has demonstrated expression of novel microsomal protein neoantigens similar to those derived from halothane (52,104) (Fig. 2). These neoantigens were expressed at markedly lower levels than the trifluoroacetylated neoantigens derived from halothane and the rank order was halothane > enflurane > isoflurane (52,104). This is consistent with the relative extents of cytochrome P450-mediated metabolism of the anesthetics (50). The neoantigens derived from enflurane and isoflurane were shown to be recognized by an anti-(trifluoroacetyl-protein) rabbit antiserum that had been raised by immunizing rabbits with trifluoroacetylated rabbit albumin (52), while the neoantigens derived from enflurane were also recognized by antibodies from patients with halothane hepatitis (104). In addition, antibodies to trifluoroacetylated protein neoantigens have been detected in sera from two patients with hepatitis presumed to be attributable to isoflurane (31,32).

It has been concluded that both enflurane and isoflurane have the potential to elicit liver injury in humans via immune processes similar to those implicated in halothane hepatitis (see Fig. 5) and that this provides a mechanistic basis for clinical cases of apparent cross-sensitization between the anesthetics (52,104). However, it is important to note that many patients who have developed halothane hepatitis have been anesthetized uneventfully with isoflurane and/or enflurane (indicating that cross-sensitization had not occurred). Presumably the relatively low levels of expression of liver neoantigens derived from the latter anesthetics are insufficient to trigger immune responsiveness in the majority of cases, regardless of whether or not sensitization to halothane (and development of halothane hepatitis) has occurred.

Antibodies that recognize trifluoroacetylated liver neoantigens have also been detected in serum from a patient with presumed desflurane hepatitis (33). The proposed mechanism of liver injury was immunological, and similar to that proposed for halothane hepatitis (see Fig. 5). In view of the chemical structure and predicted pathway of cytochrome P450–mediated metabolism of desflurane (Fig. 2), it seems likely that trifluoroacetylated neoantigens are generated in livers of animals and humans exposed to this anesthetic (33). However, this has not been demonstrated experimentally and the levels of the expression of neoantigens derived from desflurane should be extremely low, because of the very limited extent of metabolism of the compound (105). Consequently, the risk of immune-mediated liver injury in patients exposed to desflurane is likely to be extremely small.

It is unclear whether sevoflurane has the potential to elicit immune-mediated liver injury in humans. Although liver protein neoantigens might be formed via formylation, as discussed previously, this possibility has yet to be investigated experimentally. In addition, formylated liver neoantigens may not cross-react immunochemically with trifluoroacetylated neoantigens derived from halothane. Although cases of possible "sevoflurane hepatitis" have been reported in the Japanese literature, and in some instances data obtained using in vitro lymphocyte transformation tests have suggested that the patients had become sensitized to sevoflurane (34,36), the diagnostic value of the in vitro lymphocyte transformation studies is unclear. This is because lymphocytes have minimal cytochrome P450–dependent metabolic capability and the analyses were undertaken in the absence of liver proteins.

C. Hydrochlorofluorocarbon Refrigerants

The ozone-depleting chlorofluorocarbons are being replaced as industrial chemicals by hydrochlorofluorocarbons (HCFCs), which have little ozone-depleting potential. Some of the HCFCs are similar in structure to halothane and the other volatile anesthetic agents. It has been shown that several of these compounds are metabolized in the liver by CYP 2E1 to reactive species that covalently bind to proteins, thereby generating protein adducts that are immunochemically cross-reactive with the trifluoroacetylated protein adducts derived from halothane (83,106). Moreover, hepatotoxicity has been reported in guinea pigs exposed to HCFC 123 (1,1-dichloro-2,2,2-trifluoroethane) (107) and in nine humans who received repeated accidental occupational exposure to very high concentrations of a mixture of HCFC 123 and HCFC 124 (1-chloro-2,2,2,2-tetrafluoroethane) (108). Trifluoroacetylated protein adducts were detected in liver from one of the occupationally exposed human cases, while autoantibodies to two of the target proteins implicated in the mechanism of halothane hepatitis (CYP 2E1 and protein disulfide isomerase) were detected in five of the cases (108). It was concluded that humans exposed on multiple occasions to very high concentrations of certain HCFCs (most notably HCFC 123) are at risk of liver injury. It is not known whether HCFC-induced liver injury in humans is immune-mediated, or can be attributed to direct cytotoxicity. However, it is reasonable to presume that patients who have become sensitized to volatile anesthetics may become cross-sensitized to certain HCFCs.

VI. INDIVIDUAL SUSCEPTIBILITY FACTORS

Why a very small fraction of individuals exposed to volatile anesthetics sustain hepatic injury, while the vast majority do not, has yet to be established. In view of the proposed mechanism of immune-mediated liver injury (Fig. 5), both metabolic and immune factors are likely to be involved.

A. Metabolic Factors

A key metabolic susceptibility factor may be the balance between CYP 2E1-catalyzed metabolic bioactivation of the volatile anesthetics and detoxification of reactive intermediates by glutathione and other cellular nucleophiles (45).

This could vary throughout the human population (due to individual differences in CYP 2E1 activity, glutathione-S-transferase activity, and/or levels of hepatic glutathione) and thereby result in interindividual variability in levels of expression of metabolite-modified liver neoantigens (45,82). Studies undertaken with various haptenated autologous proteins have shown that the density of hapten groups and the concentrations of haptenated proteins play major roles in breaking immunological tolerance to self-proteins (109). Consequently, patients who express relatively high levels of neoantigens derived from volatile anesthetics are likely to be at greater risk of developing a neoantigen-driven immune response, and sustaining immune-mediated liver injury, than patients who express lower levels of the neoantigens.

This would explain why the incidence of liver injury in patients exposed to enflurane or isoflurane (which are metabolized to a markedly lesser extent than halothane) is markedly lower than the incidence of halothane hepatitis. It may also explain why obesity [which can enhance metabolism by inducing CYP 2E1 (110) and/or by enhancing distribution of volatile anesthetics into body fat (111)] has been identified as a risk factor in halothane hepatitis (17). In addition, existence of a metabolic susceptibility factor is supported by a report of abnormal sensitivity to electrophilic reactive metabolites derived from phenytoin in lymphocytes from 11 patients with halothane hepatitis, when compared with control lymphocytes (112). This abnormality, which implies a defective ability to detoxify the reactive intermediates, was exhibited also by lymphocytes from 19 family members of four of the patients, indicating that it is genetically inherited (112). An inherited susceptibility factor is consistent with reports of cases of halothane hepatitis in pairs of closely related women (113).

B. Immunological Factors

A consistent association between susceptibility to halothane hepatitis and HLA phenotype has not been observed (114,115). Experiments undertaken by Gut and co-workers have shown that trifluoroacetylated epitopes on proteins are very similar (both structurally and immunochemically) to the lipoyl-lysine regions contained within the E2 subunits of mitochondrial pyruvate dehydrogenase and other 2-oxoacid dehydrogenase proteins (116). The molecular mimicry was found to extend to epitopes recognized by antibodies from patients with halothane hepatitis (117,118). This structural similarity could result in immunological tolerance to trifluoroacetylated protein epitopes and may help to explain why "normal individuals" do not develop neoantigen-induced immune responses and do not sustain immune-mediated liver damage when exposed to halothane and other volatile anesthetics.

Marked interindividual variability in levels of expression of the E2 subunit of pyruvate dehydrogenase was observed in a panel of 19 human liver samples and abnormally low levels of expression of the protein were observed in liver biopsy samples from five of seven patients with halothane (119). In view of this, it has been proposed that susceptibility to halothane hepatitis (and to liver injury caused by other volatile anesthetics) may arise, at least in part, because certain individuals express unusually low levels of lipoylated E2 subunits of PDH and related proteins and so have defective immune tolerance to trifluoro-acetylated proteins epitopes (116,119).

Recently the "danger hypothesis" has been proposed by Matzinger in an attempt to provide an explanation for the loss of immune tolerance that occurs in autoimmune diseases (120). According to this hypothesis, an immune response is triggered when an antigen is presented to the immune system in the context of a "danger signal," such as cell damage, but not if a danger signal is absent. It has been suggested by other investigators that this could help to explain many immune-mediated adverse drug reactions, including liver damage due to anesthetic agents (121,122). This is an intriguing suggestion that merits further investigation, especially since several of the trifluoroacetylated neoantigens identified in livers of halothane-treated rats are stress proteins (Table 1).

VII. SUMMARY

Liver damage that can be attributed to volatile anesthetic agents is rare, but clinically well documented. This may occur following exposure to all of the volatile agents in use currently, with the possible exception of sevoflurane. Liver damage due to halothane, enflurane, isoflurane, and desflurane is a consequence of their CYP 2E1-mediated bioactivation to reactive intermediates that bind covalently to numerous different liver proteins to form neoantigens. The neoantigens elicit immune responses in susceptible patients and these immune responses have been implicated in the mechanism of anesthetic-induced liver damage. A variety of antibody assays have been described that aid diagnosis. The available evidence indicates that a complex combination of metabolic and immunological susceptibility factors explains why certain anesthetic-exposed individuals sustain liver injury, whereas the vast majority of the population do not.

REFERENCES

1. Zimmerman HJ. Anesthetic Agents. Hepatotoxicity: The Adverse Effects of Drugs and Other Chemicals on the Liver. New York: Appleton-Century-Crofts, 1978:370–394.
2. Pohl LR. Biochemical toxicology of chloroform. Rev Biochem Toxicol 1979; 1:79–107.
3. Inman WH, Mushin WW. Jaundice after repeated exposure to halothane: an analysis of Reports to the Committee on Safety of Medicines. Br Med J 1974; 1:5–10.
4. Ray DC, Drummond GB. Halothane hepatitis. Br J Anaesth 1991; 67:84–99.
5. Kenna JG, Neuberger J. Immunopathogenesis and treatment of halothane hepatitis. Clin Immunother 1995; 3:108–124.
6. Bunker JP. Final Report of the National Halothane Study. Anesthesiology 1968; 29:231–232.
7. Kenna JG, Neuberger J, Mieli-Vergani G, Mowat AP, Williams R. Halothane hepatitis in children. Br Med J (Clin Res Ed) 1987; 294:1209–1211.
8. Neuberger J, Vergani D, Mieli-Vergani G, Davis M, Williams R. Hepatic damage after exposure to halothane in medical personnel. Br J Anaesth 1981; 53:1173–1177.
9. Klion FM, Schaffner F, Popper H. Hepatitis after exposure to halothane. Ann Intern Med 1969; 71:467–477.

10. Moult PJ, Sherlock S. Halothane-related hepatitis: a clinical study of twenty-six cases. Q J Med 1975; 44:99–114.

11. Kenna JG, Neuberger J, Williams R. Specific antibodies to halothane-induced liver antigens in halothane-associated hepatitis. Br J Anaesth 1987; 59:1286–1290.

12. Benjamin SB, Goodman ZD, Ishak KG, Zimmerman HJ, Irey NS. The morphologic spectrum of halothane-induced hepatic injury: analysis of 77 cases. Hepatology 1985; 5:1163–1171.

13. Uzunalimoglu B, Yardley JH, Boitnott JK. The liver in mild halothane hepatitis. Light and electron microscopic findings with special reference to the mononuclear cell infiltrate. Am J Pathol 1970; 61:457–478.

14. Wills EJ, Walton B. A morphologic study of unexplained hepatitis following halothane anesthesia. Am J Pathol 1978; 91:11–32.

15. Martin JL, Dubbink DA, Plevak DJ, Peronne A, Taswell HF, Hay EJ, Pumford NR, Pohl LR. Halothane hepatitis 28 years after primary exposure. Anesth Analg 1992; 74:605–608.

16. Inman WH, Mushin WW. Jaundice after repeated exposure to halothane: a further analysis of reports to the Committee on Safety of Medicines. Br Med J 1978; 2:1455–1456.

17. Walton B, Simpson BR, Strunin L, Doniach D, Perrin J, Appleyard AJ. Unexplained hepatitis following halothane. Br Med J 1976; 1:1171–1176.

18. Wright R, Eade OE, Chisholm M, Hawksley M, Lloyd B, Moles TM, Edwards JC. Controlled prospective study of the effect on liver function of multiple exposures to halothane. Lancet 1975; 1:817–820.

19. Trowell J, Peto R, Smith AC. Controlled trial of repeated halothane anaesthetics in patients with carcinoma of the uterine cervix treated with radium. Lancet 1975; 1:821–824.

20. Davis M, Eddleston AL, Neuberger JM, Vergani D, Mieli-Vergani G, Williams R. Halothane hepatitis [letter]. N Engl J Med 1980; 303:1123–1124.

21. Sakaguchi Y, Inaba S, Irita K, Sakai H, Nawata H, Takahashi S. Absence of antitrifluoroacetate antibody after halothane anaesthesia in patients exhibiting no or mild liver damage. Can J Anaesth 1994; 41:398–403.

22. Lewis JH, Zimmerman HJ, Ishak KG, Mullick FG. Enflurane hepatotoxicity: a clinicopathologic study of 24 cases. Ann Intern Med 1983; 98:984–992.

23. Brown BR, Jr., Gandolfi AJ. Adverse effects of volatile anaesthetics. Br J Anaesth 1987; 59:14–23.

24. Sigurdsson J, Hreidarsson AB, Thjodleifsson B. Enflurane hepatitis: a report of a case with a previous history of halothane hepatitis. Acta Anaesthesiol Scand 1985; 29:495–496.

25. Gogus FY, Toker K, Baykan N. Hepatitis following use of two different fluorinated anesthetic agents. Isr J Med Sci 1991; 27:156–159.

26. Brunt EM, White H, Marsh JW, Holtmann B, Peters MG. Fulminant hepatic failure after repeated exposure to isoflurane anesthesia: a case report. Hepatology 1991; 13:1017–1021.

27. Sinha A, Clatch RJ, Stuck G, Blumenthal SA, Patel SA. Isoflurane hepatotoxicity: a case report and review of the literature. Am J Gastroenterol 1996; 91:2406–2409.

28. Weitz J, Kienle P, Bohrer H, Hofmann W, Theilmann L, Otto G. Fatal hepatic necrosis after isoflurane anaesthesia. Anaesthesia 1997; 52:892–895.

29. Turner GB, O'Rourke D, Scott GO, Beringer TR. Fatal hepatotoxicity after re-exposure to isoflurane: a case report and review of the literature [In Process Citation]. Eur J Gastroenterol Hepatol 2000; 12:955–959.

30. Zimmerman H. Even isoflurane [editorial]. Hepatology 1991; 13:1251–1253.

31. Gunaratnam NT, Benson J, Gandolfi AJ, Chen M. Suspected isoflurane hepatitis in an obese patient with a history of halothane hepatitis. Anesthesiology 1995; 83:1361–1364.

32. Meldrum DJ, Griffiths R, Kenna JG. Gallstones and isoflurane hepatitis. Anaesthesia 1998; 53:905–909.

33. Martin JL, Plevak DJ, Flannery KD, Charlton M, Poterucha JJ, Humphreys CE, Derfus G, Pohl LR. Hepatotoxicity after desflurane anesthesia. Anesthesiology 1995; 83:1125–1129.

34. Ogawa M, Doi K, Mitsufuji T, Satoh K, Takatori T. Drug induced hepatitis following sevoflurane anesthesia in a child. Masui 1991; 40:1542–1545.

35. Shichinohe Y, Masuda Y, Takahashi H, Kotaki M, Omote T, Shichinohe M, Namiki A. [A case of postoperative hepatic injury after sevoflurane anesthesia]. Masui 1992; 41:1802–1805.

36. Watanabe K, Hatakenaka S, Ikemune K, Chigyo Y, Kubozono T, Arai T. A case of suspected liver dysfunction induced by sevoflurane anesthesia. Masui 1993; 42:902–905.

37. Rehder K, Forbes J, Alter H, Hessler O, Stier A. Halothane biotransformation in man: a quantitative study. Anesthesiology 1967; 28:711–715.

38. Kenna JG, van Pelt FNAM. The metabolism and toxicity of inhaled anaesthetic agents. Anaesth Pharm Rev 1994; 2:29–42.

39. Cohen EN. Metabolism of the volatile anesthetics. Anesthesiology 1971; 35:193–202.

40. Gandolfi AJ, White RD, Sipes IG, Pohl LR. Bioactivation and covalent binding of halothane in vitro: studies with [^{3}H]- and [^{14}C]halothane. J Pharmacol Exp Ther 1980; 214:721–725.

41. Satoh H, Fukuda Y, Anderson DK, Ferrans VJ, Gillette JR, Pohl LR. Immunological studies on the mechanism of halothane-induced hepatotoxicity: immunohistochemical evidence of trifluoroacetylated hepatocytes. J Pharmacol Exp Ther 1985; 233:857–862.

42. Trudell JR, Ardies CM, Anderson WR. Antibodies raised against trifluoroacetyl-protein adducts bind to N-trifluoroacetyl-phosphatidylethanolamine in hexagonal phase phospholipid micelles. J Pharmacol Exp Ther 1991; 257:657–662.

43. Kharasch ED, Hankins DC, Fenstamaker K, Cox K. Human halothane metabolism, lipid peroxidation, and cytochromes P(450)2A6 and P(450)3A4. Eur J Clin Pharmacol 2000; 55:853–859.

44. Kharasch ED, Hankins D, Mautz D, Thummel KE. Identification of the enzyme responsible for oxidative halothane metabolism: implications for prevention of halothane hepatitis. Lancet 1996; 347:1367–1371.

45. Eliasson E, Gardner I, Hume-Smith H, de Waziers I, Beaune P, Kenna JG. Interindividual variability in P450-dependent generation of neoantigens in halothane hepatitis. Chem Biol Interact 1998; 116:123–141.

46. Kharasch ED, Thummel KE, Mautz D, Bosse S. Clinical enflurane metabolism by cytochrome P450 2E1. Clin Pharmacol Ther 1994; 55:434–440.

47. Kharasch ED, Hankins DC, Cox K. Clinical isoflurane metabolism by cytochrome P450 2E1. Anesthesiology 1999; 90:766–771.

48. Chase RE, Holaday DA, Fiserova-Bergerova V, Saidman LJ, Mack FE. The biotransformation of ethrane in man. Anesthesiology 1971; 35:262–267.

49. Holaday DA, Fiserova-Bergerova V, Latto IP, Zumbiel MA. Resistance of isoflurane to biotransformation in man. Anesthesiology 1975; 43:325–332.

50. Fiserova-Bergerova V, Holaday DA. Uptake and clearance of inhalation anesthetics in man. Drug Metab Rev 1979; 9:43–60.

51. Burke TR, Jr., Branchflower RV, Lees DE, Pohl LR. Mechanism of defluorination of enflurane: identification of an organic metabolite in rat and man. Drug Metab Dispos 1981; 9:19–24.

52. Christ DD, Satoh H, Kenna JG, Pohl LR. Potential metabolic basis for enflurane hepatitis and the apparent cross-sensitization between enflurane and halothane. Drug Metab Dispos 1988; 16:135–140.

53. Hitt BA, Mazze RI, Cousins MJ, Edmunds HN, Barr GA, Trudell JR. Metabolism of isoflurane in Fischer 344 rats and man. Anesthesiology 1974; 40:62–67.

54. Sutton TS, Koblin DD, Gruenke LD, Weiskopf RB, Rampil IJ, Waskell L, Eger EI. Fluoride metabolites after prolonged exposure of volunteers and patients to desflurane. Anesth Analg 1991; 73:180–185.

55. Cook TL, Beppu WJ, Hitt BA, Kosek JC, Mazze RI. Renal effects and metabolism of sevo-

flurane in Fisher 3444 rats: an in-vivo and in-vitro comparison with methoxyflurane. Anesthesiology 1975; 43:70–77.

56. Holaday DA, Smith FR. Clinical characteristics and biotransformation of sevoflurane in healthy human volunteers. Anesthesiology 1981; 54:100–106.

57. Kharasch ED. Biotransformation of sevoflurane. Anesth Analg 1995; 81:S27–S38.

58. Reynolds ES, Moslen MT. Halothane hepatotoxicity: enhancement by polychlorinated biphenyl pretreatment. Anesthesiology 1977; 47:19–27.

59. McLain GE, Sipes IG, Brown BR, Jr. An animal model of halothane hepatotoxicity: roles of enzyme induction and hypoxia. Anesthesiology 1979; 51:321–326.

60. Cousins MJ, Sharp JH, Gourlay GK, Adams JF, Haynes WD, Whitehead R. Hepatotoxicity and halothane metabolism in an animal model with application for human toxicity. Anaesth Intens Care 1979; 7:9–24.

61. Pohl LR, Gillette JR. A perspective on halothane-induced hepatotoxicity [letter]. Anesth Analg 1982; 61:809–811.

62. Clarke JB, Gandolfi AJ. Volatile anesthetics: mechanisms of potential hepatotoxicity. Clin Anesth Updates 1992; 3:1–11.

63. Berman ML, Kuhnert L, Phythyon JM, Holaday DA. Isoflurane and enflurane-induced hepatic necrosis in triiodothyronine-pretreated rats. Anesthesiology 1983; 58:1–5.

64. Rice SA, Maze M, Smith CM, Kosek JC, Mazze RI. Halothane hepatotoxicity in Fischer 344 rats pretreated with isoniazid. Toxicol Appl Pharmacol 1987; 87:411–419.

65. Lunam CA, Cousins MJ, Hall PD. Guinea-pig model of halothane-associated hepatotoxicity in the absence of enzyme induction and hypoxia. J Pharmacol Exp Ther 1985; 232:802–809.

66. Lind RC, Gandolfi AJ, Hall PD. The role of oxidative biotransformation of halothane in the guinea pig model of halothane-associated hepatotoxicity. Anesthesiology 1989; 70:649–653.

67. Farrell GC, Frost L, Tapner M, Field J, Weltman M, Mahoney J. Halothane-induced liver injury in guinea-pigs: importance of cytochrome P450 enzyme activity and hepatic blood flow. J Gastroenterol Hepatol 1996; 11:594–601.

68. Lind RC, Gandolfi AJ, Hall PM. Glutathione depletion enhances subanesthetic halothane hepatotoxicity in guinea pigs. Anesthesiology 1992; 77:721–727.

69. de Groot H, Noll T. Halothane hepatotoxicity: relation between metabolic activation, hypoxia, covalent binding, lipid peroxidation and liver cell damage. Hepatology 1983; 3:601–606.

70. Goto T, Ohwan K, Matsumoto N, Miyazaki T, Murakami Y, Ohhata M, Hori T, Shiota K. Protective effect of calcium channel blockers on the liver against halothane hepatitis in rats. Masui 1990; 39:204–209.

71. Farrell GC, Mahoney J, Bilous M, Frost L. Altered hepatic calcium homeostasis in guinea pigs with halothane-induced hepatotoxicity. J Pharmacol Exp Ther 1988; 247:751–756.

72. Van Dyke RA. Hepatic centrilobular necrosis in rats after exposure to halothane, enflurane, or isoflurane. Anesth Analg 1982; 61:812–819.

73. Harper MH, Collins P, Johnson B, Eger EId, Biava C. Hepatic Injury following halothane, enflurane, and isoflurane anesthesia in rats. Anesthesiology 1982; 56:14–17.

74. Shingu K, Eger EId, Johnson BH, Van Dyke RA, Lurz FW, Harper MH, Cheng A. Hepatic injury induced by anesthetic agents in rats. Anesth Analg 1983; 62:140–145.

75. Vergani D, Tsantoulas D, Eddleston AL, Davis M, Williams R. Sensitisation to halothane-altered liver components in severe hepatic necrosis after halothane anaesthesia. Lancet 1978; 2:801–803.

76. Vergani D, Mieli-Vergani G, Alberti A, Neuberger J, Eddleston AL, Davis M, Williams R. Antibodies to the surface of halothane-altered rabbit hepatocytes in patients with severe halothane-associated hepatitis. N Engl J Med 1980; 303:66–71.

77. Neuberger J, Gimson AE, Davis M, Williams R. Specific serological markers in the diagnosis of fulminant hepatic failure associated with halothane anaesthesia. Br J Anaesth 1983; 55: 15–19.

78. Kenna JG, Neuberger J, Williams R. An enzyme-linked immunosorbent assay for detection of antibodies against halothane-altered hepatocyte antigens. J Immunol Methods 1984; 75: 3–14.

79. Kenna JG, Neuberger J, Williams R. Identification by immunoblotting of three halothane-induced liver microsomal polypeptide antigens recognized by antibodies in sera from patients with halothane-associated hepatitis. J Pharmacol Exp Ther 1987; 242:733–740.

80. Kenna JG, Neuberger J, Williams R. Evidence for expression in human liver of halothane-induced neoantigens recognized by antibodies in sera from patients with halothane hepatitis. Hepatology 1988; 8:1635–1641.

81. Kenna JG, Satoh H, Christ DD, Pohl LR. Metabolic basis for a drug hypersensitivity: antibodies in sera from patients with halothane hepatitis recognize liver neoantigens that contain the trifluoroacetyl group derived from halothane. J Pharmacol Exp Ther 1988; 245: 1103–1109.

82. Kenna JG, Martin JL, Satoh H, Pohl LR. Factors affecting the expression of trifluoroacetylated liver microsomal protein neoantigens in rats treated with halothane. Drug Metab Dispos 1990; 18:788–793.

83. Harris JW, Pohl LR, Martin JL, Anders MW. Tissue acylation by the chlorofluorocarbon substitute 2,2-dichloro-1,1,1-trifluoroethane. Proc Natl Acad Sci USA 1991; 88:1407–1410.

84. Heijink E, De Matteis F, Gibbs AH, Davies A, White IN. Metabolic activation of halothane to neoantigens in C57Bl/10 mice: immunochemical studies. Eur J Pharmacol 1993; 248:15–25.

85. Knight TL, Scatchard KM, Van Pelt FN, Kenna JG. Sera from patients with halothane hepatitis contain antibodies to halothane-induced liver antigens which are not detectable by immunoblotting [published erratum appears in J Pharmacol Exp Ther 1995; 272(2):962]. J Pharmacol Exp Ther 1994; 270:1325–1333.

86. Ramsay LA, Eliasson E, Barnes S, Atkinson M, Smith G, Wolf CR, Kenna JG. Microsomal epoxide hydrolase is a major neoantigen and autoantigen in halothane hepatitis. Submitted.

87. Kenna JG, Martin JL, Pohl LR. The topography of trifluoroacetylated protein antigens in liver microsomal fractions from halothane treated rats. Biochem Pharmacol 1992; 44:621–629.

88. Brown AP, Gandolfi AJ. Glutathione-S-transferase is a target for covalent modification by a halothane reactive intermediate in the guinea pig liver. Toxicology 1994; 89:35–47.

89. Eliasson E, Kenna JG. Cytochrome P450 2E1 is a cell surface autoantigen in halothane hepatitis. Mol Pharmacol 1996; 50:573–582.

90. Bourdi M, Chen W, Peter RM, Martin JL, Buters JT, Nelson SD, Pohl LR. Human cytochrome P450 2E1 is a major autoantigen associated with halothane hepatitis. Chem Res Toxicol 1996; 9:1159–1166.

91. Martin JL, Reed GF, Pohl LR. Association of anti-58 kDa endoplasmic reticulum antibodies with halothane hepatitis. Biochem Pharmacol 1993; 46:1247–1250.

92. Martin JL, Kenna JG, Martin BM, Thomassen D, Reed GF, Pohl LR. Halothane hepatitis patients have serum antibodies that react with protein disulfide isomerase. Hepatology 1993; 18:858–863.

93. Satoh H, Martin BM, Schulick AH, Christ DD, Kenna JG, Pohl LR. Human antiendoplasmic reticulum antibodies in sera of patients with halothane-induced hepatitis are directed against a trifluoroacetylated carboxylesterase. Proc Natl Acad Sci USA 1989; 86:322–326.

94. Butler LE, Thomassen D, Martin JL, Martin BM, Kenna JG, Pohl LR. The calcium-binding protein calreticulin is covalently modified in rat liver by a reactive metabolite of the inhalation anesthetic halothane. Chem Res Toxicol 1992; 5:406–410.

95. Pumford NR, Martin BM, Thomassen D, Burris JA, Kenna JG, Martin JL, Pohl LR. Serum antibodies from halothane hepatitis patients react with the rat endoplasmic reticulum protein ERp72. Chem Res Toxicol 1993; 6:609–615.

96. Davila JC, Martin BM, Pohl LR. Patients with halothane hepatitis have serum antibodies directed against glucose-regulated stress protein GRP78/BiP. Toxicologist 1992; 12:255.

97. Thomassen D, Martin BM, Martin JL, Pumford NR, Pohl LR. The role of a stress protein in the development of a drug-induced allergic response. Eur J Pharmacol 1990; 183:1138–1139.

98. Amouzadeh HR, Bourdi M, Martin JL, Martin BM, Pohl LR. UDP-glucose:glycoprotein glucosyltransferase associates with endoplasmic reticulum chaperones and its activity is decreased in vivo by the inhalation anesthetic halothane. Chem Res Toxicol 1997; 10:59–63.

99. Pohl LR, Thomassen D, Pumford NR, Butler LE, Satoh H, Ferrans VJ, Perrone A, Martin BM, Martin JL. Hapten carrier conjugates associated with halothane hepatitis. Adv Exp Med Biol 1991; 283:111–120.

100. Smith GC, Kenna JG, Harrison DJ, Tew D, Wolf CR. Autoantibodies to hepatic microsomal carboxylesterase in halothane hepatitis. Lancet 1993; 342:963–964.

101. Robin MA, Descatoire V, Le Roy M, Berson A, Lebreton FP, Maratrat M, Ballet F, Loeper J, Pessayre D. Vesicular transport of newly synthesized cytochromes P4501A to the outside of rat hepatocyte plasma membranes. J Pharmacol Exp Ther 2000; 294:1063–1069.

102. Neve EP, Ingelman-Sundberg M. Molecular basis for the transport of cytochrome P450 2E1 to the plasma membrane [in Process Citation]. J Biol Chem 2000; 275:17130–17135.

103. Zhu Q, von Dippe P, Xing W, Levy D. Membrane topology and cell surface targeting of microsomal epoxide hydrolase. Evidence for multiple topological orientations. J Biol Chem 1999; 274:27898–27904.

104. Christ DD, Kenna JG, Kammerer W, Satoh H, Pohl LR. Enflurane metabolism produces covalently bound liver adducts recognized by antibodies from patients with halothane hepatitis. Anesthesiology 1988; 69:833–838.

105. Njoku D, Laster MJ, Gong DH, Eger EI, 2nd, Reed GF, Martin JL. Biotransformation of halothane, enflurane, isoflurane, and desflurane to trifluoroacetylated liver proteins: association between protein acylation and hepatic injury. Anesth Analg 1997; 84:173–178.

106. Harris JW, Jones JP, Martin JL, LaRosa AC, Olson MJ, Pohl LR, Anders MW. Pentahalo-ethane-based chlorofluorocarbon substitutes and halothane: correlation of in vivo hepatic protein trifluoroacetylation and urinary trifluoroacetic acid excretion with calculated enthalpies of activation. Chem Res Toxicol 1992; 5:720–725.

107. Marit GB, Dodd DE, George ME, Vinegar A. Hepatotoxicity in guinea pigs following acute inhalation exposure to 1,1-dichloro-2,2,2-trifluoroethane. Toxicol Pathol 1994; 22:404–414.

108. Hoet P, Graf ML, Bourdi M, Pohl LR, Duray PH, Chen W, Peter RM, Nelson SD, Verlinden N, Lison D. Epidemic of liver disease caused by hydrochlorofluorocarbons used as ozone-sparing substitutes of chlorofluorocarbons [see comments]. Lancet 1997; 350:556–559.

109. Allison AC. Theories of self tolerance and autoimmunity. In: ME Kammuller, N Bloksma, W Seinen, eds. Autoimmunity and Toxicology: Immune Dysregulation Induced by Drugs and Chemicals. Amsterdam: Elsevier, 1989:67–115.

110. O'Shea D, Davis SN, Kim RB, Wilkinson GR. Effect of fasting and obesity in humans on the 6-hydroxylation of chlorzoxazone: a putative probe of CYP2E1 activity. Clin Pharmacol Ther 1994; 56:359–367.

111. Young SR, Stoelting RK, Peterson C, Madura JA. Anesthetic biotransformation and renal function in obese patients during and after methoxyflurane or halothane anesthesia. Anesthesiology 1975; 42:451–457.

112. Farrell G, Prendergast D, Murray M. Halothane hepatitis. Detection of a constitutional susceptibility factor. N Engl J Med 1985; 313:1310–1314.

113. Hoft RH, Bunker JP, Goodman HI, Gregory PB. Halothane hepatitis in three pairs of closely related women. N Engl J Med 1981; 304:1023–1024.

114. Otsuka S, Yamamoto M, Kasuya S, Ohtomo H, Yamamoto Y, Yoshida TO, Akaza T. HLA antigens in patients with unexplained hepatitis following halothane anesthesia. Acta Anaesthesiol Scand 1985; 29:497–501.

115. Eade OE, Grice D, Krawitt EL, Trowell J, Albertini R, Festenstein H, Wright R. HLA A and B locus antigens in patients with unexplained hepatitis following halothane anaesthesia. Tissue Antigens 1981; 17:428–432.

116. Gut J, Christen U, Frey N, Koch V, Stoffler D. Molecular mimicry in halothane hepatitis: biochemical and structural characterization of lipoylated autoantigens. Toxicology 1995; 97: 199–224.

117. Christen U, Quinn J, Yeaman SJ, Kenna JG, Clarke JB, Gandolfi AJ, Gut J. Identification of the dihydrolipoamide acetyltransferase subunit of the human pyruvate dehydrogenase complex as an autoantigen in halothane hepatitis. Molecular mimicry of trifluoroacetyl-lysine by lipoic acid. Eur J Biochem 1994; 223:1035–1047.

118. Frey N, Christen U, Jeno P, Yeaman SJ, Shimomura Y, Kenna JG, Gandolfi AJ, Ranek L, Gut J. The lipoic acid containing components of the 2-oxoacid dehydrogenase complexes mimic trifluoroacetylated proteins and are autoantigens associated with halothane hepatitis. Chem Res Toxicol 1995; 8:736–746.

119. Gut J, Christen U, Huwyler J, Burgin M, Kenna JG. Molecular mimicry of trifluoroacetylated human liver protein adducts by constitutive proteins and immunochemical evidence for its impairment in halothane hepatitis. Eur J Biochem 1992; 210:569–576.

120. Matzinger P. Tolerance, danger, and the extended family. Annu Rev Immunol 1994; 12: 991–1045.

121. Park BK, Pirmohamed M, Kitteringham NR. Role of drug disposition in drug hypersensitivity: a chemical, molecular, and clinical perspective. Chem Res Toxicol 1998; 11:969–988.

122. Uetrecht JP. New concepts in immunology relevant to idiosyncratic drug reactions: the "danger hypothesis" and innate immune system. Chem Res Toxicol 1999; 12:387–395.

18

Anticonvulsant Agents

J. STEVEN LEEDER

Children's Mercy Hospital, Kansas City, Missouri, U.S.A.

MUNIR PIRMOHAMED

University of Liverpool, Liverpool, England

I. INTRODUCTION

Historically, as a therapeutic class, anticonvulsant agents have been associated with severe liver toxicity. Agents such as mephenytoin and phenacemide were removed from clinical use as a consequence of unacceptably high frequencies of liver toxicity and it is clear that a clinically significant risk of hepatotoxicity also accompanies the use of phenytoin (Dilantin, Parke-Davis, Morris Plains, New Jersey), carbamazepine (Tegretol, Novartis Pharmaceuticals, Basel, Switzerland), and valproic acid (Depakene, Abbott Laboratories, Abbott Park, Illinois), the three most commonly prescribed anticonvulsants at present. The complex pathogenesis of seizure disorders and their general refractoriness to anticonvulsant therapy often result in the use of two or more agents such that it becomes difficult to fully evaluate the hepatotoxic potential of individual agents. Nevertheless, the purpose of this chapter is to describe the clinical presentation, histopathology, mechanisms, and determinants of susceptibility of anticonvulsant-induced liver toxicity with a particular focus on the aromatic anticonvulsants phenobarbital, phenytoin, and carbamazepine, as well as lamotrigine, valproic acid, and felbamate.

II. CARBAMAZEPINE

Carbamazepine (CBZ) is a widely used anticonvulsant, and is regarded as the drug of choice for partial epilepsies (1). It is also used in trigeminal neuralgia, neuropathic pain syndromes, and bipolar depression. Since it was introduced in the 1960s, CBZ has been widely reported to adversely affect liver function. It can do this in one of three ways:

1. It leads to an increase in gamma glutamyl transferase (γ-GT), and to lesser extent in alkaline phosphatase (ALP), due to its enzyme-inducing properties. A retrospective analysis showed that 64% and 14% of users had elevations of γ-GT and ALP, respectively (2). Such an increase in liver enzymes is not an indication to stop the drug.
2. It leads to an asymptomatic mild to moderate increase in liver function tests, including transaminases. This has been observed in up to 22% of patients (3). The relationship to more severe forms of liver dysfunction is unclear.
3. It leads to clinically symptomatic hepatic injury, which is often part of a generalized hypersensitivity reaction. The exact incidence is unknown; an analysis of all adverse reactions of CBZ reported to the Swedish Regulatory Agency showed that liver disorders accounted for 10% of all reactions (4). The risk was estimated to be 16 cases per 100,000 treatment-years. Furthermore, analysis of the reports of hepatotoxicity to the Danish Committee on Adverse Drug Reactions showed that CBZ rose from ninth in frequency between 1968 and 1978 (5) to second during 1978 and 1987 (6). In a systematic review of 165 published cases of CBZ hypersensitivity up to 1998, liver involvement was observed in 47% (Pirmohamed et al., unpublished data).

A. Clinical Manifestations

Liver involvement by CBZ is often part of a hypersensitivity syndrome, although the liver can be affected on its own (3,7). In terms of severity, the effects on the liver range from an asymptomatic increase in liver enzymes (8) to fulminant hepatic failure, which has been reported to require liver transplantation (9). There is no obvious relationship with either the dose or serum levels of CBZ. The time to onset of symptomatic hepatotoxicity is about 4 weeks with a range of 1–16 weeks (10).

Hepatic injury is often accompanied by fever, rash, and eosinophilia (11–15), typical features of a hypersensitivity reaction (7). Occasionally, the hepatotoxicity is associated with hematological abnormalities (leukocytosis, agranulocytosis, pancytopenia, thrombocytopenia) (11,16,17), renal dysfunction (18), or pneumonitis (15). In some instances, the clinical picture resembles cholangitis, with jaundice, right-upper-quadrant abdominal pain, nausea, and vomiting being the predominant symptoms (19,20); the cholestasis may be prolonged in some cases (14,21). Rechallenge has been reported in a number of patients (10,11,19,22), and in accordance with an immune reaction, occurs sooner on reexposure than on the initial challenge.

Hepatic injury from CBZ usually recovers on drug withdrawal (10). However, the reactions can be fatal, with an estimated case fatality rate of 12% (23). Prognosis is worse in those with a predominantly hepatocellular pattern than in those with cholestatic injury (10,23), although it is important to note that prognosis has been derived from individual case reports or small case series, and may thus be subject to reporting bias.

Biochemical abnormalities in patients with CBZ-induced hepatic injury are variable; about 30% of patients have a cholestatic pattern with elevation of both ALP and γ-GT, about 50% have a mixed pattern where elevation of ALP and γ-GT is accompanied by an increase in transaminases, while the rest have a hepatocellular pattern where transaminases are grossly elevated with minimal changes in the cholestatic enzymes (24). There may be a rise in bilirubin levels, although the degree is variable, and is most prominent in those patients who present with cholestasis (19,20). A prolonged rise in bilirubin levels is observed in patients with vanishing bile duct syndrome (14,21). In patients with hepatocellular necrosis, the rise in bilirubin levels reflects the severity of damage (25), and may be accompanied by changes in clotting parameters.

B. Pathology

The histology, like the biochemical picture, is also variable. Granulomatous hepatitis is observed in up to three-quarters of patients (10,19,20). Granulomas, which are the predominant lesion, may be accompanied by tissue eosinophilia (24). Pericholangitis and bile duct injury are present occasionally; the vanishing bile duct syndrome has also been reported with CBZ therapy (14,21). This is characterized by disappearance of interlobular bile ducts, with or without inflammatory infiltration, and in more severe cases, cholestasis. Predominantly hepatocellular necrosis has also been reported; a case report of two children with acute liver failure demonstrated the presence of submassive necrosis on liver biopsy (9).

C. Diagnosis

Diagnosis of CBZ-induced hepatotoxicity is largely a clinical diagnosis. The onset and offset of hepatic injury are important factors to consider; in most cases, onset occurs within 12 weeks of the start of drug therapy, while improvement in liver tests is seen within 4 weeks of stopping treatment (10). Rechallenge is often positive (10,22) but is usually not possible on ethical grounds. Clearly, patients with suspected CBZ-induced liver injury should have other causes excluded by the use of appropriate virological, immunological, and radiological investigations. There are no specific diagnostic laboratory tests. Positive cytotoxicity assays (7,22) and lymphocyte transformation tests (26) have been demonstrated in some patients, while others have been shown to have circulating autoantibodies (27–30). However, these tests are largely research tools at present; they are also labor-intensive, difficult to reproduce, and may be associated with a high false-negative rate.

D. Susceptibility Factors

Older patients may be more sensitive to hepatic reactions from CBZ, while there is no sex predilection (10,31). However, it is important to note that this is based on an analysis of adverse reaction reports, and is clearly liable to be biased by vagaries of any spontaneous adverse-drug-reaction-reporting scheme. Certainly, severe reactions in children have been reported (9). It is thought that susceptibility to CBZ hypersensitivity may be genetically determined (7,32); this has been borne out by a recent case report that described the occurrence of hypersensitivity in a pair of monozygotic twins (33). Genetic case-control association studies have to date not shown any relationship to polymorphisms in genes coding for the metabolizing enzymes (34,35), although a recent study has reported an association with a TNF promoter region gene polymorphism (36) (discussed below).

E. Postulated Mechanisms

Metabolism is thought to play an important role in the pathogenesis of CBZ hypersensitivity and hepatotoxicity (Fig. 1). Although the mechanism of toxicity is poorly understood, it has been postulated that metabolites (and not the parent drug) are the causal agents (7). Evidence for this has come from in vitro studies. CBZ can be metabolized to stable, cytotoxic, and protein-reactive metabolites (37). The reactive metabolite has been suggested to be an arene oxide and an inability to detoxify may act as a predisposing factor for the toxicity observed in vivo (7,22). The metabolism of CBZ in humans, and experimental animals, is complex. The major route of metabolism both in vitro and in vivo is 10,11-epoxidation to CBZ-10,11-epoxide (which is itself a pharmacologically active drug) (38–40). Detoxication products from the postulated arene oxide have been detected in rat bile

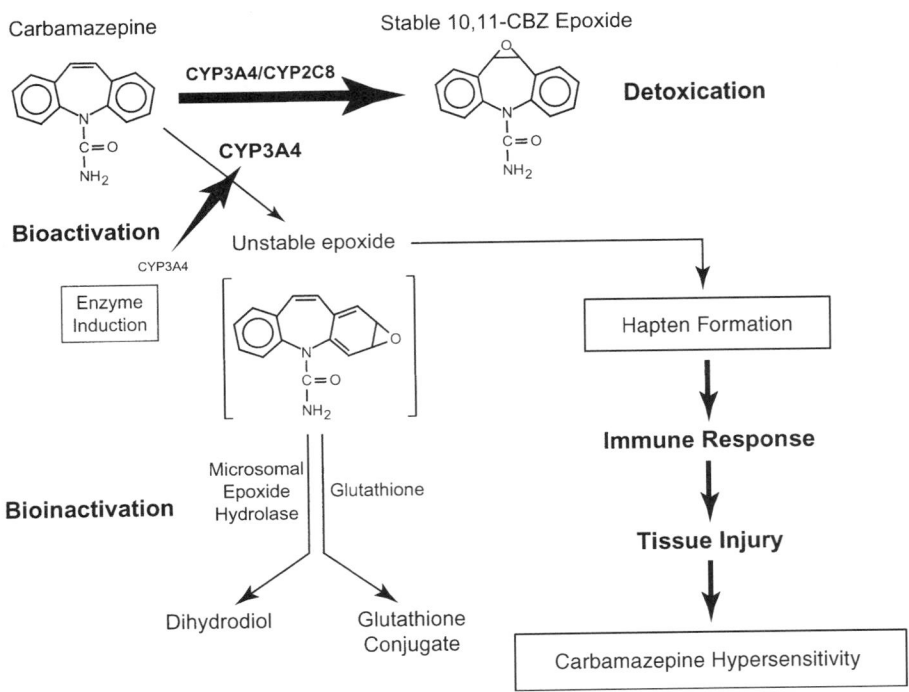

Figure 1 Mechanism of carbamazepine hypersensitivity. Bioactivation of carbamazepine to an unstable arene oxide metabolite leads to hapten formation. Subsequent involvement of the immune systems results in tissue injury at the site(s) of hapten formation, including the liver.

(41) and suggested to be present in human urine (42). In vitro metabolism studies using enzyme inhibitors and purified enzymes have indicated that both stable epoxide formation and reactive metabolite formation are, at least in part, dependent upon CYP 3A4 (43,44). In vivo, CBZ autoinduces its own metabolism by CYP 3A4 including the formation of the ring-hydroxylated metabolites 2- and 3-hydroxyCBZ, which could be generated from an unstable arene oxide intermediate (45). The arene oxide may also undergo further metabolism to catechols and quinones, as demonstrated by recent studies in mice (46). Most recently, a reactive iminoquinone intermediate has been postulated based on the appearance in patient urine of its precursor 2-hydroxyiminostilbene and degradation products of a glutathione adduct (47).

Based on the results of the in vitro cytotoxicity assay (7,22), a deficiency of microsomal epoxide hydrolase was thought to be responsible for predisposing to CBZ hypersensitivity. However, genetic analysis of the microsomal epoxide hydrolase gene has not identified specific mutations in patients with CBZ hypersensitivity (34,35). Furthermore, analysis of polymorphisms in glutathione transferases, catechol-*O*-methyl transferase, and quinone reductase has also not revealed any association with CBZ hypersensitivity (48).

Hypersensitivity reactions to CBZ are thought to have an immune basis. This is evidenced by clinical manifestation of hypersensitivity such as rash, fever, and lymphadenopathy (7), as well as rapid recurrence on rechallenge (22). Furthermore, patients with CBZ hypersensitivity have been reported to have circulating autoantibodies (27–30), drug-reactive T cells (26,49), and positive patch tests (50), all of which support an immune-mediated pathogenesis. A recent study demonstrated that serious hypersensitivity reactions (which comprised patients with varying forms of hepatotoxicity), but not mild skin reactions, showed an association with the -308 polymorphism, but not the -238 polymorphism, in the promoter region of the TNFα gene (36). This is consistent with immunohistochemical analysis of affected skin, which exhibits high TNFα levels (50). Although this is the first genetic factor that has been demonstrated in patients with CBZ hypersensitivity, it is important to note that the polymorphism was not present in all hypersensitive patients, suggesting that it is acting as a susceptibility gene. This would be consistent with the multifactorial pathogenesis of CBZ hypersensitivity reactions (51), and would suggest that predisposition to CBZ hypersensitivity is likely to be dependent on multiple genes.

III. OXCARBAZEPINE

Oxcarbazepine is a keto-analog of CBZ that has been available in Scandinavia for many years, and has only recently become licensed in the rest of Europe. It undergoes less oxidative metabolism than CBZ, and is a less potent enzyme inducer (52). There have been no literature reports of symptomatic hepatic injury with oxcarbazepine. However, there is cross-reactivity between CBZ and oxcarbazepine (22,53,54), with an estimated frequency of 25% (53). Therefore, it is possible that an individual who has suffered hepatic injury with CBZ will also develop similar injury with oxcarbazepine; in such patients, oxcarbazepine should either be used with caution or preferably not at all.

IV. PHENYTOIN

Phenytoin, like CBZ, is an aromatic anticonvulsant. It has, however, been around for much longer, and the first report of hypersensitivity to phenytoin appeared in 1941 (2). As with CBZ, phenytoin-induced hepatotoxicity is an idiosyncratic reaction and is often associated with generalized hypersensitivity phenomena (55,56). Phenytoin is also an enzyme inducer, and can lead to an asymptomatic elevation of γ-GT in almost 100% of recipients (57). A mild elevation of serum transaminases may also be present, and may normalize despite continuation of therapy (58).

More than 100 cases of symptomatic hepatic injury have been reported (23). However, the exact incidence is unknown, but has been estimated to be less than 1 in 10,000 patients. In a systematic review of 271 published cases of phenytoin hypersensitivity, liver involvement ranging from an elevation of liver enzymes to hepatic failure was present in 56% of cases (Pirmohamed et al., unpublished data).

A. Clinical Manifestations

The onset of hepatotoxicity after starting phenytoin ranges from a few days to 8 weeks (24). In accordance with the fact that this is an idiosyncratic reaction, there is no obvious relationship to dose or serum levels. Hepatic injury often occurs as part of a hypersensitivity reaction (55,56), with hepatitis being second only to rash as the most common manifestation (59). The clinical features, in fact, are very similar to those of CBZ hypersensitivity, with rash, fever, eosinophilia, and leukocytosis often accompanying the hepatic injury. Jaundice is seen in nearly half of the patients with hepatitis (24). Lymphadenopathy and splenomegaly occur in 60% of cases (56), with the constellation of symptoms mimicking infectious mononucleosis. Interstitial nephritis, pneumonitis, myositis, eosinophilic fasciitis, lupus-erythematosus-like syndrome, rhabdomyolysis, and pseudolymphoma have also been reported (55,56,60–62). Positive rechallenge has been reported in a number of patients (24).

Early reports suggested a case-fatality rate of 30–40% (2,63,64); however, this is probably an overestimate since liver involvement in most cases is mild and recovers rapidly on drug withdrawal.

An elevation of transaminases is the most common abnormality (ALT > AST), with values ranging from 2 to 100 times the upper limit of normal (56). ALP may also be elevated, although less so than the transaminases, values ranging from 2 to 8 times the upper limit of normal. Cholestasis seems to be less common than observed with CBZ. Bilirubin is variably raised, and in severe cases there may be prolongation of the prothrombin time (24).

B. Pathology

Hepatocellular injury accompanied by a prominent inflammatory infiltrate is the most common histological abnormality (56). The histological picture is, in fact, very similar to that seen in infectious mononucleosis with the exception that there is prominent eosinophil infiltration. Submassive or massive necrosis is seen in 15% of patients, and the necrosis tends to be mainly panacinar. Cholestasis has been reported in 10% of cases (65). However, cholestasis is rarely the predominant lesion as it is often accompanied by hepatocellular injury producing a mixed pattern. Granulomatous hepatitis has also been reported although it is probably less common than witnessed with CBZ (56).

C. Diagnosis

The principles of diagnosis are similar to those mentioned above for CBZ. Thus, diagnosis is largely clinical, and requires the exclusion of nondrug causes. Although positive lymphocyte cytotoxicity (7,66) and transformation tests (67) have been reported, these cannot be routinely used as diagnostic tests.

D. Susceptibility Factors

Phenytoin hepatotoxicity occurs predominantly in adults, with 80% being over the age of 20 years (23). However, phenytoin hepatotoxicity does occur in children, and indeed cholestatic hepatitis has been reported in a newborn infant (2). There appears to be no sex predilection (68). It has been suggested that American blacks are more susceptible to phenytoin reactions than Caucasians (56), including a cluster of three cases that was reported in an African-American family (69). In reviewing this issue, it has been suggested that the apparent higher incidence of reactions in blacks may reflect inaccurate epidemiological data, presumably reflecting the patient population served by inner-city hospitals (68).

Predisposition to phenytoin hypersensitivity is thought to be genetically determined: this has been suggested from the results of the in vitro cytotoxicity assay (7,66,70) and from a report of familial occurrence of phenytoin hypersensitivity (69), with two of the three affected siblings developing significant hepatitis. The nature of the genetic defect is unclear (discussed in more detail below).

E. Postulated Mechanisms

Evidence supporting the concept that phenytoin reactions are immune-mediated include the clinical features, recurrence on rechallenge, positive lymphocyte transformation tests (67), and circulating antibodies to phenytoin (71). Chemically reactive metabolites produced through cytochrome P450 (CYP)-mediated metabolism of phenytoin are again thought to be important in the pathogenesis of phenytoin hypersensitivity. It has been suggested that phenytoin is metabolized to reactive arene oxides (72), and binding of these metabolites to endogenous macromolecules initiates an immune reaction (66). In human liver microsomes, the p-hydroxylated phenytoin metabolite, 5-(4′-hydroxyphenyl)-5-phenylhydantoin (p-HPPH), is more readily converted to a covalent adduct than is the parent drug, phenytoin (73). Furthermore, the protein targets of the reactive species appear to be the members of the human CYP 2C and CYP 3A subfamilies that are responsible for their generation (74). CYP 2C9, CYP 2C19, and CYP 3A4 are also responsible for the formation of a catechol metabolite of phenytoin (75), suggesting that the protein-reactive metabolites may be the o-quinone species derived from the catechol (Fig. 2). Antibodies in patient sera recognize members of the rat CYP 2C and CYP 3A subfamilies (27), suggesting that there may be a link between the bioactivation process and immune response in the pathogenesis of phenytoin idiosyncratic toxicity.

As with CBZ, cells taken from patients with phenytoin hypersensitivity are more sensitive to toxic metabolites of phenytoin generated by a murine microsomal system than cells from controls, suggesting a detoxification deficit (7,66). Although this has been postulated to be a deficiency of microsomal epoxide hydrolase, molecular analysis of the gene has not demonstrated the presence of specific mutations in patients with phenytoin hypersensitivity (34). Whether there is a defect in the immune response genes, as demonstrated for CBZ hypersensitivity, is unknown.

V. PHENOBARBITAL

Phenobarbital is the oldest aromatic anticonvulsant, having been introduced in 1918. It is also an enzyme inducer, and thus can lead to asymptomatic increases in γ-GT and ALP

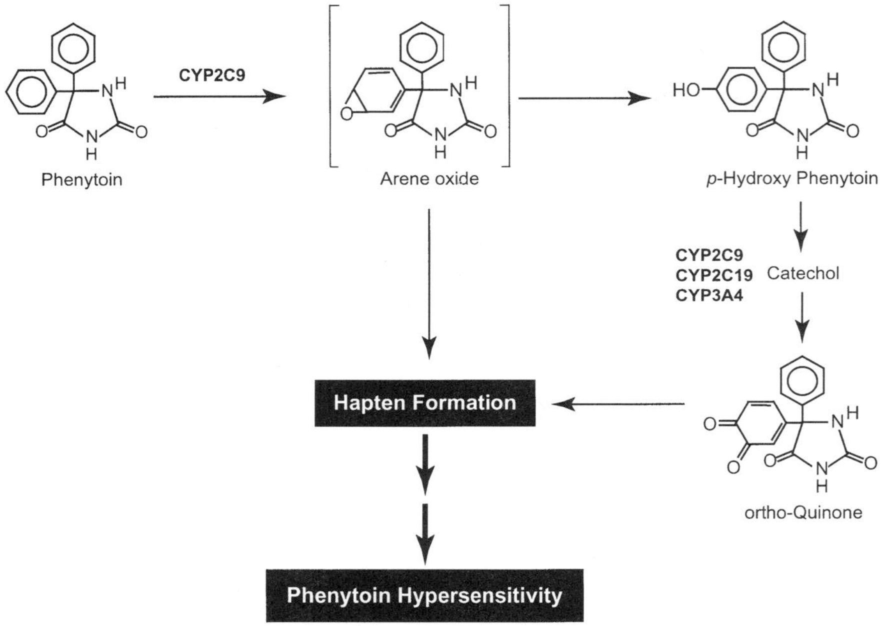

Figure 2   Mechanism of phenytoin hypersensitivity. The pathogenesis of phenytoin hypersensitivity is thought to proceed by mechanisms analogous to those described for carbamazepine. In addition to the postulated reactive arene oxide intermediate, recent evidence implicates a reactive ortho-quinone metabolite of phenytoin in hapten formation.

(57). Symptomatic hepatic injury has been reported with phenobarbital, although it is relatively rare (24). It is often associated with hypersensitivity manifestations such as rash, fever, and eosinophilia (76). Formation of chemically reactive metabolites and an inherited deficiency in the detoxication of these metabolites is thought to be involved in the pathogenesis of phenobarbital hypersensitivity (7).

A.   Cross-Sensitivity Between the Aromatic Anticonvulsants

Given the common mechanisms of aromatic anticonvulsant hypersensitivity, it is not surprising that certain patients exhibit cross-sensitivity with these drugs. Shear and Spielberg suggested that the rate of cross-sensitivity might be as high as 80% (7). A recent clinical study of 633 patients showed that 58% of patients who had a rash with phenytoin also developed a rash with CBZ, while 40% of those with a CBZ rash also developed a rash with phenytoin (77). The factors that determine whether a patient is going to exhibit cross-sensitivity are unclear.

VI.   VALPROIC ACID

Valproic acid (VPA) was introduced into clinical use in France in 1964, and eventually into the United States in 1978. It has a broad spectrum of anticonvulsant activity and is approved for the treatment of generalized absence seizures. It is also effective in the treatment of generalized tonic-clonic, myoclonic, atonic, and partial seizures with or without secondary generalization (78). In recent years, VPA has also become popular as adjunctive therapy for the treatment of bipolar disorders (78). Approval for this indication was received in 1995, and for the treatment of chronic headache in 1996. Initiation of VPA therapy is frequently associated with nausea, vomiting, and gastrointestinal disturbances that can be attenuated by gradual increases in dose, administration after meals, or use of sustained-release formulations. Excessive weight gain, hair changes, and neurological effects such as drowsiness, acute confusional states, irritability, and tremor may also be encountered (79). Most morbidity and mortality, however, is attributed to adverse events involving the liver.

A. Clinical Manifestations

The clinical manifestations of VPA hepatotoxicity cover a broad spectrum. Dose-related elevations in hepatic transaminases may occur in approximately 40% of patients without attendant symptoms of hepatic dysfunction (80). These elevations are transient and generally abate with a reduction in dose (63). Occurring less frequently, but of greater clinical concern, is the potential for fulminant hepatic failure that is irreversible in most cases. Several retrospective reviews of fatal VPA hepatotoxicity have been published from which a consistent pattern of signs and systems has emerged (81–86). Severe hepatic damage initially manifests as nausea, vomiting, abdominal pain, increased seizure frequency, lethargy, and coma. An episode of status epilepticus in close temporal proximity to the appearance of symptoms has been reported in approximately 40–60% of patients (82,83,85). More recent reviews describe the frequent occurrence of febrile illness immediately prior to the onset of hepatic failure (85). The onset of symptoms occurs within the first 6 months of therapy in 95% of affected individuals (83,85), generally within the first 2–3 months (82,84,86). However, onset as early as day 6 (87) and as late as 6 years after initiation of therapy (88) has also been reported.

Measures of hepatic function such as AST, ALT, and bilirubin may exceed three times the upper limit of normal in VPA-treated patients although fatal hepatotoxicity actually occurs in only a small number (<0.01%) of individuals (82). In fatal cases, high serum transaminase and bilirubin levels represent the consequences of extensive hepatocellular damage rather than being specific markers of VPA-associated hepatotoxicity. On the other hand, indicators of synthetic function, such as the prothrombin time and accompanying impairment of coagulation, likely provide more accurate assessment of residual hepatic function (63). Elevated ammonia levels are also present but are also observed in the absence of other indicators of compromised hepatic function. VPA has been reported to unmask latent heterozygous phenotypes of ornithine transcarbamylase deficiency leading to fatal hyperammonemic coma (89,90).

B. Pathology

The histopathology of VPA hepatotoxicity differs substantially from that associated with the aromatic anticonvulsants phenytoin, phenobarbital, and CBZ in that signs of immune involvement and eosinophilia are not present. In fatal cases, the most prominent findings reported by Zimmerman and Ishak consisted of microvesicular steatosis together with zone 3 necrosis (81). A similar picture of hepatocellular damage, including microvesicular steatosis, cellular ballooning, and single-cell or group necrosis, was observed in a series of fatal pediatric cases (85). These authors also noted proliferation of bile ducts in two patients, as has been reported by others (91).

C.   Susceptibility Factors

A series of three retrospective studies of VPA-associated hepatotoxicity in the United States delineated patient age less than 2 years, polytherapy with enzyme-inducing antiepileptic medications, developmental delay, and coincident metabolic disorders as important risk factors for developing this adverse event (82,84,86). Although VPA hepatotoxicity may occur at any age, data collected between 1978 and 1986 indicated that the risk of fatal hepatotoxicity was highest in children less than 2 years of age receiving concurrent anticonvulsant therapy in whom the incidence was estimated to be approximately $1:500$ (82,84). This represents a 16-fold increase in risk relative to children of the same age on VPA monotherapy ($1:8000$). Comparative estimates of risk for older children aged 3–10 years were $1:11,000$ in those on monotherapy and $1:6000$ in those on polytherapy. The risk of fatal hepatotoxicity was essentially unchanged ($1:600$) in children less than 2 years of age on polytherapy between 1987 and 1993 despite a trend toward decreasing use of VPA in very young children—0.8% of the studied population from 1987 to 1993 (86) compared to 2.6% in the earlier studies (82,84). Other studies have confirmed polytherapy as a risk factor but found that there was little difference in risk between younger (less than 3 years of age) and older children (3–6 years of age) (83,85).

Patients with inborn errors of metabolism or reduced hepatic mitochondrial activity also appear to be at increased risk for fatal hepatotoxicity associated with VPA (83). König et al. pointed out that a similar picture of hepatic involvement may manifest as a consequence of several metabolic defects including medium chain acyl CoA dehydrogenase deficiency, ornithine transcarbamylase deficiency, carbamoyl phosphatase synthetase deficiency, pyruvate dehydrogenase deficiency, primary carnitine deficiency, and methyl malonic acidemia, among others (85). The metabolic effects of VPA and its metabolites on mitochondrial β-oxidation (discussed in more detail below) may exacerbate existing metabolic defects or unmask latent deficiencies in susceptible individuals.

Epidemiological studies have failed to demonstrate a relationship between VPA dose and hepatotoxicity (82,84,86). However, dose cannot be separated from polytherapy as a risk factor since patients receiving concurrent antiepileptic drug therapy usually receive higher doses of VPA. The formation of putative toxic metabolites reportedly increases in proportion to serum VPA concentration (92) and with increasing VPA dose (93). It is most likely that the pathogenesis of severe VPA-associated hepatotoxicity is a multifactorial process with no single risk factor being a sole determinant of individual susceptibility. Rather, for example, low doses (and relatively low levels of toxic metabolite formation) may be sufficient for a hepatotoxic event in an individual with latent metabolic disorders whereas much larger doses would be required in less susceptible individuals.

D.   Postulated Mechanisms

Two general mechanistic hypotheses for VPA-associated hepatotoxicity have emerged over the past few years. In each, VPA biotransformation appears to be intimately involved in the process leading to hepatotoxicity although the precise mechanism remains to be elucidated. There is no clinical or laboratory evidence to implicate the immune system in the hepatic injury caused by VPA, suggesting that it may be a form of metabolic idiosyncrasy. The first hypothesis focuses on VPA interference with β-oxidation of endogenous lipids. VPA forms an ester conjugate with carnitine (94) that may lead to secondary carnitine deficiency (95). Several lines of indirect evidence and in vitro studies (96) indicate that a thioester derivative of VPA and coenzyme A may exist as a metabolic intermediate

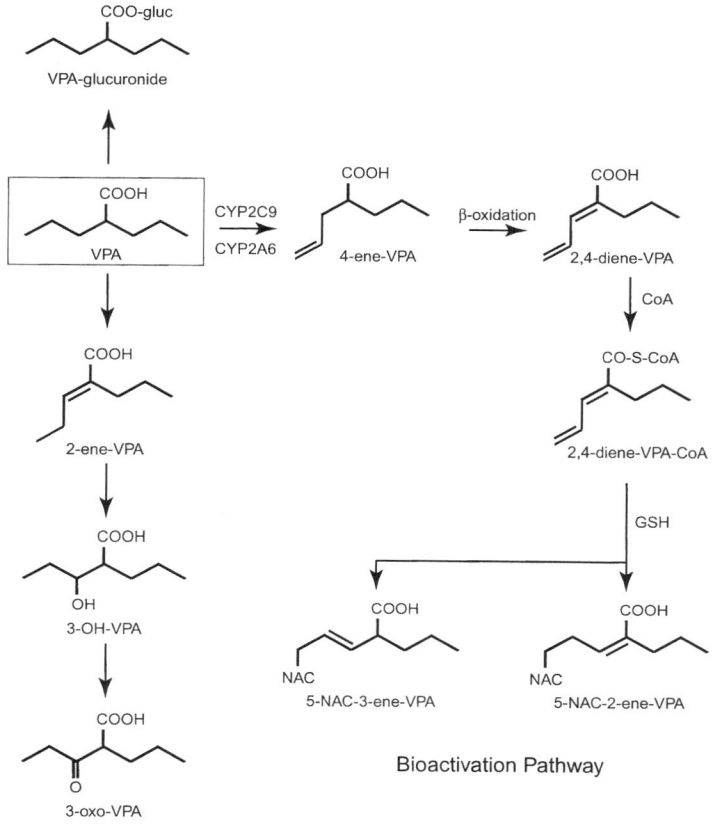

Figure 3 Major pathways for valproic acid (VPA) biotransformation. Glucuronidation of the VPA carboxyl group to form an acyl glucuronide is quantitatively the most important pathway of VPA biotransformation in humans. A significant proportion of VPA undergoes β-oxidation. Oxidation of VPA by CYP 2C9 and CYP 2A6 initiates metabolism down a "bioactivation" pathway. The extent of reactive metabolite formation can be estimated from glutathione conjugates of 2,4-diene-VPA detected in the urine as *N*-acetylcysteine adducts.

in liver tissue. Depletion of coenzyme A or the VPA-CoA ester itself could be responsible for inhibition of mitochondrial metabolism (97). VPA undergoes β-oxidation to several products (2-ene-VPA, 3-hydroxy-VPA, and 3-oxo-VPA; Fig. 3) and competes with endogenous lipids for enzymes in the β-oxidation pathway (98). Any or all of these effects could exacerbate existing latent deficiencies of mitochondrial function.

The second important hypothesis focuses on hepatotoxic unsaturated VPA metabolites. This hypothesis is based on earlier observations that the microvesicular steatosis characteristic of VPA-associated hepatotoxicity bears considerable similarity to the clinical and histological features of Jamaican vomiting sickness and Reye's syndrome. An unsaturated metabolite of the ω-oxidation pathway, 4-ene-VPA (Fig. 3), has received special attention because of its similarity to methylene cyclopropylacetic acid, the ω-oxidation product of hypoglycin A, which is responsible for microvesicular steatosis in Jamaican vomiting sickness, and 4-ene-pentanoic acid, which is used to generate experimental models of Reye's syndrome. In in vivo experimental models, 4-ene-VPA is more steatogenic than VPA in young rats (99) and is more potent as an inhibitor of β-oxidation (100). In vitro studies with cultured hepatocytes also indicate that 4-ene-VPA is more cytotoxic than the parent compound (101). Experimental evidence suggests that chemically reactive metabolites generated from 4-ene-VPA have the potential to inhibit enzymes in the β-oxidation pathway (102,103).

Hepatic microsomal cytochrome P450 (CYP) isoforms are responsible for the formation of 4-ene-VPA and this activity is inducible by phenobarbital (104). Further work has specifically implicated CYP 2C9 and, to a lesser extent, CYP 2A6 in the formation of 4-ene-VPA in humans (105). Administration of phenytoin and CBZ to adult epilepsy patients increases 4-ene-VPA formation approximately twofold under steady-state conditions (106). Induction of CYP 2A6 and CYP 2C9 activities by anticonvulsants has not been rigorously evaluated in humans although modest increases in CYP 2C immunoreactive proteins have been observed following phenobarbital treatment of cultured primary human hepatocytes (107,108). Given the comparative variabilities of CYP 2A6 activity (30-fold) and CYP 2C9 activity (<5-fold) in human liver microsomes (109), it has been proposed that CYP 2C9 may be responsible for the majority of constitutive VPA 4-ene-desaturation while CYP 2A6 plays a greater role during polytherapy with anticonvulsants (105).

The implied relationship between coadministration of inducers, increased 4-ene-VPA formation, and increased risk of hepatotoxicity in patients is analogous to the increased VPA toxicity observed in animal models following pretreatment with phenobarbital, an inducer of CYP 2A, CYP 2B, CYP 2C, and CYP 3A isoforms in rodents (110). Likewise, therapeutic drug monitoring studies of other drugs primarily metabolized by CYP 2C9 (e.g., phenytoin) indicate that CYP 2C9 activity in young children exceeds that of adults, gradually declining to adult levels during childhood (111). The fractional metabolism of VPA to the 4-ene metabolite [but not to the 2- or 3-ene metabolites) also has been shown to decline with increasing age (92,112)], providing one possible explanation for the increased incidence of VPA-associated hepatotoxicity in young children. Furthermore, indirect evidence for a causal relationship between 4-ene-VPA and hepatotoxicity is derived from the observation of relatively high levels of 4-ene-VPA in case reports and studies of patients with fulminant hepatic failure (83,113) but not in VPA-treated children free of hepatic side effects (83).

Despite these considerations, a direct causal relationship between 4-ene-VPA formation and hepatotoxicity has not been demonstrated unequivocally. For example, 4-ene-VPA has been detected in the plasma of patients with no or only minimal overt evidence of hepatic dysfunction (92), and in some studies, plasma levels of 4-ene-VPA did not appear to correlate with the degree of hyperammonemia (114) or hepatic involvement observed (115,116). Finally, in contrast to the two studies cited earlier (92,112), Siemes et al. reported lower concentrations of 4-ene-VPA in children less than 2 years of age compared to older children (116).

The apparent discrepancies in the literature regarding the role of 4-ene-VPA as a hepatotoxic metabolite and further resolution of toxic metabolites versus inhibition of β-oxidation as the primary mechanism of toxicity represent challenges for future research. The complexity of VPA metabolism obfuscates efforts to establish clear relationships between individual metabolites and the hepatotoxic process. Therefore, it may be useful

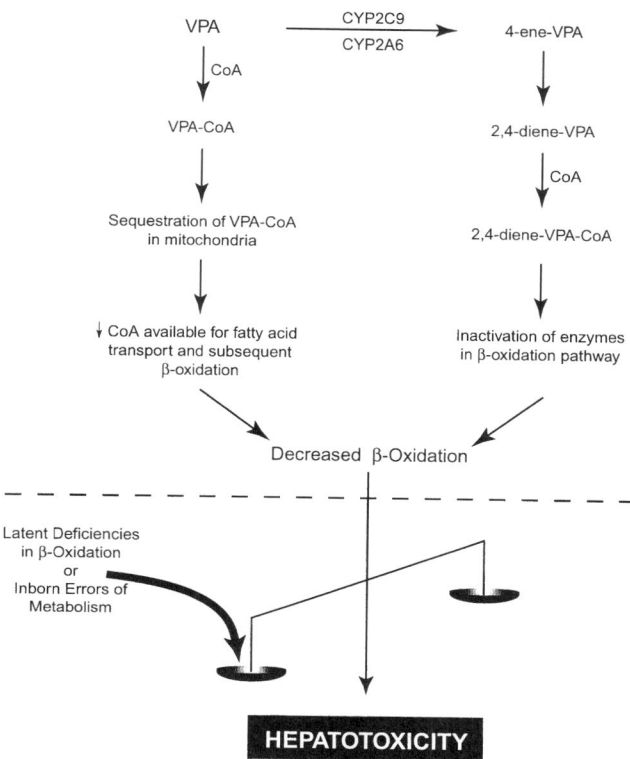

Figure 4 Hypothesis for the mechanism of VPA hepatotoxicity. Both the parent compound, VPA, and reactive metabolites from the bioactivation pathway can lead to decreased β-oxidation by various mechanisms. In patients rendered susceptible by inborn errors of metabolism or latent deficiencies in mitochondrial metabolism, the effects of VPA or its reactive metabolites on β-oxidation may tip the balance toward the manifestations of hepatotoxicity.

to conceptualize the VPA hepatotoxic process as proceeding by two parallel processes (Fig. 4): VPA itself depletes the intramitochondrial pool of CoA and thus inhibits the mitochondrial β-oxidation of long-, medium-, and short-chain natural fatty acids (117). Chemically reactive metabolites generated from 4-ene-VPA, such as 2,4-diene-VPA, have the potential to deplete mitochondrial glutathione pools (118) and, through formation of conjugates with CoA (119), inhibit enzymes in the β-oxidation pathway (102, 103). Identification of *N*-acetylcysteine conjugates of (*E*)-2,4-diene-VPA in human urine provides evidence that metabolites sufficiently reactive to form thiol adducts have been formed (120). These conjugates are potentially useful markers for future investigations assessing the relationship between reactive metabolite exposure and hepatic damage.

VII. FELBAMATE

Felbamate was approved as an antiepileptic agent in the United States in July 1993 for use as monotherapy and adjunctive therapy for partial seizures (with and without generalization) in adults and as adjunctive therapy for generalized seizures associated with Lennox-Gastaut syndrome in children. While felbamate provided significant benefits to treated patients, reports of aplastic anemia attributed to felbamate started to appear in mid-1994 as well as cases of hepatic failure, including four deaths, by the fall of 1994. The clinical use of felbamate was severely curtailed after September 1994 when the Food and Drug Administration issued a warning of a higher-than-expected incidence of aplastic anemia and hepatic failure among patients treated with the drug (121).

A. Clinical Manifestations and Pathology

The risk of hepatic failure due to felbamate was initially estimated to be 1 per 26,000–34,000 exposures (121) and has been revised to approximately 1 per 18,500–25,000 exposures (122). In one published case, a 61-year-old Caucasian woman presented with a chief complaint of nausea, vomiting, and lethargy over the previous 3.5 weeks (123). On the first day of hospitalization (day 24 of felbamate therapy), evidence of hepatic dysfunction (AST 601 U/L and γ-GT 978 U/L) and eosinophilia were present. Hepatic function continued to decline over the ensuing 2 weeks, ultimately progressing to multisystem organ failure. Massive to submassive necrosis without significant fibrosis was observed on microscopic sections and moderate inflammatory infiltrate consisting primarily of lymphocytes was present within portal tracts. Although few data are available to describe the typical presentation and clinical course, available information from seven cases of likely felbamate hepatotoxicity reveals a high incidence of females (6/7) and time to presentation of 25–181 days. Two of the seven patients were less than 12 years of age and an aromatic anticonvulsant (primidone, phenobarbital, phenytoin, or CBZ) was concomitantly administered in six cases (122).

B. Postulated Mechanisms

The mechanism of felbamate hepatotoxicity is unknown. However, considerable progress has been made over the past 5 years in identifying and characterizing potential reactive metabolites that may play a role in the pathogenesis of felbamate idiosyncratic toxicities. Evidence has been presented for an unstable aldehyde carbamate intermediate, 3-carbamoyl-2-phenylproprionaldehyde (aldehyde monocarbamate), in the pathway leading to the formation of the major metabolite in humans, 3-carbamoyl-2-phenylproprionic acid (acid monocarbamate; Fig. 5). This aldehyde carbamate metabolite predominantly undergoes reversible cyclization to form a stable cyclic structure that may serve as a "reservoir" for transport to tissues distant to the site of formation, the liver. Alternatively, it may undergo elimination to form 2-phenylpropenal (commonly called atropaldehyde), a potent electrophile that is toxic to cells in culture (124). Atropaldehyde undergoes rapid conjugation with glutathione and can be observed in urine from felbamate-treated patients as mercapturate derivatives (125). Formation of the aldehyde carbamate appears to be a "commitment step" whereby the molecule is committed to a detoxication pathway leading to 3-carbamoyl-2-phenylproprionic acid, the major urinary metabolite, or to a toxic pathway leading to atropaldehyde. The ratio of urinary mercapturate metabolites to the acid monocarbamate metabolite represents an estimate of the balance between bioactivation and detoxication, and may provide a marker for susceptibility to felbamate hepatotoxicity or aplastic anemia for future investigations (126).

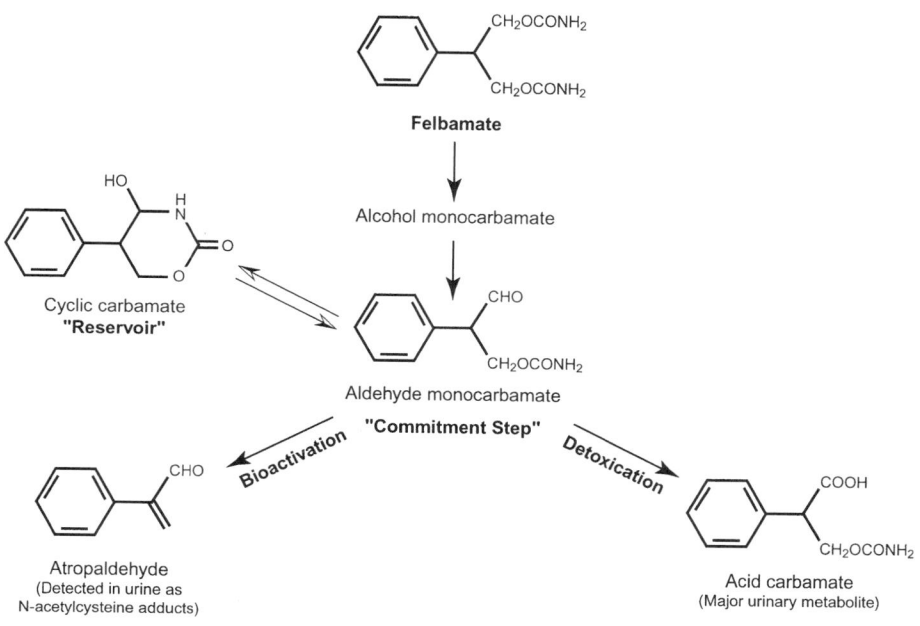

Figure 5 Proposed mechanism of felbamate bioactivation. The initial step toward felbamate bio-activation is thought to involve hydrolysis to form an alcohol monocarbamate metabolite that is further oxidized to an aldehyde monocarbamate. The aldehyde monocarbamate metabolite can cyclize to form a structure that has been proposed to function as a relatively stable "reservoir" for transport throughout the body. More importantly, the aldehyde monocarbamate metabolite represents a "commitment" step with commitment down a detoxication pathway to form the major urinary acid carbamate metabolite, or down a bioactivation pathway leading to the reactive metabolite, atro-paldehyde, which can be detected in urine as N-acetylcysteine adducts. Individual susceptibility may be determined, in part, by the relative contributions of each competing pathway.

VIII. LAMOTRIGINE

Lamotrigine, a phenyltriazine, is a broad-spectrum anticonvulsant that has been in use for about a decade. The main idiosyncratic adverse effects associated with lamotrigine use are skin rashes, which occur in 3–10% of patients (127). Children seem more to be more susceptible to cutaneous adverse reactions than adults (128). Such rashes, however, are often only one component of a generalized hypersensitivity reaction, which is also accompanied by fever and eosinophilia (129). In such cases, liver involvement is characterized by an abnormality of liver function without clinical symptoms of hepatitis (129). However, more severe liver damage from lamotrigine has also been reported; for example, there are two case reports of fulminant hepatic failure (130,131). In both patients, hepatic failure developed after introduction of lamotrigine, and was characterized by jaundice, an increase in transaminases, and coagulopathy that proved fatal in one case.

The mechanism of lamotrigine-induced hypersensitivity and hepatotoxicity is unclear. Patients started on high doses of lamotrigine and those on concomitant therapy with sodium valproate seem to be at higher risk of lamotrigine rashes; the strategy of starting at low doses and escalating the dose slowly seems to reduce the risk. The clinical symptomatology is suggestive of an immune-mediated pathogenesis, and is consistent with reports of positive lymphocyte transformation tests (132). As with the aromatic anticonvulsants, metabolism is likely to be important in the pathogenesis of the reactions. Lamotrigine largely undergoes *N*-glucuronidation with little oxidative metabolism (133,134). A recent study in a rat model has shown that lamotrigine can undergo bioactivation to an arene oxide (135), which may be important in the pathogenesis of the hypersensitivity reactions. No pharmacogenetic studies have been performed so far to investigate whether there is genetic predisposition to lamotrigine hypersensitivity.

IX. MANAGEMENT

The first and essential step in management of anticonvulsant-associated hepatotoxicity is the recognition that the drug is responsible for the hepatic injury. This is essentially a diagnosis of exclusion, and will require measurement of biochemical, immunological, and virological markers to exclude non-drug-induced diseases. If the drug is suspected, discontinuation of the offending agent is important. Subsequently, the management of severe hepatic toxicity attributed to anticonvulsant therapy is essentially supportive. Little evidence supports the use of steroids in treatment, even when the hepatic injury is thought to be immune-mediated. As a result, prevention and monitoring are more effective means of minimizing the impact of anticonvulsant-associated hepatotoxicity. In the case of VPA, risk factors are reasonably well characterized and the drug should be avoided in children less than 3 years of age and those treated with CYP-inducing aromatic anticonvulsants. Likewise, extreme caution should be exercised if a family history of fatty acid oxidation defects or urea cycle defects is present. If there has been a hepatic reaction to one aromatic anticonvulsant, then given the possibility of cross-sensitivity, the other aromatic anticonvulsants should be avoided. There is no evidence of cross-reactivity between the aromatic anticonvulsants and VPA, and this may be used for future control of seizures, although the drug should be introduced cautiously while liver function is still impaired. Routine monitoring of liver function tests is recommended by several manufacturers of the anticonvulsants reviewed; however, little evidence supports the predictive value of such monitoring. Therefore, as a general rule, clinicians should suspect and rule out hepatotoxicity in any patient who becomes ill in the first 6 months of anticonvulsant treatment.

REFERENCES

1. Chadwick D. Safety and efficacy of vigabatrin and carbamazepine in newly diagnosed epilepsy: a multicentre randomised double-blind study. Vigabatrin European Monotherapy Study Group [see comments]. Lancet 1999; 354:13–19.
2. Stricker BHC. Drug-Induced Hepatic Injury. Amsterdam: Elsevier Science Publishers, 1992.
3. Pellock JM. Carbamazepine side effects in children and adults. Epilepsia 1987; 28:S64–S70.
4. Askmark H, Wiholm B. Epidemiology of adverse drug reactions to carbamazepine as seen in a spontaneous reporting system. Acta Neurol Scand 1990; 81:131–140.
5. Døssing M, Andreasen PB. Drug-induced liver disease in Denmark: an analysis of 572 cases of hepatotoxicity reported to the Danish Board of Adverse Reactions to Drugs. Scand J Gastroenterol 1982; 17:205–211.
6. Friis H, Andreasen PB. Drug-induced hepatic injury: an analysis of 1100 cases reported to the Danish Committee on Adverse Drug Reactions between 1978 and 1987. J Intern Med 1992; 232:133–138.

7. Shear NH, Spielberg SP. Anticonvulsant hypersensitivity syndrome: in vitro assessment of risk. J Clin Invest 1988; 82:1826–1832.

8. Pirmohamed M, Park BK. Cytochromes P450 and liver injury. In: RG Cameron, G Feuer, F de la Iglesia, eds. Drug-Induced Hepatotoxicity. Vol. 121. Berlin: Springer-Verlag, 1996: 341–366.

9. Hadzic N, Portmann B, Davies ET, Mowat AP, Mieli-Vergani G. Acute liver failure induced by carbamazepine. Arch Dis Child 1990; 65:315–317.

10. Williams RJ, Ruppin DC, Grierson JM, Farrell GC. Carbamazepine hepatitis: the clinicopathological spectrum. J Gastroenterol Hepatol 1986; 1:159–168.

11. Levander HG. Granulomatous hepatitis in a patient receiving carbamazepine. Acta Med Scand 1980; 208.

12. Hopen G, Nesthus I, Laerum OD. Fatal carbamazepine-associated hepatitis: report of 2 cases. Acta Med Scand 1981; 210:333–335.

13. Soffer EE, Taylor RJ, Bertram PD, Hagitt RC, Levinson MJ. Carbamazepine-induced liver injury. South Med J 1983; 76:681–683.

14. Larrey D, Hadengue A, Pessayre D, Choudat L, Degott C, Benhamou JP. Carbamazepine-induced acute cholangitis. Dig Dis Sci 1987; 32:554–557.

15. Cox NH, Johnston SRD, Marks J, Bates D. Extensive carbamazepine eruption with eosinophilia and pulmonary infiltrate. Postgrad Med J 1988; 64:249–250.

16. Fellows WR. A case of aplastic anemia and pancytopenia with tegretol therapy. Headache 1969; 9:92–95.

17. Ponte CD. Carbamazepine-induced thrombocytopenia, rash, and hepatic dysfunction. Drug Intell Clin Pharm 1983; 17:642–644.

18. Imai H, Nakamoto Y, Hirokawa M, Akihama T, Miura AB. Carbamazepine-induced granulomatous necrotizing angiitis with acute renal failure. Nephron 1989; 51:405–408.

19. Levy M, Goodman MW, Van Dyre J, Summer HW. Granulomatous hepatitis secondary to carbamazepine. Ann Intern Med 1981; 95:64–65.

20. Mitchell MC, Boitnott JK, Arregui A, Maddrey WC. Granulomatous hepatitis associated with carbamazepine therapy. Am J Med 1981; 71:733–735.

21. Forbes GM, Jeffrey GP, Shilkin KB, Reed WD. Carbamazepine hepatotoxicity: another case of the vanishing bile duct syndrome. Gastroenterology 1992; 102:1385–1388.

22. Pirmohamed M, Graham A, Roberts P, Smith D, Chadwick D, Breckenridge AM, Park BK. Carbamazepine-hypersensitivity: assessment of clinical and in vitro chemical cross-reactivity with phenytoin and oxcarbazepine. Br J Clin Pharmacol 1991; 32:741–749.

23. Zimmerman HJ, Ishak KG. Antiepileptic drugs. In: RG Cameron, G Feuer, F de la Iglesia, eds. Drug-Induced Hepatotoxicity. Vol. 121. Berlin: Springer-Verlag, 1996:637–662.

24. Farrell GC. Drug-Induced Liver Disease. Edinburgh: Churchill Livingstone, 1994.

25. Murphy JV, Francisco CB, Roberts C. Fatal hepatorenal failure in 3 patients receiving carbamazepine. Ann Neurol 1991; 30:276–277.

26. Zakrzewska JM, Ivanyi L. In vitro lymphocyte proliferation by carbamazepine, carbamazepine-10,11-epoxide, and oxcarbazepine in the diagnosis of drug-induced hypersensitivity. J Allergy Clin Immunol 1988; 82:110–115.

27. Leeder JS, Riley RJ, Cook VA, Spielberg SP. Human anti-cytochrome P450 antibodies in aromatic anticonvulsant-induced hypersensitivity reactions. J Pharmacol Exp Ther 1992; 263: 360–367.

28. Pirmohamed M, Kitteringham NR, Breckenridge AM, Park BK. Detection of an autoantibody directed against human liver microsomal protein in a patient with carbamazepine hypersensitivity. Br J Clin Pharmacol 1992; 33:183–186.

29. Riley RJ, Smith G, Wolf CR, Cook VA, Leeder JS. Human anti-endoplasmic reticulum antibodies produced in aromatic anticonvulsant hypersensitivity reactions recognise rodent CYP3A proteins and a similarly regulated human P450 enzyme(s). Biochem Biophys Res Commun 1993; 191:32–40.

30. Leeder JS, Gaedigk A, Lu X, Cook VA. Epitope mapping studies with human anti-cytochrome P450 3A antibodies. Mol Pharmacol 1996; 49:234–243.

31. Horowitz S, Patwardhan R, Marcus E. Hepatotoxic reactions associated with carbamazepine therapy. Epilepsia 1988; 29:149–154.

32. Shear NH, Bhimji S. Pharmacogenetics and cutaneous drug reactions. Semin Dermatol 1988; 8:219–226.

33. Edwards SG, Hubbard V, Aylett S, Wren D. Concordance of primary generalised epilepsy and carbamazepine hypersensitivity in monozygotic twins. Postgrad Med J 1999; 75:680–681.

34. Gaedigk A, Spielberg SP, Grant DM. Characterization of the microsomal epoxide hydrolase gene in patients with anticonvulsant adverse drug reactions. Pharmacogenetics 1994; 4:142–153.

35. Green VJ, Pirmohamed M, Kitteringham NR, Gaedigk A, Grant DM, Boxer M, Burchell B, Park BK. Genetic analysis of microsomal epoxide hydrolase in patients with carbamazepine hypersensitivity. Biochem Pharmacol 1995; 50:1353–1359.

36. Pirmohamed M, Lin K, Chadwick D, Park BK. TNF-alpha promoter region gene polymorphisms in carbamazepine hypersensitive patients. Neurology 2001; 56:890–896.

37. Pirmohamed M, Kitteringham NR, Guenthner TM, Breckenridge AM, Park BK. An investigation of the formation of cytotoxic, protein-reactive and stable metabolites from carbamazepine in vitro. Biochem Pharmacol 1992; 43:1675–1682.

38. Tybring G, von Bahr C, Bertilsson L, Collste H, Glaumann H, Solbrand M. Metabolism of carbamazepine and its epoxide metabolite in human and rat liver in vitro. Drug Metab Dispos 1981; 9:561–564.

39. Eichelbaum M, Thomson T, Tybring G, Bertilsson L. Carbamazepine metabolism in man: induction and pharmacogenetic aspects. Clin Pharmacokin 1985; 10:80–90.

40. Kroetz DL, Kerr BM, McFarland LV, Loiseau P, Wilensky AJ, Levy RH. Measurement of in vivo microsomal epoxide hydrolase activity in white subjects. Clin Pharmacol Ther 1993; 53:306–315.

41. Madden S, Maggs JL, Park BK. Bioactivation of carbamazepine in the rat in vivo. Evidence for the formation of reactive arene oxide(s). Drug Metab Dispos 1996; 24:469–479.

42. Lertratanangkoon K, Horning MG. Metabolism of carbamazepine. Drug Metab Dispos 1982; 10:1–10.

43. Pirmohamed M, Kitteringham NR, Breckenridge AM, Park BK. The effect of enzyme induction on the cytochrome P450-mediated bioactivation of carbamazepine by mouse liver microsomes. Biochem Pharmacol 1992; 44:2307–2314.

44. Kerr BM, Thummel KE, Wurden CJ, Klein SM, Kroetz DL, Gonzalez FJ, Levy RH. Human liver carbamazepine metabolism. Role of CYP3A4 and CYP2C8 in 10,11-epoxide formation. Biochem Pharmacol 1994; 47:1969–1979.

45. Bernus I, Dickinson RG, Hooper WD, Eadie MJ. Early-stage autoinduction of carbamazepine metabolism in humans. Eur J Clin Pharmacol 1994; 47:355–360.

46. Lillibridge JH, Amore BM, Slattery JT, Kalhorn TF, Nelson SD, Finnell RH, Bennett GD. Protein-reactive metabolites of carbamazepine in mouse liver microsomes. Drug Metab Dispos 1996; 24:509–514.

47. Ju C, Uetrecht JP. Detection of 2-hydroxyiminostilbene in the urine of patients taking carbamazepine and its oxidation to a reactive iminoquinone intermediate. J Pharmacol Exp Ther 1999; 288:51–56.

48. Leeder JS. Mechanisms of idiosyncratic hypersensitivity reactions to antiepileptic drugs. Epilepsia 1998; 39(suppl 7):S8–S16.

49. Mauri-Hellweg D, Bettens F, Mauri D, Brander C, Hunziker T, Pichler WJ. Activation of drug-specific CD4$^+$ and CD8$^+$ T cells in individuals allergic to sulfonamides, phenytoin, and carbamazepine. J Immunol 1995; 155:462–472.

50. Friedmann PS, Strickland I, Pirmohamed M, Park BK. Investigation of mechanisms in toxic epidermal necrolysis induced by carbamazepine. Arch Dermatol 1994; 130:598–604.

51. Pirmohamed M, Breckenridge AM, Kitteringham NR, Park BK. Adverse drug reactions. Br Med J 1998; 316:1295–1298.

52. Isojarvi JIT, Pakarinen AJ, Rautio A, Pelkonen O, Myllyla VV. Liver enzyme induction and serum lipid levels after replacement of carbamazepine with oxcarbazepine. Epilepsia 1994; 35:1217–1220.

53. Jensen NO, Dam M, Jakobsen K. Oxcarbazepine in patients hypersensitive to carbamazepine. Irish J Med Sci 1986; 155:297.

54. Beran RG. Cross-reactive skin eruption with both carbamazepine and oxcarbazepine. Epilepsia 1993; 34:163–165.

55. Haruda F. Phenytoin hypersensitivity: 38 cases. Neurology 1979; 29:1480–1485.

56. Mullick FG, Ishak KG. Hepatic injury associated with diphenylhydantoin therapy: a clinicopathological study of 20 cases. Am J Clin Pathol 1980; 74:442–452.

57. Park BK, Wilson AC, Kaatz G, Ohnhaus EE. Enzyme induction by phenobarbitone and vitamin K1 disposition in man. Br J Clin Pharmacol 1984; 18:94–97.

58. Aiges HW, Daum F, Olson M, Kahn E, Teichberg S. The effects of phenobarbital and diphenylhydantoin on liver function and morphology. J Pediatr 1980; 97:22–26.

59. Flowers FP, Araujo OE, Hamm KA. Phenytoin hypersensitivity syndrome. J Emerg Med 1987; 5:103–108.

60. Egertonvernon JM, Fisk MJ, Snell AP. Phenytoin-induced hepatotoxicity. NZ Med J 1983; 96:467–469.

61. Masso JFM, Carrera N, Zabalza R, Bengoechea MG. Phenytoin (diphenylhydantoin) induced hepatotoxicity. Med Clin 1983; 81:320–321.

62. Smythe MA, Umstead GS. Phenytoin hepatotoxicity: a review of the literature. Drug Intell Clin Pharm 1989; 23:13–18.

63. Dreifuss FE, Langer DH. Hepatic considerations in the use of antiepileptic drugs. Epilepsia 1987; 28(suppl 2):S23–S29.

64. Bryant AE, Dreifuss FE. Hepatotoxicity associated with antiepileptic drug therapy—avoidance, identification and management. CNS Drugs 1995; 4:99–13.

65. Spechler SJ, Sperber H, Doos WG, Koff RS. Cholestasis and toxic epidermal necrolysis associated with phenytoin sodium: the role of bile duct injury. Ann Intern Med 1981; 95:455–456.

66. Spielberg SP, Gordon GB, Blake DA, Goldstein DA, Herlong HF. Predisposition to phenytoin hepatotoxicity assessed in vitro. N Engl J Med 1981; 305:722–727.

67. Tomsick RS. The phenytoin syndrome. Cutis 1983; 32:535–537.

68. Vittorio CC, Muglia JJ. Anticonvulsant hypersensitivity syndrome. Arch Intern Med 1995; 155:2285–2290.

69. Gennis MA, Vemuri R, Burns EA, Hill JV, Miller MA, Spielberg SP. Familial occurrence of hypersensitivity to phenytoin. Am J Med 1991; 91:631–634.

70. Spielberg SP. In vitro assessment of pharmacogenetic susceptibility to toxic drug metabolites in humans. Fed Proc 1984; 43:2308–2313.

71. Kleckner HB, Yakulis V, Heller P. Severe hypersensitivity to diphenylhydantoin with circulating antibodies to the drug. Ann Intern Med 1975; 83:522–523.

72. Spielberg SP, Gordon GB, Blake DA, Mellits ED, Bross DS. Anticonvulsant toxicity in vitro: Possible role of arene oxides. J Pharmacol Exp Ther 1981; 217:386–389.

73. Munns AJ, De Voss JJ, Hooper WD, Dickinson RG, Gillam EMJ. Bioactivation of phenytoin by human cytochrome P450: characterization of the mechanism and targets of covalent adduct formation. Chem Res Toxicol 1997; 10:1049–1058.

74. Cuttle L, Munns AJ, Hogg NA, Scott JR, Hooper WD, Dickinson RG, Gillam EMJ. Phenytoin metabolism by human cytochrome P450: involvement of P450 3A and 2C forms in secondary metabolism and drug-protein adduct formation. Drug Metab Dispos 2000; 28:945–950.

75. Komatsu T, Yamazaki H, Asahi S, Gillam EMJ, Guengerich FP, Nakajima M, Yokoi T.

Formation of a dihydroxy metabolite of phenytoin in human liver microsomes/cytosol: roles of cytochromes P450 2C9, 2C19, and 3A4. Drug Metab Dispos 2000; 28:1362–1368.

76. Evans WE, Self TH, Weisburst MR. Phenobarbital-induced hepatic dysfunction. Drug Intell Clin Pharm 1976; 10:439–443.

77. Hyson C, Sadler M. Cross sensitivity of skin rashes with antiepileptic drugs. Can J Neurol Sci 1997; 24:245–249.

78. Bourgeois BFD. Valproic acid: clinical use. In: RH Levy, RH Mattson, BS Meldrum, eds. Antiepileptic Drugs. 4th ed. New York: Raven Press, 1995:633–640.

79. Dreifuss FE. Valproic acid: toxicity. In: RH Levy, RH Mattson, BS Meldrum, eds. Antiepileptic Drugs. 4th ed. New York: Raven Press, 1995:641–648.

80. Sussman NM, McLain LW. A direct hepatotoxic effect of valproic acid. JAMA 1979; 242: 1173–1174.

81. Zimmerman HJ, Ishak KG. Valproate-induced hepatic injury: analysis of 23 fatal cases. Hepatology 1982; 2:591–597.

82. Dreifuss FE, Santilli N, Langer DH, Sweeney KP, Moline KA, Menander KB. Valproic acid hepatic fatalities: a retrospective review. Neurology 1987; 37:379–385.

83. Scheffner D, König S, Rauterberg-Ruland I, Kochen W, Hofmann WJ, Unkelbach S. Fatal liver failure in 16 children with valproate therapy. Epilepsia 1988; 29:530–542.

84. Dreifuss FE, Langer DH, Moline KA, Maxwell JE. Valproic acid hepatic fatalities. II. US experience since 1984. Neurology 1989; 39:201–207.

85. König SA, Siemes H, Bläker F, Boenigk E, Groß-Selbeck G, Hanefeld F, Haas N, Köhler B, Korinthenberg R, Kurek E, Lenard H-G, Penin H, Penzien JM, Schünke W, Schultze C, Stephani U, Stute M, Traus M, Weinmann H-M, Scheffner D. Severe hepatotoxicity during valproate therapy: an update and report of eight new fatalities. Epilepsia 1994; 35:1005–1015.

86. Bryant AE, Dreifuss FE. Valproic acid hepatic fatalities. III. U.S. experience since 1986. Neurology 1996; 46:465–469.

87. Kay JDS, Hilton-Jones D, Hyman N. Valproate toxicity and ornithine carbamoyltransferase deficiency. Lancet 1986; 2:1283–1284.

88. Eadie MJ, McKinnon GE, Dunston PR, McLaughlin D, Dickinson RG. Valproate metabolism during hepatotoxicity associated with the drug. Q J Med 1990; 284:1229–1240.

89. Tokatli A, Coskun S, Cataltepe S, Ozalp I. Valproate-induced lethal hyperammonemic coma in a carrier of ornithine transcarbamylase deficiency. J Inher Metab Dis 1991; 14:836–837.

90. Honeycutt D, Callahan K, Rutledge L, Wans B. Heterozygotic ornithine transcarbamylase deficiency presenting as symptomatic hyperammonemia during initiation of valproate treatment. Neurology 1992; 42:666.

91. Suchy FJ, Balistreri WF, Buchino JJ, Sondheimer JM, Bates SR, Kearns GL, Stull JD, Bove KE. Acute hepatic failure associated with the use of sodium valproate. N Engl J Med 1979; 300:962–966.

92. Kondo T, Kaneko S, Otani K, Ishida M, Hirano T, Fukushima Y, Muranaka H, Koide N, Yokoyama M. Associations between risk factors for valproate hepatotoxicity and altered valproate metabolism. Epilepsia 1992; 33:172–177.

93. Anderson GD, Acheampong AA, Wilensky AJ, Levy RH. Effect of valproate dose on formation of hepatotoxic metabolites. Epilepsia 1992; 33:736–742.

94. Millington DS, Bohan TP, Roe CR, Yergey AL, Liberato DJ. Valproylcarnitine: a novel drug metabolite identified by fast atom bombardment and thermospray liquid chromatography-mass spectrometry. Clin Chim Acta 1985; 145:69–76.

95. Krähenbühl S, Mang G, Kupferschmidt H, Meier PJ, Krause M. Plasma and hepatic carnitine and coenzyme A pools in a patient with fatal, valproate induced hepatotoxicity. Gut 1995; 37:140–143.

96. Li J, Norwood DL, Mao L-F, Schulz H. Mitochondrial metabolism of valproic acid. Biochemistry 1991; 30:388–394.

97. Ponchaut S, Draye JP, Veitch K. In vitro effects of valproate and valproate metabolites on mitochondrial oxidations: relevance of CoA sequestration to the observed inhibitions. Biochem Pharmacol 1992; 43:2435–2442.

98. Bjorge SM, Baillie TA. Inhibition of medium-chain fatty acid β-oxidation in vivo by valproic acid and its unsaturated metabolite, 2-*n*-propyl—4-pentenoic acid. Biochem Biophys Res Commun 1985; 132:245–252.

99. Kesterson JW, Granneman GR, Machinist JM. The hepatotoxicity of valproic acid and its metabolites in rats. I. Toxicologic, biochemical and histopathologic studies. Hepatology 1984; 4:1143–1152.

100. Granneman GR, Wang SI, Kesterson JW, Machinist JM. The hepatotoxicity of valproic acid and its metabolites in rats. II. Intermediary and valproic acid metabolism. Hepatology 1984; 4:1153–1158.

101. Kingsley E, Gray PD, Tolman KG, Tweedale R. The toxicity of the metabolites of sodium valproate in cultured hepatocytes. J Clin Pharmacol 1983; 23:178–185.

102. Rettenmeier AW, Prickett KS, Gordon WP, Bjorge SM, Chang SL, Levy RH, Baillie TA. Studies on the biotransformation in the perfused rat liver of 2-*n*-propyl-4-pentenoic acid, a metabolite of the antiepileptic drug valproic acid. Evidence for the formation of chemically reactive intermediates. Drug Metab Dispos 1985; 13:81–96.

103. Baillie TA. Metabolic activation of valproic acid and drug-mediated hepatotoxicity. Role of the terminal olefin, 2-*n*-propyl-4-pentenoic acid. Chem Res Toxicol 1988; 1:195–199.

104. Rettie AE, Rettenmeier AW, Howald WN, Baillie TA. Cytochrome P-450-catalyzed formation of Δ^4-VPA, a toxic metabolite of valproic acid. Science 1987; 235:890–893.

105. Sadeque AJM, Fisher MB, Korzekwa KR, Gonzalez FJ, Rettie AE. Human CYP2C9 and CYP2A6 mediate formation of the hepatotoxin 4-ene-valproic acid. J Pharmacol Exp Ther 1997; 283:698–703.

106. Levy RH, Rettemeier AW, Anderson GD, Wilensky AJ, Friel PN, Baillie TA, Acheampong A, Tor J, Guyot M, Loiseau P. Effect of polytherapy with phenytoin, carbamazepine, and stirpentol on formation of 4-ene-valproate, a hepatotoxic metabolite of valproic acid. Clin Pharmacol Ther 1990; 48:225–235.

107. Donato MT, Gómez-Lechón MJ, Castell JV. Effect of model inducers on cytochrome P450 activities of human hepatocytes in primary culture. Drug Metab Dispos 1995; 23:553–558.

108. Chang TKH, L. Y, Maurel P, Waxman DJ. Enhanced cyclophosphamide and ifosfamide activation in primary human hepatocyte cultures: response to cytochrome P-450 inducers and autoinduction by oxazaphosphorines. Cancer Res 1997; 57:1946–1954.

109. Wrighton SA, Brian WR, Sari M-A, Iwasaki M, Guengerich FP, Raucy JL, Molowa DT, Vandenbranden M. Studies on the expression and metabolic capabilities of human liver cytochrome P450IIIA5 (HLp3). Mol Pharmacol 1990; 38:207–213.

110. Waxman DJ, Azaroff L. Phenobarbital induction of cytochrome P-450 gene expression. Biochem J 1992; 281:577–592.

111. Leeder JS, Kearns GL. Pharmacogenetics in pediatrics. Implications for practice. Pediatr Clin North Am 1997; 44:55–77.

112. Shen DD, Pollack GM, Cohen ME, Duffner P, Lacey D, Ryan-Dudek P. Effect of age on the serum metabolite pattern of valproic acid in epileptic children. Epilepsia 1984; 25:674.

113. Kochen W, Schneider A, Ritz A. Abnormal metabolism of valproic acid in fatal hepatic failure. Eur J Pediatr 1983; 141:30–35.

114. Paganini M, Zaccara G, Moroni F, Campostrini R, Bendoni L, Arnetoli G, Zappoli R. Lack of relationship between sodium valproate-induced adverse effects and the plasma concentration of its metabolite 2-propylpenten-4-oic acid. Eur J Clin Pharmacol 1987; 32:219–222.

115. Tennison MB, Miles MV, Pollack GM, Thorn MD, Dupuis RE. Valproate metabolites and hepatotoxicity in an epileptic population. Epilepsia 1988; 29:543–547.

116. Siemes H, Nau H, Schultze K, Wittfoht W, Drews E, Penzien J, Seidel U. Valproate (VPA)

metabolites in various clinical conditions of probable VPA-associated hepatotoxicity. Epilepsia 1993; 34:332–346.

117. Fromenty B, Pessayre D. Inhibition of mitochondrial β-oxidation as a mechanism of hepatotoxicity. Pharmacol Ther 1995; 67:101–154.

118. Kassahun K, Farrell K, Abbott FS. Identification and characterization of the glutathione and *N*-acetylcysteine conjugates of (*E*)-2-propyl-2,4-pentadienoic acid, a toxic metabolite of valproic acid, in rats and humans. Drug Metab Dispos 1991; 19:525–535.

119. Kassahun K, Abbott FS. In vivo formation of the thiol conjugates of reactive metabolites of 4-ene-VPA and its analogue 4-pentenoic acid. Drug Metab Dispos 1993; 21:1098–1106.

120. Gopaul SV, Farrell K, Abbott FS. Identification and characterization of *N*-acetylcysteine conjugates of valproic acid in humans and animals. Drug Metab Dispos 2000; 28:823–832.

121. Pellock JM, Brodie MJ. Felbamate: 1997 update. Epilepsia 1997; 38:1261–1264.

122. Pellock JM. Felbamate. Epilepsia 1999; 40(suppl 5):S57–S62.

123. O'Neil MG, Perdun CS, Wilson MB, McGown ST, Patel S. Felbamate-associated fatal acute hepatic necrosis. Neurology 1996; 46:1457–1459.

124. Thompson CD, Kinter MT, Macdonald TL. Synthesis and in vitro reactivity of 3-carbamoyl-2-phenylproprionaldehyde and 2-phenylpropenal: putative reactive metabolites of felbamate. Chem Res Toxicol 1996; 9:1225–1229.

125. Thompson CD, Gulden PH, Macdonald TL. Identification of modified atropaldehyde mercapturic acids in rat and human urine after felbamate administration. Chem Res Toxicol 1997; 10:457–462.

126. Thompson CD, Barthen MT, Hopper DW, Miller TA, Quigg M, Hudspeth C, Montouris G, Marsh L, Perhach JL, Sofia DR, Macdonald TL. Quantification in patient urine samples of felbamate and three metabolites: acid carbamate and two mercapturic acids. Epilepsia 1999; 40:769–776.

127. Buchanan N. Lamotrigine: clinical experience in 200 patients with epilepsy with follow-up to four years. Seizure 1996; 5:209–214.

128. Dooley J, Camfield P, Gordon K, Camfield C, Wirrell E, Smith E. Lamotrigine-induced rash in children. Neurology 1996; 46:240–242.

129. Schlienger RG, Knowles SR, Shear NH. Lamotrigine-associated anticonvulsant hypersensitivity syndrome. Neurology 1998; 51:1172–1175.

130. Makin AJ, Fitt S, Williams R, Duncan JS. Fulminant hepatic failure induced by lamotrigine. Br Med J 1995; 311:292.

131. Arnon R, DeVivo D, Defelice AR, Kazlow PG. Acute hepatic failure in a child treated with lamotrigine. Pediatr Neurol 1998; 18:251–253.

132. Sachs B, Ronnau AC, von Schmiedeberg S, Ruzicka T, Gleichmann E, Schuppe HC. Lamotrigine-induced Stevens-Johnson syndrome: demonstration of specific lymphocyte reactivity in vitro. Dermatology 1997; 195:60–64.

133. Yuen AWC, Land G, Weatherley BC, Peck AW. Sodium valproate acutely inhibits lamotrigine metabolism. Br J Clin Pharmacol 1992; 33:511–513.

134. Brody MJ. Lamotrigine. Lancet 1992; 339:1397–400.

135. Maggs JL, Naisbitt DJ, Tettey JNA, Pirmohamed M, Park BK. Metabolism of lamotrigine to a reactive arene oxide intermediate. Chem Res Toxicol 2000; 13:1075–1081.

19

Hepatotoxicity of Psychotropic Drugs and Drugs of Abuse

KIA SAEIAN

Medical College of Wisconsin, Milwaukee, Wisconsin, U.S.A.

K. RAJENDER REDDY

University of Pennsylvania, Philadelphia, Pennsylvania, U.S.A.

I. INTRODUCTION

Many psychoactive medications are highly fat-soluble and require hepatic metabolism. Therefore, not surprisingly, metabolism of many these drugs is affected by hepatic dysfunction and, further, their metabolites may have hepatotoxic effects. The majority of psychotropic drugs cause a hepatitis-like illness but some may lead to a cholestatic picture. In fact, chlorpromazine's mechanism of cholestatic injury represents one of the most elegantly elucidated examples of drug-induced liver injury. A few drugs cause a mixed hepatocellular-cholestatic form of injury (Fig. 1).

The associated symptoms, particularly the prolonged pruritus due to cholestasis, may be quite distressing to the patient and frustrating to the physician but fulminant hepatic failure is uncommon. Vigilant monitoring of liver enzymes, particularly in patients with underlying liver disease, is justified. Discontinuation or dose modification is warranted if hepatic biochemical tests become elevated to >3.5 times the upper limits of normal.

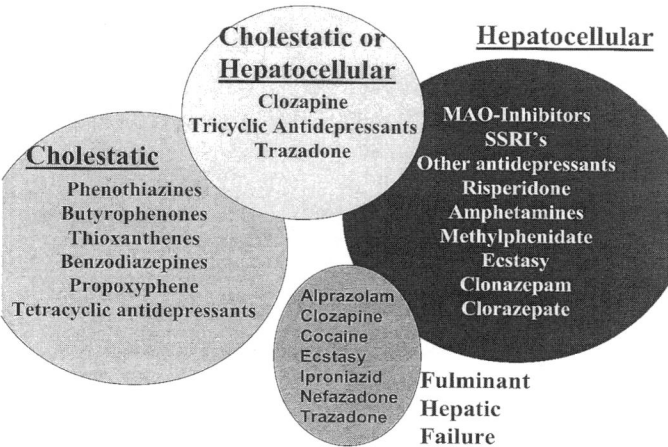

Figure 1 The predominant pattern of injury caused by psychotropic drugs is hepatocellular, but some result in cholestatic injury and a few in a mixed hepatocellular and cholestatic pattern. Only a few drugs have been noted to result in fulminant hepatic failure.

II. ANTIPSYCHOTIC MEDICATIONS (Table 1)

The most extensively studied of the psychotropic drugs appears to be the phenothiazine *chlorpromazine* (Thorazine), which was developed in 1951 as a central nervous system depressant. Partly because of its widespread use, reports of chlorpromazine's hepatotoxicity quickly followed and elegant studies of its mechanism of injury have made this medication a classic example of hepatocanalicular cholestatic injury. Overall, 1–3% of individuals on phenothiazines as well as those on haloperidol may have a hypersensitivity reaction (1). Progression to cirrhosis is rare and recovery can be expected within 2–12 months (1).

A. Phenothiazines

Although predominantly a cholestatic presentation is seen with the phenothiazines, mild hepatocellular necrosis and microscopic cholangitis in the portal tracts may also be encountered (2). Unlike many other drugs that lead to impaired bile secretion by a diffuse cytotoxic mechanism, the phenothiazines seem to selectively inhibit bile secretory function. It is not surprising, then, that the phenothiazines, chlorpromazine in particular, have been extensively studied to further elucidate the specific steps of bile secretion and to obtain more information regarding drug-induced cholestasis.

Table 1 Pattern of Injury of Antipsychotic Medications

Cholestatic	Hepatocellular
Butyrophenones (e.g., haloperidol) (30–32)	Clozapine[a] (43–46)
Clozapine[a] (48)	Loxapine (50)
Phenothiazines (e.g., chlorpromazine)[b] (3,4)	Molindone (49)
Thioxanthenes (e.g., chlorprothixene) (33–34)	Risperidone (36–38)

[a] May cause both hepatocellular and cholestatic injury.
[b] Rarely, chlorpromazine-induced injury is in a hepatocellular pattern.

In Ishak and Irey's classic review of 94 cases of presumed phenothiazine-induced toxicity referred to the Armed Forces Institute of Pathology (AFIP), more extensive evaluation determined that 47 cases resulted from other causes of liver disease (3). A total of 36 cases had good, convincing evidence of phenothiazine-induced toxicity. In the remaining 11, the relationship to the medication was uncertain. Of the group of the 36 with convincing evidence of phenothiazine-induced toxicity, 33 had received *chlorpromazine*, with one of these 33 having received *promazine* as well. The other three patients had received *prochlorperazine* (Compazine) (3).

1. Chlorpromazine

Chlorpromazine's hepatotoxicity is now well established with jaundice having been reported in 0.5–1.2% of recipients (3,4).

Clinical Presentation.   On initial presentation, the picture may be confused with extrahepatic biliary obstruction because a cholestatic illness is characterized with marked elevation of alkaline phosphatase, bilirubin, and cholesterol values. Typically aminotransferase elevations are minimal. A transient eosinophilia is present in 10–40% of cases. Accompanying agranulocytosis and/or thrombocytopenia may also be seen (3). A prodromal viral-like syndrome may be noted in approximately two-thirds of the patients. Anorexia, nausea, and abdominal pain may follow. The majority of patients develop pruritus that may be quite bothersome. Although rare, at least one case of chronic hepatitis has been attributed to chlorpromazine 4 weeks after initiation of therapy (5).

Liver biopsy findings include bile stasis, predominantly in zone 3, with some hepatocyte necrosis and portal inflammation. Eosinophils may also be seen and their presence supports a drug-induced etiology.

Course of Disease.   Most episodes of toxicity have been noted after 2–3 weeks of exposure although cases have been noted as late as 10 weeks and as early as 5 days. After cessation of the medication, the majority of patients symptomatically recover within a month of withdrawal of the medication. Liver enzyme abnormalities usually persist for a longer time with one report noting elevations in 7% after 6 months (6). Corticosteroids are of no proven benefit.

In some patients, a prolonged course may evolve. A process resembling primary biliary cirrhosis has been described and called the vanishing bile duct syndrome (7). Although classically seen with chlorpromazine, it has also been seen with other drugs including thiabendazole, tolbutamide, and cotrimoxazole among others.

Liver biopsy reveals marked paucity of bile ducts and changes of cholestasis. The disease may be self-limited but cirrhosis and complications of end-stage liver disease may ensue. In a review of 31 reported cases, the jaundice lasted anywhere from 6 to 76 months (7). Chronic jaundice, defined as lasting at least 6 months, was used for inclusion. Onset of jaundice had occurred approximately 14 days after initial exposure. Pruritus was common. No dose-related effect was reported. Examination frequently found hepatomegaly, splenomegaly, and xanthomatous skin changes. Hepatic biochemical tests are distinguished by a markedly elevated alkaline phosphatase. Despite the finding of steatorrhea, very high cholesterol levels are also found (7).

Mechanism of Toxicity.   The time course of injury, the presence of eosinophilia, and recurrence on repeat exposure all support hypersensitivity's contribution to the mechanism of chlorpromazine hepatotoxicity (8–10). The immunological reaction may be directed at chlorpromazine itself or one of its more than 170 identified metabolites. The drug is also intrinsically toxic to the liver and most treated patients experience subclinical cholestasis. It is likely that hypersensitivity and intrinsic toxicity both contribute to the frequent cholestatic injury seen with this medication.

Chlorpromazine is a cationic detergent that is highly concentrated in bile and undergoes enterohepatic circulation. In humans and experimental animals, it alters the physical properties of hepatocellular membranes and induces marked cholestasis. Multiple mechanisms of injury including impaired synthesis, secretion, and uptake of bile acids, decreased bile-salt-independent flow, altered canalicular membrane enzymes, abnormal permeability of the canalicular membranes, modified gelation and polymerization of actin, inhibition of Na^+, K^+-ATPase activity (an effect diminished by glutathione administration), accumulation of intracanalicular precipitates, and enhanced bile viscosity have been demonstrated (8–12).

Cyclooxygenase inhibitors such as indomethacin and ibuprofen prevent the decrease in chlorpromazine-induced hepatic bile flow. This finding supports the theory that arachidonic acid–derived metabolites, most notably prostanoids, may be involved in inhibition of bile flow (13).

Ultrastructural study of a perfused rat liver has demonstrated that infusion of taurodeoxycholate resolved chlorpromazine-induced changes such as dilatation of canaliculi and fragmentation or loss of canalicular microvilli (14). Taurodeoxycholate, but not taurocholate, also reverses chlorpromazine-induced cholestasis in the isolated perfused rat liver, a difference attributed to its relative hydrophobic properties (15). Ultrastructural analysis of liver biopsy tissue from a woman with acute chlorpromazine-induced hepatotoxicity showed not only swollen and damaged bile ducts but also marked proliferation of peroxisomes and mitochondria. It is unclear whether these latter changes result directly from the drug or occur as part of the liver injury and/or regeneration (16).

Susceptibility to chlorpromazine toxicity has also been evaluated. One such study postulated that individuals who were poor sulfoxidizers would be more susceptible to chlorpromazine-induced jaundice. The capacity for hydroxylation and sulfoxidation was assessed in healthy controls, subjects with chronic liver disease, and subjects with known history of chlorpromazine-induced jaundice. All of the subjects with a history of chlorpromazine-induced jaundice were poor sulfoxidizers compared to only 22% of healthy controls and 23.8% of chronic liver disease subjects. Hydroxylation capacity was intact (17). One study found that four of five patients with known chlorpromazine hepatitis as compared to 22% of controls had HLA DR6 phenotype (18). Chronic alcohol consumption also predisposes to cholestasis due to chlorpromazine (19). Thus it appears that there might be host and environmental factors that influence susceptibility to chlorpromazine hepatotoxicity.

2. Other Phenothiazines

Cyamemazine, a phenothiazine closely related to chlorpromazine in structure, has rarely been associated with hepatotoxicity. A series of six cases have been reported with one of them being a 23-year-old woman who had ingested a full bottle of cyamemazine (total dose of 4 gm) and subsequently developed pruritus 16 days after the suicide attempt and developed jaundice at day 25 (20,21). Liver biopsy showed moderate infiltration of portal tracts by lymphocytes, monocytes, neutrophils, and eosinophils. Few necrotic hepatocytes were seen but the predominant feature was of centrilobular cholestasis with canalicular bile plugs. There was slow improvement in the pruritus and subsequent normalization of liver enzymes after 2 months (20). A case report has outlined cross-hepatotoxicity between cyamemazine and the tricyclic antidepressants *desipramine* (Pertofran) and *trimipramine* (Surmontil) (22). All three drugs have a similar molecular structure.

Thioridazine (Mellaril) is felt to have a very low incidence of jaundice and/or hepatitis but at least seven cases of hepatitis (one cholestatic) have been reported (23,24). One of these cases was associated with agranulocytosis (25). *Trifluoperazine* (Stelazine) has been reported to result in jaundice (26,27). In a 26-year-old woman, jaundice was noted 2 weeks after initiation of the medication with resolution 18 days later. Subsequent haloperidol therapy was well tolerated (27). Interestingly, trifluoperazine results in calmodulin antagonism. This antagonism has been shown to be protective in animal models of acetaminophen-induced carbon tetrachloride injury (28,29).

B. Butyrophenones

Haloperidol (Haldol) is the most commonly used agent in this group and has infrequently been associated with cholestatic liver injury (30). *Bromperidol* (31) and *sulpiride* (32) have also been noted to cause reversible hepatitis after a short period of therapy.

C. Thioxanthenes

The thioxanthenes *chlorprothixene* (Taractan) and *clopenthixol* (Ordinol) have caused cholestatic jaundice and abnormal transaminases (33,34).

D. Other Antipsychotics

1. Risperidone

A novel antipsychotic agent, *risperidone* (Risperdal) has potent serotonin and dopamine antagonist properties. It is a nonphenothiazine antipsychotic (a benzisoxazole derivative) with a different structure than other antipsychotics that have been associated with hepatotoxicity. Nevertheless, cases of hepatotoxicity have been attributed to this drug. In 1996, two schizophrenic patients, one of whom had alcoholic liver disease, developed hepatotoxicity due to risperidone. One of the two patients had jaundice, which reversed upon discontinuation of the medication (35).

A number of subsequent reports have reported abnormal hepatic biochemical profile, weight gain and/or obesity, and steatosis and/or steatohepatitis (36–38). In at least one case, there was baseline obesity (37) and in another, no biopsy was done (38). A case of an 81-year-old man who developed jaundice after only two doses of risperidone has also been reported. He had mild right-upper-quadrant discomfort and no other symptoms. Repeat transaminases 2 weeks later had normalized (39).

It has been suggested based on observations of hepatotoxicity that prior to treatment with risperidone baseline liver function tests be performed and patients be followed with careful monitoring of weight and transaminases during the maintenance phase of therapy (36). A subsequent response from the manufacturer, Janssen Pharmaceuticals, questions the need for such monitoring (40).

2. Clozapine

Clozapine (Clozaril) is an atypical antipsychotic agent that is quite effective in previously treatment-resistant schizophrenia. Further, it has a low incidence of extrapyramidal symptoms. Its most feared adverse effect, however, is agranulocytosis. Clozapine has been noted to be a frequent cause of hepatic biochemical test abnormalities with reports ranging from 1 to 31% but with most of them resolving within the first 13–18 weeks (41).

In a prospective nonrandomized clozapine-drug-monitoring study, patients on clozapine were compared to a group on haloperidol (42). All patients had normal transaminases prior to treatment and were followed for 13 weeks. Patients on clozapine (37.3%) had significantly more frequent elevations of aspartate aminotransferase (AST), of at least twice the upper limit of normal, than those treated with haloperidol (16.6%). At least 60% of the cases of abnormal AST resolved within the first 13 weeks of treatment. In this study, male gender and higher plasma clozapine levels were associated with higher risk for increase in AST. In one case clozapine was discontinued because of elevated AST but subsequent reinitiation of the drug was without evidence of hepatotoxicity. In the event of persistently elevated enzymes, the investigators suggest dose reduction with concurrent monitoring of clozapine plasma levels (42). While clinically significant hepatotoxicity is infrequent, laboratory monitoring is recommended by some (43). There are reported cases of clozapine-induced hepatitis with diffuse liver damage with or without systemic symptoms as well as marked elevation of aminotransferases (43–45). One report describes two cases that resulted in elevation of liver enzymes, which subsequently necessitated discontinuation of the drug. In one of the two cases, drug rechallenge resulted in recurrence of the abnormality (43). One report outlines a case of hepatocellular damage due to clozapine in a patient with underlying hepatitis C (46). A case of fatal fulminant hepatic failure has been reported (47). In another case, cholestasis with eosinophilia was encountered (48).

3. Molindone

Molindone (Moban), an antipsychotic drug with a unique structure, has been associated with asymptomatic transaminase elevations. It has also been documented by rechallenge as the cause of hepatocellular injury in a 17-year-old schizophrenic patient 4 weeks after initiation of the drug (49).

4. Loxapine

Loxapine (Loxitane) has been implicated in one case of hepatocellular injury during the first 3 weeks of therapy (50).

III. ANTIDEPRESSANT MEDICATIONS (Table 2)

A. Tricyclic Antidepressants

Tricyclic antidepressants may lead to either a hepatocellular or cholestatic injury, with the latter being a more common finding particularly with *amitriptyline* (Elavil), *imipramine*

Table 2 Pattern of Injury of Antidepressant Medications

Cholestatic	Hepatocellular
Selective serotonin reuptake inhibitors (82–87,89–93)	Monamine oxidase inhibitors
Tetracyclic antidepressants (74–79)	Nefazodone (110)
Trazadone (114)	Nomifensine[a] (116–120)
Tricyclic antidepressants	Trazadone (112,113)
	Tricyclic antidepressants
	Zimelidine (54,122)

[a] Granulomatous liver disease noted in one report (121).

(Tofranil), and *amineptine* (Survector). Jaundice typically is seen a few weeks after initiation of therapy and recovery is rapid. Nevertheless, imipramine and amitriptyline have been associated with a prolonged disorder characterized by progressive fibrosis, portal inflammation, and ductopenia (51). The incidence of abnormal liver enzymes on tricyclic antidepressants has been reported up to 10–20% whereas the incidence of cholestatic jaundice due to imipramine is thought to be approximately 0.5–1% (52).

An in vitro study evaluating the leakage of cytoplasmic and lysosomal enzymes into the surrounding media ranked the cytotoxicity of a number of different tricyclic antidepressants. The rank order of toxicity was clomipramine (Anafranil) > nortriptyline (Pamelor) > amitriptyline > imipramine > doxepin (Sinequan, Adapin) (53). The mechanism of injury is believed to be idiosyncratic without intrinsic hepatotoxicity of these medications. Their toxicity has been documented with rechallenge in a number of cases. The cholestatic injury may resemble that of chlorpromazine and may be prolonged. Interestingly, the molecular structure of tricyclic antidepressants does have a similarity to that of phenothiazines.

Imipramine, amineptine, and *iprindole* (Prandol) have been more frequently associated with hepatotoxicity. Multiple reports of imipramine-induced liver injury (54–56) are available and a hypersensitivity mechanism is suspected at least in part due to the presence of eosinophils on liver biopsy (54). Imipramine and its metabolite *desipramine* (Norpramin) have been implicated in two cases of combined myocarditis and hepatitis (56). Isolated desipramine hepatotoxicity appears uncommon. In a study of 42 outpatient children treated with this medication, no abnormal liver function tests were found in the 24-month follow-up (57). In rats, clearance of imipramine diminished in the setting of hepatitis (58). Interestingly, in a rat model, imipramine prevented carbon tetrachloride–induced liver necrosis, an effect believed to be due to blocking of the damaging effects of calcium or modulation of protein phospholipids synthesis or degradation (59).

Amitriptyline hepatotoxicity is seen less frequently than with imipramine and presents with cholestatic jaundice both with chronic therapy and with overdose. The biopsy findings reveal a cholestatic pattern similar to that seen with chlorpromazine and may reveal eosinophilia, suggesting a hypersensitivity mechanism (60,61). In a study of a hepatocellular carcinoma cell line assessing amitriptyline and acetaminophen acute and chronic toxicity, there was no acute (24 h) toxicity but there was chronic cytotoxicity (chronic exposure of up to 10 days) (62).

Numerous European reports outline cholestasis, hepatitis, or a mixed liver injury pattern induced by amineptine (63–67). Onset of hepatotoxicity was noted 16–75 days after initiation of treatment with clinical improvement noted typically within 3 weeks of cessation although abnormalities have persisted for up to 12 weeks (63). It is believed that amineptine metabolism takes place by beta-oxidation of its side chain into a chemically reactive metabolite that may have the structure of an epoxide (65). In a study of drug oxidation capacity of nine patients with previous amineptine hepatitis, the toxicity appeared to occur in patients with extensive oxidation capacity but with increased susceptibility to amineptine's active metabolites (68).

Although cross-hepatotoxicity is quite uncommon, a case of cross-hepatotoxicity between amineptine and clomipramine was reported in 1986. In that case, the patient had previously been treated with amineptine complicated by jaundice and hepatotoxicity. Two days after cessation of the amineptine, clomipramine was started while the aminotransferases were still abnormal. One week later the patient complained of recurrent abdominal pain and liver functions were again markedly elevated. With cessation of clomipramine therapy, there was complete resolution of the pain and complete normalization of amino-transferases (66).

Clomipramine by itself has also been implicated as a cause of hepatotoxicity (67). A case report has outlined cross-hepatotoxicity between desipramine, trimipramine, and the antipsychotic *cyamemazine* (69). All three drugs have a similar molecular structure.

Tianeptine, similar in structure to amineptine, has been implicated as a cause of hepatitis (70) and of microvesicular steatosis (71), the latter being due to beta-oxidation of fatty acids in a manner similar to amineptine.

Cases of nitroxazepine (72) and lofepramine (73) hepatotoxicity have been reported. An open-label study that followed 52 elderly patients (>65 years old) prospectively during a 12-week course of treatment with lofepramine observed transient abnormalities in trans-aminases (73).

B. Tetracyclic Antidepressants

Hepatotoxicity of two tetracyclic antidepressants, *minaserine* and *maprotiline*, has also been reported. Maprotiline is thought to induce steatosis and hepatitis (74–77) in some patients following prolonged exposure. Incidents of cholestatic jaundice with both mapro-tiline and minaserine have also been observed. Isolated minaserine-induced hepatitis (78,79) as well as cross-hepatotoxicity between minaserine and a tricyclic depressant has been documented (80).

C. Serotonin Reuptake Inhibitors

The serotonin reuptake Inhibitors are now widely used. They inhibit hepatic isoenzymes function, particularly the IID6 isoenzyme system. *Paroxetine* (Paxil) is the most potent inhibitor. The concern for potential drug interactions with this class of medication goes beyond this isolated system however. Some of them appear to affect multiple isoenzyme systems [e.g., *fluoxetine* (Prozac) inhibits the CYP 2C9/19 system], which increases the number of potential drug interactions (81).

Fluoxetine results in asymptomatic increased tranaminases in approximately 0.5% of patients on long-term therapy (82,83). A Spanish group has reviewed 11 cases of hepato-toxicity, including six with clinical hepatitis (84). There have been other reports of hepato-toxicity (85–87), including one case of chronic hepatitis with positive autoimmune markers attributed to fluoxetine. In fact, the patient was treated with *prednisone* and *azathi-oprine* after fluoxetine was discontinued. Subsequently however, the patient was docu-mented to have hepatitis C by RT-PCR, which brings the contribution of fluoxetine into question (88).

Paroxetine has been implicated in both chronic and acute hepatitis (89,90). Elevation of aminotransferases is not uncommon. Severe hepatitis leading to decompensated liver disease in a man with chronic hepatitis B has been attributed to paroxetine. The patient recovered after withdrawal of the drug (91). There have been two cases of severe hepatitis in young women using both *atrium* and paroxetine. Both cases eventually resolved, one rapidly and one gradually (92). There is one report of acute hepatitis attributed to *sertraline* (Zoloft) (93). *Venlafaxine* (Effexor) is a serotonin and norepinephrine reuptake inhibitor implicated in two cases of acute hepatitis, one of which had a cholestatic component (94,95). Both patients recovered after withdrawal of venlafaxine. One case of liver injury has been attributed to the combined use of sertraline and venlafaxine (96).

D. Monamine Oxidase Inhibitors

Severe hepatic necrosis attributed to *iproniazid* (Marsilid) was first reported in 1960 (97) and eventually the drug was taken off the market. A number of similar reactions with other monamine oxidase inhibitors were subsequently reported and many of these medications were eventually abandoned. Two hydrazine monamine oxidase inhibitors still in clinical use are *phenelzine* (Nardil) and *isocarboxazid* (Marplan). Both appear to be less hepatotoxic. *Tranylcypromine* (Parnate) is a nonhydrazine monamine oxidase inhibitor in clinical use with a low incidence of hepatocellular toxicity (98).

1. Mechanism of Injury

The mechanism of injury is idiosyncratic. Some investigators believe that the idiosyncratic reaction is not immunological but rather mediated by an intermediate hepatotoxic metabolite (99), isopropylhydrazine, via a mechanism analogous to the role of acetylhydrazine in the toxicity of *isoniazid* (100). Others have postulated an immunological mechanism because of the discovery of antimitochondrial antibody 6 (anti-M6), which appears to be very specific for iproniazid toxicity (101). In one report, a patient with iproniazid toxicity was found to have an anti-M6 at a high titer. The titer progressively decreased after withdrawal of the medication and was no longer detectable at 6 months. Interestingly, anti-M6 was not found in 15 patients taking the medication but without hepatitis or in six other patients who had liver injury due to isoniazid (102). Whether the anti-M6 is a result rather than the cause of iproniazid toxicity remains unclear (103).

2. Clinical Course

Iproniazid was estimated to produce jaundice in approximately 1% of recipients (104). The onset is typically insidious, with anorexia, malaise, and fatigue. Jaundice appears after at least 1 month of exposure. Duration of illness is variable from 1 to 6 months after starting the medication. Laboratory, histological, and clinical features are consistent with a hepatocellular injury pattern. A high mortality rate of approximately 15% is reported with massive hepatic necrosis observed on a liver biopsy (105). Information on hepatotoxicity of other monoamine oxidase inhibitors is sparse. At least three cases of fatal fulminant hepatitis after administration of *iproclozide* (Sursum) have occurred. In all three cases, jaundice occurred within 7–10 days after the addition of another medication that induced microsomal enzymes (106).

Monoamine oxidase inhibitors currently in clinical use include *isocarboxazid* (Marplan), *phenelzine* (Nardil), and *tranylcypromine* (Parnate). Isocarboxazid was initially withdrawn in 1994 and reintroduced in 1999 in the United States market (107). Rather than being metabolized by hepatic microsomal cytochromes or by hepatic acetylation, isocarboxazid is a specific substrate for and is hydrolyzed by RL2 hepatic microsomal carboxylesterase, as observed in rats (108). Phenelzine was the cause of cholestatic hepatitis in a 59-year-old man after 70 days of treatment. Subsequent detailed metabolic evaluation revealed that he was a rapid acetylator. The authors propose that rapid acetylation predisposes to phenelzine-induced hepatic injury (109).

E. Remaining Antidepressants

Nefazodone (Serzone), a new antidepressant, has resulted in hepatocellular injury and subfulminant hepatic failure in three women (110). One patient recovered but the other two required liver transplantation, with one dying after transplantation (110). In another case, a woman with severe hepatocellular jaundice recovered after withdrawal of nefazo-done (111). *Trazadone* (Desyrel) has been associated with jaundice and a case of chronic hepatitis (112,113). A fatal case of hepatic necrosis occurred in a patient initially started on trazadone, *trifluoperazine*, and *lithium*. Ten weeks later, her alanine aminotransferase (ALT) was 107 and 1 week later trifluoperazine was replaced by *thioridazine*. Nine weeks later she developed jaundice and all medications were stopped. Nevertheless she developed encephalopathy and died 54 days after onset of jaundice. Postmortem liver biopsy revealed hepatic necrosis with cholestasis. The authors implicated trazadone although the impact of the neuroleptic agents cannot be excluded (114).

Chemically unrelated to other antidepressants, *bupropion hydrochloride* (Wellbu-trin) is also marketed as a nonnicotine aid for tobacco cessation (Zyban). One patient receiving bupropion hydrochloride for depression developed hepatitis 6 weeks after initiation with rapid resolution upon cessation of the drug (115). The antidepressant *nomi-fensine* was withdrawn from the market due to hemolytic anemia and granulocytopenia but was also associated with a number of cases of hepatotoxicity (116–120) including granulomatous liver disease (121). Zimelidine, another antidepressant, was withdrawn be-cause of incidents of Guillain-Barré syndrome but was also associated with hepatotoxicity (122).

IV. BENZODIAZEPINES (Table 3)

As a group, benzodiazepines are highly protein-bound agents and thus carry a small risk of hepatotoxicity. A cholestatic injury pattern has been seen with *alprazolam* (Xanax) (123,124), *chlordiazepoxide* (Librium) (125,126), *diazepam* (Valium) (127), *flurazepam* (Dalmane) (128), and *triazolam* (Halcion) (129). A hepatitis-like clinical picture has been observed with *clonazepam* (Klonopin) and *clorazepate* (Tranxene) (130).

A case of fulminant hepatitis has been attributed to alprazolam (131). *Clotiazepam*, an agent used in Europe and Asia, has been associated with a rare but nonfatal case of extensive hepatocellular necrosis 7 months after initiation (132).

Benzodiazapenes need to be used with caution in patients with underlying liver disease. Cirrhosis produces a two- to threefold increase in the half-life of both diazepam and chlordiazepoxide but does not have a significant effect on *lorazepam* (Ativan) and *oxazepam* (Serax). This impaired elimination in liver disease may lead to oversedation (133). Similarly, aging appears to lead to a significant prolongation of the half-life of diazepam and chlordiazepoxide but does not appear to have an effect on lorazepam and oxazepam (134).

Table 3   Pattern of Injury of Benzodiazepines

Cholestatic	Hepatocellular
Alprazolam (123,124)	Clonazepam (130)
Chlordiazepoxide (125,126)	Clorazepate (130)
Diazepam (127)	Clotiazepam (132)
Flurazepam (128)	
Triazolam(129)	

V. DRUGS OF ABUSE INCLUDING STIMULANTS

A. Stimulants

1. Amphetamines

Hepatotoxicity of amphetamines and metamphetamine is rare and, when present, appears to be related to the induction of hyperthermia (135,136). One particular amphetamine that is hepatotoxic is *"ecstasy"* (3,4-methylenedioxy metamphetamine), a hallucinogenic drug. This is a synthetic amphetamine that was initially developed in 1914 as an appetite suppressant but was never marketed for that purpose. Typically used illicitly as a "dance drug," it is taken for recreational purposes. Over 24 cases of hepatotoxicity have been reported (137–143). It is associated with hyperthermia, hypotension, tachycardia, disseminated intravascular coagulation, acute renal failure, rhabdomyolysis, and death. Hyperthermia may also play a role in the pathogenesis of hepatotoxicity with "ecstasy." One death has been reported and another patient required liver transplantation (144). Recovery is reported to take place in a variable amount of time from 3 weeks to 3 months (145).

2. Phencyclidine (PCP)

Known on the street as "angel dust," *phencyclidine* (PCP) is abused because of its potent psychedelic properties. It too results in hyperthermia and presumably leads to hepatic necrosis via this mechanism.

3. Cocaine

In the United States, *cocaine* abuse is a problem of enormous social, economic, and medical magnitude (146). The hepatotoxicity of cocaine is well established and may occur in conjunction with other systemic manifestations such as myocardial infarction, rhabdomyolysis, and shock (146).

Mechanism of Injury.   Animal models have shown cocaine to be a dose-dependent hepatotoxin, and a series of oxidative steps mediated primarily by the cytochrome P450 monooxygenase system are required for its hepatotoxicity (147–150). Cocaine's metabolite, norcocaine nitroxide, is thought to induce lipid peroxidation by covalently binding to cellular macromolecules with the resultant oxidative stress-inducing hepatocyte injury (151–162). Ultrastructural studies in mice indicate that first there is dilatation of the rough endoplasmic reticulum in the centrilobular hepatocytes, followed by mitochondrial membrane disruption and swelling ultimately resulting in cell death in 6–8 h (163). Such studies support the role of lipid peroxidation in cocaine's hepatotoxicity (163–164).

Concomitant ingestion of ethanol potentiates the hepatotoxicity of cocaine (165–168). This effect appears to be dependent on the cytochrome P450 monooxygenase system but is not associated with diminished intracellular glutathione (GSH) or vitamin E content (167). Nor is the effect attenuated by supplementation with antioxidants such as GSH or vitamin E (165–168).

Histopathology.   Hepatic necrosis and microvesicular steatosis are seen in humans (169). The lobular distribution of hepatic necrosis is variable with some patients exhibiting predominantly zone 1 and 2 necrosis whereas others exhibit mainly zone 3 necrosis. It appears that prolonged exposure at lower doses leads to zone 1 necrosis whereas induction by alcohol and/or higher doses lead to zone 3 necrosis. Exposure to very high doses results in panlobular necrosis.

Clinical Presentation. Those who abuse cocaine also have a high incidence of underlying chronic liver disease and/or viral hepatitis (170). The presence of underlying liver disease makes these individuals more susceptible to hepatic dysfunction related to cocaine. There is typically an early marked rise and subsequent rapid decrease of aminotransferases, mild to moderate elevation of prothrombin time, and moderate azotemia (169). Concomitant cardiac, neurological, renal, and muscular manifestations are often present.

In a retrospective evaluation of 39 consecutive patients who presented with cocaine intoxication and rhabdomyolysis over an 8-year period, 23 had biochemical evidence of hepatic dysfunction whereas 16 had severe liver injury defined by an ALT >400. Care must be taken to delineate the source of elevated AST in the setting of rhabdomyolysis (muscle vs. liver). Seven of these 16 patients died (44%). Postmortem examination of the liver revealed extensive centrilobular and midzonal necrosis in three patients and panlobular necrosis in two (171). Aggressive supportive measures may provide benefit.

4. Methylphenidate

Reversible cases of hepatocellular injury have been noted with both oral and intravenous use of *methylphenidate* (172,173) and in one case hepatocellular injury was part of multisystem organ failure that subsequently resolved (174).

B. Miscellaneous

1. Agents for Neurological Disorders

Tolcapone (Tasmar) is a reversible inhibitor of catechol-*O*-methyl transferase (COMT) that is used as an adjunct to enhance levodopa levels in the treatment of Parkinson's disease. In the premarketing studies tolcapone resulted in a threefold increase in transaminases in 1.3–3.7% of patients. Subsequently, during postmarketing surveillance, four cases of liver failure were reported (175,176). All four patients were women, three died, and at least two of the cases were consistent with fulminant hepatic failure. This resulted in issue of a "black box" warning by the Food and Drug Administration suggesting stringent monitoring requirements for patients treated with tolcapone (176). Because liver enzyme abnormalities and clinical liver dysfunction have universally occurred within the first 6 months of initiating therapy, an expert panel has recommended more frequent monitoring during the first 6 months and less frequent monitoring thereafter; withdrawal is recommended only if the transaminase elevation is two to three times the upper limit of normal (177).

Tacrine (Cognex), a cholinesterase inhibitor used in the treatment of Alzheimer's disease, has been associated with frequent elevations of liver enzymes (~50%) in treated patients (178). Increases up to 20-fold have been seen in 2% of patients (178).

The mechanism of injury remains unclear. The presence of eosinophils on biopsy raises the possibility of hypersensitivity, yet the fact that ALT levels are lower on rechallenge argues against this mechanism. The fact that tacrine is metabolized by CYP 1A2 supports the possibility of metabolic idiosyncracy (179) yet CYP 1A2 activity does not predict toxicity (180). Another proposed mechanism is uncoupling of mitochondria by tacrine (181). In a third hypothesis, tacrine induces cholinergic celiac ganglion stimulation of afferent sympathetic pathways. This is thought to result in hypoperfusion of sinusoids and subsequent reperfusion injury (182).

The hepatotoxicity typically occurs in the first 12–16 weeks of therapy, and despite the frequent liver enzyme abnormalities, the incidence of clinically detectable tacrine-associated liver disease is rare. At least one case of reversible hepatic necrosis has been noted (183) but fulminant hepatic failure has not been described. An uncontrolled study suggests that ursodeoxycholic acid supplementation may prevent moderate, but not severe, liver enzyme abnormalities associated with tacrine (184).

Riluzole (Rilutek), an antiglutamate agent approved for the therapy of amyotrophic lateral sclerosis (ALS), has been associated with two cases of acute hepatitis with variable degrees of microvesicular steatosis (185). The hepatitis occurred 25 and 48 days after initiation in the two patients with the former case confirmed by rechallenge and repeat onset of hepatitis within 15 days. Currently, the package insert recommends baseline evaluation of hepatic biochemical tests followed by monthly testing for the first 3 months and every-3-month testing for the remainder of the first year. Thereafter, "periodic" monitoring is recommended.

2. Opioids

On the whole, narcotics other than propoxyphene do not result in significant hepatotoxicity. Abuse of *heroin, methadone,* and *morphine* has been associated with elevations of transaminases (186), but this finding has typically been attributable to concomitant viral hepatitis. Sphincter of Oddi spasm as a cause of abnormal hepatic biochemical profile has also been postulated. Many illicit opioids that are injected intravenously typically contain talc (magnesium silicate), cornstarch, cotton fibers, and refractile fibers (187). The presence of talc granulomas in the liver is a common finding in patients with intravenous drug abuse.

Although methadone's half-life is slightly prolonged in patients with chronic liver disease, the maintenance dosage need not be changed (188). In humans, the kidneys eliminate morphine via glucoronidation and subsequent excretion of metabolites (morphine-3-glucoronide and morphine-6-glucoronide). After a single intravenous dose, however, no significant difference is detected between plasma levels of cirrhotic or healthy patients. Increased bioavailability of orally administered narcotics has been noted, however (189).

3. Propoxyphene (Dextropropoxyphene)

Propoxyphene, a commonly used analgesic, has been associated with multiple cases of cholestasis believed to be idiosyncratic in nature, some of which have been corroborated by rechallenge (190–193). Interestingly, a number of these patients had presented with upper abdominal discomfort and were incorrectly diagnosed with gallbladder disease (192,193). When the drug was administered to rats, both hepatomegaly and fatty infiltration of the liver have been noted (190).

4. Marijuana

The liver is the primary organ for metabolism of *tetrahydrocannabinol* (THC) and this compound is thought to inhibit liver microsomal enzymes. Although some studies have implicated marijuana as the etiology of the frequent (20–67%) liver enzyme elevations in regular users of this drug (194,195), others attribute such elevations to other causes of liver dysfunction. Four unusual cases of intravenous self-administration of this drug have indeed resulted in development of marked toxic hepatitis (196).

Table 4 Latency Period and Incidence of Hepatotoxicity due to Psychoactive Medications

Medication	Incidence	Latency period
Antidepressants		
Tricyclic antidepressants		
Amineptine	Rare	2–3 months
Amitriptyline	0.5–1%	~8 weeks
Desipramine		1–3 weeks
Imipramine	Elevated ALT ~10%	1–3 weeks
MAO Inhibitors	Rare	Weeks
SSRIs	Rare	~4 weeks
Atypicals		
Nefazadone	Rare	14–28 weeks
Trazadone	Rare	2–20 weeks
Benzodiazepines		
Diazepam	Rare	Days–months
Chlordiazepoxide		2–6 weeks
Butyrphenones		
Haldoperidol	0.002%	4–5 weeks
Cocaine	?	Hours–days
Ecstasy	?	Hours–weeks
Phenothiazines		
Chlorpromazine	0.1–1%	2–3 weeks
		Range: 5 days–10 weeks

Source: Modified from ref. 197. Used with permission.

VI. SUMMARY

A spectrum of psychoactive medications has been associated with hepatic dysfunction and liver disease. The incidence of hepatotoxicity due to these drugs and from drugs of abuse is variable and often low. The manifestations are usually evident within the first 6 months as is seen in most cases of drug-induced liver injury (197) (Table 4). Despite the frequent use of these medications and high baseline prevalence of underlying liver disease in this patient population, fulminant hepatic failure is rare (Table 5). The mechanism of hepatotoxicity in most cases appears to be intermediate metabolite-related idiosyncrasy

Table 5 Fulminant Hepatic Failure due to Psychoactive Agents

Alprazolam (131)
Clozapine (47)
Cocaine (171)
Ecstasy (3,4-MMTP) (144)
Iproniazid (105)
Nefazadone (110)
Tolcapone (175)
Trazadone[a] (116)

[a] A case report in which patient was also exposed to trifluoperazine and lithium.

that may have hypersensitivity manifestations. The syndrome of cholestatic hepatitis can be quite distressing particularly due to the prolonged nature of jaundice and the accompanying pruritus. Conservative management, monitoring with cessation of the offending medication, supportive measures, and reassurance of patients with debilitating cholestasis are likely to result in a good outcome in the majority of these patients.

REFERENCES

1. Knight ME, Roberts RJ. Phenothiazine and butyrophenone intoxication in children. Pediatr Clin North Am 1986; 33:299–309.
2. Zimmerman HJ. Hepatotoxicity: The Adverse Effects of Drugs and Other Chemicals on the Liver. 2nd ed. Philadelphia: Lippincott Williams & Wilkins, 1999.
3. Ishak KG, Irey NS. Hepatic injury associated with the phenothiazines: clinicopathologic and follow-up study of 36 patients. Arch Pathol 1972; 93:283–304.
4. Jick H, Walker AM, Porter J. Drug-induced liver disease. J Clin Pharmacol 1981; 21:359–364.
5. Russell RI, Allan JG, Patrick R. Active chronic hepatitis after chlorpromazine ingestion. Br Med J 1973; 1:655–656.
6. Larrey D, Erlinger S. Drug-induced cholestasis. Bailliere's Clin Gastroenterol 1988; 2:423–452.
7. Moradpour D, Altorfer J, Flury, Greminger P, Meyenberger C, Jost R, Schmid M. Chlorpromazine-induced vanishing bile duct syndrome leading to biliary cirrhosis. Hepatology 1994; 20:1437–1441.
8. Elias E, Boyer JL. Mechanisms of intrahepatic cholestasis. Prog Liver Dis 1979; 6:457–470.
9. Kaplowitz N, Aw TY, Simon FR, Stolz A. Drug-induced hepatotoxicity. Ann of Intern Med 1986; 104:826–839.
10. Chen EY, Lee AS. Neuroleptic-induced priapism, hepatotoxicity and subsequent impotence in a patient with depressive psychosis. Br J Psychiatry 1990; 157:759–762.
11. Keeffe EB, Blankenship NM, Scharschmidt BF. Alteration of rat liver plasma membrane fluidity and ATPase activity by chlorpromazine hydrochloride and its metabolites. Gastroenterology 1980; 79:222–231.
12. Samuels AM, Carey MC. Effects of chlorpromazine hydrochloride and its metabolites on Mg^{2+} and Na^+, K^+-ATPase activities of canalicular-enriched rat liver plasma membranes. Gastroenterology 1978; 74:1183–1190.
13. Akerboom T, Schneider I, Vom Dahl S, Sies H. Cholestasis and changes of portal pressure caused by chlorpromazine in the perfused rat liver. Hepatology 1991; 13:216–221.
14. Abernathy CO, Zimmerman HJ, Ishak KG, Utili R, Gillespie J. Drug-induced cholestasis in the perfused rat liver and its reversal by taurodeoxycholate: an ultrastructural study. PSEBM 1992; 199:54–58.
15. Utili R, Tripodi MF, Abernathy CO, Zimmerman HJ, Gillespie J. Effects of bile salt infusion of chlorpromazine-induced cholestasis in the isolated perfused rat liver. PSEBM 1992; 199:49–53.
16. Cooper PJ, Danpure CJ, Simpson KJ. Peroxisomal and mitochondrial proliferation and increased alanine:gloxylate aminotransferase activity in human liver after chlorpromazine induced cholestasis. Biochem Soc Transact 1989; 17:1071–1072.
17. Watson RGP, Olomu A, Clements D, Waring RH, Mitchell S, Elias E. A proposed mechanism for chlorpromazine jaundice-defective hepatic silphoxidation combined with rapid hydroxylation. J Hepatol 1988; 7:72–78.
18. Utili R, Abernathy CO, Zimmerman HJ, Gaeta GB, Adinolfi L, Lukacs L. Endotoxin protects against chlorpromazine-induced cholestasis in the isolated perfused rat liver. Gastroenterology 1981; 80:673–680.

19. Teschke R, Stutz, Moreno F. Cholestasis following chronic alcohol consumption: enhancement after an acute dose of chlorpromazine. Biochemi Biophys Res Commun 1980; 94:1013–1020.
20. Cardanel JF, Bonnard P, Cazier A, di Martino V, Pras V, Devergie B, Biour M. Cyamamezine-induced acute hepatitis after unique massive intake: a case report. Eur J Gastroenterol Hepatol 1999; 11:451–453.
21. Rager P, Cosculluela D, Deviers D. Drug hepatitis: possible role of cyamemazine (letter). Presse Med 1983; 12:1941.
22. Remy AJ, Larrey D, Pageaux GP, Ribstein J, Ramos J, Michel H. Cross hepatotoxicity between tricyclic antidepressants and phenothiazines. Eur J Gastroenterol Hepatol 1995; 7: 373–376.
23. Barancik M, Brandbor LL, Albion MJ. Thorazine-induced of the cholestasis. JAMA 1967; 200:69–70.
24. Urberg M. Thioridazine-induced non-icteric hepatotoxicity. J Family Pract 1990; 30:342–343.
25. Weiden PL, Buckner CD. Thioridazine toxicity. Agranulocytosis and hepatitis with encephalopathy. JAMA 1973; 224:518–520.
26. Smaga M. On the etiology of hepatitis developing during treatment with Stelazine. Vrachebnoe Delo 1967; 10:126–128.
27. Margulies AI, Berris B. Jaundice associated with administration of trifluoperazine. Can Med Associ J 1968; 98:1063–1064.
28. Dimova S, Koleva M, Rangelova D, Stoythchev. Effective nifedipine, verapamil, diltiazem and trifluoperazine on acetaminophen toxicity in mice. Arch Toxicol 1995; 70:112–118.
29. Villarruel MC, Fernandez G, De Ferreyra EC, De Fenos OM, Castro JA. Late preventive effects of trifluoperazine on carbon tetrachloride-induced hepatic necrosis. Toxicol Appl Pharmacol 1986; 83:287–93.
30. Fuller CM, Yassinger S, Donlon P, Imperato TJ, Ruebner B. Haloperidol-induced liver disease. West J Med 1977; 127:515–518.
31. Van Bellinghen M, Peuskens J, Appelmans A. Hepatotoxicity following treatment with Bromperidol (letter). J Clin Psychopharmacol 1989; 9:389–390.
32. Sarfraz A, Cook M. Sulipride-induced cholestatic jaundice. Aust NZ J Psychiatry 1996; 30: 701–702.
33. Ruddock DGS, Hoenig J. Chlorprothixene an obstructive jaundice. Br Med J 1973; 1:231.
34. Yaryura-Tobias JA, Wolpert A, White L, et al. A Clinical evaluation of clopenthixol. Curr Ther Res 1970; 12:271.
35. Fuller MA, Simon MR, Freedman L. Risperidone-associated hepatotoxicity. J Clin Psychopharmacol 1986; 16:84–85.
36. Kumra S, Herion D, Jaconbsen LK, Briguglia C, Grothe D. Case study: risperidone-induced hepatotoxicity in pediatric patients. J Am Acad Child Adolesc Psychiatry 1997; 36:701–705.
37. Landau J, Martin A. Is liver function monitoring warranted during risperidone treatment? J Am Acad Child Adolesc Psychiatry 1998; 37:1007–1008.
38. Benazzi F. Risperidone-induced hepatotoxicity. Pharmacopsychiatry 1988; 31:241.
39. Phillips EJ, Liu BA, Knowles SR. Rapid onset of risperidone-induced hepatotoxicity (letter). Ann Pharmacother 1988; 32:843.
40. Geller W, Zuiderwijk P. Risperidone-induced hepatotoxicity? J Am Acad Child Adolesc Psychiatry 1998; 37:246–247.
41. Lieberman JA. Maximizing clozapine therapy: managing side effects. J Clin Psychiatry 1998; 59(suppl 3):38–43.
42. Hummer M, Kurz M, Kurzthaler I, Oberhauer H, Miller C, Fleischhacker WW. Hepatotoxicity of clozapine. J Clin Pharmacol 1997; 17:314–317.
43. Markowitz JS, Grinberg R, Jackson C. Marked liver enzyme elevations with clozapine. J Clin Psychopharmacol 1987; 17:70–71.

44. Thatcher GW, Cates M, Bair B. Clozapine-induced toxic hepatitis. American J Psychiatry 1995; 152:296–297.

45. Kellner M, Wiedemann K, Krieg JC, Berg PA. Toxic hepatitis by clozapine treatment. Am J Psychiatry 1983; 150:985–986.

46. Worrall R, Wilson A, Cullen M. Dystonia and drug-induced hepatitis in a patient clozapine. Am J Psychiatry 1995; 152:647–648.

47. MacFarlane B, Davies S, Mannen K, et al. Fatal acute fulminant liver failure due to clozapine: a case report and review of clozapine induced hepatoxicity. Gastroenterology 1997; 112: 170–177.

48. Thompson J, Chengappa KNR, Good CB, Baker RW, Kiewe RP, Bezner J, Schooler NR. Hepatitis, hyperglycemia, pleural effusion, eosinophilia, hematuria and proteinuria occurring early in clozapine treatment. International Clin Psychopharmacol 1998; 13:95–98.

49. Bhatia SC, Banta LE, Ehrlich DW. Molindone and hepatotoxicity. Drug Intell Clin Pharm 1985; 19:744–746.

50. FDA. ADR Highlights. August 14, 1980.

51. King PD, Blitzer BL. Drug-induced cholestasis: pathogenesis and Clinical features. Semin Liver Dis 1990; 10:316–321.

52. Klerman GL, Cole JO. Clinical pharmacology of imipramine and related antidepressant compounds. Pharmacol Rev 1965; 17:101–141.

53. Yasuhara H, Dujovne CA, Ueda I, Arakawa K. Hepatotoxicity and surface activity of tricyclic antidepressants in vitro. Toxicol Appl Pharmacol 1979; 47:47–54.

54. Weaver GA, Pavlinac D, Davis JS. Hepatic sensitivity to Imipramine. Dig Dis 1977; 22: 551–553.

55. Moskovitz R, DeVane CL, Harris R, Stewart RB. Toxic hepatitis and single daily dosage imiprimamine therapy. J Clin Psychiatry 1982; 43:165–166.

56. Morrow PL, Hardin NJ, Bonadies J. Hypersensitivity myocarditis and hepatitis associated with imipramine and its metabolite, desipramine. J Forensi Sci, 1989; 34:1016–1020.

57. Hoge SK, Biedermam J. Liver function tests during treatment with desipramine in children and adolescents. J Clin Psychopharm 1987; 7:87–89.

58. Hackett AM, Shaw IC, Griffiths LA. The metabolism and excretion of [^{14}C]lipramine in an experimental hepatitis. Xenobiotica 1984; 14:491–499.

59. Fernandez G, Villarruel MC, deFerreyra EC, deFenos OM, Castro JA. Imipramine prevention of carbon tetrachloride-induced liver necrosis at late states of the intoxication process. J Appl Toxicol 1986; 6:413–418.

60. Biagi RW, Bapat BN. Intrahepatic obstructive jaundice from amitriptyline. Br J Pschiatry 1967; 113:1113–1114.

61. Yon J, Anuras S. Hepatitis caused by amitriptyline therapy. JAMA 1975; 232:833–834.

62. Hall TJ, James R, Cambridge G. Development of an in vitro hepatotoxicity assay for assessing the effects of chronic drug exposure. Res Commun Chem Pathol Pharm 1993; 79:249–256.

63. Bel A, Girard D. Hepatitis, cholestasis and amineptine (author's translation). Sem Hop 1981; 57:1992–1996.

64. Larrey D, Berson A, Habersetzer F, Tinel M, Castot A, Babany G, Letteron P, Freneaux E, Loeper J, Dansette P, Pessayre D. Genetic predisposition to drug hepatotoxicity: role in hepatitis caused by amineptine, a tricyclic antidepressant. Hepatology 1989; 10:168–173.

65. Lazaros GA, Stavrinos C, Papatheodoridis GV, Delladetsima JK, Toliopoulos A, Tassopoyulos NC. Amineptine induced liver injury: report of two cases and brief review of the literature. Hepato-Gastroenterology 1996; 43:1015–9.

66. Larrey D, Rueff B, Pessayre D, Danan G, Algard M, Geneve J, Benhamou JP. Cross hepatotoxicity between tricyclic antidepressants. Gut 1986; 27:726–727.

67. Alderman CP, Atchison MM, McNeece JI. Concurrent agranulocytosis and hepatitis secondary to clomipramine therapy. Br J Psychiatry 1993; 162:688–689.

68. Larrey D, Berson A, Habersetzer F, Tinel M, Castot A, Babany G, Letteron P, Freneaux E, Loeper J, Dansette P, Pessayre D. Genetic predisposition to drug hepatotoxicity: role in hepatitis caused by amineptine, a tricyclic antidepressant. Hepatology 1989; 10:168–173.

69. Dossing M, Andreasen PB. Drug-induced liver disease in Denmark. An analysis of 572 cases of hepatotoxicity reported to the Danish board of Adverse Reactions to Drugs. Scand J Gastroenterol 1982; 17:205–211.

70. Balleyguier C, Sterin D, Ziol M, Trinchet JC. Acute mixed hepatitis caused by tianeptine. Gastroenterol Clin Biol 1996; 20:607–608.

71. LeBricquir Y, Larrey D, Blanc P, Pageaux GP, Michel H. Tianeptine—an instance of drug-induced hepatoxicity predicted by prospective experimental studies. J Hepatol 1994; 21:771–773.

72. Chopra V. Hepatitis following nitroxazepine therapy. J Assoc Physicians India 1986; 34:305.

73. Kelly C, Roche S, Naguib M, Webb S, Roberts M, Pitt B. A prospective evaluation of the hepatotoxicity of lofepramine in the elderly. Int Clin Psychopharm 1993; 8:83–86.

74. Jean P, Rodor F, Jean-Pastor MJ, Hayek-Lanthois M, Jouglard J. Hepatitis following acute intoxication with maprotiline (Ludiomil). J Toxicol Clin Exp 1985; 5:121–123.

75. Braun JS, Geiger R, Wehner H, Schaffer S, Berger M. Hepatitis caused by antidepressive therapy with maprotiline and opipramol. Pharmacopsychiatry 1998; 31:152–155.

76. Moldawsky RJ. Hepatotoxicity associated with maprotiline therapy: case report. J Clin Psychiatry 1984; 45:178–179.

77. Aleem A. Hepatotoxicity following treatment with maprotiline. J Clin Psychopharmacol 1987; 7:54–55.

78. Zarski JP, Aubert H, Rachail M. Hepatic toxicity of new antidepressive drugs: apropos of a case. Gastro Clin Biol 1983; 7:220–221.

79. Barbare JC, Biour M, Cadot T, Latrive JP. Hepatotoxicity of minaserine: a case with positive reintroduction. Gastro Clin Biol 1992; 16:486–488.

80. Rasmussen S, Quedens JH. Possible cross hepatotoxicity between tricycylic and tetracyclic antidepressive agents. Ugeskr Laeger 1991; 153:3020–3022.

81. Burke M, Harvey AT, Preskorn SH. Pharmacokinetics of the newer antidepressants. AJM 1996; 100:119–120.

82. Cooper GL. The safety of fluoxetine—an update. Br J Psychiatry 1988; 153(suppl):77–86.

83. Gram LF. Fluoxetine (letter to editor). N Engl J Med 1995; 332(14):960–961.

84. Capella D, Bruguera M, Figueras A, Laporte JR. Fluoxetine-induced hepatitis: why is post-marking surveillance needed? Eur J Clin Pharmacol 1999; 55:545–546.

85. Cai Q, Benson MA, Talbot TJ, Devadas G, Swanson HJ, Olson JL, Kirchner JP. Acute hepatitis due to fluoxetine therapy. Mayo Clin Proc 1999; 74:692–694.

86. Bobichon R, Bernard G, Mion F. Acute hepatitis during treatment with fluoxetine. Gastroenterol Clin Biol 1993; 17:406–407.

87. Friedenberg FK, Rothstein KD. Hepatitis secondary to fluoxetine treatment. Am J Psychiatry 1996; 153:580.

88. Johnston DE, Wheeler DE. Chronic hepatitis related to use of fluoxetine. AJG 1997; 92:1225–6.

89. Helmchen C, Boerner RJ, Meyendorf R, Hegerl U. Reversible hepatotoxicity of paroxetine in a patient with major depression. Pharmacopsychiatry 1996; 29:223–226.

90. Benbow SJ, Gill G. Drug points: paroxetine and hepatotoxicity. Br Med J 1997; 314:1387.

91. deMan RA. Severe hepatitis attributed to paroxetine (Seroxat). Nederlands Tijdsch Geneeskunde 1997; 141:540–542.

92. Cadranel JF, DiMartino V, Cazier A, Pras V, Bachmeyer C, Olympio P, Gonzenbach A, Mofredj A, Coutarel P, Devergie B, Biour M. Atrium and paroxetine-related severe hepatitis. J Clin Gastroenterol 1999; 28:52–55.

93. Hautekeete ML, Cole I, VanVlieberg H, Elewant A. Symptomatic liver injury probably related to sertraline. Gastroenterol Clin Biol 1998; 22:364.

94. Horsmans Y. De Clercq M. Sempoux C. Venlafaxine-associated hepatitis. Ann Intern Med 1999; 130:944.

95. Cardona X. Avila A. Castellanos P. Venlafaxine-associated hepatitis. Ann Intern Med 2000; 132:417.

96. Kim KY. Hwang W. Narendran R. Acute liver damage possibly related to sertraline and venlafaxine ingestion. Ann Pharmacother 1999; 33:381–2.

97. Rosenblum LE, Korn RJ, Zimmerman HJ. Hepatocellular jaundice as a complication of iproniazid therapy. Arch Intern Med 1960; 105:583.

98. Bandt C, Hoffbauer FW. Liver injury associated with tranylcypromine therapy. JAMA 1964; 188:752.

99. Mitchell JR, Zimmerman HJ, Ishak KG, et al. Isoniazid liver injury: clinical spectrum, pathology and probable pathogenesis. Ann Intern Med 1976; 84:181–192.

100. Nelson SD, Mitchell JR, Snodgrass WR, et al. Hepatotoxicity and metabolism of iproniazid and isopropylhydrazine. J Pharmacol Exp Ther 1978; 206:574.

101. Homberg JC, Stelly N, Andreis I, et al. A new antimitochondrial antibody, anti-M6. Gastroenterol Clin Biol 1983; 7:529.

102. Danan G, Homber JC, Bernuau J, Roche-Sicot J, Pessayre D. Iproniazid-induced hepatitis. The diagnostic value of a new antimitochondrial antibody-M6. Gastroenterol Clin Biol 1983; 7:529–532.

103. Zimmerman HJ, Ishak KG. The hepatic injury of monamine oxidase inhibitors. J Clin Psychopharmacol 1987; 7:211–213.

104. Rosenblum LE, Korn RJ, Zimmerman HJ. Hepatocellular jaundice as a complication of iproniazid therapy. Arch Intern Med 1960; 105:583.

105. Zimmerman HJ. Update of hepatotoxicity due to classes of drugs in common clinical use: non-steroidal drugs, anti-inflammatory drugs, antibiotics, antihypertensives and cardiac and psychotropic agents. Semin Liver Dis 1990; 10:322–338.

106. Pessayre D, DeSaint-Louvent P, Degott C, Bernuau J, Rueff B, Benhamou JP. Iproclozide fulminant hepatitis; possible role of enzyme induction. Gastroenterology 1978; 75:492–496.

107. Shader RI. Greenblatt DJ. The reappearance of a monoamine oxidase Inhibitor(isocarboxazid). J Clin Psychopharmacol 1999; 19:105–106.

108. Hosokowa M, Satoh T. Differences in the induction of carboxylesterase isozymes in rat liver microsomes by perfluorinated fatty acids. Xenobiotica 1993; 23:1125–1133.

109. Bonkovsky HL, Blanchette PL, Schned AR. Severe liver injury due to phenelzine with unique hepatic deposition of extracellular material. AJM 1986; 80:689–692.

110. Aranda-Michel J. Koehler A. Bejarano PA. Poulos JE. Luxon BA. Khan CM. Ee LC. Balistreri WF. Weber FL Jr. Nefazodone-induced liver failure: report of three cases. Ann Intern Med 1999; 130:285–288.

111. Eloubeidi MA, Gaede JT, Swaim MW. Reversible nefazodone-induced liver failure. Dig Dis Sci 2000; 45:1036–1038.

112. Chu AG, Gunsolly B, Summers RW, et al. Trazadone and liver toxicity. Ann Intern Med 1983; 99:128.

113. Beck PL, Bridges RJ, Demetrick DJ, et al. Chronic active hepatitis associated with Trazadone therapy Ann Intern Med 1993; 118:791.

114. Hull M, Jones R, Bendall M. Drug points: fatal hepatic necrosis associated with trazodone and neuroleptic drugs. Br Med J 1994; 309:378.

115. Hu KQ. Tiyyagura L. Kanel G. Redeker AG. Acute hepatitis induced by bupropion. Dig Dis Sci 2000; 45:1872–1873.

116. Brades JW, Korst HA, Litmann KP. Jaundice following nomifensine. Med Welt 1980; 31: 1607–1608.

117. Thomsen F, Jensen HC, Thomsen P. Liver damage after nomifensine. Ugeskr Laeger 1981; 143:1331–1332.

118. Zarski JP, Aubert H, Rachail M. Hepatic toxicity of new antidepressive drugs: apropos of a case. Gastroenterol Clin Biol 1983; 7:220–221.

119. Vaz FG, Singh R, Nuruzzaman M. Hepatitis induced by nomifensine: hepatitis induced by nomifensine. Br Med J 1984; 289:1268.

120. Judd FK, Holwill BJ, Norman TR. Liver impairment associated with nomifensine. Aust NZ J Psychiatry 1983; 17:288–289.

121. Kummer H, Marti F. Wegmann W. Granulomas hepatitis caused by nomifensine. J Suisse Med 1985; 115:1674–1678.

122. Simpson GK. Davidson NM. Possible hepatotoxicity of zimelidine. Br Med J Clin Res Ed 1983; 287:1181.

123. Noyes R, DuPont RL, Pecknold JC, Rifkin A, Rubin RT, Swinson RP, Ballenger JC, Burrows GD. Alprazolam in panic disorder and agoraphobia: results from a multicenter trial. Arch Gen Psychiatry 1988; 45:423–428.

124. Roy-Byrne P, Vittone BM, Uhde TW. Alprazolam-related hepatotoxicity. Lancet 1983; 2: 786.

125. Kratzsch KH, Buttner W, Reinhardt G. Intrahepatic cholestasis following chlordiazepoxide—contribution to the differential diagnosis of drug jaundice. Zitschr Gesamte Innere Med Ihre Grenzgebiete. 1972; 27:408–411.

126. Lo KJ, Eastwood IR, Eidelman S. Cholestatic jaundice associated with chlordiazepoxide hydrochloride (librium) therapy. Am J Dig Dis 1967; 12:845–849.

127. Tedesco FJ, Mills LR. Diazepam (valium) hepatitis. Dig Dis Sci 1982; 27:470–472.

128. Fang MH, Ginsberg AL, Dobbins W. Cholestatic jaundice associated with flurazepam hydrochloride. Ann Intern Med 1978; 89:363–364.

129. Cobden I, Record CO, White RWB. Fatal intrahepatic cholestasis associated with triazolam. Postgrad Med J 1981; 57:730.

130. Parker JLW. Potassium clorazepate (tranxene)-induced jaundice. Postgrad Med J 1979; 55: 908.

131. Moulin CH, Rolachon A, Cohard M, Girard M, Bichard P, Pasquier D, Mallaret M, Zarski JP. Fulminant hepatitis secondary to alprazolam. Therapie 1994; 49:362–363.

132. Hebersetzer F, Larrey D, Babany G, Degott C, Corbie M, Pessayre D, Benhamou JP. Clotiazepam-induced acute hepatitis. J Hepatol 1989; 9:256–259.

133. Roberts RK, Wilkinson GR, Branch RA, Schenker S. Effect of age and parenchymal liver disease on the disposition and elimination of chlordiazepoxide (librium). Gastroenterology 1978; 75:479–485.

134. Wilkinson GR. The effects of liver disease and aging on the disposition of diazepam, chlordiazepoxide, oxazepam and lorazepam in man. Acta Psychiatri Scand 1978; 274(suppl):56–74.

135. Harvey JK, Todd CW, Howard JW. Fatality associated with Benzedrine ingestion: a case report. Del Med J 1969; 1:537.

136. Jones AL, Jarvie DR, McDermid G, et al. Hepatocellular damage following amphetamine intoxication. Clin Toxicol 1994; 34:435.

137. Tillmann HL, VanPelt FNAM, Martz W, Luecke T, Welp H, Dorries F, Veuskens A, Fischer M, Manns MP. Accidental intoxication with methylene dianiline p,p′-diaminodiphenylmethane: acute liver damage after presumed ecstasy consumption. Clin Toxicol 1997; 35:35–40.

138. Khakoo kSI, Coles CJ, Armstrong JS, Barry RE. Hepatotoxicity and accelerated fibrosis following 3,4-methylenedioxymetamphetamine ("Ecstasy") usage. J Clin Gastroenterol 1995; 20:244–247.

139. Fidler H, Dhillon A, Gertner D, Burroughs A. Chronic ecstasy (3,4-methylenedioxymetamphetamine) abuse: a recurrent and unpredictable cause of severe acute hepatitis. J Hepatol 1996; 25:563–566.

140. Giner Duran R, Flors H, Millan M, Manzanera R. Hepatitis from ecstasy. Gastroenterol Hepatol 1998; 21:158.

141. Roques V, Perney P, Beaufort P, Hanslik B, Ramos J, Durand L. LeBricquir Y, Blanc F. Acute hepatitis due to ecstasy. Presse Med 1998; 27:468–470.

142. Indart Perez A, Mendia Gorostidi A, Barrio Andres J, Arens Mirave I. Acute hepatitis induced by ecstasy. Gastroenterol Hepatol 1998; 21:499.

143. Shearman JD, Chapman RWG, Satsangi J, Ryley NG. Misuse of ecstasy. Br Med J 1992; 305:309.

144. Henry JA. Jeffreys KJ. Dawling S. Toxicity and deaths from 3,4-methylenedioxymeth-amphetamine ("ecstasy") Lancet 1992; 340:384–387.

145. Dykhuizen RS, Smith CC, Brunt PW, Atkinson P, Simpson JG. Ecstasy induced hepatitis mimicking viral hepatitis. Gut 1995; 36:939–941.

146. VanThiel DH, Perper JA. Hepatotoxicity associated with cocaine abuse. Recent Dev Alcoholism 1992; 10:335–341.

147. Thompson ML, Schuster L, Shaw K. Cocaine-induced hepatic necrosis in mice: the role of cocaine metabolism. Biochem Pharmacol 1979; 28:2389–2395.

148. Schuster L, Casey E, Welenkiwar SS. Metabolism of cocaine and norcocaine to N-hydroxy-norcocaine. Biochem Pharmacol 1983; 32:3045–3051.

149. Kloss MW, Cavagnaro J, Rosen GM, Rauckman EJ. Involvement of FAD-containing monooxygenase in cocaine-induced hepatotoxicity. Toxicol Appl Pharmacol 1982; 64:88–93.

150. Rauckman EJ, Rosen GM, Cavagnaro J. Norcocaine nitroxide: a potential hepatotoxic metabolite of cocaine. Mol Pharmacol 1982; 21:458–463.

151. Rosen GM, Kloss MW, Rauckman EJ. Initiation of in vitro lipid peroxidation by N-hydroxy-norcocaine and norcocaine nitroxide. Mol Pharmacol 1982; 22:529–531.

152. Evans MA. Role of protein binding in cocaine-induced hepatic necrosis. J Pharmacol Exp Ther 1983; 224:73–79.

153. Brittebo E. Binding of cocaine in the liver, olfactory mucosa, eye and fur of pigmented mice. Toxicol Appl Pharmacol 1988; 96:315–323.

154. Kloss MW, Rosenb GM, Rauckman EJ. Cocaine-mediated hepatotoxicity: a critical review. Biochem Pharmacol 1984; 33:169–173.

155. Freeman RW, Harbison RD. The role of Benzoylmethylecgonine in cocaine-induced hepato-toxicity. J Pharmacol Exp Ther 1981; 218:558–567.

156. Evans MA, Harbison RD. Cocaine-induced hepatotoxicity in mice. Toxicol Appl Pharmacol 1978; 45:739–754.

157. Teaf CM, Freeman RW, Harbison RD. Cocaine-induced hepatotoxicity; lipid peroxidation as a possible mechanism. Drug Chem Toxicol 1984; 7:383–396.

158. Odeleye OE, Lopen MC, Smith BT, Eskelson CD, Watson RR. Cocaine hepatotoxicity during protein undernutrition of retrovirally infected mice. Can J Physiol Pharmacol 1992; 70:338–343.

159. Kloss MW, Rosen GM, Rauckman EJ. Acute cocaine-induced hepatotoxicity in DBA/2HA male mice. Toxicol Appl Pharmacol 1982; 65:75–83.

160. Bouis P, Boelsterli UA. Modulation of cocaine metabolism in primary rat hepatocyte cultures: effects on irreversible binding and protein biosynthesis. Toxicol Appl Pharmacol 1990; 104: 429–439.

161. Bornheim LM. Effect of cytochrome P450 inducers on cocaine-mediated hepatotoxicity. Toxicol Appl Pharmacol 1998; 150:158–165.

162. Smolen TN, Smolen A. Developmental expression of cocaine hepatotoxicity in the mouse. Pharmacol Biochem Behav 1990; 36:333–338.

163. Gottfied MR, Kloss MW, Graham D, Rauckman EJ, Rosen GM. Ultrastructure of experimental cocaine hepatotoxicity. Hepatology 1986; 6:299–304.

164. Kanel GC, Cassidy W, Shuster L, Reynolds TB. Cocaine-induced liver cell injury: comparison of morphological features in man and in experimental models. Hepatology 1990; 11: 646–651.

165. Odeleye OE, Watson RR, Eskelson CD, Earnest D. Enhancement of cocaine-induced hepato-toxicity by ethanol. Drug Alcohol Depend 1993; 31:253–263.

166. Smith AD, Freeman RW, Harrison RD. Ethanol enhancement of cocaine-induced hepatotoxicity. Biochem Pharmacol 1981; 30:453–458.

167. Pirozhkov SV, Eskelson CD, Watson RR. Chronic ethanol and cocaine-induced hepatotoxicity: effects of vitamin E supplementation. Alcohol Clin Exp Res 1992; 167:904–909.

168. Boyer CS, Petersen DR. Potentiation of cocaine-mediated hepatotoxicity by acute and chronic ethanol. Alcohol Exp Res 1990; 14:28–31.

169. Wanless IR, Dore S, Gopinath N, Tan J, Cameron R, Heathcote EJ, Blendis LM, Levy G. Histopathology of cocaine hepatotoxicity; report of four patients. Gastroenterology 1990; 98:497–501.

170. Minguillan JT, Novick DM, Kreek MJ. Liver function tests in non-parenteral cocaine users. Drug Alcohol Depend 1990; 26:169–174.

171. Silva MO, Roth D, Reddy KR, Fernandez JA, Saavedra JA, Schiff ER. Hepatic dysfunction accompanying acute cocaine intoxication. J Hepatol 1991; 12:312–315.

172. Goodman CR. Hepatotoxicity due to methylphenidate hydrochloride. NY State J Med 1972; 2339–2340.

173. Mehta H, Murray B, Loludice TA. Hepatic dysfunction due to intravenous abuse of methylphenidate hydrochloride. J Clin Gastroenterol 1984; 6:149–151.

174. Stecyk O, Loludice TA, Demeter S, Jacobs J. Multiple organ failure resulting from intravenous abuse of methylphenidate hydrochloride. Ann Emerg Med 1985; 14:597–599.

175. Assal F. Spahr L. Hadengue A. Rubbia-Brandt L. Burkhard PR. Rubbici-Brandt L. Tolcapone and fulminant hepatitis. Lancet 1998; 352:958.

176. New Warnings for Parkinson's Drug Tasmar. Rockville, MD: Food and Drug Administration, November 16, 1998.

177. Olanow CW. Tolcapone and hepatotoxic effects: Tasmar Advisory Panel. Arch Neurol 2000; 57:263–267.

178. Watkins P, Zimmerman H, Knapp M, Gracon S, Lewis K. Hepatotoxic effects of tacrine administration in patients with alzheimer's disease. JAMA 1994; 271:992–998.

179. Madden S, Woolf T, Pool W, Park BK. An investigation into the formation of stable, protein-reactive and cytotoxic metabolites from tacrine in vitro. Biochem Pharmacol 1993; 46:13–20.

180. Fontana R, Turgeon D, Woolf T, Knapp M, Watkins P. Tacrine hepatotoxicity: The use of caffeine to identify potential susceptibility factors (abstract). Hepatology 1999; 19:631.

181. Berson A, Renault S, Letteron P, Robin MA, Fromenty B, Fau D, LeBot MA, et al. Uncoupling of rat and human mitochondria: a possible explanation for tacrine-induced liver dysfunction. Gastroenterology 1996; 110:1878–1890.

182. Stachlewitz R, Arteel G, Raleigh J, Connor H, Mason R, Thurman R. Development and characterization of a new model of tacrine-induced hepatotoxicity: role of the sympathetic nervous system and hypoxia-reoxygenation. J Pharmacol Exp Ther 1997; 282:1591–1599.

183. Hammel P. Larrey D. Bernuau J. Kalafat M. Freneaux E. Babany G. Degott C. Feldmann G. Pessayre D. Benhamou JP. Acute hepatitis after tetrahydroaminoacridine administration for Alzheimer's disease. J Clin Gastroenterol 1990; 12:329–331.

184. Salmon L, Montet JC, Oddoze C, Montet AM, Portugal H, Michel BF. [Ursodeoxycholic acid and prevention of tacrine-induced hepatotoxicity: a pilot study] [Author's translation]. Therapie 2001; 56:29–34.

185. Remy A, Camu W, Ramos J, Blanc P, Larrey D. Acute hepatitis after riluzole administration. J Hepatol 1999; 30:527–530.

186. Sarin SK, Malhotra V, Jiloha RC, Munjal GC, Anand BS. Liver in heroin smokers. J Assoc Physicians India 1987; 35:421–424.

187. Min KW, Gyorkey F, Cain GD. Talc granulomata in liver disease in narcotic addicts. Arch Pathol 1974; 98:331–335.

188. Novick DM, Kreek MJ, Fanizza AM, Yancovitzk SR, Gelb AM, Stenger RJ. Methadone disposition in patients with chronic liver disease. Clin Pharmacol Ther 1981; 30:353–362.

189. Sawe J. High-dose morphine and methadone in cancer patients. Clin Pharmacol 1986; 11: 87–106.
190. Lee TH, Rees PJ. Hepatotoxicity of dextropropoxyphene. Br Med J 1977; 2:296–297.
191. Klein NC, Magida MG. Propoxyphene (Darvon) hepatotoxicity. Dig Dis 1971; 16:467–469.
192. Bassendine MF, Woodhouse KW, Bennett M, James OFW. Dextropropoxyphene induced hepatotoxicity mimicking biliary tract disease. Gut 1986; 27:444–449.
193. Rosenberg WM. Ryley NG. Trowell JM. McGee JO. Chapman RW. Dextropropoxyphene induced hepatotoxicity: a report of nine cases. J Hepatol 1993; 19:470–474.
194. Hochman JS, Brill NQ. Chronic marihuana usage and liver function (letter). Lancet 1971; 2:818–819.
195. Kew MC, Bersohn I, Siew S. Possible hepatotoxicity of cannabis (letter). Lancet 1969; 1: 578–579.
196. Payne RJ, Brand SN. The toxicity of intravenously used marihuana. JAMA 1975; 233:351–354.
197. Selim K, Kaplowitz N. Hepatotoxicity of psychotropic drugs. Hepatology 1999; 29:1347–1351.

20

Antibacterials and Antifungal Agents

JEAN FREDERIC WESTPHAL and JEAN MARIE BROGARD

University Hospital, Strasbourg, France

I. INTRODUCTION

Although antimicrobial and antifungal agents are among the most widely prescribed drugs, symptomatic hepatotoxicity remains uncommon and far less frequent than other adverse effects such as gastrointestinal disorders or cutaneous reactions. However, the potential severity of the hepatotoxic reactions to some antibacterial or antifungal agents makes the issue of importance.

Antimicrobial-related liver injuries encompass most of the clinical and histopathological expressions of hepatic dysfunction, including hepatocellular necrosis, intrahepatic cholestasis, mixed hepatitis, vanishing bile duct syndrome, microvesicular steatosis, and chronic active hepatitis.

The large majority of hepatic reactions related to antimicrobial agents are idiosyncratic; liver injury occurs rarely and unpredictably. Only tetracyclines and oxypenicillins exhibit partial relationship to dose. Immunological mechanisms and a genetically determined predisposition may play a pathogenic role in acute liver injury and facilitate progression to chronic liver disease.

Establishing the clinical diagnosis of a drug-induced liver disease is often awkward because the diagnosis is based mainly on circumstantial evidence. Some confounding factors may intervene and make it difficult to identify precisely the cause of liver injury. For example, no doubt polypharmacy can render the diagnosis problematic. Also, elevated levels of liver enzymes and bilirubin during sepsis in adults without preexisting malignant neoplasms or hepatobiliary disease are common. In a prospective study including 84 patients with bacteremia, there was an abnormality of at least one of the hepatic biochemical parameters (aspartate aminotransferase, alanine aminotransferase, alkaline phosphatase, and bilirubin) in 65% of the patients (1). The elevations were usually mild (only rarely exceeded the upper limit of normal by threefold), of short duration, common to a variety of gram-positive and gram-negative infections, and of no prognostic signification.

Furthermore, jaundice in bacterial pneumonia is not rare (2) and is recognized to be of hepatocellular origin. The specific cause for the hepatic impairment in these clinical conditions is unknown.

The present chapter addresses the current knowledge of the hepatotoxic potential of commonly used antibacterial or antifungal agents.

II. ANTIBACTERIAL AGENTS

A. Beta-Lactam Antibiotics

1. Penicillins

Penicillins are a well-recognized cause of subclinical liver injury, which is more frequently cytolytic than cholestatic (3).

Hepatotoxicity is rarely associated with *natural penicillin*. Reports of benzylpenicillin and phenoxymethyl-penicillin liver injury are limited to very few case reports of acute hepatitis (4,5) or cholestasis (6).

Similarly a few single case reports of aminopenicillin-related hepatotoxicity have been described; *ampicillin* and *amoxicillin* have been involved in severe cholestasis and the vanishing bile duct syndrome (VBDS) (7,8). Rarely, cases of acute liver injury and granulomas have been attributed to amoxicillin (9). The incidence rate of developing acute liver injury related to amoxicillin has been estimated as 0.3 per 10,000 prescriptions (10).

Mild anicteric hepatitis has been described following large doses of *carbenicillin* (30 mg/day) (11). Biopsy specimens of the liver showed spotty liver cell necrosis without cholestasis. However, in another study, prolonged therapy with high daily dosage does not seem to be a risk factor for the occurrence of liver damage: no case of hepatotoxicity was recorded in a retrospective review of 35 courses of intravenous treatment with carbenicillin (12).

The semisynthetic penicillinase-resistant oxypenicillins oxacillin, (di-)cloxacillin, and flucloxacillin exhibit a well-known hepatotoxic potential. Surveys of liver reactions probably or possibly induced by oxypenicillins and spontaneously reported to some Adverse Drug Reactions Advisory Committees have allowed the clinical features and natural history to be better delineated (13,14), especially for flucloxacillin hepatotoxicity.

Flucloxacillin has been recognized as an important cause of antibacterial-induced hepatotoxicity. The risk of a patient developing flucloxacillin hepatotoxicity proves to be similar in different countries: 1 in 13,000 prescriptions in the United Kingdom, 1 in 15,000 to 1 in 26,000 in Australia, and 1 in 11,000 to 1 in 30,000 prescriptions in Sweden (13,15,16). Gender (female predominance with a sex ratio of 2:1), increasing age (odds ratio of 18 when comparing age > 55 years vs. < 30 years), duration of therapy over 14 days, and high daily doses were associated with increased risk of hepatotoxicity (13,17).

The time to onset of hepatic reaction is 1–9 weeks after starting therapy and up to 6 weeks after stopping the agent. The serum biochemical abnormalities are indicative of cholestatic hepatitis. The dominating histological feature is cholestasis, both hepatocellular and canalicular, with minimal hepatic necrosis and usually, a moderate inflammatory reaction and lymphocytic infiltration. In some cases neutrophilic and eosinophilic granulocytes may be observed. Bile ducts may be reduced in number and size, while the bile duct epithelium usually shows degenerative changes.

The course of cholestatic hepatitis is often prolonged. The tendency to protracted course in the flucloxacillin-induced cholestasis may be accounted for by the fact that some patients show continued progression of liver test abnormalities several weeks after withdrawal of the drug (13).

However, flucloxacillin is associated with an increased risk of chronic cholestasis, with 10–30% of cases continuing for more than 6 months. In these cases, histopathological pattern is characterized by paucity of smaller bile ducts and ductules, and portal tract inflammation focused on injured bile ducts. This pattern may further progress toward the VBDS or biliary cirrhosis (8,13,18–20).

The other oxypenicillins, *oxacillin*, *cloxacillin*, and *dicloxacillin*, can also cause cholestasis, with an estimated risk of developing hepatotoxicity about half that of flucloxacillin (13). The predominant pattern is cholestatic hepatitis. It usually appears after 1–4 weeks of treatment (21–27). A delay between cessation of therapy and occurrence of jaundice can be observed; it is usually about 1 week. Histological findings include portal inflammation and centrolobular cholestasis (13,24). Occasionally, granulomas may be seen (23). After discontinuation of the drug, spontaneous resolution usually occurs within 3 months (13). Oxacillin has been associated with a hepatocellular picture of liver damage (25). This is an uncommon reaction that resolves rapidly on withdrawal of the drug. High dosage and intravenous administration have been identified as risk factors (21–23,25).

Liver injury is likely to result from an idiosyncratic reaction, given the rarity of hepatotoxicity, the lack of dose dependency, and the highly variable lag period before the onset of liver abnormalities. Despite the variability of clinical symptoms indicative of allergy, other findings suggest an underlying immunoallergic process. These include the rapid recurrence of hepatic dysfunction on rechallenge, the relative frequency of mild peripheral or liver tissue eosinophilia, and the results of immunoallergic tests such as mast-cell degranulation, macrophage inhibition factor, and lymphocyte sensitization tests (27–29).

Hepatotoxicity of *amoxicillin–clavulanic acid* (ACA) has been extensively described (31–42). The liver function abnormality is mainly cholestatic (31,32,37). Less commonly, hepatocellular or mixed hepatocellular-cholestatic involvement is observed (32,42). In contrast to most adverse drug reactions, males appear to have a greater risk than females (2–4:1) (32,36,43).

The incidence rate of acute liver injury associated with ACA in a recent retrospective cohort study (10) proved to be 1.7/10,000 prescriptions. The source population was a general population registered on a single large general-practice-based computerized database. The risk increased with duration of therapy (defined as completion of two or more consecutive prescriptions) and with age. Among users of ACA combination, the risk of developing acute liver injury was more than 3 times greater after a course of two or more consecutive prescriptions than after a single one. The risk was enhanced with age: the incidence rate was 3.2/10,000 prescriptions in subjects over 65 years versus 1.3/10,000 in younger patients. Elderly people receiving repeated prescriptions of ACA appear to be the group at higher risk, with an incidence rate of 135/100,000 users, indicating substantial interaction between both risk factors.

Similar findings have been reported in a retrospective case-control study aimed at identifying risk factors for the development of ACA-associated jaundice (44): patients over 55 years had an odds ratio of 16.1 (95% confidence interval CI, 2.9–88.9) compared with patients less than 30 years. Men had an odds ratio of 2.5 (95% CI, 1.1–5.4) compared with women. Interestingly, there was no association with previous drug allergies. Furthermore, no association has been found with previous ACA exposure: some patients with ACA hepatotoxicity had taken one or more previous courses of ACA with no documented ill effect, possibly indicating the development of a hypersensitivity response.

It should be stressed, however, that adverse hepatic biochemical and histological abnormalities associated with ACA are few, considering its widespread use (45). It remains clear that elderly patients should be more closely monitored for the occurrence of ACA hepatotoxicity.

Often, there is a delay between the cessation of drug administration and the onset of jaundice; this delay can range from several days up to 8 weeks (46,47). A minority of patients develop jaundice while taking the drug.

Features of hypersensitivity, such as fever, skin rash, arthralgias, and eosinophilia, have been variably observed in approximately 30–60% of the patients. In addition, hepatitis may be accompanied by prominent extrahepatic manifestations such as acute interstitial nephritis or acute lacrimal gland inflammation and sialadenitis (42). The period of recovery proves to be variable with jaundice resolving within 1–8 weeks and complete recovery occurring over a longer period of 4–16 weeks. Although the outcome is usually good, fatalities have been reported (39,40,41,48). One case of chronic liver disease related to ACA has also been reported (46).

Histological findings include centrilobular canalicular cholestasis, variable portal edema, and mixed inflammatory infiltrate with lymphocytes, neutrophils, and eosinophils. Interlobular bile duct injury of varying degree seems to be common (42): abnormalities include irregularity of the nuclei, vacuolization of the epithelial cells, neutrophilic or lymphocytic infiltration of the epithelium, and destruction of the cells with endothelialization of the biliary epithelium (31,39,42). It appears that the presence of bile duct damage and associated bile duct proliferation in the face of cholestasis would be relatively characteristic of ACA-induced hepatotoxicity (49).

Another finding reported is the presence of a focal destructive cholangiopathy with the ducts showing extensive inflammatory infiltration and necrosis of part of the bile duct wall (46), bearing some similarities to the lesions observed in primary biliary cirrhosis or primary sclerosing cholangitis. Occasionally, granulomatous hepatitis has been described (37,38,46). Clavulanic acid is thought to account for ACA hepatotoxicity. Indeed, although amoxicillin by itself has been reported to cause abnormalities in hepatic biochemical tests and, very rarely, acute hepatitis, rechallenge with this aminopenicillin in individuals who had previously experienced ACA-related hepatotoxicity has not been associated with recurrence of liver injury; in contrast, rechallenge with ACA was positive (31,36,37,46). The results of the retrospective cohort study by Garcia Rodrigues et al. (10) also lend some support to the role of clavulanic acid: the incidence rate ratios and 95% CIs of acute liver injury for ACA compared with amoxicillin alone were 6.3 (3.2–12.7) for all cases and 8.4 (3.6–20.8) for cases presenting with jaundice. Data were derived from a cohort of 93,433 users of ACA and 360,333 users of amoxicillin alone who were followed up from 1991 through 1992.

The presence of hypersensitivity clinical manifestations suggests that an immunoallergic mechanism underlies ACA-related hepatotoxicity. This hypothesis has recently been substantiated by a HLA typing study in 35 patients with biopsy-demonstrated ACA-induced hepatitis (50). The study group was characterized by a higher frequency of DRB1 * 1501–DRB5 * 0101–DQB1 * 0602 haplotype (57% vs. 11.7% in controls, p highly significant). Those patients with this haplotype were more likely than patients without it to have a cholestatic (70% vs. 60%) or mixed (30% vs. 13%) than a hepatocellular pattern of hepatitis (0% vs. 27%). The authors conclude that ACA-induced hepatitis is associated with the DRB1 * 1501–DRB5 * 0101–DQB1 * 0602 haplotype, and that these data support the view that HLA-mediated recognition of neoantigens also plays a crucial role in the pathogenesis of drug-induced immunoallergic hepatitis. However the DRB1 * 1501–DRB5 * 0101–DQB1 * 0602 haplotype was present in 11.7% of normal controls, whereas ACA-induced hepatitis only seems to affect from 1/1000 to 1/10,000 treated patients (10,37). HLA association thus cannot be the only factor responsible to explain the pathogenesis of the disease. Other factors must act concurrently. The simultaneous existence of a metabolic idiosyncrasy is not ruled out, given the extensive metabolism of clavulanic acid in humans (51).

Transient mild elevations in liver aminotransferases have been reported in 2–5% of all patients receiving *ureidopenicillins* (52–54), but there have not been any reports of clinically evident hepatotoxicity. In isolated populations, however, higher frequencies of mild abnormalities have been observed: 21% (17 of 78 patients) AST elevation with piperacillin (53). All aminotransferase elevations were reversible and of no major clinical importance.

Safety of large doses of ureidopenicillins (mezlocillin, azlocillin, or piperacillin) given for prolonged periods for the treatment of chronic pseudomonal osteomyelitis has been assessed in a retrospective study (12). Liver damage—i.e., two- to threefold increases of aminotransferase serum levels—occurred in 19.3% (6/31) of the patients. The number and the severity of the reactions appeared to be related to the cumulative ureidopenicillin dose and/or the duration of therapy. In the subgroup of patients treated with mezlocillin, adverse reactions, including liver dysfunction, were most likely to occur with a cumulative dose of more than 250 g or when duration of therapy exceeded 2 weeks.

A review of abnormal laboratory tests noted during phase I and phase III trials assessing the antibiotic combination *piperacillin/tazobactam* showed that the most common abnormalities were related to hepatic function (55): 1.1% of patients had increased total bilirubin levels, and 5.6% had increased alanine aminotransferase levels. In comparative studies, the rates of abnormalities during administration of piperacillin/tazobactam were two- to threefold lower than those noted with imipenem/cilastatin. Laboratory test profiles observed in published clinical trials tended to parallel those described in the premarketing trials (56): rates of abnormalities in tests of hepatic function occasionally exceeded 10% among patients given piperacillin/tazobactam; these higher rates, however, were seen almost exclusively among the more seriously ill patients, including those who were bacteremic. No case of overt hepatitis was reported.

2. Other Beta-Lactam Antibiotics

Transient increases in serum aminotransferase levels and alkaline phosphatase are commonly observed in patients receiving parenteral *cephalosporins* (53,57,58). These increases have also been reported in 0.7–11% of patients on orally administered cephalosporin therapy, including ceflaclor, cefixime, and cefprozil (58). Very rarely, cholestatic hepatitis following cephalosporin therapy has been described (59–62).

Review of adverse experiences and tolerability in the first 2516 patients treated with *imipenem/cilastatin* has shown that transient elevations in hepatic enzyme levels occurred in approximately 1% of cases (63). One anecdotal case of cholestatic hepatitis related to imipenem/cilastatin has been described (64).

In a worldwide overview of 2117 patients who received *aztreonam* (65), transient increases in serum aspartate or alanine aminotransferase and alkaline phosphatase enzyme levels had occured in about 5% of patients. When such increases did occur, however, enzyme levels never increased more than three times normal and were not associated with hepatobiliary dysfunction. In all cases, when drug treatment was discontinued, enzyme levels returned to pretreatment values. Until now, no case of overt hepatitis has been reported (66).

B. Macrolide Antibiotics

1.   Epidemiology

Erythromycin has long been associated with hepatotoxicity. Earlier reports in the sixties considered erythromycin estolate as the derivative most frequently responsible for hepatitis. Other erythromycin derivatives, such as erythromycin propionate (67), erythromycin stearate (68), and erythromycin ethylsuccinate (69–71), all have also been associated with cholestatic hepatitis.

Two studies have led to the conclusion, however, that the risk of hepatotoxicity associated with erythromycin does not significantly differ from one salt to another. The first study was a prescription event monitoring in 12,208 patients (72): three cases were attributed to erythromycin stearate and no cases of jaundice were ascribed to the estolate. The second study analyzed the data from a voluntary reporting system: in 10 (0.29%) of 3422 reports erythromycins were considered to have caused hepatotoxicity; the incidence did not significantly differ between the various forms of erythromycin (73).

There are no prospective trials determining the true incidence of erythromycin-related hepatotoxicity. In a general practice-based, retrospective, cohort study, the estimated risk for erythromycin-induced cholestatic hepatitis was 3.6 per 100,000 patients (74). In a hospital-based case-control study (75), Medicaid billing data from Michigan and Florida between 1980 and 1987 were examined to determine whether erythromycin derivatives were associated with an increased risk for acute hepatitis. The 107 cases included were patients hospitalized with acute symptomatic hepatitis without an identifiable cause of liver disease noted in the medical record. Four controls per case were randomly selected. The relative risk (odds ratio) of acute liver disease associated with erythromycins was 5.2 (95% CI, 1.1–26.6). The authors concluded that the number of patients developing acute symptomatic liver disease resulting in hospitalization for each million patients treated with a 10-day course of erythromycin was 2.28 cases.

2.   Clinical and Histopathological Characteristics of Erythromycin-Related Liver Injury

In approximately three-fourths of cases, there is a lag period of about 6–20 days between initiation of therapy and the onset of clinical symptomatology. In some cases, hepatitis may be clinically obvious only after completion of erythromycin therapy, especially if the treatment has been of short duration, i.e., <8 days, or in the unusual cases where hepatitis appears within 45 days after treatment has begun (74). The clinical picture of erythromycin-induced hepatitis is similar to that of all the types of derivatives, and often resembles acute cholecystitis, including abdominal pain, nausea, jaundice, and fever (68,76). Aminotransferase serum levels are moderately increased (less than 10 times normal), and frequently associated with mild elevation of alkaline phosphatase and bilirubin serum levels, i.e., a primarily cholestatic picture. Serum eosinophilia is found in approximately 40–50% of cases. The latter, coupled with the usual lag period quoted above, prompt hepatitis after rechallenge (usually within a day), and frequent symptoms of sensitization (fever, rash), are in favor of an immunoallergic process (68,71,76,77). In addition, some cases of recurrent hepatitis due to cross-reactivity between erythromycin derivatives have been described (67,70). Keefe et al. (70) described two patients with hepatotoxicity to erythromycin estolate who developed accelerated toxicity to erythromycin ethylsuccinate many years later, including rapid recurrence of symptoms in both subjects, with eosinophilia, fever, and rash in one subject. Usually, there is complete recovery after discontinuation of the drug, but it may take several weeks. Until now, only one case of fatal hepatic coma possibly related to erythromycin hepatotoxicity (following high intravenous doses of the lactobionate derivative) has been reported (78).

Histopathological findings include centrizonal cholestasis, frequently associated with portal and lobular inflammatory infiltrate, presence of eosinophils, and mild hepatocellular necrosis (68,79). These features classify the lesions as mixed hepatic injury, predominantly cholestasis. Electron microscopy reveals dilated canaliculi, distorted or absent microvilli, diminished nuclear size, and enlargement of the endoplasmic reticulum (80).

Ductopenia as a chronic manifestation following erythromycin-induced cholestasis has been rarely reported (81,82). The absence of interlobular bile ducts in at least 50% of the portal tracts has been observed in such cases. This histopathological pattern resembles primary biliary cirrhosis. Prognosis depends on the potential of such a disease to evolve toward progressive destruction of the intrahepatic bile ducts even though the drug has been early withdrawn.

3. Hepatic Dysfunction Induced by Other Macrolides

In a review encompassing 17 multicenter comparative or noncomparative studies, less than 0.7% of 2917 patients treated with *roxithromycin* (150 mg twice a day) had changes in serum total bilirubin, ALT, AST, or alkaline phosphatase (83). Some cases of cholestatic hepatitis have been ascribed to roxithromycin (84,85).

The overall tolerability of *clarithromycin* has been assessed by compilation of data from comparative investigations conducted worldwide in a total of 4291 patients who received at least one 250- or 500-mg dose of the drug (86). The incidence of elevated AST or ALT activity was 5%.

The first cases of cholestatic hepatitis in patients who received clarithromycin therapy were reported several years ago. In a series of 13 elderly patients with chronic lung disease due to *Mycobacterium avium complex* or *Myco. abscessus*, high-dose clarithromycin monotherapy (2 g/day) elicited elevation in liver enzyme levels at weeks 1–6 of therapy in five cases (38%) and was associated with unexpectedly high serum levels of the drug (87). Three additional cases of clarithromycin-induced hepatotoxicity were subsequently reported (88,89). On the whole, the biochemical pattern was primarily cholestatic (six of eight cases) with minimal elevation of the levels of AST and ALT (seven of eight cases). In all cases the maximum absolute values for alkaline phosphatases and/or gamma glutamyl transpeptidases exceeded those for aminotransferases. The patients who developed these signs of hepatotoxicity were typically elderly or had reduced body mass, and were receiving clarithromycin doses of 2 g/day. The liver serum enzyme levels became abnormal after 4–8 weeks of therapy and were frequently asymptomatic (five of eight patients). It usually took from 1 to 3 months for levels to return to normal. Interestingly, retrial with lower dose of clarithromycin (500 mg twice a day) in four of these patients did not cause elevation of hepatic enzymes (87). Accordingly, the ability of some patients to tolerate lower dose of clarithromycin would suggest that the toxicity might be at least in part dose- and serum-level-related. In one case, however, rechallenge of clarithromycin elicited prompt recurrence of hepatic dysfunction (88), which lends some support to the possibility of hypersensitivity or an idiosyncratic reaction in some subjects.

Erythromycin acistrate is a relatively recent ester prodrug of erythromycin with a chemical structure that resembles erythromycin estolate. In toxicological studies acistrate did not determine the problems of hepatotoxicity (90). In a large postmarketing study 1549 patients with respiratory tract or skin infections were monitored for liver parameters while being treated for 7–14 days with acistrate. Ten patients (0.6%) had two or more clearly elevated liver enzyme values by the end of therapy. In only three of these cases could liver enzyme abnormalities be ascribed to acistrate therapy (91).

The tolerability profile of oral *azithromycin* has been evaluated by compilation of data from comparative studies conducted in the United States and Europe (92). A total of 3995 patients were included. Assessments of adverse events and laboratory tests were performed before beginning of treatment and approximately 7–14 days and 30 days after the start of therapy. Treatment-related biochemical abnormalities exceeding a frequency of 1% were recorded for ALT (1.7%) and AST (1.5%). In clinical trials of community-acquired pneumonia, tolerance of intravenous azithromycin has been favorable. Laboratory abnormalities, including elevated ALT or AST, were reported with an incidence of 4–6% (93), leading to discontinuation of therapy in some patients, but no case of overt acute hepatitis has been reported.

Sides and Conforti (94) reviewed the data from clinical studies over a 6-year period to assess the safety of *dirithromycin* in the treatment of a variety of acute infections. The review encompassed a total of 4263 patients treated with dirithromycin (500 mg once daily for 7–10 days). Mild elevation of ALT or AST was seen in less than 1%.

Rarely some cases of cholestatic hepatitis occurring during the course of josamycin therapy have been described (95,96).

4. Mechanism of Macrolide-Related Hepatic Injury

The mechanism for hepatotoxicity of macrolides remains relatively unknown. However, there are several lines of evidence both for toxicity and for immunoallergic processes.

Results of in vitro experiments argue for an intrinsic hepatotoxic potential of erythromycin. It has been shown to be cytotoxic against cultured hepatocytes (97), and to decrease bile secretion in the isolated perfused rat liver (98). Hepatotoxicity can also be produced in rats and dogs by administration of high doses of different esters or salts of erythromycin, suggesting a direct hepatotoxic effect (90,99).

In humans also, a number of clinical reports lend some support to such an effect: the afore-mentioned ability of certain patients to tolerate retrial of clarithromycin at lower dosage than that having previously elicited hepatotoxicity runs in favor of a toxic-type hepatic dysfunction (87).

In contrast, jaundice is frequently associated with hypersensitivity manifestations, as mentioned above.

Erythromycin is known to induce its own biotransformation by enhancing microsomal enzymes in the liver and particularly some isoenzymes of the cytochrome P450 3A subfamily with high affinity to erythromycin, especially the cytochrome P450 3A4 (CYP 3A4) (100,101). The latter demethylates and oxidizes erythromycin into unstable metabolic intermediates (so-called nitrosoalkanes), which would subsequently form inactive cytochrome P450 Fe(II)-metabolic intermediate complexes (102), thereby inhibiting CYP 3A catalytic activity. This mechanism explains largely the vast majority of pharmacokinetic drug interactions induced by the macrolides (103,104). However, unless they are stabilized through the formation of stable complexes with the iron of cytochrome P450, nitrosoalkanes are unstable, reactive metabolites that can also react with glutathione or with cysteine and might, accordingly, bind covalently to the SH groups of hepatic proteins (76). The hypothetical mechanism proposed by Pessayre et al. (76) links up all these clinical or experimental data: in some patients, the hepatotoxic potential of macrolides would produce minor liver lesions and mildy raise serum aminotransferase activity. Necrosis of a few hepatocytes would release in the circulation plasma membrane proteins modified by covalent binding of the reactive metabolites. These modified liver antigens would be recognized as foreign and might subsequently trigger immune response. In a few individuals, the immune response might be cytotoxic for the hepatocytes, eventually resulting in hepatitis.

There may be some relationship between metabolism of macrolides and their hepatotoxicity. Macrolide antibiotics differ in their abilities to bind to and inhibit cytochrome P450 isoforms. These differences allow macrolides to be classified into three groups (103,105). Group 1 agents include troleandomycin (now withdrawn) and erythromycin; these bind strongly to and inhibit CYP 3A4 by forming an inactive CYP 3A4-metabolite complex. Group 2 macrolides include clarithromycin, roxithromycin, and josamycin (100,105,106), have intermediate binding affinity to CYP 3A4, and form complexes to a lesser extent. Group 3 agents encompass spiramycin, azithromycin, and dirithromycin, which have been shown not to form nitrosoalkanes in vitro and, hence, not to inhibit CYP 3A4 (107–109). Some structural features of macrolides might account for these differences (107–110).

It has been observed that, to some extent, there is some correlation between the above-mentioned classification and the various potential of macrolides for drug interactions of metabolic type (104,105). Apparently, on the basis of the epidemiological data reported above on macrolide-induced hepatotoxicity, such a correlation might also exist between this classification and the different propensities of macrolides to cause hepatotoxicity. Indeed, erythromycins, which form nitrosoalkanes, produce hepatitis, whereas group 3 macrolides, which do not form these metabolites, have not been shown as yet to cause hepatitis. Group 2 macrolides exhibit an intermediate figure.

This apparent parallelism between the differential formation of nitrosoalkanes from the various macrolides and the propensity to cause hepatotoxicity appears therefore to be consistent with the mechanism proposed by Pessayre et al. (76) for macrolide-induced hepatotoxicity.

C. Sulfonamides

1. Clinical and Histopathological Features

Several of the sulfonamides alone or as part of a combination drug have been reported to be hepatotoxic. Those include sulfamethoxazole (111–113), trimethoprim-sulfamethoxazole (114–126), sulfamethoxypyridazine (113), sulfasalazine (127–130), pyrimethamine-sulfadoxine (131–133), and sulfamethizole (113).

Sulfonamides may cause hepatocellular injury, which usually starts within a few weeks of administration and may be accompanied by fever, skin rash, eosinophilia, and injury to other organs (68,112). Liver biopsy may show cholestasis with little or no necrosis (68,112), or prominent hepatocellular necrosis (114). The inflammatory infiltrate is usually lymphoid, sometimes with eosinophils (112–114). Infrequently, granulomatous hepatitis due to pyrimethamine-sulfadoxine, sulfasalazine, or trimethoprim-sulfamethoxazole has been observed (118,128,133). Occasionally, sulfonamide-induced liver injury may progress to chronic liver disease (113).

Although sulfonamide-induced liver injury is usually mild, massive necrosis of the liver after a short course of sulfasalazine (127) has been described, and fatal hepatotoxicity due to trimethoprim-sulfamethoxazole (114,116,122) and pyrimethamine-sulfadoxine (134,135) has been reported.

Most forms of liver dysfunction have been linked with trimethoprim-sulfamethoxazole (cotrimoxazole).

Although transient increases in aminotransferase serum levels are common, occurring in approximately 10% of patients (136), clinical hepatotoxicity is rare, except in patients with AIDS. A hospital-based case-control study has estimated that the frequency of trimethoprim-sulfamethoxazole-induced hepatitis requiring hospitalization is less than 1 in 100,000 prescriptions (75). Similarly a case history study that included approximately 280,000 patients (137) found only one case of trimethoprim-sulfamethoxazole-induced liver disease requiring hospitalization during a 5-year period.

Several cases of symptomatic hepatic injury have been reported after trimethoprim-sulfamethoxazole therapy (114–126). Most were accompanied by fever and rash, or less frequently, leukocytosis or eosinophilia.

In a number of cases, there was a multisystem reaction with lymphadenopathy, pulmonary lesions, renal insufficiency, pancreatitis, and only mild elevation of liver enzymes in the serum (68,116).

Cases where hepatitis was the predominant feature were usually cholestatic (117,124,125), but hepatocellular patterns were also reported (114). Symptoms appeared within 3 days–4 weeks of therapy, but in case of rechallenge with the sulfonamide in patients with previous hypersensitivity reactions, the latent period before adverse drug reaction is reduced and may lead to fatal outcome (122,124). The average duration of trimethoprim-sulfamethoxazole therapy before onset of symptoms of toxicity has been 2.5 weeks. Cholestasis has been of moderate severity, with serum total bilirubin <20 mg/dL. The duration of illness has varied from 1 week to 3 months, and the great majority of patients recovered. Cholestasis may be sometimes prolonged up to 6–8 months (125,126), however, and some fatal cases have been described (114,116,122).

Histopathology often showed almost pure centrilobular cholestasis, with mild to moderate portal inflammation and feathering degeneration (68,117,124,125); massive necrosis was seen in some fatal cases (114). Recently, bile duct injury with depletion of ducts and ductular proliferation has been reported with trimethoprim-sulfamethoxazole (126,138). The portal inflammatory infiltrate was mixed with a predominance of lymphocytes and small numbers of eosinophils and neutrophils. In such a pattern, ductopenia accompanies, but does not cause, the early tissue cholestasis. This may imply that the injury would be directed to both hepatocytes and duct cells and that early cholestasis would be determined by the hepatocellular injury. Subsequently, late cholestasis would be related to duct proliferation. An unusual case of hepatic phospholipidosis combined with intrahepatic cholestasis following trimethoprim-sulfamethoxazole therapy has been reported (125). The striking feature observed on electron microscopic evaluation was the presence of prominent hepatocyte lysosomal inclusions, which were characterized by concentric arrangements of lamellar membranous structures.

2. Mechanism

Several lines of evidence substantiate an immunoallergic mechanism underlying adverse reactions to sulfonamides: the relatively frequent clinical manifestations of allergy, the significant proportion of eosinophils in the inflammatory infiltrate found in liver biopsies, positive in vitro lymphocyte transformation tests in patients with trimethoprim-sulfamethoxazole-induced skin lesions, the reduced latent period before adverse drug reaction in case of rechallenge, and cross-reactions between sulfonamides (122,124,139).

However, a number of studies have recently argued in favor of an additional metabolite-dependent mechanism that would account, at least in part, for the idiosyncratic toxicity of sulfonamides.

Sulfonamides are eliminated primarily by renal excretion following N-acetylation, but a small fraction of a given sulfonamide dose undergoes hepatic oxidative metabolism by the cytochrome P450 3A4 and 2C9 isoforms (140) to a reactive metabolite, the hydroxylamine (141–143), that is toxic to peripheral blood lymphocytes (144,145).

N-Acetyltransferase activity has been demonstrated to be polymorphic, with slow and fast acetylator phenotypes (146). When the acetylator phenotype of patients with a history of sulfonamide toxicity and controls is compared, a significantly larger percentage of patients are slow acetylators compared with controls (90 vs. 55%) (147). Similar results have been subsequently reported by Wolkenstein et al. (148). These findings corroborate and substantiate the initial report by Das et al. (149), who showed that in a series of 133 patients with inflammatory bowel disease treated with sulfasalazine, 21% developed adverse reactions due to the drug. These reactions were shown to correlate with slow-acetylator phenotype. It should be stressed, however, that slow-acetylator phenotype per se is not sufficient to account for susceptibility to sulfonamide toxicity, since approximately half the population of western Europe and North America are slow acetylators (146), whereas the incidence of sulfonamide hypersensitivity reactions occur in 1/1000–1/10,000 non-AIDS patients given sulfonamides.

The role of other factors involved in the detoxification of reactive metabolites of sulfonamide has been demonstrated. When peripheral blood lymphocytes from patients who have experienced sulfonamide hypersensitivity reactions or controls are incubated with sulfonamide hydroxylamines, the lymphocytes of patients show significantly more cell death than do the cells of controls, suggesting that there are differences between patients and controls in their capacity to detoxify reactive metabolites of sulfonamides (150,151). Susceptibility to sulfonamide metabolites has also been found in some parents of the patients (150). The nature of the presumed deficiency remains unknown as yet.

This suggests that pharmacogenetic differences in the production and detoxification of reactive metabolites of sulfonamide contribute significantly to the pathophysiology of sulfonamide hypersensitivity reactions. The role of N-acetylation capacity in sulfonamide hepatoxicity may be explained as follows: in case of slow-acetylator phenotype, sulfonamides are preferentially metabolized by cytochrome-P450-mediated oxidation. This can lead to the formation of chemically reactive metabolites, in particular hydroxylamines, which need to be actively detoxified. The enhanced production of these toxic metabolites would overwhelm host defenses in patients with defective detoxification capacities for these metabolites. It is believed that these reactive metabolites would produce direct cyto-

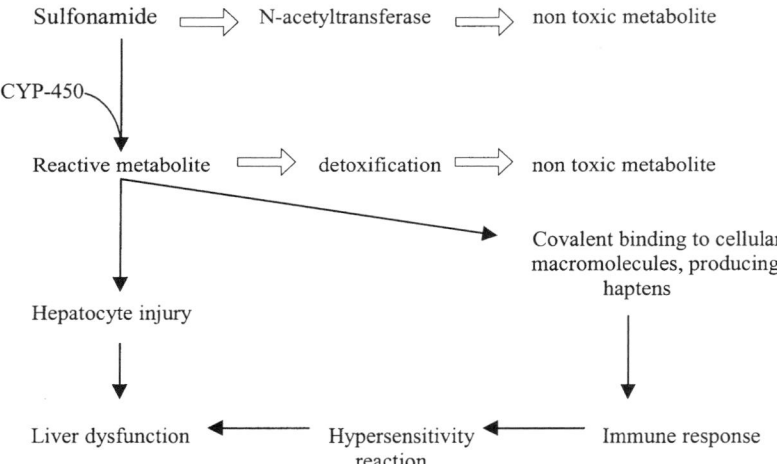

Figure 1   Pathogenesis of hypersensitivity reactions to sulfonamides.

toxic effects and, also, bind to macroproteins, producing haptens. These haptens might elicit an immune response, promoting the occurrence or the enhancement of hepatitis, as well as other idiosyncratic drug reactions observed in patients receiving sulfamethoxazole (152) (Fig. 1).

It should be stressed that some uncertainty remains, however, on the potential role of trimethoprim in trimethoprim-sulfamethoxazole hepatotoxicity. Although the sulfonamide component of the combination is suspected of causing the toxic effect (112), an anecdotal report exists of a patient who developed jaundice after trimethoprim-sulfamethoxazole exposure and had a recurrence of the jaundice when she was subsequently challenged with trimethoprim alone (153). Additionally, a retrospective study has given some epidemiological evidence that the combination of trimethoprim and sulfamethoxazole was more likely to cause hepatotoxicity than administration of the sulfonamide alone (154).

3.   Trimethoprim-Sulfamethoxazole in AIDS Patients

Sulfonamides are used as both prophylaxis and treatment for *Pneumocystis carinii* pneumonia in patients infected with the human immunodeficiency virus (HIV). The use of trimethoprim-sulfamethoxazole (cotrimoxazole) is hampered by the high incidence (24–57%) of hypersensitivity reactions in these patients (155–158). The side effects consist of rash, fever, liver and kidney damage, as well as thrombocytopenia, neutropenia, and hemolysis. These reactions typically occur during the second week of sulfonamide therapy and do not correlate with circulating levels of the sulfonamide. The incidence of hepatic injury due to trimethoprim-sulfamethoxazole appears to be especialy high, around 20%, in patients with AIDS (159–161).

The reason for the high incidence is not clear. The association of slow-acetylation phenotype with adverse reactions to sulfonamides in AIDS patients has been described repeatedly (147,162,163). It has been therefore hypothesized that the increased incidence of drug reactions to trimethoprim-sulfamethoxazole in HIV-infected patients was due to the increased production of the hydroxylamine metabolite of sulfamethoxazole. In addition, HIV-infected cells are markedly more sensitive to sulfonamide reactive metabolites than are noninfected cells (164). The increased prevalence of slow-acetylation phenotype is not due to the HIV infection per se but appears to be associated with the acute illness in advanced stages of HIV infection; indeed only the latter patients are at risk (165,166).

However, the status of acetylation phenotype does not completely explain the susceptibility of AIDS patients to trimethoprim-sulfamethoxazole (167,168). Oxidative pathways for drug metabolism are altered in AIDS patients as compared with control subjects (165). Some investigators had hypothesized that HIV-infected patients are deficient in glutathione and would therefore be more susceptible to the reactive metabolites (156,169). However, no evidence to support this hypothesis has been found in subsequent studies (170,171).

One further factor appears to modulate the risk of adverse drug reactions to trimethoprim-sulfamethoxazole. Carr et al. (172) have shown that patients with higher CD4 lymphocyte cell counts and CD4:CD8 ratios are prone to develop adverse reactions. The lack of any correlation between CD4 counts and metabolic ratios of the caffeine test (162) suggests that those two factors might be independent risk factors for trimethoprim-sulfamethoxazole-induced hypersensitivity.

D. Tetracyclines

The classic description of tetracycline hepatotoxicity was made in individuals who received high intravenous doses of tetracycline or oral doses of greater than 2 g/day (68,173). Most cases of tetracycline-induced hepatotoxic effects have been observed in women (174). Susceptibility seems to be enhanced by pregnancy and renal disease. Fatal outcome by liver failure was mainly observed with high parenteral doses. Clinical signs (nausea, vomiting, abdominal pain, mild jaundice) and biochemical disorders usually appear after 4–6 days of therapy. Values for aspartate aminotransferase rarely exceed 500 IU/L but may rise up to 1000 IU/L. High serum amylase levels have been reported in a majority of cases.

Characteristic histopathological findings of the liver usually show microvesicular steatosis with little necrosis. Portal tracts are generally spared with cellular infiltration being sparse and consisting predominantly of mononuclear cells (175). Very rarely tetracyclines have been associated with chronic cholestasis: cases of the vanishing bile duct syndrome with prolonged cholestasis have been ascribed to doxycycline and tetracycline (176).

Freneaux et al. (177) have highlighted a significant part of the involved mechanism. They showed that tetracycline inhibits the mitochondrial oxidation of fatty acids. This basic effect results in increasing precursor free fatty acid concentrations in the liver and subsequently may contribute to their increased esterification and accumulation in the form of triglycerides. As both free fatty acids and their microsomal oxidation products are toxic to the mitochondria, this toxicity might contribute to the severity of high-dose tetracycline-induced liver disease. Aside from this direct, dose-related, hepatotoxic effect common to all tetracyclines, other forms of liver injury have subsequently been recognized. In particular, minocycline, a semisynthetic tetracycline with extensive hepatic metabolism, has been associated most commonly with two types of hepatotoxicity. The first type, hypersensitivity hepatitis (178–182) has an acute onset within days to weeks after initiating minocycline. Hypersensitivity hepatitis may be associated with fever, rash, eosinophilia, and lymphadenopathy. Rarely, hypersensitivity hepatitis can result in fulminant hepatic failure (178–180). The second type, minocycline-induced hepatitis with autoimmune features

(183–186), has a delayed onset, usually a few months after initiating the drug. A series of five patients presenting with polyarthritis, positive antinuclear antibodies, and chronic hepatitis has been reported (184). The majority were young women with chronic active hepatitis on liver biopsy but negative smooth muscle antibodies. The serum aspartate aminotransferase levels ranged from 100 IU/L to nearly 2300 IU/L, while alkaline phosphatase level was elevated (twice the upper limit of normal) in only one patient. All recovered within 3 months of stopping minocycline. The reactions are unpredictable, dose independent, and features of drug hypersensitivity are prominent. A review of 16 additional cases reported to the U.K. Committee on Safety of Medicines (184) reveals that there are two predominant syndromes of autoimmunity, which overlap. The first is typical drug-induced systemic lupus erythematosus, with polyarthritis, rash, hyperglobulinemia, and positive antinuclear antibody tests. The other is hepatitis, commonly associated with rash, arthralgia, and hyperglobulinemia. Two of these patients died, one from liver failure and the other from neutropenia. A particular feature was the variable and delayed interval between starting the drug and diagnosis; indeed, it exceeded 6 months in 18 of the 21 cases reported in this review.

In a case-control study, Carson et al. (75) found that the increased risk per million patients exposed to a 10-day course of tetracycline was 1.56 cases. On the basis of the number of tetracycline prescriptions in 1991, the authors estimated that annually in the United States 31 cases of acute symptomatic liver disease resulting in hospitalization were due to tetracycline.

E. Quinolones

Cholestatic hepatitis as well as a mainly hepatocellular pattern has been described with nalidixic acid, starting within 2 weeks after the first intake (68).

Hepatotoxicity (cholestasis, hepatitis, and hepatic failure) has been reported infrequently with norfloxacin, ofloxacin, levofloxacin, and ciprofloxacin (187–193). Two reports of fatal hepatic failure have been published possibly related to ciprofloxacin treatment. In the first case, a 66-year-old man developed fulminant hepatic failure with extensive centrilobular necrosis 24 h after initiation of ciprofloxacin treatment (189). In the second case, a 92-year-old man developed progressive hepatic failure 2 days after the initiation of ciprofloxacin therapy (191). Additionally, a number of cases of ciprofloxacin-associated hepatotoxicity have been reported to the manufacturer.

Ten cases of cholestasis were observed among 10,094 patients included in phase IV studies and postmarketing surveillance of intravenous ciprofloxacin, but another report dealing with oral ciprofloxacin revealed only three cases of liver disorders among over 37,000 recipients (incidence of 0.81/100,000 recipients) (194). Arcieri et al. (195) reviewed data from 1878 courses of intravenous ciprofloxacin therapy, administered to 1869 patients in 59 clinical trials for drug safety. Over 1000 patients were treated for more than 5 days. Ciprofloxacin was administered in a unit dose of either 200 mg (68% of the patients) or 300 mg (28%) by intravenous infusion. Elevated alkaline phosphatase or ALT or AST levels were recorded in 96 cases—i.e., 39, 32, and 25, respectively (1.4, 1.7, and 2.1%, respectively). One patient who had undergone cardiac transplant was reported to have hepatic necrosis.

Similarly, the safety profile of oral ciprofloxacin (196) was established on a database (compiled through the end of 1988) of 9473 well-documented treatment courses worldwide. The daily dosage ranged between 200 mg and 2000 mg orally. The duration of treatment ranged from less than 2 days to more than 90 days. More than 38% of the patients were older than 60 years. Asymptomatic rises in alkaline phosphatase or serum aminotransferase levels amounted to 3.6% of the total number of patients. No irreversible hepatotoxicity was reported during the clinical trial period.

Minor elevations of serum aminotransferases are less common in patients treated with norfloxacin (0.1%) or ofloxacin (0.2%) (197,198).

Trovafloxacin is a new fluoroquinolone recently launched on the market. From February 1998 through early May 1999, 2.5 million prescriptions for trovafloxacin were written, and 140 patients were reported to have experienced a hepatic adverse event (incidence rate of 0.0056%). In 14 of these cases, the Food and Drug Administration (FDA) determined that liver failure was strongly associated with the concomitant administration of trovafloxacin. Four patients required liver transplantation, and five additional patients died. Some of the cases were associated with eosinophilic infiltration of the liver, suggesting a hypersensitivity hepatitis. Many of the severe cases of hepatic events seemed to be due to a hypersensitivity allergic-type reaction. Although hepatic reactions occurred between 1 and 60 days after the start of therapy, the risk of serious hepatic injury increases with exposure beyond 14 days of therapy. The development of hepatic reactions seems to be unpredictable and has occurred in some patients receiving a second or subsequent course of the drug. As a result, it has been recommended to limit the use of trovafloxacin to serious infections in hospitalized patients with monitoring of hepatic enzymes (FDA, Public Health Advisory, June 9, 1999) (199).

F. Nitrofurantoin

The incidence of symptomatic nitrofurantoin-induced liver injury has been estimated as approximately 0.02–0.003% (200).

Several types of hepatic injury have been attributed to nitrofurantoin, including acute cholestatic or cytolytic damage, granulomatous lesions, or chronic active hepatitis with or without cirrhosis after prolonged exposure to the drug (201–206).

In those instances with an acute onset, both cholestatic and cytolytic hepatitis are found (200). Cases usually present within 6 weeks of initiation of therapy and are sometimes accompanied by fever, rash, and eosinophilia. Nitrofurantoin-associated chronic liver disease is a condition seldom seen in present-day clinical practice. Typically, chronic active hepatitis has been observed in women who had been taking nitrofurantoin for extended periods of time ranging from 1 month to several years (202–205).

In a clinicopathological study of 52 reported cases of hepatic injury associated with the use of nitrofurans, Stricker et al. (200) found that nitrofurantoin-associated chronic liver disease was less common than the acute type. Both types were more frequent in women and in the elderly. Biochemically, the pattern was mainly hepatocellular (32%), whereas mixed cholestatic-hepatocellular and cholestatic patterns were unusual. HLA typing showed no increase of the HLA B8 or HLA DRw3 haplotype. HLA DR2 and HLA DR6 were more frequent than in controls, but this was not statistically significant. Prognosis is good, although recovery usually takes several months.

Nitrofurantoin hepatotoxicity is not due to direct toxicity, since the reactions are not dose-dependent and are relatively rare and unpredictable. A number of clues point to an immunoallergic mechanism: clinical manifestations of allergy are often present in acute forms of hepatic injury, and rechallenge elicits an accelerated hepatic reaction (207). Hepatotoxic manifestations related to nitrofurantoin may develop even when it is readministered after a latent period of 17 years, pointing to a long-term hepatic memory for hypersensitivity to nitrofurantoin (208). Furthermore, evidence for cross-reactivity to different nitrofuran derivatives has been reported (209). Finally, the relatively high frequency of autoantibodies (antinuclear or antismooth muscle) in chronic forms of hepatic injury also suggests the involvement of an immunoallergic process. Diagnostically, these antibodies may cause difficulties in differentiating autoimmune from nitrofurantoin-induced chronic active hepatitis. HLA B8 and HLA DRw3 have been shown to be more frequently involved in cases of autoimmune chronic active hepatitis (210), so it has been suggested that HLA typing may help in differential diagnosis (200).

As nitrofurantoin is biotransformed partly into superoxide anions (211), which are well-recognized toxic agents (212), it is possible that the immunological process involved in liver toxicity could be directed against structurally modified cellular components.

G. Rifampicin

Rifampicin may cause hyperbilirubinemia by interfering with the uptake of the unconjugated form and excretion of the conjugated form of bilirubin (213). Since rifampicin is nearly always used in combination with other antibiotics (e.g., in *Myco. avium complex* or staphylococcal infections) or with antituberculous agents, the actual hepatotoxic potential of this drug is not well defined.

In a large series of 836 patients receiving rifampicin without isoniazid (214), there was no instance of raised serum aminotransferase activity, which is consistent with the rarity of rifampicin-induced hepatotoxicity.

In fact, the risk of hepatotoxicity associated with this agent is mainly related to its combination with isoniazid. The risk of hepatotoxicity associated with the isoniazid-rifampicin combination appears to be considerably higher than with the use of rifampicin alone. Increases in serum aminotransferase activity occur in 20% of patients receiving the combination, compared with 10% in patients receiving isoniazid alone (215). Steele et al. (216) carried out a meta-analysis of 34 studies of patients taking isoniazid and/or rifampicin. The incidence of hepatotoxicity was 0.6% in 38,257 patients receiving isoniazid alone (for chemoprophylaxis), 1.6% of 2053 patients taking isoniazid with other antituberculous agents except rifampicin, 1.1% of 1264 patients receiving rifampicin but not isoniazid, and 2.5% of 6105 patients on both isoniazid and rifampicin.

Hepatitis occurs within the first 15 days of treatment with isoniazid + rifampicin, whereas the delay of occurrence is more than 1 month of therapy in patients receiving isoniazid alone. Biochemical abnormalities include a marked increase in serum aminotransferase activity and elevated serum bilirubin level. Histopathological findings comprise liver cell necrosis and hepatocellular degeneration, mild inflammatory infiltrates located mainly in the portal tracts, and, occasionally, cholestasis (215).

The hepatotoxicity associated with isoniazid or the isoniazid-rifampicin combination is caused by a metabolite-dependent direct toxicity, rather than by immune mechanisms: first, the frequency of liver dysfunction is relatively high; second, hypersensitivity manifestations such as fever, skin rash, or eosinophilia are usually absent; third, rechallenges do not lead to accelerated recurrence of hepatotoxicity (215).

Hepatic enzyme induction during rifampicin treatment enhances the hepatotoxicity of isoniazid. Rifampicin has been shown by several studies to stimulate the metabolism of isoniazid, resulting in the increased formation of hydrazine, a proven hepatotoxic agent (217–219).

Ellard and Gammon (217) demonstrated that hydrolysis of isoniazid by the isoniazid hydrolase induced by rifampicin is of greater significance in slow than in rapid acetylators. They also showed that this pathway is readily operating while the other metabolic pathway, which results in the formation of monoacetyl hydrazine, operates at a minimal level. Higher plasma levels of free hydrazine have been shown in slow acetylators as compared with rapid acetylators receiving isoniazid both before and during rifampicin administration (218). It is now generally agreed that concomitant administration of rifampicin and isoniazid results in increased levels of hydrazine, especially in slow acetylators, and that this higher amount of hydrazine can elicit hepatotoxic manifestations. This mechanistic explanation for hepatotoxicity is corroborated by the clinical findings of increased hepatotoxicity in slow acetylators (219,220). However, the role of acetylator phenotype on the occurrence of isoniazid-induced hepatotoxicity remains controversial.

Increased age, chronic liver disease, poor nutritional status, and chronic alcoholism are considered other predisposing factors in hepatitis induced by isoniazid-rifampicin treatment of tuberculosis (220–222).

Nonetheless, monitoring liver status appears necessary for prevention of serious hepatotoxicity. According to the recommendations proposed by the Joint Tuberculosis Committee of the British Thoracic Society (223), serum aminotransferase levels must be determined regularly: twice weekly during the first 2 weeks of therapy, then weekly during the rest of the first 2 months, and every month thereafter.

When serum aminotransferase levels are increased to less than three times the upper limit of normal, the treatment may be continued but the biochemical abnormalities should then be monitored at shorter intervals. When serum aminotransferase levels rise above three times the upper limit of normal, the antituberculous therapy should be stopped. After serum aminotransferase levels have return to normal, or are less than two times normal, isoniazid may be reintroduced at a lower daily dose, in combination with another antituberculous drug, except rifampicin and pyrazinamide, known to be also hepatotoxic.

H. Clindamycin

Clindamycin has been reported to result in mild to moderate elevation of aminotransferases without jaundice in up to 50% of patients receiving this antibiotic (62,224).

Hepatitis with transient jaundice during the intravenous administration of large doses of clindamycin has been described in one patient (225). The severity of concomitant sepsis, however, was a confounding factor in ascertaining the causal relationship. Biochemical presentation was both hepatocellular and cholestatic. Liver biopsy showed lobular disruption, pseudogranulomas, hepatocyte necrosis, eosinophilic bodies, and mononuclear cell infiltration of slightly widened portal tracts; parenchymal inflammatory response was minimal in comparison to the degree of hepatocellular damage and portal inflammation.

More recently one case of cholestatic liver disease with ductopenia after oral administration of clindamycin has been reported (138). The biochemical pattern was primarily cholestatic with moderate elevation of aminotransferases. Jaundice finally resolved 4 months after cessation of the drug but mild biochemical abnormalities of liver function were still present 2 years later, associated with continued duct injury and paucity on liver biopsy. An immunoallergic mechanism possibly combined with some dose-dependent toxicity [as evidenced in dogs (226)] might underlie clindamycin-associated hepatotoxicity.

III. ANTIFUNGAL AGENTS

A. Amphotericin B

Hepatotoxicity is considered a rare side effect of amphotericin B therapy (227,228). Up to now there have been only three documented cases of amphotericin B-induced hepatotoxicity. In a 32-year-old man with cryptococcal meningoencephalitis treated with amphotericin B intermittently over 1 year (total dose, 4.8 g in four separate courses) acute toxic hepatic degeneration (evidenced at autopsy) developed 4 days prior to death while the patient was receiving chlorpropamide and amphotericin B (229). There was marked centrilobular fatty infiltration with congestion but no inflammation. These findings were similar to those seen in chemical poisoning. A confounding factor in this case report, however, is that chlorpropamide is known to have hepatotoxic potential.

In another case report (230), a patient with acute myelogenous leukemia who had normal liver function was treated with amphotericin B for fungal pneumonia. While he was receiving the drug at high dosage for 18 days (cumulative dose 571 mg), asymptomatic elevation of the levels of alkaline phosphatase, aminotransferase, and bilirubin was noted. The levels returned to normal when the drug was discontinued. Rechallenge with a lower dosage prompted a rapid rise in the levels of hepatic enzymes, with subsequent return to normal when the medication was withdrawn.

A third case occurred in a 26-year-old man with life-threatening pulmonary blastomycosis who developed asymptomatic elevation of his liver enzymes after the addition of amphotericin B to the initial itraconazole therapy (231). Aminotransferases increased up to 10–20 times normal, and alkaline phosphatase was two times normal on day 10 of amphotericin B therapy, after a cumulative dose of 175 mg. The hepatotoxicity resolved rapidly with discontinuation of amphothericin B. Liver biopsy revealed a mild focal fatty change, and no evidence of acute or chronic inflammatory process.

B. Oral Antifungal Agents

These agents have been associated with different types of liver injury. A recent retrospective cohort study including 69,830 patients, 20–79 years old, free of liver and systemic disease, who had received at least one prescription of either oral ketoconazole, itraconazole, fluconazole, griseofulvin, or terbinafine was performed between 1991 and 1996 (232). This study was undertaken in the general population of the General Practice Research Database in the United Kingdom. Five cases of acute liver injury occurred during current use of oral antifungals. Two patients were using ketoconazole, another two itraconazole, and one terbinafine. Incidence rates of acute liver injury were 134.1/100,000 person-months [95% confidence interval (CI), 36.8–488] for ketoconazole, 10.4 (CI, 2.9–38.1) for itraconazole, and 2.5 (CI, 0.4–13.9) for terbinafine. The remaining case was associated with past use of fluconazole. Ketoconazole was the antifungal associated with the highest relative risk, 228 (CI, 33.9–933), when compared with the risk among nonusers, followed by itraconazole and terbinafine with relative risks of 17.7 (CI, 2.6–72.6) and 4.2 (CI, 0.2–24.9), respectively.

1. Ketoconazole

Ketoconazole appears to be implicated more frequently than the other azoles in causing hepatotoxicity, probably given its extensive metabolism in the liver (233–251). The incidence of ketoconazole-associated liver injury had been initially estimated between 1 per

1000 and 3000 patients, after taking into account the effect of underreporting in spontaneous monitoring systems (245).

The incidence, severity, and course of ketoconazole-associated liver injury have been recently assessed in a controlled cohort study (251) including 211 patients with onychomycosis. The patients were randomized to receive either ketoconazole (137 patients) or griseofulvin (74 patients). No biochemical abnormality was found before therapy, and all the patients were seronegative for hepatitis B or C. No biochemical abnormality or hepatic injury was found in patients during griseofulvin treatment. Among the patients treated with ketoconazole, 24 (17.5%) showed asymptomatic aminotransferase elevation. Four patients (2.9%) developed overt hepatitis, which resolved after discontinuation of the drug. Females and elderly patients seemed to be more prone to develop overt hepatitis, as previously observed (245). In patients with asymptomatic liver injury, the abnormal biochemical changes gradually returned to normal despite continuing ketoconazole therapy. The median duration of therapy before the recognition of hepatic dysfunction or overt hepatitis was 6 weeks (range, 2–12) and 5 weeks (range, 4–9), respectively, which were similar to the median time to onset of jaundice reported previously in some series (241,245).

Asymptomatic increase in serum aminotransferase levels occurs in 2–10% of patients (228) and is usually self-limited despite continued use of the drug (233,240,251). In contrast, maintaining ketoconazole therapy despite the occurrence of hepatitis may lead to death (246).

Biochemically, most cases of hepatitis are mainly of the hepatocellular pattern, the other pictures being of mixed hepatocellular-cholestatic or of primarily cholestatic type (238,241,251). In the 55 cases described by Stricker et al. (245), 54% of the patterns observed from liver function tests showed primarily hepatocellular pattern, 16% were cholestatic, and 25% showed mixed pattern. Recovery is usual after discontinuation of the drug, with liver function tests returning to normal within 3 months (245,246).

Histopathological findings at liver biopsy usually include preservation of normal lobular architecture, spotty necrosis, mononuclear cell infiltration in the portal area, centrilobular necrosis with central-portal bridging (233,238–241,245–247). Cholestasis, however, has been a major histological feature in some cases (241,245). An anecdotal case of granuloma formation associated with spotty necrosis has been reported (251).

The mechanism of ketoconazole-induced liver injury is not well understood. The usual absence of fever, skin rash, and eosinophilia in patients with liver injury (235,238,239,244,245), and the variable duration of ketoconazole administration before the onset of liver damage [4–270 days in the study by Lake-Bakaar et al. (246)] are consistent with a metabolic rather than a hypersensitive basis for the idiosyncratic injury. In addition, rechallenge is not followed by immediate recurrence (<48 h) of a more severe liver injury as might be expected in an allergic phenomenon (234,238,247).

Similar to a number of drugs that produce immunoallergic hepatitis in a few subjects and a mild increase in serum aminotransferase levels in a much larger proportion of patients, ketoconazole metabolism might lead to the formation of reactive metabolites that induce allergic hepatitis in the former and direct toxicity in the latter.

Since it is currently not possible to predict which individuals are susceptible to liver damage, it would seem prudent to instruct patients to stop the drug as soon as any symptoms suggestive of hepatitis (malaise, dark urine, pruritus) occur. The risk of hepatic injury is assumed to be minimal with treatment of short duration (<10 days) given that the onset of liver damage does not occur during the first week of therapy (246,251). Biochemical tests should be performed after the first 10 days of treatment and then twice a month during prolonged therapy. Indeed, given the possibility of prolonged subclinical hepatitis (for several weeks) with delayed onset of severe hepatic necrosis (246), it is warranted to monitor liver function tests regularly during prolonged treatment with ketoconazole. Asymptomatic increase in serum aminotransferase activity should alert the physician to perform a further test within 1 week, as it could signal early hepatotoxicity. If the serum aminotransferase levels increase gradually or rise significantly (greater than threefold) above normal or symptoms develop, treatment should be stopped.

2. Fluconazole

Asymptomatic elevations of hepatic enzymes may occur during fluconazole therapy; they are mild and transient and occur in <5% of patients (252). In some studies involving immunocompromised patients, the reported incidence was higher (228). However, the underlying disease or concomitant medications make causal relationship uncertain in this kind of population. Fluconazole may give rise to symptomatic hepatotoxicity only rarely. Nonfatal hepatotoxicity has been described in eight case reports (253–258). Biochemical abnormalities pointed to a mixed cytolytic-cholestatic liver injury or a prominent chole-static pattern. Five of these patients were HIV-positive and had received fluconazole for a few days to 4 months. However, drug interactions with other potentially hepatotoxic agents could have played a role in most cases. In some cases preexisting liver dysfunction might have enhanced or facilitated the occurrence of fluconazole-related liver injury (256).

Up to now, three cases of fatal hepatitis have been associated with this antifungal agent (254,259,260): onset of hepatitis emerged after 10–21 days of therapy, and two of these fatalities occurred in HIV-positive patients. The liver damage found at biopsy was a mixed hepatocellular-cholestatic pattern in one case and a widespread hepatic necrosis in another case. Granuloma, fibrosis, or inflammation of the portal tracts was not observed. In one case report of nonfatal fluconazole-related liver injury in a patient with AIDS who had received fluconazole maintenance therapy for cryptococcosis (258), electron micros-copy revealed enlarged smooth endoplasmic reticulum and megamitochondria with para-crystallin inclusions. This has been related to the prolonged duration of therapy (>3 months) rather than excessive dosage. Because the principal mechanism of action of the triazoles is to inhibit cytochrome P450 enzymes in fungal organisms, it has been hypothe-sized that the mitochondrial hepatic abnormalities could be related to some fluconazole–cytochrome P450 enzyme interaction at the level of the inner mitochondrial membrane (258). Yet the pathogenesis of fluconazole-associated liver injury remains incompletely understood.

3. Itraconazole

The safety profile of chronic itraconazole therapy has been evaluated in a prospective clinical study including 189 patients with a variety of systemic mycoses for a median of 5 months (261). Itraconazole was administered at doses of 50–400 mg/day. Asymptomatic abnormal liver function tests were seen in 7% of patients. Serum aminotransferase concen-trations were elevated in 10 patients (5%) and were <3 times the upper limit of normal in all 10 cases. Elevated serum alkaline phosphatase concentrations were seen in three patients (2%) and were >3 times the upper limit of normal in one patient. Hyperbilirubi-nemia was observed in two patients (1%) and was <2 times the upper limit of normal in both. Some retrospective studies involving a much higher number of patients have re-ported, however, quite low frequencies of itraconazole-associated liver dysfunction. In

1993 (252), the incidence of hepatic reactions associated with this azole agent was approximately 6 in almost 5 million treatments. In a review of over 4000 well-documentated patients treated with itraconazole there have been asymptomatic increases in liver enzymes in 1–2% of patients. These enzymes returned to pretreatment levels after therapy was discontinued (262). But in another study (232), the relative risk of acute hepatitis associated with itraconazole therapy in the general population has recently been estimated at 17.7 (CI, 2.6–72.6).

It remains that, up to now, only two cases of itraconazole-related symptomatic hepatitis have been reported (263,264). Biochemical abnormalities showed a mixed cholestatic-hepatocellular pattern with predominant cholestasis and returned to normal within 6 weeks following withdrawal of the drug.

The mild and transient liver enzyme elevations, the paucity of immunoallergic signs, the delayed latent period, and delayed reaction to rechallenge are compatible with metabolic idiosyncrasy to a mildly intrinsic hepatotoxicity.

Of note, itraconazole has been safely administered in a few patients with a history of hepatitis due to ketoconazole or amphotericin B (262).

4. Terbinafine

In a postmarketing surveillance study including 25,884 patients treated with terbinafine, two cases of symptomatic cholestatic hepatic injury considered potentially related to the treatment were identified (265). Asymptomatic elevations on hepatic enzymes were recorded in 38 patients (0.14%). These elevations were all reversed on discontinuation of terbinafine. The predominant indication for terbinafine treatment was onychomycosis (72%); median duration of treatment was 12 weeks, and treatment extended beyond 6 weeks in 76% of patients and for at least 12 weeks in 59%.

Hepatobiliary disorders associated with orally administered terbinafine have rarely been reported (266–268). The biochemical abnormalities observed in described cases of terbinafine-induced liver injury were indicative of a mixed cholestatic-hepatocellular pattern in three and a predominant cholestatic pattern in one. In the latter case, cholestasis was prolonged with alkaline phosphatase and gamma-glutamyl transpeptidase levels peaking about 80 days after discontinuation of the drug (268). Liver function tests returned to normal within 2–6 months after withdrawal of the drug.

The mechanism of terbinafine-induced hepatic injury remains unclear. Terbinafine binds only weakly to hepatic cytochrome P450 and does not seem to interfere with cytochrome P450 enzymes involved in drug metabolism and synthesis of steroid hormones (269). Therefore, the drug might have direct toxicity in a minority of patients. Moreover, general hypersensitivity reactions like skin rash, fever, eosinophilia, or arthritis have not been detected in the reported cases of hepatitis. Considering that terbinafine-associated liver damage has not been reported in clinical trials, an uncommon metabolically mediated idiosyncratic effect is probably involved.

5. Flucytosine

Abnormal liver function tests occur in 5–15% of patients treated with flucytosine (228). This generally includes elevation of serum aminotransferases, sometimes combined with elevation of alkaline phosphatase and bilirubin. Although most patients with flucytosine-induced hepatitis are asymptomatic, histological evidence of patchy liver necrosis has been observed, with some cases showing severe hepatic necrosis (270). The mechanism of drug-induced hepatotoxicity is unknown.

6. Griseofulvin

One case of cholestatic jaundice in a patient receiving griseofulvin has been reported (271). Onset of hepatitis occurred within 2 weeks of treatment. Liver biopsy revealed cholestasis characterized by bile canaliculi containing bile casts, associated with a slight to moderate inflammatory infiltrate in the periportal spaces. This patient recovered completely within 1 month after discontinuing the drug.

IV. CONCLUSION

There is no specific treatment for antimicrobial-induced hepatotoxicity. Management of drug-induced hepatotoxicity is usually confined to the discontinuation of the causative agent, with careful observation of the patient to make sure the expected improvement begins to occur within 2 weeks.

Supportive treatments may be needed in case of severe cholestasis or hepatocellular insufficiency. Therapy with corticosteroids may be used in patients with evident hypersensitivity but controlled trials have not proved the efficacy of such treatment. This holds true also in patients suffering from very severe acute liver disease with the potential for fulminant hepatic failure. Rarely, liver transplantation may appear as the sole therapeutic tool for some cases of fulminant hepatic failure (13,206).

Early detection of liver injury, together with prompt withdrawal of the offending agent, and delineation of high-risk groups of patients for hepatotoxicity are crucial and remain the most effective methods of prevention. Patients should be warned to report nonspecific features that may represent the onset of drug-induced hepatitis, such as fever, unexplained nausea, right-upper-quadrant abdominal pain, or asthenia. In most cases, women or the elderly seem to be at higher risk to develop hepatotoxicity related to antimicrobial agents. Patients with AIDS form another high-risk group for liver injury, especially that associated with trimethoprim-sulfamethoxazole.

Polypharmacy should be avoided when possible because drug reactions are more frequent in this condition. This is of particular relevance in the elderly: polypharmacy is usual in this population, and, as indicated earlier in several instances, advanced age by itself frequently represents a risk factor for drug-induced hepatotoxicity. Also of importance is reporting suspected adverse effects to monitoring agencies during postmarketing surveillance of new drugs because their actual hepatotoxic potential may not be recognized until after their introduction on the market.

REFERENCES

1. Sikuler E, Guetta V, Keynan A, Neumann L, Schlaeffer F. Abnormalities in bilirubin and liver enzyme levels in adult patients with bacteremia. Arch Intern Med 1989; 149:2246–2248.
2. Zimmerman HJ, Fang M, Utili R, Seef LB, Hoofnagle J. Jaundice due to bacterial infection. Gastroenterology 1979; 77:362–374.
3. Parry MF. The penicillins. Med Clin North Am 1987; 71:1093–1112.
4. Golstein LI, Ishak KG. Hepatic injury associated with penicillin therapy. Arch Pathol 1974; 98:114–117.
5. Onate J, Montejo M, Aguirrebengoa K, Ruiz-Irastorza G, Gonzales de Zarate P, Aguirre C. Hepatotoxicity associated with penicillin V therapy. Clin Infect Dis 1995; 20:474–475.

6. Williams CN, Malatjalian DA. Severe penicillin-induced cholestasis in a 91-year old woman. Dig Dis Sci 1981; 26:470–473.

7. Cavanzo FJ, Garcia CF, Botero RC. Chronic cholestasis, paucity of bile ducts, red cell aplasia and the Stevens-Johnson syndrome: an ampicillin-associated case. Gastroenterology 1990; 99:854–856.

8. Davies MH, Harrison RF, Elias E, Hubscher SG. Antibiotic-associated acute vanishing bile duct syndrome: a pattern associated with severe, prolonged, intrahepatic cholestasis. J Hepatol 1994; 20:12–116.

9. Anderson CS, Nicholis J, Rowland R, Labrooy JT. Hepatic granulomas: a 15-year experience in the Royal Adelaide Hospital. Med J Aust 1988; 148:71–74.

10. Garcia Rodriguez LA, Stricker BH, Zimmerman HJ. Risk of acute liver injury associated with the combination of amoxicillin and clavulanic acid. Arch Intern Med 1996; 156:1327–1332.

11. Wilson FM, Belamaric J, Lauter CB, Lerner AM. Anicteric carbenicillin hepatitis: eight episodes in four patients. JAMA 1975; 232:818–821.

12. Lang R, Lishner M, Ravid M. Adverse reactions to prolonged treatment with high doses of carbenicillin and ureidopenicillins. Rev Infect Dis 1991; 13:68–72.

13. Olsson R, Wiholm BE, Sand C, Zettergren L, Hultcrantz R, Myrhed M. Liver damage from flucloxacillin, cloxacillin, and dicloxacillin. J Hepatol 1992; 15:154–161.

14. Farrell GC. Drug-induced hepatic injury. J Gastroenterol Hepatol 1997; 12(Suppl):S242–S250.

15. Derby LE, Jick HJ, Henry DA, Dean AD. Cholestatic hepatitis associated with flucloxacillin. Med J Aust 1993; 158:596–600.

16. George DK, Crawford DH. Antibacterial-induced hepatotoxicity. Incidence, prevention, and management. Drug Safety 1996; 1:79–85.

17. Fairley CK, Mc Neil JJ, Desmond P, Smallwood R, Young H, Forbes A, Purcell P, Boyd I. Risk factors for development of flucloxacillin-associated jaundice. Br Med J 1993; 306:233–235.

18. Turner IB, Eckstein RP, Riley JW, Lunzer MR. Prolonged hepatic cholestasis after flucloxacillin therapy. Med J Aust 1989; 151:701–705.

19. Miros M, Welker N, Kerlin P, Harris O. Flucloxacillin-induced delayed cholestatic hepatitis. Aust NZ J Med 1990; 20:251–253.

20. Piotrowicz A, Polkey M, Wilkinson M. Ursodeoxycholic acid for the treatment of flucloxacillin-associated cholestasis. J Hepatol 1995; 22:119–121.

21. Dismukes WE. Oxacillin-induced hepatic dysfunction. JAMA 1973; 226:861–863.

22. Onorato IM, Axelrod JL. Hepatitis from intravenous high-dose oxacillin therapy: findings in an adult inpatient population. Ann Intern Med 1978; 89:497–500.

23. Bruckstein AH, Attia AA. Oxacillin hepatitis: two patients with liver biopsy, and review of the literature. Am J Med 1978; 64:519–522.

24. Tauris P, Jorgensen NF, Petersen CM, Albertsen K. Prolonged severe cholestasis induced by oxacillin derivatives: a report of two cases. Acta Med Scand 1985; 217:567–569.

25. Pollock AA, Berger SA, Simberkoff MS, Rahall JJ. Hepatitis associated with high dose oxacillin therapy. Arch Intern Med 1978; 138:915–917.

26. Kleinman MS, Presberg JE. Cholestatic hepatitis after dicloxacillin-sodium therapy. J Clin Gastroenterol 1986; 8:77–78.

27. Konikoff F, Alcalay J, Halevy J. Cloxacillin-induced cholestatic jaundice. Am J Gastroenterol 1986; 81:1082–1083.

28. Aderka D, Livni E, Salamon F, Weinberger A, Pinkhas J. Use of macrophage inhibition factor and mast-cell degranulation tests for diagnosis of cloxacillin-induced cholestasis. Am J Gastroenterol 1986; 81:1084–1086.

29. Victorino RM, Maria VA, Correia AP, Moura C. Floxacillin-induced cholestatic hepatitis with evidence of lymphocyte sensitization. Arch Intern Med 1987; 147:987–989.

30. Dowsett JF, Gillow T, Heagerty A, Radcliffe M, Toadi R, Isle I, Russell RC. Amoxycillin/clavulanic acid (Augmentin)-induced intrahepatic cholestasis. Dig Dis Sci 1989; 34:1290–1293.

31. Stricker BH, Van der Broek JW, Keuning J, Eberhardt W, Houben HG, Johnson M, Blok AP. Cholestatic hepatitis due to antibacterial combination of amoxicillin and clavulanic acid (Augmentin). Dig Dis Sci 1989; 34:1576–1580.

32. Reddy KR, Brillant P, Schiff ER. Amoxicillin-clavulanate potassium-associated cholestasis. Gastroenterology 1989; 96:1135–1141.

33. Schneider JE, Kleinman MS, Kupiec JW. Cholestatic hepatitis after therapy with amoxicillin/clavulanate potassium. NY State J Med 1989; 89:355–356.

34. Verhamme M, Ramboer C, Vanderbruaene P, Inderadjaja N. Cholestatic hepatitis due to an amoxicillin-clavulanic preparation. J Hepatol 1989; 9:260–264.

35. Michielsen PP, Vanoutryve MJ, Vanmarck EA, Demaeyer MH, Pelckmans PA, Vanmaercke YM. Amoxicillin/clavulanic acid-induced cholestasis. J Hepatol 1990; 11:392.

36. Wong FS, Ryan J, Dabkowski P, Dudley FJ, Sewell RB, Smallwood RA. Augmentin-induced jaundice. Med J Aust 1991; 154:698–701.

37. Larrey D, Vial T, Micaleff A, Babany G, Morichau-Beauchant M, Michel M, Benhamou JP. Hepatitis associated with amoxycillin-clavulanic acid combination: report of 15 cases. Gut 1992; 33:368–371.

38. Silvain C, Fort E, Levillain P, Labat-Labourdette J, Beauchant M. Granulomatous hepatitis due to combination of amoxycillin and clavulanic acid. Dig Dis Sci 1992; 37:150–152.

39. Hebbard GS, Smith KG, Gibson PR, Bathal PS. Augmentin-induced jaundice with a fatal outcome. Med J Aust 1992; 156:285–286.

40. Ragg M. MaLAM (International and Australia) and Augmentin. Lancet 1993; 342:487.

41. ADRAC. Drug-induced cholestatic hepatitis from common antibiotics. Med J Aust 1992; 157:531.

42. Hautekeete ML, Brenard R, Horsmans Y, Henrion J, Verbist L, Derue G, Druez P, Omar M, Kockx M, Hubens H, Haber I, Rahier J, Geubel AP. Liver injury related to amoxycillin-clavulanic acid: interlobular bile-duct lesions and extrahepatic manifestations. J Hepatol 1995; 22:71–77.

43. Kando JC, Yonkers AK, Cole OJ. Gender as a risk factor for adverse events to medications. Drugs 1995; 50:1–6.

44. Thomson JA, Fairley CK, Ugoni AM, Forbes AB, Purcell PM, Desmond PV, Smallwood RA, Mc Neil JJ. Risk factors for the development of amoxycillin-clavulanic acid-associated jaundice. Med J Aust 1995; 162:638–640.

45. McCaig LF, Hughes JM. Trends in antimicrobial drug prescribing among office-based physicians in the United Kingdom. JAMA 1995; 273:214–217.

46. Ryley NG, Fleming KA, Chapman RW. Focal destructive cholangiopathy associated with amoxycillin/clavulanic acid (Augmentin). J Hepatol 1995; 23:278–282.

47. Nathani MG, Mutchnick MG, Tynes DL, Ehrinpreis MN. An unusual case of amoxicillin/clavulanic acid-related hepatotoxicity. Am J Gastroenterol 1998; 93:1363–1365.

48. Limauro DL, Chan-Tompkins NH, Carter RW, Brodmerkel GJ, Agrawal RM. Amoxicillin/clavulanate hepatic failure with progression to Stevens-Johnson syndrome. Ann Pharmacother 1999; 33:560–564.

49. Stiegbauer KT, Smith C, Snoyer DC. The histological features of amoxicillin/clavulanic acid-induced hepatotoxicity. Hepathology 1994; 20:190A.

50. Hautekeete ML, Horsmans Y, Van Wayenberge C, Demanet C, Henrion J, Verbist L, Brenard R, Sempoux C, Michielsen PP, Yap PS, Rahier J, Geubel AP. HLA association of amoxicillin-clavulanate-induced hepatitis. Gastroenterology 1999; 117:1181–1186.

51. Bolton GC, Allen GD, Davies BE, Filer C, Jeffery DJ. The disposition of clavulanic acid in man. Xenobiotica 1986; 16:853–863.

52. Eliopoulos GM, Moellering RC. Azlocillin, mezlocillin, and piperacillin: new broad-spectrum penicillins. Ann Intern Med 1982; 97:755–760.

53. Parry MF. Toxic and adverse reactions encountered with new betalactam antibiotics. Bull NY Acad Med 1984; 60:358–368.

54. Drusano GL, Schimpff SC, Hewitt WL. The acylampicillins: mezlocillin, piperacillin, and azlocillin. Rev Infect Dis 1984; 6:13–32.

55. Kuye O, Teal J, DeVries VG, Morrow CA, Tally FP. Safety profile of piperacillin/tazobactam in phase I and III clinical trial studies. J Antimicrob Chemother 1993; 31(suppl A):113–124.

56. Sanders WE, Sanders CC. Pipercillin/tazobactam: a critical review of the evolving clinical literature. Clin Infect Dis 1996; 22:107–123.

57. Fekety FR. Safety of parenteral third-generation cephalosporins. Am J Med 1990; 88(suppl 4A):38S–44S.

58. Thompson JW, Jacobs RF. Adverse effects of newer cephalosporins: an update. Drug Safety 1993; 9:132–142.

59. Amman R, Neftel K, Hardmeier TH, Reinhardt M. Cephalosporin-induced cholestatic jaundice. Lancet 1982; 2:336–337.

60. Bosio M. Cholestatic jaundice and hematuria due to hypersensibility to cefaclor in a child. J Toxicol Clin Toxicol 1983; 20:79–84.

61. Eggleston SM, Belandres MM. Jaundice associated with cephalosporin therapy. Drug Intell Clin Pharm 1985; 19:553–555.

62. Stricker BH. Drug-Induced Hepatic Injury 2nd ed. Amsterdam: Elsevier, 1992.

63. Calandra GB, Brown KR, Grad LC, Ahonkhai VI, Wang C, Aziz MA. Review of adverse experiences and tolerability in the first 2,516 patients treated with imipenem/cilastatin. Am J Med 1985; 78(suppl 6A):73–78.

64. Arnaud M, Rochet N, Bonnet C, Deblois P, Bertin P, Treves R, Desproges-Gotteron R. Jaundice secondary to treatment with imipenem. Therapie 1990; 45:70.

65. Henry SA, Bendush CB. Aztreonam: worldwide overview of the treatment of patients with gram-negative infections. Am J Med 1985; 78(suppl 2A):57–64.

66. Alvan G, Nord CE. Adverse effects of monobactams and carbapenems. Drug Safety 1995; 12:305–313.

67. Tolman KG, Sannela JJ, Freston JW. Chemical structure of erythromycin and hepatotoxicity. Ann Intern Med 1974; 81:58–60.

68. Zimmerman HJ, Maddley WC. Drug-induced hepatotoxicity. In: L Schiff, ER Schiff (eds). Diseases of the Liver. 6th ed. Philadelphia: JP Lippincott, 1987.

69. Viteri AL, Greene JF, Dyck WP. Erythromycin ethylsuccinate-induced cholestasis. Gastroenterology 1979; 76:1007–1008.

70. Keefe EB, Reis TC, Berland JE. Hepatotoxicity to both erythromycin estolate and erythromycin ethylsuccinate. Dig Dis Sci 1982; 27:701–704.

71. Diehl AM, Latham P, Boitnott JK, Mann J, Maddrey WC. Cholestatic hepatitis from erythromycin ethylsuccinate. Am J Med 1984; 76:931–934.

72. Inman WH, Rawson NS. Erythromycin estolate and jaundice. Br Med J 1983; 286:1954–1955.

73. Avila P, Capella D, Laporte JR, Moreno V. Which salt of erythromycin is most hepatotoxic? Lancet 1988; 1:1104.

74. Derby LE, Jick H, Henry DA, Dean AD. Erythromycin-associated cholestatic hepatitis. Med J Aust 1993; 158:600–602.

75. Carson JL, Strom BL, Duff A, Gupta A, Shaw M, Lundin FE, Das K. Acute liver disease with erythromycins, sulfonamides, and tetracyclines. Ann Intern Med 1993; 119:576–583.

76. Pessayre D, Larrey D, Funck-Brentano C, Benhamou JP. Drug interactions and hepatitis produced by some macrolide antibiotics. J Antimicrob Chemother 1985; 16(suppl A):181–194.

77. Braun P. Hepatoxicity of erythromycin. J Infect Dis 1973; 119:300–306.

78. Gholson CF, Warren CH. Fulminant hepatic failure associated with intravenous erythromycin lactobionate. Arch Intern Med 1990; 150:215–216.

79. Zafrani ES, Ishak KG, Rudzki C. Cholestatic and hepatocellular injury associated with erythromycin esters: report of nine cases. Dig Dis Sci 1979; 24:385–396.

80. Gafter U, Mandel E, Weiss S, Djaldetti M. Erythromycin estolate-induced hepatitis: ultrastructural study of the liver. NY State J Med 1979; 20:87–89.

81. Geubel AP, Nakad A, Rahier J, Dive C. Prolonged cholestasis and disappearance of interlobular bile ducts following chlorpropamide and erythromycin ethylsuccinate: case of drug interaction? Liver 1988; 8:350–353.

82. Degott C, Feldmann G, Larrey D, Durand-Schneider AM, Grange D, Machayekhi JP, Moreau A, Potet F, Benhamou JP. Drug-induced prolonged cholestasis in adults: a histological semiquantitative study demonstrating progressive ductopenia. Hepatology 1992; 15:244–251.

83. Young RA, Gonzales JP, Sorkin EM. Roxithromycin: a review of its antibacterial activity, pharmacokinetic properties and clinical efficacy. Drugs 1989; 37:8–41.

84. Dubois A, Nakache N, Faffanel C, Balmes JL. Hépatite aiguë cholestatique après prise de roxithromycine. Gastroenterol Clin Biol 1989; 13:317–318.

85. Delcourt A, Lambert M, Brenard R, Geubel A. Reversible liver injury possibly due to roxithromycin. Acta Clin Belg 1990; 45:206.

86. Peters DH, Clissold SP. Clarithromycin. A review of its antimicrobial activity, pharmacokinetic properties and therapeutic potential. Drugs 1992; 44:117–164.

87. Wallace RJ Jr, Brown BA, Griffith DE. Drug intolerance to high-dose clarithromycin among elderly patients. Diagn Microbiol Infect Dis 1993; 16:215–221.

88. Yew WW, Chau CH, Lee J, Leung CW. Cholestatic hepatitis in a patient who received clarithromycin therapy for a *Mycobacterium chelonae* lung infection (letter). Clin Infect Dis 1994; 18:1025–1026.

89. Brown BA, Wallace RJ, Griffith DE, Girard W. Clarithromycin-induced hepatotoxicity (letter). Clin Infect Dis 1995; 20:1073–1074.

90. Viluksela M, Hanhijarvi H, Husband RF, Kosma VM, Collan Y, Mannisto PT. Comparative liver toxicity of various erythromycin derivatives in animals. J Antimicrob Chemother 1988; 21(suppl D):9–27.

91. Lehtonen L, Lankinen KS, Wikberg R, Rita H, Salmi HA, Valtonen V. Hepatic safety of erythromycin acistrate in 1549 patients with respiratory tract or skin infections. J Antimicrob Chemother 1991; 27:233–242.

92. Hopkins S. Clinical toleration and safety of azithromycin. Am J Med 1991; 91(suppl 3A): 40S–45S.

93. Garey KW, Amsden GW. Intravenous azithromycin. Ann Pharmacother 1999; 33:218–228.

94. Sides GD, Conforti PM. Safety profile of dirithromycin. J Antimicrob Chemother 1993; 31(suppl C):175–185.

95. See A, Weiffenbach E, Bouvry M. Cholestase au cours d'un traitement par la josamycine. Rev Med Interne 1986; 7:309–310.

96. Ponge A, Van Wasenhowe L, Ponge T, Cottin S. Hépatite au cours d'un traitement par la josamycine (letter). Rev Med Interne 1987; 8:117.

97. Dujovne CA. Hepatotoxic and cellular uptake interactions among surface active components of erythromycin preparations. Biochem Pharmacol 1978; 27:1926–1930.

98. Kendler J, Anuras S, Laborda O, Zimmerman HJ. Perfusion of the isolated rat liver with erythromycin estolate and other derivatives. Proc Soc Exp Biol Med 1972; 139:1272–1275.

99. Gaeta GB, Utili R, Adinolfil E, Abernathy CO, Guisti G. Characterization of the effects of erythromycin estolate and erythromycin base on the excretory function of the isolated rat liver. Toxicol Appl Pharmacol 1985; 80:185–192.

100. Larrey D, Funck Brentano C, Breil P, Vitaux J, Theodore C, Babany G, Pessayre D. Effects of erythromycin on hepatic drug-metabolizing enzymes in humans. Biochem Pharmacol 1983; 32:1063–1068.

101. Zhang XJ, Thomas PE. Erythromycin as a specific substrate for cytochrome P450 3A isoen-

zymes and identification of a high affinity erythromycin *N*-demethylase in adult female rats. Drug Metab Dispos 1996; 24:23–27.

102. Larrey D, Tinel M, Pessayre D. Formation of inactive cytochrome P-450 Fe(II)-metabolite complexes with several erythromycin derivatives but not with josamycin and midecamycin in rats. Biochem Pharmacol 1983; 32:1487–1493.

103. Periti P, Mazzei T, Mini E, Novelli A. Pharmacokinetic drug interactions of macrolides. Clin Pharmacokinet 1992; 23:106–131.

104. Von Rosenstiel NA, Adam D. Macrolide antibacterials. Drug interactions of clinical significance. Drug Safety 1995; 13:105–122.

105. Tinel M, Descatoire V, Larrey D, Loeper J, Labbe G, Letteron P, Pessayre D. Effects of clarithromycin on cytochrome P-450: comparison with other macrolides. J Pharmacol Exp Ther 1989; 250:746–751.

106. Rodrigues AD, Roberts EM, Mulford DJ, Yao Y, Ouellet D. Oxidative metabolism of clarithromycin in the presence of human liver microsomes: major role for the cytochrome P 450 3A (CYP 3A) subfamily. Drug Metab Dispos 1997; 25:623–630.

107. Delaforge M, Jaouen M, Mansuy D. Dual effects of macrolide antibiotics on rat liver cytochrome P 450. Induction and formation of metabolite-complexes: a structure-activity relationship. Biochem Pharmacol 1983; 32:2309–2318.

108. Amacher DE, Schomaker SJ, Retsema JA. Comparison of the effects of the new azalide antibiotic, azithromycin, and erythromycin estolate on rat liver cytochrome P-450. Antimicrob Agents Chemother 1991; 35:1186–1190.

109. Lindstrom TD, Hanssen BR, Wrighton SA. Cytochrome P-450 complex formation by dirithromycin and other macrolides in rat and human livers. Antimicrob Agents Chemother 1993; 37:265–269.

110. Sartori E, Delaforge M, Mansuy D. In vitro interaction of rat liver cytochromes P-450 with erythromycin, oleandomycin and erythralosamine derivatives. Importance of structural factors. Biochem Pharmacol 1989; 38:2061–2068.

111. Fries J, Siraganian R. Sulfonamide hepatitis: report of a case due to sulfamethoxazole. N Engl J Med 1966; 274:95.

112. Dujovne CA, Chan CH, Zimmerman HJ. Sulfonamide hepatic injury. Review of the literature and report of a case due to sulfamethoxazole. N Engl J Med 1967; 277:785–788.

113. Tonder M, Nordoy A, Elgjo K. Sulfonamide-induced chronic liver disease. Scand J Gastroenterol 1974; 9:93–96.

114. Colucci CF, Cicero ML. Hepatic necrosis and trimethoprim-sulfamethoxazole. JAMA 1975; 233:952–953.

115. Stevenson DK, Christie DL, Haas JE. Hepatic injury in adult caused by trimethoprim-sulfamethoxazole. Pediatrics 1978; 61:864–866.

116. Brockner J, Boisen E. Fatal multisystemic toxicity after cotrimoxazole. Lancet 1978; 1:831.

117. Nair SS, Kaplan JM, Levine LH, Geraci K. Trimethoprim-sulfamethoxazole-induced intrahepatic cholestasis. Ann Intern Med 1980; 92:511–512.

118. Steward DL, Johnson RC. Acute hepatitis caused by sulfamethoxazole-trimethoprim. Gastroenterology 1980; 78:1323.

119. Ogilvie AL, Toghill PJ. Cholestatic jaundice due to cotrimoxazole. Postgrad Med J 1980; 56:202–204.

120. Abi-Mansur P, Ardiaca MC, Allam C. Trimethoprim-sulfamethoxazole-induced cholestasis. Am J Gastroenterol 1981; 76:356–359.

121. Coto H, McGowan WR, Pierce EH, Thomas E. Intrahepatic cholestasis due to trimethoprim-sulfamethoxazole. South Med J 1981; 74:897–898.

122. Ransohoff DF, Jacobs G. Terminal hepatic failure following a small dose of sulfamethoxazole-trimethoprim. Gastroenterology 1981; 80:816–819.

123. Ghishan FK. Trimethoprim-sulfamethoxazole-induced intrahepatic cholestasis. Clin Pediatr 1983; 22:212–214.

124. Thies PW, Dull WL. Trimethoprim-sulfamethoxazole-induced cholestatic hepatitis: inadvertent rechallenge. Arch Intern Med 1984; 144:1691–1692.

125. Munoz SJ, Marinez-Hernandez A, Maddrey WC. Intrahepatic cholestasis and phospholipidosis associated with the use of trimethoprim-sulfamethoxazole. Hepatology 1990; 12:342–347.

126. Kowdley KV, Keeffe EB, Fawaz KA. Prolonged cholestasis due to trimethoprim-sulfamethoxazole. Gastroenterology 1992; 102:2148–2150.

127. Sotolongo RP, Neefe LI, Rudzki C, Ishak KG. Hypersensitivity reaction to sulfasalazine with severe hepatotoxicity. Gastroenterology 1978; 75:95–99.

128. Callen JP, Soderstrom RM. Granulomatous hepatitis associated with salicylazosulfapyridine therapy. South Med J 1978; 1159–1160.

129. Lozek JD, Werlin SL. Sulfasalazine hepatotoxicity. Am J Dis Child 1981; 135:1070–1071.

130. Smith MD, Gibson GE, Rowland R. Combined hepatotoxicity and neurotoxicity following sulfasalazine administration. Aust NZ J Med 1982; 12:76–80.

131. Koch-Weser J, Hodel C, Leimer R, Styk S. Adverse reactions to pyrimethamine/sulfadoxine. Lancet 1982; 2:1459.

132. Olsen VV, Loft S, Christensen KD. Serious reactions during malaria prophylaxis with pyrimethamine-sulfadoxine. Lancet 1982; 2:994.

133. Lazar HP, Murphy RL, Phair JP. Fansidar and hepatic granulomas. Ann Intern Med 1985; 102:722.

134. Selby CD, Ladussans EJ, Smith PG. Fatal multisystemic toxicity associated with prophylaxis with pyrimethamine and sulfadoxine (Fansidar). Br Med J 1985; 290:113–114.

135. Zitelli BJ, Alexander J, Taylor S, Miller KD, Howrie DL, Kuritsky JN, Perez TH, Van Thiel DH. Fatal hepatic necrosis due to pyrimethamine-sulfadoxine (Fansidar). Ann Intern Med 1987; 106:393–395.

136. Farrell GC. Drug-Induced Liver Disease. Edinburgh: Churchill Livingstone, 1994.

137. Beard K, Belic L, Aselton P, Perera D, Jick H. Outpatient drug-induced parenchymal liver disease requiring hospitalization. J Clin Pharmacol 1986; 26:633–637.

138. Altraif I, Lilly L, Wanless IR, Heathcote J. Cholestatic liver disease with ductopenia (vanishing bile duct syndrome) after administration of clindamycin and trimethoprim-sulfamethoxazole. Am J Gastroenterol 1994; 89:1230–1234.

139. Carr A, Tindall B, Penny R, Cooper DA. Patterns of multiple-drug hypersensitivities in HIV-infected patients. AIDS 1993; 7:1532–1533.

140. Mitra AK, Thummel KE, Kalhorn TF, Kharasch ED, Unadkat JD, Slattery JT. Inhibition of sulfamethoxazole hydroxylamine formation by fluconazole in human liver microsomes and healthy volunteers. Clin Pharmacol Ther 1996; 59:332–340.

141. Cribb AE, Spielberg SP. Hepatic microsomal metabolism of sulfamethoxazole to the hydroxylamine. Drug Metab Dispos Biol Fate Chem 1990; 18:784–787.

142. Cribb AE, Spielberg SP. Sulfamethoxazole is metabolized to the hydroxylamine in humans. Clin Pharmacol Ther 1992; 51:522–526.

143. Vree TB, Van der Ven AJ, Koopmans PP, Van Ewijk-Beneken Kolmer EW, Verwey-Van Missen CP. Pharmacokinetics of sulfamethoxazole with its hydroxy metabolites and N-4-acetyl-glucuronide, N1-glucuronide conjugates in healthy volunteers. Clin Drug Invest 1994; 9:43–53.

144. Rieder MJ, Uetrecht J, Shear NH, Spielberg SP. Synthesis and in vitro toxicity of hydroxylamine metabolites of the sulfonamides. J Pharmacol Exp Ther 1988; 244:724–728.

145. Pirmohamed M, Coleman MD, Hussain F, Breckenridge AM, Park BK. Direct and metabolism-dependent toxicity of sulphasalazine and its principal metabolites towards human erythrocytes and leucocytes. Br J Clin Pharmacol 1991; 32:303–310.

146. Weber WW, Hein DW. N-acetylation pharmacogenetics. Pharmacol Rev 1985; 37:25–79.

147. Rieder MJ, Shear NH, Kanee A, Tang BK, Spielberg SP. Prominence of slow acetylator

phenotype among patients with sulfonamide hypersensitivity reactions. Clin Pharmacol Ther 1991; 49:13–17.

148. Wolkenstein P, Carriere V, Charue D, Bastuji-Garin S, Revuz J, Roujeau JC, Beaune P, Bagot M. A slow acetylator genotype is a risk factor for sulfonamide-induced toxic epidermal necrolysis and Stevens-Johnson syndrome. Pharmacogenetics 1995; 5:255–258.

149. Das KM, Eastwood MA, McManus JP, Sircus WA. Adverse reactions during salicylazosulfa-pyridine therapy and the relation with drug metabolism and acetylator phenotype. N Engl J Med 1973; 289:491–495.

150. Shear NH, Spielberg SP, Grant DM, Tang BK, Kalow W. Differences in metabolism of sulfonamides predisposing to idiosyncratic toxicity. Ann Intern Med 1986; 105:179–184.

151. Rieder MJ, Uetrecht J, Shear NH, Spielberg SP. Diagnosis of sulfonamide hypersensitivity reactions by in vitro rechallenge with hydroxylamine metabolites. Ann Intern Med 1989; 110:286–289.

152. Rieder MJ. Mechanisms of unpredictable adverse drug reactions. Drug Safety 1994; 11:196–212.

153. Tanner AR. Hepatic cholestasis induced by trimethoprim. Br Med J 1986; 293:1072–1073.

154. Dossing M, Andreasen PB. Drug-induced liver disease in Denmark: an analysis of 572 cases of hepatotoxicity reported to the Danish board of adverse reactions to drugs. Scand J Gastroenterol 1982; 17:205–211.

155. Winston DJ, Lau WK, Gale RP, Young LS. Trimethoprim-sulfamethoxazole for the treatment of *Pneumocystis carinii* pneumonia. Ann Intern Med 1980; 92:762–769.

156. Van der Ven AJ, Koopmans PP, Vree TB, Van der Meer JW. Adverse reactions to cotrimoxazole in HIV infection. Lancet 1991; 338:431–433.

157. Caar A, Cooper DA, Penny R. Allergic manifestations of human immunodeficiency virus (HIV) infection. J Clin Immunol 1991; 11:55–64.

158. Hughes WT, Lafon SW, Scott JD, Masur H. Adverse events associated with trimethoprim-sulfamethoxazole and atovaquone during the treatment of AIDS-related Pneumocystis carinii pneumonia. J Infect Dis 1995; 171:1295–1301.

159. Gordin FM, Simon GL, Wofsy CB, Mills J. Adverse reactions to trimethoprim-sulfamethoxazole in patients with the acquired immunodeficiency syndrome. Ann Intern Med 1984; 100: 495–499.

160. Wofsy CB. Use of trimethoprim-sulfamethoxazole in the treatment of pneumocystis carinii pneumonia in patients with acquired immunodeficiency syndrome. Rev Infect Dis 1987; 9(suppl 2):S184–191.

161. Sattler FR, Cowan R, Nielsen DM, Ruskin J. Trimethoprim-sulfamethoxazole compared with pentamidine for treatment of pneumocystis carinii pneumonia in the acquired immuno-deficiency syndrome: a prospective, noncrossover study. Ann Intern Med 1988; 109:280–287.

162. Kaufmann GR, Wenk M, Taeschner W, Peterli B, Gyr K, Meyer KA, Haefeli WE. N-Acetyl-transferase-2 polymorphism in patients infected with human immunodeficiency virus. Clin Pharmacol Ther 1996; 60:62–67.

163. Smith CL, Brown I, Torraca BM. Acetylator status and tolerance of high dose trimethoprim-sulfamethoxazole therapy among patients infected with human immunodeficiency virus. Clin Infect Dis 1997; 25:1477–1478.

164. Droge W. Cysteine and glutathione deficiency in AIDS patients: a rationale for the treatment with N-acetylcysteine. Pharmacology 1993; 46:61–65.

165. Lee BL, Wong D, Benowitz NL, Sullam PM. Altered patterns of drug metabolism in patients with acquired immunodeficiency syndrome. Clin Pharmacol Ther 1993; 53:529–535.

166. O'Neil WM, Gilfix BM, Digirolano A, Tsoukas CM, Wainer IW. N-Acetylation among HIV-positive patients and patients with AIDS: when is fast, fast and slow, slow? Clin Pharmacol Ther 1997; 62:261–271.

167. Delomenie C, Grant DM, Mathelier-Fusade P, Jacomet C, Leynadier F, Jacqz-aigrin E, Rozenbaum W, Krishnamoorthy R, Dupret JM. N-acetylation genotype and risk of severe reactions to sulphonamides in AIDS patients (letter). Br J Clin Pharmacol 1994; 38:581–582.

168. Hofstede HJ, Van der Ven AJ, Koopmans PP. Drug reactions to cotrimoxazole in HIV infection: possibly not due to the hydroxylamine metabolites of sulphamethoxazole (letter). Br J Clin Pharmacol 1999; 47:571–573.

169. Staal FJ, Ela SW, Roedere M, Anderson MT, Herzenberg LA. Glutathione deficiency and human immunodeficiency virus infection. Lancet 1992; 339:909–912.

170. Van der Ven AJ, Vree TB, Kolmer EW, Koopmans PP, Van der Meer JW. Urinary recovery and kinetics of sulphamethoxazole and its metabolites in HIV-seropositive patients and healthy volunteers after a single oral dose of sulphamethoxazole. Br J Clin Pharmacol 1995; 39:621–625.

171. Pirmohamed M, Williams D, Tingle MD, Barry M, Khoo SH, O'Mahony C, Wilkins EG, Breckenridge AM, Park BK. Intracellular glutathione in the peripheral blood cells of HIV-infected patients: failure to show a deficiency. AIDS 1996; 10:501–507.

172. Carr A, Swanson C, Penny R. Clinical and laboratory markers of hypersensitivity to trimethoprim-sulfamethoxazole in patients with *Pneumocystis carinii* pneumonia and AIDS. J Infect Dis 1993; 167:180–185.

173. Burette A, Finet C, Prigogine T, De Roy G, Deltenre M. Acute hepatic injury associated with minocycline. Arch Intern Med 1984; 144:1491–1492.

174. Riely CA. Acute fatty liver of pregnancy. Semin Liver Dis 1987; 7:47–54.

175. Combes B, Whalley DJ, Adams RH, et al. Tetracycline and the liver: clinical manifestations of tetracycline toxicity. Prog Liver Dis 1972; 4:589–596.

176. Hunt CM, Washington K. Tetracycline-induced bile duct paucity and prolonged cholestasis. Gastroenterology 1994; 107:1844–1847.

177. Freneaux E, Labbe G, Letteron P, Le Dinh T, Degott C, Geneve J, Larrey D, Pessayre D. Inhibition of the mitochondrial oxidation of fatty acids by tetracycline in mice and in man: possible role in microvesicular steatosis induced by this antibiotic. Hepatology 1988; 8:1056–1062.

178. Davies MG, Kersey PJ. Acute hepatitis and exfoliative dermatitis associated with minocycline. Br Med J 1989; 298:1523–1524.

179. Min DI, Burke PA, Lewis D, Jenkins RL. Acute hepatic failure associated with oral minocycline: a case-report. Pharmacotherapy 1992; 12:68–71.

180. Boudreaux JP, Hayes DH, Mizrahi S, et al. Fulminant hepatic failure, hepatorenal syndrome and necrotizing pancreatitis after minocycline hepatotoxicity. Trans Proc 1993; 25:1073.

181. Kaufmann D, Pichler W, Beer JH. Severe episodes of high fever with rash, lymphadenopathy, neutropenia and eosinophilia after minocycline therapy for acne. Arch Intern Med 1994; 154:1983–1984.

182. Knowles SR, Shapiro L, Shear NH. Serious adverse reaction induced by minocycline. Arch Dermatol 1996; 132:934–939.

183. Malcolm A, Heap TR, Eckstein RP, Lunzer MR. Minocycline-induced liver injury. Am J Gastroenterol 1996; 91:1641–1643.

184. Gough A, Chapman S, Wagstaff K, Emery P, Elias E. Minocycline-induced autoimmune hepatitis and systemic lupus erythematus-like syndrome. Br Med J 1996; 312:169–172.

185. Golstein PE, Deviere J, Cremer M. Hepatitis and drug-related lupus induced by minocycline treatment. Am J Gastroenterol 1997; 92:143–146.

186. Bhat G, Jordan J, Sokalski S, Bajaj V, Marshall R, Berlelhammer C. Minocycline-induced hepatitis with autoimmune features and neutropenia. J Clin Gastroenterol 1998; 27:74–75.

187. Lopez-Navidad A, Domingo P, Cadafalch J, Farrerons J. Norfloxacin-induced hepatotoxicity. J Hepatol 1990; 11:277–278.

188. Blum A. Ofloxacin-induced acute severe hepatitis (letter). South Med J 1991; 84:1158.

189. Grassmick BK, Lehr VT, Sundareson AS. Fulminant hepatic failure possibly related to ciprofloxacin. Ann Pharmacother 1992; 26:636–639.
190. Levinson JR, Kumar A. Ciprofloxacin-induced cholestatic jaundice: a case-report (abstract). Am J Gastroenterol 1993; 88:1619.
191. Fuchs S, Simon Z, Brezin M. Fatal hepatic failure associated with ciprofloxacin. Lancet 1994; 34:738–739.
192. Ball P, Tillotson G. Tolerability of fluoroquinolone antibiotics: past, present, and future. Drug Safety 1995; 13:343–358.
193. Villeneuve JP, Davies C, Coté J. Suspected ciprofloxacin-induced hepatotoxicity. Ann Pharmacother 1995; 29:257–259.
194. Jick SS, Jick H, Dean AD. A follow-up safety study of ciprofloxacin users. Pharmacotherapy 1993; 13:461–464.
195. Arcieri GM, Becker N, Esposito B, Griffith E, Heyd A, Neumann C, O'Brien B. Safety of intravenous ciprofloxacin: a review. Am J Med 1989; 87(suppl 5A):92S–97S.
196. Schacht P, Hullmann R. Safety of oral ciprofloxacin: an update based on clinical trial results. Am J Med 1989; 87(suppl 5A):98S–102S.
197. Corrado ML, Struble WE, Peter C, Hoagland V, Sabbaj J. Norfloxacin: a review of safety studies. Am J Med 1987; 82(suppl 6B):22–26.
198. Halkin H. Adverse effects of the fluoroquinolones. Rev Infect Dis 1988; 10(suppl 1):S258–S261.
199. Dembry LM, Farrington JM, Andriole VT. Fluoroquinolone antibiotics: adverse effects and safety profile. Infect Dis Clin Pract 1999; 8:421–428.
200. Stricker BH, Blok AP, Claas FH, Van Parys GE, Desmet VJ. Hepatic injury associated with the use of nitrofurans: a clinicopathological study of 52 reported cases. Hepatology 1988; 8:599–606.
201. Klemola H, Penttila L, Runeberg L. Anicteric liver damage during nitrofurantoin medication. Scand J Gastroenterol 1975; 10:501–505.
202. Hatoff DE, Cohen M, Schweigert BF, Talbret WM. Nitrofurantoin: another cause of drug-induced chronic active hepatitis? A report of a patient with HLA-B8 antigen. Am J Med 1979; 67:117–121.
203. Iwarson S, Lindberg J, Lundin P. Nitrofurantoin-induced chronic liver disease: clinical course and outcome of five cases. Scand J Gastroenterol 1979; 14:497–502.
204. Sharp J, Ishak KG, Zimmerman HJ. Chronic active hepatitis and severe hepatic necrosis associated with nitrofurantoin. Ann Intern Med 1980; 92:14–19.
205. Tolman KG. Nitrofurantoin and chronic active hepatitis. Ann Intern Med 1980; 92:119–120.
206. Mollison LC, Angus P, Richards M, Jones R, Ireton J. Hepatitis due to nitrofurantoin. Med J Aust 1992; 156:347–349.
207. Golstein LI, Ishak KG, Burns W. Hepatic injury associated with nitrofurantoin therapy. Am J Dig Dis 1974; 19:987–989.
208. Paiva LA, Wright PJ, Koff RS. Long-term hepatic memory for hypersensitivity to nitrofurantoin. Am J Gastroenterol 1992; 87:891–893.
209. Engel JJ, Vogt TR, Wilson DE. Cholestatic hepatitis after administration of furan derivatives. Arch Intern Med 1975; 135:733–735.
210. Mackay IR, Tait BD. HLA associations with autoimmune-type chronic active hepatitis: identification of B8-DRw3 haplotype by family studies. Gastroenterology 1980; 72:95–98.
211. Moreno SN, Mason RP, Docampo R. Reduction of nifurtimox and nitrofurantoin to free radical metabolites by rat liver mitochondria: evidence of an outer membrane-located nitroreductase. J Biol Chem 1984; 259:6298–6305.
212. Lim LO, Bortell R, Neims AH. Nitrofurantoin inhibition of mouse liver mitochondrial respiration involving NAD-linked substrates. Toxicol Appl Pharmacol 1986; 84:493–499.
213. Capelle P, Dhumeaux D, Mora M, Feldman G, Berthelot P. Effect of rifampicin on liver function in man. Gut 1972; 13:366.

214. Emerit J, Decroix G, Chomette G, Perie C, Pessayre D. Données nouvelles sur les hépatites observées au cours des traitements antituberculeux incluant la rifampicin. Rev Fr Mal Respir 1974; 2:565–584.

215. Durand F, Jebrak G, Pessayre D, Fournier M, Bernuau J. Hepatotoxicity of antitubercular treatments. Drug Safety 1996; 15:394–405.

216. Steele MA, Burk RF, Des Prez RM. Toxic hepatitis with isoniazid and rifampicin: a meta-analysis. Chest 1991; 99:465–471.

217. Ellard GA, Gammon PT. Pharmacokinetics of isoniazid metabolism in man. J Pharmacokinet Biopharm 1976; 4:83–113.

218. Beever IW, Blair IA, Brodie MJ. Circulating hydrazine during treatment with isoniazid-rifampicin in man. Br J Clin Pharmacol 1982; 13:599P.

219. Sarma GR, Immanuel C, Kailasam S, Narayana AS, Venkatesan P. Rifampicin-induced release of hydrazine from isoniazid: a possible cause of hepatitis during treatment of tuberculosis with regimens containing isoniazid and rifampin. Am Rev Respir Dis 1986; 133:1072–1075.

220. Pande JN, Singh SP, Khilnani GC, Khilnani S, Tandon RK. Risk factors for hepatotoxicity from antituberculosis drugs: a case-control study. Thorax 1996; 51:132–136.

221. Gronhagen-Riska C, Hellstrom E, Froseth B. Predisposing factors in hepatitis induced by isoniazid-rifampin treatment of tuberculosis. Am Rev Respir Dis 1978; 118:461–466.

222. Mitchell I, Wendon J, Fitt S, Williams R. Antituberculous therapy and acute liver failure. Lancet 1995; 345:555–556.

223. Ormerod LP, Skinner C, Wales J. Hepatotoxicity of antituberculous drugs. Thorax 1996; 51:111–113.

224. Fass RJ, Saslaw S. Clindamycin: clinical and laboratory evaluation of parenteral therapy. Am J Med Sci 1972; 263:369–382.

225. Elmore M, Rissing JP, Rink L, Brooks GF. Clindamycin-associated hepatotoxicity. Am J Med 1974; 57:627–630.

226. Gray JE, Weaver RN, Bollert JA, Feenstra ES. The oral toxicity of clindamycin in laboratory animals. Toxicol Appl Pharmacol 1972; 21:516–522.

227. Gallis HA, Drew RH, Pickard WW. Amphotericin B: 30 years of clinical experience. Rev Infect Dis 1990; 12:308–329.

228. Perfect JR, Lindsay MH, Drew RH. Adverse drug reactions to systemic antifungals: prevention and management. Drug Safety 1992; 7:323–363.

229. Carnecchia BM, Kurtzke JF. Fatal toxic reaction to amphotericin B in cryptococcal meningo-encephalitis. Ann Intern Med 1960; 53:1027–1036.

230. Miller MA. Reversible hepatotoxicity related to amphotericin B. Can Med Assoc J 1984; 131:1245–1247.

231. Gill J, Sprenger HR, Ralph ED, Sharpe MD. Hepatotoxicity possibly caused by amphotericin B. Ann Pharmacother 1999; 33:683–685.

232. Garcia Rodriguez LA, Duque A, Castellsague J, Perez-Gutthann S, Stricker BH. A cohort study on the risk of acute liver injury among users of ketoconazole and other antifungal drugs. Br J Clin Pharmacol 1999; 48:847–852.

233. Petersen EA, Alling DU, Kirkpatrick CH. Treatment of chronic cutaneous candidiasis with ketoconazole: a controlled clinical trial. Ann Intern Med 1980; 93:791–795.

234. Heiberg JK, Svejgaard E. Toxic hepatitis during ketoconazole treatment. Br Med J 1981; 283:825–826.

235. Mc Nair AL, Gascoigne E, Heap J, Schuermans V, Symoens J. Hepatitis and ketoconazole therapy. Br Med J 1981; 283:1058.

236. Firebrace DA. Hepatitis and ketoconazole therapy. Br Med J 1981; 283:1058–1059.

237. Horsburgh CR, Kirkpatrick CH, Teutsch CB. Ketoconazole and the liver. Lancet 1982; 1:860.

238. Svejgaard E, Ranek L. Hepatic dysfunction and ketoconazole therapy. Ann Intern Med 1982; 96:788–789.

239. Pegram PS, Kerns FT, Wsilauskas BL, Hampton KD, Scharyj M, Burke JG. Successful keto-conazole treatment of prototothecosis with ketoconazole-associated hepatotoxicity. Arch Intern Med 1983; 143:1802–1805.

240. Rollman O, Loof L. Hepatic toxicity of ketoconazole. Br J Dermatol 1983; 143:376–378.

241. Lewis JH, Zimmerman HJ, Benson GD, Ishak KG. Hepatic injury associated with ketocona-zole therapy: analysis of 33 cases. Gastroenterology 1984; 86:503–13.

242. Svedhem A. Toxic hepatitis following ketoconazole treatment. Scand J Infect Dis 1984; 16: 123–125.

243. Duarte PA, Chow CC, Simmons F, Ruskin J. Fatal hepatitis associated with ketoconazole therapy. Arch Intern Med 1984; 144:1069–1070.

244. Bercoff E, Bernuau J, Degott C, Kalis B, Lemaire A, Tilly H, Rueff B, Benhamou JP. Keto-conazole-induced fulminant hepatitis. Gut 1985; 26:636–638.

245. Stricker BH, Block AP, Bronkhorst FB, Vanparys GE, Desmet VJ. Ketoconazole-associated hepatic injury: a clinicopathological study of 55 cases. J Hepatol 1986; 3:399–406.

246. Lake-Bakaar G, Scheuer PJ, Sherlock S. Hepatic reactions associated with ketoconazole in the United Kingdom. Br Med J 1987; 294:419–422.

247. Van Parys G, Evenepoel C, Van Damme B, Desmet VJ. Ketoconazole-induced hepatitis: a case with definite cause-effect relationship. Liver 1987; 7:27–30.

248. Benson GD, Anderson PK, Burton C, Ishak KG. Prolonged jaundice following ketoconazole-induced hepatic injury. Dig Dis Sci 1988; 33:240–246.

249. Knight TE, Shikuma CY, Knight J. Ketoconazole-induced fulminant hepatitis necessitating liver transplantation. J Am Acad Dermatol 1991; 25:398–400.

250. Klausner MA. Ketoconazole and hepatitis. J Am Acad Dermatol 1992; 26:1028–1029.

251. Chien RN, Yang LJ, Lin PY, Liaw YF. Hepatic injury during ketoconazole therapy in patients with onychomycosis: a controlled cohort study. Hepatology 1997; 25:103–107.

252. Hay RJ. Risk/benefit ratio of modern antifungal therapy: focus on hepatic reactions. J Am Acad Dermatol 1993; 29:S50–S54.

253. Franklin JM, Elias E, Hirsch C. Fluconazole induced jaundice. Lancet 1990; 336:565.

254. Munoz P, Moreno S, Berenguer J, Bernaldo de Quiros JL, Bouza E. Fluconazole related hepatotoxicity in patients with acquired immunodeficiency syndrome. Arch Intern Med 1991; 151:1020–1021.

255. Wells C, Lever AM. Dose-dependent fluconazole hepatotoxicity proved on biopsy and re-challenge. J Infect 1992; 24:111–112.

256. Gearhart MO. Worsening of liver function with fluconazole and review of azole antifungal hepatotoxicity. Ann Pharmacother 1994; 28:1117–1181.

257. Trujillo MA, Galgiani JN, Sapllner RF. Evaluation of hepatic injury arising during flucona-zole therapy. Arch Intern Med 1994; 154:102–104.

258. Guillaume MP, De Prez C, Cogan E. Subacute mitochondrial liver disease in a patient with AIDS: possible relationship to prolonged fluconazole administration. Am J Gastroenterol 1996; 91:165–168.

259. Jacobson MA, Hanks DK, Ferrell LD. Fatal acute hepatic necrosis due to fluconazole Am J Med 1994; 96:188–190.

260. Bronstein JA, Gros P, Hernandez E, Larroque P, Molinie C. Fatal acute hepatic necrosis due to dose-dependent fluconazole hepatotoxicity. Clin Infect Dis 1997; 25:1266–1267.

261. Tucker RM, Haq Y, Denning DW, Stevens DA. Adverse events associated with itraconazole in 189 patients on chronic therapy. J Antimicrob Chemother 1990; 26:561–566.

262. Grant SM, Clissold SP. Itraconazole. A review of its pharmacodynamic and pharmacokinetic properties, and therapeutic use in superficial and systemic mycoses. Drugs 1989; 37:310–344.

263. Lavrijsen AP, Balmus KJ, Nugteren Huying WM, Roldaan AC, van't Wout JW, Stricker BH. Hepatic injury associated with itraconazole. Lancet 1992; 340:251–252.

264. Gallardo-Quesada S, Luelmo-Aguilar J. Hepatotoxicity associated with itraconazole. Int J Dermatol 1995; 34:589.

265. Hall M, Monka C, Krupp P, O'Sullivan D. Safety of oral terbinafine: results of a postmarketing surveillance study in 25,884 patients. Arch Dermatol 1997; 133:1213–1219.

266. Lowe G, Gren C, Lennings P. Hepatitis associated with terbinafine treatment. Br Med J 1993; 306:248.

267. Van't Wout LW, Herrmann WA, de Vries RA, Stricker BH. Terbinafine-associated hepatic injury. J Hepatol 1994; 21:115–117.

268. Lazaros GA, Papatheodoridis GV, Delladetsima JK, Tassopoulos NC. Terbinafine induced cholestatic liver disease. J Hepatol 1996; 24:753–756.

269. Balfour JA, Faulds D. Terbinafine. A review of its pharmacodynamic and pharmaco-kinetic properties, and therapeutic potential in superficial mycosis. Drugs 1992; 43:259–284.

270. Record CO, Skinner JM, Sleight P, Speller DC. Candida endocarditis treated with 5-fluoro-cytosine. Br Med J 1971; 1:262–264.

271. Chiprut RO, Viteri A, Jamroz C, Dyck WP. Intrahepatic cholestasis after griseofulvin administration. Gastroenterology 1976; 70:1141–1143.

21

Antituberculous Agents–Induced Liver Injury

PRAMOD KUMAR GARG and RAKESH KUMAR TANDON

All India Institute of Medical Sciences, New Delhi, India

I. INTRODUCTION

Tuberculosis is a major public health problem in the developing countries and there is ample evidence for its resurgence in the developed countries during the last few years (1). However, effective treatment is available to treat most of the cases with tuberculosis. The currently recommended treatment regimen for tuberculosis includes four first-line drugs—isoniazid, rifampicin, ethambutol or streptomycin, and pyrazinamide—for a period of 3 months followed by continuation of a "core" of isoniazid and rifampicin for the next 6 months (2). The response to the treatment is generally very good and gratifying but at times it may be poor and frustrating, e.g., in patients with coexistent HIV infection, infection with resistant strains of *Mycobacterium tuberculosis*, poor drug compliance, and development of serious toxicity necessitating stoppage of drugs. The antituberculous treatment (ATT)-associated side effects may involve almost all systems in the body such as the gastrointestinal tract, liver, skin, nervous system, otovestibular apparatus, eyes, etc. Of these, drug-induced hepatotoxicity is the most important and common adverse effect observed (3,4). The underlying mechanisms of ATT-induced hepatotoxicity are not clearly understood (3,4). Development of hepatotoxicity usually has a benign course, but may result in serious morbidity and even mortality (2–5). In addition, it has important implications with regard to the treatment of the underlying tuberculosis, i.e., how to use these effective antituberculous drugs with potential hepatotoxicity in patients who have developed ATT-induced hepatotoxicity. In this review we shall discuss the incidence, course, and pathophysiology of hepatotoxicity associated with different antituberculous drugs, predisposing factors for the development of antituberculous drugs–induced hepatotoxicity, and the management of such hepatotoxicity as well as of underlying tuberculosis.

II. ISONIAZID (INH)

INH was introduced for the treatment of tuberculosis in the 1960s and is considered to be the single most effective drug against tuberculosis. Initially INH was not recognized to cause hepatotoxicity. In 1969, however, Scharer and Smith reported an alarming incidence of 10.3% of INH-induced hepatotoxicity in the form of raised transaminases and overt jaundice (6). In a large study of 2321 patients who were on INH prophylaxis, clinical hepatitis was reported to occur in 19 (1%) patients and overt jaundice in 13 patients with one death (7). After these early reports suggesting INH-induced hepatotoxicity, the U.S. Public Health Service (USPHS) conducted a large multicenter prospective study in patients receiving INH for chemoprophylaxis to determine the incidence and course of INH-induced hepatotoxicity. In that study of 13,838 patients the overall incidence of INH-induced hepatotoxicity was 10.3/1000 (1%) with a mortality rate of 0.06% (8). In addition to patients developing clinical hepatitis, a much larger proportion of patients, i.e., 10–20%, developed asymptomatic elevation of transaminases (9). However, recent data suggest that hepatotoxicity resulting in clinical hepatitis is indeed much less common. In a 7-year survey from a public health tuberculosis clinic in the United States, the incidence of INH-induced "clinical hepatitis" was 0.1% in those starting treatment and 0.15% in those completing the treatment (10). The reason for such a low incidence was that the patients were not routinely screened for a rise in transaminases and only patients with symptomatic hepatitis were included. This study underscores the point that clinically significant hepatotoxicity due to INH is very uncommon and a mere rise in transaminases does not warrant any alteration in ATT. Most of the patients with asymptomatic rise in transaminases do not develop overt hepatitis and do not usually require any alteration in their drug treatment. The usual clinical course is gradual resolution of hepatitis within 1–4 weeks after INH is discontinued. However, if the drug is continued, patients may develop severe hepatitis, including fulminant hepatic failure (11). INH alone may cause death due to hepatotoxicity. Recently, Snider and Caras, after reviewing the articles published from 1965 through 1989, identified 177 deaths from INH-induced hepatitis among persons taking INH alone for chemoprophylaxis in the United States (12). They also found that (1) deaths from INH hepatitis are less frequent now than in the 1970s; (2) an increasing proportion of deaths occur with increasing age; and (3) women may be at an increased risk of death.

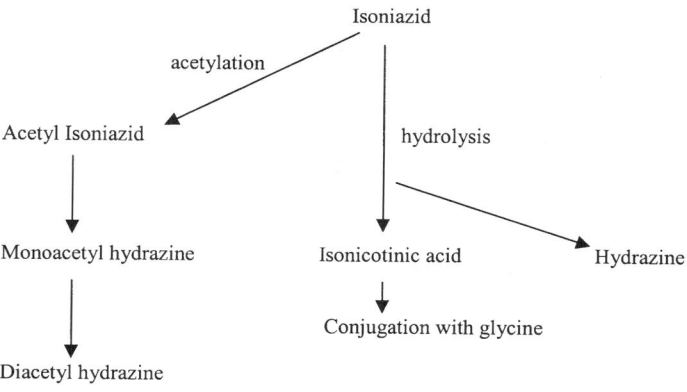

Figure 1 Metabolic pathway of INH.

III. INH METABOLISM AND POSSIBLE MECHANISM OF HEPATOTOXICITY

INH is metabolized through two important pathways, i.e., acetylation and hydrolysis (Fig. 1) (38). INH is acetylated to acetyl isoniazid. Acetyl isoniazid is then hydrolyzed to monoacetyl hydrazine and isonicotinic acid. This is known as the indirect pathway of metabolism. In the direct pathway INH is hydrolyzed by isoniazid hydrolase to isonicotinic acid and hydrazine. Isonicotinic acid formed through either the indirect or the direct pathway is conjugated with glycine and excreted by the kidneys.

The possible toxic metabolites are hydrazine and monoacetyl hydrazine. Monoacetyl hydrazine is primarily converted to diacetyl hydrazine, which is excreted by the kidneys. But monoacetyl hydrazine may also be converted to electrophilic intermediates by the P450 mixed-function oxidase enzyme system. These intermediate metabolites may cause hepatotoxicity. Hydrazine formed through the direct metabolic pathway after hydrolysis of INH has been shown to be hepatotoxic in animal studies.

The pathogenesis of INH-induced hepatotoxicity is not well understood. Both dose-related toxicity and hypersensitivity reaction have been considered. The histopathological picture resembles that of viral hepatitis and shows hepatocyte necrosis, ballooning degeneration, and inflammatory infiltrate (13). These findings may suggest dose-related toxicity. Hypersensitivity is considered unlikely because of the delayed onset of INH-induced hepatotoxicity; absence of symptoms usually associated with hypersensitivity such as rash, fever, arthralgia, and eosinophilia; and no hepatotoxicity on rechallenge in most cases (14,15). However, in some patients there is circumstantial evidence of hypersensitivity to the drug in that eosinophils are prominent on liver biopsy and there is development of hepatotoxicity on rechallenge (15). In addition, lack of direct correlation between serum drug levels and hepatotoxicity argues against a direct toxic effect (16).

IV. RIFAMPICIN

The major adverse effect of Rifampicin (RMP) therapy is hepatotoxicity. It has been reported that RMP has caused 16 deaths in 500,000 recipients of this agent (17). Minimal abnormalities in the liver function tests are common in patients receiving rifampicin and usually resolve even with continuation of the drug. Elevations of bilirubin and alkaline phosphatase levels are characteristic whereas elevations of transaminases can result from RMP, INH, or both (18). It has been observed that RMP-induced hepatotoxicity occurs earlier and produces a patchy cellular abnormality with less marked periportal inflammation compared to INH hepatitis (19). In several published studies the reported incidence of transaminase elevation and overt clinical hepatitis during RMP therapy in the absence of INH varied from 0.6 to 2.7% (20–22). On meta-analysis of these studies, the mean incidence of hepatitis in 1264 patients was 1.1%, significantly lower than that seen with INH and RMP combination (2.5%) (23). One Indian study reported jaundice in 7–8% of patients on RMP therapy (24). The mechanisms postulated to explain RMP-induced hepatitis are: (1) as a part of a systemic allergic reaction, which may be responsible for 1–3% of cases (25), and (2) unconjugated hyperbilirubinemia as a result of competition with bilirubin for uptake at the hepatocyte plasma membrane (26).

V. PYRAZINAMIDE

Hepatic injury is the most common and serious side effect of pyrazinamide (PZA) therapy. Early trials of PZA employed dosages of 40–50 mg/kg/day for prolonged periods and hepatotoxicity appeared in 15% of cases, so the use of PZA as a first-line drug was abandoned (27). Currently recommended regimens using PZA at a dosage of 20–35 mg/kg/day appear to be much safer. A large Indian study on hepatic toxicity with short-course regimens containing INH, RMP, and PZA reported that there was no indication that PZA contributed to hepatotoxicity (28). However, another case-control study from our center (29) and one recent study from the West (30) have shown that PZA contributes to the development of hepatotoxicity when it is given to patients in combination with INH and RMP. Both these studies have also reported cases of fulminant hepatic failure due to these drugs.

VI. COMBINATION OF ISONIAZID AND RIFAMPICIN AND HEPATOTOXICITY

There is evidence that drug-induced hepatitis occurs with greater frequency and may be more severe when isoniazid and rifampicin are administered in combination than when isoniazid is given alone (31,32). Some reports have suggested that hepatitis appeared sooner on INH-and-RMP combination therapy than on INH therapy alone, with prompt and major elevations of transaminase levels and hypoprothrombinemia in some patients (33,34).

Steele et al. undertook a meta-analysis to estimate the incidence of antituberculous treatment–induced hepatitis (23). A total of 34 clinical studies (22 involving adults and 12 involving children) published between 1966 and 1989 were entered into the analysis. The results showed that the incidence of clinical hepatitis in adults with INH alone was 0.6%; with multidrug INH regimens without RMP, 1.6%; and with regimens containing RMP and not INH, 1.1%. The incidence of clinical hepatitis in 6105 patients taking the INH-and-RMP combination was 2.55%, which was significantly higher than the incidence in groups of patients taking multiple drugs containing INH regimens without RMP and those taking multiple drugs containing RMP without INH. Children receiving INH plus RMP had a significantly higher incidence of hepatitis (6.9%) compared to those receiving multiple-drug INH regimens without RMP (1.6%). The authors concluded that INH-and-RMP combination caused more hepatotoxicity than either INH or RMP alone and the hepatotoxic effects of these two drugs given together were additive rather than synergistic. Why is there an increased risk of hepatotoxicity with INH-and-RMP combination? The answer probably lies in the interaction between INH and RMP metabolism. The metabolism of isoniazid is influenced by both genetic and intercurrent factors. The principal metabolite of INH, acetyl isoniazid, is converted to monoacetyl hydrazine. This in turn is metabolized by microsomal P450 enzymes to other compounds causing hepatotoxicity and this effect may be enhanced by RMP-induced enzyme induction. Because acetyl isoniazid formation occurs in larger amounts in rapid rather than slow acetylators, it was suggested that rapid acetylators might be more prone to hepatotoxicity (15). However, subsequent studies questioned the importance of this sequence to the development of hepatotoxicity as it was shown that monoacetyl hydrazine formed was rapidly converted into the less toxic diacetyl hydrazine, which was excreted rapidly (35). Both rapid and slow acetylators excreted similar proportions of monoacetyl hydrazine, suggesting that the more rapid formation of monoacetyl hydrazine was compensated by its more rapid conversion to diacetyl hydrazine and its excretion in rapid acetylators (36).

Other studies have suggested that products of hydrolysis rather than acetylation are the critical toxic metabolites of INH. Ellard and Gammon showed that a small proportion of INH is directly hydrolyzed by isoniazid hydrolase to isonicotinic acid (INA) and hydrazine, and the proportion of drug metabolized through this direct pathway is greater in slow than in rapid acetylators (37). Studies by Sarma and associates showed that the hepatotoxic action of metabolites of INH is not so much due to the monoacetyl hydrazine but to the hydrazine formed from INH (38). Rifampicin induces the metabolism of INH by isoniazid hydrolase resulting in the formation of isonicotinic acid and hydrazine (39). It has been suggested that concomitant administration of RMP and INH could result in increased levels of hydrazine and this could provoke hepatotoxicity, especially in slow acetylators (38). This hypothesis is supported by the finding of increased hepatotoxicity in slow acetylators who are given a combination of INH and rifampicin (40,41). That hydrazine, a metabolite of INH, may be responsible for INH-induced hepatotoxicity has also been suggested by a recent study. It was shown in a rabbit model that an amidase inhibitor inhibited the formation of hydrazine and decreased the measures of hepatocellular damage (42).

VII. RISK FACTORS FOR ATT-INDUCED HEPATOTOXICITY

The fact that antituberculous drugs cause hepatotoxicity in only a small percentage of patients raises the question of whether there are some predisposing factors for the development of ATT-induced hepatotoxicity. Certain such putative factors have been considered and studied. They are as follows.

A. Acetylator Status and Hepatotoxicity

As mentioned above, there is considerable confusion in the literature regarding the acetylator phenotype and hepatotoxicity. Rapid acetylators have been shown to be more susceptible to INH-induced toxic hepatitis (15). On the other hand, in patients receiving regimens containing INH and RMP, the incidence of hepatotoxicity was found to be higher in slow than in rapid acetylators (28). However, Gurumurty et al., in a study of 3000 South Indian

patients receiving various INH-containing regimens, demonstrated that there was no relationship between the acetylator phenotype and the incidence of hepatotoxicity (43). In
another study the authors also did not find any correlation between acetylator status and
development of ATT-induced hepatotoxicity (44).

B. *N*-Acetyltransferase 2 Genotype and Hepatotoxicity

A recent study has shown that slow NAT-2-genotype significantly affected the development of INH+RMP induced hepatotoxicity (45).

C. Age

INH hepatotoxicity has been correlated with age. The incidence of serious hepatotoxicity
is rare below 20 years of age—0.3% in the age group of 20–34 years, 1.2% in the 35–
39-year age group, and 2.3% in patients above the age of 50 years (46). Although a recent
Indian study claimed that age had no relation with ATT-induced hepatotoxicity (47), two
subsequent studies demonstrated once again the increased susceptibility to ATT hepatotoxicity with increasing age. A study from Belgium showed that elderly patients ($>$60 years
of age) with pulmonary tuberculosis were more likely to have raised transaminases following INH and RMP administration than younger patients (38% vs. 18%, $p < 0.05$) (48).
Another study from Denmark also found old age as a risk factor for development of ATT-
induced hepatotoxicity (49).

D. Sex

Elderly females have been reported to be at an increased risk to develop ATT-induced
hepatitis (50). However, some authors believe that the incidence of adverse hepatotoxic
reactions to antituberculous drugs is not influenced by the sex of the patients (47). In our
experience females were more susceptible to develop ATT-induced acute liver failure
(29). An 11-year study from Denmark also found females to be more susceptible to ATT-
induced liver damage (49).

E. Underlying Chronic Liver Disease

It has been shown that patients with underlying liver disease and alcoholics are more
prone to develop ATT-induced hepatotoxicity. Gronhagen-Riska et al. studied predisposing factors in isoniazid-refampicin–induced hepatitis and reported that one-half of the
patients who developed large increases in transaminases (more than 150 units/dL) were
either alcoholics or had a history of previous liver or biliary disease (50). A study from
Europe also showed that concurrent and previous biliary disorders were risk factors for
isoniazid hepatotoxicity (51). Kopanoff et al. have reported that hepatotoxicity is more
likely in alcoholics with preexisting liver damage than in nonalcoholics (8). However,
Girling observed that patients with known liver disease could be treated with isoniazid-
and-rifampicin-containing regimens without undue risk (27).

F. Hepatitis B Carrier State

There are conflicting data with regard to the risk of hepatotoxicity in patients with HBV
infection. McGlynn et al. reported that there was no evidence of increased risk of hepatotoxicity with isoniazid therapy in HBV carriers than in noncarriers (52). In another recent

study, it was observed that following isoniazid-and-rifampicin therapy, the peak transaminase and bilirubin levels were higher in patients who were HBV carriers than in others (50). Fulminant and subacute hepatic failures were seen more frequently in them, with a significantly higher mortality as compared to noncarriers (53). In a prospective study, no increased risk was noted for hepatotoxicity in patients with either underlying compensated chronic liver disease or hepatitis B carrier state (29). A recent study has, however, found that Chinese patients who were HBV carriers were more susceptible to develop ATT-induced liver injury as compared with noncarriers (34.9% vs. 9.4%, respectively) (54).

G. Hepatitis C Virus and HIV Infection

In a recent study it was shown that the relative risk of developing ATT-induced liver injury if the patient was hepatitis C or HIV positive was fivefold and fourfold, respectively. If a patient was coinfected with both hepatitis C and HIV, the relative risk was 14.4-fold (55).

H. Alcohol

Chronic alcohol consumption may be a risk factor for ATT-induced hepatotoxicity. However, the Danish study did not find alcohol consumption as an important risk factor (49).

I. Malnutrition

Mehta et al. have shown that drug-metabolizing processes in the liver, including acetylation pathways, are deranged in states of protein energy malnutrition (56,57). A significant decrease in INH metabolism has been demonstrated in kwashiorkor (58). In India, a higher incidence of rifampicin-isoniazid hepatotoxicity has been reported in patients with malnutrition (59,60). A mild degree of malnutrition in children, however, may not predispose to hepatotoxicity (61). In a study on predictive factors for the development of ATT-induced hepatotoxicity, it was observed that adult patients who were malnourished were given higher-than-normal dosages of drugs per kilogram body weight, which was probably one of the reasons for the development of hepatotoxicity in them (29).

J. ATT-Induced Hepatotoxicity and the Type of Tuberculosis

Patients with severe forms of tuberculosis are reported to be at a higher risk of hepatotoxicity than those with mild disease (49,62). Patients with tubercular meningitis have a higher incidence of hepatotoxicity as compared to those with milder disease (63). Similar findings have been reported in studies from India attributing ATT hepatotoxicity to factors such as hepatic involvement by the primary disease, malnutrition, more frequent hospitalization and parenteral therapy, and a closer biochemical monitoring in these patients and thus more chances of ATT hepatitis being diagnosed (28,64). In our experience, the site and severity of the underlying tuberculosis have no correlation with the development of ATT-induced hepatotoxicity. In fact, in our experience, 16% of patients with evident ATT hepatotoxicity did not have any definite evidence of tuberculosis (65).

VIII. CLINICAL COURSE OF ATT-INDUCED HEPATOTOXICITY

Most of the patients with ATT-induced hepatotoxicity have only asymptomatic elevation of transaminases. In about 1% of patients only overt icteric hepatitis develops. The onset

of hepatitis usually resembles that of viral hepatitis. In fact, in two studies it was emphasized that not all presumably ATT-induced hepatitis cases were due to ATT but many of
these cases were actually due to viral hepatitis (64,66). The duration of ATT-induced
hepatotoxicity has been reported to be 1–2 weeks in the majority of cases, although it
ranged from less than 1 week to 2 months. The majority of cases with ATT-induced
hepatitis resolve spontaneously following the withdrawal of the offending drugs. However,
in a substantial percentage of patients severe liver damage may occur leading to acute or
subacute liver failure with subsequent mortality. The development of ATT-induced acute
liver failure has been reported in many studies and such cases indicate the rapidity, the
severity, and the importance of ATT-induced hepatotoxicity. In a recent study, 15% of
patients with clinical ATT hepatitis developed acute and subacute liver failure, of which
nine patients died, resulting in a mortality of 75% and an overall mortality of 12% for
the whole group of patients with ATT-induced hepatotoxicity (65).

IX. MANAGEMENT OF ATT-INDUCED HEPATOTOXICITY

A. Monitoring of Liver Function Tests

All patients who are being started on ATT should have a baseline evaluation of liver
function tests (LFT). In younger patients (<35 years of age) routine monitoring of LFT
is not recommended unless patients manifest with symptoms suggestive of hepatotoxicity.
This recommendation is based on the fact that ATT-induced hepatotoxicity is rare in patients younger than 35 years. However, regular once-a-month monitoring of LFT is recommended for older patients, patients with underlying liver diseases, patients with coexistent
hepatitis B, C, or HIV infection, and malnourished patients because there are evidences
that there is an increased risk of developing ATT-induced liver injury in these groups of
patients. These recommendations are based on American Thoracic Society guidelines for
managing patients with tuberculosis (67).

B. Treatment

Once a patient develops clinical hepatitis or the liver enzymes are raised >5 times normal,
this mandates immediate stoppage of all potentially hepatotoxic drugs. A complete liver
function profile should be carried out including prothrombin time. Serology for viral hepatitis should be done. Adequate nutrition, rest, and careful clinical monitoring suffice for
the majority of patients. Serial laboratory investigations to monitor liver functions should
be done at least once a week. In patients with severe liver damage intensive medical
supportive treatment should be started. Liver transplantation may be required in certain
patients who fail to recover with conservative treatment and it has been shown to be
successful and rewarding in such cases (68).

X. TREATMENT OF UNDERLYING TUBERCULOSIS

There is a dearth of information on how best to treat the underlying tuberculosis in patients
who have developed hepatotoxicity. Treating tuberculosis in such a patient poses a difficult
clinical challenge. It is essential to first stop all potentially hepatotoxic drugs until complete clinical and biochemical resolution of hepatitis. In the interim, nonhepatotoxic drugs
such as ethambutol, streptomycin, and ciprofloxacin should be started. After complete
resolution of hepatitis, most antituberculous drugs can be safely restarted in a phased

manner. Although there exists a great deal of controversy regarding the safety and wisdom of starting the same hepatotoxic drugs that caused the hepatitis, the clinical experience has shown that the same drugs can indeed be given safely (49,70). No study is available on a systematic approach to reintroduce ATT in a patient who has had ATT hepatitis in the past. Some earlier studies have, however, shown that reintroduction of ATT may be risky (14,69). By contrast, others have shown that reintroduction of ATT (containing isoniazid and/or rifampicin) is possible in the majority of patients (27,28,70). In our experience, we could safely reintroduce INH and RMP in most of our patients (93%) after recovery from hepatitis in the appropriate dosages calculated according to body weight (65). This attempt to reintroduce potentially hepatotoxic drugs might generate some concern regarding safety. The reasons for such an attempt were that non-INH, non-RMP ATT regimens are marred with problems such as very long duration of treatment, lack of definite proof of clinical efficacy for treating tuberculosis, and development of resistance as in the case of ciprofloxacin. As a matter of caution, we reintroduced ATT in a stepwise manner with regard to both the specific drug and the dosage. In the final analysis, this strategy proved to be fairly effective and safe. Nonetheless, ATT-induced hepatotoxicity redeveloped in six of our 44 patients following reintroduction of ATT and this remained a definite and unpredictable risk. In addition, there is a small, albeit significant, subgroup of patients with ATT-induced severe liver failure and reintroduction of the same potentially hepatotoxic drugs should not be ventured in these patients following recovery.

Liver transplantation may be required for seriously ill patients with ATT-induced acute liver failure (68). Why did hepatitis not recur on rechallenge with these agents? A possible explanation could be the improved general condition after these patients had received ATT for some time with reduction of the bacterial load and toxemia. Second, these drugs were reintroduced in a phased manner and after adjustment of the dosages according to the lower body weight that was present in many of these patients. Such a cautious strategy of reintroducing ATT might have spared patients from the initial onslaught of potentially hepatotoxic drugs when given together in full dosages. It follows, therefore, that the majority of patients with ATT-induced hepatotoxicity recover completely and reintroduction of ATT is feasible and safe in them.

XI. RECOMMENDATIONS FOR REINTRODUCTION OF ATT

Based on our own and others' experiences (49,65,70), the following reintroduction strategy may be suggested. (1) After the liver enzymes and bilirubin levels have normalized, INH should be started in a small dose and then increased gradually to full dose, e.g., 50 mg/day for 3 days, then 100 mg/day for 3 days, then 200 mg/day for 3 days, and then full dose (depending on the body weight of the patient). (2) After INH has been reintroduced, pyrazinamide should be added after 1 week of observation. (3) Finally, rifampicin should be added after 1 week. The reasons for starting pyrazinamide before rifampicin are that pyrazinamide is less toxic than rifampicin and rifampicin is an enzyme inducer. During this period of ATT reintroduction, careful monitoring of liver function tests is mandatory at each step, i.e., before increasing the dose of INH and before adding another drug. If LFT shows abnormality during INH reintroduction, then INH is most likely the offending drug and should not be given to that patient. Similarly, if LFT abnormality occurs during pyrazinamide or rifampicin reintroduction, then that particular drug should not be given to the patient.

XII. CONCLUSION

ATT-induced liver injury is usually restricted to asymptomatic elevation of transaminases, which does not mandate any modification of ATT. A small number of patients (<1%) may develop clinical hepatitis that warrants modification of ATT and stoppage of all hepatotoxic drugs. The clinical course of such patients is mild and most patients recover completely. ATT can be safely restarted in most of them gradually in a phased manner. However, severe liver damage may occur in a minority of patients, which may even require liver transplantation.

REFERENCES

1. Reider HL. Misbehavior of a dying epidemic: a call for less speculation and better surveillance (editorial). Tuberc Lung Dis 1992; 73:181–182.
2. Snider DE, Jr., Cohn DL, Davidson PT, et al. Standard therapy for tuberculosis. Chest 1985; 87(suppl):117S–124S.
3. Mahashur AA, Prabhudesai PP. Hepatitis and antitubercular therapy. J Assoc Physicians India 1991; 39:595–596.
4. Gangadharam PR. Isoniazid, rifampin and hepatotoxicity (editorial). Am Rev Respir Dis 1986; 133:963–965.
5. Moulding TS, Redeker AG, Kanel GC. Twenty isoniazid associated deaths in one state. Am Rev Respir Dis 1989; 140:700–705.
6. Scharer L, Smith JP. Serum transaminase elevations and other hepatic abnormalities in patients receiving isoniazid. Ann Intern Med 1969; 71:113–120.
7. Garibaldi RA, Drusin RE, Ferebee SH, Gregg MB. Isoniazid associated hepatitis: report of an outbreak. Am Rev Respir Dis 1972; 106:357–365.
8. Kopanoff DE, Sinder DE, Caras GH. Isoniazid-related hepatitis A. U.S. Public Health Service Cooperative Surveillance Study. Am Rev Respir Dis 1978; 117:991–1001.
9. Brummer DL. Isoniazid and liver disease. Ann Intern Med 1971; 75:643.
10. Nolan CM, Goldberg SV, Buskin SE. Hepatotoxicity associated with isoniazid preventive therapy: a 7-year survey from a public health tuberculosis clinic. JAMA 1999; 281:1014–1018.
11. Cohen R, Kalser MH, Thomson RV. Fatal hepatic necrosis secondary to isoniazid therapy. JAMA 1961; 176:877–879.
12. Snider DE, Caras GH. Isoniazid associated hepatitis deaths: a review of available information. Am Rev Respir Dis 1992; 145:494–497.
13. Black M, Mitchell JR, Zimmerman HJ, Ishak KG, Epler GR. Isoniazid-associated hepatitis in 114 patients. Gastroenterology 1975; 69:289–302.
14. Meddrey WC, Boitnott JK. Isoniazid hepatitis. Ann Intern Med 1973; 70:1–12.
15. Mitchell JR, Thorgeirsson UP, Black M, et al. Increased incidence of isoniazid hepatitis in rapid acetylators: possible relation to hydrazine metabolites. Clin Pharmacol Ther 1975; 18: 70–79.
16. Mitchell JR, Long MW, Thorgeirsson UP, Jollow DJ. Acetylation rates and monthly liver function tests during one year of isoniazid preventive therapy. Chest 1975; 68:181–190.
17. Madell GL, Sande MA. Drugs used in the chemotherapy of tuberculosis and leprosy. In: AS Gilman, LS Goodman, TW Rall, et al., eds. The Pharmacological Basis of Therapeutics. 7th ed. New York: Macmillan Publishing Co., 1985:199–218.
18. Alford RH. Antimycobacterial agents. In: GL Mandell, RJ Douglas, JE Benett, eds. Principles and Practice of Infectious Diseases. 3rd ed. New York: Churchill Livingstone, 1990:350–361.
19. Thompson JE. The effect of rifampicin on liver morphology in tuberculous alcoholics. Aust NZ J Med 1976; 6:111–116.

20. Lees AW, Allan GW, Smith J. Toxicity from rifampin plus isoniazid and rifampicin plus ethambutal therapy. Tubercle 1971; 52:182–190.
21. Releigh JW. Rifampin in treatment of advanced pulmonary tuberculosis. Am Rev Respir Dis 1973; 105:397–409.
22. Hong Kong Tuberculosis Treatment Service/Brompton Hospital/British Medical Research Council. A controlled trial of daily and intermittent rifampicin plus ethambutol in the treatment of patients with pulmonary tuberculosis: results up to 30 months. Tubercle 1975; 56:79–89.
23. Steele MA, Burk RF, Desprez RM. Toxic hepatitis with isoniazid and rifampicin—a meta-analysis. Chest 1991; 99:465–471.
24. Gupta PR, Purohit JD, Mehta YR, Jain BI, Kotwal S, Sharma TN. Serum and urinary rifampicin and hepatic toxicity. Indian J Tuberc 1985; 32:86–90.
25. Mulder De Jong, Mulder RJ. Drugs used in the treatment of tuberculosis and leprosy. In: MUG Dukes, ed. Meyler's Side Effects of Drugs. Vol. 1. Oxford: Excerpta Medica, 1977:676–689.
26. Kenwright S, Levi AJ. Sites for competition in selective hepatic uptake of rifampicin SV, flavaspidic acid, billirubin and bromsalphalein. GU 1974; 15:220–226.
27. Girling DJ. The hepatic toxicity of antituberculous regimens containing isoniazid, rifampicin, and pyrazinamide. Tubercle 1978; 59:13–32.
28. Parthasarathy R, Sarma GR, Janardhanam B, et al. Hepatic toxicity in South Indian patients during treatment of tuberculosis with short course regimens containing isoniazid, rifampin and pyrazinamide. Tubercle 1986; 67:99–108.
29. Singh J, Arora A, Garg PK, Thakur VS, Pande JN, Tandon RK. Antituberculosis treatment induced hepatotoxicity: role of predictive factors. Postgrad Med J 1995; 71:359–362.
30. Mitchell I, Williams R. Liver transplantation for antituberculous drug induced acute liver failure. Lancet 1995; 345:555.
31. Lal S, Singhal SN, Burley DM, Crossley G. Effect of rifampicin and isoniazid on liver function. Br Med J 1972; 1:148–150.
32. Snider DE, Long MW, Cross PS, Farer LS. Six months isoniazid-rifampin therapy for pulmonary tuberculosis: report of a United States Health Service Cooperative Trial. Am Rev Respir Dis 1984; 129:573–579.
33. Tsagaropoulon-Stinga H, Mataki-Emmanouili T, Karida-Ka-Valioti S, Manios S. Hepatotoxic reactions in children with severe tuberculosis treated with isoniazid-rifampin. Pediatr Infect Dis 1985; 4:270–273.
34. Pessayre D, Bentata M, Degott C, Nonel O, Miguet JP, Rueff B, et al. Isoniazid-rifampin fulminant hepatitis: a possible consequence of the enhancement of isoniazid hepatotoxicity in enzyme induction. Gastroenterology 1977; 72:284–289.
35. Ellard GA, Mitchison DA, Girling DJ, Nunn AJ, Fox W. The hepatic toxicity of isoniazid among rapid and slow acetylators of the drug. Am Rev Respir Dis 1978; 118:628–629.
36. Lauterburg BH, Smith CV, Todd EL, Mitchell JR. Pharmacokinetics of the toxic hydrazine metabolites formed from isoniazid in humans. Pharmacol Exp Ther 1985; 235:566–570.
37. Ellard GA, Gammon PT. Pharmacokinetics of isoniazid metabolism in man. J Pharmacokinet Biopharm 1976; 4:83–113.
38. Sarma GR, Immanuel C, Naryana ASL, Ventakaterin P. Rifampin-induced release of hydrazine from isoniazid. A possible cause of hepatitis during treatment of tuberculosis with regimens containing isoniazid and rifampin. Am Rev Respir Dis 1986; 133:1072–1705.
39. Bevve IW, Blair IA, Brodie MJ. Circulating hydrazine during treatment with isoniazid rifampicin in man. Br J Clin Pharmacol 1982; 13:599.
40. Dickinson DS, Bailey WC, Hirschowitz BI. The effect of acetylation status on isoniazid (INH) hepatitis. Am Rev Respir Dis 1977; 115:395.
41. Wiber WW, Hein DW, Litwun A, Lower GM, Jr. Relationship of acetylator status to isoniazid toxicity, lupus erythematosus and bladder cancer. Feb Proc 1983; 42:3086–3090.
42. Sarich TC, Adams SP, Petricca G, Wright JM. Inhibition of isoniazid-induced hepatotoxicity

in rabbits by pretreatment with an amidase inhibitor. J Pharmacol Exp Ther 1999; 289:695–702.

43. Gurumurty P, Krishnamurthy MS, Nazareth O, et al. Lack of relationship between hepatic toxicity and acetylator phenotype in three thousand South Indian patients during treatment with isoniazid for tuberculosis. Am Rev Respir Dis 1984; 129:58–61.

44. Singh J, Garg PK, Thakur VS, Tandon RK. Antitubercular treatment induced hepatotoxicity: does acetylator status matter? Indian J Physiol Pharmacol 1995; 35:43–46.

45. Ohno M, Yamaguchi I, Yamamoto I, et al. Slow N-acetyltransferase 2 genotype affects the incidence of isoniazid-and-rifampicin–induced hepatotoxicity. Int J Tuberc Lung Dis 2000; 4:256–261.

46. Centers for Disease Control. National Consensus Conference on Tuberculosis. Preventive Treatment of Tuberculosis. Chest 1985; 87(suppl 2):128–132.

47. Teneja DP, Dalip K. Study of hepatotoxicity and other side effects of antitubercular drugs. J Indian Med Assoc 1990; 88:278–279.

48. van den Brande P, van Steenbergen W, Vervoort G, Demedts M. Aging and hepatotoxicity of isoniazid and rifampicin in pulmonary tuberculosis. Am J Respir Crit Care Med 1995; 152(5 Pt 1):1705–1708.

49. Dossing M, Wilcke JT, Askgaard DS, Nybo B. Liver injury during antituberculous treatment: an 11-year study. Tuberc Lung Dis 1996; 77:335–340.

50. Gronhagen-Riska C, Hellstrom PE, Froseth B. Predisposing factors in hepatitis induced by isoniazid-rifampin treatment of tuberculosis. Am Rev Respir Dis 1978; 118:461–466.

51. Riska N. Hepatitis cases in INH treated groups and in a control group. Bull Int Un Tubercle 1976; 51:203.

52. McGlynn KA, Lustbader ED, Sharma RG, Murphy EC, London WT. Isoniazid prophylaxis in hepatitis B carriers. Am Rev Respir Dis 1986; 134:666–668.

53. Wu JC, Lee SD, Yeh PF, Chan CY, et al. Isoniazid-rifampin–induced hepatitis in hepatitis B carriers. Gastroenterology 1990; 98:502–504.

54. Wong WM, Wu PC, Yuen MF, et al. Antituberculosis drug-related liver dysfunction in chronic hepatitis B infection. Hepatology 2000; 31:201–206.

55. Ungo JR, Jones D, Ashkin D, et al. Antituberculosis drug-induced hepatotoxicity: the role of hepatitis C virus and the human immunodeficiency virus. Am J Respir Crit Care Med 1998; 157(6 Pt 1):1871–1876.

56. Mehta S, Nain CK, Sharma B, Mathur VS. Metabolism of sulfadiazine in children with protein-calorie malnutrition. Pharmacology 1980; 21:369–374.

57. Mehta S, Nian CK, Sharma B, Mathur VS. Disposition of four drugs in malnourished children. Drug-Nutrient Interact 1982; 1:205–212.

58. Buchanan N, Eyberg C, Davis MD. Isoniazid pharmacokinetics in Kwashiorkor. S Afr Med J 1979; 56:299–300.

59. Rugmini PS, Mehta S. Hepatotoxicity of isoniazid and rifampin in children. Indian Pediatr 1984; 21:119–124.

60. Pande JN, Singh SPN, Khilnani GC, Khilnani S, Tandon RK. Risk factors for hepatotoxicity from antituberculous drugs: a case control study. Thorax 1996; 51:132–136.

61. Seth V, Beotra A. Hepatic function in relation to acetylator phenotype in children treated with antitubercular drugs. Indian J Med Res 1989; 89:306–309.

62. O'Brien RJ, Long MV, Floy SC, Lyle MA, Snider DE, Jr. Hepatotoxicity from isoniazid and rifampin among children treated for tuberculosis. Pediatrics 1983; 72:191–199.

63. Vasudhiphan P, Chiemanya S. Evaluation of rifampin in the treatment of tuberculous meningitis in children. J Pediatr 1975; 87:983.

64. Kumar A, Misra PK, Mehotra R, Govil YC and Rana GS. Hepatotoxicity of rifampin and isoniazid. Is it all drug induced hepatitis? Am Rev Respir Dis 1991; 16:544.

65. Singh J, Garg PK, Tandon RK. Hepatotoxicity due to antituberculous therapy: clinical profile and reintroduction of therapy. J Clin Gastroenterol 1996; 22.

66. Turktas H, Unsal M, Tulek N, Oruc O. Hepatotoxicity of antituberculous therapy (rifampicin, isoniazid and pyrazinamide) or viral hepatitis. Tuberc Lung Dis 1994; 75:58–60.

67. Treatment of tuberculosis and tuberculosis infection in adults and children. Position paper of American Thoracic Society 1994 (source-www.thoracic.org).

68. Durand F, Bernuau J, Pessayre D, et al. Deleterious influence of pyrazinamide on the outcome of patients with fulminant and subfulminant liver failure during antituberculous treatment including isoniazid. Hepatology 1995; 21:929–932.

69. Davidson PT, Le HQ. Drug treatment of tuberculosis. Drugs 1992; 43:651–673.

70. Ansari MM, Beg MH, Haleem S. Hepatitis in patients with surgical complications of pulmonary tuberculosis. Indian J Chest Dis Allied Sci 1991; 33:133–138.

22

Hepatic Injury from Antiviral Agents

MAURIZIO BONACINI

California Pacific Medical Center, San Francisco, California, U.S.A.

STAN LOUIE

University of Southern California, Los Angeles, California, U.S.A.

KEVIN WEISSMAN

King Drew Medical Center, Los Angeles, California, U.S.A.

I. INTRODUCTION

The human immunodeficiency virus (HIV) epidemic dramatically changed the way antiviral medications are administered. Patients are no longer given short courses of a single antiviral agent for symptom control, as in herpetic infections. The management of selected viral illnesses now requires prolonged administration of multiple antivirals to prevent disease progression. This paradigm shift occurred in 1995, owing to the antiretroviral management of HIV infection (1,2). Antiretroviral cocktails containing three to five antiretroviral drugs, referred to as highly active antiretroviral therapy (HAART), improved clinical outcomes by reducing morbidity and mortality associated with HIV progression (1–3). The antiviral activity of some of these agents is not limited to HIV, but includes inhibition of the hepatitis B (HBV) virus (4,5). Hepatitis C is a disease affecting close to 2% of all U.S. residents (6), and its treatment has also advanced swiftly (7). Four interferon preparations are currently approved for the treatment of chronic hepatitis C, and newer long-acting preparations have been marketed (8,9). Finally, advances have been made in the development of anti-influenza medications, which are expected to be used by an increasing number of individuals, each year (10). As a consequence, hepatic drug toxicity, sometimes detected only with extensive postmarketing experience, has been increasingly noted in some classes of drugs (11–13). Moreover, selected patients, e.g., those anti-HIV-positive, appear more prone to develop hepatotoxicity, to sulfa drugs, or oxacillin, for example (14–16). Thus, as therapy with antiviral agents becomes more common, complex, and prolonged, the potential for overt hepatotoxicity will no doubt increase (13).

II. METABOLISM OF ANTIVIRAL MEDICATIONS

Most drugs are lipophilic substances metabolized in the liver into water-soluble substances, resulting in biliary or renal elimination (17,18). The first biotransformation step is mediated by smooth endoplasmic reticulum enzymes, belonging to the cytochrome P450 (CYP) enzyme superfamily (17–19). CYP 3A4 appears to be the most important enzyme involved with the metabolism of HIV protease inhibitors (PIs) and nonnucleoside reverse transcriptase inhibitors (NNRTIs) (Table 2) (20–23). Alternative subtypes, such as CYP 2D6, are involved with ritonavir and delavirdine metabolism (Table 1) (20–23). The activity of these enzymes is determined by both gene expression and environmental induction. Genes differ between ethnic groups: for example, up to 10% of Caucasians are poor metabolizers of substrates for CYP 2D6, as compared to Asians (<1%) (19). More than 20 mutations of the CYP 3A4 gene are currently known, therefore explaining individual susceptibility to administration of the same drug (19). Thus, it is clear that the metabolism of any xenobiotic can potentially transform chemically stable compounds into toxic metabolites (17). An overview of the available data on antiviral hepatotoxicity is given in Table 2.

III. POSSIBLE MECHANISMS OF HEPATOTOXICITY

Despite advances in antiviral research, and the availability of sophisticated molecular techniques, the exact mechanisms of drug-induced hepatotoxicity (DIH) are still not clearly delineated (12). Drug-induced hepatotoxicity can be the consequence of direct chemical interaction between cellular components and either the parent agent or its metabolites (17). The injury may be dose-dependent and predictable, but is more often idiosyncratic (18). Cellular mechanisms of liver injury include: covalent binding to key cellular proteins, generation of free radicals, induction of lipid peroxidation, plasma membrane injury, mitochondrial or nuclear toxicity (12,17,18,24). Any of the above may lead to hepatocyte necrosis or apoptosis (24). Alternatively, DIH may be allergic in type, with the formation of a hapten attached to the plasma membrane, recognized by the immune system as foreign, thus initiating an intrahepatic inflammatory reaction (18).

Table 1 Overview of the Principal Antiviral Medications and Their Association with Hepatotoxicity

Drug	Abnormal liver tests > 2%	Number of hepatotoxicity cases reported	Liver failure
Abacavir	−	−	+
Delavirdine	+	−	−
Didanosine	+	4	+
Efavirenz	+	1	−
Famciclovir	+	−	−
Ganciclovir	−	5	−
Hydroxyurea	−	3	+
Indinavir	+	6	+
Interferon	+	>12	+
Lamivudine	+	5	+
Nelfinavir	+	−	−
Nevirapine	+	11	+
Ritonavir	+	12	−
Saquinavir	+	−	−
Stavudine	+	11	+
Valacyclovir	+	1	−
Zalcitabine	+	−	−
Zidovudine	+	18	+

+ = reported; − = not reported.

IV. RISK FACTORS FOR ANTIVIRAL HEPATOTOXICITY

A number of factors can increase the risk of developing hepatotoxicity due to antivirals. These include age, gender, preexisting liver disease, antioxidant status, alcohol use, baseline and HAART-induced CD4 counts changes, as well as genetic factors.

Aging results in a decline in the ability to eliminate drugs (25). The major mechanism is thought to be a decreased hepatic blood flow (26), which leads to drug accumulation and increased potential for DIH (26). In vitro, CYP activity appears to remain stable with age (26,27).

A number of antiretroviral studies have shown that women are more likely to develop drug-related toxicity when receiving HAART (28,29). Women present a complex situation owing to menstrual hormonal changes, which can theoretically affect the expression of hepatic metabolic enzymes (30). However, it appears that CYP 3A metabolism of midazolam is affected neither by gender nor by menstrual cycle phase, in white non-smokers (30). Oral contraceptives do not appear to alter the pharmacokinetics of midazolam (25) but enhance clearance of clofibrate (31).

As shown in Table 1, drugs like ritonavir and nelfinavir are mainly CYP inhibitors (20–23). Thus, one would predict that they would cause increased levels of other drugs. However, this theoretical interaction is not always noted clinically (32). In fact, ritonavir reduces ethinyl-estradiol plasma concentration by 40%, and nelfinavir reduces the levels of norethindrone by 18% (23).

Patients with preexisting liver disease, i.e., advanced fibrosis or cirrhosis, may be at higher risk for developing DIH (33). This is thought to occur mainly for drugs with

Table 2 Cytochrome P450 Metabolism and Drug-Drug Interaction of NNRTIs and PIs

Drugs	Metabolism by CYP	Inhibits CYP	Induces CYP	↑ AUC of the following drugs:	↓ AUC of the following drugs:
		HIV protease inhibitor			
Ritonavir	3A4 2D6	3A4	3A4, 2C9, 1A1	SQV 17× IDV 2–5× NFV 1.5–2.5×	—
Saquinavir	3A4	3A4	—	—	—
Amprenavir	3A4	3A4	—	—	—
Nelfinavir	3A4	3A4		IDV 50% SQV 3–7× APV 1.5–2.7×	DLV 50%
Indinavir	3A4	3A4	—	NFV 80% APV 50–60% SQV 4–7×	—
Lopinavir	3A	3A 2D6	—	RTV 50%	—
		Nonnucleoside reverse transcriptase inhibitor			
Nevirapine	3A4	—	3A	—	—
Efavirenz	3A4 2B6	3A4, 2B6, 2C9, 2C19	3A4	—	SQV 60%
Delavirdine	3A4 2D6	3A4, 2D6, 2C9, 2C19	—	RTV 70% SQV 5× NFV 2× IDV 2–5×	—

IDV = indinavir; NFV = nelfinavir; DLV = delavirdine; SQV = saquinavir; RTV = ritonavir; APV = amprenavir; AUC = area under curve.
Source: Adapted from refs. 20, 22, 23.

dose-dependent toxicity. For the majority of DIH (idiosyncratic), preexisting liver disease may place hepatocytes at risk through a decrease in defense mechanisms, e.g., low glutathione (GSH) levels (33). In addition, the use of multiple drugs in the setting of cirrhosis will complicate their pharmacodynamic interaction (33).

Patients with HIV infection are often coinfected with hepatitis B or C (34,35). In a French cohort study, three factors were significantly and independently associated with World Health Organization (WHO) grade 3 ALT elevation (greater than 5 times the upper limit of normal, ULN) after therapy with different antiretroviral agents (36). These were: prior ALT elevation, presence of HBsAg, or evidence of hepatitis C virus (HCV) infection. In another study, patients taking nucleoside analogs (NAs) were more likely to experience WHO grade 3 or 4 (greater than 5 or 10× ULN) AST or ALT elevations, if they were also anti-HCV positive (37).

Intracellular GSH is an important factor protecting hepatocytes against oxidative injury (17,38,39). A decline in cellular GSH content also may decrease the ability to eliminate reactive intermediates, allowing their accumulation (40,41), and GSH depletion has been associated with hepatotoxicity due to a number of xenobiotics, such as acetaminophen and benzene (17,18). HIV infection is associated with lower plasma GSH levels, and in these patients, hepatic GSH stores decline even in early HIV disease (41,43). Plasma and whole-blood levels of GSH are 60% and 20% lower than in controls, respectively (43,44). These findings led to the successful strategy of utilizing N-acetylcysteine supplementation to increase biosynthesis of GSH (45). However, a recent investigation suggested that the transactivatory HIV protein Tat downregulated glutamylcysteine synthetase (GCS), the rate-limiting enzyme in GSH biosynthesis (46). Intracellular levels of GSH in both liver and erythrocyte samples were significantly lower in Tat+ transgenic mice, compared to control animals (46). Patients coinfected with HIV and HCV have lower hepatic GSH stores than patients with HCV alone (41).

Chronic ethanol consumption causes an elevation in liver oxygen radical concentration, leading to oxidative damage to mitochondrial DNA (mtDNA) (47). In addition, ethanol reduces intracellular GSH stores, and decreases GSH transport into the mitochondrion (38,48). The use of alcohol by patients with either HIV or HCV infection can theoretically adversely affect the oxidant-antioxidant balance in patients receiving antiviral medications, and thus facilitate the development of liver injury (38,47). A retrospective study of 222 HIV patients showed that those who had heavy alcohol intake had 5.9 times the risk of developing grade 3 transaminase elevation compared to those who did not (47a).

In a large cohort study, patients with CD4 counts <200 had twice the likelihood of severe hepatotoxicity than patients with >200 CD4 (37), although the difference was of borderline statistical significance. Approximately two-thirds of HIV patients diagnosed with antiretroviral hepatotoxicity demonstrated baseline CD4 counts < 200/mm^3 (Table 3). Interestingly, patients whose CD4 counts increased by at least 50 cells/mm^3 had a threefold greater risk of developing grade 3 or 4 DIH, although the confidence intervals crossed the unit (0.9–10.3) (37). The latter finding may merely point to better medication compliance in patients who developed DIH (37). Two studies show that PIs were more often associated with DIH; however, these groups had lower CD4 counts than the NA group (36,37).

V. GENETIC FACTORS

Genetic variations in drug biotransformation systems modulate the risk of DIH, and antivirals should be no exception (42). There are approximately 20 different CYP isoenzymes differing in immunogenicity and catalytic activity (19,42). Deficiency in CYP 2D6 activity is found in 5–10% of Caucasians (42). CYP 2D6-deficient individuals are more likely to develop perhexiline toxicity, compared to those with normal activity (42). CYP 2C19 deficiency occurs in 5% of Caucasians and 20% of Asians and is associated with chlorpromazine and Atrium hepatotoxicity (42).

A. N-Acetylation Deficiency

The N-acetylation phenotype is determined by two alleles at a single gene locus. The prevalence of fast-acetylation phenotype ranges from 30–60% in Caucasians to >70% in Asians (42). N-Acetylation polymorphism can affect the elimination of isoniazid, sulfonamides, and caffeine, among others (42). A deficiency in N-acetyltransferase 2 activity (slow-acetylator phenotype) can lead to sulfonamide toxicity, a frequently used agent in HIV patients.

Table 3 Case Reports Detailing Antiviral Associated Liver Injury

Ref.	Drug	N =	Gender	Age	ALT	AST	ALT higher	AP	Bili	CD4	wks-peak	Hepatitis	Wks resol.	Comments
118	GCV	1	m	33	500	800		350	0.3	—	2–3	No	1–2	Positive rechallenge
117	GCV	4	—	32–37	55–110	—		61–793	—	—	Nl	—	—	
115	VAL	1	f	71	376	317	y	296	3.3	—	1	No	4	
147	HU	1	m	64	—	524		128	1.6	—	2–3	—	—	
144	HU	1	f	45	1245	1394		80	20	50	12	No	Died	Died
144	HU	1	m	42	197	196	y	166	3.8	210	8	C	9	
148	AZT	1	m	38	115	220		62	0.8	—	16	No	8 to 12	
149	AZT	1	f	34	Nl	Nl	Equal	Nl	Nl	—	48	No	died	mac
150	AZT	1	f	36	3×	3×	Equal	Nl	—	354	24	—	died	fat
151	AZT	1	m	38	873	825	y	104	9.8	—	20	No	2	
152	AZT	1	f	35	85	100		85	Nl	34	16	No	died	mac
150	AZT	1	f	40	48	220		114	0.8	104	36	—	died	mac
153	AZT	1	f	57	131	301		—	Nl	150	36	No HBV	died	mac
154	AZT	1	f	26	91	131		120	Nl	AIDS	—	B	died	mac
150	AZT	1	f	34	2.5×	8×		1.5×	0.8	114	45	—	26	
150	AZT	1	f	57	7.5×	10×		2×	2.9	150	36	—	died	mac
150	AZT	1	f	40	9.5×	25×			19.2	343	48	—	died	fat
150	AZT	1	f	31	—	—		—	—	—	—	—	—	fat
155	AZT	1	m	33	109	173		74	0.8	7%	52	No	died	fat
156	AZT	1	m	57	8×	9×		Nl	Nl	18	26	No	died	mac/mic
157	AZT	1	m	39	3×	7×		13×	6.5	—	2	no test for C	6	Positive rechallenge
155	AZT	1	m	48	109	242		207		40	48	No	died	mac
150	AZT	1	m	57	90	335			15	53	24	—	died	mac, liver = 6.8 kg
153	AZT	1	m	47	93	328		130	2.7	243	24	C	died	mac
95	d4T	1	m	43	356	115	y			—	60	—	4	steatosis-CT
92	d4T	1	f	35	43	95		46	0.7	243	52	—	4	mic/mac
95	d4T	1	f	63	92	175				192	24	—	—	
78	d4T	1	f	32	67				1.6	—	24	—	—	
95	d4T	1	f	16	120	166				239	12	—	—	
95	d4T	1	m	54	43	53				184	60	C	—	mic/mac
93	d4T/3TC	1	m	69	2414	1106	y		20.7	75	10	B	died	
92	d4T/3TC	1	m	34	41	62			2	—	40	—	—	fat

94	d4T/3TC	3	f	36-40	—	48-219		—	—	8-201	4-32	—	2 died, 1-8 wk	1 steatosis at ax
87	ddl	1	m	45	293	215	y	146	5.4	31	13	No	died	mic/mac
88	ddl	1	m	36	—	—		—	NI	—	—		died	—
87	ddl	1	m	69	54	194		186	1.3	230	13	No	died	mic
89	D4T	1	m	36	206	210		—	—	—	1		—	mac
90	ddI/d4T/1 idv	1	m	58	75	107		172	7.3	—	—		3	no fat
103	EFV	1	f	31	551	—		—	—	—	2	C	8	
107	IDV	1	m	27	807	557	y	—	—	7 to 277	20	C	—	Eosinos
106	IDV	1	m	52	1602	747	y	49	6.1	56	2	no	—	—
106	IDV	1	f	37	1875	9278		159	2.5	7	1	C	—	—
109	IDV	1	m	34	234	508		—	7.3	155	48	C	12	mic
108	IDV	1	m	46	123	—		136	12.2	10	6	no		fat
106	IDV	1	m	48	690	920		145	17.5	11	1.5	B	died	mic
100	NVP	1	f	36	7695	5391	y	777	6.2	630	8	C		738 eos
98	NVP	1	m	61	337	255	y	237	3.7	500	2	no	4	8400 eos
102	NVP	1	m	47	288	150	y	851	17.8	434	2	C	5	
102	NVP	1	m	27	3493	2365	y	266	12.3	—	2	no	6	mic
102	NVP	1	m	41	312	192	y	426	14.8	149	12	no	10	
99	NVP	1	f	31	1698	1813		10×	14.9	23	5	no	died	mac
103	NVP	1	f	31	772	—		171	—	400	5	C	4	no fat
102	NVP	1	m	49	—	555		258	31.8	569	20	C	12	no fat
109	NVP	1	m	49	348	510			8.2	32	12	C	7	
56	RTV	1	m	34	491	75	y	—	8.8	—	1	C	5	
56	RTV	10	m	33	1206	—		—	16	—	2 to 22	9/10 C	3 to 12	no fat: 1 bx, 10 patients, 1 ?acute B 9/10 taking other PI's.
110	RTV	1	f	28	254	327		—	18.1	3	5	no	8	mic, rechallenge, lactic acid, liver bx = extensive fibrosis, microvesic steatosis.

GCV = ganciclovir; AZT = zidovudine; mac = macrovesicular fat; mic = microvesicular fat; DDI = dideoxyinosine; EFV = efavirenz; EOS = eosinphils; BX = biopsy; CT = computed tomography; RTV = ritonavir; IDV = indinavir; NVP = nevirapine; D4T = stavudine; AX = autopsy; HU = hydroxyurea; VAL = valacyclovir; Nl = normal; — = not available.

B. Sulfoxidation

Sulfoxidation polymorphism has been classified into: extensive, intermediate, and deficient metabolism (42). The prevalence of deficient sulfoxidation (22% of the population) has been associated with chlorpromazine hepatotoxicity (42).

C. Glutathione Detoxification

GSH is an essential compound for the detoxification of reactive metabolites formed out of many drugs (14,17,42). GSH synthesis is achieved by a reaction catalyzed by glutathione synthetase (GS), which combines gamma-glutamyl-cysteine with glycine. In subjects with deficient GS, intracellular GSH levels can be 15% of normal values. Even low doses of acetaminophen can induce lymphocyte toxicity in these patients (42).

VI. DRUG INTERACTIONS

Patients with HIV infection may be required to take up to 15 different prescribed medications including antiretroviral, antimicrobial, nonsteroidal anti-inflammatory, and mood-altering agents used to manage the primary infection, as well as a constellation of associated disorders. More importantly, the PI and NNRTI classes, but not the NAs can significantly alter the biological activity of cytochromes (Table 2), in particular CYP 3A4 (20–23). Thus, use of multiple drugs may alter the concentration of other compounds and increase the likelihood of DIH (12,22). The combination of two protease inhibitors can increase the concentration of either one or both protease inhibitors (Table 1). In addition, approximately 40% of HIV patients in Canada or Europe take various types of complementary medicines (CAM), such as vitamins, herbs, and other nonprescription medications (49–51). The use of complementary agents is even higher in the United States and Australia, where rates are 67% and 80%, respectively (52,53). The likelihood is highest in Caucasians, college-educated patients (49–52), and southern California (50), and it is significantly lower in minority patients (50). It is unknown whether the use of CAM is associated with a proclivity to develop DIH to components of HAART. Hepatotoxicity associated with CAM appears so far to be low, but has not been prospectively studied in this patient population (49–53). On the other hand, St. John's wort can decrease plasma concentrations of indinavir, and possibly of other prescription antivirals metabolized by CYP 3A4 isoforms (54).

VII. MANIFESTATIONS OF HEPATOTOXICITY

WHO grade 3 and 4 elevations in liver enzymes occur in 6–36/100 patients/year treated with antiretrovirals. Data from three cohort studies are summarized in Table 4. Two of these cohorts (37,55) were followed more intensively (every 2–3 months) and may have led to higher prevalence of DIH. In addition, the Baltimore cohort was composed mainly of African-American patients (37), further suggesting a genetic role in the likelihood of DIH. Clinical symptoms of DIH include gastrointestinal symptoms such as nausea, vomiting, abdominal pain, and anorexia (56). In severe cases, patients may present with abnormal mental status, hepatic coma, bleeding diathesis, and portal hypertension (Table 5) (18). On the other hand, DIH is often diagnosed on routine liver enzyme testing (56). Clinical features of immune-mediated hepatotoxicity include fever, arthralgias, a skin rash, hypereosinophilia, allergic thrombocytopenia, and production of autoantibodies (18,56).

Table 4 Cohort Studies of Antiretroviral-Associated Hepatotoxicity

	French Aquitaine (36)		Baltimore, MD (37)		Italy (55)			RTV + SQV
	PI	NRTI	PI	NA	IDV	RTV	SQV	
N	748	1249	211	87				
Follow-up (days)	393	365	182	167	321	a	a	a
Age	37	37	37	36	37.1	a	a	a
CD4	144	234	109	215	253	a	a	a
Log HIV	4.0	4.2	>4	>4	—	—	—	—
HbsAg	6%	7%	3%	1%	—	—	—	—
HCV	28%	35%	48%	60%	23% had hepatitis			
ALT > 5×	7.3/100pt/yr	5.7	—	—				
or AST > 5×	—	—	36/100-year	24/100-year	2.8/100	4.0/100	1.3	5.9
Median on	23	36	10	13	—	—	—	—
Median off	8	—	—	—	—	—	—	—
% w/jaundice	20%	—	10%	—	—	—	—	—

[a] Assumed to be similar in all four groups.

Table 5 Signs and Symptoms of Nucleoside Analog–Related Lactic Acidosis

Clinical
  Fever
  Weakness, malaise
  Nausea +/− vomiting
  Anorexia
  Abdominal pain
  Diarrhea
  Dyspnea
  Myalgias
  Jaundice
  Hyperventilation
  Tender hepatomegaly
  Bleeding diathesis
  Hepatic encephalopathy
  Cardiac arrhythmias (tachycardia)
  Neuropathy
Laboratory
  Metabolic acidosis
  Elevation of serum lactate
  Elevation of serum pyruvate
  Elevation of serum lactate/pyruvate ratio
  Increased anion gap
  Increased amylase/lipase

Histologically, drugs can mimic the entire spectrum of liver pathology. Hepatic steatosis due to NAs may present as macro- or microvesicular steatosis. The most advanced form of the syndrome includes lactic acidosis, pancreatitis, and even death (57). This syndrome, similar to Reye's syndrome, has been associated with mitochondrial toxicity.

VIII. MITOCHONDRIAL TOXICITY

A systemic mitochondrial syndrome has been noted with a number of NAs, including zidovudine (AZT), didanosine (ddI), stavudine (d4T), and fialuridine (FIAU) (13,57–60). This class of analogs of naturally occurring nucleosides inhibit the HIV-1 RNA-dependent DNA polymerase (reverse transcriptase) (61). Depending on the presence or absence of a 3'-hydroxyl group on the ribose moiety, NAs result in either an abnormal DNA molecule (with the internalized analog) or a truncated DNA chain, respectively (61). In other words, they either incorporate or terminate the nascent DNA molecule (61).

The mitochondrion is unique among organelles in that it contains its own DNA, termed mtDNA, whose replication is primarily regulated by DNA (-polymerase, which is sensitive to various cytotoxic agents like NAs) (62). This class of drugs can inhibit the synthesis of both mitochondrial and nuclear DNA; however, the inhibitory concentration is much higher for nuclear DNA than for mtDNA (61), and the mitochondrion does not have the capacity to repair DNA damage (63). This leads to a decrease in mitochondrial transport chain proteins and ATP depletion (63). Anaerobic glucose metabolism ensues, leading to accumulation of pyruvate and acetyl-CoA, and lactic acidosis in the absence of cardiac disease or hypoxemia (type B lactic acidosis). Clinically, respiratory compensation may be followed by respiratory failure (Table 5). In addition, mitochondrial dysfunction leads to decreased beta-oxidation of fatty acids, leading to macro- or microvesicular steatosis and hepatomegaly. Pancreatitis, myopathy, and neuropathy also occur, all presumably due to decreased mtDNA (58,64). Typically, liver enzymes are only modestly raised (58). Fialuridine-induced liver failure occurred in humans with chronic HBV infection enrolled in an investigational protocol (58). Experiments in woodchucks, with or without woodchuck hepatitis virus, proved that FIAU hepatotoxicity was independent from the underlying viral infection (64). Mitochondrial toxicity has also been linked to the development of lipodystrophy disorders, which include HIV-related fat remodeling syndrome (65).

The first report of zidovudine-associated liver injury appeared in 1987 (66). Thereafter, other reports have associated the use of several NAs with liver disease and lactic acidosis, all thought to be related to mitochondrial toxicity (57,59). Patients at higher risk for this syndrome are women, obese patients, or those with underlying liver disease (20,21,58). It should be noted that interference with mitochondrial DNA and decreased ATP levels do not necessarily result in tissue damage, as there is a threshold above which each organ may continue to function normally (67). This may explain why not all patients receiving nucleoside analogs develop DIH.

In vitro zalcitabine, stavudine, zidovudine, and didanosine all reduce mtDNA in descending order and induce lactic acid formation (68). Recently 106 cases of NA-associated lactic acidosis were evaluated (68). In 46 cases, patients received only one NA, thus reducing confounding factors (69). Approximately 50% of the patients who developed lactic acidosis died, and all patients showed evidence of neuropathy (69). In Baltimore, serum anion gap was evaluated in 509 patients receiving a combination of NAs. The frequency of an anion gap >16 was 8% for d4T/3TC, 5% for d4T/ddI, 3% for AZT/

3TC, and 2.5% for AZT/ddI combinations (70). While patients receiving d4T/3TC were more likely to develop an abnormal anion gap, no significant correlation with the occurrence of lactic acidosis was noted (70). Likewise, 20 patients taking D4T (plus other NAs, a PI, and/or a NNRTI) developed lactic acidosis (71). Sixteen (80%) did not have combined decreased bicarbonate and increased anion gap; however, 95% had elevated ALT and of seven biopsied patients, six had hepatic steatosis (71). Therefore, when mitochondrial toxicity is suspected, lactic acid levels, rather than the anion gap, should be measured. A decline in mitochondrial to nuclear DNA ratios, measured in peripheral white cells, may be an early indication of mitochondrial toxicity and lactic acidosis in patients taking NAs combinations (71a).

IX. MANAGEMENT OF NRTI-INDUCED MITOCHONDRIAL TOXICITY

There is no etiological treatment for NA-induced mitochondrial toxicity. Immediate cessation of the drug is warranted to prevent further metabolic imbalance (58,72). Supportive care such as intravenous volume replacement, administration of bicarbonate, electrolytes replacement, and occasionally hemodialysis (even in the absence of renal failure) has been advocated (72–75). While there are no controlled trials documenting the efficacy of any therapy in this setting, there are anecdotal reports suggesting that vitamins and coenzymes may be helpful.

Coenzyme Q is an electron transporter involved in cellular respiration, and used as a scavenger for the treatment of other mitochondrial-related disorders (76). Doses of 30–60 mg given three times daily can relieve fatigue, aches, and cramps. Carnitine, a specialized amino acid derived from lysine, is usually given concomitantly with Coenzyme Q, 1–3 gr daily. Despite the fact that carnitine deficiency has not been documented, symptomatic improvements have been reported (77,78). Riboflavin is a precursor of electron-transport cofactors, and has been used to treat severe lactic acidosis. In two reported cases, cessation of NRTI and the use of riboflavin 50 mg daily (10 mg tablets) resolved lactic acidosis (79,80). Thiamine has also been used, with mixed results (75,81). Electron scavengers such as vitamins K_3 (20–60 mg/day), C (1 g b.i.d.), and E (200 IU b.i.d.) have been used (76). Other treatment modalities, such as lipoic acid and N-acetylcysteine, may theoretically provide therapeutic benefits in patients receiving NAs (44,45).

X. SPECIFIC DRUGS

We have classified antiviral drugs according to their therapeutic indications. For each medication, we have reviewed the potential toxicity according to three sources; the *Physicians' Desk Reference* (20), *Drug Facts and Comparisons* (21), and a yearly European hepatotoxicity update (82). Thus, we describe reported elevations in liver enzymes and bilirubin, as a proxy for hepatotoxicity. All doses are average adult doses. Adjustments may be needed in special circumstances (20,21). In Table 6, elevations in AST, ALT, and AP are reported as percentage of treated patients with documented grade 3 toxicity (greater than 5× ULN) unless otherwise stated (20,21,82). In addition, we have reviewed the English literature using Ovid for Medline searches and identified single or multiple cases reports of DIH associated with antiviral drugs (Table 3). Obviously, there are problems in interpreting data from case reports (13). First, not all cases of liver toxicity are reported in the published literature. Second, case reports may fail to adequately rule out other causes of hepatitis, and it may be difficult to determine or refute a cause-effect relationship

Table 6 Estimated Percentages of Treated Patients with Abnormalities >5× ULN for Serum ALT or AST, >2× ULN for Alkaline Phosphatase (AP), and >2.5× ULN for Bilirubin, Unless Otherwise Noted (20,21,82)

Drug	ALT	AST	AP	Bilirubin
Antiherpetic agent				
Acyclovir	1–2%	1–2%	—	—
Famciclovir	3.2%[a]	2.3%[a]	—	1.9%[b]
Valacyclovir	—	1–4.1%	—	—
Penciclovir	—	—	—	—
Hydroxyurea	occ	occ	—	—
Cidofovir	occ	occ	occ	—
Ganciclovir	occ	occ	—	—
Foscarnet	occ	occ	—	—
Anti-influenza drug				
Rimantadine	—	—	—	—
Amantadine	occ	occ	occ	occ
Oseltamivir	—	—	—	—
Zanmivir	occ	occ	—	—
Interferon				
IFNa2b	2–15%	4–63%	—	3–13%
IFNa2a	—	3–46%	—	Up to 11%
Alferon	—	3%	8%	4%
Interferon beta	31.2	31.2	—	—
Rebetron	—	—	—	0.9–3%[c]
Antiretroviral				
Zidovudine	11%	12.5%	occ	Mild
Didanosine	6–12.5%	7–12.5%	occ	1–2%
Stavudine	9–13%	5–11	occ	1%
Zalcitabine	5%	4–8%	1.4[e]	1%
Lamivudine	4–12.5%	2–12.5%	occ	1%
Abacavir	.2%	—	—	—
Nelfinavir	3–7.4%[d]	2–7.4%[d]	—	—
Indinavir	5.9[e]	4.0	—	12.5[c]
Ritonavir	12.5%[f]	12.5%[f]	occ	—
Lopinavir				
Amprenavir	occ	occ	—	occ
Saquinavir	5.7[e]	4.1[e]	0.5[e]	1.6[c]
Nevirapine	3.4–8.5	2–8.5	—	0.4
Delavirdine	3.8–6.7	2.1–5.6	—	0.5–1.0
Efavirenz without hepatitis	3%	3%	—	—
Efavirenz with HBV or HCV	5–8%	4–7%	—	—

— = not available or not reported; [a]>2× ULN; [b]>1.5× ULN; [c]>2× ULN; occ = occasionally reported; [d]a shift from grade 0 toxicity at baseline to grade 3 or from grade 1 to 4. This is in combination with other antiretrovirals. Placebo had a greater change; [e]>4× ULN; [f]reference 20.

between drug and liver reaction, in the absence of a rechallenge test. Third, the use of multiple medications in HIV patients makes it even more difficult to pinpoint the offending drug. Fourth, 43% of reported cases (Table 3) had coexisting hepatitis B or C: these conditions can reactivate, presenting as acute liver enzyme elevations (83–85). Finally, after a drug is FDA-approved, it is difficult to assess the total volume of usage, and consequently the relative frequency of hepatic toxicity.

Instances of severe hepatic injury reported to the FDA are rare, ranging from 0.5 to 2/10,000 prescriptions. Abacavir, didanosine, indinavir, nevirapine, ritonavir and stavudine have the highest potential (1-2/10,000), other PIs and lamivudine have intermediate potential (less than 1/10,000) and delavirdine, zalcitabine and zidovudine have the lowest potential (less than 0.5/10,000). Observational cohort studies have generated data on the prevalence of transaminase elevation (greater than 5× ULN) during ART. These percentages did not rely on spontaneous reporting, and have ranged from 4.5% to 8.2% (85a).

A. Antiretroviral Drugs

1. Nucleoside and Nucleotide Analogs

Abacavir (Ziagen, Trizivir).   Abacavir is a guanosine analog indicated in the treatment of HIV infection (20). This drug is activated to the active carbovir triphosphate by intracellular phosphotransferases (86). Abacavir competes with dGTP and inhibits the HIV-1 reverse transcriptase (RT) showing synergistic activity with AZT and nevirapine (86). Similar to other NAs, abacavir is devoid of the 3-hydroxyl ribose moiety, and thus inhibits RT by terminating viral cDNA elongation (86), in a manner similar to that of AZT, ddI, ddC, d4T, and 3TC. Like other NAs, abacavir is specific for HIV-1, and is equipotent to AZT in terms of HIV-1 inhibition. Abacavir-resistant strains remain sensitive to AZT and d4T (86). In vitro, abacavir has activity against HBV (86), and showed no CYP inhibition (20). Protein binding is about 50% (20). The average dose is 300 mg b.i.d.

The main adverse event is the development of hypersensitivity reactions, which have included liver failure (20). The prevalence of liver enzyme elevation occurring in cases of hypersensitivity reaction is not clear from the package insert. In two studies, liver enzyme elevation occurred in less than 2%, and was similar in the Abacavir group as in the AZT/3TC group (20). However, elevations in GGT were more common in the Ziagen group (19%) compared to a control group (8%). No cases of mitochondrial toxicity have been reported in the literature, despite a boxed warning in the Abacavir package insert (86).

Adefovir Dipivoxil (Preveon).   Adefovir is a nucleotide analog with a structure similar to adenine (86). The drug inhibits both HIV and HBV, by inhibiting HBV polymerase (5,86), and it is given coupled with two pivalic molecules to increase intestinal absorption. The consequence is a 50% decrease in serum carnitine, so L-carnitine, 500 mg/day must be added to the regimen (86). Adefovir dosages vary from 10 mg/day for hepatitis B to 120 mg/day for HIV therapy (5). Currently, adefovir is in phase III trials in patients with chronic hepatitis B. Infrequently, dramatic changes in liver enzymes have been noted during adefovir treatment of hepatitis B, deemed to be secondary to an immune reaction against HBV rather than DIH (86).

Didanosine (Videx).   Dideoxyinosine (ddI) is a purine dideoxynucleoside with potent activity against HIV when used in combination with other antiretroviral agents (20). ddI requires intracellular phosphorylation to the triphosphate form, which competes with dATP for viral c-DNA incorporation (20). Metabolism by CYP and drug interactions are not known (20). Plasma protein binding is less than 5% (20). Didanosine dosing is based on body weight and renal function; the usual dose is 200 mg b.i.d. (20). A delayed-release form is given at 250–400 mg daily, depending on body weight.

Grade 3 transaminase elevation occurs in up to 12.5% of patients (20,82). Other adverse effects include rash or pruritus, in 8% of patients (20). Five case reports of hepatotoxicity, two with concomitant use of d4T, have been published (Table 5). The presentation is predominantly hepatocellular, with documented hepatic steatosis, and three fatalities were reported (87–90). A combination of didanosine and stavudine has been associated with three fatal cases of lactic acidosis in pregnant women (Bristol-Myers Squibb communication). Two of the infants also died. Thus, caution is needed when considering the use of this combination in pregnant women.

Lamivudine (Epivir, Combivir, Trizivir, Epivir-HBV). Lamivudine (3TC) is a dideoxy-nucleoside analog with antiviral activity against both HIV-1 and hepatitis B virus (4,5). Lamivudine triphosphate inhibits RT by terminating cDNA chain elongation (20). The drug is poorly bound to protein (<36%) and most of it is eliminated unchanged in the urine (20,21). The usual dosage is 150 mg b.i.d. for HIV, and 100 mg/day (Epivir-HBV) for chronic hepatitis B (20). Lamivudine 150 mg is bundled with zidovudine 300 mg in a single tablet and is marketed as Combivir (20). Trizivir includes AZT and abacavir. HIV mutants emerge rapidly after the start of therapy; therefore, 3TC should not be given as monotherapy for HIV infection. HBV mutants occur as well, but usually after 6 months of treatment, and develop more commonly in HIV/HBV-coinfected patients (91).

Liver enzyme abnormalities occur as frequently as with ddI, up to 12.5% (20,82). In patients with hepatitis B treated with 3TC, discontinuation of the drug has been associated with a flare in ALT, which is thought to be due to immunity against HBV and not drug toxicity. A handful of cases of 3TC hepatotoxicity have been reported (92–94), all with concomitant use of d4T (Table 3). One of these reports may actually have represented reactivation of a HBV mutant (93).

Stavudine (Zerit). Stavudine (d4T) is a thymidine nucleoside analog indicated in the therapy of HIV infection (20). The drug terminates HIV DNA elongation by competing with dTTP (20). Stavudine binds poorly to plasma proteins and its exact metabolism has not been elucidated (20). It appears that 40% of d4T clearance is accounted for by the kidneys (21). The usual dose is 40 mg b.i.d. but adjustments need to be made for patients less than 60 kg and those with impaired creatinine clearance (20).

Grade 3 ALT elevations have been reported in 9–13% of d4T-treated patients, not different from AZT (20,21). Bilirubin abnormalities are much less common, about 1% (20,21). Nine reports of d4T-related hepatotoxicity, including one death (78,92,94,95), have been published (Table 3). The hepatic injury is predominantly hepatocellular with occasional elevations in bilirubin levels. The median time to peak injury is 32 weeks. A mixed micro- and macrovesicular liver steatosis has been documented in two cases (95). Extra caution is needed in pregnant women (see didanosine).

Zalcitabine (Hivid). Zalcitabine (ddC) is a nucleoside analog competing with dCTP for the HIV-1 RT catalytic site. The drug also inhibits β- and γ-polymerases theoretically leading to mitochondrial disease (20,67). The compound has negligible binding to proteins, is not significantly metabolized by the liver, and is mainly eliminated in the urine (20). The usual dose is 0.75 mg t.i.d., to be adjusted according to renal function (20).

Liver test abnormalities were noted in up to 8% of patients, while rash or pruritus occurred in about 3% (20). Despite the fact that in vitro, ddC induced the greatest declines in mtDNA levels (67), no case reports of hepatotoxicity have been published.

Zidovudine (Retrovir, Combivir, Trizivir). Zidovudine (AZT or Retrovir) is a synthetic analog of thymidine (20). In vitro, this compound inhibits several retroviruses by terminating DNA chain elongation (20,21). It is indicated for the treatment of adult and pediatric HIV infection and has been found to be effective in decreasing vertical transmission of HIV from mother to baby (74). AZT is 36% bound to plasma proteins and is extensively metabolized by the liver; its glucuronide metabolites are excreted by the kidneys (20,21,74). Zidovudine 300 mg is bundled with lamivudine 150 mg in a single tablet and is marketed as Combivir. The usual dose is 300 mg p.o. b.i.d. (20). Zidovudine 300 mg, lamivudine 150 mg, and abacavir 300 mg are bundled in a single formulation, Trizivir.

AZT is the NA that has been most often associated with hepatotoxicity, but is also the most prescribed antiretroviral agent. As with other NAs, AZT has been associated with a syndrome of type B lactic acidosis, pancreatitis, and hepatic steatosis. Patients at higher risk for mitochondrial toxicity are women, obese patients, or those with underlying liver disease (20,21). In adults, a grade 3 or greater increase in AST or ALT occurs in up to 12.5% of treated patients (20,21). Fifty-nine percent of reported cases occurred in women (Table 3), who represent a minority of patients with HIV, 13% at the University of Southern California. In most instances, the injury is hepatocellular with a clear predominance of AST (94%) as opposed to ALT elevation (6%) (Table 3). This may be due, in part, to muscle mitochondrial dysfunction. An elevation of AP greater than transaminases was noted in less than 10% of reported cases. Jaundice was noted in three (17%) of 18 reported cases. Peak enzyme elevation occurred after a median of 36 weeks. Resolution occurred between 2 and 26 weeks. Most reported cases had a fatal outcome, mostly in association with lactic acidosis. The majority of histological reports noted macro- rather than microvesicular (73% vs. 7%) steatosis (Table 3). In one case a massively enlarged liver weighed 6.8 kg (150).

2. Nonnucleoside Reverse-Transcription Inhibitors (NNRTIs)

Nevirapine (Viramune). Nevirapine is a NNRTI that acts by binding to and disrupting the RT catalytic site (20). It is indicated in the treatment of HIV infection, in combination with other antiretroviral agents (20). Human DNA polymerases, including the mitochondrial DNA polymerase, are not affected (20). The drug is 60% bound to proteins and peak concentrations are achieved 4 h after oral administration (20). Nevirapine is metabolized by CYP 3A4 and is considered to induce CYP 3A activity (20). Cimetidine and macrolides, known CYP 3A inhibitors, result in higher nevirapine levels (20). The usual dose is 200 mg daily for 2 weeks to assess the possible occurrence of cutaneous side effects; then it is increased to 200 mg b.i.d. (96). Recently, a more cautious increase (starting at 100 mg/day) was found to be associated with fewer cutaneous rashes (97).

Grade 3 ALT elevations occur in up to 8.5% of patients (20). Patients must be monitored during therapy and if ALT or AST increase >5× ULN, the drug must be discontinued (20). Bilirubin elevations > 2.5 mg% were less frequent in the nevirapine group compared with a control group (20). However, three cases of hepatic failure associated with nevirapine therapy have been reported so far (98–101). One patient was successfully treated with corticosteroids (100). We have seen four cases of possible or probable nevirapine toxicity (102). All cases were accompanied by cutaneous rash and jaundice. Most reported cases (71%) had a predominant ALT elevation (Table 2). The peak serum bilirubin was 31.8 mg% (101). Two patients with underlying cirrhosis developed ascites and both improved after drug withdrawal (98,102). Four of nine reported cases had peripheral hypereosinophilia, implying an allergic-type reaction (98–103). Of patients developing a skin rash, a substantial number (30–75%) also develop hepatitis (104,105). Recently, two severe cases of hepatitis occurred in health care workers who took nevirapine as prophylaxis for HIV after occupational exposure (105). In a review by the Food and Drug Administration, it appears that 8/12 patients classified as "hepatotoxic reaction" developed clinical hepatitis (105). The median time to onset of the hepatic reaction was 3 weeks (105). On the other hand, a one-time dose administered at the onset of labor was efficacious in decreasing vertical transmission by 50%, and led to no instances of hepatic injury (105a).

Delavirdine (Rescriptor).   Delavirdine is a NNRTI with a mechanism of action and indication similar to nevirapine (20). Delavirdine is 98% protein-bound, and is metabolized primarily by CYP 3A and additionally by CYP 2D6 (20). The drug inhibits several CYP isozymes, chiefly CYP 3A (Table 1). The typical dose is 400 mg t.i.d. (20). An elevated ALT, AST, or bilirubin appears to be somewhat less common with delavirdine than with other drugs (Table 6). There are no reported cases of symptomatic hepatitis.

Efavirenz (Sustiva).   Efavirenz is a HIV-1-specific NNRTI (20). This drug is highly bound to proteins (>99%) and its half-life is long, allowing a once-daily dosage of 600 mg (20). The major enzymes involved in the metabolism of efavirenz are CYP 3A4 and CYP 2B6 (20). This compound has inhibitory effects on CYP 2C9, 2C19, and 3A4 isozymes (20). In patients without serological evidence of chronic hepatitis, AST and ALT elevations occur no more often in the efavirenz treated-group (3%), compared to the control group. Patients with hepatitis B or C are more likely to develop liver enzyme elevations with efavirenz (up to 8%), compared to control regimens (up to 5%) (20). One case of reversible hepatotoxicity has been reported (103).

3.   Protease Inhibitors (PIs)

Amprenavir, indinavir, lopinavir, nelfinavir, ritonavir, and saquinavir are compounds indicated for the treatment of HIV-1 infection in combination with other antiretrovirals (20). All these peptide-like drugs inhibit HIV-1 protease by binding to its active site, and render the enzyme incapable of processing the viral gag-pol polyprotein precursor into smaller, functional proteins (20). This leads to production of noninfectious HIV-1 particles.

Amprenavir (Agenerase).   In vitro, amprenavir exhibits synergistic HIV-1 activity in combination with abacavir, AZT, ddI, and saquinavir and additive anti-HIV-1 activity in combination with indinavir, nelfinavir, and ritonavir. Resistance due to HIV-1 protease mutations is less likely when the drug is used in combination with other antiviral agents (20). Protein binding is about 90% and the average dose is 1200 mg b.i.d. (20). Amprenavir is metabolized in the liver by CYP 3A4, which is also inhibited by the drug. Amprenavir is not known to affect other CYP enzymes. Patients with impaired liver function require dosage adjustments. Caution should be used when coadministering drugs that are substrates, inducers, or inhibitors of CYP 3A4. In two studies, no increased frequency of grade 3 or 4 AST, ALT, or bilirubin elevations was seen, compared to controls (20).

Indinavir (Crixivan).   Indinavir has synergistic activity with AZT and ddI in vitro (20). Cross-resistance exists between indinavir and ritonavir, and varying degrees of resistance between indinavir and other PIs. Indinavir is approximately 60% protein-bound (20). CYP

3A4 is the major enzyme responsible for its metabolism. The dosage is 800 mg t.i.d., with adequate hydration to prevent nephrolithiasis.

Indinavir causes asymptomatic unconjugated hyperbilirubinemia, which occurs more frequently above 2.4 g/day. Jaundice, cholecystitis, and cholestasis were reported in less than 2% of patients in clinical trials (20). In 1–8% of patients receiving indinavir alone, ALT and AST rose to >5× ULN, mostly in a reversible manner. Six published cases of severe hepatitis indicate that steatosis, including microvesicular steatosis, occurred with this drug, in two patients with associated peripheral eosinophilia (106–109). One fatal case has been reported (106).

Nelfinavir (Viracept). Nelfinavir is active against HIV-1 and several isolates of HIV-2 (20). In combination with NAs, nelfinavir demonstrates additive to synergistic antiviral activity in vitro, without enhanced cytotoxicity. Nelfinavir is 98% protein-bound, and its usual dose is 1250 mg (5 tablets) twice daily (20). Multiple CYP enzymes are involved in nelfinavir metabolism, CYP 3A being the most significant. To date, there are no specific reports of clinical hepatitis.

Ritonavir (Norvir). Ritonavir inhibits both HIV-1 and HIV-2 proteases (20). CYP 3A is the major isoform involved in ritonavir metabolism, although CYP 2D6 also contributes to its metabolism (20). Ritonavir should be used cautiously with drugs metabolized by CYP 3A, because ritonavir inhibits CYP 3A and CYP 2D6. Ritonavir can also induce CYP 3A, CYP 1A2, and possibly CYP 2C9 (20). Affinity for CYP enzymes occurs in the following order CYP 3A > CYP 2D6 > CYP 2C9. The usual dose is 600 mg twice daily.

Elevations in liver transaminases and GGT were reported in 2–15% of patients (20). Acute hepatitis occurred in 10 (7%) of 141 patients (56). In two large prospective databases, ritonavir appeared to have more potential for liver enzyme elevation, compared to other PIs (37,55). Ten of 12 (83%) reported cases of ritonavir toxicity occurred in patients with HCV infection (56,109,110). Two-thirds of cases were associated with a bilirubin > 3 mg% (Table 3).

Saquinavir (Fortovase, Invirase). Saquinavir is additive to synergistic with AZT, 3TC, ddC, ddI, d4T, and nevirapine (20). Saquinavir is approximately 97% protein-bound. The usual dose is 1200 mg t.i.d. In vitro studies show that approximately 90% of saquinavir is metabolized by CYP 3A4. Grade 3 (or greater) elevations in alkaline phosphatase, ALT, and bilirubin occur in up to 0.5%, 5.7%, and 1.6%, respectively (20). No clinical case reports of hepatotoxicity are published in the literature.

Lopinavir/Ritonavir (Kaletra). At steady state, lopinavir is approximately 98% protein-bound and is extensively and almost exclusively metabolized by CYP 3A. Ritonavir inhibits lopinavir metabolism, thereby increasing its plasma levels (Abbott Laboratories package insert). Lopinavir/ritonavir inhibits CYP 2D6 in vitro, but to a lesser extent than CYP 3A. The recommended dosage for this combination is 400 mg/100 mg b.i.d. The liquid formulation at a total daily dose of 10 mL contains approximately 3.4 g of alcohol. No reports of hepatotoxicity have been published to date.

B. Antiherpetic Drugs

1. Acyclovir (Zovirax)

Acyclovir is a NA requiring intracellular phosphorylation to the active triphosphate form (20,21). It has virustatic properties against several herpes viruses, including herpes viruses-

1 and -2 (HSV-1, HSV-2), varicella zoster (VZV), cytomegalovirus (CMV), and Epstein-Barr virus (EBV) (21,111). Plasma binding is less than 33% (21) and the major route of elimination is urinary (21). The usual dose is 200 mg 5 times a day (21). For severe cases of herpetic infection, e.g., esophagitis or colitis, the dose is IV, 5 mg/kg q8h. A higher dose of 10 mg/kg q8h is used for encephalitis (21). Acyclovir has no major effects on liver enzymes and clinical hepatotoxicity has not been reported (13,20,111).

2. Famciclovir (Famvir)

Famciclovir is a prodrug that is biotransformed in the liver into the active agent, penciclovir (112,113). Similar to other nucleoside analogs, penciclovir requires intracellular phosphorylation to penciclovir triphosphate, a competitive inhibitor of dGTP (21,112). The first phosphorylation step is carried out by a viral thymidine kinase, so that the enzyme-deficient mutants may be resistant to the drug. Famciclovir is active against several herpes viruses, including HSV-1, HSV-2, and VZV (21). It is indicated for the acute therapy of herpes zoster (shingles) and for recurrent genital herpes simplex (112,113). The drug has been used with some success in patients with chronic hepatitis B. The usual dose is 500 mg t.i.d. (20). Pruritus and abnormal liver tests have been reported (20,111), but no cases of hepatotoxicity have been described in the literature (111–113).

3. Penciclovir (Denavir)

Penciclovir has a structure similar to DHPG (ganciclovir) and antiviral activity parallel to acyclovir. The drug is used as a 1% cream for the treatment of herpes labialis (111). Penciclovir is less than 20% bound to plasma proteins and is mostly eliminated in the urine (20,113). Liver enzyme elevations have not been noted (20).

4. Valacyclovir (Valtrex)

Valacyclovir is a prodrug of acyclovir (21,111). Its indications are similar to those of Famvir (21). Valtrex has better activity against HSV than against VZV (21). Plasma protein binding is <20% and there is no CYP metabolism (21). The majority of the drug is excreted in the urine (21). The usual dose is 1 gr orally t.i.d. Elevations of liver enzymes have been reported in up to 4% of treated patients (21). Reversible hepatotoxicity has been reported (111,114,115).

5. Foscarnet (Foscavir)

Foscarnet is an inorganic pyrophosphate analog with activity against HSV, VZV, CMV, EBV, and influenza viruses (111). This virustatic agent does not require phosphorylation, and is active against thymidine kinase-deficient (resistant) strains of HSV and CMV (111). Unlike NAs, foscarnet acts as a noncompetitive inhibitor of several viral RNA and DNA polymerases as well as HIV-1 RT (21). Foscarnet is indicated in the treatment of CMV retinitis and resistant mucocutaneous herpes in immunosuppressed patients (111).

    The usual induction dose is 40 mg/kg IV q12h for HSV, and 90 mg/kg q12h for CMV, to be adjusted for renal function. Maintenance dose for CMV is 90–120 mg/kg daily (21). In clinical trials, abnormal liver tests were seen in 1–5% of patients receiving foscarnet (20). In some series, an elevated bilirubin occurred in 12% and ALT in 5% of treated patients (116). However, no case reports of hepatotoxicity have been published (13).

6. Ganciclovir (Cytovene)

Ganciclovir (DHPG) is an acyclic guanosine analog, structurally related to acyclovir (111). This virustatic agent is effective against several herpes viruses, especially CMV (111). Ganciclovir triphosphate is incorporated into the viral DNA chain as it possesses a 3'-OH group (111).

The medication may be given orally, intravenously, and intravitreally, its main indication being the treatment of CMV retinitis in immunocompromised hosts and the prevention of CMV disease (111). The usual dose is 5 mg/kg IV every 12 h as induction, and 5 mg/kg/day as maintenance (21). Oral ganciclovir is given at a dose of 1 gr p.o. t.i.d. with food (21). In clinical trials, hepatitis occurred in up to 1% of AIDS patients or transplant recipients. Liver enzyme abnormalities were reported in 2% (20,117). One report noted an ALT increase confirmed by rechallenge in one patient (118). In all reported cases, liver injury appeared mild and reversible (117,118). Two additional cases of severe hepatotoxicity with bilirubin up to 49 mg% have been reported with the use of a combination mycophenolate and oral ganciclovir in patients who received a combined renal and pancreatic transplant. The relative contribution of mycophenolate, ganciclovir, or an opportunistic infection was unclear (119).

7. Cidofovir (Vistide)

Cidofovir is an acyclic nucleotide phosphonate derivative with potent activity against HSV-1 and -2, VZV, EBV, and CMV (111). Since cidofovir does not require activation by viral thymidine kinase, it may have a role in the treatment of thymidine-kinase-deficient HSV (111). Cidofovir is indicated for CMV retinitis in patients with AIDS. It has unlabeled uses in CMV pneumonia or gastroenteritis, and congenital or neonatal CMV disease. Renal effects, bone marrow toxicity, and lactic acidosis are the main side effects (111). Increased alkaline phosphatase, ALT, and AST have been reported but there are no specific reports of clinical hepatitis (21).

C. Antiinfluenza Drugs

1. Oseltamivir (Tamiflu)

Oseltamivir is a selective neuraminidase inhibitor of influenza A and B (20,111). It prevents the detachment of virions from the host cells and thus prevents its spread (21). Oseltamivir must be hydrolyzed in the liver into its active form, oseltamivir carboxylate (21). The drug is active against both A and B influenza strains and is approved for the treatment of flu symptoms when taken within 48 h of their onset (21). The binding of the active compound to plasma proteins is 3% (21). The drug appears not to induce or inhibit CYP, and elimination is predominantly urinary (20,21). The usual dosage is 75 mg p.o. b.i.d. for 5 days (20). The oseltamivir package insert reveals no hepatotoxicity (20).

2. Zanamivir (Relenza)

Zanamivir has activity against influenza A and B and its mode of action is similar to oseltamivir (20). Zanamivir has <10% plasma protein binding (21) and is excreted unchanged in the urine (20). This drug is administered via inhalation and the dose is two disks (10 mg) inhaled q12h (20). Although liver enzyme elevations have been recorded, they were similar to controls (20).

3. Amantadine (Symadine, Amantadine, Symmetrel)

Amantadine is indicated in the treatment of influenza A (but not B) and is also used as an anti-Parkinsonism agent (21). The mode of action of this drug is not well understood (21). It appears to interfere with viral entry and with the release of infectious virions from the host cell (21).

   This drug does not alter immune response to the flu vaccine and may be given for 2–3 weeks to cover patients after vaccine administration (21). Amantadine is not metabolized and is excreted in the urine; thus adjustments are needed in patients with renal insufficiency (21). The usual dose is 100 mg b.i.d. (21). Elevated liver enzymes and bilirubin have both been reported but there are no specific reports of clinical hepatitis (13,20).

4. Rimantadine (Flumadine)

Rimantadine is a synthetic antiviral agent whose action is not well known (21). It may interfere with the uncoating of influenza A (but not B) virus (21). This drug is indicated for decreasing influenza symptoms when taken within 48 h after their onset (21). It has also been used to prevent clinical illness for the 4 weeks following flu vaccination (21).

   Plasma protein binding is about 40%. The drug is metabolized in the liver and eliminated in the kidneys (21). The recommended dose is 100 mg b.i.d. (21). There are no reported liver test abnormalities with the use of rimantadine (20). However, owing to decreased clearance the dosage must be adjusted in patients with liver disease (21).

D. Interferons

Interferons (IFNs) are glycoproteins divided into three major families: α-, β-, γ-interferons. IFNs were discovered when lymphocytes exposed to inactivated viruses produced an antiviral factor. This ability to "interfere" with viral replication became the basis for the name of these factors. IFNs produced by activated lymphocytes and macrophages are classified as IFN-α, while IFN-β is derived from fibroblasts and epithelial cells, and leukocytes produce IFN-γ (120–122). IFNs have a number of properties, including: stimulation of 2′5′-oligoadenylate synthetase, stimulation of α_2-microglobulin, increased expression of MHC-I and II molecules on the surface of effector cells, and antifibrotic and antiproliferative effects (20,111,120–122). These properties are utilized in the treatment of viral and neoplastic disease processes (111,121,122). Interferons are not directly virucidal but appear to promote resistance of the target cell to the infecting virus by inducing the intracellular production of substances that hinder viral replication and release (111).

   Among the most common indications for interferon therapy are chronic viral hepatitis B and C. In these groups, detection of hepatotoxicity is difficult because of the underlying liver disease (18). In a 1989 review of the side effects of α-interferon, hepatotoxicity was not described (120). However, interferon treatment of cancer patients, presumably without hepatitis, results in 25–80% of patients developing liver enzyme abnormalities, depending on the dose used. In the majority of cases AST or ALT elevations do not exceed $5\times$ ULN (121–124). Less frequently seen are increases in alkaline phosphatase or LDH (121). In mice, interferon preparations cause hepatic necrosis and steatosis; however, doses of mouse interferon were 1000 times higher (per unit of body weight) than those used in humans (125). Three cancer patients who developed liver test abnormalities developed

Table 7 Transaminase Elevations Associated with Interferon Therapy

1. Mild to moderate elevations, in patients with solid tumors (steatosis) (121–123)
2. Granulomatous hepatitis (126,127)
3. Severe elevations, in patients with hepatitis C, may be associated with viral clearance (due to immune stimulation) (137,138)
4. Severe elevations, in patients with undiagnosed autoimmune hepatitis with or without coexistent HCV infection (133–136)
5. Fulminant hepatitis, in patients with solid tumors (140)
6. Fulminant hepatitis, in patients with HBV- or HCV-associated cirrhosis (limited residual liver capacity) (139)

biopsy-proven steatosis (121). In addition, three cases of reversible granulomatous hepatitis associated with interferon therapy have been described (126,127). In very few cases, interferon, used as therapy for viral hepatitis, has been associated with liver failure (0.04%), invariably in patients with cirrhosis or advanced fibrosis (128–132). Patients with chronic autoimmune hepatitis (AIH), whether of type 1, 2, or 3, should not be treated with α-interferon as severe exacerbations of liver disease, presumably due to its immuno-modulatory effects, have been described (133–135). In fact, interferon has been associated with the unmasking of underlying AIH, in cases where autoimmune markers were negative before therapy, and became detectable after the start of interferon (136). In these cases, interferon should be stopped and immunosuppression should be considered (136). Interferons have also been associated with hepatic damage in patients clearing serum HCV RNA, probably as an immune reaction to HCV (137,138). Finally, interferon has been associated with hyperthyroidism in 0.4% of treated patients (128), and this complication is known to induce elevated liver enzymes, up to $10\times$ ULN (129). The different clinical situations where interferon therapy has been associated with hepatic damage are summarized in Table 7.

1. Interferon α-2a (Roferon)

Roferon is a 165 AA sequence of naturally occurring interferon alpha-2a produced by *Escherichia coli* bacteria (20). The major route of elimination of Roferon is renal (20). This drug is indicated in the treatment of chronic hepatitis C, HIV-related Kaposi's sarcoma, hairy cell leukemia, and as an adjunct to chemotherapy in Philadelphia-positive CML (20). Doses range from 3 MU SQ t.i.w. upward (20). A pegylated form (Pegasys) is forthcoming and will be given at a dose of 180 µg SQ weekly.

AST and alkaline phosphatase elevations were reported in non–hepatitis C studies, where severe elevations occurred in up to 46% and up to 11% of patients, respectively (20). Three cases of severe hepatitis (ALT > 500) with varying degrees of bilirubin abnormalities and coagulopathy have been described (136,137). All three were associated with HCV RNA becoming negative, and therefore may have represented immune clearance induced by interferon, rather than intrinsic hepatotoxicity (136,137). Similarly, one patient with both HBV and HCV infection was treated with 3 MU t.i.w. and as HCV RNA became negative, HBV DNA became detectable and was associated with an ALT flare (180 IU/L) (139). This case illustrates the fact that interferon may alter the equilibrium between two viruses and lead to immune-mediated liver damage (139).

2. Interferon Alfa-n3 (Alferon N)

Alferon contains a number of proteins, each approximately 166 AA, derived from human leukocytes (20). Human donors are screened for infectious process and the leukocyte products are processed to inactivate any model pathogenic viruses (20). This particular IFN is indicated in the treatment of condylomata acuminata and is administered intralesionally twice weekly at a maximum dose of 2.5 MU per session (20). The administration of Alferon to patients with cancer led to grade 3 and 4 AST, bilirubin, and alkaline phosphatase elevations in 3%, 4%, and 8% of patients, respectively (20). No cases of overt hepatitis have been reported.

3. Interferon Alfacon-1 (Infergen)

Infergen is a 166-AA consensus sequence of several naturally occurring interferon-α, produced by *E. coli* cells (20). Biologically, this product is similar to other interferons, except that its dosage units are micrograms (9–15 µg SQ t.i.w.) instead of international units (21). Infergen is indicated for the treatment of patients with chronic hepatitis C, either naive or prior nonresponders to interferon monotherapy (21). Because hepatitis C is characterized by wide fluctuations of ALT, it is difficult to determine the prevalence of interferon-induced hepatotoxicity in these patients. There are no specific reports of clinical hepatitis with Infergen, interferon-α2b (IntronA), peginterferon-α2b (PEG-Intron), or interferon-α2b plus ribavirin (Rebetron).

Intron A shares the same mode of activity of other interferons (111). It is indicated for the treatment of chronic hepatitis B at a dose of 5 MU SQ daily (21,111). PEG-Intron, dosed at 1.5 µg/kg weekly, is indicated in the treatment of patients with hepatitis C, and a contraindication to ribavirin. Either interferon with ribavirin has the best chance to eradicate HCV (7–9). Intron A is also approved for the treatment of melanoma, hairy cell leukemia, follicular lymphoma, Kaposi's sarcoma, and papillomavirus infections (21). In patients treated for hepatitis B, IntronA resulted in elevated ALT (greater than 2× ULN) in 60% of responders and in 30% of nonresponders (21). It is believed that these ALT elevations reflect an immune response to HBV antigens, rather than DIH per se. In patients treated for other indications, AST elevations occur in up to 63% (Table 4). Rebetron is twice as likely as monotherapy to induce pruritus, noted in as many as 21% of patients (21). A bilirubin >3× ULN was noted in 0.9–3% of HCV patients compared to 0.4% of patients on monotherapy (21). The latter fact most likely reflects ribavirin-induced hemolysis (21).

4. Ribavirin (Virazole, Rebetol)

Ribavirin is a purine nucleoside analog (111). Its mode of action is uncertain, but it is thought to inhibit IMP dehydrogenase, thereby depleting the intracellular pool of dGTP and subsequently dATP (21,141). It is also postulated that the drug acts as a guanosine analog (21,111), thereby inhibiting viral RNA polymerase or reverse transcriptase. Ribavirin is active, in vitro, against a number of viruses (111). Ribavirin is only licensed for the treatment of severe respiratory syncytial virus (Virazole), given as an aerosol at a dose of 20 mg/mL (20), and as an adjunct to interferon (Rebetol in Rebetron) for the treatment of hepatitis C (111). However, the drug may have clinical utility in Lassa fever and Hantavirus infections (111). The metabolism of ribavirin is not well understood (21). In Rebetron, the drug is given at a dose of 800–1200 mg for the treatment of hepatitis C. No adverse hepatic events were reported in the treatment of RSV (21,142).

E. Other Antivirals

1. Hydroxyurea (Hydrea, Droxia)

Hydroxyurea is an antimetabolite that has antiretroviral effects, in combination with NAs (143–145). The drug has been used for over 35 years to treat chronic myelocytic leukemia (CML) and polycythemia vera, and is also useful in adult sickle-cell anemia (20,145). Hydroxyurea depletes the intracellular pool of deoxyribonucleotides and inhibits DNA repair (143,145). The drug is believed to be metabolized primarily by the liver, although renal elimination also occurs (145). Indications include adjuvant therapy for HIV infection, melanoma, resistant and recurrent CML, and advanced ovarian carcinoma (20). The dosage in HIV patients is 500 mg b.i.d. (146). In rats with hepatic steatosis and in dogs, hepatic iron accumulation occurs (20). In humans, elevated liver enzymes have been reported, but no more frequently than with placebo (20,146). Three cases of presumed hydroxyurea-induced hepatitis have been reported (144,147). The injury is mainly hepatocellular but a bilirubin as high as 20 mg% has been recorded (144). A fatal outcome in a patient with HIV and HBV coinfection was reported (146).

XI. CONCLUSIONS

The majority of hepatotoxicity cases associated with antiviral medications have been noted with the use of antiretroviral agents. The drugs most commonly implicated appear to be ritonavir, followed by AZT, D4T, and other NAs. NNRTIs such as nevirapine and efavirenz are emerging as probable causes of hepatitis, which can occasionally be severe. Patients at higher risk are women, those with concomitant hepatitis B or C, and those with CD4 counts < 200 cells/mm^3. Based on this experience, all newer antiretrovirals will need to undergo postmarketing surveillance for hepatotoxicity. All clinicians should be familiar with the incidence, severity, and management of drug-induced hepatotoxicity, especially mitochondrial toxicity, which carries a particularly severe prognosis. In addition, liver enzyme levels in patients with underlying viral hepatitis need to be closely monitored while HAART is being administered.

REFERENCES

1. Palella F, Delaney K, Moorman A, et al. Declining morbidity and mortality among patient with advanced human immunodeficiency virus infection. N Engl J Med 1998; 448:854–860.
2. Temesgen Z, Wright AJ. Antiretrovirals. Mayo Clin Proc 1999; 74:1284–1401.
3. Mauskopf JA, Tolson JM, Simpson KN, et al. Impact of zidovudine-based triple combination therapy on an AIDS drug assistance program. J AIDS 2000; 23:302–313.
4. Dienstag JL, Schiff ER, Wright TL, et al. Lamivudine as initial treatment for chronic hepatitis B in the US. N Engl J Med 1999; 341(17):1256–1263.
5. Gilson RJC, Chopra K, Newell AM, et al. A placebo-controlled phase I/II study of adefovir dipivoxil in patients with chronic hepatitis B virus infection. J Vir Hep 1999; 6(5):387–395.
6. Alter MJ, Kruszon-Moran D, Nainan OV, et al. Prevalence of hepatitis C virus infection in the United States, 1988 through 1994. N Engl J Med 1999; 341:556–562.
7. Liang TJ. Combination therapy for hepatitis C infection. N Engl J Med 1998; 339:1549.
8. Manns M, McHutchison JG, Gordon S, et al. Peginterferon alfa-2B plus ribavirin compared to interferon alfa-2B plus ribavirin for the treatment of chronic hepatitis C: 24-week treatment analysis of a multicenter multinational phase III randomized controlled trial. Hepatology 2000; 32:297A.

9. Trepo C, Lindsay K, Niederau C, et al. Pegylated interferon ALFA-2B (PEG-Intron) mono-
    therapy is superior to Interferon ALFA-2b (INTRON A) for the treatment of chronic hepatitis.
    J Hepatol 2000; 32(suppl 2):29.

10. Hayden FG. Update on influenza and rhinovirus infections. Adv Exp Med Biol 1999; 458:
    55–76.

11. Wood AJJ. Thrombotic thrombocytopenic purpura and clopidogrel-a need for new ap-
    proaches to drug safety. N Engl J Med 2000; 342:1824–1826.

12. Larrey D. Drug-induced liver diseases. J Hepatol 2000; 32(suppl 1):77–82.

13. Styrt B, Freiman JP. Hepatoxicity of antiviral drugs. Gastrointest Clin North Am 1995; 24:
    839–852.

14. Levy M. Role of viral infections in the induction of adverse drug reactions. Drug Safety
    1997; 16:1–8.

15. Ungo JR, Jones D, Ashkin D, et al. Antituberculosis drug-induced hepatotoxicity: the role
    of hepatitis C virus and the human immunodeficiency virus. Am J Respir Crit Care Med
    1998; 157:1871–1876.

16. Saliba B, Herbert PN. Oxacillin hepatotoxicity in HIV-infected patients [letter]. Ann Intern
    Med 1994; 120:1048.

17. DeLeve L, Kaplowitz N. Mechanisims of drug-induced liver disease. Gastroenterol Clin
    North Am 1995; 24(4):787–810.

18. Zimmermann HJ. The spectrum of hepatotoxicity. In: HJ Zimmermann, ed. Hepatotoxicity.
    2nd ed. Philadelphia: Lippincott, Williams & Wilkins, 1999.

19. Tanaka E. Update: genetic polymorphism of drug metabolizing enzymes in humans. J Clin
    Pharm Ther 1999; 24:424–429.

20. Physicians' Desk Reference. 54th ed. Montclair, NJ: Medical Economics, 2000.

21. Drug Facts and Comparisons. 54th ed. St Louis, MO: Facts and Comparisons, 1999.

22. Barry M, Mulachy F, Merry C, Gibbions S, Back D. Pharmacokinetics and potential interac-
    tions amongst antiretroviral agents used to treat patients with HIV infections. Clin Phamaco-
    kinet 1999; 36(4):289–304.

23. Bartlett JG, Gallant JE. 2000–2001 Medical Management of HIV Infection. Baltimore: Johns
    Hopkins University, 2000:81–89.

24. Kaplowitz N. Mechanisms of liver cell injury. J Hepatol 2000; 32:39–47.

25. Holazo AA, Winkler MB, Patel IH. Effects of age, gender, and oral contraceptives on intra-
    muscular midazolam pharmacokinetics. J Clin Pharm 1988; 28:1040–1045.

26. Mayersohn M. Considerations in the elderly. In: WE Evans, JJ Schentag, W Juska, eds.
    Applied Pharmakotherapeutics. 3rd ed. Vancouver, WA: 1992.

27. Hunt C, Westerkam W, Stave G. Effects of age and gender on the activity of human hepatic
    CYP3A. Biochem Pharmacol 1992; 44(2):275–283.

28. Fletcher CV, Acosta EP, Strykoski JM. Gender differences in human pharmacokinetics and
    pharmacodynamics. J Adolesc Health 1994; 15:619–629.

29. Tanaka E. Gender-related differences in pharmacokinetics and their clinical significance. J
    Clin Pharm Ther 1999; 24:339–346.

30. Kashuba AD, Bertino JS, Rocci ML, et al. Quantification of 3-month intraindividual variabil-
    ity and the influence of sex and menstrual cycle phase on CYP3A activity as measured by
    phenotyping with intravenous midazolam. Clin Pharmacol Ther 1998; 64:269–277.

31. Miners JO, Robson RA, Birkett DJ. Gender and oral contraceptive steroids as determinants
    of drug glucuronidation: effects of clofibric acid elimination. Br J Clin Pharmacol 1984; 18:
    240–243.

32. Villani P, Regazzi MB, Castelli F. Pharmacokinetics of efavirenz (EFV) alone and in combi-
    nation therapy with nelfinavir (NFV) in HIV-I infected patients. Br J Clin Pharmacol 1999;
    48:712–715.

33. Schenker S, Martin RR, Hoyumpa AM. Antecedent liver disease and drug toxicity. J Hepatol
    1999; 41:1098–1105.

34. Bonacini M, Puoti M. Hepatitis C in patients with human immunodeficiency virus infection: diagnosis, natural history, meta-analysis of sexual and vertical transmission, and therapeutic issues. Arch Intern Med 2000; 160:3365–3373.

35. Ockenga J, Tillmann HL, Trautwein C, et al. Hepatitis B and C in HIV-infected patients. J Hepatol 1997; 27:18–24.

36. Saves M, Vandentorren S, Daucourt V, et al. Severe hepatic cytolysis: incidence and risk factors in patients treated by antiretroviral combinations Aquitaine cohort, France, 1996–1998. AIDS 1999; 13:F115–F121.

37. Sulkowski M, Thomas DL, Chaisson RE, Moore RD. Hepatotoxicity associated with antiretroviral therapy in adults infected with human immunodeficiency virus and the role of hepatitis C or B virus infection. JAMA 2000; 284:74–80.

38. Ookhtens M, Kaplowitz N. Role of the liver in interorgan homeostasis of glutathione and cyst(e)ine. Semin Liver Dis 1998; 18:414–429.

39. Barbaro G, DiLorenzo G, Asti A, et al. Hepatocellular mitochondrial alterations in patients with chronic hepatitis C: ultrastructural and biochemical findings. Am J Gastroenterol 1999; 94:2198–2205.

40. Loguercio C, Clot P, Albano E, et al. Free radicals and not acetaldehyde influence the circulating levels of glutathione after acute or chronic alcohol abuse in vivo and in vitro studies. Ital J Gastroenterol Hepatol 1997; 29:168–173.

41. Barbaro G, Di Lorenzo G, Soldini M, et al. Hepatic glutathione in chronic hepatitis C: quantitative evaluation in patients who are HIV positive and HIV negative and correlations with plasma and lymphocytic concentrations and with the activity of liver disease. Am J Gastroenterol 1996; 91:2569–2574.

42. Larrey, D, Pageaux P. Genetic predisposition to drug-induced hepatotoxicity. J Hepatol 1997; 26(suppl 2);12–21.

43. Herzenberg LA, De Rosa SC, Dubs JG, et al. Glutathione deficiency is associated with impaired survival in HIV disease. Proc Natl Acad Sci USA 1997; 94:1967–1972.

44. Walmsley SL, Winn LM, Harrison ML, Uetrecht JP, Wells PG. Oxidative stress and thiol-disulfide depletion in plasma and peripheral blood lymphocytes from HIV infected patients: toxicological and pharmacological implications. AIDS 1997; 11:1689–1697.

45. De Rosa SC, Zaretsky MD, Dubs JG, et al. N-Acetylcysteine replenished glutathione in HIV infection. Eur J Clin Invest 2000; 30:915–929.

46. Choi J, Liu RM, Kundu RK, et al. Molecular mechanism of decreased glutathione content in human immunodeficiency virus type 1 Tat-transgenic mice. J Biol Chem 2000; 275:4694–4698.

47. Fromenty B, Pessayre D. Impaired mitochondrial function in microvesicular steatosis: effects of drugs, ethanol, hormones, and cytokines. J Hepatol 1997; 26:43–53.

47a. Nunez M, Lana R, Mendoza JL, Martin-Carbonero L, Soriano V. Risk factors for severe hepatic injury after introduction of highly active antiretroviral therapy. J AIDS 2001; 27: 426–431.

48. Fernadez-Checa JC, Kaplowitz N, Garcia-Ruiz C, et al. GSH transport in mitochondria: defense against TNF-induced oxidative stress and alcohol-induced defect. Am J Physiol 1997; 274:G7–G17.

49. Smith SR, Boyd EL, Kirking DM. Nonprescription and alternative medication use by individuals with HIV disease. Ann Pharmacother 1999; 44:294–400.

50. Strader D, Bacon B, Hoofnagle J, LaBrecque D, Morgan T, Lindsay K. Use of CAM by patients in liver disease clinics [abstract]. Natcher Conference Center, Bethesda, MD, August 1999.

51. Ostrow MJ, Cornelisse PGA, Heath KV, et al. Determinants of complementary therapy use in HIV-infected individuals receiving antiretroviral or anti-opportunistic agents. J AIDS 1997; 15:115–120.

52. Fairfield KM, Eisenberg DM, Davis RB, Libman H, Phillips RS. Patterns of use, expendi-

tures, and perceived efficacy of complementary and alternative therapies in HIV-infected patients. Arch Intern Med 1998; 158:2257–2264.

53. McKnight I, Scott M. Managing HIV: HIV and complementary medicine. Med J Aust 1996; 165:144–145.

54. Piscitelli SC, Burstein AH, Chaitt D, Alfaro RM, Falloon J. Indinavir concentrations and St. John's wort. Lancet 2000; 355:547–548.

55. Bonfanti P, Valsecchi L, Parazzini F, et al. Incidence of adverse reactions in HIV patients treated with protease inhibitors: a cohort study. J AIDS 2000; 23(3):236–245.

56. Arribas JR, Ibanez C, Ruiz-Antoran B, et al. Acute hepatitis in HIV-infected patients during ritonavir treatment. AIDS 1998; 12:1722–1724.

57. Carr A, Miller J, Law M, Cooper DA. A syndrome of lipoatrophy, lactic acidaemia and liver dysfunction associated with HIV nucleoside analogue therapy: contribution to protease inhibitor-related lipodystrophy syndrome. AIDS 2000; 14(3):F25–32.

58. McKenzie, Fried MW, Sallie R, et al. Hepatic failure and lactic acidosis due to fialuridine (FIAU) an investigational nucleoside analogue for chronic hepatitis B. N Engl J Med 1995; 444:1099–1105.

59. Arnaudo E, Dalakas M, Shanke S, et al. Depletion of muscle mitochondria DNA in AIDS patients with zidovudine-induced myopathy. Lancet 1991; 447:508–510.

60. Styrt BA, Piazza-Hepp TD, Chikami GK. Clinical toxicity of antiretroviral nucleoside analogs. Antiviral Res 1996; 41:121–145.

61. Lewis W, Dalakas MC. Mitochondrial toxicity of antiviral drugs. Nature Med 1995; 1:417–422.

62. Rusanen H, Majamaa K, Hassinen IE. Increased activities of antioxidant enzymes and decreased ATP concentration in cultured fibroblasts with the 3243AB to G mutation in mitochondrial DNA. Biochim Biophys Acta 2000; 1500:10–16.

63. De La Asuncion JG, del Olmo ML, Sastre J, et al. AZT treatment induces molecular and ultrastructural oxidative damage to muscle mitochondria. Prevention by antioxidant vitamins. J Clin Invest 1998; 102:4–9.

64. Tennant BC, Baldwin BH, Graham LA, et al. Antiviral activity and toxicity of fialuridine in the woodchuck model of hepatitis B infection. Hepatology 1998; 28:179–191.

65. Brinkman K, Smeitink JA, Romijin JA, Reiss P. Mitochondrial toxicity induced by nucleoside–analogue reverse–transcriptase inhibitors is a key factor in the pathogenesis of antiretroviral-therapy-related lipodystrophy. Lancet 1999; 354:1112–1115.

66. Melamed A, Muller RJ, Gold, J, et al. Possible Zidovudine-induced Hepatotoxicity. JAMA 1987; 258:2063.

67. Wallace DC. Diseases of mitochondrial DNA. Annu Rev Biochem 1992; 61:1175–1212.

67a. Collins AR, Duthie SJ, Fillion L, et al. Oxidative DNA damage in human cells: the influence of antioxidants and DNA repair. Biochem Soc Trans 1997; 25:426–441.

68. Chen CH, Vazquez-Padua M, Cheng YC. Effect of anti-human immunodeficiency virus nucleoside analogs on mitochondrial DNA and its implication for delayed toxicity. Mol Pharmacol 1991; 39(5):625–628.

69. Boxwell DE, Styrt BA. Lactic acidosis (LA) in patients receiving nucleoside reverse transcriptase inhibitors (NRTIs). 39th ICAAC, San Francisco, September 26–29, 1999. Abstract 1284.

70. Moore R, Keruly J, Chaisson R. Difference in anion gap with different RTI combinations. 7th Conference on Retroviruses and Opportunistic Infections, San Francisco, January 2000. Abstract 55.

71. Lonergan JT, Havlir D, Behling C, Pfander H, Hassanein T, Mathews WC. Hyperlactatemia in 20 patients receiving NRTI combination regimens. 7th Conference on Retroviruses and Opportunistic Infections, San Francisco, January 2000. Abstract 56.

71a. Cote HG, Brumme ZL, Craib KJ, et al. NEJM 2002; 346:811–820.

72. Saint-Marc T, Touraine JL. The effects of discontinuing stavudine therapy on clinical and

metabolic abnormalities in patients suffering from lipodystrophy. AIDS 1999; 13(15):2188–2189.

73. Chodock R, Mylonakis E, Shemin D, Runarsdottir V, Yodice P, Renzi R, Tashima K, Towe C, Rich JD. Survival of a human immunodeficiency patient with nucleoside-induced lactic acidosis—role of haemodialysis treatment. Nephrol Dial Transplant 1999; 14(10):2484–2486.

74. Scalfaro P, Chesaux JJ, Buchwalder PA, Biollaz J, Micheli JL. Severe transient neonatal lactic acidosis during prophylactic zidovudine treatment. Intens Care Med 1998; 24:247–250.

75. Roy PM, Gouello JP, Pennison-Besnier I, Chennebault JM. Severe lactic acidosis induced by nucleoside analogues in an HIV-infected man. Ann Emerg Med 1999; 34(2):282–284.

76. Peterson PL. The treatment of mitochondrial myopathies and encephalomyopathies. Biochim Biophys Acta 1995; 1271:275–280.

77. Claessens YE, Cariou A, Chiche JD, Dauriat G, Dhainaut JF. L-Carnitine as a treatment of life-threatening lactic acidosis induced by nucleoside analogues. AIDS 2000; 14(4):472–473.

78. Lenzo NP, Garas BA, French MA. Hepatic steatosis and lactic acidosis associated with stavudine treatment in a HIV patient: a case report. AIDS 1997; 11(10):1294–1296.

79. Fouty B, Frerman F, Reves R. Riboflavin to treat nucleoside analogue-induced lactic acidosis. Lancet 1998; 352(9124):291–292.

80. Luzzati R, Del Bravo P, Di Perri G, Luzzani A, Concia E. Riboflavine and severe lactic acidosis. Lancet 1999; 353(9156):901–902.

81. Schramm C, Wanitschke R, Galle PR. Thiamine for the treatment of nucleoside analogue-induced severe lactic acidosis. Eur J Anaesthesiol 1999; 16(10):733–735.

82. Biour M, Poupon R, Grange JD, Chazouilleres O, Jaillon P. Hepatotoxicite des medicaments. Gastroenterol Clin Biol 2000; 24:1310–1351.

83. Rodriguez-Rosado R, Garcia-Samaniego J, Soriano V. Hepatotoxicity after introduction of highly active antiretroviral therapy. AIDS 1998; 122:1256.

84. Vento S, Garofano T, Renzini C, Casali F, Ferraro T, Concia E. Enhancement of hepatitis C virus replication and liver damage in HIV-coinfected patients on antiretroviral combination therapy. AIDS 1998; 12:116–117.

85. Rutschmann OT, Negro F, Hirschel A, Hadengue A, Anwar D, Perrin LH. Impact of treatment with human immunodeficiency virus protease inhibitors on hepatitis C viremia in patients coinfected HIV. J Infect Dis 1998; 177:783–785.

85a. Monforte A, Bugarini R, Pezzotti P, et al. Low frequency of severe hepatotoxicity and association with HCV coinfection in HIV-positive patients treated with HAART. AIDS 2001; 28:114–123.

86. Crowe S. New reverse transcriptase inhibitors. Adv Exp Med Biol 1999; 458:183–197.

87. Bissuel F, Habersetzer F, Chassard D, et al. Fulminant hepatitis with severe lactate acidosis in HIV-infected patients on didanosine therapy. J Intern Med 1994; 235:367–372.

88. Lai KK, Gang DL, Zawacki JK, Cooley TP. Fulminant hepatic failure associated with 2′, 3′-dideoxyinosine (ddI). Ann Intern Med 1991; 115:283–284.

89. Brivet FG, Nion I, Megarbane B, et al. Fatal lactic acidosis and liver steatosis associated with didanosine and stavudine treatment: a respiratory chain dysfunction. J Hepatol 2000; 32:364–365.

90. Allaouchiche B, Duflo F, Cotte I, et al. Acute pancreatitis with severe lactic acidosis in an HIV-infected patient on didanosine therapy. J Antimicrob Chemother 1999; 44:137–138.

91. Benhamou Y, Bochet M, Thibault V, et al. Long-term incidence of hepatitis B virus resistance to lamivudine in human immunodeficiency virus-infected patients. Hepatology 1999; 30:1302–1306.

92. Mokrzycki M, Harris C, May H, et al. Lactic acidosis associated with stavudine administration: a report of five cases. Clin Infect Dis 2000; 30:198–200.

93. Schiano TD, Lissoos TW, Ahmed A, et al. Lamivudine-induced liver failure in hepatitis B cirrhosis. Am J Gastroenterol 1997; 92:1563–1564.

94. Johri S, Alkhuja S, Siviglia G, Soni A. Steatosis-lactic acidosis syndrome associated with stavudine and lamivudine therapy. AIDS 2000; 14(9):1286–1287.

95. Miller K, Cameron M, Wood L, et al. Lactic acidosis and hepatic steatosis associated with use of stavudine: report of four cases. Ann Intern Med 2000; 133:192–196.

96. Ho TT, Wong KH, Chan KC, Lee SS. High incidence of lipodystrophy on a protease inhibitor-sparing highly antiretroviral therapy regimen. AIDS 2000; 14(4):468–469.

97. Anton P, Soriano V, Jimenez-Nacher I, et al. Incidence of rash and discontinuation of nevirapine using two different escalating initial doses. AIDS 1999; 13:524–525.

98. Cattelan AM, Erne E, Salatino A, et al. Severe hepatic failure related to nevirapine treatment. Clin Infect Dis 1999; 29(2):455–456.

99. Langlet P, Guillaume MP, Devriendt J, et al. Fatal liver failure associated with nevirapine in a pregnant HIV patient: the first reported case [abstract]. Gastroenterology 2000; 118: A6623.

100. Leitze Z, Nadeem A, Choudhary A, Saul Z, Roberts I, Manthous CA. Nevirapine-induced hepatitis treated with corticosteroids? AIDS 1998; 12:1115–1117.

101. Clarke S, Harrington P, Condon C, Kelleher D, Smith OP, Mulcahy F. Late onset hepatitis and prolonged deterioration in hepatic function associated with nevirapine therapy. Intern J STD AIDS 2000; 11:336–337.

102. Prakash M, Poreddy V, Tiyyagura L, Bonacini M. Jaundice and hepatocellular damage associated with nevirapine therapy. Am J Gastroenterol 2001; 46:1571–1574.

103. Piroth L, Grappin M, Sgro C, Buisson M. Recurrent NNRTI-induced hepatotoxicity in an HIV-HCV-coinfected patient. 2000; 34:534–535.

104. Ho TTY, Wong KH, Chan KCW, Lee SS. High incidence of nevirapine-associated rash in HIV-infected Chinese. AIDS 1998; 12(15):2082–2083.

105. Serious adverse events attributed to nevirapine regimens for postexposure prophylaxis after HIV exposures—worldwide, 1997–2000. MMWR 2001; 49(51):1153–1156.

105a. Guay LA, Musoke P, Fleming T, et al. Intrapartum and neonatal single-dose nevirapine compared with zidovudine for prevention of mother-to-child transmission of HIV-1 in Kampala, Uganda: HIVNET 012 randomised trial. Lancet 1999; 354:795–803.

106. Brau N, Leaf HL, Wieczorek RL, Margolis DM. Severe hepatitis in three AIDS patients treated with indinavir. Lancet 1997; 449:924–925.

107. Matsuda J, Gonani K, Yamanaka M. Severe hepatitis in patients with AIDS and hemophilia B treated with indinavir [letter]. Lancet 1997; 450:464.

108. Vergis E, Paterson L and Singh N. Indinavir-associated hepatitis in patients with advanced HIV infection. Int J STD AIDS 1998; 9:54.

109. Benveniste O, Longuet P, Duval X, et al. Two episodes of acute renal failure, rhabdomyolysis and severe hepatitis in an AIDS patient successively treated with ritonavir and indinavir. Clin Infect Dis 1999; 28:1180–1181.

110. Picard O, Rosmordue O, Cabane J. Hepatotoxicity associated with ritonavir. Ann Intern Med 1998; 129:670–671.

111. Keating MR. Antiviral agents for non-human immunodeficiency virus infections. Mayo Clin Proc 1999; 74:1266–1283.

112. Wedemeyer H, Boker KHW, Pethig K, et al. Famciclovir treatment of chronic hepatitis B in heart transplant recipients: a prospective trial. Transplantation 1999; 68:1503–1511.

113. Sacks SL, Wilson B. Famciclovir/penciclovir. Adv Exp Med Biol 1999; 458:135–147.

114. Ball AR. Valaciclovir update. Adv Exp Med Biol 1999; 458:149–157.

115. Renkes P, Trechot Ph, Blain H. Valaciclovir-induced hepatitis. Acta Clin Belg 1999; 54:17–18.

116. Aschan J, Ringden O, Ljungman P, Lonnqvist B, Ohlman S. Foscarnet for treatment of cytomegalovirus. Scand J Infect Dis 1992; 24:143–150.

117. Figge HL, Bailie GR, Briceland LL, Kowalsky SF. Possible ganciclovir-induced hepatotoxicity in patients with AIDS. Clin Pharm 1992; 11:432–434.

118. Shea BF, Hoffman S, Sesin GP, Hammer SM. Ganciclovir hepatotoxicity. Pharmacotherapy 1987; 7:223–226.

119. Kuypers D, Lau SG, Chapmen JR, Allen RDM. Hepatotoxicity in combined renal and pancreas allograft recipients treated with ganciclovir [abstract]. Immunol Cell Biol 1998; 76: A10.

120. Renault PF, Hoofnagle JH. Side effects of alpha interferon. Semin Liver Dis 1989; 9:273–277.

121. Quesada JR, Talpaz M, Rios A, Kurzrock R, Gutterman JU. Clinical toxicity of interferon in cancer patients: a review. J Clin Oncol 1986; 4:234–243.

122. Atzpodien J, Lopez Hanninen E, Kirchner H, et al. Multiinstitutional home-therapy trial of recombinant human interleukin-2 and interferon alfa-2 in progressive metastatic renal cell carcinoma. J Clin Oncol 1995; 13:497–501.

123. Gasparini G, Dal Fior S, Pozza F, et al. Phase I study of escalating dose mitoxantrone in combination with a-2-interferon in patients with advanced solid tumor. Invest New Drug 1991; 9:245–252.

124. Schomburg A, Kirchner H, Lopez-Hanninen E, et al. Hepatic and serologic toxicity of systemic interleukin-2 and/or interferon-α. Am J Clin Oncol 1994; 17:199–209.

125. Gresser et al. Electrophoretically pure mouse interferon inhibits growth, induces liver and kidney lesions, and kills suckling mice. Am J Pathol 1981; 102:396–402.

126. Propst A, Propst T, Dietze O, Kathrein H, Judmeier G, Vogel W. Development of granulomatous hepatitis during treatment with interferon alfa-2b. Dig Dis Sci 1995; 40:2117–2118.

127. Veerabagu M, Finkelstein S, Rabinovitz M. Granulomatous hepatitis in a patient with chronic hepatitis C treated with interferon. Dig Dis Sci 1997; 42:(7)1445–1448.

128. Fattovich G, Giustina G, Favarato S, et al. A survey of adverse events in 11,241 patients with chronic viral hepatitis treated with alfa interferon. J Hepatol 1996; 24:38–47.

129. Berris B, Feinman SV. Thyroid dysfunction and liver injury following alpha-interferon treatment of chronic viral hepatitis. Dig Dis Sci 1991; 36:1657–1660.

130. Marcellin P, Colin J-F, Boyer N, et al. Fatal exacerbation of chronic hepatitis B induced by recombinant alpha-interferon. Lancet 1991; 338:828.

131. Hoofnagle JH, Di Bisceglie AM, Waggoner JG, Park Y. Interferon alfa for patients with clinically apparent cirrhosis due to chronic hepatitis B. Gastroenterology 1993; 104:1116–1121.

132. Laskus T, Radkowski M, Slusarczyk J, Cianciara J. Severe exacerbation of chronic active hepatitis B during interferon alpha therapy. Digestion 1992; 52:61–64.

133. Ruiz-Moreno M, Rua MJ, Carreno V, et al. Autoimmune chronic hepatitis type 2 manifested during interferon therapy in children. J Hepatol 1991; 12:265–266.

134. Papo T, Marcellin P, Bernuau J, Durand F, Poynard T, Benhamou J-P. Autoimmune chronic hepatitis exacerbated by alpha-interferon. Ann Intern Med 1992; 116:1.

135. Gschwantler M, Schrutka-Kolbl C, Weiss W. Acute exacerbation of antiliver cytosol antibody-positive autoimmune chronic hepatitis by α-interferon. Am J Gastroenterol 1995; 90:12.

136. Vento S, DiPerri G, Garofano T, et al. Hazards of interferon therapy for HBV-seronegative chronic hepatitis. Lancet 1989; 2:926.

137. Cervoni J-P, Degos F, Marcellin P, et al. Acute hepatitis induced by α-interferon, associated with viral clearance, in chronic hepatitis C. J Hepatol 1997; 27:1113–1116.

138. Shimizu Y, Shuji J, Akiharu W, et al. Hepatic Injury after interferon therapy for chronic hepatitis C [letter]. Ann Intern Med 1994; 121:723.

139. Villa E, Grottola A, Trande P, et al. Reactivation of hepatitis B virus infection induced by interferon (IFN) in HBsAg-positive, antiHCV-positive patients. Lancet 1993; 341:1413.

140. Durand JM, Kaplanski G, Portal I, Scheiner C, Berland Y, Soubeyrand J. Liver failure due to recombinant alpha interferon. Lancet 1991; 338:1268–1269.
141. Zoulim F, Trepo C. Nucleoside analogs in the treatment of chronic viral hepatitis: efficiency and complications. J Hepatol 1994; 21:142–144.
142. Mills J. Prevention and treatment of respiratory syncitial virus infections. Adv Exp Med Biol 1999; 458:39–53.
143. Lori F, Malykh A, Cara A, et al. Hydroxyurea as an inhibitor of human immunodeficiency virus-type 1 replication. Science 1994; 266:801–805.
144. Weissman SB, Sinclair GI, Green CL, Fissell WH. Hydroxyurea-induced hepatitis in human immunodeficiency virus-positive patients. J Infect Dis 1999; 29:223–224.
145. Gwilt PR, Tracewell WG. Pharmacokinetics and pharmacodynamics of hydroxyurea. Clin Pharmacokin 1998; 34:347–358.
146. Rutschmann OT, Opravil M, Iten A, et al. A placebo-controlled trial of didanosine plus stavudine, with and without hydroxyurea for HIV infection. AIDS 1998; 12:F71–77.
147. Heddle R, Calvert AF. Hydroxyurea induced hepatitis. Med J Aust 1980; 1:121.
148. Chen SCA, Barker SM, Mitchell DH, et al. Concurrent zidovudine-induced myopathy and hepatoxicity in patients treated for human immunodeficiency virus (HIV) infection. Pathology 1992; 24:109–111.
149. Acosta B, Grimsley EW. Zidovudine-associated type B lactic acidosis and hepatic steatosis in an HIV-infected patient. South Med J 1999; 92:421–423.
150. Freiman J, Helfert K, Hamrell M, et al. Hepatomegaly with severe steatosis in HIV-seropositive patients. AIDS 1993; 7:379–385.
151. Gradon JD, Chapnick EK, Sepkowitz DV. Zidovudine-induced hepatitis. J Intern Med 1992; 231:317–318.
152. Olano J, Borucki M, Wen J, et al. Massive hepatic steatosis and lactic acidosis in a patient with AIDS who was receiving zidovudine. Clin Infect Dis 1995; 21:973–976.
153. Krishnamurthy S, Miguel S, Petra B, et al. Zidovudine-induced fatal lactic acidosis and hepatic failure in patients with acquired immunodeficiency. Crit Care Med 1997; 25:1425–1430.
154. Jolliet P, Widmann J-J. Reyes syndrome in an adult with AIDS. Lancet 1990; 335:1457.
155. Fortgang H, Belitsos PC, Chaisson RE, et al. Hepatomegaly and Steatosis in HIV-infected patients receiving nucleoside analog antiretroviral therapy. Am J Gastroenterol 1995; 90: 1433–1436.
156. Chariot P, Drogou I, de-Lacroix-Szmania I, et al. Zidovudine-induced mitochondrial disorder with massive liver steatosis, myopathy, lactic acidosis and mitochondrial DNA depletion. J Hepatol 1999; 30:156–160.
157. Dubin G, Braffman MN. Zidovudine induced hepatotoxicity. Ann Intern Med 1989; 110: 85–86.

23

Hepatotoxicity of Cardiovascular and Antidiabetic Drugs

FELIX A. DE LA IGLESIA

University of Michigan Medical School, Ann Arbor, Michigan, U.S.A.

JEFFREY R. HASKINS

Cellomics, Inc., Pittsburgh, Pennsylvania, U.S.A.

GEORGE FEUER

University of Toronto, Toronto, Canada

I. INTRODUCTION

Cardiovascular disease and diabetes are among the leading causes of mortality and morbidity in the civilized world. Therapeutic approaches to these diseases in general require a significant number of drugs and concomitant administration of a large group of medications that in many instances leads to significant drug interactions and target organ toxicity (1). One of the challenges facing physicians today is the assimilation of new developments in health care to follow treatment guidelines and awareness of potential side effects of an increasing number of new medications. Drugs designed for cardiovascular diseases or diabetes have effects on the liver in addition to those in other organs. For example, hypolipidemic agents can induce systemic adverse reactions in addition to hepatic changes. Nicotinic acid in a sustained-release formulation caused severe or fatal liver injury among other symptoms (2). Elevated phospholipid levels were reported in the serum and liver, and generalized phospholipidosis developed in patients receiving a coronary vasodilator agent (diethylaminoethoxyhexestrol) or an antiarrhythmic agent (3,4). Amiodarone exerts thyroid and corneal injury apart from or in addition to the phospholipidosis seen in the liver and other organs (2). Diabetics taking captopril developed abnormal liver function, cholelithiasis, and lymphocyte infiltration. In general, adverse drug reactions to cardiovascular or antidiabetic drugs may affect numerous organs, and this chapter will focus on drug effects causing impairment of hepatic function.

Impaired hepatic function can emerge as a result of many drugs taken either singly or in combination (5). Thus, it is often difficult to establish a causal relationship between the applied drug and the development of liver injury. However, the relationship can be established with certainty when the same liver reaction is observed after a repeat administration of the drug (6,7). When the response pattern is characteristic, such as phospholipidosis or nonalcoholic steatohepatitis in response to a vasodilator (3) or antiarrhythmic (8,9), the hepatotoxicity can be clearly established. Unwanted or unanticipated effects may complicate the treatment of patients and restrict the use of a drug essential to the management of the disease, be it an antihypertensive, an antiarrhythmic, a hypolipidemic, or an antidiabetic drug. If the drug producing the hepatotoxicity is absolutely essential to control a life-threatening situation, then the potential for hepatic toxicity may be acceptable until a proper pharmacological balance is achieved.

Liver impairment due to pharmacological agents is in most cases not due to a single entity. The observed lesions depend not only on the drug involved but also on the duration of exposure and preexisting hepatic pathology. Determining preexisting liver disease as a contributory cause of hepatotoxicity represents a major challenge to hepatologists. Following acute exposure, hepatocellular steatosis, cholestasis, hepatitis, necrosis, or other dysfunction can occur in graded steps. The result of chronic insidious exposure may be cirrhosis or neoplastic changes irrespective of the drug administered chronically. The morphological, biochemical, and clinical signs of the liver injury brought about by cardiovascular or antidiabetic drug ranges from mild to severe with acute to chronic pathological response including steatosis (10,11), cholestasis (12–14), hepatitis (15–19), granulomatous hepatitis (20–23), cholelithiasis and fibrosis (24), and cirrhosis (11,25). Drugs also can cause one or more of these changes simultaneously. Drug-induced hepatic alterations have been reported in 5–35% of patients receiving cardiovascular or antidiabetic medications. There is a significant number of heart disease patients in North America and 42.6% of men and 28.5% of women were hospitalized for cardiovascular causes during 1996 or 1997. The number of diabetic patients in the United States and Canada for the same period was 3.5% of males and 2.9% of females, notwithstanding that 50% of diabetics are not diagnosed and morbidity in the adult population is increasing at alarming rates (26,27). These figures strongly emphasize the importance of recognizing drug-induced adverse reactions as early as possible in these disease groups. The information below will integrate clinical, biochemical, and pathological aspects and mechanism of actions associated with the hepatotoxicity of cardiovascular and antidiabetic drugs.

II. CARDIOVASCULAR DRUGS

The definition of cardiovascular drugs in a broad sense includes antiarrhythmics, coronary vasodilators, antihypertensive agents (angiotensin-converting enzyme inhibitors, alpha-adrenergic agonists, beta-adrenergic blocking agents, calcium channel blockers), and lipid-regulating agents (hypolipidemic and cholesterol-lowering drugs).

Cardiovascular drugs are biologically potent agents from a wide range of chemical structures and occasional effects can be linked to the intended pharmacology. Antiarrhythmic drugs reaching high plasma concentrations enhance the risk of sinoatrial and atrioventricular block, and toxic concentrations may induce tachycardia (28–30). Systemic side effects reported after administration of either antiarrhythmic drugs or angiotensin-converting enzyme inhibitors include angioedema, bradycardia, hypotension, agranulocytosis and bone marrow suppression, renal failure, and pulmonary toxicity characterized by pneumonitis. Hepatic toxicity may precede or follow the appearance of some of these clinical reactions.

A. Antiarrhythmics

1. Amiodarone

Amiodarone is an effective antiarrhythmic drug limited to the treatment of refractory ventricular tachyarrhythmias and the limitation is due to the potential for serious hepatotoxicity (31–36). Amiodarone is also useful for the restoration and maintenance of normal sinus rhythm and prevention of thromboembolic complications from stroke (37). Major noncardiac side effects include corneal microdeposits, photosensitivity, blue-gray skin discoloration, hepatotoxicity, gastrointestinal problems, thyroid abnormalities, and peripheral neuropathy (37–42).

The most serious, life-threatening nonhepatic adverse reaction is pulmonary toxicity, interstitial pneumonitis, and fibrosis (43,44). Hepatic changes due to amiodarone have been described histologically (40,45–53). There are features of alcoholic hepatitis, fatty change, fibrosis, and cirrhosis, mostly related to the length of treatment and extent of dosage (8,54–57). Patients taking amiodarone may show evidence of phospholipidosis, and liver cells contain characteristic concentric, lamellar inclusions with high osmiophilic density, and greatly expanded lysosomes by electron microscopy (8,46,58,59). The phospholipid-laden lysosomal lamellar bodies are characteristic of amiodarone hepatotoxicity and represent the distinguishing features from alcoholic liver disease (60). The concentric, lamellar inclusions in secondary lysosomes resemble the primary phospholipidosis inclusions from inborn errors of lipid metabolism, such as Tay-Sachs, Niemann-Pick, and Fabry's disease (8,61–63). Similar hepatic inclusion bodies develop with other amphiphilic drugs (3,33,56,61,64). This condition was originally described due to the effects of a coronary vasodilator in Japan (64,65). Phospholipid fatty liver was definitively attributed to amiodarone (8,46,58,63). Amiodarone causes changes resembling alcoholic liver injury, including macro- and microvesicular steatosis, cell enlargement, Mallory bodies, and fibrosis (56). These pseudoalcoholic hepatitis changes were found in asymptomatic, anicteric patients who took amiodarone for more than 1 year and had mild transaminase (less than 1.5–2 times the upper limit of normal), alkaline phosphatase, and serum bilirubin elevations.

Amiodarone effects include elevations of alanine (ALT) and aspartate (AST) aminotransferases and gamma-glutamyl transpeptidase. Patients with immediate life-threatening ventricular tachycardia or ventricular fibrillation are likely to have these enzyme elevations. Elevated AST can be difficult to interpret, because this enzyme may be increased in myocardial infarction, defibrillation, or congestive heart failure. Amiodarone hepatic effects are related to the highly variable systemic availability of oral doses, which influence the biotransformation of the drug. The major active metabolite of amiodarone in humans is N-desethylamiodarone (Fig. 1). The enzyme responsible for N-desethylation is cytochrome

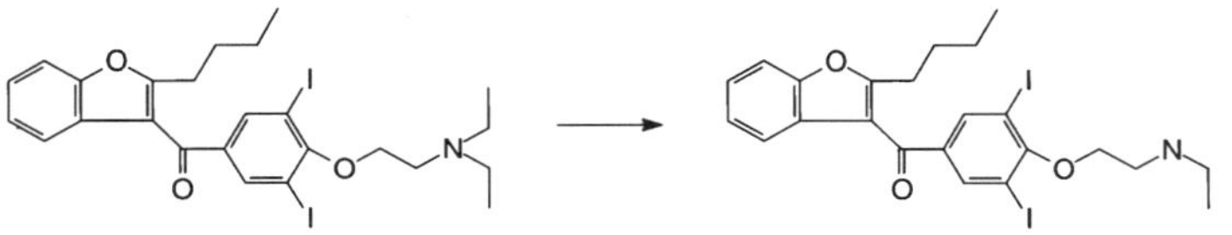

Figure 1   *N*-Desethyl metabolism of amiodarone.

P450 3A4 present in liver and gut. Individual sensitivity to amiodarone and hepatic effects can be related to different expression levels of CYP 3A4 activity.

The mechanism of toxicity relates to the inability of lysosomes to eliminate the drug or its metabolites, resulting in the accumulation of phospholipid-containing membranes in the hepatocyte cytoplasm (39,66,67). There is also mitochondrial dysfunction (4,68,69). Symptomatic hepatitis results from amiodarone treatment (19), and the drug modulates polymorphic variants of drug metabolism by interaction with cytochrome P450 enzymes, hence the possibility of interactions with other drugs that share the same metabolism (70,71).

Amiodarone alcoholic-like hepatitis incidence is approximately 1% similar to the occurrence in long-term studies (51,72–75). The amiodarone liver injury with alcoholic hepatitis symptoms is unpredictable, cytotoxic, and represents an unusually increased susceptibility rather than chemical toxicity. Although there is a close resemblance to alcohol-induced liver disease, amiodarone-induced hepatic lesions have different zonal disposition in the liver lobule (76). Acute foamy cytoplasmic change with massive accumulation of microvesicular cytoplasmic lipid is common in amiodarone hepatitis and reflects the composition of lipid accumulated (3,77). Amiodarone-induced lysosomal inclusions accumulate gradually in the hepatocyte cytoplasm as shown by human liver cell cultures (78), and the phospholipid fatty liver is reversible in experimental animals (48,79). In humans, lysosomal phospholipids may persist for several months after the drug administration has been discontinued.

Severe hepatitis and fatal outcomes from amiodarone injury have been reported (31,32,45,49,80). Fatal hepatocellular necrosis has been reported with amiodarone at high doses (19,81,82). Long-term amiodarone treatment may evoke mild hepatic lesions or more severe liver dysfunction unrelated to the degree of increases in transaminases, alkaline phosphatase, or bilirubin (83,84). Amiodarone causes asymptomatic elevations of serum transaminases between 1.5- and fourfold above the upper limit of normal in about 4–25% of the patients (51,85). Up to a 100-fold increase in serum transaminase has been reported (84,86), and cardiac patients receiving amiodarone have abnormal transaminases (51). The transaminase levels returned to normal after the dose was reduced or the treatment stopped. Fibrosis or cirrhosis (8), acute confluent, necrotizing hepatitis (19), and infrequent fatal hepatic injury suggests a wide range of hepatotoxic presentations (8,46,51,58,80,87,88). Acute intravenous amiodarone can cause hepatic necrosis or acute hepatitis (50,89). Death can follow amiodarone-induced hepatic failure (47–49,81).

Hepatic tissue levels of amiodarone and desethylamiodarone can be detected several months after treatment has been stopped; the presence of the drug or its metabolite may account for the persistent hepatic injury due to strong lipid-binding affinity (90,91). Phospholipid fatty liver may develop as early as 2 months of treatment (46,92). The phospholipid accumulation in lysosomes may inhibit phospholipase A_1 or other enzymes (93–96).

A Reye's syndrome–like illness after amiodarone intake was reported (49,97), and increased transaminases and ammonia levels were followed by coma and death. Although the symptoms may resemble Reye's syndrome, the histological appearance of the liver did not show the characteristic microvesicular fatty change. Other reports suggested that amiodarone can induce Reye's syndrome in children, similarly to aspirin, including the characteristic hepatic injury (97–99). Experimental effects of amiodarone on mitochondria are discussed in another chapter.

2. Aprindine

Aprindine is effective for the control of arrhythmias in patients with ischemic heart disease (100–102) and has caused a low incidence of side effects, with liver reactions that included lobular hepatitis and cholestasis (16,103,104). Cases of acute hepatitis caused by aprindine have been reported (16,105,106), and symptoms and pathology were mild, with onset about 3 weeks after drug therapy was started and subsiding rapidly after drug withdrawal. Rechallenge caused mild hepatitis with subsequent recovery, without evidence of hypersensitivity (16,105). Asymptomatic elevations in serum transaminases and alkaline phosphatase levels with slightly increased bilirubin were observed about 3 weeks after initiation of aprindine therapy. The mechanism of aprindine toxicity is not known, and cholestasis may accompany the hepatitic reaction (102).

3. Quinidine

Quinidine is an essential drug for the treatment of cardiac arrhythmias. Clinical symptoms of quinidine-induced hepatotoxicity include weakness, nausea or vomiting, anorexia, myalgia, and abdominal pains. Frequently observed clinical signs within 6–12 days of treatment were fever and hepatomegaly, occasionally splenomegaly, and rarely jaundice (107–110). No deaths have been reported following quinidine hepatotoxic reactions, and normal hepatic function returned after discontinuation of the drug in all cases.

Rechallenge at small doses of the drug leads to prompt recurrence of fever and hepatic dysfunction. By light microscopy, liver changes included distinct centrilobular or spotty hepatocellular necrosis and degeneration, periportal subacute inflammatory reaction, and sinusoid dilatation (108,109). Electron microscopy revealed viable cells neighboring necrotic hepatocytes with many lysosomes and fat droplets in the centrilobular zone. Mitochondria had size and shape variations and endoplasmic reticulum membranes were increased and dilated. Kupffer cells in necrotic areas were hyperplastic with marked proliferation of microvilli and cytoplasmic clumps of darkly stained lysosome-like material (109). Approximately 1 month from the beginning of quinidine therapy, transaminases and alkaline phosphatase activities increased and then fell rapidly to baseline levels. Biochemical function tests were altered, but returned to normal approximately 4 days after rechallenge (107,109,110). These data suggest a hypersensitivity mechanism for quinidine hepatotoxicity. In all cases there was a relatively uniform sensitization period followed by fever and hepatic dysfunction with eosinophilic infiltration of the liver parenchyma. The centrilobular lesions may represent hepatocellular damage by reactive metabolites upon interaction with a specific cytochrome P450 (111,112).

Reversible granulomatous hepatitis can be observed in quinidine-induced hepatotoxicity (20–23). Clinical toxicity included weakness, dizziness, diaphoresis, fever, urticaria, and increased serum enzymes. The formation of granulomata in the liver was detected as early as 3 days after readministration of quinidine. Light microscopy of liver biopsies showed hepatitis with noncaseating granulomata scattered throughout the parenchyma with few or no necrotic changes. By means of electron microscopy, granulomata contained histiocytes, lymphocytes, and engulfed hepatocytes with alteration of cytoplasmic organelles and dilated smooth endoplasmic reticulum. Immunofluorescence showed slightly positive polyvalent antihuman γ-globulin and monovalent antihuman IgG in the granulomata (23).

Disopyramide has antiarrhythmic effects similar to those of quinidine. The toxicity is probably associated with a mechanism similar to that described for quinidine (113). Disopyramide hepatotoxicity can be complicated with disseminated intravascular coagulopathy (114).

4. Procainamide

Procainamide is an aminobenzamide for the management of cardiac arrhythmias, and about half of a single dose undergoes biotransformation into N-acetylprocainamide (115). N-Acetylprocainamide may have fewer side effects than the parent drug (116). Excessive dosage leads to blockade of cardiac electrical conduction leading to ventricular arrhythmias. Side effects include central nervous system disorders, agranulocytosis, gastrointestinal distress and systemic lupus erythematosus–like syndrome (117–119). Procainamide-induced liver abnormalities have been reported, but do not appear to be frequent and include intrahepatic cholestasis, granulomatous hepatitis, and increased transaminases and bilirubin levels (120–126).

Hepatitis is uncommon as a result of procainamide insult. Clinical symptoms include fever, chills, and granulomatous hepatitis upon liver biopsy. The liver changes may develop rapidly, since they were observed within 1 week after initiation of procainamide regimen (125). The aggregate of clinical symptoms and liver biopsy findings strongly suggested a hypersensitivity mechanism. Symptoms subsided within 24 h after the drug was withdrawn and repeat liver biopsy 12 months later showed normal liver. Rechallenge caused reappearance of fever together with mild transaminases and bilirubin increases that receded quickly. Allergic reaction to procainamide was suspected on account of positive results from in vitro mast cell degranulation tests. Other immune cell function tests were negative in response to procainamide, including lymphocyte stimulation, and macrophage migration tests. A parenchymal granulomatous reaction similar to that seen with quinidine has been observed.

Procainamide-induced intrahepatic cholestasis is associated with serum alkaline phosphatase, γ-glutamyltranspeptidase, transaminases, and bilirubin elevations. A hypersensitivity reaction with acute hepatic dysfunction was reported with procainamide after a large single intravenous dose was administered during cardiac electrophysiology studies (126). Clinical features were rash, fever, arthralgia, and myalgia, followed by increased serum creatine phosphokinase, indicating episodic rhabdomyolysis. Acute hepatocellular injury was evidenced by increased serum bilirubin and transaminases. Hepatic enzymes continued to rise after procainamide administration was discontinued and peaked at 11 days slowly receding over several weeks, with no improvement in γ-glutamyltranspeptidase (120,121).

Phenotypic characteristics influence the acetylation of procainamide and other drugs, like hydralazine. Poor acetylators develop lupus erythematosus reactions and are at risk of hepatic damage since prolonged exposures may lead to reactive metabolism and DNA damage (127). Dose titration and genotyping determination of acetylator polymorphisms constitute viable pharmacogenetic measures to reduce the risk of hepatotoxicity (128–130).

B. Antihypertensives

1. Hydralazine and Dihydralazine

Hydralazine is widely prescribed for controlling hypertension. It is well tolerated, but patients may develop headache, flushing, palpitations, and electrocardiographic abnormalities (18). Fatal hepatotoxicity attributed to hydralazine has been reported (131). One major side effect of this drug is the occurrence of a systemic lupus erythematosus–like syndrome, related to the polymorphic recessive trait for acetylation (132–135). Reports of hydralazine-related liver injury include hepatitis, intrahepatic cholestasis, centrilobular necrosis, and granuloma formation in the parenchyma (17,18,87,136–141). Dihydralazine administration causes hepatitis (135,136,142). Hypersensitivity reactions occurred when hydralazine was taken for the treatment of hypertension concomitant with epilepsy drugs such as primidone, phenytoin, and phenobarbital. Most clinical manifestations of hydralazine liver reactions returned to normal shortly after drug discontinuation (134).

Hepatitis can occur after 2–6 months of hydralazine treatment (17,134) and in some reports the onset was from 6 to 9 months and up to 1 year (138,142,143). Highly elevated transaminases and slightly increased alkaline phosphatase activities are observed together with increased bilirubin. Microscopy revealed submassive to massive necrosis, hemorrhage, reticulum collapse, inflammatory cell infiltration, ductular cell proliferation, and infrequent cytoplasmic fat droplets. Cholestasis was seen in periportal areas (18). These microscopic findings were consistent with drug-induced toxic hepatitis. In one case the liver showed severe inflammation with bridging necrosis, also termed subacute necrosis (17). Complete remission was established approximately 6 months after discontinuation of hydralazine therapy.

The major pathway of hydralazine biotransformation in humans is hepatic acetylation, and the enzyme *N*-acetyltransferase controls the rate of acetylation (Fig. 2) (144). The expression of this enzyme has genotypic control and the recessive polymorphisms result in a poor acetylator phenotype (145,146). Nonspecific arylamidase is reduced in drug-induced or alcoholic liver injury and contributes to poor metabolism exacerbating the lack of acetylation (139). The liver showed various degrees of centrilobular necrosis together with low arylamidase activity (18). A relationship may exist between the endo-

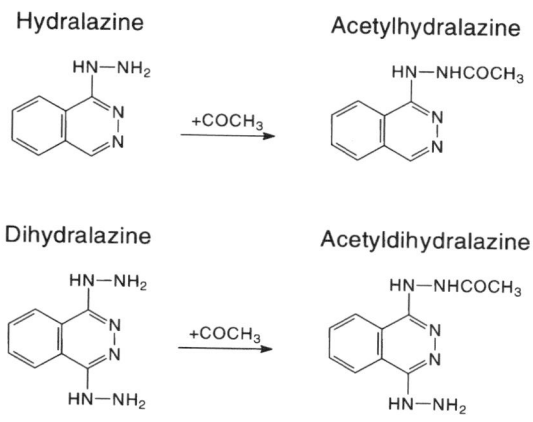

Figure 2   Acetylation pathway of hydralazine and dihydralazine.

plasmic reticulum function changes, reduced acetylation, and hepatic cell necrosis with hydralazine-induced liver injury related to smooth endoplasmic reticulum dysfunction (147).

Dihydralazine is a hydralazine analog and caused hepatitis in a small number of cases (136,142,143). Hepatitis following dihydralazine administration reversed quickly after drug administration was interrupted and worsened upon rechallenge. The dihydralazine liver reaction appears to be similar to hydralazine hepatitis (18,139–141). The onset of dihydralazine hepatitis may vary from a few weeks to several months after drug therapy is initiated. Significant increases of serum transaminase activities were observed, and encephalopathy and prolonged prothrombin time may accompany the clinical presentation. Most studies reported either centrilobular or severe bridging necrosis as the main lesion, leading occasionally to fibrosis. Dihydralazine induced several cytochrome P450 isoenzymes, and antiliver microsome autoantibodies reacting specifically against some cytochrome P450 species were found in patients with dihydralazine-induced hepatitis (148,149).

2. Labetalol

Labetalol hydrochloride is an α/β-adrenergic-receptor-blocking drug that lowers blood pressure in hypertensive patients. Labetalol reduces blood pressure by partially blocking the α-adrenoceptors in peripheral arterioles causing vasodilatation at the expense of reduced peripheral resistance. At the same time, the β-adrenoceptor blockade in the myocardium prevents reflex tachycardia that otherwise would have increased cardiac output. Following oral labetalol to resting or exercising hypertensive patients, plasma renin activity and aldosterone concentrations decreased, particularly when these parameters were elevated before treatment. Undesirable effects due to the receptor pharmacology include bronchial constriction, postural hypertension, disturbance of peripheral circulation, heart failure, and hepatotoxicity.

Mild hepatocellular and cholestatic injury has been reported with labetalol and severe hepatocellular injury has been rarely found (150). Liver abnormalities, however, occurred after short-term or long-term treatment and were progressive. In severe cases, hepatic related effects were pruritus, dark urine, and jaundice. The hepatic injury is usually completely reversible but hepatic necrosis, cholangitis, and death due to liver failure have been reported (151,152).

3. α-Methyldopa

α-Methyldopa was introduced in 1960 and has been one of the most frequently prescribed drugs for the treatment of moderate or severe hypertension (115,153,154). The molecular mechanisms of the liver effects have not been clearly established. Considering the extent of α-methyldopa use, the drug is generally safe, although clinical symptoms and biochemical changes have been reported (154a,154b). These included sedation, vertigo, lactation from prolactin release, extrapyramidal signs, and depression. Various digestive tract symptoms and postural hypotension have also occurred. Edema may result from salt and water retention. Allergic reactions included fever, autoimmune hemolytic anemia, granulocytopenia, and thrombocytopenia. Positive tests for systemic lupus erythematosus, rheumatoid factors, and Coombs' antiglobulin may be found (155–157).

Knowledge of α-methyldopa-induced liver toxicity is mainly from case reports and epidemiological investigations (6,158–163). Hepatic symptoms develop within 6–10 weeks or up to 4–6 months after initiation of α-methyldopa therapy. Signs of hepatic injury can become manifest after 2–11 years of exposure (11,159,164–166). This difference in onset suggests that liver toxicity can be short-term or long-term based on exposure time and each has a particular subset of biochemical findings, liver histopathology, and clinical symptoms.

Patients exposed for short-term periods to α-methyldopa show acute illness, general malaise, weakness, abdominal pain, nausea, and occasionally jaundice and fever (15,164). Hepatic dysfunction is mild, and the clinical symptoms and biochemical abnormalities return to normal upon drug discontinuation, although approximately one-third of the short-term patients develop persistently high transaminase levels even after being withdrawn from α-methyldopa therapy (15,164,166). Long-term patients developed hepatic injury and had a more protracted course of disease. Clinical symptoms indicative of liver effects were initially mild, gradually worsened, and included severe discomfort, chronic nausea, weakness, epigastric pain, colic, and dyspepsia.

More than 80 cases of α-methyldopa hepatitis have been reported and the administered dose varied between 0.25 mg and 1g/day, with a patient median age of about 57 years (167). Symptoms are difficult to differentiate from those of viral hepatitis (168). Prodromal symptoms include chills, fever, headaches, fatigue, malaise, anorexia, nausea, diarrhea, and vomiting. Hepatitis is frequently accompanied by fever and other symptoms after 1–4 weeks from the start of drug therapy and frank jaundice may follow a few days later. Hepatic dysfunction and jaundice may occur between 8 to 10 weeks (6) or 6 to 7 months (169) of α-methyldopa therapy. Upon rechallenge, hepatic reactions occur shortly thereafter (163). Several deaths due to hepatic coma were reported following prolonged α-methyldopa intake (15,159,160).

Underlying disease conditions, such as serological abnormalities, arthritis, and lupus erythematosus, can contribute to α-methyldopa hepatotoxicity. The liver is often enlarged and tender, and clinical symptoms include marked jaundice and cholestasis in almost half of cases. Liver function tests suggest parenchymal cell damage. Increased bilirubin is a frequent finding with elevated transaminases frequently exceeding 1000 units. Alkaline phosphatase may be normal or increased. The albumin-to-globulin ratio is usually within normal limits, but sometimes globulins, particularly the gamma fraction, are increased (7,159).

Histopathological changes ranged from acute hepatitis to chronic active hepatitis (164,170). Morphological alterations included parenchymal cell degeneration, focal, confluent or massive necrosis, and inflammation with portal tracts infiltrated by lymphocytes and mononuclear cells. Occasionally, eosinophils and plasma cells were present, and slight to moderate portal fibrosis could be observed (7,154,169). Central perivenous inflammation is a characteristic change. Massive panlobular necrosis, steatosis, and reticulum collapse have been observed in severe liver damage. Nonspecific changes in hepatocytes and sinusoidal cells are seen by electron microscopy. Degraded plasma membranes in the vascular and biliary poles and nuclear inclusions in liver cells with increased activity of mesenchymal cells were found in chronic active hepatitis (170–173).

α-Methyldopa-induced hepatic damage is also attributable to hypersensitivity rather than to direct liver cell toxicity (174). The immune reaction is evident by positive Coombs' tests, antinuclear antibodies, and lupus erythematosus cells. The onset and severity of the hepatic injury showed no clear relationship to dose or duration of treatment. A relatively small numbers of patients with allergic hypersensitivity background exposed to α-methyldopa (prone to hypersensitivity liver injury) may be most at risk. The hypersensitivity lesion has not been reproduced in experimental animals. Thus, a specific, immunologically mediated hypersensitivity reaction may be responsible for α-methyldopa hepatic toxicity (159,160). Sera from patients with α-methyldopa hepatotoxicity were cytotoxic to isolated rabbit hepatocytes pretreated with α-methyldopa and a cytochrome P450 inducer (175). Antibody-positive sera localized specific fluorescence at the plasma membrane of hepatocytes from patients on α-methyldopa. These findings support the hypothesis that immune-mediated mechanisms are involved in hepatic damage and that metabolic activation may be necessary in the generation of metabolites that can react antigenically. α-Methyldopa has been associated with immune, drug-induced hemolytic anemia that may or may not occur concomitantly with hepatitis (155,157,176,177).

Following long-term α-methyldopa exposures ranging from 1 to 11 years with a mean of 5 years, patients developed mild and gradually increasing discomfort, dyspepsia, nausea, weakness, and epigastric pain. Chronic hepatitis-like reactions appeared to be the main finding in liver biopsies from long-term patients (11,25). Liver function tests showed increased serum bilirubin, transaminases, and alkaline phosphatase activities, but were less pronounced than those changes in acute α-methyldopa hepatitis. Mild to moderate focal necrosis, hepatocyte pleomorphism, and variations in nuclear size were seen. In addition, there was infiltration of neutrophils, lymphocytes, eosinophils, plasma cells, and histiocytes. Kupffer cell proliferation with diastase-resistant granules, an indication of necrosis and phagocytic activity, was also present. Fatty change was a common finding after chronic exposure to α-methyldopa, although the mechanism is not yet established (11,25), but may involve factors such as uncoupling of oxidative phosphorylation or inhibition of triglyceride secretion. Compounds that bind to macromolecules, especially in the endoplasmic reticulum, may inhibit protein synthesis and hence interfere with lipoprotein assembly and transport (4,10,165).

Excess α-methyldopa metabolites deplete the glutathione content of liver cells. Antipyrine elimination improves following withdrawal of α-methyldopa in subjects with normal liver function tests, suggesting covalent binding and cytochrome P450 inhibition. The decreased metabolic capacity returns to normal levels about 6 months after α-methyldopa withdrawal (178). In animals, α-methyldopa is oxidized to semiquinone and quinone via cytochrome P450 and reactive metabolites bind covalently with cytoplasmic macromolecules (112). The large functional reserve for drug metabolism by the liver may account for the delay of symptoms or lesions development over prolonged periods (174). Fatty change, increased collagen deposition, impaired drug metabolism, and decreased cytochrome P450 and lowered glutathione concentrations contribute to hepatic dysfunction and eventual chronic liver damage by α-methyldopa.

Acute liver necrosis is an unusual complication of α-methyldopa therapy. This serious condition may develop within a short period of treatment, even within 8–10 weeks of α-methyldopa therapy. Isolated instances of submassive necrosis appear to have repaired after withdrawal from the drug. The most remarkable histological feature during the acute reaction phase was extensive periportal necrosis. Rechallenge with α-methyldopa resulted in increased serum transaminases within 8 days and fatal submassive hepatic necrosis (179). The protracted effects of the drug after discontinuation of therapy have been studied, and liver scans 6–9 months after treatment was stopped revealed generalized mottling and hypertrophic left lobe; broad periportal fibrosis and collapsed stroma were noted with microscopic evaluation (161,180).

Cholestasis is a rare consequence of α-methyldopa hepatotoxicity (12,166,181). α-Methyldopa exposures up to 250 mg daily for 6 years resulted in severe cholestatic liver disease without evidence of extrahepatic biliary obstruction (14). The liver architecture was preserved, although with marked cholestasis. Edema and lymphocytic and neutrophilic infiltration of the portal tracts were seen. Mild ductular proliferation was noted in periportal areas. Withdrawal from the drug resulted in normal transaminase and bilirubin levels within 6 weeks, and alkaline phosphatase returned to normal 22 weeks after α-methyldopa therapy was stopped.

Cirrhosis or hepatic failure due to α-methyldopa administration has been reported in patients receiving the drug from 7 weeks to 3 months (162,166,177). Increased bilirubin, transaminases, alkaline phosphatase, and globulin with reduced albumin were shown by laboratory tests, and liver histology included hepatocellular necrosis, cytoplasmic vacuolation, and collapse in portal tracts. Necrotic areas were lined with inflammatory cells and ballooned cells were scattered throughout the parenchyma (162). Hepatic failure followed by death after 7 weeks of α-methyldopa treatment was reported (166).

4. Papaverine

The benzylisoquinoline alkaloid papaverine has smooth-muscle-depressant properties, causing relaxation of peripheral arterioles and coronary arteries, with resulting low systemic blood pressure. Papaverine has been widely used in the treatment of cardiac or cerebral circulatory disorders. Other indications for papaverine have been to control smooth muscle spasms in intestinal, urinary, and biliary tracts. Clinical side effects are rare and mild (182–185).

Hypersensitivity-type hepatitis occurred 1–4 weeks after papaverine treatment. Fever, eosinophilia, and eosinophilic infiltration of liver parenchyma were observed (185). The eosinophilic infiltration was marked in portal areas and patchy throughout the liver lobule. Serum transaminases and alkaline phosphatase levels were highly elevated. In general, liver function tests were within normal limits 2 weeks after papaverine was discontinued. Rechallenge 2 months later resulted in immediate increase of transaminases and alkaline phosphatase together with moderate eosinophilia, confirming the drug toxicity (185).

5. Angiotensin-Converting-Enzyme Inhibitors

Inhibitors of the angiotensin-converting enzyme affect the renin-angiotensin system controlling the regulation of blood pressure. Several ACE inhibitors are used in antihypertensive therapy including benazepril, captopril, enalapril, lisinopril, perindopril, quinapril, and others (186–189). The renin-angiotensin system is a complex neuroendocrine system regulating water and electrolyte balance related to hemodynamics. The angiotensin-converting enzyme (ACE) is a peptidyldipeptide carboxyhydrolase that catalyzes the conversion of angiotensin I to angiotensin II. ACE inhibitors suppress production of angiotensin II, the most vasoactive substance in the renin-angiotensin system. Impaired liver function can develop during therapy with some ACE inhibitors (190). The impairment of function is reflected in increased serum liver enzymes and bilirubin, cholestatic jaundice, and hepatocellular injury with or without cholestasis in the tissue. These findings occur even in clinically asymptomatic patients without preexisting liver disorder. The laboratory changes were reversible when drug treatment was discontinued. The fact that these agents are frequently prescribed together with diuretics or calcium antagonists may add to potential liver toxicity due to unanticipated interactions (188).

Captopril, enalapril, quinapril, and lisinopril are ACE inhibitors used in the treatment of hypertension and heart failure. The main adverse effects are hyperkalemia, and liver or renal impairment. The clinical liver dysfunction resembles viral infection (malaise, fever, muscle pain, or rash) and can be considered hypersensitivity or a reaction to increased bradykinins. Loss of appetite, nausea, and abdominal pain also occurred during captopril or enalapril therapy. Enalapril, quinapril, and fosinopril may undergo microsomal bioactivation via cytochrome P450 3A, but captopril is thought to cause non-cytochrome-P450-dependent toxicity (191). Metabolism of quinapril results in quinaprilat that is biologically active in several tissues (186).

In terms of hepatotoxicity, consistent cholestatic and hepatocellular lesions have been found with captopril, enalapril, and lisinopril (192–203). Therefore, patients treated with ACE inhibitors may develop impaired hepatic function, including elevations of liver enzymes and bilirubin, increases of serum albumin, and hepatocellular or cholestatic jaundice and hepatitis.

Given the availability of several drugs of different chemical structures in this class, patients can alternate safely from one to another, and the high level of reported events are related to excessive dosage (188). Captopril-dependent toxicity developed after treatment for congestive heart failure. Replacement of captopril with lisinopril for 3 weeks was without events and hepatotoxicity developed after returning to captopril. When captopril was discontinued, liver enzymes returned to normal levels within 2 weeks and clinical signs resolved within the same time frame (204).

Cross-reactivity for ACE inhibitor hepatotoxicity was reported between enalapril and captopril (24). Elevated transaminases and alkaline phosphatase followed low doses of enalapril and laboratory abnormalities returned to normal level upon discontinuation. When captopril was given at low incremental doses over 2 months, liver enzymes became abnormal. Liver biopsy showed dense lymphocytic infiltration, scattered polymorphs, and eosinophils in the portal tracts with some degree of portal fibrosis. Liver function gradually improved after captopril was discontinued.

C. Lipid Regulators

Upon establishment of the relationship of altered lipid metabolism and cardiovascular degenerative disease, regulation or control of lipid profiles has characterized the growth of pharmacotherapy in this area. Atherosclerosis contributes to 50% of all mortality in the United States (205). In terms of risk reduction, a 1% decrease in cholesterol levels results in a 2% reduction in coronary artery disease morbidity (206,207). Traditionally, dietary control, physical exercise, and significant lifestyle modification were recognized as fundamental paradigms in the control of dyslipidemias. Emerging knowledge on lipoprotein metabolism suggested strong genetic control, and receptor-mediated interactions determined the phenotype most likely to respond to therapy. Thus, lipid regulation by agents affecting specific cell surface receptors or specific metabolic or enzyme inhibitors constitutes contemporary pharmacotherapy, encompassing homozygous or heterozygous, familial combined, or polygenic dyslipoproteinemias. Therapeutic approaches aimed at modifying basic lipid metabolism might eventually elicit unexpected toxicity, considering the significant role of the liver in lipid and lipoprotein metabolism. Paradoxically, there are not many reports characterizing liver structure in patients receiving hypolipidemics considering the large number undergoing lipid-regulating therapy. This probably reflects trends for reliance on biochemical or phenotypic markers. Modulation of hepatic lipid metabolism and the prolonged exposure of patients to these therapeutic agents prompted the review of lipid-regulating effects on liver function. Much of the unanswered questions in hyperlipoproteinemias concern liver structure and function to distinguish liver changes due to the disease from alterations caused by drugs (208).

Early approaches to the treatment of dyslipidemias employed resins, probucol, and nicotinic acid either alone or in combination with fibrates (209). These agents influenced preferentially triglycerides with minor effects on cholesterol metabolism or lipoprotein production. Inhibition of 3-hydroxy-e-methylglutaryl coenzyme A reductase (HMG-CoA), the rate-limiting enzyme of cholesterol biosynthesis, was made possible by compactin or mevinolin. Cholesterol control, mainly decreasing the low-density lipoprotein (LDL)-cholesterol fraction, became a significant therapeutic approach, and therapeutic regimens for dyslipidemias now include fibrates, statins, or the association of both, depending on clinical response. Most commonly used fibrates include clofibrate, etofibrate, fenofibrate, bezafibrate, and gemfibrozil. Statins are lovastatin, simvastatin, fluvastatin, mevastatin, pravastatin, atorvastatin, and others.

Changes in serum proteins from hypercholesterolemic patients consist of elevated LDL (210). Dyslipidemias occur in later stages of life at a time when several drugs may be administered concurrently, antihypertensives, antirheumatics, and sedatives being the most frequent association. An early study described the ultrastructure of hepatocytes in two different hyperlipidemias (211), recognizing fatty change as a principal landmark (212). Some degree of underlying hepatic pathology may be present in response to exogenous factors such as diet, alcohol intake, or even superimposed drug-related effects by other distinct agents (213). Nicotinic acid induced ultrastructural changes in the liver within a background of preexisting changes (214,215). Several reports have described the liver structure after the administration of other lipid regulators, including clofibrate (216–218), fenofibrate (219), and gemfibrozil. (208). In most of these studies, however, the lack of baseline structural data somewhat diminished the value of the observations.

1. Nicotinic Acid

Nicotinic acid or niacin and close derivatives are useful lipid-lowering agents; however, nicotinic acid causes marked peripheral vasodilatation, flushing, gastrointestinal irritation, and hepatotoxicity (76,220–222). The mechanism of this hepatic reaction has not been defined. There are, however, major frequent and limiting clinical effects aside from flushing that include nausea, vomiting, and hyperpigmentation of the skin. Large or medium doses of nicotinic acid sometimes cause hepatotoxicity and jaundice, particularly slow-release forms in excess of 3 g/day (115,223–225). Clinical effects of intrahepatic cholestasis during nicotinic acid therapy are marked pruritus, jaundice, increased serum bilirubin, and alkaline phosphatase (226–228).

2. Fibrates

Clofibrate was the first agent in this class for the control of dyslipidemia and was approved more than 25 years ago. Administration of clofibrate to experimental animals caused significant hepatomegaly and induced hepatic drug-metabolizing enzymes (229), together with increased peroxisomes and liver tumors. The unknown cause of hepatomegaly, the peroxisome proliferation phenomenon, and the tumor formation formed a quizzical triad with relevance for human risk (230,231). Fibrates available for use in the last decades were clofibrate, gemfibrozil, fenofibrate, bezafibrate, and others, but most of these drugs are now directed to the control of severe hypertriglyceridemia and pancreatitis. The prominent animal findings, together with some of the clinical effects observed, created doubts about the long-term safety of fibrates. Like other agents in this class, asymptomatic trans-aminase elevations over a range of multiples of the upper limit of normal have been recognized (5,232). Most fibrate-related clinical reactions are related to the gastrointesti-nal, central nervous, and tegumentary systems (233). No deaths and recovery from these effects other than in liver and muscle were reported in an extensive surveillance study after administration of fenofibrate, ciprofibrate, gemfibrozil, and bezafibrate (234). One report included a case of fatal hepatitis during treatment with perhexiline maleate and bezafibrate (235).

Biopsy data from fibrate-exposed liver and from naïve hyperlipidemics show pre-dominantly fatty change, although it may be different from the steatosis of obesity (236). Reports described the long-term effects of clofibrate in liver biopsies from dyslipoprotein-emic patients (216–218,237,238) and confirmed the lack of significant changes in subcel-lular organelles, including peroxisomes. The number and volume density of peroxisomes increased by 50% and 23%, respectively, during the first few months of treatment, and subsequently the values returned to normal limits perhaps due to adaptation. Although morphometric data revealed increase volume and numerical density, contemporary evalua-tion criteria indicate that more than twofold increases in the number of peroxisomes are necessary to consider this finding as biologically relevant (239). Long-term administration of gemfibrozil was studied in liver biopsies from hyperlipoproteinemic patients (208). Hepatic fatty change was present irrespective of the pattern of dyslipidemia. The number of peroxisomes was not increased based on the results of a limited morphometric study (240).

Fenofibrate has been studied for liver toxicity (219), and there are isolated reports of hepatitis (238,241,242). Organelle antibodies were found against smooth muscle, nu-cleus, and mitochondria in about 70% of drug-induced hepatitis attributed to a heteroge-neous group of drugs that included clometacin, fenofibrate, oxyphenysatin, and papaverine (243). Most events were moderate, including asymptomatic transaminase elevations (244). Liver biopsies from hyperlipidemic patients taking fenofibrate showed no significant he-patic alterations compared to a cohort group (219), and fatty change was also reported. A morphometric study of liver biopsies from fenofibrate patients showed no changes in peroxisomes (245,246). Taking all the liver biopsy data together it could be concluded that the peroxisome proliferation seen in rodents does not happen in humans. It is plausible that effects would be seen in humans at higher doses, but species differences in peroxisome ontogenesis are remarkable (247).

3. Statins

HMG-CoA reductase inhibitors constitute a class of drugs widely used in contemporary therapy for cholesterol and atherosclerosis control (248). Atorvastatin, cerivastatin, flu-vastatin, lovastatin, pravastatin, and simvastatin appear to have different kinetics of HMG-CoA reductase inhibition, and thus are the basis of different therapeutic modalities (249). Atorvastatin ablates atherosclerotic lesions in mouse models (250), in rabbits (251–253), and in pigs (254). Lovastatin and pravastatin lower cholesterol and triglycerides in very-low-density lipoproteins (VLDL), LDL, and apoprotein B (ApoB), with minor increases in high-density lipoproteins (HDL) and no changes in Apo-1 (255–258). The extent of LDL modulation has been studied comparing lovastatin and atorvastatin (259). Statins have been coadministered with fibrates, to obtain a more pronounced VLDL decrease and HDL increase. However, these beneficial effects have been contrasted with a higher risk of myopathy (260,261).

Atorvastatin is a second-generation statin that shares the mechanism of the class while causing prolonged inhibition of HMG-CoA reductase together with ApoB reduction (262,263). Owing to the significant LDL-lowering properties (40–60%) it is effective in heterozygous familial hypercholesterolemia (264). Mild liver transaminase elevations are frequently observed with HMG-GoA inhibitors and these increases usually resolve after withdrawal from therapy. No record of permanent liver damage has been documented (232). In a study including 4271 patients on atorvastatin, 0.7% had transaminases higher than 3 times the upper limit of normal (265,266). Pravastatin, fluvastatin, lovastatin, or simvastatin caused transaminase elevations above 3 times the upper limit of normal in a small percentage of patients, usually 1–4% in clinical trials (267–274). The low rate of hepatic adverse events with pravastatin may have been the result of the single-daily-dose mode of administration (255). However, the adverse event rates may not be comparable, since the evaluation criteria may not be uniform among investigators and also subject to different regulatory interpretation worldwide. The International Conference of Harmonization is guiding standardization efforts in adverse reaction reporting (275).

In experimental studies, lovastatin caused marked hepatocellular atypia and foci of cellular alteration in rats, and bile duct hyperplasia and centrilobular hepatocyte necrosis in rabbits. Transaminase elevation in dogs abated while treatment was continued, and there were no changes in primates (276–278). Fluvastatin caused hepatocellular necrosis in rodents in a carcinogenicity study (279). An experimental HMG-CoA inhibitor, GR 95030X, increased transaminases and creatine phosphokinase, but no histological changes in the liver of marmosets (280). Nonhuman primates do not show liver morphological changes with pravastatin (281), and dogs given simvastatin had transaminase increases greater than 10 times the control values without hepatocellular morphological changes upon biopsy at the crest of the transaminase elevation (282).

Most of these experimental studies used very high, systemic toxic doses that could have resulted in blood levels intolerable in humans. The pathogenesis of elevated transaminases upon HMG-CoA inhibition is not known. Dogs receiving atorvastatin for up to 2 years had transaminase and alkaline phosphatase elevations with reversible hepatic lesions including lipofuscin deposition (283). Proposed, but not definitely established, mechanisms have been attributed to the extent of inhibitor exposure and to cellular toxicity because of persistent mevalonate synthesis inhibition. The elevated transaminases in humans appear to resolve regardless of whether or not therapy is discontinued. The average increases are modest and not accompanied by elevated bilirubin or alkaline phosphatase. To our knowledge, there are no literature reports of liver damage confirmed by biopsy accompanying these transaminase elevations. Considering the experimental evidence reflected in the intense enzyme induction and the metabolic enzyme inhibition, the transaminase elevation may not represent direct liver cell toxicity. Changes in the clearance or metabolism of transaminases might contribute to the high levels observed. Marmosets may represent a good model for studying transaminase elevations, as seen with some experimental compounds (280).

Overall, statins as a class of lipid-regulating agents do not appear to pose significant hepatotoxicity risk, based on the extent of universal use and the low frequency of reported, documented reactions over the past decade or more. Squalene synthase inhibitors, such as ER 27856 and ER 28448 (284), show promise as potent hypercholesterolemics in the laboratory, but there is little evidence as to their safety and lack of liver effects.

D. Vasodilators

1. Organic Nitrates

Organic nitrates are useful therapeutic agents for the symptomatic treatment of angina pectoris. Their onset and duration of activity may be related to their prerequisite metabolism to show the circulatory effects. Organic nitrate biotransformation was ablated by cytochrome P450 inhibitors and biotransformation of glyceryl trinitrate was catalyzed by isoenzymes induced by phenobarbital (285). Organic nitrates are classified into short-acting (amyl nitrate, isosorbide dinitrite) and long-acting (erythrityl tetranitrate, penta-erythritol tetranitrate). Nitroglycerine may be short- or long-acting based on the pharmaceutical formulation. Most of the clinical toxicity of nitrates is derived from circulatory effects, including methemoglobinemia (286–289). Significant paucity of liver toxicity is reported with these agents. However, since these are combined usually with other vasodilators, including calcium channel blockers or beta-adrenoceptor antagonists (290), hepatic reactions may emerge due to metabolic interactions.

There is hepatic cytochrome P450-dependent biotransformation of organic nitrates. When glyceryl trinitrate (GTN) was incubated with aortic supernatant and rat hepatic microsomes, there were concentration-dependent increases in guanylyl cyclase activity pointing to a role of nitric oxide (NO) (291). The guanylyl cyclase was increased with phenobarbital-induced microsomes and reduced by metabolic inhibitors (292). Glyceryl trinitrate is mutagenic to *Salmonella* TA1535 and the mechanism of DNA damage may be via NO generation due to metabolic reduction (293). GTN also induces hepatocellular carcinoma in rats (294). No p53 mutations were found in the tumors but K-ras point mutations occurred in half of the tumors. Sodium nitrate given to Wistar rats caused liver tumors including hepatocellular carcinoma and hemangiosarcoma (295), whereas in another study in F-344 rats, sodium nitrite did not cause tumors (296). In contrast, pentaerythritol tetranitrate administered to F344 rats and B6C3F1 mice was essentially nontoxic and did not induce liver neoplasia (297). These studies do not provide sufficient evidence to affirm a liver neoplastic potential upon long-term use of these agents.

III. ANTIDIABETIC DRUGS

The treatment of diabetes, particularly diabetes resulting from insulin resistance, is a major challenge. The drug armamentarium was static for more than a decade until the advent of the thiazolidinediones, or "insulin sensitizers," and the aldose reductase inhibitors that showed significant promise. The search for the treatment of diabetes or its complications in the United States is intense, as evidenced by the number of clinical trials underway. Thanks to Internet access (http://www.centerwatch.com/studies/listing.htm) and as of this writing, there are over 500 clinical trials in progress addressing diabetes type 1 and 2 treatments, prevention, and approaches to different complications, such as foot ulcers, gastroparesis, neuropathy, nephropathy, retinopathy, and macular disease. Most of the treatments get individualized and adjusted according to the patient response, contributing to a heterogeneous matrix of polytherapy (1). Part of the heterogeneity in treatment responses has been attributed to the polygenic and polyphenotypic characteristic of type 2 diabetes, and genomic studies may hold promise for the future in the design of new therapeutic interventions (298–301).

A. Hormones

1. Insulin

In diabetes mellitus, the administration of insulin or oral hypoglycemic agents constitutes standard treatment. The use of insulin, as with any hormone, is for replacement therapy owing to the patient's insufficient production of own insulin. In chronic use of insulin, some undesired side effects occur such as hypoglycemic reactions, local lipodystrophy, and presbyopia. Oral hypoglycemics include sulfonylureas, biguanides, α-glucosidase inhibitors, and thiazolidinedione derivatives. These drugs cause release or better utilization of endogenous insulin. Toxic clinical reactions of these drugs most commonly encountered are nausea and vomiting; occasionally flareup of peptic ulcer and epigastric distress are reported. In some patients cholestatic jaundice has been found.

B. Sulfonylureas

These drugs are orally active hypoglycemic agents acting in part by stimulating insulin secretion from the β cells of the pancreas. Members of this group include acetohexamide, chlorpropamide, glipizide, glyburide, and tolbutamide. Major side effects are usually associated with overdose that can induce hypoglycemia. Jaundice has been reported rarely as a hepatic side effect.

1. Acetohexamide

Acetohexamide is an oral antidiabetic agent that stimulates insulin release from the pancreas and reduces glucose output from the liver. Side effects are hypoglycemic reactions (302–304). Cholestatic jaundice has been found in rare cases (305,306).

2. Chlorpropamide

Chlorpropamide reduces blood sugar concentration by stimulating insulin secretion from pancreatic islets. The drug is readily absorbed from the gastrointestinal tract and slowly excreted by the kidneys as unchanged chlorpropamide. Prolonged treatment with chlorpropamide and by all sulfonylurea drugs can cause severe hypoglycemia, particularly in elderly patients with reduced plasma clearance and impaired liver or kidney function (307). Usually the dose-related side effects are transient, reducing the dose level, or complete withdrawal results in regression of the symptoms. Adverse reactions are associated with idiosyncrasy or hypersensitivity, which include jaundice and skin eruption (308–311).

3. Glipizide

Glipizide is rapidly absorbed, extensively metabolized, and improves insulin secretion from the β cells of the pancreas. Side effects include various manifestations of hypoglycemia, nervousness, weakness, and paresthesia (312–314). Hepatic or renal disease may be a predisposing factor.

4. Glyburide and Tolbutamide

The major action of glyburide and tolbutamide is an increased release of insulin from the pancreatic β cells. Glyburide also affects some other mechanisms leading to decreased blood glucose. Glyburide is highly bound to plasma proteins and it is completely metabolized in the liver and eliminated mainly via the kidney. Tolbutamide is also readily absorbed and bound to plasma proteins after absorption from the gastrointestinal tract. It is metabolized in the liver and kidney. In patients treated with glyburide or tolbutamide hypoglycemia may develop (312,314). With glyburide treatment, hepatic porphyria has been reported (315); very rarely, elevated liver enzymes were found and in isolated cases cholestasis, jaundice, and hepatitis (316–322). Liver function normalizes after withdrawal of these drugs.

C. Oligosaccharides

1. Acarbose

Acarbose is a complex oligosaccharide produced by fermentation of *Actinoplanes utahensio*, and competitively inhibits pancreatic α-amylase and α-glucosidase activity in the brush border membrane of the small intestine. This effect delays the absorption of carbohydrates resulting in a lowering of blood glucose concentration (323). Acarbose does not enhance insulin secretion, but lowers postprandial hyperglycemia, resulting in an improved blood glucose control. Gastrointestinal disturbances are the most frequently observed side effects of acarbose (324,325) and clinically significant hepatotoxicity is rare (326).

Acarbose at high doses increases serum transaminases and sometimes causes hyperbilirubinemia (189,327). Severe hepatotoxicity occurred with acarbose and concomitant administration of glyburide. Liver enzymes and bilirubin were highly elevated at discontinuation and laboratory values returned to normal within 2 months. Liver enzymes increased within 1 week after a rechallenge dose and enzymes were within normal limits at 1–4 months (328).

D. Thiazolidinediones

These novel antidiabetic agents constitute a different chemical class with different pharmacological effects from sulfonylureas, biguanides, or alpha-glucosidase inhibitors (329,330) and are prescribed for the management of type 2 diabetes mellitus (Fig. 3). Thiazolidinediones act primarily through a PPAR-γ-receptor-mediated signal enhancing the responsiveness in muscle or adipose tissues, or decreasing insulin resistance by increasing insulin sensitivity of insulin-dependent tissues and inhibiting hepatic gluconeogenesis (331,332). Cholesterol biosynthesis inhibition by glitazones appears to be independent of the PPAR-γ mechanism (333). These drugs are indicated in type 2 diabetes, but they are not effective in the absence of insulin as is the case with diabetes type 1. The glycemic control takes place in the presence of insulin, reducing the dose of the exogenous hormone (insulin rescue). Patients receiving thiazolidinediones in combination with either insulin or other oral hypoglycemic compounds may have a risk of hypoglycemia due to the adjunct therapy.

Experimental animals, including mice and rats but not nonhuman primates, develop cardiac hypertrophy, interscapular brown fat hyperplasia, and endothelial cell proliferation (334–337). The cardiac enlargement is preventable by the coadministration of ACE inhibitors, indicating an indirect participation of the renin-angiotensin system (338). Extensive animal studies did not reveal abnormalities in safety evaluation models (334–336,339–341). The adipose tissue of rodents undergoes significant metabolic or morphological changes with glitazones (342,343), while exerting significant effects on adipocyte differentiation (344,345). The significance of these findings is not clear over the long term in diabetics (346).

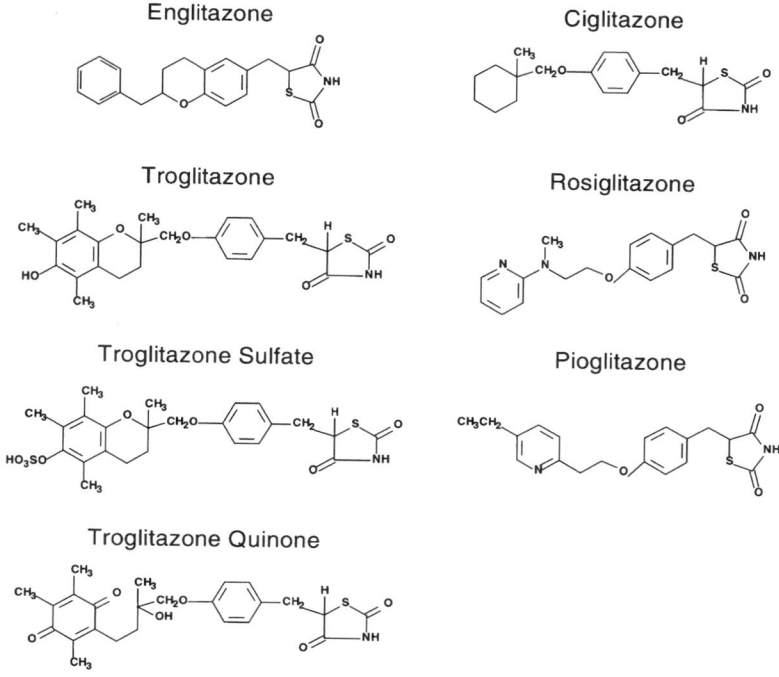

Figure 3 Molecular structure of thiazolidinediones and major troglitazone metabolites.

1. Troglitazone

This is an oral antihyperglycemic agent that normalizes blood glucose by increasing target cell responses to insulin. This compound was discovered by Japanese researchers in the 1980s and is the same group that developed the first HMG-CoA inhibitor about the same era (329) (Fig. 3). Troglitazone reduces hepatic glucose output and enhances insulin-dependent glucose disposition in skeletal muscle. Its mechanism of action is related to binding to peroxisome-proliferator-activated receptor in the nucleus that regulates the transcription of a number of insulin-responsive genes required for the control of glucose and lipid metabolism. The troglitazone molecule contains two chiral centers and each of the four stereoisomers shows similar pharmacological effects; the tocopherol group appears to confer antioxidant activity (347).

Clinical trials with troglitazone included 2510 patients and 5% had transaminases greater than 1.5 times the upper limit of normal, 48 patients (1.9%) had transaminases 3 times above that limit, and 10% of those had enzyme elevations 20 times above the upper limit of normal and two patients had overt jaundice (326,348). Among other reactions within a short time after approval, reversible jaundice, idiosyncratic drug reaction, liver failure, and death were reported in the United States (82,349–355,399,400), eventually leading to withdrawal of the drug.

Troglitazone hepatotoxicity is a complex manifestation of clinical and organ changes leading to toxic hepatitis, cholestatic injury, and fulminant hepatitis with or without massive necrosis, none of which are predictable. The diversity of onset periods, heterogeneous liver pathology, and number of concomitant medications contribute little to defining clearly the severe troglitazone hepatic syndrome (Table 1). In terms of fulminant hepatitis, the interaction of glibenclamide and troglitazone was identified in three of four patients with fulminant hepatitis (354).

2. Rosiglitazone

This oral thiazolidinedione increases insulin sensitivity similarly to other glitazones. It improves glycemic control together with reduced circulating insulin levels at lower doses than troglitazone. Rosiglitazone is a highly selective and potent agonist of peroxisome-proliferator-activated receptor γ that is found in key target tissues for insulin action such as liver, skeletal muscle, and adipose tissue. The dosage is lower than that of troglitazone, but the overall effects on glycemic control are similar. The specific mechanism by which rosiglitazone exerts increased sensitivity to insulin in these tissues is not known. Rosiglitazone has clinical activity when used as monotherapy or in combination with other agents, such as metformin (82,356).

Available clinical trial data showed no firm evidence of hepatotoxicity with only sporadic increases of liver enzymes (357). In controlled trials, 0.2% of patients had reversible transaminases elevations above 3 times the upper limit of normal, no different than controls (358). A 69-year-old man receiving 4 mg of rosiglitazone daily developed hepatic failure after 21 days of therapy (359). However, the patient was severely hypotensive and recovery followed supportive care and withdrawal from the drug. A second case of severe hepatocellular damage after 2 weeks on drug recovered after therapy discontinuation. This patient received Accolate, a recently identified hepatotoxin. The investigator recommended earlier and more frequent liver enzyme monitoring, and discontinuation is advised when transaminases elevations are higher than 3 times the upper limit (358,360). Clinical experience postmarketing has not identified any cases of acute liver failure with death or liver transplant in over one million patients who received the drug.

3. Pioglitazone

Pioglitazone monohydrochloride is used to treat type 2 diabetes, and chemically it is a racemic mixture with both enantiomers of equal pharmacological activity. Pioglitazone is extensively metabolized by the hepatic cytochrome P450 system mainly by CYP 2C8 and CYP 3A4 and to some extent by the mainly extrahepatic CYP 1A1. Pioglitazone is an inducer of CYP 3A4 and in in vitro studies the hepatic metabolism was inhibited 85% by ketoconazole. It is difficult to predict the interaction with other drugs, and caution will be needed when it is coadministered with inducers of competing substrates (356). When glipizide, digoxin, warfarin, or metformin was coadministered individually with pioglitazone, no pharmacokinetic interactions were found (361).

In clinical studies with pioglitazone, there was no evidence of drug-induced hepatotoxicity or elevation of serum alanine aminotransferase levels (82,356,362). During controlled trials in the United States, four of 1526 diabetics (0.26%) had transaminases elevations greater than 3 times the upper limit of normal, not different from controls (361). No cases of acute liver failure have been reported in the literature.

4. Other

Other thiazolidinediones include ciglitazone (363,364) and englitazone (365), but no reports were found regarding liver reactions with these drugs. NC-2100 is a thiazolidinedione with a different receptor activation profile than other compounds in this class. Whether

Table 1 Age, Sex, Treatment Duration, Laboratory Findings,[a] and Outcome of Severe Hepatic Reactions to Troglitazone

Patient	1	2	3	4	5	6	7	8	9	10	11	12	13
Age/sex	51F	51F	44F	65F	59F	85M	58M	48F	61F	64F	55F	48F	50F
Dose, mg	200	200	200–400	400	400	200–400	400	400	400	400	?	200–400	400
Treated days	153	176	138	63	105	140	100	≈100	120	120	?	≈180	140
Bilirubin	8	6	29	20	16	16	8	0.7	8	11	6	105	29
ALT	718	1230	606	1164	405	6081	1655	826	1367	3000	1661	653	1227
ALKP	410	182	2940	240	345	?	378	333	174	167	?	?	216
Outcome[b]	R	R	R	R	T	F	F	R	T	F	T/F	R	F
Ref.	412	412	352	352	349	353	354	389	400	400	400	351	355

[a] Rounded values, either peak or at presentation.

[b] F, fatal; R, reversible; T, transplant.

? = not available.

the weak PPAR-γ activation of this drug translates into lesser hepatotoxicity is not clear (366).

5. Oxadiazolidinediones

Similarly to thiazolidinediones, experimental studies with this chemical class show efficacy in diabetes models. However, no adipocyte differentiation effects are seen, indicating different biological properties and perhaps a distinct clinical profile. The oxadiazole YM440 from Yamanouchi in Japan has been proposed as a useful agent from this class (367). Given the concerns with thiazolidinediones, focus will be on the lack of clinical liver effects.

E. Biguanides

1. Metformin

Metformin exerts glycemic control only when there is functional insulin secretion. This drug exerts no effect on the pancreatic beta cells, so its mechanism of action is not fully understood. The compound increases the effect of insulin on peripheral receptor sites or potentiates the action of insulin by increasing the number of insulin receptors on cell surface membranes (368). Metformin, buformin, and phenformin are biguanides introduced in the late fifties to treat insulin-resistant diabetes type 2. Phenformin and buformin were withdrawn from use because of lactic acidosis (1). Metformin causes lactic acidosis if not properly prescribed (369). Metformin is effective as a monotherapy agent or in combination with sulfonylureas. The glucose utilization in tissues is via oxidative metabolism whereas nonoxidative metabolism mediates glucose utilization by the intestine. As a result, extra lactate enters the liver to maintain gluconeogenesis and biguanides inhibit gluconeogenesis from alanine (370). This balance mechanism is a safeguard against excessive glucose lowering.

The absorption of metformin is relatively slow and it is excreted in the urine in unchanged form. It is not metabolized, although its use is contraindicated in the presence of liver disease or renal impairment. In some cases acute clinically significant hepatic dysfunction might develop during metformin therapy (189,371,372).

F. Insulinotropic Agents

Insulinotropic agents are also recognized as insulin secretion enhancers or insulin secretagogues that stimulate insulin release from β cells and other depots. This mechanism is similar to sulfonylureas, perhaps with some differences at the molecular level. Drugs in this category are repaglinide and nateglinide (373–375). The liver toxicity is not established owing to limited clinical experience. These drugs are also being studied in combination with other antidiabetics, such as glyburide, and no liver reactions have been reported (375).

G. Progress in Hepatotoxicity by Cardiovascular or Antidiabetic Drugs

With every significant event that leads to the identification of a new drug-induced hepatotoxicity, new approaches are fueled to advance knowledge and to take advantage of new, enabling technologies usually available after drugs have been developed or before they reach commercialization and widespread use. The heterogeneous clinical presentations of diabetes or cardiovascular disease indicate major background differences and phenotypic outcomes representing the interaction of several, if not many, determinant genetic effects. Screening for genetic traits in diabetics poses logistic intellectual and ethical challenges. In addition, the genetic control of liver-detoxifying mechanisms as well as markers of injury can modulate the extent of the underlying pathology as well as the expression of the liver injury markers. Several genetic polymorphisms have been characterized in diabetes and in cardiovascular disease, and these can cause different pharmacological or toxic reactions to drugs (129,146). Variable pharmacodynamics can evolve from gene effects, differences in receptor structure or population, membrane transporters, and other basic cellular functions (376). Hence, pharmacogenetic interventions will improve the management of diabetes or cardiovascular disease while anticipating or preventing liver reactions. A clinical trial on type 2 diabetes and troglitazone covered 4079 patients screened for transaminases and genotyped for *diabetes disease* and *toxicity* genes (301) (Table 2). These gene panels were selected from a group of candidate genes based on a functional expression. The study identified a small subset of genes combining phase II drug metabolism, glucose transport, and PPAR-γ single-point mutations. These gene mutations occurred in a small group of diabetics and this occurrence was beyond mere chance (Table 3). The same profile of gene mutations was found in one of the fatal outcomes. The study could be hindered from many vantages since it included a small number of genes as well as the lack of an age-matched cohort. Nevertheless, by pursuing genetic modulations by sulfotransferase polymorphisms (377), transaminase variants (378), and other predispositions, such as race, a profile or cluster may emerge. Targeted studies showed that diabetics possess impaired sulfotransferase activity among other functional decrements (379) and glitazones are predominantly metabolized via phase II conjugation and quinone oxidative reductions (380,381). These reactions occur in hepatocytes or blood white cells (382) and a hypothesis was tested observing liver cell and peripheral blood cells reactions in parallel, making this approach simpler and amenable to minimally invasive techniques, such as flow cytometry of blood samples.

Mechanisms of hepatic cell toxicity have been studied closely in recent years, and sensitive parameters of functional changes have been identified, such as mitochondrial transmembrane potential changes (383). Protracted impairment of beta-oxidation in mitochondria leads to many different liver changes from exposures to anticonvulsants, antibiotics, and anti-inflammatory agents. Amiodarone, perhexiline, and diethylaminoethoxy-

Table 2 Genetic Polymorphisms Common in the Genotype of Diabetics at Risk of Liver Injury

Polymorphism found	Functional change
CYP 450 1A1 wt/v	Drug interaction
CYP 450 2C19m1 wt/v	Drug interaction
CYP 450 2D6 wt/v	Drug interaction
NQO1 (DT diaphorase)	2/3 decreased metabolic activity
GLUT-1	Increased NIDDM risk
PPAR γ-892	Reduced fasting glucose/BMI Increased insulin sensitivity
PPAR γ-1431	Increased leptin levels

Source: Shi et al. (301).

Table 3 Serum Transaminases and Bilirubin from Diabetics with Heterozygous Gene Polymorphisms

Parameter	All patients			Patients with 4 polymorphisms[a]			Patients with 5 polymorphisms[b]	
	A	B	C	A	B	C	A	C
Patients	2393	60	18	34	3	1[d]	11	1[4]
Alanine aminotransferase (U/L)	20 ± 0[c]	252 ± 34	551 ± 77	19 ± 1	494 ± 388	1270	18 ± 2	1270
Aspartate aminotransferase (U/L)	19 ± 0	148 ± 25	336 ± 66	18 ± 1	428 ± 383	1194	18 ± 2	1194
Bilirubin (mg/dL)	0.7 ± 0.0	1.0 ± 0.2	1.7 ± 0.5	0.6 ± 0.0	3.3 ± 2.7	8.8	0.7 ± 0.1	8.8

[a] Patients with four concurrent polymorphisms were heterozygous for GLUT-1 (associated with increased risk for type 2 diabetes), PPARγ-892 (increased insulin sensitivity, reduced fasting glucose), PPARγ-1431 (increased leptin levels), and NQO1 (65% reduced metabolic activity).

[b] Patients with five concurrent polymorphisms were heterozygous for GLUT-1, PPARγ-892, PPARγ-1431, NQO1, and CYP1A1 (increased propensity for drug interactions).

[c] Values represent mean ± SEM.

[d] Only one patient had elevations above 10X ULN and four or five heterozygous unusual gene associations at the time troglitazone treatment was discontinued. Enzyme levels grouped as <3X ULN (A), ≥3X ULN (B), and ≥10X ULN (C).

Source: Adapted from Shi et al. (301).

hexestrol are cardiovascular drug examples that also affect oxidative phosphorylation (69,384). Severe detriments in oxidative phosphorylation lead to liver damage and fatal organ failure (385). French investigators proposed that every drug under clinical development should be studied for effects on mitochondria (69). Studies using coherent multiprobe fluorescence with isolated liver cells monitored simultaneously the effects of tacrine on mitochondrial transmembrane potential, cell membrane permeability, calcium traffic, and cytoskeletal integrity in real time (386). Diabetic mitochondria appear to be in a relative state of uncoupling that paradoxically is ameliorated by troglitazone (387). This approach was used to study mitochondrial transmembrane potential effects in response to three thiazolidinediones (388,389). The transmembrane potential "lesion" can be observed with troglitazone and rosiglitazone in vitro (Fig. 4).

This coherent fluorescent multiprobe assay will be useful to study drug interactions in normal or diabetic hepatocytes, yielding useful data for the prediction of drug combination effects. It is not difficult to predict that decoding of these reactions at the subcellular and molecular level will take place in the near future in most clinical laboratory settings.

In diabetics, peripheral blood cells, like platelets, are altered in the diabetic state (390) and different phenolsulfotransferase genotypes are expressed in liver, lung, other organs, and platelets, resulting in variations in therapeutic activity, biotransformation, and toxicity in drugs that undergo sulfate conjugation. Thiazolidinediones are metabolized via sulfate conjugation and the impairment of this metabolic capacity might therefore result in toxicity (391). Thiazolidinediones also affect ATP consumption (388), which might

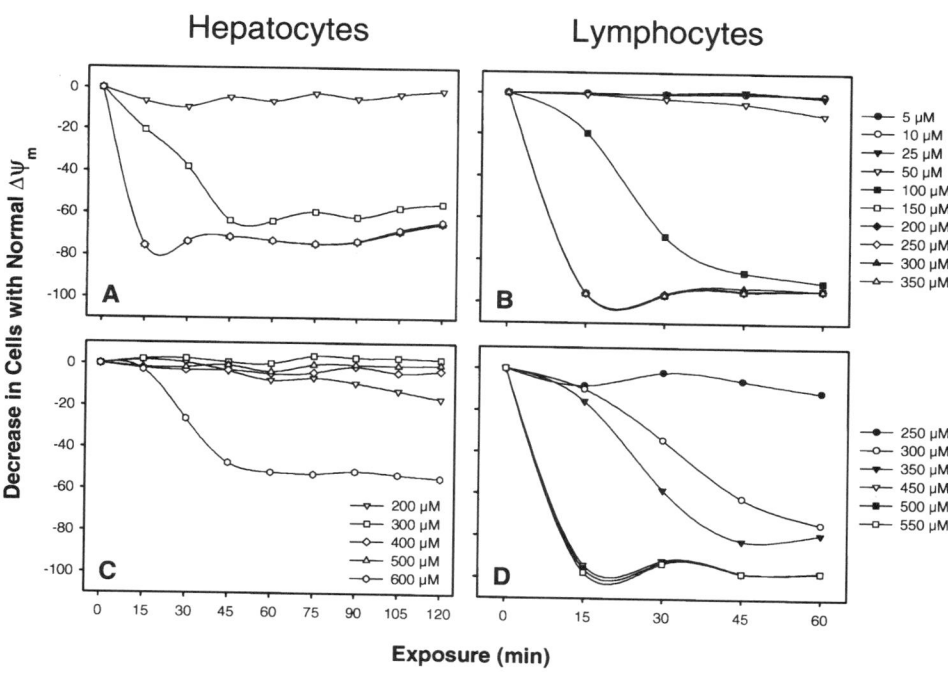

Figure 4 Changes in mitochondrial transmembrane potential ($\Delta\psi_m$) with thiazolidinediones. Troglitazone (A,B) and rosiglitazone (C,D) exert similar profiles in either hepatocytes or peripheral lymphocytes. Adapted from Haskins et al. (388).

lead to decreased capacity for glucuronidation due to altered redox state (392). Contributing factors might include disruptions in glucose transporter 4 (393), PPAR-γ receptor mutations (394), as well as reduced quinone reductase activity (395). The disruption of the DT diaphorase gene, reducing the effectiveness of quinone detoxification mechanisms, increases the risk of anticoagulant toxicity and might enhance the toxicity of the antidiabetic agent. DT diaphorase is found in the liver but more abundantly in extrahepatic tissues. The reduction of quinones to hydroquinones is a detoxifying pathway that protects against oxidation products; however, some hydroquinones may auto-oxidize and generate reactive oxygen species or even alkylate DNA (396). The use of supportive therapy that employs anticoagulants that undergo reductive metabolism may precipitate a liver reaction already initiated by the main therapeutic agent. To this date, no studies have been reported employing *NQO1-null* mutant mice that have increased sensitivity to menadione toxicity (expressed by increased lethality and elevated transaminases when compared to the wild type) with thiazolidinediones.

IV. CONCLUDING REMARKS

This review has attempted to critically assess the hepatic side effects of cardiovascular and antidiabetic drugs and to update the knowledge base from a previous work (397). Hepatotoxicity has been ascertained on the basis of biochemical, morphological, and clinical findings and the fact that liver abnormalities subside after withdrawal of the drug in question. This may be difficult to accomplish in a framework of polytherapy. Rechallenge quickly confirms the source of liver injury, causing similar symptoms as found in the original reaction. Although very practical, this approach may cascade into more severe reactions and the damage may become irreparable. Several cardiovascular and antidiabetic drugs have hepatotoxic potential since many of them undergo metabolic biotransformation in the liver or some possess intrinsic strong lipid-binding affinity. Although hepatotoxicity has been documented in many studies by means of clinical, morphological, and laboratory evaluations, the conclusions could have been better supported by control or baseline data.

Unexpected drug reactions affect the liver at early stages, and on occasion, fulminant hepatic injury may result (76,398). Should the effects not be recognized at an early stage, irreversible changes and death may be the outcome (353,355). Liver reactions, either mild or severe, develop with cardiovascular drugs including antiarrhythmics, antihypertensives, and hypolipidemics. Among diabetics, adverse hepatic reactions can develop following intake of sulfonylureas, biguanides, α-glucosidase inhibitors, or thiazolidinediones, indicating no specific relationship of the hepatic side effect with the chemical structure or therapeutic group. An important component of the patient response may be preexisting pathology or altered phenotype. Overall, morphological, biochemical, and clinical data documented hepatic changes consisting of elevated liver enzymes, cholestasis, fatty change, granulomatous reactions, hepatitis, necrosis, fibrosis, and cirrhosis. The cellular or molecular basis of the liver reactions in every instance cannot always be ascertained. Liver injury, whether or not dependent on a particular drug or metabolite, is frequently associated with immunological effects that have not been characterized unequivocally. Increased transaminases in the absence of elevated bilirubin or other liver function tests in patients on cardiovascular or antidiabetic drugs are associated with a range of hepatic morphological changes that can resolve or evolve into significant liver injury. Although elevated transaminases may represent an important index of deranged liver function, the degree of the elevation does not usually parallel the extent of parenchymal cell damage at early stages of the disease. It follows that hepatotoxicity of any drug could be confirmed by morphology, and that uncertainty or lack of cause-effect relationships can be diminished if the biopsy is taken as close as possible to the apogee of the clinical course. In life-threatening situations liver biopsy represents an essential component in the management of the patient. The results of a biopsy may indicate the need for liver transplantation and conclusions derived on the potential hepatotoxicity of cardiovascular or antidiabetic drugs emphasize the importance of this procedure.

The diagnosis of hepatotoxicity due to drugs or their actions is very important since it leads to immediate withdrawal of the causative agent. Elevated serum transaminases are fairly frequent during the course of disease and may not relate exclusively to a liver effect, but severe hepatitis or other type of inflammatory reaction during therapy is rare. Treatment with cardiovascular drugs may cause hepatitis, and among antidiabetics only glyburide and troglitazone appeared to have caused severe, but occasionally fatal, hepatitis. Understanding the complex nature and extent of liver injury and improving the prediction of the outcomes in treatment and prognosis will be important elements for advances in the knowledge and prevention of hepatic reactions to cardiovascular and antidiabetic drugs.

DEDICATION

Drs. de la Iglesia and Haskins regret the untimely passing away of Dr. Feyer, their friend and colleague of many years. This chapter is dedicated to his memory.

REFERENCES

1. Scheen AJ, Lefebvre PJ. Antihyperglycaemic agents. Drug interactions of clinical importance. Drug Safety 1995; 12:32–45.
2. Lahoti S, Lee WM. Hepatotoxicity of anticholesterol, cardiovascular, and endocrine drugs and hormonal agents. Gastroenterol Clin North Am 1995; 24:907–922.
3. de la Iglesia FA, Feuer G, Takada A, Matsuda Y. Morphologic studies on secondary phospholipidosis in human liver. Lab Invest 1974; 30:539–549.
4. Pessayre D, Larrey D. Acute and chronic drug-induced hepatitis. Baillieres Clin Gastroenterol 1988; 2:385–422.
5. Zimmerman HJ. Update of hepatotoxicity due to classes of drugs in common clinical use: nonsteroidal drugs, anti-inflammatory drugs, antibiotics, antihypertensives, and cardiac and psychotropic agents. Semin Liver Dis 1990; 10:322–338.
6. Elkington SG, Schreiber WM, Conn HO. Hepatic injury caused by L-alpha-methyldopa. Circulation 1969; 40:589–595.
7. Eliastam M, Holmes AW. Hepatitis, arthritis and lupus cell phenomena caused by methyldopa. Am J Dig Dis 1971; 16:1014–1018.
8. Poucell S, Ireton J, Valencia-Mayoral P, Downar E, Larratt L, Patterson J, Blendis L, Phillips MJ. Amiodarone-associated phospholipidosis and fibrosis of the liver. Light, immunohistochemical, and electron microscopic studies. Gastroenterology 1984; 86:926–936.
9. Guigui B, Perrot S, Berry JP, Fleury-Feith J, Martin N, Metreau JM, Dhumeaux D, Zafrani ES. Amiodarone-induced hepatic phospholipidosis: a morphological alteration independent of pseudoalcoholic liver disease. Hepatology 1988; 8:1063–1068.
10. Kremer GJ, Kossling FK, Lange HJ, Victor N. Determination of lipids in the liver. Chemical and histological studies on 150 liver punctures. Dtsch Med Wochenschr 1969; 94:163–166 passim.
11. Arranto AJ, Sotaniemi EA. Morphologic alterations in patients with alpha-methyldopa-

induced liver damage after short- and long-term exposure. Scand J Gastroenterol 1981; 16: 853–863.

12. Hoffbrand BI, Fry W, Bunton GL. Cholestatic jaundice due to methyldopa. Br Med J 1974; 3:559.

13. Fisher MM. Mechanisms of drug-induced choleostatis. Semin Liver Dis 1980; 1:151–156.

14. Moses A, Zahger D, Amir G. Cholestatic liver injury after prolonged exposure to methyldopa. Digestion 1989; 42:57–60.

15. Rodman JS, Deutsch DJ, Gutman SI. Methyldopa Hepatitis. A report of six cases and review of the literature. Am J Med 1976; 60:941–948.

16. Herlong HF, Reid PR, Boitnott JK, Maddrey WC. Aprindine hepatitis. Ann Intern Med 1978; 89:359–361.

17. Bartoli E, Massarelli G, Solinas A, Faedda R, Chiandussi L. Acute hepatitis with bridging necrosis due to hydralazine intake: report of a case. Arch Intern Med 1979; 139:698–699.

18. Itoh S, Ichinoe A, Tsukada Y, Itoh Y. Hydralazine-induced hepatitis. Hepatogastroenterology 1981; 28:13–16.

19. Kalantzis N, Gabriel P, Mouzas J, Tiniakos D, Tsigas D, Tiniakos G. Acute amiodarone-induced hepatitis. Hepatogastroenterology 1991; 38:71–74.

20. Chajek T, Lehrer B, Geltner D, Levij IS. Quinidine-induced granulomatous hepatitis. Ann Intern Med 1974; 81:774–776.

21. Geltner D, Chajek T, Rubinger D, Levij IS. Quinidine hypersensitivity and liver involvement: a survey of 32 patients. Gastroenterology 1976; 70:650–652.

22. Gelb A, Grazenas N, Sussman H. Acute granulomatous disease of the liver. Dig Dis 1979; 15:842–847.

23. Bramlet DA, Posalaky Z, Olson R. Granulomatous hepatitis as a manifestation of quinidine hypersensitivity. Arch Intern Med 1980; 140:395–397.

24. Hagley MT, Benak RL, Hulisz DT. Suspected cross-reactivity of enalapril- and captopril-induced hepatotoxicity. Ann Pharmacother 1992; 26:780–781.

25. Arranto AJ, Sotaniemi EA. Histologic follow-up of alpha-methyldopa-induced liver injury. Scand J Gastroenterol 1981; 16:865–872.

26. Surveillance Online: Laboratory Centre for Disease Control, Health Canada, Statistics Canada, Ottawa, Canada, 1998.

27. Diabetes in Canada National Statistics: Health Canada, Statistics Canada, Ottawa, Canada, 1997.

28. Reimold SC. Avoiding drug problems: the safety of drugs for supraventricular tachycardia. Eur Heart J 1997; 18(suppl C):C40–44.

29. Nygaard TW, Sellers TD, Cook TS, DiMarco JP. Adverse reactions to antiarrhythmic drugs during therapy for ventricular arrhythmias. Jama 1986; 256:55–57.

30. Rotmensch HH, Belhassen B, Swanson BN, Shoshani D, Spielman SR, Greenspon AJ, Greenspan AM, Vlasses PH, Horowitz LN. Steady-state serum amiodarone concentrations: relationships with antiarrhythmic efficacy and toxicity. Ann Intern Med 1984; 101:462–469.

31. McGovern B, Garan H, Kelly E, Ruskin JN. Adverse reactions during treatment with amiodarone hydrochloride. Br Med J 1983; 287:175–180.

32. McGovern B, Garan H, Ruskin JN. Serious adverse effects of amiodarone. Clin Cardiol 1984; 7:131–137.

33. Shenasa M, Vaisman U, Wojciechowski M, Denker S, Murthy V, Akhtar M. Abnormal abdominal computerized tomography with amiodarone therapy and clinical significance. Am Heart J 1984; 107:929–933.

34. de Korwin JD, Gagey S, Paille F, Zannad F, Schmitt J. Acute hepatitis attributed to amiodarone. Gastroenterol Clin Biol 1986; 10:688–689.

35. Mason JW. Amiodarone. N Engl J Med 1987; 316:455–466.

36. Vrobel TR, Miller PE, Mostow ND, Rakita L. A general overview of amiodarone toxicity: its prevention, detection, and management. Prog Cardiovasc Dis 1989; 31:393–426.

37. Howard PA. Amiodarone for the maintenance of sinus rhythm in patients with atrial fibrillation. Ann Pharmacother 1995; 29:596–602.

38. Reasor MJ, Kacew S. An evaluation of possible mechanisms underlying amiodarone-induced pulmonary toxicity. Proc Soc Exp Biol Med 1996; 212:297–304.

39. Reasor MJ, Kacew S. Amiodarone pulmonary toxicity: morphologic and biochemical features. Proc Soc Exp Biol Med 1991; 196:1–7.

40. Raeder EA, Podrid PJ, Lown B. Side effects and complications of amiodarone therapy. Am Heart J 1985; 109:975–983.

41. Wilson JS, Podrid PJ. Side effects from amiodarone. Am Heart J 1991; 121:158–171.

42. Fornaciari G, Monducci I, Barone A, Bassi C, Beltrami M, Tomasi C. Amiodarone-induced acute hepatitis: case report. J Clin Gastroenterol 1992; 15:271–273.

43. Martin WJd, Rosenow ECd. Amiodarone pulmonary toxicity: recognition and pathogenesis (Part I). Chest 1988; 93:1067–1075.

44. Martin WJd, Rosenow ECd. Amiodarone pulmonary toxicity: recognition and pathogenesis (Part II). Chest 1988; 93:1242–1248.

45. Fogoros RN, Anderson KP, Winkle RA, Swerdlow CD, Mason JW. Amiodarone: clinical efficacy and toxicity in 96 patients with recurrent, drug-refractory arrhythmias. Circulation 1983; 68:88–94.

46. Rigas B, Rosenfeld LE, Barwick KW, Enriquez R, Helzberg J, Batsford WP, Josephson ME, Riely CA. Amiodarone hepatotoxicity: a clinicopathologic study of five patients. Ann Intern Med 1986; 104:348–351.

47. Rinder HM, Love JC, Wexler R. Amiodarone hepatotoxicity. N Engl J Med 1986; 314:318–319.

48. Tordjman K, Katz I, Bursztyn M, Rosenthal T. Amiodarone and the liver [letter]. Ann Intern Med 1985; 102:411–412.

49. Yagupsky P, Gazala E, Sofer S, Maor E, Abarbanel J. Fatal hepatic failure and encephalopathy associated with amiodarone therapy. J Pediatr 1985; 107:967–970.

50. Pye M, Northcote RJ, Cobbe SM. Acute hepatitis after parenteral amiodarone administration. Br Heart J 1988; 59:690–691.

51. Lewis JH, Ranard RC, Caruso A, Jackson LK, Mullick F, Ishak KG, Seeff LB, Zimmerman HJ. Amiodarone hepatotoxicity: prevalence and clinicopathologic correlations among 104 patients. Hepatology 1989; 9:679–685.

52. Flaharty KK, Chase SL, Yaghsezian HM, Rubin R. Hepatotoxicity associated with amiodarone therapy. Pharmacotherapy 1989; 9:39–44.

53. Anastasiou-Nana MI, Anderson JL, Nanas JN, Lutz JR, Smith RA, Anderson KP, Crapo RO, Call NB. High incidence of clinical and subclinical toxicity associated with amiodarone treatment of refractory tachyarrhythmias. Can J Cardiol 1986; 2:138–145.

54. Simon JB, Manley PN, Brien JF, Armstrong PW. Amiodarone hepatotoxicity simulating alcoholic liver disease. N Engl J Med 1984; 311:167–172.

55. Verma RR, Troup PJ, Komorowski RA, Sarna T. Clinical and morphologic effects of amiodarone on the liver. Gastroenterology 1985; 88:1091–1093.

56. Lewis JH, Mullick F, Ishak KG, Ranard RC, Ragsdale B, Perse RM, Rusnock EJ, Wolke A, Benjamin SB, Seeff LB, et al. Histopathologic analysis of suspected amiodarone hepatotoxicity. Hum Pathol 1990; 21:59–67.

57. Goldman IS, Winkler ML, Raper SE, Barker ME, Keung E, Goldberg HI, Boyer TD. Increased hepatic density and phospholipidosis due to amiodarone. Am J Roentgenol 1985; 144:541–546.

58. Shepherd NA, Dawson AM, Crocker PR, Levison DA. Granular cells as a marker of early amiodarone hepatotoxicity: a pathological and analytical study. J Clin Pathol 1987; 40:418–423.

59. Adams PC, Bennett MK, Holt DW. Hepatic effects of amiodarone. Br J Clin Pract Suppl 1986; 44:81–95.

60. Uchida T, Kao H, Quispe-Sjogren M, Peters RL. Alcoholic foamy degeneration—a pattern of acute alcoholic injury of the liver. Gastroenterology 1983; 84:683–692.

61. Lullmann H, Lullmann-Rauch R, Wassermann O. Drug-induced phospholipidoses. II. Tissue distribution of the amphiphilic drug chlorphentermine. CRC Crit Rev Toxicol 1975; 4:185–218.

62. Hruban Z. Pulmonary and generalized lysosomal storage induced by amphiphilic drugs. Environ Health Perspect 1984; 55:53–76.

63. Dake MD, Madison JM, Montgomery CK, Shellito JE, Hinchcliffe WA, Winkler ML, Bainton DF. Electron microscopic demonstration of lysosomal inclusion bodies in lung, liver, lymph nodes, and blood leukocytes of patients with amiodarone pulmonary toxicity. Am J Med 1985; 78:506–512.

64. Matsuda Y, Ikegami F, Kobayashi K, Hasumura Y, Takada A. Phospholipidosis caused by diethylaminoethoxyhexestrol. Saishin Igaku 1971; 26:2263–2267.

65. Oda T, Shikata T, Naito C, Suzuki H, Kanetaka T. Phospholipid fatty liver: a report of three cases with a new type of fatty liver. Jpn J Exp Med 1970; 40:127–140.

66. Reasor MJ. A review of the biology and toxicologic implications of the induction of lysosomal lamellar bodies by drugs. Toxicol Appl Pharmacol 1989; 97:47–56.

67. Schmitz G, Muller G. Structure and function of lamellar bodies, lipid-protein complexes involved in storage and secretion of cellular lipids. J Lipid Res 1991; 32:1539–1570.

68. Berson A, De Beco V, Letteron P, Robin MA, Moreau C, El Kahwaji J, Verthier N, Feldmann G, Fromenty B, Pessayre D. Steatohepatitis-inducing drugs cause mitochondrial dysfunction and lipid peroxidation in rat hepatocytes. Gastroenterology 1998; 114:764–774.

69. Fromenty B, Pessayre D. Impaired mitochondrial function in microvesicular steatosis. Effects of drugs, ethanol, hormones and cytokines. J Hepatol 1997; 26:43–53.

70. Funck-Brentano C, Jacqz-Aigrain E, Leenhardt A, Roux A, Poirier JM, Jaillon P. Influence of amiodarone on genetically determined drug metabolism in humans. Clin Pharmacol Ther 1991; 50:259–266.

71. Saal AK, Werner JA, Greene HL, Sears GK, Graham EL. Effect of amiodarone on serum quinidine and procainamide levels. Am J Cardiol 1984; 53:1264–1267.

72. Plomteux G, Heusghem C, Ernould H, Vandeghen N. Long-term hepatic tolerance of amiodarone in the clinic. Eur J Pharmacol 1969; 8:369–376.

73. Rumessen JJ. Hepatotoxicity of amiodarone. Acta Med Scand 1986; 219:235–239.

74. Harris L, McKenna WJ, Rowland E, Holt DW, Storey GC, Krikler DM. Side effects of long-term amiodarone therapy. Circulation 1983; 67:45–51.

75. Harris L, McKenna WJ, Rowland E, Krikler DM. Side effects and possible contraindications of amiodarone use. Am Heart J 1983; 106:916–923.

76. Ishak KG. The liver. In: RH Riddell, ed. Pathology of Drug-Induced and Toxic Disease. London: Churchill Livingstone, 1982:457–513.

77. Robinson K, Mulrow JP, Rowland E, McKenna WJ. Long-term effects of amiodarone on hepatic function. Am J Cardiol 1989; 64:95–96.

78. Yap SH, Rijntjes PJ, Moshage HJ, Croes H, Jap PH. Amiodarone-induced lysosomal inclusions in primary cultures of human hepatocytes. Gastroenterology 1987; 92:272–273.

79. Svensson CK, Chong MT. Effect of amiodarone on the disposition of acetaminophen in the rat. J Pharm Sci 1989; 78:900–902.

80. Lim PK, Trewby PN, Storey GC, Hole DW. Neuropathy and fatal hepatitis in a patient receiving amiodarone. Br Med J 1984; 288: 1638–1639.

81. Gilinsky NH, Briscoe GW, Kuo CS. Fatal amiodarone hepatoxicity. Am J Gastroenterol 1988; 83:161–163.

82. Steadman's Physicians' Desk Reference. Montvale, NJ: Medical Economics, 2000.

83. Morelli S, Guido V, De Marzio P, Aguglia F, Balsano F. Early hepatitis during intravenous amiodarone administration. Cardiology 1991; 78:291–294.

84. Rhodes A, Eastwood JB, Smith SA. Early acute hepatitis with parenteral amiodarone: a toxic effect of the vehicle? Gut 1993; 34:565–566.

85. Hilleman D, Miller MA, Parker R, Doering P, Pieper JA. Optimal management of amiodarone therapy: efficacy and side effects. Pharmacotherapy 1998; 18:138S–145S.

86. Snir Y, Pick N, Riesenberg K, Yanai-Inbar I, Zirkin H, Schlaeffer F. Fatal hepatic failure due to prolonged amiodarone treatment. J Clin Gastroenterol 1995; 20:265–266.

87. Stevenson RN, Nayani TH, Davies JR. Acute hepatic dysfunction following parenteral amiodarone administration. Postgrad Med J 1989; 65:707–708.

88. Babany G, Mallat A, Zafrani ES, Saint-Marc Girardin MF, Carcone B, Dhumeaux D. Chronic liver disease after low daily doses of amiodarone: report of three cases. J Hepatol 1986; 3: 228–232.

89. Lupon-Roses J, Simo-Canonge R, Lu-Cortez L, Permanyer-Miralda G, Allende-Monclus H. Probable early acute hepatitis with parenteral amiodarone. Clin Cardiol 1986; 9:223–225.

90. Seydel JK, Wassermann O. NMR-studies on the molecular basis of drug-induced phospholipidosis. II. Interaction between several amphiphilic drugs and phospholipids. Biochem Pharmacol 1976; 25:2357–2364.

91. Ruben Z, Rorig KJ, Kacew S. Perspectives on intracellular storage and transport of cationic-lipophilic drugs. Proc Soc Exp Biol Med 1993; 203:140–149.

92. Capron-Chivrac D, Reix N, Quenum C, Capron JP. Acute hepatopathy caused by amiodarone. Study of a case and review of the literature. Gastroenterol Clin Biol 1985; 9:535–539.

93. Shaikh NA, Downar E, Butany J. Amiodarone—an inhibitor of phospholipase activity: a comparative study of the inhibitory effects of amiodarone, chloroquine and chlorpromazine. Mol Cell Biochem 1987; 76:163–172.

94. Reasor MJ, Ogle CL, Walker ER, Kacew S. Amiodarone-induced phospholipidosis in rat alveolar macrophages. Am Rev Respir Dis 1988; 137:510–518.

95. Hostetler KY, Giordano JR, Jellison EJ. In vitro inhibition of lysosomal phospholipase A1 of rat lung by amiodarone and desethylamiodarone. Biochim Biophys Acta 1988; 959:316–321.

96. Hostetler KY, Reasor MJ, Walker ER, Yazaki PJ, Frazee BW. Role of phospholipase A inhibition in amiodarone pulmonary toxicity in rats. Biochim Biophys Acta 1986; 875:400–405.

97. Jones DB, Mullick FG, Hoofnagle JH, Baranski B. Reye's syndrome-like illness in a patient receiving amiodarone. Am J Gastroenterol 1988; 83:967–969.

98. Waldman RJ, Hall WN, McGee H, Van Amburg G. Aspirin as a risk factor in Reye's syndrome. JAMA 1982; 247:3089–3094.

99. Starko KM, Mullick FG. Hepatic and cerebral pathology findings in children with fatal salicylate intoxication: further evidence for a causal relation between salicylate and Reye's syndrome. Lancet 1983; 1:326–329.

100. Fasola AF, Carmichael R. The pharmacology and clinical evaluation of aprindine a new antiarrhythmic agent. Acta Cardiol 1974; 18(suppl):317–333.

101. Reid PR, Greene HL, Varghese PJ. Suppression of refractory arrhythmias by aprindine in patients with the Wolff-Parkinson-White syndrome. Br Heart J 1977; 39:1353–1360.

102. Stoel I, Hagemeijer F. Aprindine: a review. Eur Heart J 1980; 1:147–156.

103. Elisaf M, Stefanaki-Nikou S, Voulgarelis M, Masalas C, Tsianos EV. Aprindine-induced hepatic granulomata. J Hepatol 1992; 14:276–279.

104. van Leeuwen R, Meyboom RH. Agranulocytosis and aprindine [letter]. Lancet 1976; 2:1137.

105. Elewaut A, Van Durme JP, Goethals L, Kauffman JM, Mussche M, Elinck W, Roels H, Bogaert M, Barbier F. Aprindine-induced liver injury. Acta Gastroenterol Belg 1977; 40: 236–243.

106. Brandes JW, Schmitz-Moormann P, Lehmann FG, Martini GA. Jaundice after aprindin. Dtsch Med Wochenschr 1976; 101:111–113.

107. Deisseroth A, Morganroth J, Winokur S. Quinidine-induced liver disease. Ann Intern Med 1972; 77:595–597.

108. Handler SD, Hirsch NR, Haas K, Davidson FZ. Quinidine hepatitis. Arch Intern Med 1975; 135:871–872.

109. Koch MJ, Seeff LB, Crumley CE, Rabin L, Burns WA. Quinidine hepatotoxicity: a report of a case and review of the literature. Gastroenterology 1976; 70:1136–1140.

110. Murphy PJ, Rymer W. Quinidine-induced liver disease? Ann Intern Med 1973; 78:785–786.

111. McLean AE, McLean E, Judah JD. Cellular necrosis in the liver induced and modified by drugs. Int Rev Exp Pathol 1965; 4:127–157.

112. Mitchell JR, Jollows DJ. Progress in hepatology. Metabolic activation of drugs to toxic substances. Gastroenterology 1975; 68:392–410.

113. Meinertz T, Langer KH, Kasper W, Just H. Disopyramide-induced intrahepatic cholestatis. Lancet 1977; 2:828–829.

114. Doody PT. Disopyramide hepatotoxicity and disseminated intravascular coagulation. South Med J 1982; 75:496–498.

115. Kalant H, Roschlau WH, Sellers EM. Principles of Medical Pharmacology, 4th ed. Toronto: University of Toronto, 1985:207–208.

116. Harron DW, Brogden RN. Acecainide (N-acetylprocainamide): a review of its pharmacodynamic and pharmacokinetic properties, and therapeutic potential in cardiac arrhythmias. Drugs 1990; 39:720–740.

117. Adams LE, Sanders CE, Jr., Budinsky RA, Donovan-Brand R, Roberts SM, Hess EV. Immunomodulatory effects of procainamide metabolites: their implications in drug-related lupus. J Lab Clin Med 1989; 113:482–492.

118. Amadio P, Jr., Cummings DM, Dashow L. Procainamide, quinidine, and lupus erythematosus. Ann Intern Med 1985; 102:419.

119. Lawson DH, Jick H. Adverse reactions to procainamide. Br J Clin Pharmacol 1977; 4:507–511.

120. Ahn CS, Tow DE. Intrahepatic cholestasis due to hypersensitivity reaction to procainamide. Arch Intern Med 1990; 150:2589–2590.

121. Chuang LC, Tunier AP, Akhtar N, Levine SM. Possible case of procainamide-induced intrahepatic cholestatic jaundice. Ann Pharmacother 1993; 27:434–437.

122. Hellman E. Allergy to procainamide. JAMA 1952; 149:1393–1394.

123. King JA, Blount REJ. An unexpected reaction to procainamide. JAMA 1963; 186:603–604.

124. Leibowitz S. Chills and fever following oral use of procainamide. N Engl J Med 1951; 245:1006.

125. Rotmensch HH, Yust I, Siegman-Igra Y, Liron M, Ilie B, Vardinon N. Granulomatous hepatitis: a hypersensitivity response to procainamide. Ann Intern Med 1978; 89:646–647.

126. Worman HJ, Ip JH, Winters SL, Tepper DC, Gomes AJ. Hypersensitivity reaction associated with acute hepatic dysfunction following a single intravenous dose of procainamide. J Intern Med 1992; 232:361–363.

127. Lemke LE, McQueen CA. Acetylation and its role in the mutagenicity of the antihypertensive agent hydralazine. Drug Metab Dispos 1995; 23:559–565.

128. Okumura K, Kita T, Chikazawa S, Komada F, Iwakawa S, Tanigawara Y. Genotyping of N-acetylation polymorphism and correlation with procainamide metabolism. Clin Pharmacol Ther 1997; 61:509–517.

129. Nebert DW. Polymorphisms in drug-metabolizing enzymes: what is their clinical relevance and why do they exist? Am J Hum Genet 1997; 60:265–271.

130. Aw T, Hanna P, Petrini J, Kaplowitz N. Hepatic Drug Metabolism and Drug-Induced Liver Injury. In: G Gitnick, ed. Current Hepatology. Vol. 5. Chicago: Yearbook Medical Publishers, 1985:113–196.

131. Stumpf JL. Fatal hepatotoxicity induced by hydralazine or labetalol. Pharmacotherapy 1991; 11:415–418.

132. Alarcon-Segovia D, Wakim KG, Worthington JW, Ward LE. Clinical and experimental studies on the hydralazine syndrome and its relationship to systemic lupus erythematosus. Medicine 1967; 46:1–33.

133. Batchelor JR, Welsh KI, Tinoco RM, Dollery CT, Hughes GR, Bernstein R, Ryan P, Naish PF, Aber GM, Bing RF, Russell GI. Hydralazine-induced systemic lupus erythematosus: influence of HLA-DR and sex on susceptibility. Lancet 1980; 1:1107–1109.

134. Irias JJ. Hydralazine-induced lupus erythematosus-like syndrome. Am J Dis Child 1975; 129: 862–864.

135. Wechsler B, Brion NO, Colau C, Ximenes H, Godeau P. Lupus erythematosus induced by dihydralazine. Nouv Presse Med 1979; 8:3754–3755.

136. Pariente EA, Pessayre D, Bernuau J, Degott C, Benhamou JP. Dihydralazine hepatitis: report of a case and review of the literature. Digestion 1983; 27:47–52.

137. Shaefer MS, Markin RS, Wood RP, Shaw BW, Jr. Hydralazine-induced cholestatic jaundice following liver transplantation. Transplantation 1989; 47:203–204.

138. Jori GP, Peschile C. Hydralazine disease associated with transient granulomas in the liver. A case report. Gastroenterology 1973; 64:1163–1167.

139. Itoh S, Yamaba Y, Ichinoe A, Tsukada Y. Hydralazine-induced liver injury. Dig Dis Sci 1980; 25:884–887.

140. Forster HS. Hepatitis from hydralazine. N Engl J Med 1980; 302:1362.

141. Barnett DB, Hudson SA, Golightly PW. Hydrallazine-induced hepatitis? Br Med J 1980; 280:1165–1166.

142. Knoblauch M, Cueni B, Spycher M, Schmid M. [Dihydralazine-induced acute hepatitis with IgM deficiency]. Schweiz Med Wochenschr 1977; 107:651–656.

143. Enat R, Rader G, Barzilai D. [Liver damage caused by adelphan]. Schweiz Med Wochenschr 1977; 107:657–658.

144. Koch-Weser J. Medical intelligence drug therapy. N Engl J Med 1976; 295:320–323.

145. Weber WW, Hein DW. *N*-Acetylation pharmacogenetics. Pharmacol Rev 1985; 37:25–79.

146. Weber WW. Populations and genetic polymorphisms. Mol Diagn 1999; 4:299–307.

147. Hutterer F, Klion FM, Wengraf A, Schaffner F, Popper H. Hepatocellular adaptation and injury: structural and biochemical changes following dieldrin and methyl butter yellow. Lab Invest 1969; 20:455–464.

148. Nataf J, Bernau J, Larry D, Guillin MC, Ruff B, Benhamou JP. A new anti-liver microsome antibody: a specific marker of dihydralazine-induced hepatitis. Gastroenterology 1986; 90: 1751.

149. Bourdi M, Gautier JC, Mircheva J, Larrey D, Guillouzo A, Andre C, Belloc C, Beaune PH. Antiliver microsomes autoantibodies and dihydralazine-induced hepatitis: specificity of autoantibodies and inductive capacity of the drug. Mol Pharmacol 1992; 42:280–285.

150. Clark JA, Zimmerman HJ, Tanner LA. Labetalol hepatotoxicity. Ann Intern Med 1990; 113: 210–213.

151. Rahn KH. Clinical experience with dual-acting drugs in hypertension. Clin Invest 1992; 70: S39–42.

152. Douglas DD, Yang RD, Jensen P, Thiele DL. Fatal labetalol-induced hepatic injury. Am J Med 1989; 87:235–236.

153. Irvine RO, O'Brien KP, North JDK. Alpha methyldopa in treatment of hypertension. Lancet 1962; 1:300–303.

154. Gillmore BL, Freis ED. Methyldopa in the treatment of hypertension. Med Ann DC 1965; 34:13–18.

154a. Kalant H, Roschlau WH, Sellers EM. Principles of Medical Pharmacology. 4th ed. Toronto: University of Toronto Press, 1985; 207–208.

154b. Beanlands DS, Allard PP, Wilson M, Orbeck KW, Helman AB, Lefebvre R. Comparison of efficacy and safety of pindolol and alpha-methyldopa in treatment of mild to moderate hypertension: results of a double-blind evaluative study. Clin Invest Med 1978; 1(3–4):139–145.

155. Pai RG, Pai SM. Methyldopa-induced reversible immune thrombocytopenia. Am J Med 1988; 85:123.

156. Manohitharajah SM, Jenkins WJ, Roberts PD, Clarke RC. Methyldopa and associated thrombocytopenia. Br Med J 1971; 1:494.

157. Breland BD, Hicks GS, Jr. Hepatitis and hemolytic anemia associated with methyldopa therapy. Drug Intell Clin Pharm 1982; 16:489–492.

158. Goldstein GB, Lam KC, Mistilis SP. Drug-induced active chronic hepatitis. Am J Dig Dis 1973; 18:177–184.

159. Hoyumpa AM, Jr., Connell AM. Methyldopa hepatitis: report of three cases. Am J Dig Dis 1973; 18:213–222.

160. Maddrey WC, Boitnott JK. Severe hepatitis from methyldopa. Gastroenterology 1975; 68: 351–360.

161. Schweitzer IL, Peters RL. Acute submassive hepatic necrosis due to methyldopa: a case demonstrating possible initiation of chronic liver disease. Gastroenterology 1974; 66:1203–1211.

162. Thomas E, Bhuta S, Rosenthal WS. Methyldopa-induced liver injury: rapid progression to fatal postnecrotic cirrhosis. Arch Pathol Lab Med 1976; 100:132–135.

163. Tysell JE, Jr., Knauer M. Hepatitis induced by methyldopa (aldomet): report of a case and a review of the literature. Am J Dig Dis 1971; 16:848–855.

164. Seggie J, Saunders SJ, Kirsch RE, Campbell JA, Gitlin N, Clain D, Terblanche J. Patterns of hepatic injury induced by methyldopa. S Afr Med J 1979; 55:75–83.

165. Sotaniemi EA, Hokkanen OT, Ahokas JT, Pelkonen RO, Ahlqvist J. Hepatic injury and drug metabolism in patients with alpha-methyldopa-induced liver damage. Eur J Clin Pharmacol 1977; 12:429–435.

166. Toghill PJ, Smith PG, Benton P, Brown RC, Matthews HL. Methyldopa liver damage. Br Med J 1974; 3:545–548.

167. Furhoff AK. Adverse reactions with methyldopa—a decade's reports. Acta Med Scand 1978; 203:425–428.

168. Thomas E, Rosenthal WS, Zapiach L, Micci D. Spectrum of methyldopa liver injury. Am J Gastroenterol 1977; 68:125–133.

169. Williams ER, Khan MA. Liver damage in patients on methyldopa. J Ther Clin Res 1967; 1:5–7.

170. Balazs M, Kovach G. Chronic aggressive hepatitis after methyldopa treatment: case report with electron-microscopic study. Hepatogastroenterology 1981; 28:199–202.

171. Balazs MS, Varkonyi S, Juhasz J. Electronmikroskopische Untersuchungen in fällen von chronisch-aggressiver hepatitis. Acta Hepatogastroenterol 1973; 20:399–409.

172. Gerlach U, Manitz G, Themann H. Fine structural studies in active chronic hepatitis with special reference to the mesenchyma. Acta Hepatosplenol 1969; 16:90–105.

173. Schmid M. Laboratory findings in chronic hepatitis. Dtsch Med Wochenschr 1967; 92:305–309.

174. Sherlock S. Diseases of the Liver and Biliary System. Oxford: Blackwell Scientific, 1987: 390–424.

175. Neuberger J, Kenna JG, Nouri Aria K, Williams R. Antibody mediated hepatocyte injury in methyl dopa induced hepatotoxicity. Gut 1985; 26:1233–1239.

176. Kirtland HHd, Mohler DN, Horwitz DA. Methyldopa inhibition of suppressor-lymphocyte function: a proposed cause of autoimmune hemolytic anemia. N Engl J Med 1980; 302:825–832.

177. Myer SL, Knell AJ. Cirrhosis and haemolysis complicating methyldopa treatment. Br Med J 1977; 1:879.

178. Ylikallio A, Sotaniemi EA. Drug metabolism and liver function after methyldopa withdrawal. Br J Clin Pharmacol 1980; 10:115–119.

179. Rehman OU, Keith TA, Gall EA. Methyldopa-induced submassive hepatic necrosis. JAMA 1973; 224:1390–1392.

180. Puppala AR, Steinheber FU. Fulminant hepatic failure associated with methyldopa. Am J Gastroenterol 1977; 68:578–581.

181. Sataline L, Lowell D. Letter: Methyldopa toxicity. Gastroenterology 1976; 70:148–149.

182. Gilliss MR. Papaverine—safety in use. J Am Geriatr Soc 1973; 21:200–201.

183. Ronnov-Jessen V, Tjernlund A. Hepatotoxicity due to treatment with papaverine: report of four cases. N Engl J Med 1969; 281:1333–1335.

184. Pathy MS, Reynolds AJ. Papaverine and hepatotoxicity. Postgrad Med J 1980; 56:488–490.

185. Kiaer HW, Olsen S, Ronnov-Jessen V. Hepatotoxicity of papaverine. Arch Pathol 1974; 98: 292–296.

186. Materson BJ. Adverse effects of angiotensin-converting enzyme inhibitors in antihypertensive therapy with focus on quinapril. Am J Cardiol 1992; 69:46C–53C.

187. Kuhn M. Angiotensin-converting enzyme inhibitors. AACN Clin Issues Crit Care Nurs 1992; 3:461–471.

188. McAreavey D, Robertson JI. Angiotensin converting enzyme inhibitors and moderate hypertension. Drugs 1990; 40:326–345.

189. Compendium of Pharmaceuticals and Specialties. Vol. 33. Canadian Pharmaceutical Association, Toronto, 1998.

190. Hagley MT, Hulisz DT, Burns CM. Hepatotoxicity associated with angiotensin-converting enzyme inhibitors [see comments]. Ann Pharmacother 1993; 27:228–231.

191. Jurima-Romet M, Huang HS. Comparative cytotoxicity of angiotensin-converting enzyme inhibitors in cultured rat hepatocytes. Biochem Pharmacol 1993; 46:2163–2170.

192. Vandenburg M, Parfrey P, Wright P, Lazda E. Hepatitis associated with captopril treatment. Br J Clin Pharmacol 1981; 11:105–106.

193. Ryckelynck JP, Batho JM, Peny J, Beuve-Mery P. Hepatitis due to captopril. Nouv Presse Med 1982; 11:1950–1951.

194. Rahmat J, Gelfand RL, Gelfand MC, Winchester JF, Schreiner GE, Zimmerman HJ. Captopril-associated cholestatic jaundice. Ann Intern Med 1985; 102:56–58.

195. Lunel F, Grippon P, Cadranel JF, Victor N, Opolon P. Acute hepatitis after taking enalapril maleate (Renitec). Gastroenterol Clin Biol 1987; 11:174–175.

196. Hurault de Ligny B, Mariot A, Kessler M, Caraman PL, Netter P. Hepatitis during captopril combination therapy. Therapie 1982; 37:698–700.

197. Hagley MT, Hulisz DT, Burns CM. Hepatotoxicity associated with angiotensin-converting enzyme inhibitors. Ann Pharmacother 1993; 27:228–231.

198. Bellary SV, Isaacs PE, Scott AW. Captopril and the liver. Lancet 1989; 2:514.

199. Bailer SO, Isaac DE. Captopril and the liver. Lancet 1989; 2:154–156.

200. Todd P, Levison D, Farthing MJ. Enalapril-related cholestatic jaundice. J R Soc Med 1990; 83:271–272.

201. Shionoiri H, Nomura S, Oda H, Kimura K, Takasaki I, Takagi N. Hepatitis associated with captopril and enalapril but not delapril in a patient with congestive heart failure receiving chronic hemodialysis. Curr Ther Res 1986; 42:1171–1176.

202. Larrey D, Babany G, Bernuau J, Andrieux J, Degott C, Pessayre D, Benhamou JP. Fulminant hepatitis after lisinopril administration. Gastroenterology 1990; 99:1832–1833.

203. Hagley MT. Captopril-induced cholestatic jaundice. South Med J 1991; 84:100.

204. Daniels DA, Bayliff CD, Paterson NA, Massel D. Angiotensin-converting enzyme inhibitor associated hepatotoxicity. Can J Hosp Pharm 1996; 49:36–38.

205. Ross R. The pathogenesis of atherosclerosis: a perspective for the 1990s. Nature 1993; 362: 801–809.

206. Furberg CD, Byington RP, Crouse JR, Espeland MA. Pravastatin, lipids, and major coronary events. Am J Cardiol 1994; 73:1133–1134.

207. Todd PA, Ward A. Gemfibrozil. A review of its pharmacodynamic and pharmacokinetic properties, and therapeutic use in dyslipidaemia. Drugs 1988; 36:314–339.

208. de la Iglesia FA, Lewis JE, Buchanan RA, Marcus EL, McMahon G. Light and electron

microscopy of liver in hyperlipoproteinemic patients under long-term gemfibrozil treatment. Atherosclerosis 1982; 43:19–37.

209. Gotto AM, Jr. Dyslipidemia and atherosclerosis. A forecast of pharmaceutical approaches. Circulation 1993; 87:III54–59.

210. Statistics NCfH. Total Serum Cholesterol Levels of Adults 20 to 74 Years of Age: United States, 1976–1980. Washington DC: Department of Health and Human Services, 1986.

211. Ancla M, Beaumont V. Etude du foie au microscope electronique dans deux variétés d'hyperlipidemies majeures. Pathol Biol 1966; 14:1167–1177.

212. Kovacs K, Lee R, Little JA. Ultrastructural changes of hepatocytes in hyperlipoproteinaemia. Lancet 1972; 1:752–753.

213. Ma MH, Goldfisher S, Biempica L. Morphology of the normal liver cell. Prog Liver Dis 1972; 4:1–17.

214. Baggenstoss AH, Christensen NA, Berge KG, Baldus WP, Spiekerman RE, Ellefson RD. Fine structural changes in the liver in hypercholesteremic patients receiving long-term nicotinic acid therapy. Mayo Clin Proc 1967; 42:385–399.

215. Kohn RM, Montes M. Hepatic fibrosis following long acting nicotinic acid therapy: a case report. Am J Med Sci 1969; 258:94–99.

216. Kemmer C, Hanefeld M. Ultrastructural results in liver biopsies of patients with hyperlipoproteinaemia. Zentralbl Allg Pathol 1977; 121:243–253.

217. Hanefeld M, Kemmer C, Leonhardt W, Kunze KD, Jaross W, Haller H. Effects of p-chlorophenoxyisobutyric acid (CPIB) on the human liver. Atherosclerosis 1980; 36:159–172.

218. Voss KS, Kemmer C. Image processing in pathology part 8: internal structure of mitochondria during treatment of HLP-patients with regadrin. Exp Pathol 1987; 15:311–318.

219. Blumcke S, Schwartzkopff W, Lobeck H, Edmondson NA, Prentice DE, Blane GF. Influence of fenofibrate on cellular and subcellular liver structure in hyperlipidemic patients. Atherosclerosis 1983; 46:105–116.

220. Winter SL, Boyer JL. Hepatic toxicity from large doses of vitamin B3 (nicotinamide). N Engl J Med 1973; 289:1180–1182.

221. Etchason JA, Miller TD, Squires RW, Allison TG, Gau GT, Marttila JK, Kottke BA. Niacin-induced hepatitis: a potential side effect with low-dose time-release niacin. Mayo Clin Proc 1991; 66:23–28.

222. Christensen NA, Anchor RW, Berge KG. Nicotinic acid treatment of hypercholesterolemia. JAMA 1961; 177:546.

223. Riven AV. Jaundice occurring during nicotinic acid therapy for hypercholesterolemia. JAMA 1959; 170:2088–2089.

224. Henkin Y, Johnson KC, Segrest JP. Rechallenge with crystalline niacin after drug-induced hepatitis from sustained-release niacin. JAMA 1990; 264:241–243.

225. Dalton TA, Berry RS. Hepatotoxicity associated with sustained-release niacin. Am J Med 1992; 93:102–104.

226. Einstein N, Baker A, Galper J, Wolfe H. Jaundice due to nicotinic acid therapy. Am J Dig Dis 1975; 20:282–286.

227. Patel SD, Taylor HC. Intrahepatic cholestasis during nicotinic acid therapy. Cleve Clin J Med 1994; 61:70–75; quiz 80–72.

228. Rader JI, Calvert RJ, Hathcock JN. Hepatic toxicity of unmodified and time-release preparations of niacin. Am J Med 1992; 92:77–81.

229. Boiteux-Antoine AF, Magdalou J, Fournel-Gigleux S, Siest G. Comparative induction of drug-metabolizing enzymes by hypolipidaemic compounds. Gen Pharmacol 1989; 20:407–412.

230. Reddy JK, Azarnoff DL, Hignite CE. Hypolipidaemic hepatic peroxisome proliferators form a novel class of chemical carcinogens. Nature 1980; 283:397–398.

231. de la Iglesia FA, Farber E. Hypolipidemics carcinogenicity and extrapolation of experimental results for human safet assessments. Toxicol Pathol 1982; 10:152–174.

232. Blum CB. Comparison of properties of four inhibitors of 3-hydroxy-3-methylglutaryl-coenzyme A reductase. Am J Cardiol 1994; 73:3D–11D.

233. Monk JP, Todd PA. Bezafibrate. A review of its pharmacodynamic and pharmacokinetic properties, and therapeutic use in hyperlipidaemia. Drugs 1987; 33:539–576.

234. Sgro C, Escousse A. Side effects of fibrates (except liver and muscle). Therapie 1991; 46: 351–354.

235. Valmalle R, Bacq Y, Furet Y, Dorval E, Barbieux JP, Metman EH. Fatal acute hepatitis during treatment with perhexiline maleate and bezafibrate. Gastroenterol Clin Biol 1989; 13: 530–531.

236. Bacon BR, Farahvash MJ, Janney CG, Neuschwander-Tetri BA. Nonalcoholic steatohepatitis: an expanded clinical entity. Gastroenterology 1994; 107:1103–1109.

237. Hanefeld M, Kemmer C, Kadner E. Relationship between morphological changes and lipid-lowering action of p-chlorphenoxyisobutyric acid (CPIB) on hepatic mitochondria and peroxisomes in man. Atherosclerosis 1983; 46:239–246.

238. Schwandt P, Klinge O, Immich H. Clofibrate and the liver. Lancet 1978; 2:325.

239. Gray RH, de la Iglesia FA. Quantitative microscopy comparison of peroxisome proliferation by the lipid-regulating agent gemfibrozil in several species. Hepatology 1984; 4:520–530.

240. de la Iglesia FA, Pinn SM, Lucas JA, McGuire EJ. Quantitative stereology of peroxisomes in hepatocytes from hyperlipoproteinemic patients receiving gemfibrozil. Micron 1981; 12: 97–107.

241. Vachon JM. Hepatitis caused by procetofen. Nouv Presse Med 1980; 9:2740.

242. Chatrenet P, Regimbeau C, Ramain JP, Penot J, Bruandet P. Chronic active cirrhogenic hepatitis induced by fenofibrate. Gastroenterol Clin Biol 1993; 17:612–613.

243. Homberg JC, Abuaf N, Helmy-Khalil S, Biour M, Poupon R, Islam S, Darnis F, Levy VG, Opolon P, Beaugrand M, et al. Drug-induced hepatitis associated with anticytoplasmic organelle autoantibodies. Hepatology 1985; 5:722–727.

244. Roberts WC. Safety of fenofibrate—US and worldwide experience. Cardiology 1989; 76: 169–179.

245. Gariot P, Barrat E, Mejean L, Pointel JP, Drouin P, Debry G. Fenofibrate and human liver. Lack of proliferation of peroxisomes. Arch Toxicol 1983; 53:151–163.

246. Gariot P, Barrat E, Drouin P, Genton P, Pointel JP, Foliguet B, Kolopp M, Debry G. Morphometric study of human hepatic cell modifications induced by fenofibrate. Metabolism 1987; 36:203–210.

247. de la Iglesia FA, Gray RH, McGuire EJ. Subcellular organelle biogenesis and dynamics in peroxisome proliferation. J Am Coll Toxicol 1992; 11:343–348.

248. Blumenthal RS. Statins: effective antiatherosclerotic therapy. Am Heart J 2000; 139:577–583.

249. Burnett JR, Wilcox LJ, Telford DE, Kleinstiver SJ, Barrett PH, Newton RS, Huff MW. The magnitude of decrease in hepatic very low density lipoprotein apolipoprotein B secretion is determined by the extent of 3-hydroxy-3-methylglutaryl coenzyme A reductase inhibition in miniature pigs. Endocrinology 1999; 140:5293–5302.

250. Johnston TP, Baker JC, Hall D, Jamal S, Palmer WK, Emeson EE. Regression of poloxamer 407–induced atherosclerotic lesions in C57BL/6 mice using atorvastatin. Atherosclerosis 2000; 149:303–313.

251. Bocan TM, Mazur MJ, Mueller SB, Brown EQ, Sliskovic DR, O'Brien PM, Creswell MW, Lee H, Uhlendorf PD, Roth BD, et al. Antiatherosclerotic activity of inhibitors of 3-hydroxy-3-methylglutaryl coenzyme A reductase in cholesterol-fed rabbits: a biochemical and morphological evaluation. Atherosclerosis 1994; 111:127–142.

252. Bocan TM, Mueller SB, Brown EQ, Lee P, Bocan MJ, Rea T, Pape ME. HMG-CoA reductase and ACAT inhibitors act synergistically to lower plasma cholesterol and limit atherosclerotic lesion development in the cholesterol-fed rabbit. Atherosclerosis 1998; 139:21–30.

253. Bustos C, Hernandez-Presa MA, Ortego M, Tunon J, Ortega L, Perez F, Diaz C, Hernandez

G, Egido J. HMG-CoA reductase inhibition by atorvastatin reduces neointimal inflammation in a rabbit model of atherosclerosis. J Am Coll Cardiol 1998; 32:2057–2064.

254. Burnett JR, Wilcox LJ, Telford DE, Kleinstiver SJ, Barrett PH, Newton RS, Huff MW, Barrett P. Inhibition of HMG-CoA reductase by atorvastatin decreases both VLDL and LDL apolipoprotein B production in miniature pigs. Arterioscler Thromb Vasc Biol 1997; 17: 2589–2600.

255. Jones PH, Farmer JA, Cressman MD, McKenney JM, Wright JT, Proctor JD, Berkson DM, Farnham DJ, Wolfson PM, Colfer HT, et al. Once-daily pravastatin in patients with primary hypercholesterolemia: a dose-response study. Clin Cardiol 1991; 14:146–151.

256. Vega GL, Grundy SM. Management of primary mixed hyperlipidemia with lovastatin. Arch Intern Med 1990; 150:1313–1319.

257. Vega GL, Krauss RM, Grundy SM. Pravastatin therapy in primary moderate hypercholesterolaemia: changes in metabolism of apolipoprotein B-containing lipoproteins. J Intern Med 1990; 227:81–94.

258. Grundy SM, Vega GL, Garg A. Use of 3-hydroxy-3-methylglutaryl coenzyme A reductase inhibitors in various forms of dyslipidemia. Am J Cardiol 1990; 66:31B–38B.

259. Krause BR, Newton RS. Lipid-lowering activity of atorvastatin and lovastatin in rodent species: triglyceride-lowering in rats correlates with efficacy in LDL animal models. Atherosclerosis 1995; 117:237–244.

260. Pierce LR, Wysowski DK, Gross TP. Myopathy and rhabdomyolysis associated with lovastatin-gemfibrozil combination therapy. JAMA 1990; 264:71–75.

261. Bottorff M. 'Fire and forget?'—pharmacological considerations in coronary care. Atherosclerosis 1999; 147(Suppl 1):S23–30.

262. Carpentier Y, Ducobu J, Sternon J. Atorvastatin (Lipitor). Rev Med Brux 1999; 20:427–433.

263. Lea AP, McTavish D. Atorvastatin. A review of its pharmacology and therapeutic potential in the management of hyperlipidaemias. Drugs 1997; 53:828–847.

264. Wierzbicki AS, Lumb PJ, Semra YK, Crook MA. High-dose atorvastatin therapy in severe heterozygous familial hypercholesterolaemia. QJ Med 1998; 91:291–294.

265. Black DM, Bakker-Arkema RG, Nawrocki JW. An overview of the clinical safety profile of atorvastatin (lipitor), a new HMG-CoA reductase inhibitor. Arch Intern Med 1998; 158: 577–584.

266. Nawrocki JW, Weiss SR, Davidson MH, Sprecher DL, Schwartz SL, Lupien PJ, Jones PH, Haber HE, Black DM. Reduction of LDL cholesterol by 25% to 60% in patients with primary hypercholesterolemia by atorvastatin, a new HMG-CoA reductase inhibitor. Arterioscler Thromb Vasc Biol 1995; 15:678–682.

267. Stalenhoef AF, Mol MJ, Stuyt PM. Efficacy and tolerability of simvastatin (MK-733). Am J Med 1989; 87:39S–43S.

268. Walker JF. Simvastatin: the clinical profile. Am J Med 1989; 87:44S–46S.

269. The Pravastatin Multinational Study Group for Cardiac Risk Patients. Effects of pravastatin in patients with serum total cholesterol levels from 5.2 to 7.8 mmol/liter (200 to 300 mg/dl) plus two additional atherosclerotic risk factors. Am J Cardiol 1993; 72:1031–1037.

270. Walker JF. HMG CoA reductase inhibitors. Current clinical experience. Drugs 1988; 36:83–86.

271. Tobert JA. Efficacy and long-term adverse effect pattern of lovastatin. Am J Cardiol 1988; 62:28J–34J.

272. Strauss WE, Lapsley D, Gaziano JM. Comparative efficacy and tolerability of low-dose pravastatin versus lovastatin in patients with hypercholesterolemia. Am Heart J 1999; 137:458–462.

273. Ceska R. Fluvastatin in the treatment of hyperlipoproteinemia, initial experience. Vnitr Lek 1996; 42:533–536.

274. Bilheimer DW. Long-term clinical tolerance of lovastatin and simvastatin. Cardiology 1990; 77:58–65.

275. International Conference on Harmonisation; Guidance on data elements for transmission of individual case safety reports; availability. Fed Reg 1998; 60:2396–2404.

276. Alberts AW, MacDonald JS, Till AF, Tobert JA. Lovastatin. Cardiovasc Drug Rev 1989; 7:89–109.

277. Gerson RJ, MacDonald JS, Alberts AW, Kornbrust DJ, Majka JA, Stubbs RJ, Bokelman DL. Animal safety and toxicology of simvastatin and related hydroxy-methylglutaryl-coenzyme A reductase inhibitors. Am J Med 1989; 87:28S–38S.

278. MacDonald JS, Gerson RJ, Kornbrust DJ, Kloss MW, Prahalada S, Berry PH, Alberts AW, Bokelman DL. Preclinical evaluation of lovastatin. Am J Cardiol 1988; 62:16J–27J.

279. Robison RL, Suter W, Cox RH. Carcinogenicity and mutagenicity studies with fluvastatin, a new, entirely synthetic HMG-CoA reductase inhibitor. Fundam Appl Toxicol 1994; 23:9–20.

280. Owen K, Pick CR, Libretto SE, Adams MJ. Toxicity of a novel HMG-CoA reductase inhibitor in the common marmoset (*Callithrix jacchus*). Hum Exp Toxicol 1994; 13:357–368.

281. Manabe S, Sudo S, Yamashita K, Miyakoshi N, Matsunuma N, Tanase H, Masuda H. Subacute toxicological study in monkeys treated orally with pravastatin sodium for 5 weeks. J Toxicol Sci 1989; 14 Suppl 1:57–83.

282. Gerson RJ, Allen HL, Lankas GR, MacDonald JS, Alberts AW, Bokelman DL. The toxicity of a fluorinated-biphenyl HMG-CoA reductase inhibitor in beagle dogs. Fundam Appl Toxicol 1991; 16:320–329.

283. Walsh KM, Rothwell CE. Hepatic effects in beagle dogs administered atorvastatin, a 3-hydroxy-3-methylglutaryl coenzyme A reductase inhibitor, for 2 years. Toxicol Pathol 1999; 27:395–401.

284. Hiyoshi H, Yanagimachi M, Ito M, Ohtsuka I, Yoshida I, Saeki T, Tanaka H. Effect of ER-27856, a novel squalene synthase inhibitor, on plasma cholesterol in rhesus monkeys. Comparison with 3-hydroxy-3-methylglutaryl-CoA reductase inhibitors. J Lipid Res 2000; 41:1136–1144.

285. McDonald BJ, Bennett BM. Cytochrome P-450 mediated biotransformation of organic nitrates. Can J Physiol Pharmacol 1990; 68:1552–1557.

286. Ellis M, Hiss Y, Shenkman L. Fatal methemoglobinemia caused by inadvertent contamination of a laxative solution with sodium nitrite. Isr J Med Sci 1992; 28:289–291.

287. Gowans WJ. Fatal methaemoglobinaemia in a dental nurse. A case of sodium nitrite poisoning. Br J Gen Pract 1990; 40:470–471.

288. Tanen DA, LoVecchio F, Curry SC. Failure of intravenous *N*-acetylcysteine to reduce methemoglobin produced by sodium nitrite in human volunteers: a randomized controlled trial. Ann Emerg Med 2000; 35:369–373.

289. Haley TJ. Review of the physiological effects of amyl, butyl, and isobutyl nitrites. Clin Toxicol 1980; 16:317–329.

290. Talbert RL, Bussey HI. Update on calcium-channel blocking agents. Clin Pharm 1983; 2:403–416.

291. Bennett BM, McDonald BJ, St. James MJ. Hepatic cytochrome P-450-mediated activation of rat aortic guanylyl cyclase by glyceryl trinitrate. J Pharmacol Exp Ther 1992; 261:716–723.

292. McDonald BJ, Monkewich GJ, Long PG, Anderson DJ, Thomas PE, Bennett BM. Effect of dexamethasone treatment on the biotransformation of glyceryl trinitrate: cytochrome P450 3A1 mediated activation of rat aortic guanylyl cyclase by glyceryl trinitrate. Can J Physiol Pharmacol 1994; 72:1513–1520.

293. Maragos CM, Andrews AW, Keefer LK, Elespuru RK. Mutagenicity of glyceryl trinitrate (nitroglycerin) in Salmonella typhimurium. Mutat Res 1993; 298:187–195.

294. Tamano S, Ward JM, Diwan BA, Keefer LK, Weghorst CM, Calvert RJ, Henneman JR, Ramljak D, Rice JM. Histogenesis and the role of p53 and K-ras mutations in hepatocarcinogenesis by glyceryl trinitrate (nitroglycerin) in male F344 rats. Carcinogenesis 1996; 17:2477–2486.

295. Aoyagi M, Matsukura N, Uchida E, Kawachi T, Sugimura T, Takayama S, Matsui M. Induction of liver tumors in Wistar rats by sodium nitrite given in pellet diet. J Natl Cancer Inst 1980; 65:411–414.

296. Maekawa A, Ogiu T, Onodera H, Furuta K, Matsuoka C, Ohno Y, Odashima S. Carcinogenicity studies of sodium nitrite and sodium nitrate in F-344 rats. Food Chem Toxicol 1982; 20: 25–33.

297. Bucher JR, Huff J, Haseman JK, Eustis SL, Lilja HS, Murthy AS. No evidence of toxicity or carcinogenicity of pentaerythritol tetranitrate given in the diet to F344 rats and B6C3F1 mice for up to two years. J Appl Toxicol 1990; 10:353–357.

298. Guillausseau PJ, Tielmans D, Virally-Monod M, Assayag M. Diabetes: from phenotypes to genotypes. Diabetes Metab 1997; 23 Suppl 2:14–21.

299. Sacks DB, McDonald JM. The pathogenesis of type II diabetes mellitus. A polygenic disease. Am J Clin Pathol 1996; 105:149–156.

300. Turner RC, Hattersley AT, Shaw JT, Levy JC. Type II diabetes: clinical aspects of molecular biological studies. Diabetes 1995; 44:1–10.

301. Shi MM, Bleavins MR, Thompson RG, Chin JF, de la Iglesia FA. Candidate gene profiles for liver toxicity and metabolism in NIDDM patients receiving troglitazone. Unpublished data.

302. Harris EL. Adverse reactions to oral antidiabetic agents. Br Med J 1971; 3:29–30.

303. Seltzer HS. Drug-induced hypoglycemia: a review based on 473 cases. Diabetes 1972; 21: 955–966.

304. Kitabchi AE, Goodman RC. Hypoglycemia. Pathophysiology and diagnosis. Hosp Pract 1987; 22:45–56, 59–60.

305. Goldstein MJ, Rothenberg AJ. Jaundice in a patient receiving acetohexamide. N Engl J Med 1966; 275:97–99.

306. Rank JM, Olson RC. Reversible cholestatic hepatitis caused by acetohexamide. Gastroenterology 1989; 96:1607–1608.

307. Jackson JE, Bressler R. Clinical pharmacology of sulphonylurea hypoglycaemic agents: part 1. Drugs 1981; 22:211–245.

308. Gupta R, Sachar DB. Chlorpropamide-induced cholestatic jaundice and pseudomembranous colitis. Am J Gastroenterol 1985; 80:381–383.

309. Baciewicz AM, Dattilo R, Willis SE, Kershaw JL. Jaundice and rash associated with chlorpropamide. Diabetes Care 1985; 8:200–201.

310. Gill MJ, Ratliff DA, Harding LK. Hypoglycemic coma, jaundice, and pure RBC aplasia following chlorpropamide therapy. Arch Intern Med 1980; 140:714–715.

311. Frier BM, Stewart WK. Cholestatic jaundice following chlorpropamide self-poisoning. Clin Toxicol 1977; 11:13–17.

312. Harrower AD. Comparative tolerability of sulphonylureas in diabetes mellitus. Drug Safety 2000; 22:313–320.

313. Kilo C, Meenan A, Bloomgarden Z. Glyburide versus glipizide in the treatment of patients with non-insulin-dependent diabetes mellitus. Clin Ther 1992; 14:801–812.

314. Prendergast BD. Glyburide and glipizide, second-generation oral sulfonylurea hypoglycemic agents. Clin Pharm 1984; 3:473–485.

315. Fujii S, Nakashima T, Kaneko T. Glibenclamide-induced photosensitivity in a diabetic patient with erythropoietic protoporphyria. Am J Hematol 1995; 50:223.

316. Haider Z, Obaidullah S, Fayyaz ud D. Comparative study of glibenclamide & chlorpropamide in newly diagnosed maturity onset diabetics. J Pak Med Assoc 1976; 26:23–26.

317. Awadallah R, El-Dessoukey EA. Serum enzyme changes in experimental diabetes before and after treatment with some hypoglycaemic drugs. Z Ernahrungswiss 1977; 16:235–240.

318. van Basten JP, van Hoek B, Zeijen R, Stockbrugger R. Glyburide-induced cholestatic hepatitis and liver failure. Case-report and review of the literature. Neth J Med 1992; 40:305–307.

319. Saw D, Pitman E, Maung M, Savasatit P, Wasserman D, Yeung CK. Granulomatous hepatitis associated with glyburide. Dig Dis Sci 1996; 41:322–325.
320. Rumboldt Z, Bota B. Favorable effects of glibenclamide in a patient exhibiting idiosyncratic hepatotoxic reactions to both chlorpropamide and tolbutamide. Acta Diabetol Lat 1984; 21: 387–391.
321. Meadow P, Tullio CJ. Glyburide-induced hepatitis [letter]. Clin Pharm 1989; 8:470.
322. Goodman RC, Dean PJ, Radparvar A, Kitabchi AE. Glyburide-induced hepatitis. Ann Intern Med 1987; 106:837–839.
323. Lebovitz HE. Oral antidiabetic agents. The emergence of alpha-glucosidase inhibitors. Drugs 1992; 44:21–28.
324. Coniff RF, Shapiro JA, Seaton TB, Hoogwerf BJ, Hunt JA. A double-blind placebo-controlled trial evaluating the safety and efficacy of acarbose for the treatment of patients with insulin-requiring type II diabetes. Diabetes Care 1995; 18:928–932.
325. Hollander P. Safety profile of acarbose, an alpha-glucosidase inhibitor. Drugs 1992; 44:47–53.
326. Lee WM. Drug-induced hepatotoxicity. N Engl J Med 1995; 333:1118–1127.
327. Andrade RJ, Lucena M, Vega JL, Torres M, Salmeron FJ, Bellot V, Garcia-Escano MD, Moreno P. Acarbose-associated hepatotoxicity. Diabetes Care 1998; 21:2029–2030.
328. Carrascosa M, Pascual F, Aresti S. Acarbose-induced acute severe hepatotoxicity. Lancet 1997; 349:698–699.
329. Horikoshi H, Yoshioka T. Troglitazone—a novel antidiabetic drug for treating insulin resistance. Drug Discov Today 1998; 3:79–88.
330. Saltiel AR, Olefsky JM. Thiazolidinediones in the treatment of insulin resistance and type II diabetes. Diabetes 1996; 45:1661–1669.
331. Adams MD, Raman P, Judd RL. Comparative effects of englitazone and glyburide on gluconeogenesis and glycolysis in the isolated perfused rat liver. Biochem Pharmacol 1998; 55: 1915–1920.
332. Chen C. Troglitazone: an antidiabetic agent. Am J Health Syst Pharm 1998; 55:905–925.
333. Wang M, Wise SC, Leff T, Su TZ. Troglitazone, an antidiabetic agent, inhibits cholesterol biosynthesis through a mechanism independent of peroxisome proliferator-activated receptor-gamma. Diabetes 1999; 48:254–260.
334. de la Iglesia FA, Herman JR, McGuire EJ, Gough AW, Masuda H. Chronic toxicity study of the antidiabetic troglitazone in Wistar rats. Toxicol Sci 1998; 42:50 (Abstr 246).
335. Herman JR, McGuire EJ, de la Iglesia FA, Walsh KM, Masuda H. Carcinogenicity study of the antidiabetic troglitazone in Wistar rats. Toxicol Sci 1998; 42:71 (Abstr 351).
336. Herman JR, Metz AL, McGuire EJ, de la Iglesia FA, Masuda H. Subchronic toxicity of the antidiabetic troglitazone in Wistar rats. Fundam Appl Toxicol 1997; 36:273 (Abstr 1387).
337. Breider MA, Gough AW, Haskins JR, Sobocinski G, de la Iglesia FA. Troglitazone-induced heart and adipose tissue cell proliferation in mice. Toxicol Pathol 1999; 27:545–552.
338. Nakano N, Moriguchi A, Morishita R, Kida I, Tomita N, Matsumoto K, Nakamura T, Higaki J, Ogihara T. Role of angiotensin II in the regulation of a novel vascular modulator, hepatocyte growth factor (HGF), in experimental hypertensive rats. Hypertension 1997; 30:1448–1454.
339. McGuire EJ, Dethloff LA, Parker RF, de la Iglesia FA, Gough AW, Masuda H. Carcinogenicity study of the antidiabetic troglitazone in B6C3F1 mice. Toxicol Sci 1998; 42:50 (Abstr 247).
340. McGuire EJ, Dethloff LA, Walsh KM, de la Iglesia FA, Masuda H. Subchronic toxicity of the antidiabetic troglitazone in B6C3F1 mice. Fundam Appl Toxicol 1997; 36:273 (Abstr 1388).
341. Rothwell C, E, Bleavins MR, McGuire EJ, de la Iglesia FA, Masuda H. 52-Week oral toxicity study of troglitazone in cynomolgus monkeys. Fundam Appl Toxicol 1997; 36:273 (Abstr 1386).

342. Okuno A, Tamemoto H, Tobe K, Ueki K, Mori Y, Iwamoto K, Umesono K, Akanuma Y, Fujiwara T, Horikoshi H, Yazaki Y, Kadowaki T. Troglitazone increases the number of small adipocytes without the change of white adipose tissue mass in obese Zucker rats. J Clin Invest 1998; 101:1354–1361.

343. Rothwell NJ, Stock MJ, Tedstone AE. Effects of ciglitazone on energy balance, thermogenesis and brown fat activity in the rat. Mol Cell Endocrinol 1987; 51:253–257.

344. Tafuri SR. Troglitazone enhances differentiation, basal glucose uptake, and Glut1 protein levels in 3T3-L1 adipocytes. Endocrinology 1996; 137:4706–4712.

345. Tai TAC, Jennermann C, Brown KK, Oliver BB, MacGinnitie MA, Wilkison WO, Brown HR, Lehmann JM, Kliewer SA, Morris DC, Graves RA. Activation of the nuclear receptor peroxisome proliferator-activated receptor gamma promotes brown adipocyte differentiation. J Biol Chem 1996; 271:29909–29914.

346. Himms Hagen J. Brown adipose tissue metabolism and thermogenesis. Annu Rev Nutr 1985; 5:69–94.

347. Inoue I, Katayama S, Takahashi K, Negishi K, Miyazaki T, Sonoda M, Komoda T. Troglitazone has a scavenging effect on reactive oxygen species. Biochem Biophys Res Commun 1997; 235:113–116.

348. Misbin RI. Troglitazone-associated hepatic failure. Ann Intern Med 1999; 130:330.

349. Neuschwander-Tetri BA, Isley WL, Oki JC, Ramrakhiani S, Quiason SG, Phillips NJ, Brunt EM. Troglitazone-induced hepatic failure leading to liver transplantation: a case report. Ann Intern Med 1998; 129:38–41.

350. Watkins PB, Whitcomb RW. Hepatic dysfunction associated with troglitazone. N Engl J Med 1998; 338:916–917.

351. Kohlroser J, Mathai J, Reichheld J, Banner BF, Bonkovsky HL. Hepatotoxicity due to troglitazone: report of two cases and review of adverse events reported to the United States Food and Drug Administration. Am J Gastroenterol 2000; 95:272–276.

352. Gitlin N, Julie NL, Spurr CL, Lim KN, Juarbe HM. Two cases of severe clinical and histologic hepatotoxicity associated with troglitazone. Ann Intern Med 1998; 129:36–38.

353. Vella A, de Groen PC, Dinneen SF. Fatal hepatotoxicity associated with troglitazone. Ann Intern Med 1998; 129:1080.

354. Shibuya A, Watanabe M, Fujita Y, Saigenji K, Kuwao S, Takahashi H, Takeuchi H. An autopsy case of troglitazone-induced fulminant hepatitis. Diabetes Care 1998; 21:2140–2143.

355. Herrine SK, Choudhary C. Severe hepatotoxicity associated with troglitazone [letter; comment]. Ann Intern Med 1999; 130:163–164.

356. Brown MN. The thiazolidinediones or "glitazones" a treatment option for type 2 diabetes mellitus. Med Health RI 2000; 83:118–120.

357. Goldstein BJ. Rosiglitazone. Int J Clin Pract 2000; 54:333–337.

358. Avandia (rosiglitazone maleate) prescribing information, Smith Kline Beecham, 1999.

359. Forman LM, Simmons DA, Diamond RH. Hepatic failure in a patient taking rosiglitazone. Ann Intern Med 2000; 132:118–121.

360. Al-Salman J, Arjomand H, Kemp DG, Mittal M. Hepatocellular injury in a patient receiving rosiglitazone: a case report. Ann Intern Med 2000; 132:121–124.

361. Actos (pioglitazone hydrochloride) prescribing information, Takeda Pharmaceuticals, 1999.

362. Gillies PS, Dunn CJ. Pioglitazone. Drugs 2000; 60:333–343; discussion 344–345.

363. Fujita T, Sugiyama Y, Taketomi S, Sohda T, Kawamatsu Y, Iwatsuka H, Suzuoki Z. Reduction of insulin resistance in obese and/or diabetic animals by 5-[4-(1-methylcyclohexylmethoxy)benzyl]-thiazolidine-2,4-dione (ADD-3878, U-63,287, ciglitazone), a new antidiabetic agent. Diabetes 1983; 32:804–810.

364. Chang AY, Wyse BM, Gilchrist BJ. Ciglitazone, a new hypoglycemic agent. II. Effect on glucose and lipid metabolisms and insulin binding in the adipose tissue of C57BL/6J-ob/ob and −+/? mice. Diabetes 1983; 32:839–845.

365. Stevenson RW, Hutson NJ, Krupp MN, Volkmann RA, Holland GF, Eggler JF, Clark DA,

McPherson RK, Hall KL, Danbury BH, et al. Actions of novel antidiabetic agent englitazone in hyperglycemic hyperinsulinemic ob/ob mice. Diabetes 1990; 39:1218–1227.

366. Fukui Y, Masui S, Osada S, Umesono K, Motojima K. A new thiazolidinedione, NC-2100, which is a weak PPAR-gamma activator, exhibits potent antidiabetic effects and induces uncoupling protein 1 in white adipose tissue of KKAy obese mice. Diabetes 2000; 49:759–767.

367. Shimaya A, Kurosaki E, Nakano R, Hirayama R, Shibasaki M, Shikama H. The novel hypoglycemic agent YM440 normalizes hyperglycemia without changing body fat weight in diabetic db/db mice. Metabolism 2000; 49:411–417.

368. Kanigur-Sultuybek G, Guven M, Onaran I, Tezcan V, Cenani A, Hatemi H. The effect of metformin on insulin receptors and lipid peroxidation in alloxan and streptozotocin induced diabetes. J Basic Clin Physiol Pharmacol 1995; 6:271–280.

369. Bailey CJ. Biguanides and NIDDM. Diabetes Care 1992; 15:755–772.

370. Hotta N, Komori T, Kobayashi M, Sakakibara F, Koh N, Sakamoto N. The inhibitory action of buformin, a biguanide on gluconeogenesis from alanine and its transport system in rat livers. Diabetes Res Clin Pract 1993; 19:49–58.

371. Babich MM, Pike I, Shiffman ML. Metformin-induced acute hepatitis. Am J Med 1998; 104: 490–492.

372. Swislocki AL, Noth R. Case report. Pseudohepatotoxicity of metformin [letter]. Diabetes Care 1998; 21:677–678.

373. Fuchtenbusch M, Standl E, Schatz H. Clinical efficacy of new thiazolidinediones and glinides in the treatment of type 2 diabetes mellitus. Exp Clin Endocrinol Diabetes 2000; 108:151–163.

374. Uwai Y, Saito H, Hashimoto Y, Inui K. Inhibitory effect of anti-diabetic agents on rat organic anion transporter rOAT1. Eur J Pharmacol 2000; 398:193–197.

375. Wolffenbuttel BH, Landgraf R. A 1-year multicenter randomized double-blind comparison of repaglinide and glyburide for the treatment of type 2 diabetes. Dutch and German Repaglinide Study Group. Diabetes Care 1999; 22:463–467.

376. Evans WE, Relling MV. Pharmacogenomics: translating functional genomics into rational therapeutics. Science 1999; 286:487–491.

377. Shi MM, Sinz M, Rose K, Myrand SP, Bleavins MR, de la Iglesia FA. Human phenol sulfotransferase 1A1*2 genetic polymorphism in type 2 diabetic patients. Am J Hum Genet 2000; 67(suppl 2) (Abstr 2024).

378. Heard PL, Bleavins MR, Johnson KJ, Shi MM, de la Iglesia FA. Induction of alanine aminotransferase gene expression by tacrine in HEPG2 cells. Toxicol Sci 2000; 54:387.

379. Silverman JF, O'Brien KF, Long S, Leggett N, Khazanie PG, Pories WJ, Norris HT, Caro JF. Liver pathology in morbidly obese patients with and without diabetes. Am J Gastroenterol 1990; 85:1349–1355.

380. Loi CM, Alvey CW, Vassos AB, Randinitis EJ, Sedman AJ, Koup JR. Steady-state pharmacokinetics and dose proportionality of troglitazone and its metabolites. J Clin Pharmacol 1999; 39:920–926.

381. Yamazaki H, Shibata A, Suzuki M, Nakajima M, Shimada N, Guengerich FP, Yokoi T. Oxidation of troglitazone to a quinone-type metabolite catalyzed by cytochrome P-450 2C8 and P-450 3A4 in human liver microsomes. Drug Metab Dispos 1999; 27:1260–1266.

382. Fromenty B, Letteron P, Fisch C, Berson A, Deschamps D, Pessayre D. Evaluation of human blood lymphocytes as a model to study the effects of drugs on human mitochondria. Effects of low concentrations of amiodarone on fatty acid oxidation, ATP levels and cell survival. Biochem Pharmacol 1993; 46:421–432.

383. Lemasters JJ, Qian T, Bradham CA, Brenner DA, Cascio WE, Trost LC, Nishimura Y, Nieminen AL, Herman B. Mitochondrial dysfunction in the pathogenesis of necrotic and apoptotic cell death. J Bioenerg Biomembr 1999; 31:305–319.

384. Fromenty B, Pessayre D. Inhibition of mitochondrial beta-oxidation as a mechanism of hepatotoxicity. Pharmacol Ther 1995; 67:101–154.

385. Bioulac-Sage P, Parrot-Roulaud F, Mazat JP, Lamireau T, Coquet M, Sandler B, Demarquez JL, Cormier V, Munnich A, Carre M, et al. Fatal neonatal liver failure and mitochondrial cytopathy (oxidative phosphorylation deficiency): a light and electron microscopic study of the liver. Hepatology 1993; 18:839–846.

386. Plymale DR, Haskins JR, de la Iglesia FA. Monitoring simultaneous subcellular events in vitro by means of coherent multiprobe fluorescence. Nat Med 1999; 5:351–355.

387. Haskins JR, Johnson JH, de la Iglesia FA. Ex vivo functional assessment of mitochondrial transmembrane potential from lean and diabetic Zucker rats with or without troglitazone. Diabetes 1999; 48 (Abstr).

388. Haskins JR, Rowse PE, Rahbari R, de la Iglesia FA. Thiazolidinedione toxicity to isolated hepatocytes revealed by coherent multiprobe fluorescence microscopy and correlated with multiparameter flow cytometry of peripheral leukocytes. Arch Toxicol, 2001; 75:425–438.

389. Haskins JR, Rowse PE, Rahbari R, de la Iglesia FA. Comparative toxicity of thiazolidine-diones in isolated rat hepatocytes. Toxicol Sci 2000; 54:43.

390. Mazzanti L, Mutus B. Diabetes-induced alterations in platelet metabolism. Clin Biochem 1997; 30:509–515.

391. Raftogianis RB, Wood TC, Otterness DM, Van Loon JA, Weinshilboum RM. Phenol sulfo-transferase pharmacogenetics in humans: association of common SULT1A1 alleles with TS PST phenotype. Biochem Biophys Res Commun 1997; 239:298–304.

392. Braun L, Kardon T, Puskas F, Csala M, Banhegyi G, Mandl J. Regulation of glucuronidation by glutathione redox state through the alteration of UDP-glucose supply originating from glycogen metabolism. Arch Biochem Biophys 1997; 348:169–173.

393. Zisman A, Peroni OD, Abel ED, Michael MD, Mauvais-Jarvis F, Lowell BB, Wojtaszewski JF, Hirshman MF, Virkamaki A, Goodyear LJ, Kahn CR, Kahn BB. Targeted disruption of the glucose transporter 4 selectively in muscle causes insulin resistance and glucose intoler-ance. Nat Med 2000; 6:924–928.

394. Barroso I, Gurnell M, Crowley VE, Agostini M, Schwabe JW, Soos MA, Maslen GL, Wil-liams TD, Lewis H, Schafer AJ, Chatterjee VK, O'Rahilly S. Dominant negative mutations in human PPAR gamma associated with severe insulin resistance, diabetes mellitus and hy-pertension. Nature 1999; 402:880–883.

395. Radjendirane V, Joseph P, Lee YH, Kimura S, Klein-Szanto AJ, Gonzalez FJ, Jaiswal AK. Disruption of the DT diaphorase (NQO1) gene in mice leads to increased menadione toxicity. J Biol Chem 1998; 273:7382–7389.

396. Cadenas E. Antioxidant and prooxidant functions of DT-diaphorase in quinone metabolism. Biochem Pharmacol 1995; 49:127–140.

397. Cameron RG, de la Iglesia FA, Feuer G. Hepatotoxicity of Cardiovascular Drugs. In: RG Cameron, G Feuer, FA de la Iglesia, eds. Drug-Induced Hepatotoxicity. Berlin: Springer Verlag, 1996:477–513.

398. Clementz GL, Holmes AW. Nicotinic acid-induced fulminant hepatic failure. J Clin Gas-troenterol 1987; 9:582–584.

399. Hirose S, Kamoi K, Sasaki H. A case of severe troglitazone-induced liver injury in a non-insulin-dependent diabetes mellitus patient. J Jpn Diab Soc 1998; 41:295–299.

400. Murphy EJ, Davern TJ, Shakil AO, Shick L, Masharani U, Chow H, Freise C, Lee WM, Bass NM. Troglitazone-induced fulminant hepatic failure. Acute Liver Failure Study Group. Dig Dis Sci 2000; 45:549–553.

24

Cancer Chemotherapy

LAURIE D. DELEVE

University of Southern California, Los Angeles, California, U.S.A.

I. INTRODUCTION

This chapter is comprised of three sections. The first section examines the factors that alter liver metabolism and how this can affect efficacy and toxicity from anticancer drugs. The second section reviews liver toxicity in hematopoietic stem cell transplantation; this topic warrants its own section, since several of the conditioning regimens for stem cell transplantation have a high incidence of liver toxicity and a high case-fatality rate. The final section is the more traditional review of hepatotoxicity listed for individual anticancer drugs.

II. HEPATIC METABOLISM OF ANTICANCER DRUGS

Most anticancer drugs are potentially toxic compounds with a narrow therapeutic index. Thus changes in pharmacokinetics or drug metabolism that effect the disposition of these drugs may easily alter efficacy or cause toxicity. This section describes how variability in hepatic metabolism will affect disposition of anticancer drugs and how this may predispose to liver toxicity.

A. Drug Interactions

1. Drug Interactions and Drug Disposition

In general, the incidence of adverse drug reactions increases exponentially with the number of drugs prescribed. This is partially because individuals on multiple drugs tend to have more severe underlying illness and partially due to falsely attributing disease symptoms to drug toxicity. However, drug interactions contribute to the disproportionate rise in adverse reactions due to polypharmacy. Cancer patients are at particular risk because of the narrow therapeutic index of anticancer drugs, the use of anticancer drugs in combination regimens, and the many supportive drugs used in this population. Supportive drugs used in patients on antineoplastic regimens include antiemetics, antipyretics, analgesics, antihistamines, antifungals, antivirals, and antibacterial antibiotics, many of which are potential hepatotoxins.

Drug interactions that affect drug metabolism by the liver may inhibit detoxification, induce metabolic activation, or inhibit excretion and thereby increase efficacy or toxicity. Conversely, inhibition of metabolic activation or induction of detoxification pathways may diminish efficacy of anticancer drugs. These interactions are more important when a drug is more extensively metabolized and when the affected pathway contributes a large share to overall metabolism.

Increased Efficacy and/or Toxification. *Inhibition of detoxification* by oxidative metabolism and/or conjugation reactions by concomitant medication may lead to drug toxicity. CYP 3A4 is the most abundant P450 in the liver (around 30% of total hepatic P450); it is inducible and it is responsible for the metabolism of over 50% of xenobiotics. Inhibition of CYP 3A4 is responsible for many clinically significant interactions. Vinca alkaloids (vincristine, vinblastine, vindesine, vinorelbine) and docetaxel are mainly detoxified by CYP 3A4-catalyzed metabolism and are predominantly excreted into bile. Ketoconazole, itraconazole, and fluconazole—antifungals frequently used in this population—are P450 3A4 inhibitors and should be avoided during therapy with these vinca alkaloids or docetaxel, since the unmetabolized parent compound may reach toxic levels. Indeed, there are several case reports of neurotoxicity from the combination of vincristine with itraconazole that have been attributed to inhibition of CYP 3A4 by itraconazole.

6-Mercaptopurine, 6-thioguanine, and azathioprine are prodrugs (see Fig. 1). When orally administered these thiopurines are subjected to first-pass metabolism by xanthine oxidase in the liver and intestine. When 6-mercaptopurine is given orally, e.g., in maintenance therapy for acute lymphoblastic leukemia, inhibition of xanthine oxidase by allopurinol inhibits first-pass metabolism in the intestine and liver, increases bioavailability, and can precipitate toxicity (1). Allopurinol has little effect on the area-under-the-curve (AUC) when these thiopurines are given intravenously (1). The mechanism of hepatotoxicity of these drugs will be discussed more in depth in the last section of this chapter.

The liver extensively metabolizes paclitaxel: around 90% of the dose is converted to metabolites. Total fecal excretion is approximately 70% of the dose and the largest component by far is 6α-hydroxypaclitaxel, a detoxification product. Given the extensive metabolism, paclitaxel might be expected to be prone to toxicity through interaction with inhibitors of metabolism. In humans, CYP 2C8 is responsible for the formation of the major metabolite, 6α-hydroxypaclitaxel, whereas CYP 3A4 catalyzes formation of 2-hydroxylation products that are minor metabolites in most individuals. Several compounds inhibit paclitaxel metabolism in vitro in human microsome studies, but major

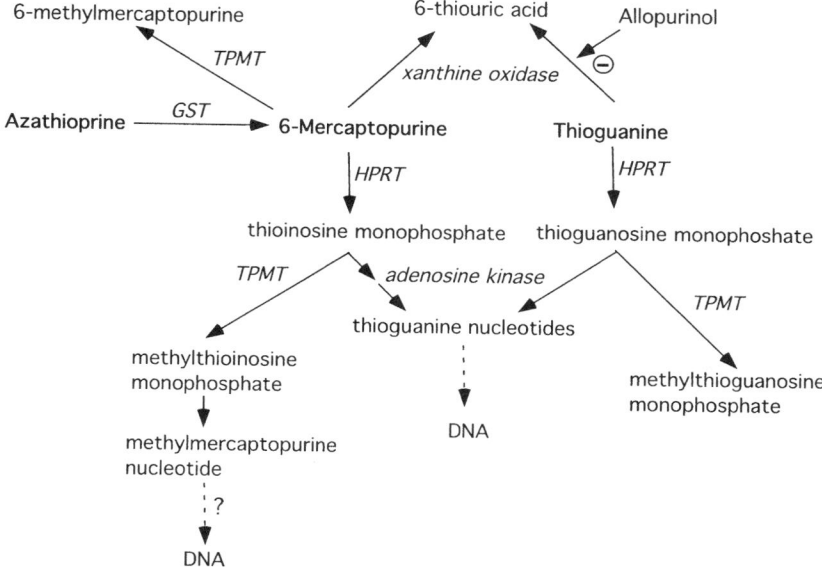

Figure 1 Thiopurine metabolism. A simplified schematic of 6-mercaptopurine, 6-thioguanine, and azathioprine metabolism. Thioguanine nucleotides are the presumptive toxic metabolites. HPRT, hypoxanthine phosphoribosyltransferase; TPMT, thiopurine *S*-methyltransferase; GST, glutathione-*S*-transferase.

effects have not been reported clinically. This is likely because of the lack of clinically used drugs that inhibit CYP 2C8.

Irinotecan is now a component in the chemotherapy of advanced colorectal cancer. It is metabolized by carboxylesterase-2 (2) to SN-38 (7-ethyl-10-hydroxy camptothecin), the putative active metabolite, which is conjugated by uridine diphosphate glucuronosyl transferase 1A1 (3) (UGT-1A1) to the glucuronide, SN-38-glucuronide (Fig. 2). Irinotecan and its metabolites are actively excreted in bile (4) and fecal excretion accounts for elimination of two-thirds of the dose (5). Increased concentrations of SN-38 in the intestine are thought to be the cause of the delayed-onset diarrhea associated with irinotecan, whereas glucuronidation of SN-38 protects against this toxicity. Valproate inhibits UGT (6) and

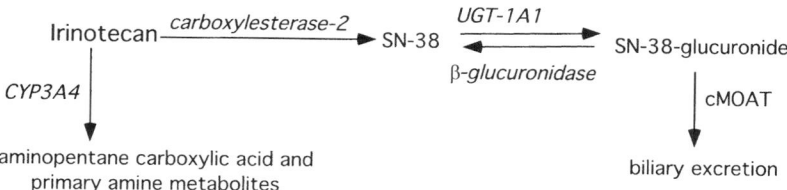

Figure 2 Irinotecan metabolism. Irinotecan is metabolized by carboxylesterase-2 to the toxic metabolite, SN-38. SN-38-glucuronide is a detoxified metabolite that can be excreted into bile via cMOAT. Intestinal toxicity may be due to bacterial deconjugation of the glucuronide with regeneration of SN-38.

inhibits formation of SN-38-glucuronide experimentally (7). Thus treatment with valproate may increase the risk of intestinal toxicity from irinotecan.

Induction of metabolic activation by P450 will enhance efficacy and could potentially cause toxicity. Cyclophosphamide requires metabolic activation by CYP 3A4/5 at the higher range of therapeutic concentrations and by CYP 2C9 at low concentrations to form 4-hydroxycyclophosphamide (8). 4-Hydroxycyclophosphamide is an intermediate metabolite in the formation of phosphoramide mustard, the active metabolite, and acrolein, the metabolite responsible for much of its toxicity. Phenobarbital induces P450 activation of cyclophosphamide, which will increase both efficacy and toxicity. A similar mechanism would apply to ifosfamide.

Drug-induced *inhibition of biliary excretion* may occur at the level of the active transporters on the canalicular pole of the hepatocyte (mechanical obstruction of the biliary tree is discussed below). P-glycoprotein, the multidrug resistance drug efflux pump that is overexpressed in some cancer cells, is present at the canalicular pole of the hepatocyte. This transmembrane-spanning protein is responsible for biliary excretion of hydrophobic cationic antineoplastic drugs (see Table 1; also discussed in another chapter). Inhibition of P-glycoprotein at the canalicular pole of hepatocytes will block excretion of substrates into bile and increase drug levels. Verapamil and cyclosporin are both inhibitors of P-glycoprotein, but through different mechanisms. Verapamil is a substrate for P-glycoprotein and is a competitive inhibitor of this pump, whereas cyclosporin inhibits transport function by interfering with substrate recognition and ATP hydrolysis (9). Experimental studies have demonstrated that decreased clearance of drugs through inhibition of P-glycoprotein translates clinically into increased AUC (10,11) and an increase in toxicity (11). Examples of this type of drug interaction are the decrease in vincristine clearance in the presence of verapamil (10), of paclitaxel or etoposide clearance in the presence of Cremophor (a drug solubilizer used in the formulation of paclitaxel) (12,13), and of etoposide (11) or doxorubicin clearance in the presence of cyclosporin (see review in ref. 10). The effect on biliary excretion is only part of the pharmacokinetic change that occurs with inhibition of P-glycoprotein. Inhibition of P-glycoprotein on renal tubular epithelium will inhibit urinary excretion, analogous to the effect on the hepatocyte. Also, P-glycoprotein pumps drugs from the enterocyte back into the intestinal lumen, so inhibition of P-glycoprotein may increase intestinal uptake of orally administered drugs. The toxicity due to decreased excretion of the drug needs to be taken into account when pharmacological inhibition of P-glycoprotein is used to overcome drug resistance in tumor cells that express P-glycoprotein: expression of P-glycoprotein allows the tumor cell to efflux the chemotherapeutic agent, whereas pharmacological inhibition of P-glycoprotein-mediated transport allows intracellular accumulation of drug in cells.

Table 1   Selected Substrates of P-Glycoprotein

Vinca alkaloids (vincristine, vinblastine)
Anthracyclines (doxorubicin, daunorubicin, epirubicin, idarubicin)
Epipodophyllotoxin (etoposide, teniposide)
Taxanes (paclitaxel, docetaxel)
Actinomycin D
Topotecan
Mithramcyin

Inhibition of P450 or P-glycoprotein in the small intestine may *increase bioavailability* of orally administered drugs through decreased first-pass metabolism (see previous discussion and below).

Decreased Efficacy and/or Toxicity. Fluconazole causes a significant reduction in plasma clearance of cyclophosphamide due to *inhibition of P450 activation* that is presumably accompanied by reduced formation of 4-hydroxycyclophosphamide. The effect of this interaction on clinical efficacy has not been established (14).

Induction of detoxification by P450 may decrease efficacy. Vincristine is partially metabolized by CYP 3A4. Concomitant use of carbamazepine or phenytoin increases vincristine clearance (15). Docetaxel is detoxified by CYP 3A4. In liver microsomes prepared from patients who had been treated with phenobarbital, docetaxel hydroxylation is induced (16).

Experimentally, phenobarbital pretreatment reduces the AUC of irinotecan and the active metabolite, SN-38, with an increase in the SN-38-glucuronide (7) (Fig. 2). This is most likely due to induction of CYP 3A4 and UGT. The relevance of this is demonstrated by a comparison of irinotecan pharmacokinetics in patients with colorectal cancer versus those with malignant glioma (17). Ninety-one percent of the patients with malignant glioma were on phenytoin, carbamazepine, or phenobarbital. Enhanced irinotecan clearance and reduced concentrations of SN-38 and SN-38-glucuronide are consistent with induction of CYP 3A4 metabolism of irinotecan. The low incidence of severe toxicity in the malignant glioma patients in conjunction with the low plasma concentrations of irinotecan suggests that treatment with anticonvulsants has a significant effect on irinotecan disposition.

2. Drug Interactions and Liver Toxicity

Patients treated with combination chemotherapy commonly develop mild to moderate transient elevations of liver tests, although the individual drugs have little or no risk of liver injury. Interactions of drugs may lead to such abnormalities. For example, a large retrospective study of patients with breast cancer treated with cyclophosphamide, doxorubicin, and 5-FU reported liver test abnormalities in around 85% of patients without known liver metastases (18). The abnormal liver tests did not require discontinuation of the treatment regimen and 90% of patients had normal liver tests 1 year after discontinuing the therapy. Each of these drugs individually has a low incidence of liver test abnormalities at conventional doses, suggesting an interaction between the drugs in this regimen. The underlying mechanism for these interactions is unknown.

Similarly, although the individual drugs rarely cause toxicity, some conditioning regimens for stem cell transplantation have a high incidence of hepatic veno-occlusive disease. This is likely due to additive or synergistic toxicity of the drugs, as will be discussed below.

B. Underlying Liver Disease

1. Underlying Liver Disease and Hepatic Metabolism

In general, underlying liver disease may affect hepatic metabolism. A special consideration in this setting is the involvement of the liver by the underlying neoplasm. Infiltrative liver disease by primary or metastatic tumor may lead to liver dysfunction through several mechanisms. Extensive replacement of normal liver tissue can lead to a decrease in metabolic capacity. Impairment of biliary drug excretion may occur due to compression of intrahepatic bile ductules or the extrahepatic biliary tree. Tumor invasion may compromise normal hepatic blood flow and impair clearance of drugs by the liver.

Given the narrow therapeutic range of most anticancer drugs, there is a heightened awareness of the need to alter dosing when drug clearance may be impaired. Attempts to modify dosing of anticancer drugs based on changes in a single liver test, regardless of the type of underlying liver disease, have led to empirical decisions about dose reduction of anticancer drugs that have not always been confirmed by experimental data. A better approach, when possible, is to correlate abnormal disposition of a drug to the severity of a specific type of liver disease, rather than to changes of a single liver test independent of the underlying pathology. Some clinical research has correlated clearance of anticancer drugs with tests of liver function. Both antipyrine and lidocaine are metabolized by P450 and are measures of liver function, with the distinction that the former is flow-independent and the latter flow-dependent. Similarly, the erythromycin breath test is a measure of hepatic CYP 3A4 activity that has been used in clinical research to predict toxicity or to correlate liver function with drug disposition.

A limitation in the oncology literature is that patients with liver test abnormalities are often excluded from the early clinical trials of new anticancer drugs. Thus the disposition of a drug in patients with liver disease may not be known until phase III clinical trials are completed and the drug has been made more widely available.

The tubulin acting drugs—vincristine, vinblastine, vindesine, vinorelbine, paclitaxel, and docetaxel—are predominantly detoxified in the liver and mainly excreted into bile. The vinca alkaloids and docetaxel are mainly metabolized by CYP 3A4 (19–21), whereas paclitaxel is predominantly metabolized by CYP 2C8 and, to a lesser degree, by CYP 3A4 (22). Cancer patients with underlying liver disease may have decreased clearance of these drugs, due either to decreased hepatic function or to decreased biliary excretion. For example, patients with extensive liver metastases have reduced vinorelbine clearance, and clearance of the drug correlates with lidocaine clearance (23).

Ondansetron, one of the newer antinauseants used in oncology, is extensively metabolized by P450. The major metabolites are formed by CYP 1A2, CYP 1A1, and CYP 2D6. First-pass metabolism of orally administered ondansetron is impaired in cirrhotic patients, with a significant increase in bioavailability (24). AUC after intravenous administration was also significantly higher than in healthy controls. Ondansetron clearance was closely correlated to antipyrine clearance. There are conflicting reports as to whether systemic concentrations of 5-hydroxytryptamine receptor 3 antagonists correlate with effect, so that it is unclear whether changes in clearance will alter the therapeutic response.

2. Underlying Liver Disease and Liver Toxicity

Preexistent liver disease is the main risk factor for progressive liver disease due to methotrexate. Portal fibrosis in the pretreatment liver biopsy or risk factors for steatohepatitis, such as chronic alcohol abuse, obesity, and diabetes mellitus, predispose to progressive liver disease with chronic low-dose methotrexate.

In children treated with methotrexate and/or 6-mercaptopurine for acute lymphoblastic leukemia, viral hepatitis is a risk factor for elevated serum transaminases during therapy, but there appears to be little, if any, increased risk of persistent elevation of serum aminotransferase (25–27). It is unclear whether treatment with these drugs adds to the risk of hepatitis C–related fibrosis and/or cirrhosis in children with acute lymphoblastic leukemia. In a large cohort of children with childhood leukemia treated with unspecified regimens of chemotherapy, none of the patients had developed evidence of severe chronic liver disease 13–27 years after the estimated time of infection (25).

Hepatitis C is a risk factor for hepatotoxicity for some drugs (28–32). Prevalence of hepatitis C exposure is 1.8%, or 3.9 million individuals nationwide; 65% of these individuals are between 30 and 49 years old, with a prevalence in this age group of 3–3.9% (33). As this cohort of individuals ages, the number of cancer patients with concomitant hepatitis C will rise. Thus liver injury due to the interaction between anticancer drugs and hepatitis C is likely to increase in the coming decades.

Withdrawal of chemotherapy can lead to reactivation of hepatitis B in carriers and exacerbation of chronic active hepatitis B. The presumptive mechanism is increased viral synthesis during immunosuppression with consequent hepatocyte infection. Withdrawal of chemotherapeutic or immunosuppressive drugs is accompanied by restoration of immune function with rapid destruction of infected hepatocytes. The course of hepatitis in such patients can be fulminant and there is a high incidence of liver failure and death. This has been most commonly described for patients with hepatitis B and hematological malignancies, but has also been described for hepatitis C and for solid tumors. Reactivation of hepatitis is much less common in patients who receive steroid-free chemotherapy (34).

C. Aging

1. Aging and Hepatic Metabolism

With the aging of the population, the median age for cancer is now 70 years. This has stimulated an interest in the effect of aging on disposition of and response to anticancer drugs in the elderly. Although there is no direct correlation between physiological change and increasing chronological age, most individuals sustain some decrease in liver function with aging. Although it has never been felt to be an entirely satisfactory explanation, age-related changes in hepatic metabolism have often been attributed to the 25–35% decrease in liver blood flow, liver mass, antipyrine clearance, and P450 content that is seen, on average, in the elderly (35,36). A recent in vivo study in rats has provided an attractive alternative hypothesis (37). This study demonstrated pseudocapillarization of the liver, i.e., thickening of sinusoidal endothelial cells with reduction in endothelial fenestration as well as an increase in extracellular matrix in the space of Disse. These changes in the sinusoidal lining would create a diffusional barrier to drugs, in particular protein-bound drugs, and to oxygen. The morphological findings were accompanied by changes in high-energy phosphate (ATP, ATP/Pi, etc.) detected by ^{31}P magnetic resonance spectroscopy, which could indicate hepatocyte hypoxia. If pseudocapillarization occurs with aging in humans, this could diminish both hepatic clearance and oxidative metabolism of drugs.

In univariate analysis, 5-fluorouracil clearance is significantly reduced with age (38) and age is an independent risk factor for 5-fluorouracil toxicity (39). 5-Fluorouracil is metabolized by hepatic dihydropyrimidine dehydrogenase (DPD), but hepatic DPD activity does not change with age (40). Mitomycin is primarily metabolized in the liver and excreted in the bile (41). AUC of mitomycin increases with age in patients with normal hepatic, renal, cardiac, and bone marrow function (42). Epirubicin is a stereoisomer of doxorubicin that is predominantly cleared by the liver. Epirubicin clearance decreases with age in females, but the study that demonstrated this did not have sufficient males to determine whether this applied to males as well (43). Daunorubicin clearance decreases and AUC and cardiotoxicity increase in rats with age (44,45). The mechanism for the age-related changes in pharmacokinetics of 5-fluorouracil, mitomycin, epirubicin, and daunorubicin has not been defined, but may relate to changes in the liver described in the preceding paragraph.

2. Aging and Liver Toxicity

It is sometimes stated that age is a risk factor for methotrexate toxicity. However, age has not been found to be an independent risk factor for methotrexate-induced aminotransferase elevation (46). It remains to be established whether age per se predisposes to fibrosis in chronic methotrexate therapy. However, the age-related decline in renal function is a risk factor for methotrexate hepatotoxicity.

D. Gender

Anthracycline metabolism occurs mainly in the liver. Females have significantly lower clearance of doxorubicin and epirubicin than males (43,47). Females also have an incidence of cardiotoxicity that is twice as high as males (48) and lower clearance may play a role in this. This increased risk of cardiac dysfunction in females is already apparent in childhood (49,50).

Females have increased risk of toxicity from 5-fluorouracil (39,51,52). This is consistent with the finding that 5-fluorouracil clearance is significantly lower in females than in males (53). However, current data have not determined why clearance is lower in females. 5-Fluorouracil is metabolized by hepatic dihydropyrimidine dehydrogenase (DPD) and low levels of DPD or DPD deficiency (see below) predispose to decreased 5-fluorouracil clearance and toxicity. Interestingly, females with 5-fluorouracil toxicity are more likely to have low DPD levels than males with toxicity (52). Thus one would speculate that the increased incidence of toxicity and the decreased clearance in females is due to lower DPD levels in the female population. However, two prospective studies, i.e., not in patients with 5-fluorouracil toxicity, did not find an effect of gender on DPD activity in peripheral blood mononuclear cells and liver (40,54). Hormonal status does not appear to affect DPD activity and the gene for DPD is on chromosome 1, an autosomal chromosome. It has been observed that patients with breast cancer have lower DPD activity than healthy controls (55), so underlying disease or nutritional status may be confounders in the studies done in patients with 5-fluorouracil toxicity. Clearly more studies are needed to reconcile these findings.

E. Nutrition

1. Nutrition and Hepatic Metabolism

Undernourishment is common in patients with advanced cancer. Protein-calorie malnutrition or a low daily intake of protein can decrease oxidative metabolism by 20–40% (56). Protein depletion also causes a significant decrease in hepatic DPD activity in rats that is associated with significantly decreased hepatic metabolism and clearance of 5-fluorouracil and increased morbidity and mortality (57). Doxorubicin clearance is decreased and AUC is increased in rabbits fed a low-protein diet (58).

2. Nutrition and Liver Toxicity

Protein malnourishment is a risk factor in the human epidemics of hepatic veno-occlusive disease due to pyrrolizidine alkaloids. However, it has not been identified as a risk factor for hepatic veno-occlusive disease due to high-dose chemotherapy for hematopoietic stem cell transplantation. However, protein deprivation depletes hepatic glutathione levels and experimental data suggest that decreased hepatic glutathione levels may predispose to hepatic veno-occlusive disease (59,60). A low-protein diet also increases liver toxicity due to irradiation in rats (61).

F. Genetic Polymorphisms

The reader is referred to a review on the impact of metabolic polymorphisms on the efficacy and toxicity of various anticancer drugs (62).

The therapeutic effect of 5-fluorouracil is through formation of nucleotides that block normal nucleic acid formation. This is balanced by catabolism by dihydropyrimidine dehydrogenase (DPD) in the liver. More than 85% of 5-fluorouracil is broken down by DPD and DPD activity is therefore a major determinant of 5-fluorouracil activity and toxicity. DPD enzyme activity follows a Gaussian distribution with up to a sixfold inter-individual variation. In addition to the normal variation of DPD activity, there are also mutations in the DPD gene that can lead to DPD deficiency, which occurs in less than 3% of the population. Low DPD levels and DPD deficiency reduce 5-fluorouracil clearance and can lead to severe or life-threatening toxicity. There is a relatively weak correlation between DPD activity in peripheral blood mononuclear cells and in the liver (54), yet low DPD activity in peripheral blood mononuclear cells is a strong predictor of reduced 5-fluorouracil clearance (38).

In Gilbert's syndrome there is a longer TATAA element in the upstream promoter region of the gene encoding for UDP-glucuronosyltransferase 1 (UGT-1) that is associated with decreased transcription (63). Up to 16% of the population may be homozygous for this abnormality, although only 3–10% of the population is diagnosed clinically with Gilbert's syndrome. Gilbert's syndrome results in decreased bilirubin glucuronidation, which may enhance toxicity of drugs that require conjugation by UGT-1 for detoxification. As described earlier and in Fig. 2, irinotecan is metabolized by carboxyesterase-2 to the active metabolite, SN-38. SN-38 is detoxified to SN-38-glucuronide by UGT-1. Both SN-38 and the detoxified conjugate, SN-38-glucuronide, are actively excreted into bile (4). Unconjugated SN-38 in the intestine is thought to be the cause of delayed-onset intestinal toxicity in patients treated with irinotecan. Case reports have described severe intestinal toxicity in two patients with Gilbert's syndrome who were treated with irinotecan (64). In vitro studies with liver microsomes showed that individuals homozygous for the longer TATAA element formed less SN-38-glucuronide than individuals who are heterozygous, and heterozygous individuals formed less SN-38-glucuronide than homozygous individuals with the normal-length TATAA element (65). Thus Gilbert's syndrome may be a risk factor for delayed-onset diarrhea, but this remains to be confirmed in clinical studies.

III. LIVER TOXICITY AND HEMATOPOIETIC STEM CELL TRANSPLANTATION

Hematopoietic stem cell transplantation, the new name for what used to be referred to as bone marrow transplantation, is commonly complicated by drug-induced and non-drug-related forms of liver disease. The drug-induced complications include hepatic sinusoidal obstruction syndrome (SOS), the new name for what used to be referred to as hepatic veno-occlusive disease, and nodular regenerative hyperplasia. These need to be differentiated from other liver diseases frequently seen in this setting, notably graft-versus-host disease, viral hepatitis, fungal liver disease, tumor infiltration of the liver, cholestasis of sepsis, and liver injury due to total parenteral nutrition (see the recent review in ref. 66). This section provides an extensive discussion of hepatic SOS, since it has the highest mortality of any chemotherapy-induced liver disease.

A. Hepatic Sinusoidal Obstruction Syndrome

SOS, or "bush tea disease," was first recognized in humans in the early twentieth century as a complication of pyrrolizidine alkaloids ingested as herbal teas or contaminating the food supply (67). Sporadic cases have been described in patients treated with a wide variety of antineoplastic drugs at conventional doses. At present the most common cause of SOS in North America and western Europe is the preparative regimen used for hemato-poietic stem cell transplantation.

In hematopoietic stem cell transplantation, SOS is caused by synergistic toxicity between the drugs used in high-dose combination chemotherapy or high-dose chemother-apy plus total-body irradiation, the so-called conditioning regimen in transplantation. There is no evidence to suggest that the transplantation itself contributes to the disease. In studies that included more than 100 patients transplanted to treat malignancies and nonmalignant conditions, the incidence of SOS has varied between 1 and 54% (68). The risk is particularly high when the transplantation is done for the treatment of malignancy, because of the higher doses of chemotherapy as well as patient-related factors. The wide range in risk of SOS between transplant units is largely due to differences in patient selection criteria, choice of chemotherapy/irradiation regimen, and criteria to diagnose SOS.

1. Diagnosis of SOS

SOS presents clinically with tender hepatomegaly, fluid retention, weight gain, and jaun-dice. The diagnosis of SOS in the setting of stem cell transplantation is based on these clinical features, and diagnostic criteria have been published by investigators in Seattle and Baltimore (69,70). The Seattle criteria require two of three findings occurring within 20 days of transplantation: bilirubin > 2 mg/dL, hepatomegaly or right-upper-quadrant pain of liver origin, and greater than 2% weight gain due to fluid accumulation. The Baltimore criteria require hyperbilirubinemia plus two of three other findings: bilirubin >2 mg/dL (usually painful), hepatomegaly, greater than 5% weight gain, and ascites. In addition to these criteria, it is necessary to first rule out competing causes such as (hyper) acute graft-versus-host disease, sepsis, cardiac failure, and tumor infiltration. Retrospec-tive comparison of these criteria found that more patients fulfilled the Seattle criteria and that the Baltimore criteria identified a sicker population (71). Although the Baltimore criteria identify a more clinically relevant population, the patients identified by these crite-ria may be further along in their course by the time they fulfill the criteria. SOS may be classified as mild, moderate, or severe. Mild disease is clinically apparent but resolves without therapy; moderate disease requires diuretics or pain medication, but resolves com-pletely; and severe disease requires treatment but does not resolve before death or day 100. Published graphs derived from retrospective data allow prediction of severity of disease for patients treated with regimens that contain cyclophosphamide (72).

Diagnosis is usually based on the diagnostic criteria above. The most useful addi-tional diagnostic tool is transvenous liver biopsy. This may be required to differentiate

SOS from hyperacute graft-versus-host disease. The transvenous approach also allows measurement of the hepatic venous pressure gradient: if higher than 10 mmHg this has a 90% specificity for SOS, although only a 50% sensitivity. Ultrasound can confirm hepatomegaly, may exclude tumor infiltration of the hepatic parenchyma and vasculature, and will detect biliary tract disease. However, two prospective studies in patients before and after stem cell transplantation did not support the usefulness of ultrasound in establishing the diagnosis of SOS (73,74).

2. Drugs that Cause SOS

Anticancer drugs may cause SOS at conventional doses, but the risk is substantially higher at the high doses used for stem cell transplantation. Even at high doses, the components of the conditioning regimen by themselves are not particularly hepatotoxic, but exhibit toxicity in combination regimens. Thus high-dose cyclophosphamide by itself rarely causes SOS (75), high-dose busulfan did not cause SOS in the small number of patients treated with it as a single agent (76), melphalan has little or no effect on liver tests (77–79), and total-body irradiation used alone within the dose range used in stem cell transplantation is not hepatotoxic (80).

The highest incidence of SOS occurs with combination regimens such as cyclophosphamide–total-body irradiation, busulfan-cyclophosphamide, BCNU-cyclophosphamide-etoposide, and carboplatin-cyclophosphamide-BCNU. The common element in these regimens, cyclophosphamide, is particularly toxic to sinusoidal endothelial cells in vitro (59). In contrast, patients treated with regimens combining busulfan and melphalan have a much lower incidence of SOS compared to the cyclophosphamide-containing regimens listed above (81,82).

Busulfan may predispose to SOS by depletion of glutathione in hepatocytes and sinusoidal endothelial cells (83). In the case of the busulfan-cyclophosphamide regimen, this then sets the stage for cyclophosphamide, which is given after busulfan, in two ways. Glutathione depletion in the sinusoidal endothelial cells increases susceptibility to the toxicity of acrolein, the proximate toxic metabolite derived from cyclophosphamide (59) (see Fig. 3). Glutathione depletion in the hepatocyte increases export of the cyclophosphamide metabolite, 4-hydroxycyclophosphamide, from the hepatocyte (L.D. DeLeve and J.T. Slattery, unpublished observation), which would increase the concentration of acrolein in the space of Disse, further endangering the sinusoidal endothelial cell. Consistent with this concept, in regimens with busulfan-cyclophosphamide, the risk is higher when busulfan is given before rather than after cyclophosphamide (84). It has not been practical in

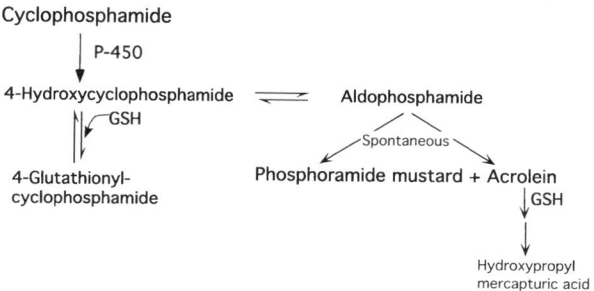

Figure 3 Simplified scheme of cyclophosphamide metabolism.

the past to give cyclophosphamide first, because nausea and emesis from cyclophospha-mide therapy complicated the oral administration of busulfan. However, with the advent of an intravenous formulation of busulfan, it will need to be confirmed whether the risk of SOS is lower if cyclophosphamide is given first. Busulfan may have a similar effect when it is given prior to melphalan, since glutathione depletion sensitizes to melphalan toxicity (85).

It has been shown in several studies that busulfan toxicity and efficacy benefit from dosage adjustment through therapeutic drug monitoring (86). Similarly, SOS associated with high-dose cyclophosphamide may be more common in individuals with higher con-centrations of cyclophosphamide metabolites (87), so therapeutic monitoring may prove to be of value. Lower doses of total-body irradiation decrease the risk of SOS, but increase the risk of leukemic relapse.

Mylotarg (gemtuzumab ozogamicin) is a new drug for acute myeloid leukemia that causes SOS. To date only a limited number of studies have reported on the liver toxicity from Mylotarg. The incidence and overall mortality vary in the few published studies, but the case-fatality rate appears to be high. Among 142 patients treated with Mylotarg, 23% had bilirubin elevations, mainly 1.5–3 times the upper limit of normal (88); it was not stated in this study whether patients with hyperbilirubinemia had other criteria for a diagnosis of SOS. In a series of 119 patients who had not received stem cell transplanta-tion, 14 patients (12%) developed SOS and eight died from SOS, for a case-fatality rate of 57% and an overall mortality rate from SOS of 6.7% (89). In a series of 23 patients treated with Mylotarg for acute myeloid leukemia that had relapsed after stem cell trans-plantation, 11 patients developed SOS and seven of 11 died, for a case-fatality rate of 64% and an overall mortality rate from SOS of 30% (90). In a series of 27 patients who underwent stem cell transplantation after Mylotarg treatment, three died of SOS for an overall mortality rate of 11% (88). Based on this limited information, it is not possible to determine whether exposure to both Mylotarg and stem cell transplantation is a risk for SOS or whether patients who have relapsed and need to cross over to the other treat-ment are at higher risk for SOS. The mechanism of Mylotarg cytotoxicity and genotoxicity will be discussed later.

B. Mechanism of Disease

Two clinical features provide clues to the mechanisms involved in SOS. First, in other intrinsic liver diseases parenchymal disease precedes the development of portal hyperten-sion. However, in SOS the signs and symptoms of portal hypertension precede evidence of parenchymal damage. In SOS, disruption of the liver circulation is the cause and not the consequence of the parenchymal disease. Second, veno-occlusive lesions of the hepatic veins are not essential to the development of the clinical picture: 45% of patients with mild or moderate disease and 25% of patients with severe SOS did not have occluded hepatic venules at autopsy (91). In-depth examination of the changes in the experimental model (see below) has established that the essential change occurs at the level of the sinusoid. Occlusion of central veins is associated with more severe disease and the devel-opment of ascites (91,92), which suggests that veno-occlusive lesions may add to the impairment of the circulation that occurs at the level of the sinusoid. The original name accorded to this disease, hepatic veno-occlusive disease, reflects the fact that the veno-occlusive lesion is easily recognized on light microscopy. The more recent recognition that involvement of the vein is not essential has led to the name change from hepatic veno-occlusive disease to hepatic sinusoidal obstruction syndrome.

Experimental studies have confirmed that changes in the hepatic sinusoid are the earliest changes in SOS. In vitro studies have shown that sinusoidal endothelial cells are more susceptible than hepatocytes to drugs that cause SOS (59,93,94). This is consistent with studies done in the rat using monocrotaline, a pyrrolizidine alkaloid that is one of the best-studied toxins involved in SOS. In this model the first morphological change noted by electron microscopy is loss of sinusoidal endothelial cell fenestration and the appearance of gaps in the sinusoidal endothelial cell barrier (95). The gaps increase in size over time and at the same time there is a decrease in the number of Kupffer cells and loss of venous endothelium. Studies with in vivo microscopy and confirmation by electron microscopy have shown that blood cells begin to track under sinusoidal endothelial cells that round up. The accumulation of blood in the space of Disse dissects off the sinusoidal lining, which creates an embolus of sinusoidal lining cells downstream that obstructs flow (96). By the time hepatocyte necrosis is observed, there is extensive sloughing of the sinusoidal lining, i.e., Kupffer cells, sinusoidal endothelial cells, and stellate cells. At this time point there is also a significant influx of monocytes within the sinusoids, which exacerbates the obstruction of sinusoidal flow by the embolized sinusoidal lining cells. These studies demonstrate that rounding up or swelling of sinusoidal endothelial cells is the initiating event in this experimental model of SOS and that this leads to dissection and embolization of sinusoidal lining cells that block the microcirculation.

The SOS-inducing drugs and toxins examined to date all profoundly deplete sinusoidal endothelial cell glutathione prior to cell death, and support of sinusoidal endothelial cell glutathione will prevent cell death (59,93,94). A continuous infusion of glutathione or N-acetylcysteine into the portal vein prevents the rounding up of the sinusoidal endothelial cells and the subsequent events that lead to the development of SOS in the monocrotaline model (60). If the glutathione infusion is discontinued several days after monocrotaline has been eliminated, full-blown SOS develops rapidly. Although glutathione protection may occur (partially) by preventing profound glutathione depletion, another mechanism for protection must be invoked to explain glutathione protection several days after monocrotaline has been eliminated. Since full-blown SOS in this model normally takes 72 h to develop, the accelerated development of SOS within 24 h after discontinuation of glutathione indicates that glutathione is suppressing a persistent change in the sinusoid.

One possible explanation for the rounding up of the sinusoidal endothelial cells may be increased activity of matrix metalloproteinases (MMPs) that allows the cells to let loose from the extracellular matrix in the space of Disse. In the experimental model, de novo synthesis of MMP-9 (gelatinase B) and increased MMP-9 activity occur 12 h after monocrotaline, which coincides with rounding up of the SEC (97). Furthermore, inhibition of MMP activity completely prevents SOS. MMP expression and activity are regulated by redox status and can be suppressed by glutathione and N-acetylcysteine (98–101). Thus the protective effect of glutathione and N-acetylcysteine may be (partially) due to inhibition of MMP activity.

An additional biochemical change that has been observed experimentally in SOS relates to nitric oxide. In the in vivo model hepatic vein nitric oxide decreases in parallel with the changes in the sinusoidal lining (102). Manipulations of nitric oxide production experimentally also suggest that decreased nitric oxide contributes to the development of

SOS (102). Analogous to glutathione, continuous infusion of nitric oxide prevents the rounding up of the sinusoidal endothelial cells and the subsequent steps involved in SOS (DeLeve and McCuskey, unpublished observations), further supporting the importance of this morphological change in the sinusoidal endothelial cell in the pathogenesis of this disease. Interestingly, tonic release of NO by endothelial cells reduces MMP-9 expression, whereas inhibition of NO synthesis increases cytokine-stimulated MMP-9 expression (103).

Although the disease is defined as a nonthrombotic obstruction of flow, the issue of clotting has been a recurring topic of research interest. The reader is referred to an in-depth review of this topic (104). Many of the observed changes interpreted to indicate a procoagulant state may have been sequelae of functional impairment and damage to the liver in SOS: hepatic dysfunction with decreased synthesis of anticoagulants (protein C, FVII, and ATIII), endothelial damage with release of membrane and intercellular proteins (vWF, FVIII, PAI-1, and tPA), and increased synthesis of acute-phase reactants (fibrinogen). Immunohistochemical studies in livers of patients with SOS have detected factor VIII and fibrinogen in the wall of the central veins, but not in the sinusoids or vascular lumen (105). Platelet glycoproteins could not be detected by immunostaining in the livers of patients with SOS (105). Electron microscopy of pyrrolizidine alkaloid-induced SOS in humans did not detect clotting (106). Sequential observations during the development of SOS in the experimental model by in vivo microscopy and electron microscopy have not demonstrated any evidence of clotting (95). Thus a role for coagulation has not been ruled out, but current studies do not provide evidence to support a role for activation of coagulation and local excess fibrin production as essential elements of SOS.

C. Nodular Regenerative Hyperplasia

In two case series, liver biopsy or autopsy material from patients within 100 days of stem cell transplantation has shown nodular regenerative hyperplasia in 8 and 23% of cases, respectively (91,107). Although the symptoms of nodular regenerative hyperplasia, i.e., hepatomegaly, ascites, and mild elevations of serum bilirubin, are the same symptoms used to diagnose SOS, the time of onset of symptoms is usually much later (66). The lesions may or may not be detectable with diagnostic imaging and the features are nondiagnostic. Double-spiral computerized tomography may aid in differentiating nodular regenerative hyperplasia from hepatocellular carcinoma.

A widely cited hypothesis for nodular regenerative hyperplasia is that it is due to local variation in blood flow within the liver: impairment of sinusoidal perfusion leading to atrophy with compensatory regeneration in adjacent areas (108–111). If this is true, heterogeneity of flow in the microcirculation could be due to impaired circulation at either the venular or sinusoidal level. Semiquantitative evaluation of the histology in a large autopsy study of patients with nodular regenerative hyperplasia showed that the most common vascular abnormality was obliteration of portal veins (112). Changes at the level of the sinusoids were demonstrated by ultrastructural studies of biopsies from three renal transplant patients who developed nodular regenerative hyperplasia, SOS, sinusoidal fibrosis, and/or peliosis hepatis due to azathioprine (113). This study demonstrated damage to and loss of sinusoidal endothelial cells, consistent with the selective toxicity of azathioprine for sinusoidal endothelial cells noted by in vitro studies (94). Since damage to sinusoidal endothelial cells is also the postulated mechanism of injury for SOS, it is not surprising that chemotherapy that causes SOS would also cause nodular regenerative hyperplasia.

D. Cyclosporin-Induced Cholestasis

Clinically significant liver toxicity from cyclosporin is uncommon. The most common form is bland cholestasis. Cyclosporin impairs canalicular function by inhibiting several of the canalicular transporters, with impairment of both bile-acid-dependent and bile-acid-independent bile flow (114–123).

IV. HEPATOTOXICITY BY ANTICANCER THERAPY

A. Diagnosis

Mild or moderate transient elevations of liver tests without clinical toxicity are common in patients treated with anticancer therapy and these may often be ignored. However, when clinical toxicity occurs, early diagnosis and discontinuation of the offending drug from the anticancer regimen is imperative. The diagnosis of drug-induced liver toxicity is often difficult in any clinical setting. The difficulty of diagnosis in cancer patients is compounded by a variety of other causes of liver disease related to the underlying cancer or cancer therapy (Table 2). There are systematic approaches to the diagnosis of drug-induced liver disease (124,125), but these do not lend themselves to drugs given cyclically in chemotherapy regimens. As in any setting, diagnosis is based on knowledge of the type of liver injury previously observed with a particular drug, the temporal relationship between drug exposure and evidence of liver toxicity, recurrent or exacerbated response upon reexposure, histological appearance if a biopsy is warranted, and exclusion of competing causes of liver disease.

B. Hepatotoxicity Due to Specific Anticancer Drugs

The majority of anticancer drugs in use today were first tested fairly long ago, many in the 1950s–1970s. Much of our information on the type and frequency of liver injury is

Table 2   Causes of Abnormal Liver Tests in Cancer Patients

Toxicity of anticancer drugs
Toxicity of supportive medications
Drug interactions
Radiation-induced liver disease
Tumor infiltration of the liver
Budd-Chiari syndrome (hypercoagulable state, tumor obstruction)
Paraneoplastic syndrome (Stauffer's syndrome)
Graft-versus-host disease (stem cell transplantation)
Total parenteral nutrition
Viral hepatitis
Fungal liver disease
Sepsis
Hemolysis
Congestive hepatopathy

Table 3 Conventional Dose Chemotherapy: Effect on Liver Tests and Liver Injury

Drug	Transient liver test abnormalities	Liver injury
6-Mercaptopurine		Numerous reports of either hepato-cellular or cholestatic liver disease
6-Thioguanine		Case reports of VOD; 1 case of peliosis hepatis when given with cytarabine; case reports of nodular regenerative hyperplasia when given with busulfan
Actinomycin D		VOD, particularly for right-sided Wilm's tumors
Busulfan		2 case reports of cholestatic liver injury; VOD in high-dose combination regimens
Carmustine (BCNU)	Up to 25% (232,233)	Case reports of liver injury, some fatalities. VOD
Chlorozotocin	Up to 25% elevations of amino-transferases (234)	3 case reports of severe cholestatic liver injury in 1 series
2-Chloro-3'-deoxyadenosine		1 case report peliosis hepatis in hairy cell leukemia
Cisplatin		Rare cases of steatosis and cholestasis; case reports of hepatocellular injury at high doses
Cyclophosphamide	Uncommon; see text for high dose	Rare case reports at conventional doses; VOD with high dose
Cytarabine	Frequent in one series but confounders obscure true causality; high dose may give transient abnormalities.	Case reports of cholestatic jaundice; case report of peliosis when given with 6-thioguanine
Dacarbazine	Mild, transient elevation of aminotransferases in up to 50% (235)	>15 case reports of VOD
Etoposide	Low incidence of moderate, transient liver test abnormalities (236)	Case reports of hepatocellular injury
Fluorodeoxyuridine (into hepatic art.)		Sclerosing cholangitis
Gemcitabine	Aminotransferase elevations WHO grade I–II[a] in 60% of patients, grade III/IV in 5–10% (237–240)	1 case report of fatal, fulminant liver failure
L-asparaginase	Abnormalities in >50% of patients in older literature; considerably less in recent years	Steatosis (40–90% incidence on autopsy); occasional hepatocellular necrosis
Lomustine (CCNU)	Uncommon (241)	Rare case reports of liver injury, some fatalities. VOD with high dose
Methotrexate	Aminotransferase elevation is common at high doses (139–141)	Steatosis, fibrosis and cirrhosis with maintenance therapy; case reports of hepatocellular carcinoma following fibrosis/cirrhosis

Table 3 Continued

Drug	Transient liver test abnormalities	Liver injury
Mitoxantrone	Transient abnormalities in bilirubin or aminotransferases (242,243)	
Mylotarg	Bilirubin elevations, 1.5–3 times ULN in 23% (88)	Incidence of SOS ranges from 12 to 48% with a case fatality rate of 60% (88–90)
Paclitaxel		One published case of fatal hepatic coma in patient with multiple liver metastases (244)
Streptozotocin	Up to 67% in 1973 study, but most patients had liver metastases (245)	
Flutamide	Aminotransferase elevations	By 1996, 46 reported cases of severe cholestatic hepatitis (3/10,000 users) with 20 fatalities (229)
Cyproterone acetate	10% with alkaline phosphatase and 3% with aminotransferase elevations (223)	13 case reports of hepatocellular injury with 8 fatalities; a series of 96 cases with 33 fatalities and 5 additional case reports with 2 fatalities not available to author for review
Tamoxifen		Steatosis; case reports of nonalcoholic steatohepatitis, some with cirrhosis; case report of peliosis; sinusoidal dilatation (also seen in experimental animals) (246)
Megestrol acetate		Case report of bland cholestasis
Mithramycin	Uncommon with dosing for hypercalcemia; frequent with daily dosing	Frequent liver injury with daily dosing

[a] See Table 4.

Unless stated, these findings pertain to conventional-dose rather than high-dose chemotherapy. Toxicity of high-dose treatment is discussed in the text.

derived from an era prior to hepatitis C testing and, in many cases, prior to testing for hepatitis B or even hepatitis A. A good example of this is methotrexate. In a frequently cited report from 1960, there was a very significant increase in the percentage of children with fibrosis noted on autopsy after aminopterin and methotrexate were introduced in 1948 (see details below). The extremely high incidence of liver injury seen in that era is not observed in the high-dose regimens today. Given the liberal use of transfusions in a period prior to hepatitis testing, viral hepatitis was likely a major confounder.

During much of the period when many of the currently used anticancer drugs were first tested, liver-imaging modalities were often inadequate to rule out occult involvement of the liver by tumor. Even current imaging modalities may not always detect tumor infiltration (126). Thus the bulk of the case reports, which are the major source for determining patterns of liver injury in humans, occurred in an era when jaundice due to liver metastases could easily have been attributed to chemotherapy.

The most clear-cut evidence of hepatotoxicity comes from studies using a drug as a single agent, since attribution of causality in a multidrug regimen may be difficult and toxicity may be due to an interaction of two or more drugs. Most anticancer drugs will be incorporated into a multidrug regimen once initial safety testing is complete. Thus our information on hepatotoxicity due to single drug exposure will often be 20 or more years old for many drugs. Thus much of the information of these drugs as single agents was reported prior to availability of diagnostic studies for viral hepatitis and of current imaging modalities. A final complication in cancer patients is the multitude of factors that may affect the liver (Table 2).

Although a high frequency of case reports may reliably link toxicity to a given drug, the bulk of our knowledge base for anticancer drugs comes from sporadic reports in the older literature, which is fraught with the difficulties described in the preceding paragraphs. This is particularly problematic for host-dependent, dose-independent toxicity (idiosyncratic reactions): these reactions usually occur with low frequency and the only reported cases may have occurred several decades ago. Thus, before one assumes that an anticancer drug does indeed cause hepatocellular injury, jaundice, or fibrosis, it is imperative to note the year of publication of the case reports that describe the injury.

Chemotherapeutic agents commonly cause transient increases in liver test abnormalities without evidence of clinically significant liver injury. Table 3 lists causes of transient liver test abnormalities at conventional doses of chemotherapy (as opposed to high-dose regimens used in stem cell transplantation and some experimental regimens). The right-hand column of Table 3 provides descriptions of the type of clinically apparent liver injury, which is mostly derived from case reports.

The relative infrequency of significant liver injury by chemotherapeutic agents is somewhat unexpected. The liver may be relatively protected since many of these compounds target rapidly proliferating cells, whereas liver cells have a slow turnover. As with other categories of drugs, the liver is also protected because of the relative strength of the detoxification pathways within the hepatocyte that protect it from electrophilic metabolites and drug-induced oxidative stress.

V. SELECTED ANTICANCER DRUGS AND MODALITIES

A. Alkylating Agents

1. Cyclophosphamide

Cyclophosphamide at standard doses is an uncommon cause of liver toxicity, with few reported cases of liver test abnormalities and rare case reports of clinically significant hepatocellular necrosis (127). SOS is seen almost exclusively at high doses of cyclophosphamide and in conjunction with synergistic agents, such as busulfan, total-body irradiation, or BCNU. The incidence of SOS in high-dose regimens that contain cyclophosphamide is often in the range of 20–40%.

Cyclophosphamide metabolism (see Fig. 3) by CYP 2C9 and 3A4 (8) in hepatocytes yields 4-hydroxycyclophosphamide, which appears in the circulation. 4-Hydroxycyclophosphamide equilibrates with aldophosphamide, which follows two pathways: spontaneous decomposition to phosphoramide mustard and acrolein, and metabolism by aldehyde dehydrogenase 1 (ALD1) to carboxyethyl phosphoramide mustard. Phosphoramide mustard is the putative antineoplastic moiety and acrolein is the proximate toxic metabolite.

There is wide interindividual variation in metabolism of intravenously administered cyclophosphamide and this variability may contribute to the risk of SOS (87). The presumptive mechanism of toxicity in SOS is through hepatocyte metabolism of cyclophosphamide and formation of acrolein, the proximate toxic metabolite (59). Acrolein is toxic to endothelial cells in general (128,129), but toxicity is greatest in the sinusoidal endothelial cells owing to their proximity to hepatocytes.

2. Busulfan

As a single agent, liver toxicity due to high-dose busulfan is described as cholestatic (76), but only two case reports have described cholestatic liver disease at standard chemotherapeutic doses. A large case series found that patients treated with the combination of busulfan plus 6-thioguanine had a significant incidence of noncirrhotic portal hypertension and/or of nodular regenerative hyperplasia (130). The literature on high-dose busulfan as a single agent is too limited to comment on whether it can induce SOS at all, but the risk seems to be low (76) and it is certainly less than with dimethylbusulfan alone (131,132). This may reflect differences in cellular toxicity. Busulfan is equally toxic to hepatocytes and sinusoidal endothelial cells, whereas dimethylbusulfan toxicity is selective for sinusoidal endothelial cells as is seen with other drugs closely linked to SOS (L.D. DeLeve, unpublished observation).

Busulfan is a weak alkylating agent. Experimental in vitro studies of busulfan toxicity and genotoxicity have been difficult to interpret as the doses needed to induce either interstrand crosslinking or toxicity have been significantly higher than therapeutic plasma concentrations in most of the studies. Busulfan toxicity requires glutathione-S-transferase-mediated conjugation to glutathione, which leads to oxidative stress (83). There are two mechanisms of oxidative stress. In an environment high in glutathione (e.g., within the hepatocyte) the busulfan-glutathione conjugate itself causes oxidative stress. In a low-glutathione environment, busulfan conjugation to glutathione further depletes intracellular glutathione, and the glutathione depletion causes oxidative stress.

Busulfan significantly depletes whole-liver glutathione levels in vivo at doses comparable to those used in hematopoietic stem cell transplantation (83). In vitro, both hepatocyte and sinusoidal endothelial cell glutathione are diminished to a similar degree. The synergistic effect of busulfan on liver toxicity by hematopoietic stem cell transplantation conditioning regimens may be due to glutathione depletion, oxidative stress, or both. Busulfan is synergistic with both cyclophosphamide and melphalan, which are both glutathione detoxified.

3. Dacarbazine

Dacarbazine-induced SOS has been reported in at least 15 case reports. The disease varies from the usual presentation of SOS in that it is associated with peripheral eosinophilia and thrombosis of the central venules and veins. The peripheral eosinophilia has been seen after the first exposure to dacarbazine (133), which suggests that this is related to the toxicity rather than implicating a hypersensitivity reaction.

The only site of microsomal activation of dacarbazine is the liver. The initial microsomal metabolite transforms spontaneously through several steps to the proximate methyl-donating metabolite, either a methylcarbonium or a methyldiazonium ion (134). This drug is selectively toxic to sinusoidal endothelial cells, which can metabolically activate it, and it is detoxified by glutathione (93).

4. Melphalan

At standard chemotherapeutic doses, melphalan is not hepatotoxic. As a single agent, high-dose melphalan (140 mg/m²) has been associated with either mild, transient elevations of serum aminotransferase and bilirubin (77,135) or no abnormalities at all (78,79). In high-dose multidrug conditioning regimens, melphalan is associated with SOS. However, it has been reported that the incidence and severity of SOS following the busulfan-melphalan regimen was lower than that seen historically due to the busulfan-cyclophosphamide regimen (81).

Melphalan, or L-phenylalanine mustard, is a bifunctional alkylating agent. Conjugation of melphalan to glutathione (GSH) requires glutathione-S-transferase and the glutathionyl conjugate is a noncompetitive inhibitor of GSH (136). Efflux of the GSH conjugate by MRP1 should determine ongoing conjugation of the parent compound, since efflux from the cell reduces the concentration of intracellular conjugate available to inhibit glutathione-S-transferase (136,137). The evidence that GSH conjugation detoxifies melphalan is not entirely straightforward: depletion of GSH exacerbates toxicity, but the addition of GSH or the GSH precursor N-acetylcysteine does not attenuate toxicity (85).

B. Antimetabolites

1. Methotrexate

Concern about methotrexate-induced fibrosis was raised by a much-cited 1960 study of 273 children treated for acute leukemia (138). The study described a 31% incidence of fibrosis in autopsy cases prior to the use of chemotherapy between 1940 and 1947 and an increase to 78% incidence of fibrosis between 1948 and 1951 when the folic acid antagonists aminopterin and methotrexate were used. No information was provided about the frequency of transfusion before and after the introduction of chemotherapy, and testing for viral hepatitis was, of course, not available. More recent studies have not found a significant incidence of liver injury (see below).

In high-dose methotrexate therapy for osteosarcoma, childhood acute lymphocytic leukemia, and adult non-Hodgkin's lymphomas, methotrexate may be infused in doses of 3–15 g/m². During maintenance therapy, weekly oral doses of low-dose methotrexate may be interspersed with additional infusions of high-dose methotrexate. Thus very large cumulative doses can be achieved. Although high-dose methotrexate has a high incidence of transient elevation of aminotransferase, the current literature suggests that this does not result in chronic liver disease (26,139–141). However, the incidence of fibrosis in this population may be underestimated. Liver tests correlate poorly with histological abnormalities and clinical studies using high-dose methotrexate have not routinely performed liver biopsies after treatment with significant cumulative doses of methotrexate. Thus clinically asymptomatic fibrosis likely goes undiagnosed.

Given the significant numbers of long-term disease-free survivors, long-term toxicity is a concern. Two case reports of hepatocellular carcinoma following methotrexate-induced fibrosis were reported in 1977 and 1987 (142,143); it should be noted that these reports preceded hepatitis C testing in leukemia patients, a population with a high incidence of hepatitis C. In a large meta-analysis, patients with psoriasis and rheumatoid arthritis have a 7% chance of progression of histological abnormalities on liver biopsy for every gram of methotrexate (144). Even if one assumes that asymptomatic fibrosis goes undiagnosed if systematic biopsies are not done, given the very high cumulative doses of methotrexate administered in cancer therapy, the incidence of significant liver injury would seem to be much lower than that suggested by the literature for rheumatoid arthritis and psoriasis.

2. Thiopurines

Liver injury from 6-mercaptopurine usually presents with jaundice that may be accompanied by pruritus. The injury is most commonly cholestatic, but hepatocellular necrosis may also be present. Although liver injury due to 6-mercaptopurine has frequently been reported, the actual incidence of toxicity is difficult to estimate but may be lower than suggested by early studies. In 1952, 6-mercaptopurine was first incorporated into the treatment for leukemia. Between 1954 and 1959, 6-mercaptopurine (typically 2.5 mg/kg/day, but as high as 5 mg/kg/day) was reported to induce jaundice in 6–14% of leukemic patients (145–147). The incidence in a 1964 study of 38 patients was reported to be as high as 42% (148). In current regimens for acute lymphoblastic leukemia, 6-mercaptopurine is used within multidrug regimens, usually with other potential hepatotoxins such as L-asparaginase, cytarabine, and methotrexate. Liver injury is not singled out as a major toxicity in most of the larger studies, and when it does occur, cannot be attributed to any particular drug in the regimen. Only one clear-cut case of drug-induced cholestatic hepatitis was found in an 18-year follow-up study of 396 patients with inflammatory bowel disease treated with 6-mercaptopurine (50 mg/day or 1.5 mg/kg) (149).

Metabolism of 6-mercaptopurine, 6-thioguanine, and azathioprine is shown in Fig. 3. Oral administration of thiopurines leads to extensive first-pass metabolism in the intestine and liver by xanthine oxidase. Cytotoxicity is due to formation of thioguanine nucleotides. In target tissues the effect of thiopurines is determined by the balance between detoxification by thiopurine S-methyltransferase (TPMT) and toxification by hypoxanthine phosphoribosyltransferase (HPRT): HPRT initiates formation of thioguanine nucleotides, whereas methylation reactions by TPMT shunt drug away from thioguanine nucleotide formation. There is a genetic polymorphism of TPMT activity with a trimodal distribution: 90% of persons have wild type, which confers high activity, 10% are heterozygotes with intermediate activity, and 0.3% are homozygous mutants with little or no detectable TPMT activity. Since TPMT shunts metabolites away from the activation pathway, low TPMT activity confers increased risk for hematopoietic toxicity (see review in ref. 150) and perhaps also for secondary malignancies, including brain tumors and acute myelogenous leukemia (151). However, hepatotoxicity from these thiopurines may be due to a different mechanism, namely high first-pass metabolism in the liver by TPMT to 6-methylmercaptopurine. What evidence is there to suggest this? TPMT mRNA is highly expressed in the liver (150) and hepatotoxicity is more frequent among individuals with higher TPMT activity (152). Studies that compared patients with and without 6-mercaptopurine hepatotoxicity demonstrated pharmacokinetics consistent with increased first-pass metabolism in the patients with toxicity, notably delayed time to peak concentrations, lower peak levels, and lower AUCs (153). High erythrocyte 6-methylmercaptopurine levels have been reported to correlate with hepatotoxicity (154). Alternatively or additionally, TPMT may contribute to toxicity through formation of methylmercaptopurine nucleotides derived from methylthioinosine monophosphate (see Fig. 3) (155).

An injury described as VOD has been linked to 6-thioguanine, often in combination with cytarabine (156–159). These cases have most often resembled radiation-induced liver disease (RILD) in some of the clinical and histological features. Patients present with hepatomegaly that is sometimes described as painful, and ascites, but without jaundice.

Bilirubin is often normal or marginally elevated, as is seen in RILD. There are veno-occlusive lesions and centrilobular congestion, but centrilobular hepatocyte atrophy is described rather than necrosis. Several of the patients also had underlying cirrhosis.

6-Thioguanine with busulfan has been linked to nodular regenerative hyperplasia (130,160). There is also a case report of peliosis hepatis associated with 6-thioguanine plus cytarabine (161).

It is not surprising that this group of liver injuries is linked to one drug, such as 6-thioguanine. SOS, nodular regenerative hyperplasia, peliosis hepatis, and sinusoidal dilatation often share similar causes and in some cases up to all four have been described within the same liver. Azathioprine (all four lesions), urethane (peliosis and SOS), heroin (sinusoidal dilatation, sinusoidal and perivenular fibrosis), thorotrast (peliosis, veno-occlusive lesions with hepatocyte atrophy), and oral contraceptives (sinusoidal dilatation and peliosis hepatis) cause an overlap of these injuries. Damage to sinusoidal endothelial cells and sometimes to hepatic venular endothelial cells seems to be the common link in these four types of liver injury (94,113,162–165). Azathioprine, another thiopurine, has been shown to be selectively toxic to sinusoidal endothelial cells (94), but this has not been examined specifically for 6-thioguanine.

3. Fluorodeoxyuridine

Fluorodeoxyuridine or floxuridine (FUDR) may be infused into the hepatic artery to treat hepatic metastases. This may cause liver test abnormalities and, in more serious cases, sclerosing cholangitis. High-grade obstruction of the common hepatic duct may extend into the left and right hepatic ducts and there are usually also multiple strictures of the intrahepatic ducts. The incidence varies widely in the literature; in a recent study of 32 patients who received an average of 7.3 cycles of chemotherapy, the incidence of liver test abnormalities was 15.6% and of severe biliary sclerosis was 9.3% (166). In another recent study in which 38 patients received two cycles of FUDR plus dexamethasone, 22% had elevations of AST and/or alkaline phosphatase and 7% had bilirubin elevations greater than 3 times the upper limit of normal (167). Concomitant treatment with dexamethasone has been suggested to reduce liver injury from intra-arterial FUDR, but this has not been well established (167–169). Progressive elevation of bilirubin levels, pruritus, or sepsis in patients with sclerosing cholangitis may be successfully palliated with percutaneous transhepatic biliary drainage (170). There are histological changes in the hilar vessels that suggest organization of occlusive thrombi (171). The biliary duct strictures of sclerosing cholangitis may therefore be due to circulatory impairment secondary to drug-induced damage to the peribiliary vascular plexus.

C. Monoclonal Antibodies

Mylotarg (gemtuzumab ozogamicin) is a new drug for acute myeloid leukemia that seems to have a significant incidence of SOS (88,89,172). In one case series, the overall mortality rate due to SOS in patients treated with Mylotarg who did not undergo stem cell transplantation was 7% (89). In patients who underwent stem cell transplantation after Mylotarg, the reported overall mortality from SOS was 11% (88). In patients who first underwent stem cell transplantation and later received Mylotarg, the overall mortality rate from SOS was 30% (90). Mylotarg has not been on the market long and future studies will need to more clearly define the incidence of SOS and risk factors.

Mylotarg is a conjugate of calicheamicin linked to the "humanized" monoclonal anti-CD33 antibody. CD33 is a myeloid surface antigen that is expressed on more than 90% of blast cells in acute myeloid leukemia, but not on hematopoietic stem cells or lymphoid cells. The presumptive mechanism of action of Mylotarg is preferential binding to cells with the CD33 antigen, internalization of the conjugate, and release of the calicheamicin moiety by acid hydrolysis within lysosomes (173,174). Calicheamicin has a methyltrisulfide group that is reduced by glutathione. The resulting diradical species binds to the minor groove of double-stranded DNA and causes sequence-selective oxidation of deoxyribose leading to DNA strand breaks (175,176). The mechanism leading to Mylotarg-induced SOS is undefined. Since both sinusoidal endothelial cells and Kupffer cells are of bone marrow origin (177,178), it is possible that one or both may have CD33 surface antigen that binds Mylotarg.

D. Miscellaneous Anticancer Drugs

L-Asparaginase is used in the treatment of acute lymphoblastic leukemia. It is a microbial product derived from *Escherichia coli* or from *Erwinia chrysanthemi*. Interference with liver function is manifested by decreased serum albumin, coagulation factors, and lipoproteins. Liver toxicity is thought to be due to inhibition of protein synthesis by asparaginase and glutaminase activity (179,180). In the past a particularly high incidence of liver toxicity was described with elevated alkaline phosphatase and serum aminotransferase and depression of liver synthetic function. A total of 40–87% of patients were found to have hepatic steatosis on autopsy and this could be detected up to 9 months after the last dose of L-asparaginase (181,182). The incidence of liver test abnormalities and of frank liver disease is considerably lower in the recent literature, although severe and fatal cases are still reported. In adults the incidence of transient WHO grade I or II liver test abnormalities (WHO grades listed in Table 4) is around 50% (183) with few cases of significant liver test abnormalities (183,184). A recent study of 245 patients with acute lymphoblastic leukemia randomized to conventional-dose or high-dose L-asparaginase as part of a multi-drug regimen found antithrombin III levels less than 50% in 0 and 2.5%, antithrombin III levels of 50–70% in 1.7 and 10.3%, and fibrinogen less than 100 mg/dL in 8.4 and 10.3% of patients, respectively, in the conventional- and high-dose L-asparaginase treatment groups (185). Liver test abnormalities and liver injury were not listed among the major toxicity reactions. In another recent study of 377 patients with acute lymphoblastic leukemia treated with a regimen that included L-asparaginase, liver test abnormalities and

Table 4 WHO Grades of Liver Test Abnormalities (247)

Grade 0	≤1.25× ULN
Grade 1	1.26–2.5× ULN
Grade 2	2.6–5× ULN
Grade 3	5.1–10× ULN
Grade 4	>10× ULN

The WHO grades apply to aminotransferases, alkaline phosphatase, and bilirubin. ULN, upper limit of normal.

liver injury were not listed among the more frequent toxicities; among a subgroup of 43 patients in this study who did not complete the full 30-week treatment regimen, 2% developed hepatitis (186).

Actinomycin D (or dactinomycin) has been associated with SOS. There may be some synergistic toxicity with abdominal irradiation or vincristine. The risk may correlate with the dose of radiation and perhaps also the dose of actinomycin D (187).

Most of the reported cases of actinomycin D have been in patients with right-sided Wilms' tumors (188). The risk of SOS may be greater when the right-sided tumors are large (189). The incidence of actinomycin D–induced SOS is low for left-side Wilms' tumors and for rhabdomyosarcoma (188,190). One potential explanation is that external vascular compression from these large right-sided nephroblastomas is impeding hepatic venous outflow, i.e., causing a Budd-Chiari syndrome. Another contributing factor may be intravascular extension of the nephroblastoma, causing Budd-Chiari syndrome, which may be underdiagnosed in the older literature (191). In one study, intravascular extension of tumor was diagnosed by ultrasonography in only 40% of cases, perhaps owing to the lesser imaging quality of older ultrasonography equipment in the early cases of the series (191). Budd-Chiari syndrome and SOS share many of the same clinical and histological features. The unanswered question is whether the increased incidence of SOS with right-sided Wilms' tumors is due to hepatic venous outflow obstruction acting in concert with actinomycin D–induced SOS, due to undiagnosed Budd-Chiari syndrome, or due to some other unidentified risk factor.

E. Radiation

Radiation-induced liver disease (RILD), or radiation hepatitis, occurs after hepatic irradiation. With conventional fractionation of irradiation, RILD occurs at doses in excess of 30–35 Gy in adults. Children or adults who have recently undergone partial hepatectomy may develop RILD at lower doses.

The signs and symptoms of RILD resemble Budd-Chiari syndrome or SOS, with hepatomegaly, weight gain, and varying amounts of ascites. Common histological features are sinusoidal congestion, sinusoidal fibrosis, and subendothelial and adventitial fibrosis of the central veins. However, RILD differs from SOS due to stem cell transplantation conditioning therapy in several ways (192) (see Table 5): (1) The diagnostic criteria for SOS in stem cell transplantation include elevations of bilirubin > 2 mg/dL and tenderness of the liver, whereas in RILD bilirubin elevations are usually minimal and right-upper-

Table 5 Differences Between Sinusoidal Obstruction Syndrome (SOS) and Radiation-Induced Liver Disease (RILD)

	SOS in stem cell transplantation	RILD
Time of onset	Day 0–30	2 Weeks–4 months (usually 1–2 months)
Resolution of signs/symptoms	30–60 Days	Months
RUQ pain	Marked	Mild
Bilirubin	>2 mg/dL, often markedly elevated	Normal or minimal elevation
Histology	Centrilobular necrosis	Centrilobular atrophy

quadrant pain is much less pronounced (192,193). (2) A characteristic histological feature of SOS is centrilobular necrosis, whereas in RILD there is atrophy of the centrilobular cords and coagulative necrosis is uncommon (192–194). The presence of atrophy rather than necrosis may reflect the fact that RILD becomes clinically apparent at a much later time point. (3) In RILD fibrin has been identified within the central vein by electron microscopy, but fibrin has not been demonstrated by electron microscopic examination of SOS. (4) In SOS onset of the first clinical signs can occur as early as day 0, the day of stem cell infusion, or as late as 30 days after exposure to the conditioning regimen. Onset of RILD typically occurs 1–2 months after irradiation, although it may occur as early as 2 weeks or as late as 7 months afterward (192). (5) Signs of SOS resolve within 30–60 days of onset in patients who survive the disease, whereas in RILD evidence of liver injury can persist for months after the insult has been discontinued (193,195). Thus clinical presentation, histology, and time course of disease distinguish RILD from SOS.

Historically, RILD has limited use of hepatic irradiation in the treatment of intra-hepatic cancers. However, with the advent of three-dimensional radiation therapy treatment planning, much higher doses of radiation can be delivered to the liver with a low incidence of RILD (196).

Hepatic irradiation can also act synergistically with chemotherapy to cause liver toxicity. Total-body irradiation contributes to the risk of SOS in hematopoietic stem cell transplantation, although the doses of irradiation used (10–16 Gy) are well below the hepatotoxic dose for radiation alone. In combination with cyclophosphamide, the incidence of SOS is higher in single-dose than in hyperfractionated total-body irradiation (197). Higher doses of total body irradiation, i.e., >12 Gy, may also increase the risk (69). Doses of irradiation > 20 Gy may also contribute to the incidence of SOS when used in conjunction with L-asparaginase for Wilms' tumor. No features have been identified that distinguish SOS due to high-dose combination chemotherapy (i.e., chemotherapeutic drugs without irradiation) from that resulting from hepatic irradiation plus high-dose chemotherapy.

Long-term radiation damage in various tissues may be due to damage to microvascular endothelial cells (198–203), with apoptosis of the microvascular endothelial cells (204–206). Irradiation significantly depletes mitochondrial glutathione and causes oxidative damage to mitochondrial and nuclear DNA (207). Glutathione depletion enhances toxicity of radiation in vitro and in vivo (61,207). Changes in the endothelial cell glutathione pool may explain the synergistic toxicity of total-body irradiation and chemotherapy in stem cell conditioning regimens.

F. Hormones

1. Tamoxifen

Tamoxifen, a nonsteroidal drug with antiestrogenic and estrogenic properties, is widely used in the chemoprevention of breast cancer. Reported liver injury from tamoxifen includes nonalcoholic fatty liver disease (208–213), peliosis hepatis (214), acute hepatitis (215), and hepatocellular cancer (216,217).

Nonalcoholic fatty liver disease (NAFLD) is the most common form of liver injury due to tamoxifen. A Japanese study that screened 105 women on tamoxifen by annual abdominal computerized-tomography examination found a 38% incidence of fatty liver, which developed during the first 2 years of therapy in 35 of the 40 cases (85%) (213). Forty percent of the patients with fatty liver (16 of 40 patients) had sustained elevations of aminotransferases. In addition, there have been three reported cases of cirrhosis in the presence of steatohepatitis by liver biopsy (209,211). Future studies will need to determine whether the risk of severe steatohepatitis in tamoxifen users warrants routine screening for nonalcoholic fatty liver disease.

Rats treated with tamoxifen develop nodular regenerative hyperplasia, hepatic adenomas, and hepatocellular carcinomas (218). Tamoxifen is metabolized by CYP 3A4. There are substantial differences between rats and humans in the rate of tamoxifen metabolism and in the metabolites formed. To achieve clinically relevant serum concentrations, rats must be given high doses, which result in very high liver concentrations of tamoxifen and its metabolites (219,220). Rats are also more susceptible to liver DNA damage from tamoxifen, albeit at liver concentrations that are much higher than those seen in humans (220,221). The propensity for hepatocellular cancer in rats may be very species specific, since liver tumors are not found in mice or hamsters. There is currently no epidemiological evidence in humans of a significant increase in the incidence of liver cancer (see review in ref. 218), but there have been case reports of hepatocellular cancer after long-term use of tamoxifen (216,217). Given the expanded indications for use of tamoxifen, future clinical studies will undoubtedly carefully monitor the risk of hepatocellular carcinoma.

2. Cyproterone Acetate

Cyproterone acetate is a synthetic progesterone derivative with antiandrogenic and progesterone-like activity, used in the treatment of advanced prostate cancer. It is marketed in the United Kingdom and Germany, but is not approved by the Food and Drug Administration. In a large surveillance study of 1685 patients receiving cyproterone acetate for indications other than prostate cancer, elevated liver tests were noted in 10% of patients treated with 50 mg/day and 20% of those receiving >100 mg/day (222). A retrospective analysis of 78 patients receiving 50 mg/day of cyproterone acetate for advanced prostate cancer reported elevation of alkaline phosphatase in 14% of patients without known liver involvement and elevated aminotransferases in 2.5% (223). There have been 18 case reports of cyproterone-associated hepatitis with six fatalities. A review article (222) cited a report of 96 hepatotoxic events with 33 fatalities attributed to cyproterone acetate (224); however, I have been unable to obtain this report to date. There has also been one report of cirrhosis in a pediatric patient treated for precocious puberty (225).

Cyproterone acetate is mitogenic, tumorigenic, and induces DNA adducts and DNA-repair synthesis in rat liver (see reviews in refs. 226, 227). High levels of DNA adducts are also formed in human hepatocytes. It has been suggested that formation of the reactive metabolite is catalyzed by hydroxysteroid-sulfotransferases. Although long-term exposure to cyproterone acetate at high doses may potentially induce hepatocellular carcinomas, this is unlikely to be clinically relevant given the current life expectancy for advanced prostate cancer.

3. Flutamide

Liver injury from flutamide presents with marked elevations of bilirubin and a wide range in elevation of serum aminotransferases. The predominant histological feature determined on autopsy is marked to massive hepatic necrosis. In a multicenter study of 905 patients treated with flutamide, liver tests with elevations greater than 4 times the upper limit of normal occurred in 0.8% of patients (228). According to postmarketing surveillance, severe liver disease due to flutamide has occurred in 46 patients with 20 fatalities (229).

The rate of serious liver injury is estimated to be 3 per 10,000 flutamide users, based on the number of prescriptions written.

Flutamide is a synthetic nonsteroidal that is a competitive antagonist of the androgen receptor. After oral administration, flutamide undergoes extensive first-pass metabolism with formation of several oxidized metabolites. Formation of electrophilic metabolites is catalyzed via CYP 3A and CYP 1A (230). Experimental studies in rat hepatocytes (231) suggest that toxicity from the electrophilic metabolites occurs through depletion of hepatocyte glutathione, which is accompanied by oxidative stress. Toxicity to mitochondria is manifested by depression of mitochondrial respiration and ATP formation, but the study did not report whether mitochondrial toxicity was due to depletion of mitochondrial glutathione.

VI. CONCLUSIONS

Transient liver test abnormalities are a common occurrence in cancer chemotherapy. Our knowledge of chemotherapy-induced liver injury is confounded by the injurious effects of a variety of insults to the liver in cancer patients as well as by the limitations in the older literature. Nevertheless it is clear that liver injury is a relatively frequent complication in some of the current treatments for hematological malignancies, but that clinically apparent liver injury occurs much less frequently with conventional-dose chemotherapy.

REFERENCES

1. Zimm S, Colins JM, O'Neill D, Chabner BA, Poplack DG. Inhibition of first-pass metabolism in cancer chemotherapy: interaction of 6-mercaptopurine and allopurinol. Clin Pharmacol Ther 1983; 34:810–817.
2. Humerickhouse R, Lohrbach K, Li L, Bosron WF, Dolan ME. Characterization of CPT-11 hydrolysis by human liver carboxylesterase isoforms hCE-1 and hCE-2. Cancer Res 2000; 60:1189–1192.
3. Iyer L, King CD, Whitington PF, Green MD, Roy SK, Tephly TR, Coffman BL, Ratain MJ. Genetic predisposition to the metabolism of irinotecan (CPT-11). Role of uridine diphosphate glucuronosyltransferase isoform 1A1 in the glucuronidation of its active metabolite (SN-38) in human liver microsomes. J Clin Invest 1998; 101:847–854.
4. Sugiyama Y, Kato Y, Chu X. Multiplicity of biliary excretion mechanisms for the camptothecin derivative irinotecan (CPT-11), its metabolite SN-38, and its glucuronide: role of canalicular multispecific organic anion transporter and P-glycoprotein. Cancer Chemother Pharmacol 1998; 42(suppl):S44–S49.
5. Slatter JG, Schaaf LJ, Sams JP, Feenstra KL, Johnson MG, Bombardt PA, Cathcart KS, Verburg MT, Pearson LK, Compton LD, Miller LL, Baker DS, Pesheck CV, Lord RS, 3rd. Pharmacokinetics, metabolism, and excretion of irinotecan (CPT-11) following I.V. infusion of [(14)C]CPT-11 in cancer patients. Drug Metab Dispos 2000; 28:423–433.
6. Anderson GD. A mechanistic approach to antiepileptic drug interactions. Ann Pharmacother 1998; 32:554–563.
7. Gupta E, Wang X, Ramirez J, Ratain MJ. Modulation of glucuronidation of SN-38, the active metabolite of irinotecan, by valproic acid and phenobarbital. Cancer Chemother Pharmacol 1997; 39:440–444.
8. Ren S, Yang JS, Kalhorn TF, Slattery JT. Oxidation of cyclophosphamide to 4-hydroxycyclophosphamide and dechloroethylcyclophosphamide in human liver microsomes. Cancer Res 1997; 57:4229–4235.

9. Ambudkar SV, Dey S, Hrycyna CA, Ramachandra M, Pastan I, Gottesman MM. Biochemical, cellular, and pharmacological aspects of the multidrug transporter. Annu Rev Pharmacol Toxicol 1999; 39:361–398.

10. Kivistö KT, Kroemer HK, Eichelbaum M. The role of human cytochrome P450 enzymes in the metabolism of anticancer agents: implications for drug interactions. Br J Clin Pharmacol 1995; 40:523–530.

11. Lum BL, Kaubisch S, Yahanda AM, Adler KM, Jew L, Ehsan MN, Brophy NA, Halsey J, Gosland MP, Sikic BI. Alteration of etoposide pharmacokinetics and pharmacodynamics by cyclosporine in a phase I trial to modulate multidrug resistance. J Clin Oncol 1992; 10:1635–1642.

12. Ellis AG, Webster LK. Inhibition of paclitaxel elimination in the isolated perfused rat liver by Cremophor EL. Cancer Chemother Pharmacol 1999; 43:13–18.

13. Ellis AG, Crinis NA, Webster LK. Inhibition of etoposide elimination in the isolated perfused rat liver by Cremophor EL and Tween 80. Cancer Chemother Pharmacol 1996; 38:81–87.

14. Yule SM, Walker D, Cole M, McSorley L, Cholerton S, Daly AK, Pearson AD, Boddy AV. The effect of fluconazole on cyclophosphamide metabolism in children. Drug Metab Dispos 1999; 27:417–421.

15. Villikka K, Kivisto KT, Maenpaa H, Joensuu H, Neuvonen PJ. Cytochrome P450-inducing antiepileptics increase the clearance of vincristine in patients with brain tumors. Clin Pharmacol Ther 1999; 66:589–593.

16. Royer I, Monsarrat B, Sonnier M, Wright M, Cresteil T. Metabolism of docetaxel by human cytochromes P450: interactions with paclitaxel and other antineoplastic drugs. Cancer Res 1996; 56:58–65.

17. Friedman HS, Petros WP, Friedman AH, Schaaf LJ, Kerby T, Lawyer J, Parry M, Houghton PJ, Lovell S, Rasheed K, Cloughsey T, Stewart ES, Colvin OM, Provenzale JM, McLendon RE, Bigner DD, Cokgor I, Haglund M, Rich J, Ashley D, Malczyn J, Elfring GL, Miller LL. Irinotecan therapy in adults with recurrent or progressive malignant glioma. J Clin Oncol 1999; 17:1516–1525.

18. Larroquette CA, Hortobagyi GN, Buzdar AU, Holmes FA. Subclinical hepatic toxicity during combination chemotherapy for breast cancer. JAMA 1986; 256:2988.

19. Zhou-Pan XR, Seree E, Zhou XJ, Placidi M, Maurel P, Barra Y, Rahmani R. Involvement of human liver cytochrome P450 3A in vinblastine metabolism: drug interactions. Cancer Res 1993; 53:5121–5126.

20. Zhou XJ, Zhou-Pan XR, Gauthier T, Placidi M, Maurel P, Rahmani R. Human liver microsomal cytochrome P450 3A isozymes mediated vindesine biotransformation: metabolic drug interactions. Biochem Pharmacol 1993; 45:853–861.

21. Kajita J, Kuwabara T, Kobayashi H, Kobayashi S. CYP3A4 is mainly responsible for the metabolism of a new vinca alkaloid, vinorelbine, in human liver microsomes. Drug Metab Dispos 2000; 28:1121–1127.

22. Rahman A, Korzekwa KR, Grogan J, Gonzalez FJ, Harris JW. Selective biotransformation of taxol to 6 alphahydroxytaxol by human cytochrome P450 2C8. Cancer Res 1994; 54:5543–5546.

23. Robieux I, Sorio R, Borsatti E, Cannizzaro R, Vitali V, Aita P, Freschi A, Galligioni E, Monfardini S. Pharmacokinetics of vinorelbine in patients with liver metastasis. Clin Pharmacol Ther 1996; 59:32–40.

24. Figg WD, Dukes GE, Pritchard JF, Herman DJ, Lesesne HR, Carson SW, Songer SS, Powell JR, Hak LJ. Pharmacokinetics of ondansetron in patients with hepatic insufficiency. J Clin Pharmacol 1996; 36:206–215.

25. Locasciulli A, Testa M, Pontisso P, Benvegnu L, Fraschini D, Corbetta A, Noventa F, Masera G, Alberti A. Prevalence and natural history of hepatitis C infection in patients cured of childhood leukemia. Blood 1997; 90:4628–4633.

26. Farrow AC, Buchanan GR, Zwiener RJ, Bowman WP, Winick NJ. Serum aminotransferase elevation during and following treatment of childhood acute lymphoblastic leukemia. J Clin Oncol 1997; 15:1560–1566.

27. Meir H, Balawi I, Nayel H, El Karaksy H, El Haddad A. Hepatic dysfunction in children with acute lymphoblastic leukemia in remission: relation to hepatitis infection. Med Pediatr Oncol 2001; 36:469–473.

28. Horina JH, Wirnsberger GH, Kenner L, Holzer H, Krejs GJ. Increased susceptibility for CsA-induced hepatotoxicity in kidney graft recipients with chronic viral hepatitis C. Transplantation 1993; 56:1091–1094.

29. Zylberberg H, Carnot F, Mamzer M-F, Blancho G, Legendre C, Pol S. Hepatitis C virus-related fibrosing cholestatic hepatitis after renal transplantation. Transplantation 1997; 63: 158–160.

30. Ungo JR, Jones D, Ashkin D, Hollender ES, Bernstein D, Albanese AP, Pitchenik AE. Antituberculosis drug-induced hepatotoxicity. The role of hepatitis C virus and the human immunodeficiency virus. Am J Respir Crit Care Med 1998; 157:1871–1876.

31. Strasser SI, Myerson D, Spurgeon CL, Sullivan KM, Storer B, Schoch HG, Kim S, Flowers ME, McDonald GB. Hepatitis C virus infection and bone marrow transplantation: a cohort study with 10-year follow-up. Hepatology 1999; 29:1893–1899.

32. Sulkowski MS, Thomas DL, Chaisson RE, Moore RD. Hepatotoxicity associated with antiretroviral therapy in adults infected with human immunodeficiency virus and the role of hepatitis C or B virus infection. JAMA 2000; 283:74–80.

33. Alter MJ, Kruszon-Moran D, Nainan OV, McQuillan GM, Gao F, Moyer LA, Kaslow RA, Margolis HS. The prevalence of hepatitis C virus infection in the United States, 1988 through 1994. N Engl J Med 1999; 341:556–562.

34. Cheng AL. Steroid-free chemotherapy decreases the risk of hepatitis flare-up in hepatitis B virus carriers with non-Hodgkin's lymphoma [letter]. Blood 1996; 87:1202.

35. Durnas C, Loi CM, Cusack BJ. Hepatic drug metabolism and aging. Clin Pharmacokinet 1990; 19:359–389.

36. Sotaniemi EA, Arranto AJ, Pelkonen O, Pasanen M. Age and cytochrome P450-linked drug metabolism in humans: an analysis of 226 subjects with equal histopathologic conditions. Clin Pharmacol Ther 1997; 61:331–339.

37. Le Couteur DG, Cogger VC, Markus AM, Harvey PJ, Yin ZL, Annselin AD, McLean AJ. Pseudocapillarization and associated energy limitation in the aged rat liver. Hepatology 2001; 33:537–543.

38. Etienne MC, Chatelut E, Pivot X, Lavit M, Pujol A, Canal P, Milano G. Co-variables influencing 5-fluorouracil clearance during continuous venous infusion: a NONMEM analysis. Eur J Cancer 1998; 34:92–97.

39. Stein BN, Petrelli NJ, Douglass HO, Driscoll DL, Arcangeli G, Meropol NJ. Age and sex are independent predictors of 5-fluorouracil toxicity. Cancer 1994; 75:11–17.

40. Lu Z, Zhang R, Diasio RB. Population characteristics of hepatic dihydropyrimidine dehydrogenase activity, a key metabolic enzyme in 5-fluorouracil chemotherapy. Clin Pharmacol Ther 1995; 58:512–522.

41. den Hartigh J, McVie JG, van Oort WJ, Pinedo HM. Pharmacokinetics of mitomycin C in humans. Cancer Res 1983; 43:5017–5021.

42. Miya T, Sasaki Y, Karato A, Saijo N. Pharmacokinetic study of mitomycin C with emphasis on the influence of aging. Jpn J Cancer Res 1992; 83:1382–1385.

43. Wade JR, Kelman AW, Kerr DJ, Robert J, Whiting B. Variability in the pharmacokinetics of epirubicin: a population analysis. Cancer Chemother Pharmacol 1992; 29:391–395.

44. Cusack BJ, Mushlin PS, Johnson CJ, Vestal RE, Olson RD. Aging increases the cardiotoxicity of daunorubicin and daunorubicinol in the rat. J Gerontol. Series A, Biol Sci Med Sci 1996; 51:B376–B384.

45. Cusack BJ, Young SP, Vestal RE, Olson RD. Age-related pharmacokinetics of daunorubicin

and daunorubicinol following intravenous bolus daunorubicin administration in the rat. Cancer Chemother Pharmacol 1997; 39:505–512.

46. Anonymous. The effect of age and renal function on the efficacy and toxicity of methotrexate in rheumatoid arthritis: Rheumatoid Arthritis Clinical Trial Archive Group. J Rheumatol 1995; 22:218–223.

47. Dobbs NA, Twelves CJ, Gillies H, James CA, Harper PG, Rubens RD. Gender affects doxorubicin pharmacokinetics in patients with normal liver biochemistry. Cancer Chemother Pharmacol 1995; 36:473–476.

48. Grenier MA, Lipshultz SE. Epidemiology of anthracycline cardiotoxicity in children and adults. Semin Oncol 1998; 25:72–85.

49. Lipshultz SE, Lipsitz SR, Mone SM, Goorin AM, Sallan SE, Sanders SP, Orav EJ, Gelber RD, Colan SD. Female sex and higher drug dose as risk factors for late cardiotoxic effects of doxorubicin therapy for childhood cancer. N Engl J Med 1995; 332:1738–1743.

50. Silber JH, Jakacki RI, Larsen RL, Goldwein JW, Barber G. Increased risk of cardiac dysfunction after anthracyclines in girls [see comments]. Med Pediatr Oncol 1993; 21:477–479.

51. Zalcberg J, Kerr D, Seymour L, Palmer M. Haematological and non-haematological toxicity after 5-fluorouracil and leucovorin in patients with advanced colorectal cancer is significantly associated with gender, increasing age and cycle number: Tomudex International Study Group. Eur J Cancer 1998; 34:1871–1875.

52. Milano G, Etienne MC, Pierrefite V, Barberi-Heyob M, Deporte-Fety R, Renee N. Dihydropyrimidine dehydrogenase deficiency and fluorouracil-related toxicity. Br J Cancer 1999; 79:627–630.

53. Bressolle F, Joulia JM, Pinguet F, Ychou M, Astre C, Duffour J, Gomeni R. Circadian rhythm of 5-fluorouracil population pharmacokinetics in patients with metastatic colorectal cancer. Cancer Chemother Pharmacol 1999; 44:295–302.

54. Chazal M, Etienne MC, Renée N, Bourgeon A, Richelme H, Milano G. Link between dihydropyrimidine dehydrogenase activity in peripheral blood mononuclear cells and liver. Clin Cancer Res 1996; 2:507–510.

55. Lu Z, Zhang R, Carpenter JT, Diasio RB. Decreased dihydropyrimidine dehydrogenase activity in a population of patients with breast cancer: implication for 5-fluorouracil-based chemotherapy. Clin Cancer Res 1998; 4:325–329.

56. Walter-Sack I, Klotz U. Influence of diet and nutritional status on drug metabolism. Clin Pharmacokin 1996; 31:47–64.

57. Davis LE, Lenkinski RE, Shinkwin MA, Kressel HY, Daly JM. The effect of dietary protein depletion on hepatic 5-fluorouracil metabolism. Cancer 1993; 72:3715–3722.

58. Cusack BJ, Young SP, Loseke VL, Hurty MR, Beals L, Olson RD. Effect of a low-protein diet on doxorubicin pharmacokinetics in the rabbit. Cancer Chemother Pharmacol 1992; 30:145–148.

59. DeLeve LD. Cellular target of cyclophosphamide toxicity in the murine liver: role of glutathione and site of metabolic activation. Hepatology 1996; 24:830–837.

60. Wang X, Kanel GC, DeLeve LD. Support of sinusoidal endothelial cell glutathione prevents hepatic veno-occlusive disease in the rat. Hepatology 2000; 31:428–434.

61. Geraci JP, Mariano MS, Jackson KL. Radiation hepatology of the rat: microvascular fibrosis and enhancement of liver dysfunction by diet and drugs. Radiat Res 1992; 129:322–332.

62. Iyer L, Ratain MJ. Pharmacogenetics and cancer chemotherapy. Eur J Cancer 1998; 34:1493–1499.

63. Bosma PJ, Roy Chowdhury J, Bakker C, Gantla S, De Boer A, Oostra BA, Lindhout D, Tytgat GNJ, Jansen PLM, Oude Elferink RPJ, Roy Chowdhury N. The genetic basis of the reduced expression of bilirubin UDP-glucuronosyltransferase I in Gilbert's syndrome. N Engl J Med 1998; 333:1171–1175.

64. Wasserman E, Myara A, Lokiec F, Goldwasser F, Trivin F, Mahjoubi M, Misset JL,

Cvitkovic E. Severe CPT-11 toxicity in patients with Gilbert's syndrome: two case reports. Ann Oncol 1997; 8:1049–1051.

65. Iyer L, Hall D, Das S, Mortell MA, Ramirez J, Kim S, Di Rienzo A, Ratain MJ. Phenotype-genotype correlation of in vitro SN-38 (active metabolite of irinotecan) and bilirubin glucuronidation in human liver tissue with UGT1A1 promoter polymorphism. Clin Pharmacol Ther 1999; 65:576–582.

66. Strasser SI, McDonald GB. Gastrointestinal and hepatic complications. In: ED Thomas, KG Blume, SJ Forman, eds. Hematopoietic Cell Transplantation. Cambridge, MA: Blackwell Scientific Publications, 1999:627–658.

67. Willmot FC, Robertson GW. Senecio disease, or cirrhosis of the liver due to senecio poisoning. Lancet 1920; 2:848–849.

68. Bearman SI. The syndrome of hepatic veno-occlusive disease after marrow transplantation. Blood 1995; 85:3005–3020.

69. McDonald GB, Hinds MS, Fisher LD, Schoch HG, Wolford JL, Banaji M, Hardin BJ, Shulman HM, Clift RA. Veno-occlusive disease of the liver and multiorgan failure after bone marrow transplantation—a cohort study of 355 patients. Ann Intern Med 1993; 118:255–267.

70. Jones RJ, Lee KSK, Beschorner WE, Vogel VG, Grochow LB, Vogelsang GB, Sensenbrenner LL, Santos GW, Saral R. Veno-occlusive disease of the liver following bone marrow transplantation. Transplantation 1987; 44:778–783.

71. Blostein MD, Paltiel OB, Thibault A, Rybka WB. A comparison of clinical criteria for the diagnosis of veno-occlusive disease of the liver after bone marrow transplantation. Bone Marrow Transplant. 1992; 10:439–443.

72. Bearman SI, Anderson GL, Mori M, Hinds MS, Shulman HM, McDonald GB. Venoocclusive disease of the liver: development of a model for predicting fatal outcome after marrow transplantation. J Clin Oncol 1993; 11:1729–1736.

73. Hommeyer SC, Teefey SA, Jacobson AF, Higano CS, Bianco JA, Colacurcio CJ, McDonald GB. Venoocclusive disease of the liver: prospective study of US evaluation. Radiology 1992; 683:686.

74. Teefey SA, Brink JA, Borson RA, Middleton WD. Diagnosis of venoocclusive disease of the liver after bone marrow transplantation: value of duplex sonography. AJR 1995; 164:1397–1401.

75. Deeg HJ, Shulman HM, Schmidt E, Yee GC, Thomas ED, Storb R. Marrow graft rejection and veno-occlusive disease of the liver in patients with aplastic anemia conditioned with cyclophosphamide and cyclosporine. Transplantation 1986; 42:497–501.

76. Peters WP, Henner WD, Grochow LB, Olsen G, Edwards S, Stanbuck H, Stuart A, Gockerman J, Moore J, Bast RC, Jr., Seigler HF, Colvin OM. Clinical and pharmacological effects of high dose single agent busulfan with autologous bone marrow support in the treatment of solid tumors. Cancer Res 1987; 47:6402–6406.

77. Ayash LJ, Elias A, Wheeler C, Reich E, Schwartz G, Mazanet R, Tepler I, Warren D, Lynch C, Gonin R, Schnipper L, Frei E, III, Antman K. Double dose-intensive chemotherapy with autologous marrow and peripheral-blood progenitor-cell support for metastatic breast cancer: a feasibility study. J Clin Oncol 1994; 12:37–44.

78. Singhal S, Powles R, Treleaven J, Horton C, Swansbury GJ, Mehta J. Melphalan alone prior to allogeneic bone marrow transplantation from HLA-identical sibling donors for hematologic malignancies: alloengraftment with potential preservation of fertility in women. Bone Marrow Transplant 1996; 18:1049–1055.

79. Moreau P, Fiere D, Bezwoda WR, Facon R, Attal M, Laporte JP, Colombat P, Haak HL, Monconduit M, Lockhorst H, Girault D, Harousseau JL. Prospective randomized placebo-controlled study of granulocyte-macrophage colony-stimulating factor without stem-cell transplantation after high-dose melphalan in patients with multiple myeloma. J Clin Oncol 1997; 15:660–666.

80. Fajardo LF, Berthrong M. Radiation injury in surgical pathology. Am J Surg 1978; 2:159–199.

81. Lee JL, Gooley T, Bensinger W, Schiffman K, McDonald GB. Veno-occlusive disease of the liver after busulfan, melphalan, and thiotepa conditioning therapy: incidence, risk factors, and outcome. Biol Blood Marrow Transplant 1999; 5:306–315.

82. Srivastava A, Bradstock KF, Szer J, de Bortoli L, Gottlieb DJ. Busulphan and melphalan prior to autologous bone marrow transplantation. Bone Marrow Transplant 1993; 12:323–329.

83. DeLeve LD, Wang X. Role of oxidative stress and glutathione in busulfan toxicity in cultured murine hepatocytes. Pharmacology 2000; 60:143–154.

84. Méresse V, Hartmann O, Vassal G, Benhamou E, Valteau-Couanet D, Brugieres L, Lemerle J. Risk factors for hepatic veno-occlusive disease after high-dose busulfan-containing regimens followed by autologous bone marrow transplantation: a study in 136 children. Bone Marrow Transplant 1992; 10:135–141.

85. Vahrmeijer AL, van Dierendonck JH, Schutrups J, van de Velde CJ, Mulder GJ. Effect of glutathione depletion on inhibition of cell cycle progression and induction of apoptosis by melphalan (L-phenylalanine mustard) in human colorectal cancer cells. Biochem Pharmacol 1999; 58:655–664.

86. McCune JS, Gibbs JP, Slattery JT. Plasma concentration monitoring of busulfan: does it improve clinical outcome? Clin Pharmacokinet 2000; 39:155–165.

87. McDonald GB, Ren S, Bouvier ME, Risler L, Kalhorn TF, Cole SL, Gooley TA, Schoch HG, Batchelder AL, McDonald SJ, Linterman R, Ellis S, Slattery JT. Venooclusive disease of the liver and cyclophosphamide pharmacokinetics: a prospective study in marrow transplant patients. Hepatology 1999; 30:314A.

88. Sievers EL, Larson RA, Stadtmauer EA, Estey E, Lowenberg B, Dombret H, Karanes C, Theobald M, Bennett JM, Sherman ML, Berger MS, Eten CB, Loken MR, van Dongen JJ, Bernstein ID, Appelbaum FR, Mylotarg Study G. Efficacy and safety of gemtuzumab ozogamicin in patients with CD33-positive acute myeloid leukemia in first relapse. J Clin Oncol 2001; 19:3244–3254.

89. Giles FJ, Kantarjian HM, Kornblau SM, Thomas DA, Garcia-Manero G, Waddelow TA, David CL, Phan AT, Colburn DE, Rashid A, Estey EH. Mylotarg (gemtuzumab ozogamicin) therapy is associated with hepatic venoocclusive disease in patients who have not received stem cell transplantation. Cancer 2001; 92:406–413.

90. Rajvanshi P, Shulman HM, Sievers EL, McDonald GB. Hepatic sinusoidal obstruction following Gemtuzumab ozogamicin (Mylotarg). Blood 2002; 2310–2314.

91. Shulman HM, Fisher LB, Schoch HG, Henne KW, McDonald GB. Venooclusive disease of the liver after marrow transplantation: histological correlates of clinical signs and symptoms. Hepatology 1994; 19:1171–1180.

92. Rollins BJ. Hepatic veno-occlusive disease. Am J Med 1986; 81:297–306.

93. DeLeve LD. Dacarbazine toxicity in murine liver cells: a novel model of hepatic endothelial injury and glutathione defense. J Pharmacol Exp Ther 1994; 268:1261–1270.

94. DeLeve LD, Wang X, Kuhlenkamp JF, Kaplowitz N. Toxicity of azathioprine and monocrotaline in murine sinusoidal endothelial cells and hepatocytes: the role of glutathione and relevance to hepatic venooclusive disease. Hepatology 1996; 23:589–599.

95. DeLeve LD, McCuskey RS, Wang X, Hu L, McCuskey MK, Epstein RB, Kanel G. Characterization of a reproducible rat model of hepatic veno-occlusive disease. Hepatology 1999; 29:1779–1791.

96. DeLeve LD, Ito Y, Machen NW, McCuskey MK, Wang X, McCuskey RS. Embolization by sinusoidal lining cells causes the congestion of hepatic venooclusive disease. Gastroenterology 2000; 118:A2345.

97. DeLeve LD, Wang X, Tsai J, Kanel G, Tokes Z. Prevention of hepatic venoocclusive disease in the rat by inhibition of matrix metalloproteinases. Gastroenterology 2001; 120:A54.

98. Cai T, Fassina GF, Morini M, Aluigi MG, Masiello L, Fontanini G, D'Agostini F, De Flora S, Noonan DM, Albini A. N-Acetylcysteine inhibits endothelial cell invasion and angiogenesis. Lab Invest 1999; 79:1151–1159.

99. Tyagi SC, Ratajska A, Weber KT. Myocardial matrix metalloproteinase(s): localization and activation. Mol Cell Biochem 1993; 126:49–59.

100. Tyagi SC, Kumar S, Borders S. Reduction-oxidation (redox) state regulation of extracellular matrix metalloproteinases and tissue inhibitors in cardiac normal and transformed fibroblast cells. J Cell Biochem 1996; 61:139–151.

101. Upadhya GA, Strasberg SM. Glutathione, lactobionate, and histidine: cryptic inhibitors of matrix metalloproteinases contained in University of Wisconsin and histidine/tryptophan/ketoglutarate liver preservation solutions. Hepatology 2000; 31:1115–1122.

102. DeLeve LD, Wang X. Decrease in nitric oxide production contributes to hepatic venoocclusive disease. Hepatology 1999; 30:218A.

103. Eberhardt W, Beeg T, Beck KF, Walpen S, Gauer S, Bohles H, Pfeilschifter J. Nitric oxide modulates expression of matrix metalloproteinase-9 in rat mesangial cells. Kidney Int 2000; 57:59–69.

104. Korte W. Veno-occlusive disease of the liver after bone marrow transplantation: is hypercoagulability really part of the problem? Blood Coagul Fibrinol 1997; 8:367–381.

105. Shulman HM, Gown AM, Nugent DJ. Hepatic veno-occlusive disease after bone marrow transplantation-immunohistochemical identification of the material within occluded central venules. Am J Pathol 1987; 127:549–558.

106. Brooks SEH, Miller CG, McKenzie K, Audretsch JJ, Bras G. Acute veno-occlusive disease of the liver. Arch Pathol 1970; 89:507–520.

107. Snover DC, Weisdorf S, Bloomer J, McGlave P, Weisdorf D. Nodular regenerative hyperplasia of the liver following bone marrow transplantation. Hepatology 1989; 9:443–448.

108. Wanless IR, Godwin TA, Allen F, Feder A. Nodular regenerative hyperplasia of the liver in hematologic disorders: a possible response to obliterative portal venopathy. A morphometric study of nine cases with an hypothesis on the pathogenesis. Medicine 1980; 59:367–379.

109. Thomas PA, McCusker JJ, Merrigan EH, Conte NF. Lobar cirrhosis with nodular hyperplasia (hamartoma) of the liver treated by left hepatic lobectomy. Am J Surg 1966; 112:831–834.

110. Whelan TJ, Baugh JH, Chandor S. Focal nodular hyperplasia of the liver. Ann Surg 1973; 177:150–158.

111. Travers H, D'Amato NA. Vascular alterations in focal nodular hyperplasia of the liver. Milit Med 1978; 143:96–101.

112. Wanless IR. Micronodular transformation (nodular regenerative hyperplasia) of the liver: a report of 64 cases among 2,500 autopsies and a new classification of benign hepatocellular nodules. Hepatology 1990; 11:787–797.

113. Haboubi NY, Ali HH, Whitwell HL, Ackrill P. Role of endothelial cell injury in the spectrum of azathioprine-induced liver disease after renal transplant: light microscopy and ultrastructural observations. Am J Gastroenterol 1988; 83:256–261.

114. Böhme M, Müller M, Leier I, Jedlitschky G, Keppler D. Cholestasis caused by inhibition of the adenosine triphosphate-dependent bile salt transport in rat liver. Gastroenterology 1994; 107:255–265.

115. Kadmon M, Klünemann C, Böhme M, Ishikawa T, Gorgas K, Otto G, Herfarth C, Keppler D. Inhibition by cyclosporin A of adenosine triphosphate-dependent transport from the hepatocyte into bile. Gastroenterology 1993; 104:1507–1514.

116. Böhme M, Büchler M, Müller M, Keppler D. Differential inhibition by cyclosporins of primary-active ATP-dependent transporters in the hepatocyte canalicular membrane. FEBS Lett 1993; 333:193–196.

117. Moran D, De Buitrago JM, Fernandez E, Galan AI, Munoz ME, Jimenez R. Inhibition of biliary glutathione secretion by cyclosporine A in the rat: possible mechanisms and role in the cholestasis induced by the drug. J Hepatol 1998; 29:68–77.

118. Yasumiba S, Tazuma S, Ochi H, Chayama K, Kajiyama G. Cyclosporin A reduces canalicular membrane fluidity and regulates transporter function in rats. Biochem J 2001; 354:591–596.

119. Azer SA, Stacey NH. Differential effects of cyclosporin A on the transport of bile acids by human hepatocytes. Biochem Pharmacol 1993; 46:813–819.

120. Mosely RH, Johnson TR, Morrissette JM. Inhibition of bile acid transport by cyclosporine A in rat liver plasma membrane vesicles. J Pharmacol Exp Ther 1990; 253:974–980.

121. Tamai I, Safa AR. Competitive inhibition of cyclosporins with the vinca alkaloid-binding site of P-glycoprotein in multidrug-resistant cells. J Biol Chem 1990; 265:16509–16513.

122. Román ID, Monte MJ, Gonzalez-Buitrago JM, Esteller A, Jimenez R. Inhibition of hepatocytary vesicular transport by cyclosporin A in the rat: relationship with cholestasis and hyperbilirubinemia. Hepatology 1990; 12:83–91.

123. Román ID, Coleman R. Disruption of canalicular function in isolated rat hepatocyte couplets caused by cyclosporin A. Biochem Pharmacol 1994; 48:2181–2188.

124. Maria VA, Victorino RM. Development and validation of a clinical scale for the diagnosis of drug-induced hepatitis. Hepatology 1997; 26:664–669.

125. Danan G, Benichou C. Causality assessment of adverse reactions to drugs—I. A novel method based on the conclusions of international consensus meetings: application to drug-induced liver injuries. J Clin Epidemiol 1993; 46:1323–1330.

126. Mori T, Sugita K, Suzuki T, Ishikawa T, Kurosawa H, Matsui A. Histopathologic features of the biopsied liver at onset of childhood B-precursor acute lymphoblastic leukemia presenting as severe jaundice. J Pediatr Gastroenterol Nutr 1997; 25:354–357.

127. Modzelewski JR, Jr., Daeschner C, Joshi VV, Mullick FG, Ishak KG. Veno-occlusive disease of the liver induced by low-dose cyclophosphamide. Mod Pathol 1994; 7:967–972.

128. Patel JM, Block ER. Acrolein-induced injury to cultured pulmonary artery endothelial cells. Toxicol Appl Pharmacol 1993; 122:46–53.

129. Kachel DL, Martin WJ, II. Cyclophosphamide-induced lung toxicity: mechanism of endothelial cell injury. J Pharmacol Exp Ther 1994; 268:42–46.

130. Shepherd PC, Fooks J, Gray R, Allan NC. Thioguanine used in maintenance therapy of chronic myeloid leukaemia causes non-cirrhotic portal hypertension. Results from MRC CML. II. Trial comparing busulphan with busulphan and thioguanine. Br J Haematol 1991; 79:185–192.

131. Shulman HM, McDonald GB, Matthews D, Doney KC, Kopecky KJ, Gauvreau JM, Thomas ED. An analysis of hepatic venoocclusive disease and centrilobular hepatic degeneration following bone marrow transplantation. Gastroenterology 1980; 79:1178–1191.

132. Kanfer EJ, Petersen FB, Buckner CD, Stewart P, Storb R, Hill RS, Appelbaum FR, Clift RA, Doney KC, Shulman HM, Thomas ED. Phase I study of high-dose dimethylbusulfan followed by autologous bone marrow transplantation in patients with advanced malignancy. Cancer Treat Rep 1987; 71:101–102.

133. Paschke R, Heine M. Pathophysiological aspects of dacarbazine-induced human liver damage. Hepatogastroenterology 1985; 32:273–275.

134. Hill DL. Microsomal metabolism of triazenylimidazoles. Cancer Res 1975; 35:3106–3110.

135. Lazarus HM, Herzig RH, Graham-Pole J, Wolff SN, Phillips GL, Strandjord S, Hurd D, Forman W, Gordon EM, Coccia P, Gross S, Herzig GP. Intensive melphalan chemotherapy and cryopreserve autologous bone marrow transplantation for the treatment of refractory cancer. J Clin Oncol 1983; 1:359–367.

136. Awasthi S, Bajpai KK, Piper JT, Singhal SS, Ballatore A, Seifert WE, Jr., Awasthi YC, Ansari GA. Interactions of melphalan with glutathione and the role of glutathione S-transferase. Drug Metab Dispos 1996; 24:371–374.

137. Paumi CM, Ledford BG, Smitherman PK, Townsend AJ, Morrow CS. Role of multidrug resistance protein 1 (MRP1) and glutathione S-transferase A1-1 in alkylating agent resistance: kinetics of glutathione conjugate formation and efflux govern differential cellular sensitivity to chlorambucil versus melphalan toxicity. J Biol Chem 2001; 276:7952–7956.

138. Hutter RVP, Shipkey FH, Tan CTC, Murphy ML, Chowdhury M. Hepatic fibrosis in children with acute leukemia: a complication of therapy. Cancer 1960; 13:288–307.

139. Weber BL, Tanyer G, Poplack DG, Reaman GH, Feusner JH, Miser JS, Bleyer WA. Transient acute hepatotoxicity of high-dose methotrexate therapy during childhood. NCI Monogr 1987: 207–212.

140. Schmiegelow K, Pulczynska M. Prognostic significance of hepatotoxicity during maintenance chemotherapy for childhood acute lymphoblastic leukaemia. Br J Cancer 1990; 61: 767–772.

141. Rask C, Albertioni F, Bentzen SM, Schroeder H, Peterson C. Clinical and pharmacokinetic risk factors for high-dose methotrexate-induced toxicity in children with acute lymphoblastic leukemia—a logistic regression analysis. Acta Oncol 1998; 37:277–284.

142. Ruymann FB, Mosjczuk AD, Sayers RJ. Hepatoma in a child with methotrexate-induced hepatic fibrosis. JAMA 1977; 238:2631–2633.

143. Fried M, Kalra J, Ilardi CF, Sawitsky A. Hepatocellular carcinoma in a long-term survivor of acute lymphocytic leukemia. Cancer 1987; 60:2548–2552.

144. Whiting-O'Keefe QE, Fye KH, Sack KD. Methotrexate and histologic hepatic abnormalities: a meta analysis. Am J Med 1991; 90:711–716.

145. Frei E, III, Holland JF, Schneiderman MA, Pinkel D, Selkirk G, Freireich EJ, Silver RT, Gold GL, Regelson W. A comparative study of two regimens of combination chemotherapy in acute leukemia. Blood 1958; 13:1126–1148.

146. Farber S. Summary of experience with 6-mercaptopurine. Ann NY Acad Sci 1954; 60:412–414.

147. McIlvanie SK, MacCarthy JD. Hepatitis in association with prolonged 6-mercaptopurine therapy. Blood 1959; 14:80–90.

148. Einhorn M, Davidsohn I. Hepatotoxicity of mercaptopurine. JAMA 1964; 188:802–806.

149. Present DH, Meltzer SJ, Krumholz MP, Wolke A, Korelitz BI. 6-Mercaptopurine in the management of inflammatory bowel disease: short- and long-term toxicity. Ann Intern Med 1989; 111:641–649.

150. Krynetski EY, Evans WE. Pharmacogenetics as a molecular basis for individualized drug therapy: the thiopurine S-methyltransferase paradigm. Pharm Res 1999; 16:342–349.

151. McLeod HL, Krynetski EY, Relling MV, Evans WE. Genetic polymorphism of thiopurine methyltransferase and its clinical relevance for childhood acute lymphoblastic leukemia. Leukemia 2000; 14:567–572.

152. Relling MV, Hancock ML, Rivera GK, Sandlund JT, Ribeiro RC, Krynetski EY, Pui CH, Evans WE. Mercaptopurine therapy intolerance and heterozygosity at the thiopurine S-methyltransferase gene locus [see comments]. J Natl Cancer Inst 1999; 91:2001–2008.

153. Berkovitch M, Matsui D, Zipursky A, Blanchette VS, Verjee Z, Giesbrecht E, Saunders EF, Evans WE, Koren G. Hepatotoxicity of 6-mercaptopurine in childhood acute lymphocytic leukemia: pharmacokinetic characteristics. Med Pediatr Oncol 1996; 26:85–89.

154. Dubinsky MC, Lamothe S, Yang HY, Targan SR, Sinnett D, Theoret Y, Seidman EG. Pharmacogenomics and metabolite measurement for 6-mercaptopurine therapy in inflammatory bowel disease. Gastroenterology 2000; 118:705–713.

155. Dervieux T, Blanco JG, Krynetski EY, Vanin EF, Roussel MF, Relling MV. Differing contribution of thiopurine methyltransferase to mercaptopurine versus thioguanine effects in human leukemic cells. Cancer Res 2001; 61:5810–5816.

156. Merino JM, Casanova F, Sáez-Royuela F, Velasco A, Gonzalez JB. Veno-occlusive disease of the liver associated with thiopurines in a child with acute lymphoblastic leukemia. Pediatr Hematol Oncol 2000; 17:429–431.

157. Griner PF, Elbadawi A, Packman CH. Veno-occlusive disease of the liver after chemotherapy of acute leukemia: report of two cases. Ann Intern Med 1976; 85:578–582.

158. D'Cruz CA, Wimmer RS, Harcke HT, Huff DS, Naiman JL. Veno-occlusive disease of the

liver in children following chemotherapy for acute myelocytic leukemia. Cancer 1983; 52: 1803–1807.

159. Satti MB, Weinbren K, Gordon-Smith EC. 6-Thioguanine as a cause of toxic veno-occlusive disease of the liver. J Clin Pathol 1982; 35:1086–1091.

160. Key NS, Kelly PM, Emerson PM, Chapman RW, Allan NC, McGee JO. Oesophageal varices associated with busulphan-thioguanine combination therapy for chronic myeloid leukaemia. Lancet 1987; 2:1050–1052.

161. Larrey D, Freneaux E, Berson A, Babany G, Degott C, Valla D, Pessayre D, Benhamou JP. Peliosis hepatis induced by 6-thioguanine administration. Gut 1988; 29:1265–1269.

162. de Araujo MS, Gerard F, Chossegros P, Porto LC, Barlet P, Grimaud JA. Vascular hepato-toxicity related to heroin addiction. Virchows Arch A Pathol Anat Histopathol 1990; 417: 497–503.

163. Trigueiro de Araujo MS, Gerard F, Chossegros P, Guerret S, Grimaud JA. Lack of hepatocyte involvement in the genesis of the sinusoidal dilatation related to heroin addiction: a morpho-metric study. Virchows Arch A Pathol Anat Histopathol 1992; 420:149–153.

164. Zafrani ES, Cazier A, Baudelot AM, Feldmann G. Ultrastructural lesions of the liver in human peliosis. A report of 12 cases. Am J Pathol 1984; 114:349–359.

165. DeLeve LD. Glutathione defense in non-parenchymal cells. Semin Liver Dis 1998; 18:403–413.

166. Porta C, Danova M, Accurso S, Tinelli C, Girino M, Riccardi A, Palmeri S. Sequential intrahepatic and systemic fluoropyrimidine-based chemotherapy for metastatic colorectal cancer confined to the liver: a phase II study. Cancer Chemother Pharmacol 2001; 47:423–428.

167. Kemeny N, Gonen M, Sullivan D, Schwartz L, Benedetti F, Saltz L, Stockman J, Fong Y, Jarnagin W, Bertino J, Tong W, Paty P. Phase I study of hepatic arterial infusion of floxuri-dine and dexamethasone with systemic irinotecan for unresectable hepatic metastases from colorectal cancer. J Clin Oncol 2001; 19:2687–2695.

168. Campos LT. A randomized trial of intrahepatic infusion of fluorodeoxyuridine with dexa-methasone versus fluorodeoxyuridine alone in the treatment of metastatic colorectal cancer [letter; comment]. Cancer 1993; 71:875–876.

169. Kemeny N, Seiter K, Niedzwiecki D, Chapman D, Sigurdson E, Cohen A, Botet J, Oderman P, Murray P. A randomized trial of intrahepatic infusion of fluorodeoxyuridine with dexa-methasone versus fluorodeoxyuridine alone in the treatment of metastatic colorectal cancer. Cancer 1992; 69:327–334.

170. Brown KT, Kemeny N, Berger MF, Getrajdman GI, Napp T, Fong Y, Herman S, Kurtz RC, Botet J, Blumgart LH. Obstructive jaundice in patients receiving hepatic artery infusional chemotherapy: etiology, treatment implications, and complications after transhepatic biliary drainage. J Vasc Interv Radiol 1997; 8:229–234.

171. Ludwig J, Kim CH, Wiesner RH, Krom RA. Floxuridine-induced sclerosing cholangitis: an ischemic cholangiopathy? Hepatology 1989; 9:215–218.

172. Neumeister P, Eibl M, Zinke-Cerwenka W, Scarpatetti M, Sill H, Linkesch W. Hepatic veno-occlusive disease in two patients with relapsed acute myeloid leukemia treated with anti-CD33 calicheamicin (CMA-676) immunoconjugate. Ann Hematol 2001; 80:119–120.

173. Press OW, Shan D, Howell-Clark J, Eary J, Appelbaum FR, Matthews D, King DJ, Haines AM, Hamann P, Hinman L, Shochat D, Bernstein ID. Comparative metabolism and retention of iodine-125, yttrium-90, and indium-111 radioimmunoconjugates by cancer cells. Cancer Res 1996; 56:2123–2129.

174. van Der Velden VH, te Marvelde JG, Hoogeveen PG, Bernstein ID, Houtsmuller AB, Berger MS, van Dongen JJ. Targeting of the CD33-calicheamicin immunoconjugate Mylotarg (CMA-676) in acute myeloid leukemia: in vivo and in vitro saturation and internalization by leukemic and normal myeloid cells. Blood 2001; 97:3197–3204.

175. Nicolaou K, Smith A, Yue E. Chemistry and biology of natural and designed enediynes. Proc Natl Acad Sci USA 1993; 90:5881–5888.

176. Dedon PC, Goldberg IH. Free-radical mechanisms involved in the formation of sequence-dependent bistranded DNA lesions by the antitumor antibiotics bleomycin, neocarzinostatin, and calicheamicin. Chem Res Toxicol 1992; 5:311–332.

177. Gao Z, McAlister VC, Williams GM. Repopulation of liver endothelium by bone-marrow-derived cells. Lancet 2001; 357:932–933.

178. Takezawa RI, Watanabe Y, Akaike T. Direct evidence of macrophage differentiation from bone marrow cells in the liver: a possible origin of Kupffer cells. J Biochem 1995; 118: 1175–1183.

179. Durden DL, Salazar AM, Distasio JA. Kinetic analysis of hepatotoxicity associated with antineoplastic asparaginases. Cancer Res 1983; 43:1602–1605.

180. Villa P, Corada M, Bartosek I. L-asparaginase effects on inhibition of protein synthesis and lowering of the glutamine content in cultured rat hepatocytes. Toxicol Lett 1986; 32:235–241.

181. Land VJ, Sutow WW, Fernbach DJ, Lane DM, Williams TE. Toxicity of L-asparaginase in children with advanced leukemia. Cancer 1972; 30:339–347.

182. Pratt CB, Johnson WW. Duration and severity of fatty metamorphosis of liver following L-asparaginase therapy. Cancer 1971; 28:361–364.

183. Chim CS, Kwong YL, Chu YC, Chan CH, Chan YT, Liang R. Improved treatment outcome in adult acute lymphoblastic leukemia using the intensive German protocol, a preliminary report. Hematol Oncol 1997; 15:19–26.

184. Wiernik PH, Dutcher JP, Paietta E, Gucalp R, Markus S, Weinberg V, Azar C, Garl S, Benson L. Long-term follow-up of treatment and potential cure of adult acute lymphocytic leukemia with MOAD: a non-anthracycline containing regimen. Leukemia 1993; 7:1236–1241.

185. Rizzari C, Valsecchi MG, Arico M, Conter V, Testi A, Barisone E, Casale F, Lo Nigro L, Rondelli R, Basso G, Santoro N, Masera G, Associazione Italiano Ematologia Oncologia P. Effect of protracted high-dose L-asparaginase given as a second exposure in a Berlin-Frankfurt-Münster-based treatment: results of the randomized 9102 intermediate-risk childhood acute lymphoblastic leukemia study—a report from the Associazione Italiana Ematologia Oncologia Pediatrica. J Clin Oncol 2001; 19:1297–1303.

186. Silverman LB, Gelber RD, Dalton VK, Asselin BL, Barr RD, Clavell LA, Hurwitz CA, Moghrabi A, Samson Y, Schorin MA, Arkin S, Declerck L, Cohen HJ, Sallan SE. Improved outcome for children with acute lymphoblastic leukemia: results of Dana-Farber Consortium Protocol 91-01. Blood 2001; 97:1211–1218.

187. Flentje M, Weirich A, Potter R, Ludwig R. Hepatotoxicity in irradiated nephroblastoma patients during postoperative treatment according to SIOP9/GPOH. Radiother Oncol 1994; 31: 222–228.

188. Tornesello A, Piciacchia D, Mastrangelo S, Lasorella A, Mastrangelo R. Veno-occlusive disease of the liver in right-sided Wilms' tumours. Eur J Cancer 1998; 34:1220–1223.

189. Ludwig R, Weirich A, Hofmann WJ, Waldherr R. Veno-occlusive disease as hepatotoxic side effect of the nephroblastoma SIOP-9 treatment protocol: preliminary results of the German group. Med Pediatr Oncol 1992; 20:434.

190. Ortega JA, Donaldson SS, Ivy SP, Pappo A, Maurer HM. Venoocclusive disease of the liver after chemotherapy with vincristine, actinomycin D, and cyclophosphamide for the treatment of rhabdomyosarcoma. Cancer 1997; 79:2435–2439.

191. Mushtaq I, Carachi R, Roy G, Azmy A. Childhood renal tumours with intravascular extension. Br J Urol 1996; 78:772–776.

192. Lawrence TS, Robertson JM, Anscher MS, Jirtle RL, Ensminger WD, Fajardo LF. Hepatic toxicity resulting from cancer treatment. Int J Radiat Oncol Biol Phys 1995; 31:1237–1248.

193. Ingold JA, Reed GB, Jr., Kaplan HS, Bagshaw MA. Radiation hepatitis. AJR 1965; 93:200–208.

194. Reed GB, Jr., Cox AJ, Jr. The human liver after radiation injury: a form of veno-occlusive disease. Am J Pathol 1966; 48:597–611.

195. Selzer G, Parker RGF. Senecio poisoning exhibiting as Chiari's syndrome: a report on twelve cases. Am J Pathol 1950; 27:885–907.

196. McGinn CJ, Ten Haken RK, Ensminger WD, Walker S, Wang S, Lawrence TS. Treatment of intrahepatic cancers with radiation doses based on a normal tissue complication probability model. J Clin Oncol 1998; 16:2246–2252.

197. Grinsky T, Benhamou E, Bourhis JH, Dhermain F, Guillot-Valls D, Ganansia V, Luboinski M, Perez A, Cosset J-M, Socie G, Baume D, Bouaouina N, Briot E, Beaudre A, Bridier A, Pico JL. Prospective randomized comparison of single-dose versus hyperfractionated total-body irradiation in patients with hematologic malignancies. J Clin Oncol 2000; 18:981–986.

198. Hopewell J, Withers HR. Proposition: long-term changes in irradiated tissues are due principally to vascular damage in the tissues. Med Phys 1998; 25:2265–2268.

199. Cicciarello R, d'Avella D, Gagliardi ME, Albiero F, Vega J, Angileri FF, D'Aquino A, Tomasello F. Time-related ultrastructural changes in an experimental model of whole brain irradiation. Neurosurgery 1996; 38:772–779; discussion 779–780.

200. Rezvani M, Hopewell JW, Robbins ME. Initiation of non-neoplastic late effects: the role of endothelium and connective tissue. Stem Cells 1995; 13:248–256.

201. Hopewell JW, Calvo W, Jaenke R, Reinhold HS, Robbins ME, Whitehouse EM. Microvasculature and radiation damage. Recent Results Cancer Res 1993; 130:1–16.

202. Jaenke RS, Robbins ME, Bywaters T, Whitehouse E, Rezvani M, Hopewell JW. Capillary endothelium. Target site of renal radiation injury. Lab Invest 1993; 68:396–405.

203. Reinhold HS. The influence of radiation on blood vessels and circulation. Chapter II. Cell viability of the vessel wall. Curr Topics Radiat Res Q 1974; 10:9–28.

204. Langley RE, Bump EA, Quartuccio SG, Medeiros D, Braunhut SJ. Radiation-induced apoptosis in microvascular endothelial cells. Br J Cancer 1997; 75:666–672.

205. Pena LA, Fuks Z, Kolesnick RN. Radiation-induced apoptosis of endothelial cells in the murine central nervous system: protection by fibroblast growth factor and sphingomyelinase deficiency. Cancer Res 2000; 60:321–327.

206. Paris F, Fuks Z, Kang A, Capodieci P, Juan G, Ehleiter D, Haimovitz-Friedman A, Cordon-Cardo C, Kolesnick R. Endothelial apoptosis as the primary lesion initiating intestinal radiation damage in mice. Science 2001; 293:293–297.

207. Morales A, Miranda M, Sanchez-Reyes A, Biete A, Fernandez-Checa JC. Oxidative damage of mitochondrial and nuclear DNA induced by ionizing radiation in human hepatoblastoma cells. Int J Radiat Oncol Biol Phys 1998; 42:191–203.

208. Saibara T, Onishi S, Ogawa Y, Yoshida S, Enzan H. Non-alcoholic steatohepatitis. Lancet 1999; 354:1299–1300.

209. Van Hoof M, Rahier J, Horsmans Y. Tamoxifen-induced steatohepatitis [letter]. Ann Intern Med 1996; 124:855–856.

210. Pratt DS, Knox TA, Erban J. Tamoxifen-induced steatohepatitis [letter]. Ann Intern Med 1995; 123:236.

211. Oien KA, Moffat D, Curry GW, Dickson J, Habeshaw T, Mills PR, MacSween RN. Cirrhosis with steatohepatitis after adjuvant tamoxifen [letter]. Lancet 1999; 353:36–37.

212. Cortez Pinto H, Baptista A, Camilo ME, Bruno de Costa E, Valente A, Carneiro de Moura M. Tamoxifen-associated steatohepatitis-report of three cases. J Hepatol 1995; 23:95–97.

213. Murata Y, Ogawa Y, Saibara T, Nishioka A, Fujiwara Y, Fukumoto M, Inomota T, Enzan H, Onishi S, Yoshida S. Unrecognized hepatic steatosis and non-alcoholic steatohepatitis in adjuvant tamoxifen for breast cancer patients. Oncol Reports 2000; 7:1299–1304.

214. Loomus GN, Aneja P, Bota RA. A case of peliosis hepatis in association with tamoxifen therapy. Am J Clin Pathol 1983; 80:881–883.

215. Storen EC, Hay JE, Kaur J, Zahasky K, Hartmann L. Tamoxifen-induced submassive hepatic necrosis. Cancer J 2000; 6:58–60.

216. Moffat DF, Oien KA, Dickson J, Habeshaw T, McLellan DR. Hepatocellular carcinoma after long-term tamoxifen therapy. Ann Oncol 2000; 11:1195–1196.

217. Law CH, Tandan VR. The association between tamoxifen and the development of hepatocellular carcinoma: case report and literature review. Can J Surg 1999; 42:211–214.

218. Wilking N, Isaksson E, von Schoultz E. Tamoxifen and secondary tumours: an update. Drug Safety 1997; 16:104–117.

219. Dragan YP, Fahey S, Street K, Vaughan J, Jordan VC, Pitot HC. Studies of tamoxifen as a promoter of hepatocarcinogenesis in female Fischer F344 rats. Breast Cancer Res Treat 1994; 31:11–25.

220. Carthew P, Martin EA, White IN, De Matteis F, Edwards RE, Dorman BM, Heydon RT, Smith LL. Tamoxifen induces short-term cumulative DNA damage and liver tumors in rats: promotion by phenobarbital. Cancer Res 1995; 55:544–547.

221. Martin EA, Rich KJ, White IN, Woods KL, Powles TJ, Smith LL. 32P-postlabelled DNA adducts in liver obtained from women treated with tamoxifen. Carcinogenesis 1995; 16: 1651–1654.

222. Rabe T, Feldmann K, Heinemann L, Runnebaum B. Cyproterone acetate: is it hepato- or genotoxic? Drug Safety 1996; 14:25–38.

223. Hinkel A, Berges RR, Pannek J, Schulze H, Senge T. Cyproterone acetate in the treatment of advanced prostatic cancer: retrospective analysis of liver toxicity in the long-term follow-up of 89 patients. Eur Urol 1996; 30:464–470.

224. Anonymous. Hepatic reactions with cyproterone acetate (Cyprostat, Androcur). Curr Problems Pharmacovigilance 1995; 21:1.

225. Garty BZ, Dinari G, Gellvan A, Kauli R. Cirrhosis in a child with hypothalamic syndrome and central precocious puberty treated with cyproterone acetate. Eur J Pediatr 1999; 158: 367–370.

226. Werner S, Topinka J, Kunz S, Beckurts T, Heidecke CD, Schwarz LR, Wolff T. Studies on the formation of hepatic DNA adducts by the antiandrogenic and gestagenic drug, cyproterone acetate: 1. adduct levels in various species including man and 2. persistence and accumulation in the rat. Adv Exp Med Biol 1996; 387:253–257.

227. Schwarz LR, Werner S, Topinka J, Andrae U, Neumann I, Wolff T. The liver as origin and target of reactive intermediates exemplified by the progesterone derivative, cyproterone acetate. Adv Exp Med Biol 1996; 387:243–251.

228. Oosterlinck W, Casselman J, Mattelaer J, Van Velthoven R, Kurjatkin O, Schulman C. Tolerability and safety of flutamide in monotherapy, with orchiectomy or with LHRH-a in advanced prostate cancer patients: a Belgian multicenter study of 905 patients. Eur Urol 1996; 30:458–463.

229. Wysowski DK, Fourcroy JL. Flutamide hepatotoxicity. J Urol 1996; 155:209–212.

230. Berson A, Wolf C, Chachaty C, Fisch C, Fau D, Loeper J, Gauthier JC, Beaune P, Pompon D, Maurel P, Pessayre D. Metabolic activation of the nitroaromatic antiandrogen flutamide by rat and human cytochrome P-450, including forms belonging to the 3A and 1A subfamilies. J Pharmacol Exp Ther 1983; 265:366–372.

231. Fau D, Eugene D, Berson A, Letteron P, Fromenty B, Fisch C, Pessayre D. Toxicity of the antiandrogen flutamide in isolated rat hepatocytes. J Pharmacol Exp Ther 1994; 269:954–962.

232. De Vita VT, Carbone PP, Owens AH, Jr., Gold GL, Krant MJ, Edmonson J. Clinical trials with 1,3-*bis*(2-chloroethyl)-1-nitrosourea, NSC-409962. Cancer Res 1965; 25:1876–1881.

233. Phillips GL, Fay JW, Herzig GP, Herzig RH, Weiner RS, Wolff SN, Lazarus HM, Karanes C, Ross WE, Kramer BS. Intensive 1,3-bis(2-chloroethyl)-1-nitrosourea (BCNU), NSC: 4366650 and cryopreserved autologous marrow transplantation for refractory cancer: a phase I–II study. Cancer 1983; 52:1792–1802.

234. Hoth D, Woolley P, Green D, Macdonald J, Schein P. Phase I studies on chlorozotocin. Clin Pharmacol Ther 1978; 23:712–722.

235. Johnson RO, Metter G, Wilson W, Hill G, Krementz E. Phase I evaluation of DTIC (NSC-45388) and other studies in malignant melanoma in the Central Oncology Group. Cancer Treat Rep 1976; 60:183–187.

236. Chard RL, Jr., Krivit W, Bleyer WA, Hammond D. Phase II study of VP-16-213 in childhood malignant disease: a Children's Cancer Study Group Report. Cancer Treat Rep 1979; 63: 1755–1759.

237. Abratt RP, Bezwoda WR, Falkson G, Goedhals L, Hacking D, Rugg TA. Efficacy and safety profile of gemcitabine in non-small-cell lung cancer: a phase II study. J Clin Oncol 1994; 12:1535–1540.

238. Anderson H, Lund B, Bach F, Thatcher N, Walling J, Hansen HH. Single-agent activity of weekly gemcitabine in advanced non-small-cell lung cancer: a phase II study. J Clin Oncol 1994; 12:1821–1826.

239. Catimel G, Vermorken JB, Clavel M, de Mulder P, Judson I, Sessa C, Piccart M, Bruntsch U, Verweij J, Wanders J, et al. A phase II study of Gemcitabine (LY 188011) in patients with advanced squamous cell carcinoma of the head and neck. EORTC Early Clinical Trials Group. Ann Oncol 1994; 5:543–547.

240. Lund B, Hansen OP, Theilade K, Hansen M, Neijt JP. Phase II study of gemcitabine (2′,2′-difluorodeoxycytidine) in previously treated ovarian cancer patients. J Natl Cancer Inst 1994; 86:1530–1533.

241. Hoogstraten B, Gottlieb JA, Caoili E, Tucker WG, Talley RW, Haut A. CCNU (1-(2-chloroethyl)-3-cyclohexyl-1-nitrosourea, NSC-79037) in the treatment of cancer: phase II study. Cancer 1973; 32:38–43.

242. Paciucci PA, Ohnuma T, Cuttner J, Silver RT, Holland JF. Mitoxantrone in patients with acute leukemia in relapse. Cancer Res 1983; 43:3919–3922.

243. Feldman EJ, Alberts DS, Arlin Z, Ahmed T, Mittelman A, Baskind P, Peng YM, Baier M, Plezia P. Phase I clinical and pharmacokinetic evaluation of high-dose mitoxantrone in combination with cytarabine in patients with acute leukemia. J Clin Oncol 1993; 11:2002–2009.

244. Feenstra J, Vermeer RJ, Stricker BH. Fatal hepatic coma attributed to paclitaxel [letter]. J Natl Cancer Inst 1997; 89:582–584.

245. Broder LE, Carter SK. Pancreatic islet cell carcinoma. II. Results of therapy with streptozotocin in 52 patients. Ann Intern Med 1973; 79:108–118.

246. Coe JE, Ishak KG, Ross MJ. Estrogen-induced hepatic toxicity and hepatic cancer: differences between two closely related hamster species. Liver 1998; 18:343–351.

247. Miller AB, Hoogstraten B, Staquet M, Winkler A. Reporting results of cancer treatment. Cancer 1981; 47:207–214.

25

Immunomodulating Agents and the Transplant Situation

MARY F. HEBERT

University of Washington School of Pharmacy, Seattle, Washington, U.S.A.

SHARI L. TAYLOR

GI Pathology Partners, P.C., Memphis, Tennessee, U.S.A.

ROBERT L. CARITHERS, JR.

University of Washington School of Medicine, Seattle, Washington, U.S.A.

I. INTRODUCTION

Many adverse reactions are seen with the immunosuppressive agents commonly used in transplantation. However, hepatotoxicity is infrequently reported. Of greater concern are the many drug interactions associated with immunosuppressive agents. Drug interactions are particularly common in patients receiving cyclosporin, tacrolimus, or sirolimus. Each of these agents is metabolized by the cytochrome P450 IIIA enzyme (CYP3A) in the liver and small intestine (1–4). In addition, they are all substrates for *p*-glycoprotein (a countertransport pump) in the gastrointestinal tract and liver (5,6). The major drug interactions for these agents occur via effects on CYP3A and *p*-glycoprotein.

Other drug interactions can be of critical importance in transplant recipients. Azathioprine is converted to 6-mercaptopurine (6-MP) by glutathione-*S*-transferase. Detoxification of 6-MP to thiouric acid occurs via xanthine oxidase. Inhibition of xanthine oxidase, a major site for drug interactions with azathioprine by agents such as allopurinol, can result in accumulation of 6-MP and fatal bone marrow suppression (7–10). The metabolism of the corticosteroids is not fully understood. In general, their metabolism involves sequential hydroxylation followed by conjugation. Drug interactions with the corticosteroids in most cases involve nonspecific enzyme inducers or inhibitors. Mycophenolate mofetil is rapidly hydrolyzed to its active form, mycophenolic acid, by gut and blood esterases. Mycophenolic acid is subsequently conjugated and then undergoes enterohepatic recirculation. The major site of drug interactions for this agent appears to be the gastrointestinal tract through decreased absorption and possibly inhibition of enterohepatic recirculation (11).

The clinical implications of drug interactions with immunosuppressive agents are great. Agents that increase the levels of the immunosuppressive medications are associated with significant and potentially life-threatening toxicities. In contrast, use of agents that decrease the levels of immunosuppressive agents often results in allograft rejection. This chapter will discuss the rare hepatotoxicity of commonly used immunosuppressive agents as well as the most frequent drug interactions seen with these medications.

Determination of hepatotoxicity for the immunosuppressive agents, particularly in the transplant setting, can be difficult. Isolating the potential culprit in a suspected case of drug-induced hepatotoxicity is difficult enough in patients receiving multiple medications. In addition, concomitant illnesses, such as viral infections, may contribute to or mask drug-induced hepatotoxicity in the transplant setting (12–15). Early in the history of transplantation, there were few immunosuppressive agents. Azathioprine and prednisone were the mainstay of rejection prophylaxis, with cyclophosphamide available as an alternative. At that time, there were few choices available if a patient developed toxicity to one agent or another. As a result, there was a great deal of reluctance to discontinue any immunosuppressive drug for risk of losing the transplant to rejection.

Cyclosporin increased the success of transplantation and provided an additional immunosuppressive choice. Initially, therapeutic monitoring of cyclosporin was not readily available at all centers and higher doses typically were used. Most reports of cyclosporin-induced hepatotoxicity were published during that era. Increased accessibility to drug level monitoring and clinical experience has resulted in lower doses and concentrations of cyclosporin and very few reports of hepatotoxicity.

In the past several years, additional immunosuppressive agents have been approved for clinical use. The mechanisms of these various immunosuppressives differ. As a result, various combinations can be used to achieve the same desired effect. Azathioprine, cyclophosphamide, and mycophenolate mofetil all can be used to inhibit proliferation of lymphocytes. Substitution of one of these agents for another can be utilized to optimize and individualize immunosuppressive efficacy and to minimize toxicity. Cyclosporin and tacrolimus primarily inhibit interleukin-2 production and can be interchanged for efficacy and safety. Sirolimus inhibits interleukin-2 activity and has been used in various combinations with the other immunosuppressives to optimize transplant outcomes. Antibody preparations (muromonab CD3, antilymphocyte preparations, daclizumab, and basiliximab) that are used for prevention and/or treatment of rejection will not be discussed in this chapter.

II. CORTICOSTEROIDS

Corticosteroids have been in widespread use since the initiation of clinical transplantation and their toxicity has been well recognized. Acute administration of corticosteroids can result in adverse effects ranging from hyperglycemia and sodium retention to psychosis. Chronic administration is associated with adverse effects on the gastrointestinal tract, skin, eyes, and bone. However, it is very uncommon for patients to develop clinical manifestations of corticosteroid-induced hepatotoxicity. Most information on hepatotoxicity of the corticosteroids was published 30–40 years ago and is quite limited.

A. Mechanism of Toxicity

Corticosteroids are well known to enhance the mobilization and redistribution of fat. In animals, corticosteroids are associated with increased plasma free fatty acids (16,17). In addition, steroids have been shown to decrease esterification of fatty acids in the liver (17). It is thought that these mechanisms may lead to the development of corticosteroid-induced hepatic steatosis (16,18).

B. Risk Factors

Although there are no documented risk factors for corticosteroid-induced hepatotoxicity, other illnesses that can cause fatty liver may mask or may be exacerbated by the administration of corticosteroids.

C. Histological Characteristics

Corticosteroids are generally associated with macrovesicular steatotic liver injury. Large triglyceride globules fill the hepatocytes leading to displacement of the nucleus and other intracellular constituents (Fig. 1). The hepatocytes take on an appearance similar to adipose cells (19). Other more severe liver damage, noted histologically in animals, has not been seen in humans.

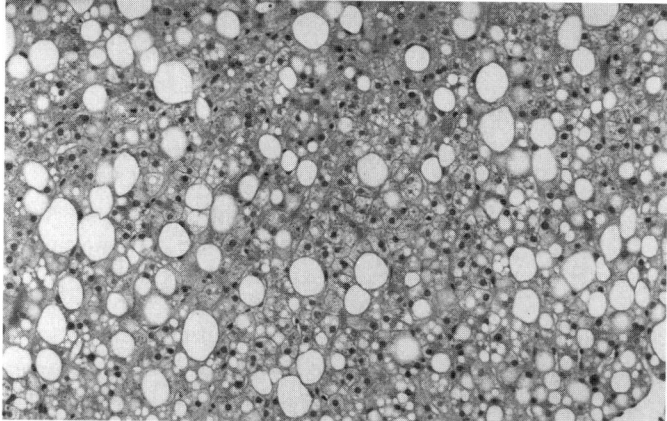

Figure 1   Corticosteroid-induced macrovesicular steatosis. Single, large droplets of fat are present within hepatocytes, displacing the nucleus to one side.

D. Clinical Manifestations

Generally, liver function is well preserved in patients with corticosteroid-induced fatty liver. The most common clinical finding is hepatomegaly (20–22). Rare cases of fat embolism have been reported (23,24).

E. Drug Interactions

Drugs that alter corticosteroid levels are often not clinically recognized because the concentrations of these agents are not routinely monitored. However, significant changes in corticosteroid concentrations are seen with drugs that inhibit or induce a wide range of enzymes. Both ketoconazole and oral contraceptives can increase prednisolone levels (25–27). In addition, nonspecific enzyme inducers such as rifampin, phenobarbital, carbamazepine, and phenytoin have all been shown to induce the metabolism of corticosteroids (28–31).

III. AZATHIOPRINE

Of all the immunosuppressive drugs used clinically, there are more reports of hepatotoxicity from azathioprine than from any other agent. Despite this, there has been some controversy as to whether azathioprine actually causes liver injury. Many case reports of putative azathioprine hepatotoxicity do not include viral hepatitis serologies (hepatitis A, B, C, or CMV) and are complicated by the concomitant administration or simultaneous cessation of other potentially hepatotoxic agents (32–38). On the other hand, there are many complete case reports that have excluded other potential etiologies for the liver disease, have documented improvement or resolution with discontinuation of azathioprine, and have demonstrated recurrence with azathioprine rechallenge (32,39–42). Based on these reports, it is clear that there is a causal relationship between azathioprine and hepatotoxicity. However, the incidence of azathioprine hepatotoxicity is unclear.

The three most commonly reported forms of azathioprine hepatotoxicity include veno-occlusive disease, nodular regenerative hyperplasia, and peliosis hepatis (35–38, 40,41,43–46). Other less specific forms of hepatotoxicity have also been reported (32, 33,39,47).

A. Mechanism of Toxicity

The exact mechanism of azathioprine-induced hepatotoxicity has yet to be clearly defined. Azathioprine, a chemical analog of the purines, undergoes extensive metabolism. The parent compound is rapidly converted in vivo to 6-mercaptopurine (48–52). Subsequently, 6-MP is metabolized by different pathways to thiouric acid (51,53), thiopurine nucleotides (50–52,54,55), and via methylation of the thiol group (56,57). There is evidence to suggest that metabolites may be major contributors to the hepatotoxicity of azathioprine (58–65). 6-Mercaptopurine has been associated with intrahepatic cholestasis, hepatocellular necrosis, dilated sinusoids, and intrahepatic collections of red blood cells (61–64). 6-Thioguanine has been associated with veno-occlusive disease (65). All of these reactions are consistent with the reports of azathioprine-induced hepatotoxicity. It is possible that patients who develop azathioprine hepatotoxicity have unusually high levels of the hepatotoxic metabolites. However, such correlations have not been reported. It is also possible that certain individuals are more susceptible to the development of idiopathic reactions despite having normal azathioprine and metabolite levels. DeLeve et al. (66) found that in an in vitro murine cell culture model, azathioprine led to an 80% reduction in glutathione in sinusoidal endothelial cells and a 54% reduction in hepatocytes. This profound depletion of glutathione in sinusoidal endothelial cells may in part explain azathioprine's hepatotoxicity.

Haboubi et al. (36) have suggested that the three types of azathioprine-induced hepatotoxicity (veno-occlusive disease, nodular regenerative hyperplasia, and peliosis hepatis) are due to the same basic mechanism with the location and severity of injury dictating the histological manifestation. They suggest that the initial injury is damage to the sinusoidal and terminal hepatic venular endothelial cells. The histological manifestations of endothelial cell damage include leaking of red blood cells into the space of Disse and progressive fibrosis. This theory is supported by sequential biopsies that demonstrate progression from peliosis hepatis to nodular regenerative hyperplasia (36). Peliosis may result from damage to the sinusoidal endothelial cells with liver cell necrosis being a secondary phenomenon. Progressive fibrosis can cause narrowing and even obliteration and capillarization of the sinusoids, ultimately leading to increased sinusoidal pressure and portal hypertension. Veno-occlusive disease appears to result from damage to the terminal hepatic venule endothelial cells with subsequent subendothelial edema and narrowing of the lumen. Nodular regenerative hyperplasia may be the end result of the sinusoidal lesion, which leads to hypoperfusion, hepatocellular injury, and necrosis of some areas and regenerative hyperplasia in normally perfused areas (45,67).

B. Risk Factors

The most frequently reported clinical setting of azathioprine-induced hepatotoxicity is among male renal transplant recipients (35,36,40,41,43–45). There are infrequent reports of azathioprine-induced hepatotoxicity in female patients (41,42). In addition, there are multiple reports of azathioprine hepatotoxicity among patients with other underlying diseases such as systemic lupus erythematosus (47), bone marrow transplant recipients with graft-versus-host disease (45), inflammatory bowel disease (45), panuveitis (43), and liver transplant recipients (42). CMV and dialysis also may play a role in the development of veno-occlusive disease, peliosis hepatis, and nodular regenerative hyperplasia (44,68).

C. Histological Characteristics

Azathioprine-induced veno-occlusive disease, nodular regenerative hyperplasia, and peliosis hepatis can occur separately or simultaneously. The characteristic lesion of veno-occlusive disease is subintimal fibrous proliferation and edema of the small hepatic veins, with progressive luminal narrowing. In the acute stages, centrilobular congestion, hepatocyte dropout, and sinusoidal dilatation (changes of acute venous outflow tract obstruction) are also observed (Fig. 2). With time, the veno-occlusive lesions become more densely fibrotic, and the changes of chronic venous outflow tract obstruction appear: perivenular and pericellular fibrosis with eventual central-central bridging. Nodular regenerative hyperplasia can be seen in some cases, and is characterized by diffuse nodularity of the liver in the absence of fibrosis. The centers of the nodules are paler and composed of hepatocytes that are slightly enlarged, while the periphery of the nodules are more deeply eosinophilic and are composed of atrophic hepatocytes (Fig. 3). The nodularity is best highlighted with a reticulin stain. In some cases, thrombosis or obliteration of portal veins may be evident. Peliosis hepatis is characterized by cystic, blood-filled spaces in the liver.

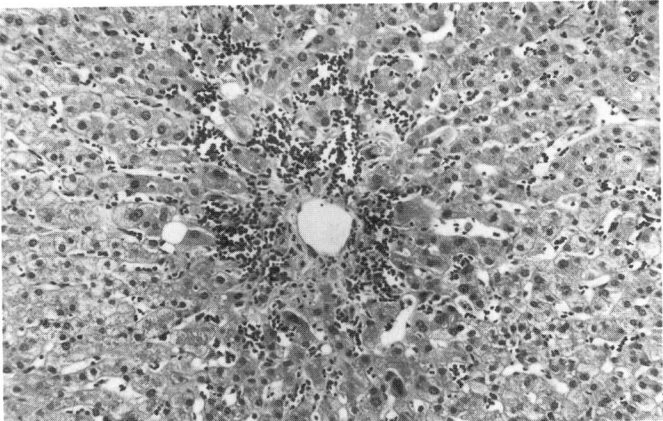

Figure 2 Azathioprine-induced hepatotoxicity. Centrilobular congestion and hepatocyte dropout associated with azathioprine.

D. Clinical Manifestations

The majority of cases of azathioprine-induced hepatotoxicity have occurred between 6 months and 5 years after initiation of treatment, although there are a few reports of hepatotoxicity occurring as early as 17 days following the institution of therapy (35,36,40–45).

Presenting symptoms have included one or more of the following: malaise, arthralgias, fatigue, fever, abdominal pain, anorexia, nausea, vomiting, diarrhea, weight loss, pruritus, scleral icterus, and jaundice. In severe cases ascites, esophageal varices, hepatomegaly, splenomegaly, and coagulopathy have been described. Peak serum bilirubin values have ranged from normal to 33.8 mg/dL, AST from normal to 2965 U/L, ALT from normal to 790 U/L, alkaline phosphatase from normal to 1525 U/L, and GGT from normal to 344 U/L. On presentation, serum bilirubin concentrations typically are in the 1.5–7

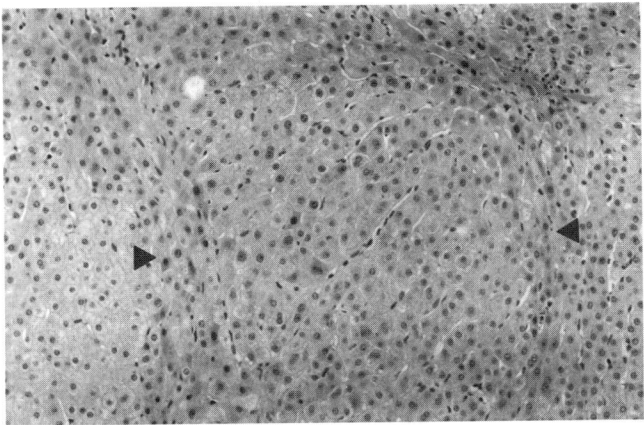

Figure 3 Nodular regenerative hyperplasia. The nodules are composed of hyperplastic hepatocytes with zones of hepatocyte atrophy (arrowheads) at the periphery.

mg/dL range, AST and ALT 1.5–2 times the upper limit of normal, and alkaline phosphatase 450–700 U/L.

Outcomes for patients experiencing azathioprine-induced hepatotoxicity have depended on the extent and manifestations of the toxicity. In general, most patients manifesting nonspecific cholestasis without veno-occlusive disease, peliosis hepatis, or nodular regenerative hyperplasia have had a complete recovery within a few months after discontinuation of azathioprine, but several developed the same hepatotoxic reaction on rechallenge (32,39,47).

Patients who have developed peliosis hepatis or nodular regenerative hyperplasia typically have a less severe course than those who develop veno-occlusive disease. Some patients with nodular regenerative hyperplasia have done well with a reduced dose of azathioprine (44). Others have continued to decline or developed stable hepatic dysfunction until azathioprine was discontinued (35,44). Still others have had continued symptoms of portal hypertension or death despite discontinuation of azathioprine (36,38,45).

Patients who develop veno-occlusive disease from azathioprine have a very high mortality rate with or without discontinuation of azathioprine (36,37,40,41,43,44,46). A few patients with azathioprine-induced veno-occlusive disease have survived. Some of these patients were left with significant hepatic dysfunction despite discontinuation of azathioprine, while others had complete resolution of clinical manifestations of liver damage (36,37,40,41,43).

E. Management

Patients requiring long-term treatment with azathioprine should be followed regularly. All patients who develop abnormal liver function tests, symptoms of hepatic dysfunction, or jaundice should be evaluated for liver biopsy. Although it seems prudent to discontinue azathioprine at the first signs of hepatotoxicity, confounding variables may make it difficult to determine whether or not a particular case is due to drug-induced hepatic injury.

Improvement in hepatotoxicity or complete resolution has been reported in some cases after discontinuation of azathioprine and initiation of cyclophosphamide (40,41). With the availability of agents such as mycophenolate mofetil, switching to one of the newer immunosuppressive agents may prove to be a better option than cyclophosphamide in solid-organ transplant patients. Patients with significant portal hypertension have been treated with supportive care, anticoagulation, portacaval shunts, and hepatic transplantation with variable results (37,43,45).

F. Drug Interactions

Allopurinol is a well-known inhibitor of xanthine oxidase, which has been shown to cause increased levels of 6-mercaptopurine (9,10). The concomitant administration of allopurinol with azathioprine has been associated with severe, and in some cases fatal, bone marrow suppression (7,8). Anticipatory dose reduction of azathioprine does not always eliminate this problem (7). Since there are many immunosuppressive alternatives, avoiding this interaction altogether is recommended.

IV. CYCLOSPORIN

Cyclosporin has many adverse effects including nephrotoxicity, hypertension, and neurotoxicity, which are commonly seen following transplantation. However, clinically significant hepatotoxicity is quite uncommon. Most reports of hepatotoxicity describe a relatively benign increase in AST, ALT, and bilirubin, which are generally associated with elevated cyclosporin levels (69–77). In addition, there is some evidence that cyclosporin increases the incidence of cholelithiasis (76). The number of reports of cyclosporin-induced hepatotoxicity has declined over the last 10 years, probably due to the lower doses and target concentrations of cyclosporin currently used.

A. Mechanism of Toxicity

The mechanism of cyclosporin hepatotoxicity and the relative contribution of the parent compound and its various metabolites to this reaction are unknown. However, cyclosporin's ability to impair bile flow and decrease excretion of biliary solutes through inhibition of hepatic vesicular transport may be important (78). In animal models, cyclosporin has been shown to induce cholestasis by interfering with bile-salt-dependent and -independent bile flow as well as by decreasing bile salt secretion (79–81). Another proposed mechanism of cholestasis and potential hepatotoxicity is via cyclosporin's alteration of membrane calcium permeability and inhibition of bile acid uptake and release (82,83).

  Cyclosporin administration has been associated with increased serum cholesterol and triglyceride levels (84–86). Lipid regulation is a very complex process involving multiple enzymes such as HMG-CoA reductase (involved in the rate limiting step of cholesterol synthesis), cholesterol 7α-hydroxylase (involved in the primary pathway of cholesterol metabolism), lipoprotein lipase (involved in triglyceride clearance), and various receptors for products such as LDL, HDL, and VLDL. In the in vivo animal model, cyclosporin does not appear to affect HMG-CoA reductase activity, LDL receptor expression, or HDL receptor expression; however, it does decrease hepatic cholesterol 7α-hydroxylase and skeletal muscle/adipose tissue lipoprotein lipase content (Fig. 4) (87). Other investigators have found that cyclosporin decreases LDL receptor expression in vitro (88). This difference may be related to the complex feedback loops involved in the in vivo cholesterol regulation process.

B. Risk Factors

There are no clear risk factors for cyclosporin-induced hepatotoxicity. Because cyclosporin is known to have a very large number of drug interactions, agents that increase cyclosporin concentration (e.g., ketoconazole, erythromycin, grapefruit) potentially will increase adverse events. Since there appears to be a dose relationship with cyclosporin and hepatotoxicity (69–77,89), the use of inhibitors of CYP 3A and/or p-glycoprotein in theory may increase the risk for hepatotoxicity.

  Diabetic patients have been reported to have an increased incidence of cholelithiasis compared to the nondiabetic control patients receiving cyclosporin (90). Further work in this area is needed to clarify the relationship between diabetes and cyclosporin-induced cholelithiasis.

C. Histological Characteristics

Few data have been published on the histological changes associated with cyclosporin hepatotoxicity in humans. In rats, cyclosporin hepatotoxicity is associated with centrilobular fatty change, hepatocyte necrosis, dilated endoplasmic reticulum, increased autophagic

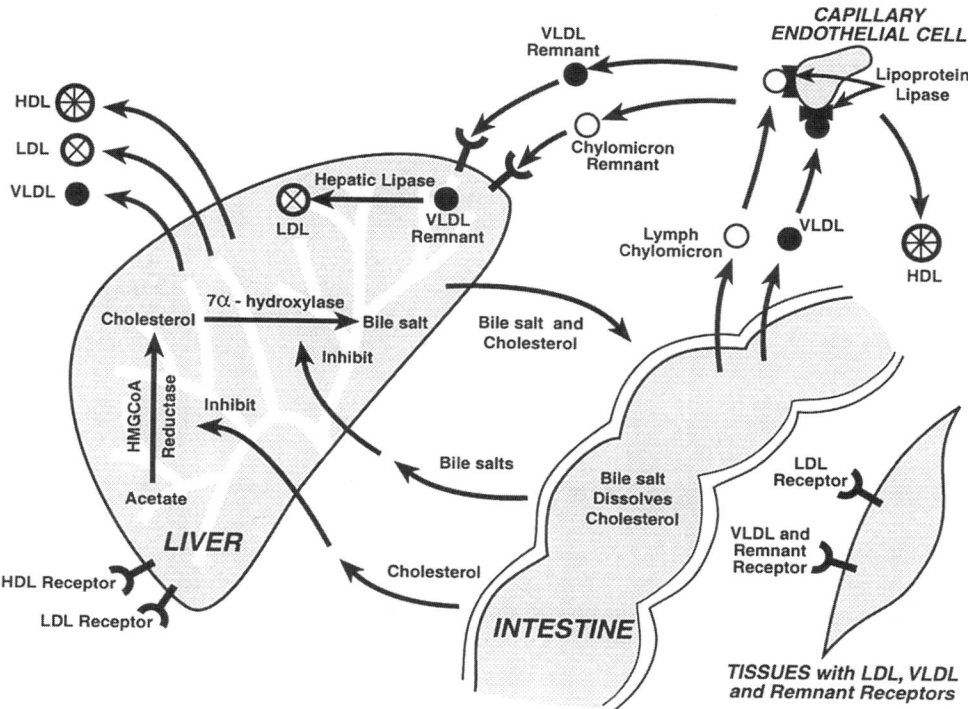

Figure 4 Lipid regulation. This is a simplified diagram of lipid regulation. Acetate is converted to cholesterol in the liver via a multistep process. HMG CoA reductase is involved in the rate-limiting step in cholesterol synthesis. The primary pathway for cholesterol metabolism is via 7α-hydroxylase. Triglycerides are hydrolyzed from very-low-density lipoproteins (VLDL) and chylomicron remnants by lipoprotein lipase. Although low-density-lipoprotein (LDL) receptors are most abundant on the adrenal gland, liver, and intestine, they are also found on skeletal muscle and adipose tissue. Cyclosporin has been shown to inhibit hepatic 7α-hydroxylase and decrease skeletal muscle/adipose tissue lipoprotein lipase content.

vacuoles, and granulomatous hepatitis (91–93). In dogs, histological examination of jaundiced animals who received cyclosporin revealed focal areas of necrosis and cholestasis (94). Wisecarver et al. found bile duct epithelial hypertrophy, cytoplasmic vacuoles, and "foamy" droplets within the hepatic sinusoids in seven liver transplant patients with high cyclosporin levels (89).

D. Clinical Manifestations

In a study of 59 patients treated with cyclosporin for autoimmune uveitis, 58% developed at least one liver function test abnormality. Abnormalities in liver function tests occurred between 1 and 13 months (mean 5.5 months) following initiation of cyclosporin. The usual pattern was a mild increase in alkaline phosphatase, which was occasionally accompanied by slight increases in bilirubin and aminotransferases. Alkaline phosphatase elevations peaked at 1.5–2.5 times normal. Of the patients with a reaction to cyclosporin, 44% had an elevation in liver function tests on a single observation or elevations that lasted less than 2 weeks. The other 56% had a prolonged course lasting more than 2 weeks and up to 4 years (70). Similar findings have been reported in heart transplant patients (74).

Lorber et al. (77) reported that from a total of 466 renal allograft patients receiving cyclosporin and prednisone, 49% developed at least one episode of hepatotoxicity. Of the patients developing hepatotoxicity, 48% developed hyperbilirubinemia, 47% increased AST, 73% increased ALT, 84% increased LDH, and 59% increased alkaline phosphatase. Ninety-four percent of patients developed elevated liver function tests within 90 days of starting cyclosporin. The few patients who developed late increases in liver function tests (>90 days), all had single events that responded to cyclosporin dose reduction.

Development of biliary sludge or gallstones has been reported in 2.4–30% of patients receiving cyclosporin following transplantation (76,77,90,95). Lowell et al. (90) found that up to 30% of diabetic pancreas and kidney transplant patients receiving cyclosporin developed cholelithiasis, an incidence significantly higher than in nondiabetic control patients.

E. Management

Reports of cyclosporin-induced hepatotoxicity have declined dramatically over the last 10 years. Furthermore, reported cases rarely result in clinically significant sequelae (69,77). Most cases of hepatotoxicity resolve without discontinuation of cyclosporin, but may require dose reduction (70,94). Patients receiving cyclosporin who develop cholestasis, particularly those with elevated blood levels, should be evaluated for cyclosporin-induced hepatotoxicity. After other potential causes are ruled out, decreasing the cyclosporin dose or switching to tacrolimus may be helpful. Mathieu et al. (96) reported one case of a patient who developed cyclosporin hepatotoxicity 9 days after heart transplantation manifested as increased bilirubin and slightly increased aminotransferases. The patient's liver function tests nearly normalized within 1 week of conversion to tacrolimus. It has been suggested that ursodiol may be of benefit in cyclosporin-induced cholestasis (97). However, no studies or case reports have shown ursodiol to be effective in cyclosporin-induced hepatotoxicity.

F. Drug Interactions

Cyclosporin is an 11-amino-acid cyclic polypeptide that undergoes extensive metabolism in the liver and small bowel. Over 30 metabolites of cyclosporin have been identified (98–100). Cyclosporin is metabolized primarily by CYP3A4 and to a lesser extent by CYP3A5 (1–3). It also is a known substrate for p-glycoprotein (Fig. 5) (5). In addition, cyclosporin has been shown to inhibit both CYP3A and the ABC transporters (101,102). Because of these characteristics, cyclosporin undergoes many drug interactions. In the transplant setting, many adverse events such as hypertension, infections, and seizures require treatment with concomitant medications. Many medications typically used to treat these transplant complications interact with cyclosporin and lead to increased or decreased levels, thus putting the patient at risk for cyclosporin toxicity or allograft rejection. Table 1 lists several agents associated with clinically significant increases or decreases in cyclosporin levels through their effects on CYP3A or p-glycoprotein. Avoiding these agents when equally effective and safe alternatives are available simplifies patient management. Certain situations require the concomitant administration of agents that interact with cyclo-

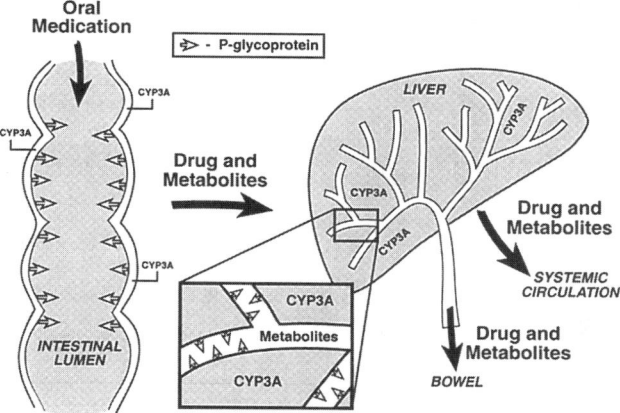

Figure 5 Intestinal and hepatic CYP 3A and *p*-glycoprotein. Cyclosporin, tacrolimus, and sirolimus are all metabolized by CYP 3A and are substrates for *p*-glycoprotein. *p*-Glycoprotein and the direction of transport are represented by the arrows. Intestinal CYP3A and *p*-glycoprotein are expressed in highest quantities in the villus tip of enterocytes in the proximal (duodenum–jejunum) and with a lesser amount in the distal (ileum) portion of the small bowel. Intestinal *p*-glycoprotein acts as a countertransport pump moving drug and metabolites back into the intestinal lumen. This process maximizes drug exposure to intestinal CYP 3A. Once the drug and metabolites make it to the liver, they are again exposed to CYP 3A and undergo further metabolism. Hepatic *p*-glycoprotein most likely pumps primarily metabolites into the bile. Drugs that inhibit or induce CYP 3A and/ or *p*-glycoprotein will substantially increase or decrease systemic concentrations of the drugs metabolized or transported by these, respectively.

sporin. In these cases, careful monitoring of cyclosporin blood levels and dosage adjustment may be necessary.

V. TACROLIMUS

A causal relationship between tacrolimus and hepatotoxicity is controversial. Although some have reported cases of presumed tacrolimus hepatotoxicity (103), others have sug-

Table 1 Commonly Used Agents that Increase or Decrease Cyclosporin Concentrations (106–119)

Increase cyclosporin levels	Decrease cyclosporin levels
Amiodarone	Carbamazepine
Clarithromycin	Phenobarbital
Diltiazem	Phenytoin
Erythromycin	Rifampin
Fluconazole	
Grapefruit juice	
Intraconazole	
Ketoconazole	
Nicardipine	
Verapamil	

gested that the histological lesions described may have represented rejection rather than drug toxicity (104). However, improvement in the hepatotoxicity with tacrolimus dose reduction or discontinuation is not consistent with this explanation. Nonetheless, differentiation between rejection and tacrolimus hepatotoxicity will be extremely difficult in liver transplant patients.

A. Histological Characteristics

Tacrolimus hepatotoxicity is reported to be associated with perivenular hepatocellular dropout and sinusoidal congestion (103).

B. Clinical Manifestations

Fisher et al. (103) described tacrolimus hepatotoxicity in five liver allograft recipients. Hepatotoxicity developed 6–24 weeks after initiation of tacrolimus and appeared to respond to a decrease in dose. Biochemical abnormalities ranged from mild to moderate increases in ALT (166–744 U/L) and alkaline phosphatase (68–1293 U/L). Significant improvement was noted in the liver enzymes of two patients within 7 days of tacrolimus dose reduction and in all five patients by 1 month. Although most patients required only dose reduction, one patient had an initial improvement with dose reduction, but required discontinuation of tacrolimus to normalize aminotransferase values.

C. Management

Since most patients thought to have tacrolimus-induced hepatotoxicity responded to dose reduction, this is the suggested approach. If no response or an inadequate response is seen, switching to another immunosuppressive agent should be considered.

D. Drug Interactions

Like cyclosporin, tacrolimus is metabolized by CYP3A4 and transported via p-glycoprotein (4,6). Therefore, agents that inhibit or induce CYP3A or p-glycoprotein will increase or decrease tacrolimus levels and potentially increase the risk of toxicity or rejection. It is anticipated that all the agents that interact with cyclosporin will also interact with tacrolimus (Table 1).

VI. MYCOPHENOLATE MOFETIL

There are no published reports of mycophenolate mofetil–induced hepatotoxicity. Product labeling information describes increased liver function tests (LDH, AST, ALT, GGT), hepatitis, and liver damage in 3–23% of kidney or heart transplant patients receiving the drug (11). The two most problematic drug interactions currently reported with mycophenolate mofetil are antacids and cholestyramine, both of which are associated with significant decreases in mycophenolic acid levels.

VII. SIROLIMUS

There is no published information on the hepatotoxicity of sirolimus. Package labeling information mentions increases in lactic dehydrogenase and serum aminotransferases in more than 3% but less than 20% of patients (105). Elevations in alkaline phosphatase and serum aminotransferases greater than 5–10 times normal were not significantly different between the sirolimus groups (2–5 mg/day) and either the placebo or azathioprine groups in clinical trials (M. Buttaro, personal communication, 2000). Since sirolimus is metabolized by CYP3A and p-glycoprotein, it is expected that agents that interact with cyclosporin will also interact with sirolimus (Table 1) (4,105).

VIII. SUMMARY

Hepatotoxicity from immunosuppressive agents is uncommon. When hepatotoxicity does occur, it can be difficult to diagnose owing to administration of other medications and the presence of concomitant illnesses. If a patient develops potential hepatotoxicity from an immunosuppressive agent, the overall immunosuppressive regimen should be assessed before decisions are made on the best approach to management. In some cases, dose reduction or discontinuation of the suspected hepatotoxic immunosuppressive may be the best plan of action. Other cases may require initiation of one or more additional immunosuppressive agents. The optimum approach depends on the individual patient, the duration posttransplantation, rejection history, concomitant immunosuppression, and the patient's ability to tolerate each of the agents.

Azathioprine-induced hepatotoxicity, in particular, requires timely evaluation and response. In some cases, delay in discontinuation of azathioprine has resulted in progression of liver damage and mortality. It is recommended that patients with suspected azathioprine-induced hepatotoxicity undergo liver biopsy. If the diagnosis is confirmed, immediate discontinuation of the azathioprine is recommended. Typically, cyclosporin and tacrolimus hepatotoxic reactions respond rapidly to dose reduction. However, some cases may require discontinuation to see complete resolution of hepatic dysfunction. Corticosteroids are associated with steatosis, which generally does not have any clinical manifestations. Continuation of the corticosteroids is usually possible. Finally, mycophenolate mofetil and sirolimus do not have any published information implicating hepatotoxicity.

A more frequently encountered problem in transplantation is the large number of drug interactions seen with the immunosuppressive agents. Prior to initiating any agent in a patient following transplantation requires careful evaluation of the medication profile for drug interactions. In particular, agents that alter CYP3A or p-glycoprotein with cyclosporin, tacrolimus, or sirolimus; generalized enzyme inhibitors or inducers with corticosteroids; inhibitors of xanthine oxidase with azathioprine and antacids/cholestyramine with mycophenolate mofetil are all problematic.

REFERENCES

1. Lown KS, Kolars JC, Thummel KE, Barnett JL, Kunze KL, Wrighton SA, Watkins PB. Interpatient heterogeneity in expression of CYP3A4 and CYP3A5 in small bowel. Lack of prediction by the erythromycin breath test. Drug Metab Dispos 1994; 22:947–955.
2. Watkins PB. Drug metabolism by cytochromes P450 in the liver and small bowel. Gastroenterol Pharmacol 1992; 21:511–526.
3. Aoyama T, Yamano S, Waxman DJ, Lapenson DP, Meyer UA, Fischer V, Tyndale R, Inaba T, Kalow W, Gelboin HV, Gonzalez FJ, et al. Cytochrome P-450 hPCN3 a novel cytochrome P-450 IIIA gene product that is differentially expressed in human liver. cDNA and deduced amino acid sequence and distinct specificities of cDNA-expressed hPCN1 and hPCN3 for the metabolism of steroid hormones and cyclosporine. J Biol Chem 1989; 264:10388–10395.

4. Sattler M, Guengerich FD, Yun C-H, Christians U, Sewing K-F. Cytochrome p-450 3A enzymes are responsible for biotransformation of FK506 and rapamycin in man and rat. Drug Metab Dispos 1992; 20:153–761.

5. Lown KS, Mayo RR, Leichtman AB, Hsiano HL, Turgeon DK, Schmiedlin-Ren P, Brown MB, Guo W, Rossi SJ, Benet LZ, Watkins PB. Role of intestinal p-glycoprotein (mdr 1) in interpatient variation in the oral bioavailability of cyclosporine. Clin Pharmacol Ther 1997; 62:248–260.

6. Saeki T, Ueda K, Tanigawara Y, Hori R, Komano T. Human p-glycoprotein transports cyclosporin A and FK506. J Biol Chem 1993; 268:6077–6080.

7. Cummins D, Sekar M, Halil O, Banner N. Myelosuppression associated with azathioprine-allopurinol interaction after heart and lung transplantation. Transplantation 1996; 61:1661–1662.

8. Kennedy DT, Hayney MS, Lake KD. Azathioprine and allopurinol: the price of an avoidable drug interaction. Ann Pharmacother 1996; 30:951–954.

9. Watts RWE, Watts JEM, Seegmiller JE. Xanthine oxidase activity in human tissues and its inhibition by allopurinol. J Lab Clin Med 1965; 66:688–697.

10. Zimm S, Collins JM, O'Neill D, Chabner BA, Poplack DG. Inhibition of first-pass metabolism in cancer chemotherapy: interaction of 6-mercaptopurine and allopurinol. Clin Pharmacol Ther 1983; 34:810–816.

11. Roche Laboratories Inc. CellCept, mycophenolate mofetil package insert, Nutley, 1998:1–12.

12. Anuras S, Piros J, Bonney WW, Forker EL, Colville DS, Corry RJ. Liver disease in renal transplant recipients. Arch Intern Med 1977; 137:42–48.

13. Horina JH, Wirnsberger GH, Kenner L, Holzer H, Krejs GJ. Increased susceptibility for CsA-induced hepatotoxicity in kidney graft recipients with chronic viral hepatitis C. Transplantation 1993; 56:1091–1094.

14. Degos F, Degott C, Bedrossian J, Camilieri JP, Barbanel C, Duboust A, Rueff B, Benhamou JP, Kreis H. Is renal transplantation involved in post-transplantation liver disease? A prospective study. Transplantation 1980; 29:100–102.

15. Delgado J, Munoz de Bustillo E, Ibarrola C, Colina F, Morales JM, Rodriguez E, Aguado JM, Fuertes A, Gomez MA. Is azathioprine a contributory factor? J Heart Lung Transplant 1999; 18:607–610.

16. Hill RB, Droke WE, Hays AP. Hepatic lipid metabolism in the cortisone-treated rat. Exp Mol Pathol 1965; 4:320–327.

17. Jeanrenaud B. Effect of glucocorticoid hormones on fatty acid mobilization and reesterification in rat adipose and tissue. Biochem J 1967; 103:627–633.

18. Bhagwat AG, Deodhar SD. Experimental hepatic injury produced in the rabbit by glucocorticoids. Arch Pathol 1968; 85:346–356.

19. Popper H. Morphologic and biochemical aspects of fatty liver. Acta Hepto Splenolog 1961; 8:279–292.

20. Soffer LJ, Iannaccone A, Gabrilove JL. Cushing's syndrome: study of fifty patients. Am J Med 1961; 30:129–146.

21. Steinberg H, Webb WM, Rafsky HA. Hepatomegaly with fatty infiltration secondary to cortisone therapy: case report. Gastroenterology 1952; 21:304–309.

22. Stollerman GH. Rheumatic fever. Arch Intern Med 1956; 98:211–220.

23. Hill RB. Fatal fat embolism from steroid-induced fatty liver. N Engl J Med. 1961; 265:318–320.

24. Jones JP, Engleman EP, Najarian JS. Systemic fat embolism after renal homotransplantation and treatment with corticosteroids. N Engl J Med 1965; 273:1453–1458.

25. Zucher RM, Frey BM, Frey FJ. Impact of ketoconazole on metabolism of prednisolone. Clin Pharmacol Ther 1989; 45:366–372.

26. Boekenoogen SJ, Szefler SJ, Jusko WJ. Prednisolone disposition and protein binding in oral contraceptive users. J Clin Endocrinol Metab 1983; 56:702–709.

27. Legler UF, Benet LZ. Marked alterations in dose-dependent prednisolone kinetics in women taking oral contraceptives. Clin Pharmacol Ther 1986; 39:425–429.

28. Buffington GA, Dominguez JH, Piering WF, Hebert LA, Kauffman HM, Lemann J. Interaction of rifampin and glucocorticoids. JAMA 1976; 236:1958–1960.

29. Hendrickse W, McKiernan J, Pickup M, Lowe J. Rifampicin-induced nonresponsiveness to corticosteroid treatment in nephrotic syndrome. Br Med J 1979; 1:306.

30. Ohnhaus EE, Park BK. Measurement of urinary 6-β-hydroxycortisol excretion as an in vivo parameter in the clinical assessment of the microsomal enzyme-inducing capacity of antipyrine, phenobarbitone and rifampicin. Eur J Clin Pharmacol 1979; 15:139–145.

31. Choi Y, Thrasher K, Werk EE, Sholiton LJ, Olinger C. Effect of diphenylhydantoin on cortisol kinetics in humans. J Pharmacol Exp Ther 1971; 176:27–34.

32. Ramalho HJ, Terra EG, Cartapatti E, Barberato JB, Alves VAF, Gayotto LCC, Abbud-Filho M. Hepatotoxicity of azathioprine in renal transplant recipients. Transplant Proc 1989; 21: 1716–1717.

33. Sparberg M, Simon N, Del Greco F. Intrahepatic cholestasis due to azathioprine. Gastroenterology 1969; 57:439–441.

34. Zarday Z, Veith FJ, Gliedman ML, Soberman R. Irreversible liver damage after azathioprine. JAMA 1972; 222:690–691.

35. Hankey GJ, Saker BM. Peliosis hepatis in a renal transplant recipient and in a haemodialysis patient. Med J Aust 1987; 146:102–105.

36. Haboubi NY, Ali HH, Whitwell HL, Ackrill P. Role of endothelial cell injury in the spectrum of azathioprine-induced liver disease after renal transplant: light microscopy and ultrastructural observations. Am J Gastroenterol 1988; 83:256–261.

37. Eisenhauer T, Hartmenn H, Rumpf KW, Helmchen U, Scheler F, Creutzfeldt W. Favourable outcome of hepatic veno-occlusive disease in a renal transplant patient receiving azathioprine, treated by portacaval shunt. Digestion 1984; 30:185–190.

38. Jones MC, Best PV, Catto GRD. Is nodular regenerative hyperplasia of the liver associated with azathioprine therapy after renal transplantation? Nephrol Dial Transplant 1988; 3:331–333.

39. Small P, Lichter M. Probable azathioprine hepatotoxicity: a case report. Ann Allergy 1989; 62:518–520.

40. Katzka DA, Saul SH, Jorkasky D, Sigal H, Reynolds JC, Soloway RD. Azathioprine and hepatic venoocclusive disease in renal transplant patients. Gastroenterology 1986; 90:446–454.

41. Read AE, Wiesner RH, LaBrecque DR, Tifft JG, Mullen KD, Sheer RL, Petrelli M, Ricanati ES, McCullough AJ. Hepatic veno-occlusive disease associated with renal transplantation and azathioprine therapy. Ann Intern Med 1986; 104:651–655.

42. Sterneck M, Wiesner RH., Ascher N, Roberts J, Ferrell L, Ludwig J, Lake J. Azathioprine hepatotoxicity after liver transplantation. Hepatology 1991; 14:806–810.

43. Weitz H, Gokel JM, Loeschke K, Possinger K, Eder M. Veno-occlusive disease of the liver in patients receiving immunosuppressive therapy. Virchows Arch 1982; 395:245–256.

44. Buffet C, Cantarovitch M, Pelletier G, Fabre M, Martin E, Charpentier B, Etienne JP, Fries D. Three cases of nodular regenerative hyperplasia of the liver following renal transplantation. Nephrol Dial Transplant 1988; 3:327–330.

45. Duvoux C, Kracht M, Lang P, Vernant J-P, Safrani E-S, Dhumeaux D. Hyperplasie nodulaire regenerative du foie associée à la prise d'azathioprine. Gastroenterol Clin Biol 1991; 15: 968–973.

46. Marubbio AT, Danielson B. Hepatic veno-occlusive disease in a renal transplant patient receiving azathioprine. Gastroenterology 1975; 69:739–743.

47. DePinho RA, Goldberg CS, Lefkowitch JH. Azathioprine and the liver, evidence favoring idosyncratic, mixed cholestatic-hepatocellular injury in humans. Gastroenterology 1984; 86: 162–165.

48. Lin S-N, Jessup K, Floyd M, Wang TP, van Buren CT, Caprioli RM, Kahan BD. Quantitation of plasma azathioprine and 6-mercaptopurine levels in renal transplant patients. Transplantation 1980; 29:290–294.

49. Odlind B, Hartvig P, Lindstrom B, Lonnerholm G, Tufveson G, Grefberg N. Serum azathioprine and 6-mercaptopurine levels and immunosuppressive activity after azathioprine in uremic patients. Int J Immunopharmacol 1986; 8:1–11.

50. Lennard L, Brown CB, Fox M, Maddocks JL. Azathioprine metabolism in kidney transplant recipients. Br J Clin Pharmacol 1984; 18:693–700.

51. Chan GLC, Erdmann GR, Gruber SA, Matas AJ, Canafax DM. Azathioprine metabolism: pharmacokinetics of 6-mercaptopurine, 6-thiouric acid and 6-thioguanine nucleotides in renal transplant patients. J Clin Pharmacol 1990; 30:358–363.

52. Lennard L, Maddocks JL. Assay of 6-thioguanine nucleotide, a major metabolite of azathioprine, 6-mercaptopurine and 6-thioguanine in human red blood cells. J Pharm Pharmacol 1983; 35:15–18.

53. Elion GB, Callahan S, Nathan H, Bieber S, Rundles RW, Hitchings GH. Potentiation by inhibition of drug degradation: 6-substituted purines and xanthine oxidase. Biochem Pharmacol 1963; 12:85–93.

54. Bergan S, Rugstad HE, Bentadal O, Stokke O. Monitoring of azathioprine treatment by determination of 6-thioguanine nucleotide concentrations in erythrocytes. Transplantation 1994; 58:803–808.

55. Lennard L, Harrington CI, Wood M, Maddocks JL. Metabolism of azathioprine to 6-thioguanine nucleotides in patients with pemphigus vulgaris. Br J Clin Pharmacol 1987; 23:229–233.

56. Remy CN. Metabolism of thiopyrimidines and thiopurines: S-methylation and S-adenosylmethionine transmethylase and catabolism in mammalian tissue. J Biol Chem 1963; 238: 1078–1084.

57. Woodson LC, Weinshilbaum RM. Human kidney thiopurine methyltransferase: purification and biochemical properties. Biochem Pharmacol 1983; 32:819–826.

58. Philips FS, Sternberg SS, Hamilton L, Clarke DA. The toxic effects of 6-mercaptopurine and related compounds. Ann NY Acad Sci 1954; 60:283–296.

59. Gross R. Hepatotoxicity of 6-mercaptopurine and azathioprine. Mayo Clin Proc 1994; 69: 498–500.

60. Einhorn M, Davidsohn I. Hepatotoxicity of mercaptopurine. JAMA 1964; 188:802–806.

61. Clark PA, Hsia YE, Huntsman RG. Toxic complications of treatment with 6-mercaptopurine, two cases with hepatic necrosis and intestinal ulceration. Br Med J 1960; 1:383–395.

62. McIlvanie SK, MacCarthy JD. Hepatitis in association with prolonged 6-mercaptopurine therapy. Blood 1958; 14:80–90.

63. Shorey J, Schenker S. Hepatotoxicity of mercaptopurine. Arch Intern Med 1968; 122:54–58.

64. Minow RA, Stern MH, Casey JH, Rodriguez V, Luna MA. Clinico-pathologic correlation of liver damage in patients treated with 6-mercaptopurine and adriamycin. Cancer 1976; 38: 1524–1528.

65. Griner PF, Elbadawi A, Packman CH. Veno-occlusive disease of the liver after chemotherapy of acute leukemia, report of two cases. Ann Intern Med 1976; 85:578–582.

66. DeLeve LD, Wang X, Kuhlenkamp JF, Kaplowitz N. Toxicity of azathioprine and monocrotaline in murine sinusoidal endothelial cells and hepatocytes: the role of glutathione and relevance to hepatic venoocclusive disease. Hepatology 1996; 23:589–599.

67. Wanless IR, Godwin TA, Allen F, Feder A. Nodular regenerative hyperplasia of the liver in hematologic disorders: a possible response to obliterative portal venopathy: a morphomet-

ric study of nine cases with an hypothesis on the pathogenesis. Medicine 1980; 59:367–379.

68. Mourad G, Bories P, Berthelemy C, Barneon G, Michel H, Mion C. Peliosis hepatis and nodular regenerative hyperplasia of the liver in renal transplants: is cytomegalovirus the cause of this severe disease? Transplant Proc 1987; 19:3697–3698.

69. Klintmalm GBG, Iwatsuki S, Starzl TE. Cyclosporin A hepatotoxicity in 66 renal allograft recipients. Transplantation 1981; 32:488–489.

70. Kassianides C, Nussenblatt R, Palestine AG, Mellow SD, Hoofnagle JH. Liver injury from cyclosporine A. Dig Dis Sci 1990; 35:693–697.

71. Atkinson K, Biggs J, Dodds A, Concannon A. Cyclosporin-associated hepatotoxicity after allogeneic marrow transplantation in man: differentiation from other causes of post transplant liver disease. Transplant Proc 1983; 15:s2761–2767.

72. McKenzie FN, Moses GC, Henderson AR. Routine "cardiac" and "hepatic" serum enzyme profiles in cardiac transplant patients treated with cyclosporine A: operative and postoperative findings. Clin Chem 1985; 31:822–825.

73. Laupacis A, Keown PA, Ulan RA, Sinclair NR, Stiller CR. Hyperbilirubinemia and cyclosporin A levels. Lancet 1981; 2:1426–1427.

74. Schade RR, Guglielmi A, Van Thiel DH, Thompson ME, Warty V, Griffith B, Sanghvi A, Bahnson H, Hardesty R. Cholestasis in heart transplant recipients treated with cyclosporine. Transplant Proc 1983; 15:2757–2760.

75. Loertscher R, Wenk M, Harder F, Brunner F, Follath F, Thiel G. Hyperbilirubinemia and cyclosporin A levels in renal transplant patients. Lancet 1981; 2:635–636.

76. Kahan BD, Flechner SM, Lorber MI, Golden D, Conley S, Van Buren CT. Complications of cyclosporine-prednisone immunosuppression in 402 renal allograft recipients exclusively followed at a single center from one to five years. Transplantation 1987; 43:197–204.

77. Lorber MI, Van Buren CT, Flechner SM, Williams C, Kahan BD. Hepatobiliary and pancreatic complications of cyclosporine therapy in 466 renal transplant recipients. Transplantation 1987; 43:35–40.

78. Roman ID, Monte MJ, Gonzalez-Buitrago JM, Esteller A, Jimenez R. Inhibition of hepatocytary vesicular transport by cyclosporin A in the rat: relationship with cholestasis and hyperbilirubinemia. Hepatology 1990; 12:83–91.

79. Stone BG, Udani M, Sanghvi A, Warty V, Plocki K, Bedetti CD, Van Thiel DH. Cyclosporin A–induced cholestasis: the mechanism in a rat model. Gastroenterology 1987; 93:344–351.

80. Rotolo FS, Branum GD, Bowers BA, Meyers WC. Effect of cyclosporine on bile secretion in rats. Am J Surg 1986; 151:35–40.

81. Cadranel JF, Dumont M, Mesa VA, Degott C, Touchard D, Erlinger S. Effect of chronic administration of cyclosporin A on hepatic uptake and biliary secretion of bromosulfophthalein in rat. Dig Dis Sci 1991; 36:221–224.

82. Nicchitta CV, Kamoun M, Williamson JR. Cyclosporin augments receptor-mediated cellular Ca fluxes in isolated hepatocytes. J Biol Chem 1985; 260:13613–13618.

83. Stacey NH, Kotecka B. Inhibition of taurocholate and ouabain transport in isolated rat hepatocytes by cyclosporin A. Gastroenterology 1988; 95:780–786.

84. Ballantyne CM, Podet EJ, Patsch WP, Harati Y, Appel V, Gotto AM, Young JB. Effects of cyclosporine therapy on plasma lipoprotein levels. JAMA 1989; 262:53–56.

85. Drueke TB, Abdulmassih Z, Lacour B, Bader C, Chevalier A, Kreis H. Atherosclerosis and lipid disorders after renal transplantation. Kidney Int 1991; 31(suppl):24–28.

86. Kuster GM, Drexel H, Bleisch JA, Rentsch K, Pei P, Binswanger U, Amann FW. Relation of cyclosporine blood levels to adverse effects on lipoproteins. Transplantation 1994; 57:1479–1483.

87. Vaziri ND, Liang K, Azad H. Effect of cyclosporine on HMG-CoA reductase, cholesterol 7α-hydroxylase, LDL receptor, HDL receptor, VLDL receptor and lipoprotein lipase expressions. J Pharmacol Exp Ther 2000; 294:778–783.

88. Rayyes OA, Wallmark A, Floren CH. Cyclosporine inhibits catabolism of low-density lipo-proteins HepG2 cells by about 25%. Hepatology 1996; 24:613–619.

89. Wisecarver JL, Earl RA, Haven MC, Timmins PW, Shaw BW, Stratta RJ, Langnas AN, Zetterman RK, Donovan JP, Shaefer MS, Markin RS. Histologic changes in liver allograft biopsies associated with elevated whole blood and tissue cyclosporine concentrations. Modern Pathol 1992; 5:611–616.

90. Lowell JA, Stratta RJ, Taylor RJ, Bynon JS, Larsen JL, Nelson NL. Cholelithiasis in pancreas and kidney transplant recipients with diabetes. Surgery 1993; 114:863–864.

91. Kahan BD. Cyclosporine. N Engl J Med 1989; 321:1725–1738.

92. Whiting PH, Simpson JG, Davidson RJL, Thomson AW. Pathological changes in rats receiving cyclosporin A at immunotherapeutic dosage for 7 weeks. Br J Exp Pathol 1983; 64:437–444.

93. Farthing MJG, Clark ML. Nature of the toxicity of cyclosporin A in the rat. Biochem Pharmacol 1981; 30:3311–3316.

94. Calne RY, White DJG, Pentlow BD, Rolles DK, Syrakos T, Ohtawa T, Smith DP, McMaster P, Evans DB, Herbertson BM, Thiru S. Cyclosporin A: preliminary observations in dogs with pancreatic duodenal allografts and patients with cadaveric renal transplants. Transplant Proc 1979; 11:860–864.

95. Steck TB, Costanzo-Nordin MR, Keshavarizian A. Prevalence and management of cholelithiasis in heart transplant patients. J Heart Lung Transplant 1991; 10:1029–1032.

96. Mathieu P, Carrier M, White M, Pellerin M, Perrault LP, Pelletier G, Pelletier LC. Conversion of cyclosporine A to tacrolimus following heart transplantation. Can J Cardiol 1999; 15:1229–1232.

97. Kowdley KV, Keeffe EB. Hepatotoxicity of transplant immunosuppressive agents. Gastroenterol Clin North Am 1995; 24:991–1001.

98. Maurer G, Loosli HR, Schreier E, Keller B. Disposition of cyclosporin in several animal species and man. I. Structural elucidation of its metabolites. Drug Metab Dispos 1984; 12:120–126.

99. Maurer G, Lemaire M. Biotransformation and distribution in blood of cyclosporin and its metabolites. Transplant Proc 1986; 18:25–34.

100. Christians U, Schlitt HJ, Bleck JS, Schiebel HM, Kownatzki R, Maurer G, Strohmeyer SS, Schottmann R, Wonigeit K, Pichlmayr R, Sewing KF. Measurement of cyclosporine and 18 metabolites in blood, bile and urine by high-performance liquid chromatography (HPLC). Transplant Proc 1988; 20:609–613.

101. Lampen A, Christians U, Guengerich FP, Watkins PB, Kolars JC, Bader A, Gonschior A-K, Dralle H, Hackbarth I, Sewing K-F. Metabolism of the immunosuppressant tacrolimus in the small intestine: cytochrome P450, drug interactions, and interindividual variability. Drug Metab Dispos 1995; 23:1315–1324.

102. Naito M, Tsuruo T. Competitive inhibition by verapamil of ATP-dependent high affinity vincristine binding to the plasma membrane of multidrug-resistant K562 cells without calcium ion involvement. Cancer Res 1989; 49:1452–1455.

103. Fisher A, Mor E, Hytiroglou P, Emre S, Boccagni P, Chadoff L, Sheiner P, Schwartz M, Thung SN, Miller C. FK506 hepatotoxicity in liver allograft recipients. Transplantation 1995; 59:1631–1632.

104. Tsamandas AC, Jain AB, Felekouras ES, Fung JJ, Demetris AJ, Lee RG. Central venulitis in the allograft liver. Transplantation 1997; 64:252–257.

105. Wyeth-Ayerst Pharmaceuticals. Rapamune (sirolimus) oral solution product labeling. Philadelphia, 2000:1–4.

106. Nicolau DP, Uber WE, Crumbley AJ, Strange C. Amiodarone-cyclosporine interaction in heart transplant patient. J Heart Lung Transplant 1992; 11:564–568.

107. Gersema LM, Proter CB, Russell EH. Suspected drug interaction between cyclosporine and clarithromycin. J Heart Lung Transplant 1994; 13:343–345.

108. Neumayer HH, Wagner K. Diltiazem and economic use of cyclosporin. Lancet 1986; 2:523.

109. Gupta SK, Bakran A, Johnson RWG, Rowland M. Cyclosporin-erythromycin interaction in renal transplant patients. Br J Clin Pharmacol 1989; 27:475–481.

110. Lopez-Gil JA. Fluconazole-cyclosporine interaction: a dose-dependent effect? Ann Pharmacother 1993; 27:427–430.

111. Ducharme MP, Warbasse LH, Edwards DJ. Disposition of intravenous and oral cyclosporine after administration with grapefruit juice. Clin Pharmacol Ther 1995; 57:485–491.

112. Trenk D, Brett W, Jahnchen E, Birnbaum D. Time course of cyclosporin/itraconazole interaction. Lancet 1987; 2:1335–1336.

113. Gomez DY, Wacher VJ, Tomlanovich SJ, Hebert MF, Benet LZ. The effects of ketoconazole on the intestinal metabolism and bioavailability of cyclosporine. Clin Pharmacol Ther 1995; 58:15–19.

114. Hebert MF, Roberts JP, Prueksaritanont T, Benet LZ. Bioavailability of cyclosporine with concomitant rifampin administration is markedly less than predicted by hepatic enzyme induction. Clin Pharmacol Ther 1992; 52:453–457.

115. Sketris IS, Methot ME, Nicol D, Belitsky P, Knox MG. Effect of calcium-channel blockers on cyclosporine clearance and use in renal transplant patients. Ann Pharmacother 1994; 28:1227–1231.

116. Bourbigot B, Guiserix J, Airiau J, Bressollette L, Morin JF, Cledes J. Nicardipine increases cyclosporin blood levels. Lancet 1986; 1:1447.

117. Cooney GF, Mochon M, Kaiser B, Dunn SP, Goldsmith B. Effects of carbamazepine on cyclosporine metabolism in pediatric renal transplant recipients. Pharmacotherapy 1995; 15:353–356.

118. Carstensen H, Jacobsen N, Dieperink H. Interaction between cyclosporin A and phenobarbitone. Br J Clin Pharmacol 1986; 21:550–551.

119. Freeman DJ, Laupacis A, Keown PA, Stiller CR, Carruthers SG. Evaluation of cyclosporin-phenytoin interaction with observations on cyclosporin metabolites. Br J Clin Pharmacol 1984; 18:887–893.

26

Methotrexate Controversies

ADRIAN REUBEN

Medical University of South Carolina, Charleston, South Carolina, U.S.A.

I. INTRODUCTION

Methotrexate (MTX), a classic antimetabolite that inhibits folic acid metabolism, has been licensed in the United States since 1953 and commercially available since 1955. An analog of both folic acid and the antecedent folic acid antagonist aminopterin (withdrawn because of toxicity), MTX competes with 5-methyltetrahydrofolate (the major folate in serum) and with folinic acid (5-formyltetrahydrofolate) for uptake into cells. Once inside the cell, MTX is polyglutamylated by folylpolyglutamate synthetase, and it is likely that this conversion, which impairs MTX egress from the cell, determines MTX's cytotoxicity. Intracellularly, MTX inhibits tetrahydrofolate reductase leading to a reduced supply of tetrahydrofolates (especially folinic acid), which in turn impairs synthesis of thymidylate (a pyrimidine precursor) and purines and stops DNA biosynthesis, thereby causing cell death (1).

Folic acid antagonists were originally used for childhood leukemia but soon aminopterin, and later methotrexate (amethopterin), was shown to improve arthritic symptoms in patients with psoriasis and rheumatoid arthritis (2–4). Over successive decades, the oncological indications for MTX grew to cover the treatment of a variety of solid tumors including head and neck cancers, breast cancer, gestational and trophoblastic diseases, non-Hodgkin's lymphoma, pediatric tumors, and sarcoma—especially osteosarcoma. MTX has been used in both conventional and high-dose regimens, often in combination with leucovorin (folinic acid) "rescue" and other chemotherapeutic agents. Similarly, MTX treatment of inflammatory disorders has expanded beyond psoriasis and rheumatoid arthritis. MTX is used now for connective tissue disorders, such as Reiter's syndrome, polymyositis/dermatomyositis, and Wegener's granulomatosis, as well as for uveitis, asthma, and sarcoidosis.

MTX has been known to be hepatotoxic almost since its introduction into clinical practice (5). Thus, because of the seriousness of its hepatotoxic and other adverse effects (bone marrow toxicity, alopecia, mucositis, erythematous skin rashes, nephrotoxicity, interstitial pneumonitis, osteopenia, and neurotoxicity), MTX use is restricted to situations in which less hazardous remedies fail. In this context, there are two main controversies in MTX therapy; the first concerns the stringency of monitoring for hepatotoxicity, while the second is whether MTX is an effective and safe treatment for certain liver diseases per se, notably primary biliary cirrhosis (PBC). The controversy over the need for pre-MTX liver biopsies and the appropriate surveillance of patients on long-term MTX therapy for various inflammatory disorders has largely been resolved, especially for the treatment of rheumatoid arthritis and to a certain extent for the treatment of psoriasis. Guidelines have been published for hepatotoxicity monitoring in the treatment of rheumatoid arthritis (6) and psoriasis (7,8), but adherence to these published guidelines may not be universally consistent (9). Guidelines are also emerging for monitoring MTX therapy for more recent indications such as Crohn's disease, based on careful clinical, biochemical, and liver histological follow-up (10). In contrast to this growing consensus, a lively debate still continues between protagonists and antagonists of MTX therapy for PBC and other liver disorders (11–18).

II. ACUTE LIVER INJURY CAUSED BY MTX

As with many other drugs, reversible elevations of aminotransferases are quite common following initiation of MTX therapy, with a prevalence of approximately 14% in one report (19). In patients treated with cyclical therapy the enzymes rise with each course— usually higher the more frequent the dosing—but subside within a month. With high-dose therapy (with or without leucovorin rescue), aminotransferases may rise up to 40-fold above normal, sometimes accompanied by hyperbilirubinemia (20,21) and with an occasional clinical presentation of "acute hepatitis" (22,23). The injury is acute, and even when there is deep jaundice and dramatic increases in alanine aminotransferase (ALT) and aspartate aminotransferase (AST) levels (24), these abnormalities resolve within a few weeks of stopping MTX almost invariably without long-term sequelae (25). Liver biopsy may show steatosis but not fibrosis or cirrhosis (25). Indeed, the severity of acute hepatotoxicity induced by MTX is thought to predict for a good oncological therapeutic response (26). Rare cases of reversible liver failure have been described (27) but incrimination of MTX as the sole culprit in these cases was not unequivocal. A case of rapidly progressive subfulminant liver failure requiring transplantation has been reported (28).

III. CHRONIC LIVER INJURY CAUSED BY MTX

A. High-Dose MTX

The most significant long-term side effect of chronic MTX therapy is hepatic fibrosis leading to cirrhosis. High-dose daily MTX, whether given for leukemia in children (5,

29,30) or for psoriasis in adults (31–33), was associated with the development of hepatic fibrosis or cirrhosis. One impediment to assessing the true role of MTX in causing cirrhosis in adults with psoriasis had been the lack of baseline pre-MTX liver biopsies in many of the older studies. This was an especially important omission since it is known that liver histological abnormalities are present in psoriatic patients, even before MTX therapy (34). Preexisting liver abnormalities in patients with psoriasis, mostly steatosis (35), may be related to the systemic dermatological condition itself and/or comorbid conditions such as alcohol excess, obesity, exposure to other hepatotoxins, hepatitis C, and so forth. Portal inflammation, steatosis, and portal fibrosis are also found in patients with rheumatoid arthritis (36,37). In some series, fibrosis has been reported in up to 22% and cirrhosis in 0–2% of psoriatic patients without MTX therapy (38). The prevalence of cirrhosis in psoriatics was reported in another series as being 0.6% without MTX therapy and as high as 25% after 5 years of 50 mg weekly bolus MTX treatment (39). In those patients with more than mild fibrosis, alcohol abuse and other causes of liver injury could be identified in most cases. Notwithstanding the difficulties in estimating the absolute fibrogenic potential of MTX (because of uncertainty about underlying preexisting liver pathology and other variables causing liver injury), there is little doubt that high-dose MTX, whether daily or weekly, does cause hepatic fibrosis and cirrhosis that may even deteriorate to warrant liver transplantation (40).

B. Histological Changes Due to MTX

Mindful of the pitfalls in interpretation alluded to above, there is agreement about the histopathological changes caused by MTX. The earliest changes are ultrastructural and include lysosomal and mitochondrial injury, endoplasmic reticulum hypertrophy, autophagic vacuole formation, and desmosomal injury (41,42). There is bile duct damage (43) and stellate cell (Ito cell, lipocyte, or fat-storing cell) hyperplasia (41,44). It is the latter, presumably, that leads to deposition of collagen in the space of Disse (45), causing fibrosis and ultimately cirrhosis (46). A propensity for periportal inflammation to proceed to periportal, sinusoidal, and bridging fibrosis has been suggested (47), but it is dubious that MTX causes bona fide chronic hepatitis (27). Other lesions attributed to MTX include marked macrovesicular steatosis, zone 3 focal hepatocyte degeneration, hepatocyte nuclear pleomorphism, and Kupffer cell proliferation (48). Roenigk et al. have classified these light microscopic changes into five levels of severity (7), to permit ease of comparison both within and between patients (see Table 1). Although this grading system is subjective, insensitive to small changes, and only semiquantitative (especially for fibrosis), it is still widely used to grade liver histopathology in psoriatic patients on MTX treatment (8,49), especially when deciding whether to continue or discontinue treatment. Other grading systems have not supplanted the Roenigk scheme (50), including quantitative estimates of collagen content by image analysis (51).

The fibrosis caused by MTX is typically periportal with extensions into the parenchyma in a sinusoidal or "chicken-wire" pattern, reminiscent of the fibrosis of alcoholic and nonalcoholic fatty liver disease. MTX cirrhosis is usually micronodular (47).

C. Mechanism of MTX-Induced Liver Injury

The mechanism of MTX-induced liver injury, especially chronic injury, is unknown but has been attributed to the intracellular buildup of polyglutamylated MTX and the toxic effects of 7-hydroxymethotrexate, the major MTX metabolite (52). However, it is unclear

Table 1 Roenigk Classification of Liver Histology in Chronic MTX Therapy

| | Histology | | | |
Classification	Fatty change	Nuclear pleomorphism	Fibrosis	Necroinflammatory change
Grade I	Mild or none	Mild or none	None	Mild portal tract inflammation
Grade II	Moderate to severe	Moderate to severe	None	Portal tract inflammation, moderate to severe Hepatocellular necrosis, moderate to severe
Grade IIIa	0/+	0/+	Mild; fibrotic septa Extending into lobule	0/+
Grade IIIb	0/+	0/+	Moderate to severe	0/+
Grade IV	0/+	0/+	Cirrhosis	0/+

0/+ denotes absent/present.
Source: Roenigk et al. (7,49).

whether the fibrosis is initiated by hepatocyte or bile duct injury, or by independent activation of hepatic stellate cells. One of the earliest changes seen in MTX-treated patients before light microscopic abnormalities occur is the increased appearance of matrix proteins, several collagens, and transforming growth factor (53), suggesting a primary role for the stellate cell.

Unfortunately there is no animal model that mimics human MTX liver injury well. Acute MTX toxicity in the rat is cholestatic and appears to be caused by 7-hydroxymethotrexate precipitation in bile (52), Chronic daily oral administration of MTX to rats causes zone 3 necrosis and Kupffer cell enlargement and, in some animals, fibrosis (54). MTX-induced steatosis appears to result from interference with methionine metabolism and transmethylation reactions, as the striking steatogenic effect of MTX in rats can be mitigated by choline administration (55).

D. Low-Dose MTX Therapy

1. Psoriasis

The enthusiasm for MTX as effective therapy for proliferative and inflammatory conditions like psoriasis and rheumatoid arthritis, respectively, was soon tempered by its toxicity in patients dosed daily, notably the advent of advanced hepatic fibrosis. Many years later, low-dose weekly regimens of MTX were introduced and found to be effective but there was disagreement over safety and, in particular, the risk of advanced fibrosis and cirrhosis. MTX should be reserved for patients with moderate to severe psoriasis, meaning psoriatic erythroderma, moderate to severe psoriatic arthritis, more than 20% body surface involvement, localized pustular psoriasis, lack of response to phototherapy, PUVA, and retinoids, or psoriasis that affects certain areas of the body so that normal function and employment are prevented. In short, for MTX use the psoriasis should be life-ruining physically, emotionally, or economically.

The results of numerous biopsy studies, in both psoriasis (24 studies) and rheumatoid arthritis patients (20 studies) taking long-term weekly MTX, are listed in detail in a recent review by West (38). In psoriatics on MTX, the prevalence of fibrosis ranged from 14 to 34% and of cirrhosis from 0 to 21%, but conclusions from these studies are compromised by the lack of baseline biopsies. Unfortunately, even when studies were done of paired pretreatment and on-treatment histology, there was poor agreement over the risk of MTX causing fibrosis. In some series, clinically significant fibrosis that dictated cessation of therapy was rare (56) even when cumulative doses of 5.1 g were used (57). At the other extreme (39), 13% of patients who ingested a 2.2-g cumulative dose and 26% who ingested 4 g developed cirrhosis. Excluding extremes, the likely cirrhosis rate for psoriatics treated with MTX is approximately 7–10% (56–61) and one estimate predicts 6.7% increased risk of progression of fibrosis for every additional gram of drug ingested (62). Although the reasons for those discrepancies are not proven, it seems likely that comorbid clinical variables influence the risk of developing MTX-associated fibrosis and cirrhosis. The most important of these appears to be alcohol. For example, previous or ongoing heavy alcohol use increases the risk of MTX-induced fibrosis 2.5–5-fold (62). It seems that weekly alcohol ingestion of as little as 100 g is sufficient to increase the risk of progression to cirrhosis (62). Obesity and diabetes together enhance the fibrogenic potential of MTX (63,64), but it is unclear whether either does so alone (60,65,66). Other potentiating factors are preexisting liver disease (34,59), excessive vitamin A ingestion (39), and renal failure (39,67), presumably because the latter raises MTX blood levels. Historically, prior arsenical therapy potentiated MTX hepatotoxicity (39), but this is no longer a consideration. Whether advancing years aggravate MTX-induced liver damage is unclear (34,59,65,66, 68) but neither severity of psoriasis (65), gender (63), HLA phenotype (69), nor corticosteroid treatment (65) appears to influence MTX liver damage. Aside from comorbid conditions, the single most important factor in MTX-induced liver fibrosis in psoriasis is the dosing regimen, and arguably the cumulative dose. We have recently performed a liver transplant in a patient who had received daily MTX doses for 3 years; there were no other risk factors for liver disease. Daily dosing has not been the standard of care in psoriasis and rheumatoid arthritis since the 1970s, when the change from daily to weekly dosing was adopted. Daily dosing should be avoided.

The unanswered question whether MTX hepatotoxicity in psoriasis is related directly to cumulative dose and/or duration of therapy is important, as the answer will dictate the intensity of monitoring and, in particular, the frequency of liver biopsy.

Liver Biopsy. In patients with risk factors for liver disease, it is recommended that a baseline biopsy be done. However, since a small percentage of psoriasis patients may not continue to take MTX after the initial 2–4 months of therapy (because of adverse effects, lack of efficacy, etc.), the first liver biopsy can be postponed for this period until it is certain that long-term treatment is needed. In patients with risk factors for liver disease, namely those with a prior or current history of alcohol excess, abnormal liver test results, chronic hepatitis B or C infection, obesity or diabetes, other hepatotoxin exposure, or a family history of an inheritable liver disease, the baseline biopsy should be done early (i.e., before MTX is started or within the first 2–4 months of therapy). In psoriatics without these risk factors, the first biopsy can be postponed until the patient has consumed 1–1.5

g of drug, since it is rare for serious liver disease to develop below that cumulative dose. Some studies have shown a correlation between the degree of liver injury and cumulative dose (32,39,59,65,70,71) while others have not (33,35,57,58,60,61,63,68). It has been suggested that continuation of MTX following demonstration of fibrosis or cirrhosis actually may not lead to disease progression (35,39,59) and, contrary to expectation, only rarely to liver decompensation (72). These latter experiences have prompted some authorities to question the need for frequent liver biopsy in MTX-treated psoriasis, except in high-risk patients. Rather they suggest reducing the frequency of biopsy and substituting monitoring by serial measurement of serum amino-terminal propeptide of type III procollagen (PIIIP) or dynamic hepatic scintigraphy nuclear medicine scanning (73,74). Notwithstanding, consensus opinion (49) still recommends follow-up biopsy every 1–1.5 g of incremental cumulative dose of MTX as long as the baseline liver biopsy was normal. If liver chemistries (aminotransferases, alkaline phosphatase, bilirubin, and albumin) are abnormal (49,74), then repeat biopsy should be done after the next cumulative dose of 0.5–1 g (or approximately after 6 months of further therapy).

Patients showing Roenigk grade I or II changes (Table 1) may continue on therapy. Those with grade IIIa changes should undergo repeat liver biopsy approximately 6 months later (or change to alternative therapy), whilst those with grade IIIb and IV changes should not be given further MTX therapy. Unfortunately, for some patients discontinuing MTX is unacceptable because of the medically, emotionally, or economically disabling nature of their uncontrolled psoriasis. The decision not to interrupt MTX in those circumstances can only be taken if the patient is made fully aware of the risks of decompensated liver disease and signs an informed consent to continue with therapy. MTX treatment for psoriasis and psoriatic arthritis usually consists of a single weekly oral, intramuscular, or subcutaneous dose, ordinarily 7.5–30 mg (rarely as high as 50 mg/week), or an intermittent weekly oral schedule of three divided doses over a 24-h period (i.e., three 12-hourly doses) not to exceed 30 mg/week.

Toxicity Monitoring.   The recommended monitoring protocol consists of baseline and interval blood testing, baseline and interval urinalysis, and liver biopsy, as shown in Table 2. In contrast, the conclusion of a retrospective study of serial liver biopsies in patients with psoriasis treated with MTX (presented recently) was that such biopsy monitoring has little impact on clinical management (74a). Several noninvasive tests have been proposed for MTX monitoring but none have proved reliable enough to replace liver biopsy as a means of detecting significant fibrosis. Liver enzymes are poor predictors of liver injury in psoriatics, as 30–50% of patients will have normal aminotransferases despite significant histological abnormalities (7,65). Certainly, elevated bilirubin and/or enzymes or decreased serum albumin (75) are causes for concern. The diagnostic benefit of frequent hepatic panel monitoring, say every 4–6 weeks, has not been tested although it would certainly add to the cost of care. In patients with rheumatoid arthritis, 4–8-weekly hepatic panel monitoring is advocated (see below) and is thought to be useful in early detection of significant liver injury. Some authors recommend 4–8-weekly hepatic panel testing in psoriatics, too (74). Fasting serum bile salt concentrations (76), aminopyrine breath tests (77), galactose tolerance tests (78), and antipyrine clearance (79) have all failed as screening tests for MTX hepatotoxicity. More recently, measurements of serum levels of extracellular matrix derivatives and indicators of cytokine activation have been explored as surrogate tests for liver fibrosis. Results for individual markers often show overlap among patients with normal and fibrotic liver, especially at early stages of fibrogenesis before

Table 2 Monitoring of MTX Therapy in Psoriasis

A. Baseline or prior to MTX therapy
   (i) Blood tests
      Complete blood count (CBC)
      Basic metabolic panel (BMP; i.e., BUN, creatinine, electrolytes, calcium, glucose)
      Hepatic panel (total bilirubin, AST, ALT, alkaline phosphatase, albumin)
      HBsAg, anti-HCV
      HIV antibodies (in high-risk patients)
   (ii) Urinalysis
   (iii) Liver biopsy
      (a) High-risk patients—before or within 2–4 months of initiation of MTX therapy
      (b) Low-risk patients—within 1–1.5 g of initiation of MTX therapy
B. During MTX therapy
   (iv) Blood tests
      CBC weekly for 2 weeks, biweekly for next month, then approximately monthly
      BMP at 3–4-monthly intervals
      Hepatic panel—every 3–4 months (or more frequently until first liver biopsy is done—
      see A (iii))
   (v) Urinalysis
      3–4-monthly intervals
   (vi) Liver biopsy
      (a) High-risk patients—after initial biopsy, at MTX cumulative doses of 1.5, 3, 4 g and
         each additional 1–1.5-g increments
      (b) Low-risk patients—at MTX cumulative doses of 1–1.5 (?baseline biopsy), 3, 4 g
         and each additional 1–1.5-g increments
      (c) Abnormal hepatic panel—follow-up biopsy after incremental 0.5–1 g or after a
         further 6 months MTX

Source: Psoriasis Task Force Guidelines: Roenigk et al., Arch Dermatol 1972; 105:363; Roenigk et al., Arch Dermatol 1973; 108:363; Roenigk et al. (7); Roenigk et al. (49).

cirrhosis is established (80,81). PIIIP, one of the most promising markers thus far, does indeed rise during MTX therapy (82,83), but this occurs equally when liver histology is normal, only steatotic, or distinctly abnormal (84). Unfortunately PIIIP does not correlate with the degree of fibrosis (85). Nonetheless, advocates of PIIIP monitoring claim that persistent normality over repeated testing excludes a degree of liver injury more severe than Roenigk grade I. Older studies show that colloid-isotope liver-spleen scans (86), computed tomography (87), magnetic resonance imaging (88), and isotope hepatobiliary scans (89) do not predict for significant early liver injury, and none are recommended for patient monitoring. Whereas liver sonography detects fat and fibrosis fairly reliably (89), it cannot distinguish between them. An early vote for dynamic hepatic scintography (90) has yet to be seconded, especially since a later study did not show quite the same reliability for excluding serious disease (91).

Neither patients (92) nor their physicians (9) are enthusiastic about liver biopsy, so the development of a noninvasive screening test for early hepatic fibrosis would be an advantage. Recently, a fibrosis index based on the analysis of five serum components (alpha$_2$-macroglobulin, haptoglobin, apolipoprotein A-1, γ-glutamyl transpeptidase, and total bilirubin) that relate to hepatic extracellular matrix metabolism and fibrogenic cytokine upregulation has been shown to be useful in following the progression of hepatic fibrosis in patients with chronic hepatitis C, and may eliminate the need for liver biopsy in 50% of patients (93). If this index is not seriously perturbed by inflammation and fibrosis in extrahepatic sites (e.g., skin and joints in patients with psoriasis, arthritis, etc.), it may prove valuable in monitoring methotrexate hepatic fibrosis, too.

Hepatotoxic MTX Drug Interactions.   Nowadays physicians must actively look for potential interactions between therapeutic drugs (either prescribed or over-the-counter), herbal remedies, complementary ("alternative") medicines, and foodstuffs that can interfere with the absorption, pharmakokinetics, metabolism, and disposal of other drugs they are prescribing. Such interactions can blunt or enhance the therapeutic action of prescribed drugs, and also cause toxicity. Additive and synergistic drug toxicity can also occur at the target organ level. The primary route of elimination of MTX is via the kidneys. Drugs that decrease renal clearance of MTX, and thereby enhance its toxicity, include recognized nephrotoxins (e.g., aminoglycosides, cyclosporin, and tacrolimus), some antibiotics (e.g., penicillins, cephalosporins, and sulfonamides), and many agents used for arthritis (salicylates, other nonsteroidal anti-inflammatory drugs, and colchicine). Ethanol has already been discussed as a synergistic hepatotoxin. Many drugs increase free blood levels of MTX by displacing it from protein binding in the serum (salicylates, probenecid, phenytoin, retinoids, sulfonylureas, and tetracycline) whereas others, such as dipyridamole, potentiate the intracellular accumulation of MTX and enhance its cytotoxicity. Other folate antagonists may act synergistically with MTX but this is more likely to cause bone marrow depression than hepatotoxicity. A full list of such interactions may be found in a review by Evans and Christensen (94), which clearly needs updating, especially with respect to interference with MTX metabolism.

2.   Rheumatoid Arthritis and Other Rheumatic Diseases

Rheumatoid Arthritis.   Many of the conclusions that were drawn from the extensive yet often disparate data on MTX therapy of psoriasis were originally applied to MTX therapy of rheumatoid arthritis. Rheumatologists initially endorsed and adopted the monitoring protocol used in MTX treatment of psoriasis (95). The data in patients with rheumatoid disorders seemed consistent with that in psoriatics. First, it was found that many patients with rheumatoid arthritis have some degree of underlying liver pathology that must be taken into account when judging lesions attributed to MTX. Next, some rheumatoid arthritis patients appear to be at greater risk than others of suffering MTX liver damage. As in psoriasis, conditions that predispose to hepatic steatosis and fibrosis, especially heavy alcohol use and diabetes combined with obesity, contribute to and even potentiate MTX hepatotoxicity. Similarly, underlying liver diseases, such as chronic hepatitis B and C, are also risk factors that may lead to fibrosis. Third, liver injury in patients with rheumatoid arthritis is arguably related to the extent of MTX exposure in terms of cumulative dose and possibly duration of therapy. However, an important and widely accepted difference between MTX therapy of psoriatic and rheumatoid patients is that hepatotoxicity appears to be less frequent in rheumatoid arthritis—possibly 2.5–5-fold lower—than in psoriasis (62). Thus, less aggressive monitoring is now recommended for uncomplicated MTX-treated rheumatoid arthritis, compared to psoriasis (97) (Table 3).

Although liver histological abnormalities are common in rheumatoid arthritis, fibrosis is now considered to be either uncommon or absent, unless there are comorbid causes of liver injury. Mild fibrosis (Roenigk grade IIIa) occurred in a maximum of 15% of rheumatoid arthritis patients in one series (37), in which two-thirds of all the patients had only Roenigk grade I changes and 17% had grade II. Most series that examined liver

Table 3 Monitoring of MTX Therapy in Rheumatoid Arthritis

A. Baseline or prior to MTX therapy
   (i) Blood tests
       CBC
       BMP
       HBsAg, anti-HCV
   (ii) Liver biopsy
       High-risk patients only
           Prior excessive alcohol consumption
           Persistently abnormal baseline AST values
           Chronic hepatitis B or C infection
           ?Obesity and/or insulin-dependent diabetes
B. During MTX therapy
   (i) Blood tests
       AST, ALT, and albumin levels—all at 4–8 week intervals
   (ii) Liver biopsy
       Either when 5 of 9 AST values are abnormal in a given 12-month interval
       or when 6 of 12 AST values are abnormal with monthly testing
       or when serum albumin is decreased, despite good rheumatoid arthritis control
   (iii) For the following liver biopsy results
       (a) Roenigk grades I, II, III
           resume MTX and monitor as in B(i) and (ii)
       (b) Roenigk grade IIIb, IV
           discontinue MTX
   (iv) Discontinue MTX
       if AST or albumin abnormalities persist and the patient refuses liver biopsy

histology in untreated rheumatoid arthritis patients are devoid of cirrhosis, with rare exceptions (96,97). Similarly, the frequency of severe liver disease is low in rheumatoid arthritis patients on long-term MTX treatment (98). Admittedly, mild hepatic fibrosis can be seen with MTX therapy (97) and progression can occur, but MTX-induced cirrhosis is distinctly unusual. Stability of liver histology is the rule with MTX therapy in rheumatoid patients and even histological improvement has been reported (36,38,98–100). The worst estimate reported for cirrhosis in MTX-treated rheumatoid arthritis is a 5-year cumulative incidence of 0.94% (98). In those instances in which cirrhosis occurs in MTX-treated rheumatoid arthritis, a potentiating cause such as obesity with diabetes (99–101) or alcohol abuse (62,100) can usually be found (102).

On the whole, MTX is well tolerated in rheumatoid arthritis patients and its toxicity profile compares favorably with that of other disease-modifying antirheumatic drugs (103). Although liver enzyme elevation occurs commonly with MTX use, it is rare for this to necessitate cessation of therapy (104). Concomitant therapy with folate supplements ameliorates aminotransferase elevations (105). Hydroxychloroquine may reduce MTX hepatotoxicity (106) by reducing MTX bioavailability (107), whereas aspirin (106) and other nonsteroidal anti-inflammatory drugs (NSAIDs) (108) may exacerbate it.

Kremer has analyzed the reasons why MTX-treated rheumatoid arthritis patients seem to fare better than their psoriasis counterparts (109). He proposes that lessons learned from the treatment of psoriasis were used to the advantage of rheumatoid patients, specifically by enforcing a strict ban on alcohol use (110–112) and by reducing the use of potential hepatotoxins (like steroids and NSAIDs), which was feasible because of a favorable response to MTX therapy. Kremer further stresses the benefit of frequent hepatic panel testing that was practiced by rheumatologists, who would reduce MTX doses whenever AST values rose or albumin levels fell. In earlier studies in MTX-treated psoriatic patients, doses of MTX were not lowered unless aminotransferases were 2–3 times elevated above normal. This difference in MTX dose regulation probably accounts partly for the low prevalence of MTX hepatotoxicity experienced by rheumatoid arthritis patients.

The hypothesis that frequent blood testing is useful in managing MTX therapy was tested in a prospective study of 94 MTX-treated rheumatoid arthritis patients (in three cohorts), in whom very frequent AST and ALT testing was done at intervals as often as 2-weekly preceding liver biopsy (113). A total of 354 follow-up liver biopsies were done in these patients. The investigators found that the prevalence of abnormal ASTs and ALTs in the interval before liver biopsy correlated with the degree of histological injury, judged by the Roenigk grade. MTX doses were reduced when AST and albumin results were abnormal. There were no instances of bridging fibrosis (Roenigk grade IIIb) or cirrhosis (Roenigk grade IV) in these three cohorts of "teetotal" patients. Whereas the sensitivity of an elevated AST value to detect mild early fibrosis (Roenigk grade IIIa) was only 12%, if ASTs were elevated on less than half the occasions tested there was 97% certainty of having normal liver histology. The authors attributed the absence of severe lesions to their insistence on strict alcohol abstinence, and frequent adjustments of weekly MTX dose when they observed abnormalities of aminotransferases and serum albumin (109). Alkaline phosphatase elevations occurred in about one-third of the treated patients but were thought to be too sensitive to be of any value in MTX management. Of interest, the authors found that the probability of missing an elevated AST by infrequent sampling ranged from 9% for 30-day sampling to as high as 68% with 3-month sampling. From these and other data are derived the latest (revised) guidelines for monitoring MTX treatment of rheumatoid arthritis (6,97), as shown in Table 3. Presumably these data have persuaded some dermatologists to suggest that 4–8-weekly blood testing intervals be applied to MTX monitoring in psoriasis (74).

As in psoriasis, there is disagreement over whether the magnitude of the cumulative MTX dose has any impact on hepatotoxicity. Although the results of some studies have shown that AST elevations are more frequent in rheumatoid patients taking up to 25 mg MTX weekly compared with those on 10–15 mg weekly (114,115), this is not reproducible (116,117). There are, nonetheless, many published examples of extremely high cumulative MTX doses and prolonged durations of therapy in rheumatoid arthritis that did not lead to cirrhosis. In one study of 23 patients, up to 10 g of MTX was administered for over 10 years (99), yet only two patients progressed to Roenigk grade IIIb (bridging fibrosis) when therapy was continued after Roenigk grade IIIa changes (mild fibrosis) were found. In two other prospective studies, only one of 10 patients treated for 6 years (118) and seven of 18 patients receiving 2–7 g MTX (109) developed mild fibrosis at worst, and none had cirrhosis. Whether it can really be proved that rheumatoid patients are inherently less susceptible to MTX toxicity then psoriatics, as some authors claim (119), is doubtful. However, it is clear that alcohol abstinence and minimizing MTX doses (whether guided by frequent AST monitoring or not) are safe strategies in treating both psoriatics and patients with rheumatoid arthritis.

Liver Biopsy.   In contrast to patients with psoriasis, baseline liver biopsies are recommended by the American College of Rheumatology (ACR) only for rheumatoid patients embarking on MTX therapy who are at high risk for underlying liver disease (97,120).

This includes those with a history of extensive alcohol consumption, with hepatitis B or C infection, or with persistently elevated AST (and/or ALT). Similarly, follow-up liver biopsy on treatment is recommended only if AST elevation of any magnitude persists (i.e., five of nine abnormal ASTs in a given 12-month interval or six of 12 when AST is tested monthly) *or* if a subnormal serum albumin cannot be explained on the basis of uncontrolled rheumatoid disease or, by implication, by proteinuria or another nonhepatic cause (Table 3). Guidelines from the Health and Public Policy Committee of the American College of Physicians (ACP) (121) support the ACR ruling that restricts baseline liver biopsies to high-risk patients, whereas the American College of Gastroenterology (ACG) recommends baseline biopsies in patients with rheumatoid arthritis and psoriasis alike, before starting MTX (8). The ACG recommendation was based on data available at the time, which showed that significant yet unsuspected fibrotic liver disease was common in rheumatoid patients (37,61,66,96).

If follow-up liver biopsy shows Roenigk grade IIIa changes or less, MTX therapy can continue and standard monitoring is resumed. This contrasts with the recommended care of MTX-treated psoriatics, in whom the finding of grade IIIa change prompts a repeat biopsy after 6 months of further therapy (Table 3). If the biopsy in rheumatoid patients shows Roenigk grade IIIb or IV on MTX treatment, the drug is discontinued.

Toxicity Monitoring. The ACR protocol for laboratory testing (97,120) in rheumatoid arthritis is more intense and stringent than that of the ACP (121) and the ACG (8). ACR guidelines state that aminotransferases and albumin should be measured at 4–8-weekly intervals, and *any* elevation of AST or ALT or reduction in albumin is considered significant. ACP recommends monthly laboratory testing but considers enzyme rises significant only if they are threefold elevated above normal; ACG recommends 1–2-monthly testing.

Although the utility of serial AST, ALT, and albumin testing of rheumatoid patients taking MTX has been challenged (122), this protocol is well defended by its principal author (123) as being derived from the largest data set ever published in which the effect of a potential hepatotoxin (MTX) on liver histology and simultaneously measured liver enzymes were examined (112,113). Moreover, in a study designed to test the usefulness and cost savings of the ACR guidelines for monitoring MTX hepatotoxicity (124), 112 MTX-treated rheumatoid patients were followed prospectively using the strict guidelines recommended for psoriatics on MTX (as shown in Table 2). The results of applying ACR guidelines retrospectively were then examined using the same data. With ACR guidelines (which advocate more frequent hepatic panel testing and less frequent liver biopsy), 15 instead of 66 patients underwent biopsy, on 18 instead of 110 occasions, respectively. Biopsy complications occurred in two patients, neither of whom would have been biopsied under ACR guidelines. Of the five patients who had Roenigk grade IIIb or IV liver histology, four would have been biopsied under ACR guidelines. This included two patients whose pre-MTX laboratory results did not indicate a biopsy, but who developed frequent AST elevations on MTX and would therefore have been biopsied on therapy. One patient with obesity and poorly controlled insulin-dependent diabetes had persistently normal AST and albumin values, yet the baseline biopsy showed grade IIIa changes that progressed to cirrhosis during therapy. Neither of these two biopsies was mandated by the ACR protocol. The authors estimated that applying ACR instead of psoriasis guidelines avoided 92 biopsies in 51 patients (including two complications) and saved almost $100,000. They further reasoned that adding poorly controlled diabetes to the indications for pretreatment liver biopsy would have given the ACR guidelines 100% sensitivity. A study that has so far appeared only in abstract form (125) does not endorse the ACR guidelines. On the other hand, a decision-analysis study (126) that compared the monitoring strategy of "no biopsy versus biopsy," after 5 and 10 years of MTX therapy in rheumatoid arthritis, concluded that biopsy was not cost-effective after 5 years and even 10 years of therapy, since the cost-effectiveness ratios were 1.9 million dollars and $52,000 per year of life saved, respectively.

Aside from hepatic panel monitoring [and here ALT is as effective as AST (97)], noninvasive monitoring appears to be no better than in MTX-treated psoriasis. Studies on fibrogenesis markers in MTX-treated rheumatoid arthritis patients are limited. PIIIP is elevated in untreated rheumatoid arthritis and normalizes with MTX therapy (127), but it is not known whether PIIIP rises again in this setting when hepatic fibrosis starts. In a study (128) whose objectives were to determine quantitative liver function prospectively and to assess the relationship between such testing and liver histology, neither galactose elimination, aminopyrine breath tests, liver enzymes, γ-glutamyl transpeptidase (transferase), serum bile acids, bilirubin, nor albumin was of any practical use. In particular, no relationship was found between changes in results of galactose elimination, aminopyrine breath tests, and MTX dose, age, enzyme elevation, alcohol intake, or liver histology.

Ideal monitoring guidelines cannot be fully evidence-based until a large prospective study is done in which patients are stratified according to the indication for MTX therapy (e.g., psoriasis, psoriatic arthritis, rheumatoid arthritis, etc.), and clinical variables such as obesity, diabetes, alcohol intake, and age and laboratory variables such as liver enzymes, albumin, serological tests for fibrogenesis, fibrogenic and inflammatory cytokine levels in the serum, and modern liver imaging are correlated with liver histology (129). As yet, liver biopsy is still the most reliable means of diagnosing fibrosis in MTX-treated patients and will be the standard until better noninvasive testing [such as automated assays of multiple serum markers of liver fibrosis (130)] are available and shown to be helpful. It remains to be seen whether more sensitive histological measures of fibrosis, such as the semiquantitative scoring system that was recently tested in MTX-treated rheumatoid arthritis patients (131), will enhance understanding of the natural history of MTX hepatotoxicity and its management, as has been the case with the grading and staging systems now used regularly for the assessment of liver histology in chronic hepatitis.

Other Rheumatic and Inflammatory Conditions.   Data are limited on hepatotoxicity in other conditions for which MTX is prescribed, mostly because the number of patients being reported is small and large prospective series are not available for analysis. Of these conditions, juvenile rheumatoid arthritis is a common indication for MTX. In two series of patients who had liver biopsy monitoring, only two of 63 discontinued therapy because of fibrosis (132,133), whereas in two other series combined none of 21 patients developed fibrosis or cirrhosis with cumulative doses of up to 3 g (134,135). In a later study (136), only modest liver histological changes (Roenigk grade I or II) were seen in 13 of 14 patients who also had modest enzyme abnormalities (which exceeded threefold elevation in five patients). Irrespective, none of the patients developed any significant fibrosis and no significant clinical consequences were apparent, despite doses that were either greater than 3 or 4 g/1.73 m² body surface area. The addition of folinic acid (2.5–7.5 mg daily) to the regimen for children on low-dose weekly MTX (10–20 mg/m²) who had already experienced aminotransferase elevations and gastrointestinal symptoms dramatically ameliorated both hepatotoxicity and gastrointestinal toxicity without affecting the clinical efficacy of MTX (137). Finally, in a recent study of the relationship between hepatotoxic risk factors and liver histology in 25 patients with juvenile rheumatoid arthritis (138), only two patients (6%) had grade IIIa liver changes at worst. The only risk factors that correlated with liver histology were the frequency of serum biochemical abnormalities and the degree of obesity (body mass index). Neither age, gender, disease duration, arthritis subtype, course, duration of MTX treatment, cumulative dose, route of administration, concurrent use of other medications (including folic acid), or other potential hepatotoxicity played any role in liver injury. Thus the hepatotoxic effect of MTX in juvenile rheumatoid arthritis parallels that seen in adult rheumatoid arthritis. It is therefore suggested that similar guidelines should be used to follow these children on MTX therapy.

Studies on the hepatotoxicity of MTX therapy of other disorders such as dermatomyositis (139), sarcoidosis, and asthma are either largely anecdotal or retrospective (140). When hepatic fibrosis occurs it is usually mild and may often be ascribed to comorbid states, such as diabetes (139). Wider experience is awaited. In sarcoidosis, liver involvement with the primary disease process is common, and when MTX has been used in both children and adults, liver toxicity has rarely been reported. In one study, however, in which liver biopsies were done in 33 of 50 patients, six had to discontinue therapy for hepatic reactions that were considered to be due to MTX (141). MTX appears to benefit idiopathic granulomatous hepatitis, including loss of granulomas (142). Overall, however, MTX appears to be well tolerated in many inflammatory (10) and connective tissue disorders, in a manner comparable to that seen in rheumatoid arthritis.

Hepatotoxic Drug Reactions. These reactions are the same in MTX-treated rheumatic disorders as they are in MTX-treated psoriasis, except that there is a higher likelihood that patients with rheumatic disorders use analgesics, especially NSAIDs. Thus if there is any additive or synergistic effect between MTX and NSAIDs, it should be seen in this group of patients. Some authors have reported such interactions (108) but, in general, it has been difficult to implicate concurrent NSAID use as a significant cofactor in MTX hepatotoxicity. Concurrent use of a wide variety of NSAIDs does not appear to affect MTX pharmacokinetics (including the area under the curve following ingestion, total systemic clearance, distribution volume, or the half-life of MTX) but does lead to an increased interpatient variability of MTX blood levels, which may not be clinically important (143).

Concomitant use of sulfasalazine and cyclosporin does not appear to enhance MTX hepatotoxicity (144,145) although there may be bone marrow, skin rash, and renal interactions. The demonstration that insulin augments MTX polyglutamate synthesis in human tumor cell lines (146) has not been correlated with any clinical interaction between insulin and MTX. It is intriguing to speculate that with insulin-resistant states (such as obesity and type II diabetes), in which insulin levels are high, or during insulin administration, there may be another mechanism for enhancing MTX toxicity. Insulin apparently also suppresses gamma-glutamyl hydrolase, the enzyme that degrades polyglutamates, and this would enhance intracellular MTX levels (147).

IV. OVERVIEW OF MTX HEPATOTOXICITY AND MONITORING

MTX use, which is so effective in treating many difficult inflammatory disorders, does have the propensity to cause liver fibrosis and even cirrhosis. The risk of MTX-induced cirrhosis has been assuaged greatly over the past two decades by dosing patients weekly rather than daily and monitoring them carefully with repeated liver biopsy or frequent simple laboratory testing. Until proved otherwise, it appears that rheumatology patients may be less susceptible to MTX-induced hepatic fibrosis than psoriasis patients.

The guidelines for MTX monitoring of rheumatoid arthritis patients should be applied prospectively, in a study, to MTX-treated psoriatics, controlling for dose and risk factors such as alcohol. Such a study could show that psoriatics react no differently than rheumatoid patients to methotrexate. Until truly reliable markers of fibrogenesis in MTX-treated patients are available, a liver biopsy should be done when there is any doubt about the safety of methotrexate therapy. Guidelines are just that, *guidelines*, and are not infallible. Physicians must exercise common "clinical" sense in the care of their patients. Thus, patients on MTX therapy should be followed carefully, because when this is neglected, avoidable decompensated cirrhosis can develop leading to death or the need for liver transplantation (40). Physicians should be vigilant about restricting alcohol use in MTX-treated patients and should also look for other causes of liver disease (such as hepatitis C and, the increasingly prevalent, nonalcoholic steatohepatitis) as well as hidden causes of liver injury such as occupational and environmental exposure to nondrug hepatotoxins, at work and at home (148). In contrast to the monitoring of psoriasis patients, MTX therapy of uncommon conditions such as juvenile rheumatoid arthritis, other inflammatory skin conditions, Crohn's disease, and sarcoidosis can probably be monitored safely using the currently recommended guidelines for rheumatoid arthritis, unless the patient is known or suspected to have underlying liver disease. In the United Kingdom, monitoring of Crohn's disease treated with MTX is recommended to be closer to that used for psoriatics than for patients with rheumatoid arthritis (149). Although the data are not yet conclusive, it should be feasible to adopt a monitoring scheme that can be customized to the patient's needs, until better evidence-based guidelines become available.

V.   MTX THERAPY OF LIVER DISEASE

The controversy over the use of MTX to treat PBC is a classic in the genre of debates in clinical science. Acknowledged experts in the field, seasoned investigators, take diametrically opposed positions that they champion with fervor bordering on passion, using plausible data that somehow do not jibe with the evidence presented by the opposition. In this, as with other similar debates in hepatology, it is likely that the truth lies between the two views (150).

A.   Primary Sclerosing Cholangitis

The stimulus for using MTX to treat cholestatic liver disease was a serendipitous observation. When MTX was used to treat a patient with a life-threatening skin disorder, the coexistent primary sclerosing cholangitis (PSC) appeared to improve and not deteriorate as feared. This unexpected, but encouraging experience was repeated in several other similar patients (151) and in an open-labeled study (152) of at least 1 year of MTX therapy in 10 patients with early-stage PSC. All symptomatic patients became asymptomatic, liver enzymes improved (but not bilirubin), and six of nine patients who had repeat biopsies after 1 year of MTX had improvement in necroinflammatory liver histology. Even repeat cholangiograms in six patients either improved (2) or stabilized (4). Unfortunately, a follow-up double-blind, placebo-controlled randomized trial of MTX in 24 patients with PSC (of whom 50% already had cirrhosis) did not show efficacy (152); neither did a pilot study in five patients in which MTX was combined with ursodeoxycholic acid (UDCA) treatment (153). In the latter study, there were frequent extrahepatic complications of MTX, and a case report also documented life-threatening *Pneumocystis carinii* pneumonia in a PSC patient on MTX therapy (154). MTX is not a treatment option for PSC.

B. Primary Biliary Cirrhosis

MTX was evaluated initially in nine symptomatic patients with PBC (155), some but not all of whom showed slow improvement in symptoms, liver enzymes, and liver histology. Transient aminotransferase elevations occurred that seemed to predict a favorable response to MTX. The positive responses to MTX were seen primarily in those patients who had precirrhotic PBC, and this was confirmed later in five more patients who experienced remission of symptoms, biochemical amelioration, and histological improvement (156). A pilot study conducted at the National Institutes of Health in nine PBC patients (157) also showed improvement in symptoms, alkaline phosphatase elevation, and histological inflammatory activity, but patients with more advanced disease did not benefit and fibrosis progressed. Fibrosis progression, despite improvement in inflammation, was also reported by Bach et al. (158) in a primarily histopathological study of MTX-treated PBC patients.

The early positive results of MTX therapy in PBC have been criticized for the relatively short-term and uncontrolled nature of the studies in a disease that is notoriously slow to progress and sometimes shows periods of stability (12). An interim (24 month) analysis of a randomized double-blind trial comparing MTX with colchicine in 83 PBC patients showed greater symptomatic, biochemical, and possible histological improvement in the MTX-treated patients than those on colchicine (159). In contrast, the long-term results of a completed placebo-controlled trial did not show any efficacy for MTX in PBC (160). In that study (160) there was even a trend toward a threefold increase in the rate of death or liver transplantation as a result of liver disease during or after the trial in MTX-treated patients compared to placebo-treated controls (in a Cox multivariate regression analysis). In contrast to an earlier report of severe interstitial pneumonitis complicating MTX therapy in 14% of patients (161), the MTX-treated patients in the trial by Hendrickse et al. (160) had few side effects (which were readily reversible). The results of a smaller trial in precirrhotic PBC patients in Argentina showed MTX to be ineffective in preventing progression to cirrhosis despite symptomatic improvement and a biochemical response (162). The lack of benefit of adding MTX to UDCA treatment of PBC in Chile (163) contrasts with the observation in Boston that MTX improves liver biochemical tests, and some histology too, in PBC patients who respond incompletely to UDCA (164). How can we explain the differences in outcomes among these many studies and others (165)? While arguments go back and forth over which dose of MTX is best, how likely are intolerable side effects to occur, how long is a reasonable follow-up period, and what constitutes a "favorable response" (11–18), it is clear that MTX may be beneficial in some precirrhotic PBC patients (but probably not in cirrhotics), that side effects cannot be ignored and may be risky, and that some patients who do not respond to other, more benign therapy, such as UDCA and colchicine, may experience slowing of liver disease progression with MTX. The answers will clearly lie in controlled trials of MTX (and other therapies) for those patients who do not respond to UDCA, when the end-points are not only symptomatic relief (albeit an important benefit for the patient), biochemical results, and liver histology, but definitely rates of death and/or transplantation. Such studies are in progress and their results are awaited. Until then, most authorities in the field do not recommend MTX therapy outside of clinical trials, unless in the hands of experts skilled in the care of PBC and the careful use of MTX (166–169).

REFERENCES

1. Bertino JR. The general pharmacology of methotrexate. In: WS Wilke, ed. Methotrexate Therapy in Rheumatic Disease. New York: Marcel Dekker, 1989:11–23.
2. Gubner R, August S, Ginsberg V. Therapeutic suppression of tissue reactivity. II. Effect of aminopterin in rheumatoid arthritis and psoriasis. Am J Med Sci 1951; 221:176–182.
3. O'Brien WM, Van Scott EJ, Black RL, Auerbach R, Eisen AZ, Bunim JJ. Clinical trial of amethopterin (methotrexate) in psoriatic and rheumatoid arthritis (preliminary report). Arthritis Rheum 1962; 5:312.
4. Black RL, O'Brien WM, Van Scott EJ, Auerbach R, Eisen AZ, Bunim JJ. Methotrexate therapy in psoriatic arthritis: double-blind study on 21 patients. JAMA 1964; 189:743–747.
5. Colsky J, Greenspan EM, Warren TN. Hepatic fibrosis in children with acute leukemia after therapy with folic acid antagonists. Arch Pathol 1955; 59:198–206.
6. American College of Rheumatology Ad Hoc Committee on Clinical Guidelines for monitoring drug therapy in rheumatoid arthritis. Arthritis Rheum 1996; 39:723–731.
7. Roenigk HH, Auerbach R, Maibach HI, Weinstein GD. Methotrexate in psoriasis: revised guidelines. J Am Acad Dermatol 1988; 19:145–146.
8. Lewis J, Schiff E. Methotrexate-induced chronic liver injury: guidelines for detection and prevention. Am J Gastroenterol 1988; 88:1337–1345.
9. Petrazzuoli M, Rothe MJ, Grin-Jorgensen C, Ramsey WH, Grant-Kels JM. Monitoring patients taking methotrexate for hepatotoxicity. J Am Acad Dermatol 1994; 31:969–977.
10. Te HS, Schiano TD, Kuan SF, Hanauer SB, Conjeevaram HS, Baker AL. Hepatic toxic effects of long-term methotrexate use in the treatment of inflammatory bowel disease. Am J Gastroenterol 2000; 95:3150–3156.
11. Lindor KD. Primary biliary cirrhosis: questions and promises [editorial]. Ann Intern Med 1997; 120:733–735.
12. LaRusso N. Search for medical treatment for primary biliary cirrhosis [letter]. Lancet 1997; 351:1046.
13. Kaplan MM. Primary biliary cirrhosis [letter]. Lancet 1998; 351:216.
14. Dufour J-FJ, Kaplan MM. Methotrexate and liver disease [letter]. N Engl J Med 1996; 335:898–899.
15. Bonis PAL, Kaplan MM. Low-dose methotrexate in primary biliary cirrhosis [letter]. Gastroenterology 1999; 117:1510–1511.
16. Gleeson D, Underwood JCE, Hendrickse MT, Giaffer MH. Low-dose methotrexate in primary biliary cirrhosis [letter]. Gastroenterology 1999; 118:1512.
17. Angulo P, Dickson ER. Methotrexate in the treatment of primary biliary cirrhosis: the hype and the hope [editorial]. Gastroenterology 1999; 117:492–495.
18. Angulo P, Dickson ER. Low-dose methotrexate in primary biliary cirrhosis. [letter]. Gastroenterology 1999; 117:1512–1513.
19. Berkowitz RS, Goldstein DP, Bernstein MR. Ten years' experience with methotrexate and folinic acid as primary therapy for gestational trophoblastic disease. Gynecol Oncol 1986; 23:111–118.
20. Hersh EM, Wong VG, Henderson ES, Freireich EJ. Hepatotoxic effects of methotrexate. Cancer 1996; 19:600–606.
21. Jaffe N, Traggis D. Toxicity of high-dose methotrexate (NSC-740) and citrovorum factor (NSC-3590) in osteogenic sarcoma. Cancer Chemother Rep 1975; 6:31–36.
22. Taft LI. Methotrexate-induced hepatitis in childhood leukemia. Isr J Med Sci 1965; 1:823.

23. Banerjee AK, Lakhani S, Vincent M, Selby P. Dose-dependent acute hepatitis associated with administration of high dose methotrexate. Hum Toxicol 1988; 7:561–562.

24. Chan H, Evans WE, Pratt CB. Recovery from toxicity with high-dose methotrexate: prognostic factors. Cancer Treat Rep 1977; 61:797–804.

25. Weber BL, Tanyer G, Poplack DG, Reaman GH, Feusner JM, Miser JS, Bleyer WA. Transient acute hepatotoxicity of high-dose methotrexate therapy during childhood. NCI Monogr 1987; 5:207–212.

26. Schmiegelow K, Pulczynska M. Prognostic significance of hepatotoxicity during maintenance chemotherapy of childhood acute leukemia. Br J Cancer 1990; 61:767–772.

27. Clegg DO, Furst DE, Tolman KG, Payne R. Acute, reversible hepatic failure associated with methotrexate treatment of rheumatoid arthritis. J Rheumatol 1989; 16:1123–1126.

28. Hakim NS, Kobienia B, Benedetti E, Bloomer J, Payne WD. Methotrexate-induced hepatic necrosis requiring liver transplantation in a patient with rheumatoid arthritis. Int Surg 1998; 83:224–225.

29. Hutter RVP, Shipkey FH, Tan CTC, Murphy ML, Chowdhury M. Hepatic fibrosis in children with acute leukaemia: a complication of therapy. Cancer 1960; 13:288–307.

30. McIntosh S, Davidson DL, O'Brien RT, Pearson HA. Methotrexate hepatotoxicity in children with leukemia. J Pediatr 1977; 90:1019–1021.

31. Coe RO, Bull FE. Cirrhosis associated with methotrexate treatment of psoriasis. JAMA 1968; 206:1515–1520.

32. Dahl MGC, Gregory MM, Scheuer PJ. Methotrexate in psoriasis—comparison of different dose regimens. Br Med J 1972; 1:654–656.

33. Podurgiel BJ, McGill DB, Ludwig J, Taylor WF, Muller SA. Liver injury associated with methotrexate therapy for psoriasis. Mayo Clin Proc 1973; 48:787–792.

34. Nyfors A, Poulsen H. Liver biopsy from psoriatics related to methotrexate therapy. II. Findings before and after methotrexate therapy in 88 patients: a blind study. Acta Pathol Microbiol Scand. Section A Pathol 1976; 84:262–270.

35. Nyfors A, Poulsen H. Liver biopsy from psoriatics related to methotrexate therapy. T. Findings in 123 consecutive non-methotrexate-treated patients. Acta Pathol Microbial Scand 1976; 84:253–251.

36. Lanse SB, Arnold GL, Goweens JD, Kaplan MM. Low incidence of hepatotoxicity associated with long-term, low-dose oral methotrexate in treatment of refractory psoriasis, psoriatic arthritis and rheumatoid arthritis: an acceptable risk/benefit-ratio. Dig Dis Sci 1985; 30:104–109.

37. Rau R, Karger T, Herborn G, Frenzel H. Liver biopsy findings in patients with rheumatoid anthritis undergoing longterm treatment with methotrexate. J Rheumatol 1989; 16:489–493.

38. West SG. Methotrexate hepatotoxicity. Rheum Dis Clin North Am 1997; 23:883–915.

39. Zachariae H, Kragbelle IT, Sogaard H. Methotrexate induced liver cirrhosis. Studies including serial liver biopsies during continued treatment. Br J Dermatol 1980; 102:407–412.

40. Gilbert SE, Klintmalm G, Mentor A, Silverman A. Methotrexate-induced cirrhosis requiring liver transplantation in three patients with psoriasis: a word of caution in light of the expanding use of this "steroid" sparing agent. Arch Intern Med 1990; 150:889–891.

41. Nyfors A, Hopwood D. Liver ultrastructure in psoriatics related to methotrexate therapy. I. A prospective study of findings in hepatocytes from 24 patients before and after methotrexate treatment. Acta Pathol Microbiol Scand Section A Pathol 1977; 85:787–800.

42. Horvath E, Kovacs K, Ross RC, Saibil F, Kerenyi NA. Desmosomal abnormalities in the liver of methotrexate-treated psoriatics. Experientia 1977; 33:1202–1204.

43. Hopwood D, Nyfors A. Liver ultrastructure in psoriatics related to methotrexate therapy. II. Findings in bile ducts from 11 methotrexate treated psoriatics and 2 controls. Acta Pathol Microbiol Scand Section A Pathol 1977; 85:801–811.

44. Horvath E, Saibil FG, Kovacs K, Kerenyi NA, Ross RC. Fine ultrastructural changes in the liver of methotrexate-treated psoriatics. Digestion 1978; 17:488–502.

45. Bjorkman DJ, Hammon EH, Lee RG, Clegg DO, Tolman KG. Hepatic ultrastructure after methotrexate therapy for rheumatoid arthritis. Arthritis Rheum 1988; 31:1465–1472.

46. Albanis E, Friedman SL. Hepatic fibrosis. Clin Liver Dis 2001; 5:315–334.

47. Nyfors A, Poulsen H. Morphogenesis of fibrosis and cirrhosis in methotrexate-treated patients with cirrhosis. Am J Surg Pathol 1977; 1:235–243.

48. Kevat S, Ahern M, Hall P. Hepalolotoxicity of methotrexate in rheumatic diseases. Med Toxicol 1988; 3:197–208.

49. Roenigk HH Jr, Auerbach R, Maibach H, Weinstein G, Lebwohl M. Methotrexate in psoriasis: consensus conference. J Am Acad Dermatol 1998; 38:478–485.

50. Hall PD, Ahern MJ, Jarvis LR, Stoll P, Jenner MA, Harley H. Two methods of assessment of methotrexate hepatotoxicity in patients with rheumatoid arthritis. Ann Rheum Dis 1991; 50:471–476.

51. Nohlgard C, Rubio CA, Kocky Hammar H. Liver fibrosis quantified by image analysis in methotrexate-treated patients with psoriasis. J Am Acad Dermatol 1993; 28:40–45.

52. Bremnes RM, Smeland E, Huseby NE, Eide JJ, Aarbakke J. Acute hepatotoxicity after high dose methotrexate administration to rats. Pharmacol Toxicol 1991; 69:132–139.

53. Jaskewicz K, Voigt H, Blakolmer K. Increased matrix proteins, collagen and transforming growth factor are early markers of hepatotoxicity in patients on long-term methotrexate therapy. J Toxicol Clin Toxicol 1996; 34:301–305.

54. Hall PD, Jenner MA, Ahern MJ. Hepatotoxicity in a rat model caused by orally administrated methotrexate. Hepatology 1991; 14:906–910.

55. Freeman-Narrod M. Choline antagonism of methotrexate liver toxicity in the rat. Med Pediatr Oncol 1997; 3:9–14.

56. Warin AP, Landells JW, Levene GM, Baker H. A prospective study of the effects of weekly oral methotrexate on liver biopsy: findings in severe psoriasis. Br J Dermatol 1975; 93:321–327.

57. Boffa MJ, Chalmers RJ, Haboubi NY, Shomaf M, Mitchell DM. Sequential liver biopsies during long-term methotrexate treatment for psoriasis: a reappraisal. Br J Dermatol 1995; 133:774–778.

58. Ashton RE, Millward-Sadler GH, White JE. Complications in methrotrexate treatment of psoriasis with particular reference to liver fibrosis. J Invest Dermatol 1982; 79:229–232.

59. Robinson JIT, Baughman RD, Auerbach R, Cimis RJ. Methotrexate hepatotoxicity in psoriasis: consideration of liver biopsies at regular intervals. Arch Dermatol 1980; 116:413–415.

60. Newman M, Auerbach R, Feiner H, Holzman RS, Shupack J, Migdal P, Culubret M, Camuto P, Tobias H. The role of liver biopsies in psoriatic patients receiving long-term methotrexate treatment: improvement in the abnormalities after cessation of treatment. Arch Dermatol 1989; 125:1218–1224.

61. Themido R, Loureiro M, Pecegueiro M, Brandao M, Campos MC. Methotrexate hepatotoxicity in psoriatic patients submitted to long-term therapy. Acta Dermatol Venerol 1992; 72: 361–364.

62. Whiting-O'Keefe QE, Fye KM, Sack KD. Methotrexate and histologic hepatic abnormalities: a meta-analysis. Am J Med 1991; 90:711–716.

63. Roenig KHH Jr, Bergfeld WF, St. Jaques R, Owens FJ, Hawk WA. Hepatotoxicity of methotrexate. Arch Dermatol 1971; 103:250–261.

64. Weinstein GD, Cox JW, Suringa DWR, Millard MM, Kalser M, Frost. Evolution of possible chronic hepatotoxicity from methotrexate for psoriasis. Arch Dermatol 1970; 102:613–618.

65. Psoriasis-liver-methotrexate interactions. Arch Dermatol 1973; 108:36–42.

66. O'Connor GT, Olmstead EM, Zug K, Baughman RD, Beck JR, Dunn JL, Seal P, Lewandowski JF. Detection of hepatotoxicity associated with methotrexate therapy for psoriasis. Arch Dermatol 1989; 125:1209–1217.

67. Reese LT, Grisham TW, Aach RD, Elsen AZ. Effects of methotrexate on the liver in psoriasis. J Invest Dermatol 1974; 62:597–602.

68. Van De Kerkhof PC, Hoefnagels WH, Van Haelst UJ, Mali JW. Methotrexate maintenance therapy and liver damage in psoriasis. Clin Exp Dermatol 1955; 10:194–200.

69. Pestana A, Halprin KM, Taylor JR, Schiff ER, Esquenazi V, Comerford M, Gomez C. Predictive value of HLA antigens for methotrexate-induced liver damage in patients with psoriasis. J Am Acad Dermatol 1985; 12:26–29.

70. Tobias H, Auerbach R. Hepatotoxicity of long-term methotrexate therapy for psoriasis. Arch Intern Med 1973; 132:391–396.

71. Almeyda J, Barnado D, Baker H, Levene GM, Landells JW. Structural and functional abnormalities of the liver in psoriasis before and during methotrexate therapy. Br J Dermatol 1972; 87:625–631.

72. Zachariae H, Sogaard H, Heickendorff L. Methotrexate-induced liver cirrhosis: clinical, histological and serological studies—a further 10-year follow-up. Dermatology 1996; 192:343–346.

73. Zachariae H. Liver biopsies and methorexate: a time for reconsideration? J Am Acad Dermatol 2000; 42:531–534.

74. Cuellar ML, Espinoza LR. Methotrexate use in psoriasis and psoriatic arthritis. Rheum Dis Clin North Am 1997; 23:797–809.

74a. Aithal GP, Haug KB, Gumustop B, Burt AD, Record CO. Hepatology 2001; 34:342A.

75. Reynolds FS, Lee WM. Hepatotoxicity after long-term methotrexate therapy. South Med J 1986; 79:536–539.

76. Lawrence CM, Srange RC, Summerly RA, Scriven AJ, Elmahallawy M, Wood A, Fletcher PJ, Beckett GJ. Assessment of liver function using fasting bile salt concentrations in psoriasis prior to and during methotrexate therapy. Clin Chim Acta 1983; 129:341–351.

77. Williams CN, McCauley D, Malatjalian DO, Turnbull GK, Ross JB. The aminopyrine breath test, an inadequate early indicator of methotrexate-induced liver disease in patients with psoriasis. Clin Invest Med 1987; 10:54–58.

78. Lenler-Petersen P, Sogard H, Thestrup-Pederson H, Zarchariae H. Galactose tolerance test and methorexate-induced liver fibrosis and cirrhosis in patients with psoriasis. Acta Dermato-Venereol (Stockh) 1982; 62:448–550.

79. Palmer HM. Hepatic toxicity of methotrexate treatment of psoriasis. Practitioner 1973; 211: 324–328.

80. Wu J, Danielsson A. Detection of hepatic fibrogenesis: a review of available techniques. Scand J Gastroenterol 1995; 30:817–825.

81. Hayasaka A, Saisho H. Serum markers as tools to monitor liver fibrosis. Digestion 1998; 59:381–384.

82. Boffa MJ, Smith A, Chalmers RJG, Mitchell DM, Rowan B, Wanes TW, Shomaf H, Haboubi NY. Serum type III procollagen aminopeptide for assessing liver damage in methotrexate-treated psoriasis patients. Br J Dermatol 1996; 135:538–544.

83. Zachariae H, Aslam HM, Bjerring P, Sogaard H, Zachariae E, Heickendorff L. Serum aminoerminal propeptide of type III precollagen in psoriasis and psoriatic arthritis: relation to liver fibrosis and arthritis. J Am Acad Dermatol 1991; 25:50–53.

84. Mitchell D, Smith A, Rowan B, Warnes TW, Haboubi NY, Lucas SB, Chalmers RJ. Serum type III precollagen peptide, dynamic liver function tests and hepatic fibrosis in psoriatic patients receiving methotrexate. Br J Dermatol 1990; 122:1–7.

85. Oogarah PK, Rowland PC, Mitchell DM, Smith A, Chalmers RJ, Rowan B, Haboubi NY. Abnormalities of serum type III procollagen aminoterminal peptide in methotrexate-treated psoriatic patients with normal liver histology do not correlate with hepatic ultrastructural changes. Br J Dermatol 1995; 133:512–518.

86. Geronemus RG, Auerbach R, Tobias H. Liver biopsies versus liver scans in methotrexate-treated patients with psoriasis. Arch Dermatol 1982; 118:649–651.

87. Magnetic resonance imaging of parenchymal liver disease: a comparison with ultrasound, radionuclide scintigraphy and X-ray computer tomography: the Clinical NMR Group. Clin Radiol 1987; 38:495–502.

88. Rademaker M, Webb JA, Lowe DG, Meynck-Thomas RH, Kirby JD, Munro DD. Magnetic resonance imaging as a screening procedure for methorexate-induced liver damage. Br J Dermatol 1987; 117:311–316.

89. Arias JM, Morton KA, Albro TE, Patch GG, Valdiva S, Greenberg HE, Christian PE, Datz PL. Comparison of methods for identifying early methotrexate-induced hepatotoxicity in patients with rheumatoid arthrisis. J Nucl Med 1993; 34:1905–1909.

90. McHerney PM, Bingham EA, Callender ME, Delvin PB, O'Hare MD, Ferguson WR, Laird JD, Burrows D. Dynamic hepatic scintigraphy in the screening of patients for methotrexate-induced hepatotoxicity. Br J Dermatol 1992; 127:122–125.

91. Van Dooren-Greebe R, Kuijpers A, Buijs W, Kniest PH, Coistens FH, Nagengast FM, dee Boo T, Willems JC, Duller P, van de Kerkhof PC. The value of dynamic hepatic scintigraphy and serum aminoterminal propeptide of type III procollagen for early detection of methorexate-induced hepatic damage in psoriasis patients. Br J Dermatol 1996; 134:481–487.

92. Ferraz MB, Ciconelli RM, Vilar MJ. Patient's preference regarding the option of performing unselective liver biopsy following methotrexate treatment in rheumatoid arthritis. Clin Exp Rheumatol 1994; 12:621–625.

93. Imbert-Bismut F, Ratziu V, Pieroni L, Charlotte F, Benhamon Y, Poynard T. Biochemical markers of liver fibrosis in patients with hepatitis C virus infection: a prospective study. Lancet 2001; 357:1069–1075.

94. Evans WE, Christensen ML. Drug interactions with methotrexate. J Rheumatol 1985; 12(suppl 12):15–20.

95. Furst DE, Kremer JM. Methotrexate in rheumatoid arthritis. Arthritis Rheum 1988; 81:305–314.

96. Brick JE, Morland LW, Al-Kawas F, Chang WWL, Layne RD, DiBartolomeo AG. Prospective analysis of liver biopsies before and after methotrexate therapy in rheumatoid arthritis patients. Semin Arthritis Rheum 1989; 19:31–44.

97. Kremer JM, Alarcon GS, Lightfott RW Jr, Willkens RF, Furst DE, Williams HJ, Dent PB, Weinblatt ME. Methotrexate for rheumatoid arthritis: suggested guidelines for monitoring liver toxicity. Arthritis Rheum 1994; 37:316–328.

98. Chandran G, Ahern MJ, Pall PD, Geddes R, Smith MD, Hill W, Harley JH. Cirrhosis in patients with rheumatoid arthritis receiving low-dose methotrexate. Br J Rheumatol 1994; 33:981–984.

99. Aponte J, Petrelli M. Histopathologic findings in the liver of rheumatoid arthritis patients treated with long-term bolus methotrexate. Arthritis Rheum 1988; 12:1457–1464.

100. Shergy WJ, Polisson RP, Caldwell DS, Rice JR, Pisetsky DS, Allen NB. Methotrexate-associated hepatotoxicity: retrospective analysis of 210 patients with rheumatoid arthritis. Am J Med 1988; 85:771–774.

101. Minocha A, Dean HA, Pittsley RA. Liver cirrhosis in rheumatoid arthritis patients with long-term methotrexate. Vet Hum Toxicol 1993; 35:45–48.

102. Walker AM, Funch D, Dreyer NA, Tolman KG, Kremer JM, Alarcon GS, Lee RG, Weinblatt ME. Determinants of serious liver disease among patients receiving low-dose methotrexate for rheumatoid arthritis. Arthritis Rheum 1993; 36:329–335.

103. Singh G, Fries JF, Williams CA, Zatarain E, Spitz P, Bloch DA. Toxicity profiles of disease modifying antirheumatic drugs in rheumatoid arthritis. J Rheumatol 1991; 18:188–194.

104. Leonard PA, Clegg DO, Carson CC, Canon GW, Egger MJ, Ward JR. Low-dose pulse methotrexate in rheumatoid arthritis: an 8-year experience with hepatotoxicity. Clin Rheumatol 1987; 6:575–582.

105. Morgan SL, Baggott JE, Vaughn WH, Austin JS, Veitch TA, Lee JY, Koopman WJ, Krumdieck CL, Alarcon GS. Supplementation with folic acid during methotrexate therapy for rheumatoid arthritis: a double-blind placebo-controlled trial. Ann Intern Med 1994; 121:833–841.

106. Fries JF, Singh A, Lenert L, Furst DE. Aspirin, hydroxychloroquine, and hepatic enzyme

abnormalities with methotrexate in rheumatoid arthritis. Arthritis Rheum 1990; 33:1611–1619.

107. Seideman P, Albertioni F, Beck O, Esksborg S, Peterson C. Chloroquine reduces the bioavailability of methotrexate in patients with rheumatoid arthritis. A possible mechanism of reduced hepatotoxicity. Arthritis Rheum 1994; 37:830–833.

108. Rabinovitz M, Van Thiel DH. Hepatotoxicity of nonsteroidal anti-inflammatory drugs. Am J Gastroenterol 1992; 87:1696–1704.

109. Kremer JM. Liver toxicity does not have to follow methotrexate therapy of patients with rheumatoid arthritis. Am J Gastroenterol 1997; 92:184–196.

110. Kremer JM, Lee RG, Tolman KG. Liver histology in rheumatoid arthritis patients receiving long-term methotrexate therapy: a prospective study with baseline and sequential biopsy samples. Arthritis Rheum 1989; 31:305–314.

111. Kremer JM, Kaye GI. Electron microscopic analysis of sequential liver biopsies from patients with rheumatoid arthritis: correlation with light microscopic findings. Arthritis Rheum 1992; 32:1202–1213.

112. Kremer JM, Kaye GI, Kaye NW, Ishak KG, Axiotis CA. Light and electron microscopic analysis of sequential liver biopsy samples from patients with rheumatoid arthritis receiving long-term therapy: follow-up over prolonged treatment intervals and correlation with clinical and laboratory variables. Arthritis Rheum 1995; 38:1194–1203.

113. Kremer JM, Furst DE, Weinblatt ME, Blotner SD. Significant changes in AST across hepatic histological biopsy grades: prospective analysis of 3 cohorts receiving methotrexate therapy for rheumatoid arthritis. J Rheumatol 1996; 23:459–461.

114. Gabriel S, Cregsen E, O'Fallon WM, Jaquith J, Bunch T. Treatment of rheumatoid arthritis with higher dose intravenous methotrexate. J Rheumatol 1990; 17:460–465.

115. Schnabel A, Reinhold-Keller E, Willmann V, Gross WL. Tolerability of methotrexate starting with 15 or 25 mg/week for rheumatoid arthritis. Rheumatol Int 1994; 14:33–38.

116. Furst DE, Koehnke R, Burmeister LF, Kohler J, Cargill I. Increasing methotrexate effect with increasing dose in the treatment of resistant rheumatoid arthritis. J Rheumatol 1989; 16:313–320.

117. Thompson RN, Watts C, Edelman J, Esdaile J, Russell AS. A controlled two-center trial of parenteral methotrexate therapy for refractory rheumatoid arthritis. J Rheumatol 1984; 11:760–763.

118. Weinblatt ME, Weissman BN, Holdsworth DE, Fraser PA, Maier AL, Falchuk KR, Coblyn JS. Long-term prospective study of methotrexate in the treatment of rheumatoid arthritis. Arthritis Rheum 1992; 35:129–137.

119. Weinstein A, Marlowe S, Korn J, Farouhar F. Low-dose methotrexate treatment of rheumatoid arthritis: long-term observations. Am J Med 1985; 79:331–337.

120. Guidelines for monitoring drug therapy in rheumatoid arthritis: American College of Rheumatology Ad Hoc Committee on Clinical Guidelines. Arthritis Rheum 1996; 39:723–731.

121. Health and Public Policy Committee, American College of Physicians. Methotrexate in rheumatoid arthritis. Ann Intern Med 1987; 107:418–419.

122. Levin DM. Re: JM Kremer—editorial [letter] Am J Gastroenterol 1997; 92:1402–1403.

123. Kremer JM. Response to Dr. Levin [letter]. Am J Gastroenterol 1997; 92:1402–1403.

124. Erickson AR, Reddy V, Vogelgesang SA, West SG. Usefulness of the American College of Rheumatology recommendations for liver biopsy in methotrexate-treated rheumatoid arthritis. Arthritis Rheum 1995; 38:1115–1119.

125. Jackson CG, Sawitzke Clegg DO. Monitoring methotrexate toxicity in rheumatoid arthritis: failure of ACR guidelines to predict hepatic fibrosis. Arthritis Rheum 1994; 37:S361 (abstr).

126. Berquist SR, Felson DT, Prashker MJ, Freedberg KA. The cost-effectiveness of liver biopsy in rheumatoid arthritis patients treated with methotrexate. Arthritis Rheum 1995; 38:326–333.

127. Biasi D, Bambara LM, Carletto A, Casaril M, Capra F, Caramaschi P, Corrocher R. Effects

on fibrogenesis markers of rheumatoid arthritis therapy with methotrexate. J Rheumatol 1996; 23:453–454.

128. Beyeler C, Richen J, Thomann SR, Lauterberg BM, Gerber NJ. Quantitative liver function in patients with rheumatoid arthritis treated with low-dose methotrexate: a longitudinal study. Br J Rheumatol 1997; 36:338–344.

129. Oberti F, Valsesia E, Pilette C, Rousselet MC, Bedossa P, Aube C, Gallois Y, Rifflet H, Maiga MY, Penneau-Fontbonne D, Cales P. Noninvasive diagnosis of hepatic fibrosis or cirrhosis. Gastroenterology 1997; 113:1609–1616.

130. McRosenberg W, Burt A, Becka M, Voelker M, Arthur MJ. European Liver Fibrosis Consortium. Automated assays of serum markers of liver fibrosis predict histological hepatic fibrosis. Hepatology 2000; 32:183 (abstr).

131. Richard S, Guerret S, Gerard F, Tebib JG, Vignon E. Hepatic fibrosis in rheumatoid arthritis patients treated with methotrexate: application of a new semiquantitative scoring system. Rheumatology 2000; 39:50–54.

132. Danao T, Steinbrunner J, Medendorp SV. Methotrexate in juvenile rheumatoid arthritis. Arthritis Rheum 1989; 32(suppl 9):28.

133. Keim D, Ragsdale C, Heidelberger K, Sullivan D. Hepatic fibrosis with the use of methotrexate for juvenile rheumatoid arthritis. J Rheumatol 1990; 17:846–848.

134. Graham LD, Myones BL, Rivas-Chacon RF, Pachman LM. Morbidity associated with long-term methotrexate therapy in juvenile rheumatoid arthritis. J Pediatr 1992; 120:468–473.

135. Kugathasan S, Newman AJ. Liver biopsy findings in patients with juvenile rheumatoid arthritis receiving long-term weekly methotrexate therapy. J Pediatr 1996; 128:149–151.

136. Hashkes PJ, Balistreri WF, Bove KE, Ballard ET, Passo MH. The long-term effect of methotrexate therapy on the liver in patients with juvenile rheumatoid arthritis. Arthritis Rheum 1997; 40:2226–2230.

137. Ravelli A, Migliavacca D, Viola S, Ruperto N, Pistorio A, Martini A. Efficacy of folinic acid in reducing methotrexate toxicity in juvenile idiopathic arthritis. Clin Exp Rheumatol 1999; 17:625–627.

138. Hashkes PJ, Balistreri WF, Bove KE, Ballard ET, Passo MH. The relationship of hepatotoxic risk factors and liver histology in methotrexate therapy for juvenile rheumatoid arthritis. J Pediatr 1999; 134:47–52.

139. Zieglschmid-Adams ME, Pandya AG, Cohen SB, Sontheimer RD. Treatment of dermatomyositis with methotrexate. J Am Acad Dermatol 1995; 32:754–757.

140. Davies H, Olson L. Gibson P. Methotrexate as a steroid-sparing agent for asthma in adults. Cochrane Database Syst Rev 2000 CD000391.

141. Lower EE, Baughman RP. Prolonged use of methotrexate for sarcoidosis. Arch Intern Med 1995; 155:846–851.

142. Knox TA, Kaplan MM, Gelfand JA, Wolff SM. Methotrexate treatment of granulomatous hepatitis. Ann Intern Med 1995; 122:592–595.

143. Iqbal MP, Baig JA, Ali AA, Niazi SK, Mehboobali N, Hussain MA. The effects of nonsteroidal anti-inflammatory drugs on the disposition of methotrexate in patients with rheumatoid arthritis. Biopharm Drug Dispos 1998; 19:163–167.

144. Nisar M, Carlisle L, Amos RS. Methotrexate and sulphasalzine as combination therapy in rheumatoid arthritis. Br J Rheumatol 1994; 33:651–654.

145. Stein CM, Pincus T, Yocum D, Tugwell P, Wells G, Gluck O, Kraag G, Torley H, Tesser J, McKendry R, Brooks RH. Combination treatment of severe rheumatoid arthritis with cyclosporine and methotrexate for forty-eight weeks: an open-label extension study: the Methotrexate-Cyclosporine Combination Study Group. Arthritis Rheum 1997; 40:1843–1851.

146. Schilsky RL, Ordway FS. Insulin effects on methotrexate polyglutamate synthesis and enzyme binding in cultured human breast cancer cells. Cancer Chemother Pharmacol 1985; 15:272–277.

147. Galivan J, Rees MS. Insulin-dependent suppression in glutamyl hydrolase activity and elevated cellular methotrexate polyglutamates. Biochem Pharmacol 1995; 50:1659–1663.

148. Redlich CA, Cullen MR. Nonalcoholic steatohepatitis [letter]. Ann Intern Med 1997; 127: 410.

149. Rampton DS. Therapy update: methotrexate in Crohn's disease. Gut 2001; 48:790–791.

150. Tang H, Neuberger J. Methotrexate in gastroenterology—dangerous villain or simply misunderstood? Aliment Pharmacol Ther 1996; 10:851–858.

151. Kaplan MM, Arora S, Pincus SH. Primary sclerosing cholangitis and low dose oral pulse methotrexate. Ann Intern Med 1987; 106:231–235.

152. Knox TA, Kaplan MM. Treatment of primary sclerosing cholangitis with oral methotrexate. Am J Gastroenterol 1991; 86:546–552.

153. Lindor KD, Jorgensen RA, Anderson ML, Gores GJ, Hofmann AF, La Russo NF. Ursodeoxycholic acid and methotrexate for primary sclerosing cholangitis: a pilot study. Am J Gastroenterol 1996; 91:511–515.

154. Duerkson DR, Blondell-Hill E, Bailey RJ. *Pneumocystis carinii* pneumonia complicating methotrexate treatment of primary sclerosing cholangitis. Am J Gastroenterol 1995; 90: 1886–1887.

155. Kaplan MM, Knox TA. Treatment of primary biliary cirrhosis with low-dose weekly methotrexate. Gastroenterology 1991; 101:1332–1338.

156. Kaplan MM, De Lellis RA, Wolfe HJ. Sustained biochemical and histologic remission of primary biliary cirrhosis in response to medical treatment. Ann Intern Med 1997; 126:682–688.

157. Bergasa NV, Jones EA, Kleiner DE, Rabin L, Park Y, Wells MC, Hoofnagle JH. Pilot study of low-dose oral methotrexate treatment for primary biliary cirrhosis. Am J Gastroenterol 1996; 91:295–299.

158. Bach N, Thung SN, Schafner F. The histologic effect of low-dose methotrexate therapy for primary biliary cirrhosis. Arch Pathol Lab Med 1998; 122:342–345.

159. Kaplan MM, Schmid C, Provenzale D, Sharma A, Dickstein G, McKusick A. A prospective trial of colchicine and methotrexate in the treatment of primary biliary cirrhosis. Gastroenterology 1999; 117:1173–1180.

160. Hendrickse MT, Rigney E, Giaffer MH, Soomro I, Triger DR, Underwood JCE, Gleeson D. Low-dose methotrexate is ineffective in primary biliary cirrhosis: long-term results of a placebo-controlled trial. Gastroenterology 1999; 117:400–407.

161. Sharma A, Provenzale D, McKusick A, Kaplan MM. Interstitial pneumonitis after low-dose methotrexate therapy in primary biliary cirrhosis. Gastroenterology 1994; 107:266–270.

162. Sorda J, Findor J. Methotrexate therapy in primary biliary cirrhosis. Acta Gastroenterol Latinoam 2000; 30:221–225.

163. Gonzalez-Koch A, Brahm J, Antezana C, Smok G, Cumsille MA. The combination of ursodeoxycholic acid and methotrexate for primary biliary cirrhosis is not better then ursodeoxycholic acid alone. J Hepatol 1997; 27:143–149.

164. Bonis PAL, Kaplan MM. Methotrexate improves biochemical tests in patients with primary biliary cirrhosis who respond incompletely to ursodiol. Gastroenterology 1999; 117:395–399.

165. Lindor KD, Dickson ER, Jorgensen RA. The combination of ursodeoxycholic acid and methotrexate for patients with primary biliary cirrhosis: the results of a pilot study. Hepatology 1995; 22:1158–1162.

166. Heathcote EJ. Evidence-based therapy of primary biliary cirrhosis. Eur J Gastroenterol Hepatol 1999; 11:607–615.

167. Angulo P, Lindor KD. Management of primary biliary cirrhosis and autoimmune cholangitis. Clin Liver Dis 1998; 2:333–351.

168. Poupon R, Poupon RE. Treatment of primary biliary cirrhosis. Best Pract Res Clin Gastroenterol 2000; 14:615–628.

169. Gish RG, Mason A. Autoimmune liver disease: current standards, future directions. Clin Liver Dis 2001; 5:287–314.

27

Adverse Effects of Hormones and Hormone Antagonists on the Liver

MUHAMMAD NAEEM and STEVEN SCHENKER

University of Texas Health Science Center at San Antonio, San Antonio, Texas, U.S.A.

I. INTRODUCTION

This chapter discusses the adverse effects on the hepatobiliary system of hormonal agents used to enhance or inhibit various endocrine effects. This includes female sex hormones and anabolic steroids, as well as antithyroid and oral hypoglycemic drugs.

II. FEMALE SEX HORMONES AND ORAL CONTRACEPTIVES

A. Normal Physiology

Estrogens are 18-carbon steroids derived from cholesterol. Naturally occurring estrogens have an aromatic A ring, a phenolic hydroxyl group at C_3, and either a ketone (estrone) or a hydroxyl group (estradiol) at C_{17} (Fig. 1) (1). The C_{17} site (as discussed later) has a major role in the cholestatic properties of these hormones. Estrogen (as estradiol), as well

677

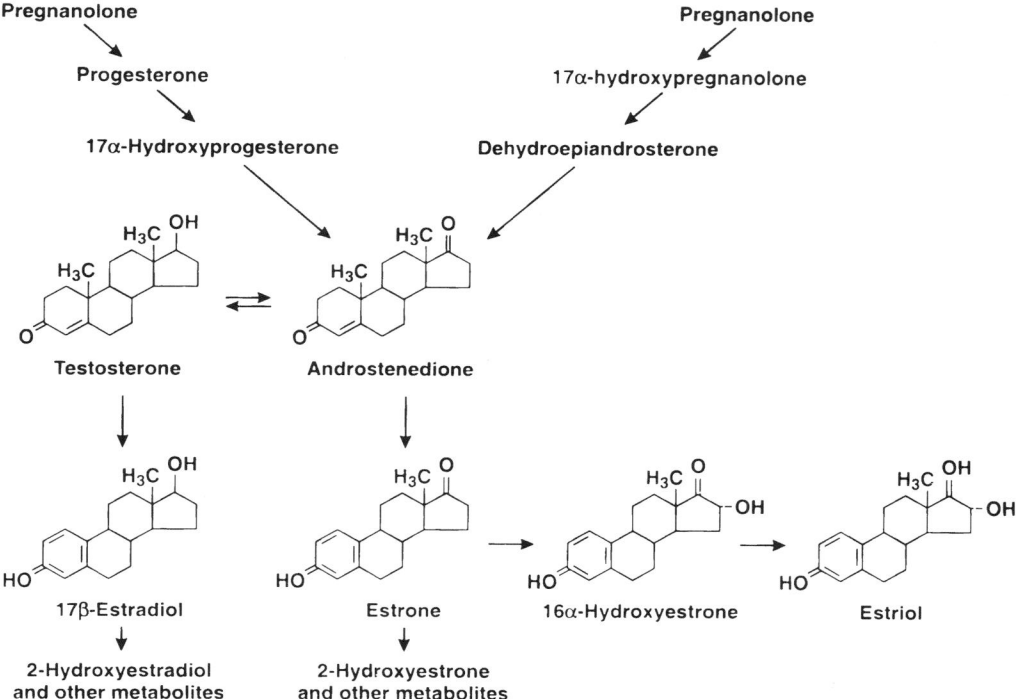

Figure 1   Synthesis and metabolism of estrogens (1).

as progesterone, is a secretory product of the ovaries. Most estrone and estriol are formed from estradiol in the liver or in peripheral tissues from androstenedione and other androgens. Synthetic estrogens have subtle alterations in native chemical structure. Estrone and estriol are metabolized in liver to hydroxylated and conjugated derivatives that are excreted in bile and may subsequently undergo intestinal hydrolysis and an enterohepatic circulation.

The cellular and intracellular effects of estrogens depend on their binding to estrogen receptors complexed to heat shock proteins (HSP). HSP is dissociated from the receptor ligand complex, which, in turn, binds to estrogen response elements (ERE) genes. ERE then interact with specific cellular proteins (transacting factors) to activate transcription and regulate the formation of specific mRNAs (1,2). Some of the effects of estrogens appear to be mediated by paracrine effects of growth factors and cytokines released by adjacent cells.

The physiological effects of estrogens are many, including the development of primary and secondary sexual characteristics, increase in the level of various proteins, such as transcortin and ceruloplasmin, as well as various clotting factors, changes in plasma lipids with an increase in high-density lipoprotein, and a reduction in low-density lipoprotein, modification in the renin-angiotensin system, and of bone growth (3,4).

B.   Adverse Effects on the Hepatobiliary System

The multiple discrete, possibly adverse effects of these agents on the liver and biliary tract are cited in Table 1, and will be discussed sequentially below.

Table 1 Adverse Effects of
Estrogenic Hormones on the Liver and
Biliary System

Intrahepatic cholestasis
    Oral contraceptives, pregnancy
Gallbladder disease
Tumor formation
    Adenoma/carcinoma
    ? Focal nodular hyperplasia
    ? Angiosarcoma
Vascular effects
    Hepatic vein thrombosis
    Hemangioma growth
    Peliosis hepatis
Effects on other liver disorders
Effects on hepatic drug metabolism
    Oxidation
    Glucuronidation
    Alcoholic liver disease

C. Intrahepatic Cholestasis

1. Clinical Features

Abnormal liver tests and jaundice associated with oral contraceptives (OCs) were reported more than 50 years ago (5), and a large body of literature is available on this subject. The reported incidence of cholestatic jaundice with these agents is $1:10,000$ worldwide (6), but the actual prevalence is likely to be higher. Since liver test abnormalities may develop early in the course of hormonal drug use, they are easily missed if not monitored (7,8). Both genetic predisposition and total dose and structure dependence (see below) seem to play a part. Thus, some ethnic groups are more susceptible to cholestatic effects of OCs (6). Estrogen-induced cholestasis has been reported in Scandinavian families (9). Chilean females of Araucanian descent have a particularly high incidence of jaundice (10). In a study of three generations of blood relatives, the susceptibility to OC-induced cholestasis, jaundice of pregnancy, or both were common and seemed to be transmitted as a dominant trait (11). Other studies have also documented jaundice with the use of OCs in women with a family history of cholestasis of pregnancy.

    The disorder may be preceded by mild malaise, anorexia, nausea, and pruritus, the latter sometimes severe. Jaundice usually develops early, but has been reported to be delayed for up to 9 months after start of drug use (6,12). Pruritus and jaundice are the two key features. Bilirubin increase usually is modest (below 10 mg/dL) (6,13), and transaminases are increased in about 70% of cases, but usually to less than 3 times normal (14). In terms of markers of cholestasis, alkaline phosphatase is increased only modestly (threefold) and γ-glutamyl transferase (GGT) is usually normal (15,16). The few references to high transaminases (in excess of 10 times normal) may represent a coincidental hepatic injury (6,12), as has been suggested (17).

2. Pathology

Biopsy of the liver on light microscopy shows canalicular bile plugs and cholestasis, predominantly in zone 3, and absence of significant inflammation (6,12). The parenchyma usually shows only mild injury, with some acidophilic bodies likely representing apoptosis (9). This has been termed "bland cholestasis."

Electron microscopy shows dilated canaliculi with blunted and fragmented microvilli (6,18). This is a nonspecific finding, seen with other forms of cholestasis. Mitochondria are often misshapen and the endoplasmic reticulum is dilated with vesiculation (6,19).

3. Pathogenesis

The mechanism(s) of OC-induced cholestasis appears to be multifactorial, likely involving the dose and type (structure) of the estrogen, as well as a genetic susceptibility to the agent [either sensitivity at the basolateral or canalicular bile acid transporter level (Fig. 2) and/or the metabolism of the estrogenic compound]. It is generally appreciated that estrogenic hormones and their derivatives selectively inhibit the excretion of sulfobromophthalein (BSP) and bilirubin in rats (20) and humans (6,21–23), if sensitive monitoring measures are used. This may be a dose-dependent phenomenon similar to that seen with C_{17}-alkylated anabolic steroids (24). Moreover, some structural changes in the estrogen molecule seem to promote cholestasis and others inhibit it. Thus, an oxygen group at C_3 (25), a glucuronide at C_{17} on the D ring (26,27), and a decreased excretion of A-ring glucuronides (28) may promote cholestasis. The issue of decreased sulfation versus glucuronidation as a factor in cholestasis of OC use is unresolved (29). These data and the proclivity of some ethnic or genetically related women to a higher incidence of OC-induced jaundice strongly suggest individual susceptibility in addition to intrinsic "toxicity" of estrogenic substances to the biliary canalicular apparatus. In contrast to the estrogenic component of OC, few data incriminate the progestational contribution to cholestasis, except perhaps in large doses and as an additive to estrogens (17).

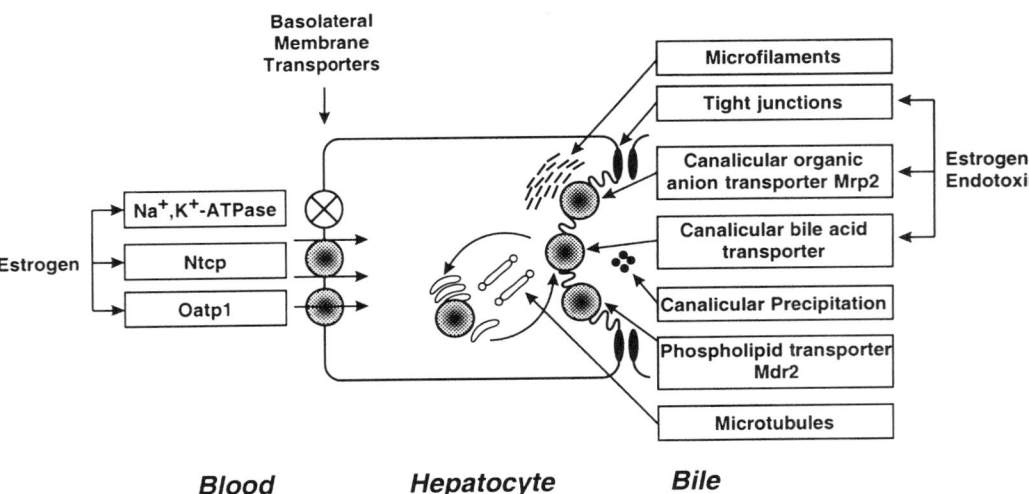

Figure 2   Main sites of action of estrogen for causing experimental cholestasis. (Modified from ref. 16.)

The adverse effects of estrogens (and/or their derivatives) appear to be exerted primarily both at the basolateral membrane and the canalicular level, and affect bile secretion (Fig. 2). Information as to the precise biochemical and anatomical sites of estrogen effect has evolved with better characterization of the bile acid secretory process. Nevertheless, despite the use of isolated hepatocytes and perfused rat liver (30–32) and recent characterization of bile acid transporters (33–37), the mechanism(s) are incompletely defined. It appears, however, that estrogen (by altering membrane lipids) decreases the fluidity of the basolateral membrane, alters the conformation of Na^+K^+-ATPase at that site, and impairs the activity of transporters for bile acid uptake (38–42). It is not certain, however, whether the changes in membrane fluidity actually cause or merely coexist with the impaired bile acid uptake (43,44). Moreover, other effects of estrogen are likely exerted on the canalicular bile acid transporters (37,45). In a recent study on Sprague-Dawley and Mrp2-deficient TR rats, it was shown that the estrogen metabolite estradiol-17β (β-D-glucuronide) ($E_2$17G) induces cholestasis by a canalicular anion Mrp2-dependent mechanism independent of transport (46). $E_2$17G, following secretion by MRP2 into canaliculus, appears to trans-inhibit the transport of bile acids by the bile salt excretory pump. Additional effects of estrogen may be on bile-acid-independent bile flow (30,47–49). The earlier concept that estrogen primarily alters tight junctions, thus causing regurgitation of bile, appears to have been abandoned (21,38).

4. Prognosis and Treatment

In most cases, jaundice resolves within a month of stopping the agent and the overall outcome is favorable. No residual effects on liver histology or function have been reported after discontinuation of the estrogenic compound.

Treatment consists of stopping the provoking agent, avoiding unnecessary surgery, and addressing the symptoms. Acutely the major concern is pruritus and this is treated with cholestyramine, and if not tolerated or effective, with other agents such as nightly phenobarbital, rifampicin, antihistamines, and skin care such as avoidance of heat and use of starch baths. Opioid antagonists are still in the research realm (50).

Two other drugs have been suggested for the treatment of the cholestasis, per se, as the patient is recovering. One is ursodeoxycholic acid, which may not only improve bile flow, but also relieve pruritus. It is believed to be cytoprotective by displacing less polar bile salts from liver cell membranes (51). While its benefit remains to be confirmed, it does not appear to have toxic effects, other than diarrhea at higher doses.

The other agent is S-adenosyl-L-methionine (SAMe). This derivative of methionine has an important role in transsulfuration and transmethylation reactions in hepatocytes; it improves membrane fluidity and mitochondrial-reduced glutathione (an antioxidant) concentration and may also enhance bile flow (43) (Fig. 3). It does not appear to have toxic effects, and has been used in rats to prevent the cholestatic effects of ethinyl estradiol (52). It has been used in the cholestasis of pregnancy (see below), without apparent problems for the fetus (53). Variable benefit has been obtained with SAMe, perhaps owing to different severity of the disease; hence, more data on the therapeutic value of this agent are needed (44,53,54).

5. Cholestasis of Pregnancy

Inasmuch as the major increase in estrogen in pregnancy is felt to be the cause of cholestasis seen in pregnancy, and this entity differs in some respects from the effects of OCs, some discussion of this syndrome seems warranted here.

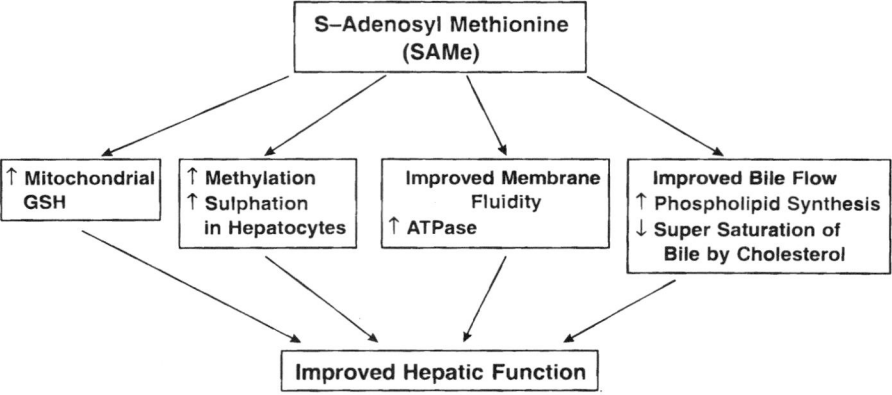

Figure 3 Proposed mechanisms of action of SAMe in cholestasis.

This syndrome clinically resembles cholestasis seen with OCs and the laboratory test derangements are similar (55). The onset is usually in the third trimester when estrogens peak. Cholestasis resolves soon after delivery and may recur with subsequent pregnancies and with the use of OCs. Hence, it is felt that estrogens are responsible for the cholestasis. The mechanism(s) likely are similar to those discussed earlier, except that here the estrogen load is much higher. Some researchers have also suggested that progesterone metabolites may have a cholestatic role (56). Since the problem is seen in only a small minority of pregnancies, it is evident that hypersensitivity of some women must contribute. Indeed, a mutation of the *multi-drug-resistant-3* (*MDR-3*) gene has been reported in those families (57). Hence, heterozygous defects in membrane transporters or genetic polymorphism may play a role in this disorder in predisposing the liver to the cholestatic effects of estrogens. Treatment options are similar to those cited earlier for OC-induced cholestasis, except that transfer of drugs to the fetus and the possible consequences of this always need to be considered.

Importantly, cholestasis in pregnancy enhances preterm birth rate (13%) and fetal death rate (4%) (58–60). This may relate, at least in part, to altered placental metabolism of steroids. Thus, decreased fetal adrenal production of dehydroepiandrosterone (a substrate for placental estrogens) has been reported in such patients (61). The mechanism is unknown, but bile acids, which are increased in these patients (62), also have strong vasoconstrictive properties (63).

D. Effects of Estrogen on Gallbladder Dysfunction

A key aspect of the diagnosis (and treatment) of estrogen-induced intrahepatic cholestasis is to differentiate it from extrahepatic cholestasis. Such a distinction is especially important as estrogens promote gallbladder dysfunction and cholestasis. Thus, long-term OC use is associated with greater prevalence of gallstones (64,65), and this is true also in pregnancy. A prospective study of 272 pregnant women showed an incidence of gallbladder sludge (31%) and stone formation (2%) that was respectable. However, most patients with biliary sludge remain asymptomatic and it resolves spontaneously after delivery. Biliary colic was rarely seen in association with gallstones in this group (66). The mechanisms of this effect seem to be both an increased lithogenic effect (increased cholesterol/decreased bile acids in bile) (67,68), and decreased gallbladder motility (i.e., greater bile stasis) (69,70). The latter has an important contribution from progesterone (70). Thus, gallbladder dysfunction must be added to the list of adverse effects of estrogen on the hepatobiliary system.

E. Tumor Formation

1. Hepatocellular Adenoma

Epidemiology. This solid liver tumor is seen in women of childbearing age; otherwise, it is a rare lesion. Prior to 1960, reports of adenoma were exceedingly rare (71). After the introduction of OCs in the 1960s, the incidence rose sharply, and subsequently some 300 cases were diagnosed yearly in the United States (72). The incidence of these lesions increases with the dose and duration of estrogen use (73). Thus, the risk of developing an adenoma increases 100-fold in patients taking OCs for more than 5 years, and 500-fold with more than 7 years' usage (72) (Fig. 4). In 10% of cases, however, the exposure may only be 6–12 months and, of course, the lesion may be diagnosed after OCs are stopped (74). Occasionally, older patients on replacement hormonal therapy have been reported to develop this tumor (72,75). Case-controlled studies in 1979 showed an incidence of 3.4 cases per 100,000 OC users (72), but now with a decrease in estrogen concentration in OC preparations, this number has declined (73).

Clinical Features. Clinical presentations of hepatic adenoma are of four types: an asymptomatic lesion found incidentally on imaging or at surgery, a mass found on physical examination, pain, and/or bleeding into the mass with possible hemoperitoneum (75–79). The distribution of these presentations varies considerably among reports, but is, on average, similar with pain generally highest on the list (Fig. 5). The pain is in the right upper quandrant or epigastrium, may radiate to the subscapular area, and is accompanied often by tenderness and evidence of blood loss. There may be a hemoperitoneum and shock with severe bleeding. Jaundice may be seen due to compression of the intrahepatic bile ducts by the tumor (75,80).

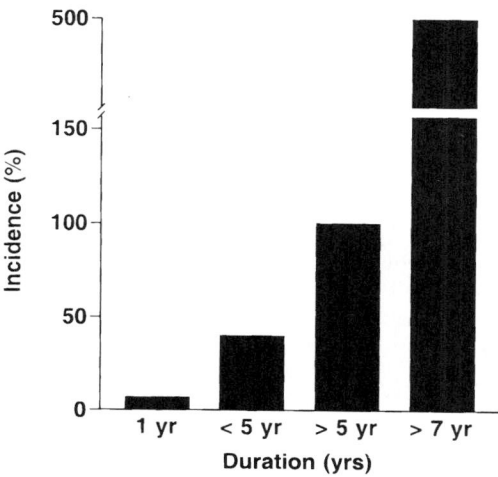

Figure 4 Duration of OC use and incidence of hepatocellular adenoma. (Modified from ref. 72.)

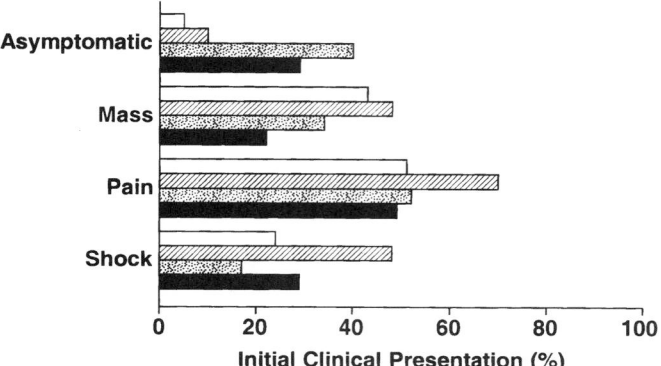

Figure 5   Presentation of hepatic adenoma in four case series. (Modified from ref. 17: *open bar*: ref. 77; *lined bar*: ref. 78; *dotted bar*: ref. 79; *solid bar*: ref. 75.)

Diagnosis depends first on consideration of possible presence of this entity, a careful history of contraceptive use, physical examination, which may detect a mass, and ultimately an imaging study. Liver tests usually remain normal; however, an elevated alkaline phosphatase and GGT may be seen (79). Adenomas larger than 3 cm in diameter are usually diagnosed by ultrasound, computed tomography (CT) scan, or radionucleotide scan. The former two modalities usually define the presence of a mass, but are not specific for adenomas unless bleeding into the lesion is shown (favoring an adenoma). Decreased labeled sulfur colloid uptake has generally been reported for adenomas and has been attributed to decrease in Kupffer cell number or function. However, accumulation of colloid has been described in adenomas, similar to that seen with focal nodular hyperplasia (FNH) (81,82). Hepatic arteriography may show a filling defect with clear margins and increased vascularity, which strongly suggests the presence of adenoma. However, difficulties in differentiating FNH from adenoma may remain in up to 25% of patients (83) (Table 2). Recently a characteristic magnetic resonance imaging appearance has been suggested for the diagnosis of FNH (see below) (Table 3), which may help in this regard (84). Liver biopsy of these lesions may be hazardous owing to enhanced bleeding and may not be diagnostic if the sample is small or confounded by fibrosis due to a prior bleed (83).

Pathology.   Hepatic adenomas consist of encapsulated hepatocytes and are devoid of portal tracts. Kupffer cells are missing or scanty. The vascularity is high with poor connective tissue support. Adenomas may contain fat (73,85).

Pathogenesis.   The pathogenesis of this disorder is not defined. In view of the association with OC use, it has been proposed that estrogen transforms normal hepatocytes into adenoma via induction of estrogen receptors (86,87), but the experimental evidence is not conclusive (88). In patients with underlying glycogen storage disease, an imbalance of insulin and glucagon may have a role (89). The vascularity of these lesions may be a clue to the pathogenesis.

Prognosis and Treatment.   Hepatic adenomas regress and may disappear after OCs are discontinued (90,91–93). On occasion, however, they may continue to grow and rupture even after OCs are stopped (94). There are also reports of transformation of these benign lesions into cancer, even after OCs are stopped (93,95). Hence, as suggested recently, the

Table 2 Comparison of Diagnostic and Clinical Characteristics of FNH and Hepatic Adenoma

	FNH	Hepatic adenoma
Clinical	Any age group	Women of childbearing age
	Mostly asymptomatic (80%)	Abdominal pain/mass (65%)
	OC use in 60%	OC use in 90%
	Usually less than 5 cm	>5 cm
	Normal enzymes	Normal enzymes unless hemorrhage
Histology	Fibrosis 4+	+/−
	Central scar >95%	—
	Septa formation	—
	Ductule proliferation (+)	—
Diagnostic imaging		
US	Nonspecific	Nonspecific
Dopplers	Arterial flow	Venous flow
CT	Iso or hypodense	Peripheral arterial enhancement, hyper or hypodense areas precontrast
	Arterial enhancement of stellate scar	
Angiography	Hypervascular/dense blush, central vascular supply	Hypervascular tumor, peripheral vascular supply
Scintigraphy		
Colloids	↑ or normal	Focal defect

FNH, focal nodular hyperplasia.
Source: Modified with permission from *Schiff's Diseases of the Liver*, 1999.

index of suspicion should be high and lesions with irregular borders, continuing enlargement, and any increase in α-fetoprotein should be referred for surgical removal (96). Pregnancy may be associated with adenoma growth and rupture (with fetal complications) and thus, pregnancy should be avoided if the adenoma had not been resected.

As to treatment, clearly significant discomfort and bleeding are indications for resection. Many feel that even uncomplicated lesions are best resected, if technically feasible (92,97), to avoid future bleeding or possibility of malignant transformation. Elective surgical resection usually accomplishes removal of the adenoma with minimal mortality (1%) (98). Laparoscopic resection is another option, if technically feasible (83). Orthotopic liver transplantation may be needed for multifocal lesions (99,100), especially with evidence of cancer formation. In patients with inoperable tumors, arterial embolization has been

Table 3 MRI Criteria for Diagnosis of FNH

Slightly hyperintense or isointense on T_2-weighted images
Homogeneous signal intensity
Presence of a central stellate area hyperintense on T_1-weighted images
Marked enhancement of the lesion at the arterial phase
Accumulation of gadolinium chelates within the central area on delayed contrast-enhanced T_1 weighted image
Absence of tumor capsule

Source: Used with permission from Mathieu et al. (84).

used to reduce tumor size (92,101), preoperatively, or to control bleeding (102). In the older literature, mortality is high, up to (21%) with intraperitoneal bleeding (72), and emergency resection of the bleeding liver lesion also carries a significant mortality of up to 8%.

Another option, which we favor less, for small (<5 cm), uncomplicated adenomas is a brief (2 year) follow-up after OCs are stopped (103). These patients require careful monitoring for decrease in lesion size, as even adenomas that appear to have regressed may rarely (two case reports) present later with cancer (92,104).

2. Focal Nodular Hyperplasia

FNH is a common benign solid tumor of the liver, with an autopsy incidence of about 0.3–0.6% (105,106). Nevertheless, it will be discussed only briefly here as its relationship to OCs is in considerable doubt. Thus, its female/male ratio is only 2:1 (vs. 9:1 for adenoma), its incidence has not increased since the use of OCs, and information as to growth, bleeding, and regression of the lesions in relation to OCs is controversial (107–110). However, differentiation of FNH from adenoma is important as the treatment for the former is conservative owing to absence of life-threatening complications and cancerous transformation.

FNH consists of single or multiple nodules of hyperplastic hepatocytes with Kupffer cells and atypical bile ducts, usually containing a central stellate scarred area containing large vessels. There usually is no capsule (111). The hyperplasia is felt to be likely due to hyperperfusion or anomalous circulation (106,112,113).

Patients with FNH usually have no complaints (114), with lesions identified only during imaging or at surgery. Pain and hemorrhage are very unusual, and a normal physical examination is noted in the large majority. Some may present with hepatomegaly, abdominal tenderness, or a mass. Liver tests are usually normal. A series of imaging techniques have been used for diagnosis. A radionucleotide scan with increased uptake by the Kupffer cells is typical, but is not always seen. A central scar by CT is also helpful, if seen. An MRI with 98% specificity has been described (110) (Table 3). Biopsy may be diagnostic; however, interpretation may be difficult.

The prognosis of FNH is excellent in most patients. Malignant transformation does not occur (115–117). Asymptomatic patients may be followed expectantly but the rare symptomatic (or diagnostically uncertain) lesions should be excised, if feasible. It is uncertain whether lesions increase in size during pregnancy (110,118,119). A recent large study (216 women with FNH) with tumor size followed by MRI suggested that neither OCs nor pregnancy influenced FNH (110).

3. Cancer

Although some 100 cases of hepatocellular carcinoma (HCC) have been reported in the setting of OC use (79,94,120–140), the causal relationship has not been firmly established. Nevertheless, while HCC is rare in young individuals, and in the absence of underlying cirrhosis, HCC in association with OCs occurs in young women who are not cirrhotic (131,132,136). These tumors tend to be well differentiated, often fibrolamellar, occur without an increase in α-fetoprotein, and tend to be slow growing, although they may metastasize very rarely (21). Recipients of the synthetic steroid diethylstilbesterol also may have a higher risk of developing HCC (142–144). Case reports also have alleged a higher risk of HCC with prolonged OC use (131–133,136), and adenoma has been related to cancer development (see above). The carcinogenic effect of OCs, if present, is considered small

(138). In addition to HCC, several cases of angiosarcoma and hemangioepithelioma have been reported in association with estrogen use (145–147).

4. Vascular Abnormalities

Hepatic Vein Thrombosis (HVT). Many cases of HVT in association with OC use have been reported (148), and the number is likely higher. While association does not prove causality, a large case-control study has shown that OC use increased the risk of HVT twofold as compared to matched controls (149). Many of the OC users also had an underlying overt or subtle myeloproliferative state (150). It is believed that the increase in HVT is due to the thrombogenic effects of the OCs (148,151), possibly aided by the presence of polycythemia. The presence of inherited rare thrombogenic risk factors, such as factor V Leiden, and possibly minor abdominal trauma, may be additive to the OC effects (152). Clearly some "sensitizing" factor(s) is essential, as this problem is very rare despite the extensive use of OCs.

Clinical features of HVT characteristically include abdominal pain and hepatic tenderness, ascites, and often jaundice. The completeness and severity of these features depends on the rapidity and completeness of hepatic vein occlusion. Physical findings consist primarily of the presence of a large, tender liver and free fluid in the abdomen. Liver tests are characteristic of hepatic cellular damage. Imaging studies (Doppler ultrasound, CT scan, and ultimately percutaneous venography) confirm the diagnosis. A nucleotide scan may show sparing of the caudate lobe, which drains separately into the vena cava. A liver biopsy (when possible) shows centrilobular congestion and necrosis.

Prognosis depends on the rate and completeness of occlusion of hepatic veins. A complete HVT, left untreated, has a serious prognosis. Treatment options (in addition to OC removal and diuretics) include thrombolytic drugs (if used early) or a surgical side-to-side portacaval shunt to permit decompressive hepatic venous drainage (153). This should be combined with anticoagulation to prevent continuing thrombosis and diuretics for management of ascites. A transjugular intrahepatic portasystemic shunt has been employed successfully (154). Another option is hepatic transplantation with anticoagulation, especially if cirrhosis is already established and/or less drastic treatment fails (155).

Hemangiomas and Related Lesions. The role of estrogen (whether with OC use or in pregnancy) is to increase the growth of hemangiomas (156). These changes are often reversible and rarely require surgery.

OC use can also produce sinusoidal dilatation, selective for zones 1 and 2 (151,157), and peliosis hepatis (158).

F. Effects of Estrogen on Various Liver Diseases

There is extensive epidemiological evidence that the liver in women is more sensitive to adverse effects of alcohol. In other words, a similar exposure to ethanol results in earlier and/or greater liver damage in women than in men (159–161). It is, in part, for this reason that one drink per day has been established as a safe alcohol intake in nonpregnant women versus twice that much for men (162,163). These effects of gender have been reproduced in one experimental model of alcoholic liver injury in rats (164). There was clear evidence of greater biochemical and pathological injury in female rats given ethanol in the Tsukamoto-French model of alcohol administration. Other studies suggested that this gender effect may be due to estrogen, which both enhances ethanol-induced endotoxin permeability via the gut (165) and promotes greater binding of endotoxin to Kupffer cells with subsequent release of tumor necrosis factor-α (TNFα) (166,167). Thus, estrogen may enhance the adverse effects of ethanol on the liver. Whether this hormone may also alter significantly other types of liver injury remains to be seen. There is anecdotal data that cholestasis may be enhanced by OC use in patients with acute viral hepatitis. Also, female sex hormones may decrease mitochondrial fatty acid oxidation (168,169) and, thus, may contribute to the fatty liver of pregnancy.

G. Effects of Female Sex Hormones on Hepatic Drug Metabolism

Estrogenic hormones are known to inhibit oxidative metabolism of some agents (i.e., tacrine) (170) or caffeine (171), while they seem to enhance the glucuronidation of others (i.e., acetaminophen) (172). These types of drug-drug interactions may have clinical significance.

III. ANABOLIC STEROIDS

A. General Comments

These agents are synthetic or semisynthetic C_{17}-alkylated steroids and have been used considerably less than OCs. However, they have been employed for treatment of aplastic anemia, impotence, and transsexualism in females, as well as most recently for body building among athletes.

Two general types of hepatic dysfunction may occur with these drugs: cholestatic jaundice, which develops after a short period of drug use and which is largely dose-dependent, and the less common neoplastic and vascular disorders that may ensue after a long duration of drug use. The former problem was described initially some 50 years ago (173). In patients with aplastic anemia given high therapeutic doses of these steroids, the incidence of jaundice may reach up to 17% (174), and usually appears within a few months (175). The vascular and neoplastic lesions are less common and may take 2–15 years to manifest (176).

B. Cholestasis

1. Clinical Features

The rate and degree of development of hepatic dysfunction with anabolic steroids depends in large measure on the dose of the drug (175). With low therapeutic doses, jaundice is rare, although elevated transaminases (40–200 IU) are common. With high doses of the drug, jaundice is common and serum bilirubin may even reach 20 mg/dL. Alkaline phosphatase is characteristically only mildly (up to threefold) elevated (177), and remains normal in one-third of patients (21). These abnormal liver tests are often preceded by mild systemic symptoms of malaise, anorexia, and/or nausea. Pruritus is variable, but usually not striking (178). Physical examination is normal except for modest hepatomegaly, at times.

Liver biopsy shows cholestasis mainly in zone 3 and the parenchyma shows only very mild changes in the hepatocytes without significant inflammation in the portal areas (177,179). This, together with only mild increase in alkaline phosphatase, is characteristic of anabolic-steroid-induced (or OCs-caused) canalicular disease and has been termed "bland cholestasis" (17). Indeed, electron microscopy shows blunting and loss of microvilli in canaliculi with degenerative changes in the lysozomes (180). Similar changes can be seen in rats given norethandrolone, with injury to pericanalicular filaments (181).

2. Pathogenesis

The anabolic steroids appear to produce cholestasis primarily (if not completely) due to the intrinsic (predictable) adverse effects of the agent on the liver. Thus, damage is dependent on the dose and duration of drug use (8,24,182–184), is reproducible in most animal species (185), has a rapid onset, a high incidence, and depends on the particular structure of the steroid molecule (186). Anabolic steroids that induce jaundice have an alkyl group in the C_{17} position (175). In addition, a methyl substituent on the C_{17} position or a keto group on C_3 appears to enhance toxicity of the agent (185). Other structural modifications appear to mitigate the cholestasis. The toxic effect is independent of the androgenic action.

The toxic effects of these agents are at the excretory step of bile secretion and likely involve both the bile-salt-dependent and the bile-salt-independent fraction of bile flow (187). The structures affected seem to be the basolateral and canalicular membranes (18,21,188), and perhaps the pericanalicular microfibrillar network, which can alter canalicular contraction and, thus, bile flow (181). Much of the data on the mechanisms of anabolic-steroid-induced cholestasis derives from and parallels the information cited earlier for estrogenic compounds. The similarity in the structure of these substances and of some bile acids suggests possible competitive interaction. Whether genetic predisposition affects the toxicity of these agents in humans is uncertain, but there certainly are differences among various species in their adverse response (189,190), and jaundice due to norethisterone has been described in two sisters (191,192).

3. Prognosis and Treatment

With discontinuation of these drugs, recovery from cholestasis is usually complete, but in the presence of jaundice this may take weeks or months (175,178). There are a few reports of biliary cirrhosis in the setting of anabolic steroid use, but this may be coincidental and on an immune basis. Several deaths have been cited in elderly patients with other medical problems (193). No treatment is necessary, other than early diagnosis and stopping the drug.

C. Vascular and Neoplastic Lesions

Anabolic steroids have been reported to cause peliosis hepatis with hepatomegaly and occasional hepatic dysfunction related to this (151,194). This may have a different pathogenesis than cholestasis, as it has a lower frequency, seems to be independent of dose and duration of use, and may be caused by steroids lacking a C_{17} alkyl group (195). Diagnosis of this entity is usually at autopsy, although imaging studies have been successful at times (196). A liver biopsy, with a suspected lesion, is likely hazardous (17). There are a few reports of reversal of these lesions after cessation of anabolic steroid therapy (197,198).

Anabolic steroids have also been incriminated in the development of hepatic nodular regenerative hyperplasia, adenomas, and cancer (177). Although the number of reported lesions is not large and a coincidence could be argued (199), there are data on about 60 patients with hepatocellular cancer who had been taking anabolic steroids (200). Moreover, there have been reports of regression of some of these lesions after withdrawal of the drug (201,202), and androgen receptors have been found in normal hepatocytes and hepatocellular carcinoma (203,204). Thus, the evidence, while not conclusive, is suggestive.

The clinical course of these lesions is relatively benign. Thus, contrary to adenomas due to OCs, lesions caused by anabolic steroids seldom rupture, usually are asymptomatic, and often are multiple (205). Also, patients with hepatocellular cancer associated with these drugs often tend to have a more benign course, usually with a normal α-fetoprotein (206). More studies to characterize these lesions are needed.

IV. ANTIHORMONAL AGENTS

These agents have low hormonal activity per se, but bind to the receptors for the active hormones and this appears to inhibit their endocrine effect.

A. Antiestrogens

The three agents definitively incriminated in hepatic dysfunction are tamoxifen, toremifene, and cyclofenil. Tamoxifen and toremifene are used in the prevention and treatment of estrogen-dependent breast cancer. Cyclofenil is used in Europe to induce ovulation. Various forms of liver disease have been attributed to tamoxifen—hepatocellular (207–209), cholestatic (210), and mixed (211) (Table 4). Of interest, steatohepatitis with Mallory bodies has been reported in three patients (208,209,212). A similar case has been attributed to toremifene, an analog of tamoxifen (213). Occasional cases of peliosis have been seen. These few cases and diversity of damage make it difficult to assess the mechanism(s) involved. By contrast, cyclofenil-induced liver injury appears to be more frequent (214) and is primarily hepatocellular (214).

B. Antiandrogens

These agents (flutamide, nilutamide, and cyproterone) are used for the treatment of prostatic cancer. All have been reported to lead to hepatocellular injury, including fulminant hepatic failure (215–217). The liver disease caused by these agents appears to be idiosyncratic and is rare, except for cyproterone, where a higher incidence has been reported (218).

C. Antigonadotropins

Danazol has anabolic properties in addition to inhibiting anterior pituitary function. It is now used only for the latter indication. The chemical structure of the drug resembles that

Table 4   Hepatic Injury
Associated with Tamoxifen

Jaundice
   Cholestatic
   Hepatocellular
   Mixed
Benign cyst
Peliosis hepatis
Fatty liver (steatosis)
Steatohepatitis

of estrogens. Both cholestasis and hepatocellular jaundice have been described in patients (219–221). The mechanism(s) of danazol hepatotoxicity is uncertain, with both intrinsic and idiosyncratic theories considered.

V. ORAL HYPOGLYCEMIC AGENTS

A. General Concepts

The main groups of oral agents that lower blood sugar are the sulfonylureas, the biguanides (metformin), and the new class of thiazolidinedione drugs (i.e., troglitozone). In addition, acarbose (an α-glucosidase inhibitor) is available.

Numerous sulfonylureas are available; all appear to lower blood sugar by stimulating functioning β cells in the pancreatic islets. They are well absorbed and most reach peak plasma concentrations within 2–4 h. All bind strongly to albumin and, hence, may be displaced by other competing drugs. Most sulfonylureas (or their active metabolites) are excreted in urine; hence, their action may be increased in the presence of renal disease or in the elderly with lesser renal function. Changes in drug structure, in addition to the sulfonylurea moiety, alter the pharmacokinetics and, hence, duration of drug action. None of these agents are recommended in pregnancy, owing to the risk of blood sugar fluctuation for the fetus.

Metformin, a biguanidine, does not require functioning β cells, as it decreases blood sugar by inhibiting hepatic sugar release from gluconeogenesis. This agent has a short half-life, about 3 h, does not stimulate appetite, and causes no hypoglycemia. It is not bound to serum proteins, and as it is excreted unchanged in the urine, it should not be used in the presence of renal failure. Its main toxic effect is the very rare lactic acidosis, and [except for one reported case (222)] it does not cause hepatic dysfunction. Hence, it is cited here only because it is an alternative therapy for other drugs that may result in liver damage. Any lactic acidosis present, however, may be enhanced by severe hepatic disease, as lactate is metabolized by the liver.

The first of the thiazolidonedione class of antidiabetic agents was troglitazone (Rezulin). These agents act by decreasing insulin resistance by improving sensitivity to insulin in muscle and adipose tissue, as well as inhibiting hepatic gluconeogenesis. Troglitazone is metabolized to sulfate and glucuronide conjugates and is oxidized also to a quinone metabolite (223,224). Surprisingly, troglitazone concentrations were not increased in patients with liver disease, but the elimination of metabolites was decreased (225). Two other agents in this class, pioglitazone (Actose) and rosiglitazone (Avandia), are also metabolized in the liver to pharmacologically active derivatives. The former agent is oxidized primarily by cytochromes P450 3A4 and 2C8, while the metabolism of rosiglitazone is via cytochrome P450 2C8. The clearance of these agents, therefore, may be decreased in the presence of liver disease, but is not altered by renal dysfunction.

B. Sulfonlyureas

Diabetic patients may manifest abnormal liver tests (usually mildly increased transaminases) and a fatty liver, sometimes progressing to nonalcoholic steatohepatitis (226–228). Fatty liver is especially common in type II diabetes and is independent of drug use. This clearly needs to be distinguished from liver injury patterns caused by sulfonlylurea (or other drug) therapy.

Table 5 Liver Injury due to Sulfonylureas

Sulfonylureas	Type of hepatic injury
First generation	
Acetohexamide	Hepatocellular: cholestatic
Azapinamide	Hepatocellular (rare)
Carbutamide	Hepatocellular with features of cholestasis: withdrawn
Chlorproamide	Cholestatic, granulomas
Methohexamide	Hepatocellular, 0.5–1.0% withdrawn
Tolozamide	Cholestatic (rare)—chronic cholestasis similar to PBC
Tolbutamide	Cholestatic (rare)—chronic cholestasis similar to PBC
Second generation	
Glyburide	Hepatocellular and cholestatic jaundice granulomas
Glipizide	↑ Aminotransferases—cholestatic (rare)
Gliclazide	No reported toxicity
Glisoxepide	↑ Aminotransferases (rare)—jaundice (rare)
Glymidine	↑ Aminotransferases

Source: Modified with permission from HJ Zimmerman. In: *Hepatotoxicity: The Adverse Effects of Drugs and Other Chemicals of the Liver*. 2nd ed. Chap. 20. Philadelphia: Lippincott Williams & Wilkins, 1999.

Liver injury due to sulfonylureas has varied in incidence and presentation with the specific drug used (Table 5). Glyburide, glypizide, and chlorpropamide are metabolized in the liver; hence they may accumulate and may produce hypoglycemia in patients with liver disease. The first-generation drugs tended to produce hepatocellular damage (metahexamide, carbutamide, azaprinamide) or mixed parenchymal/cholestatic disease (glyburide), and some of these have been withdrawn. Evidence of liver injury for these drugs is usually seen in the first 4–6 weeks of their initial use and certainly within 6 months. Hepatic dysfunction may be heralded by the development of nonspecific gastrointestinal symptoms, rash, and fever, but this is variable. The nature of the hepatic illness depends on the drug taken, but more recently has been cholestatic (tolbutamide, diabinese, tolazamide) or mixed (glyburide, glipizide) (229). Liver pathology also depends on the drug, but usually shows cholestasis with some cell injury, and at times granulomas (230,231). Cholestatic injury usually resolves, albeit slowly, after withdrawal of the drug. Occasional progression to a form of biliary cirrhosis has been reported (232,233). In summary, the presently used sulfonylurea antidiabetic drugs rarely cause hepatic dysfunction, and when this occurs it is usually a cholestatic or mixed injury.

As to pathogenesis of the liver injury, its rarity must imply primarily an idiosyncratic mechanism. The occasional presence of rash and fever, as well as granulomas in both liver and bone marrow (234–236), supports this view, and suggests that the unpredictable reaction has features of immune hypersensitivity. On the other hand, there is some evidence of underlying intrinsic toxicity of these agents. Thus, some of these agents (i.e., glybuthiazole) had a very high incidence of hepatotoxicity before being withdrawn, and some (i.e., chlorpropamide) appeared to cause dose-dependent injury (237). However, some species seemed to be more susceptible to liver damage than others (238). Nitrophenyl-containing sulfonylureas (carbutamide, metahexaminde, glybuthiazole) seemed to exert greater toxicity than drugs with other chemical groups (239). It seems, therefore, that these agents have some mild intrinsic toxic potential that, in the presence of host sensitivity, translates into liver injury.

C. Biguanidines and Acarbose

The key agent in the biguanidine group is metformin. As indicated earlier, there is no solid evidence that this drug causes hepatic dysfunction. Other than transient gastrointestinal disturbances, the main toxic concern is the rarely encountered lactic acidosis. Whether underlying liver disease may enhance this metabolic disturbance is uncertain, but this has been suggested (240), and it is our policy not to use this drug in patients with severe underlying hepatic dysfunction. Of interest, it has been suggested that metformin (and perhaps other hypoglycemic agents that improve insulin resistance) may benefit nonalcoholic steatohepatitis. Indeed, this appeared to be the case for metformin in an experimental model of fatty liver in genetically obese mice (241). Preliminary studies suggest that this may also be true in patients (241a).

As regards acarbose, several patients with increased transaminase and two instances of jaundice have been reported in patients using this agent (242–244).

D. Troglitazone and Other Thiazolidene Class Agents

Troglitazone (Rezulin) was approved for the treatment of type II diabetes in 1997 and rapidly gained acceptance as a valuable therapeutic agent alone or with other hypoglycemic drugs. However, the drug has been shown to cause hepatocellular disease in some patients. The onset of hepatic dysfunction is usually within 7 months of starting therapy (mean 147 days), and this may be preceded or accompanied by the nonspecific symptoms of malaise, anorexia, and nausea. In one instance only a few doses of the drug appeared to precipitate liver damage (245). The injury may be severe, especially if the drug is not stopped expeditiously, and it has led to the need for hepatic transplantation and to death in a number of patients (246–250).

The mechanism(s) of troglitazone-induced liver injury is uncertain but seems to be primarily idiosyncratic, and likely due to a metabolic sensitivity. It has been suggested that the quinone metabolite may be a culprit, based on liver toxicity of other quinones, such as that derived from acetaminophen. Such quinones may alkylate cellular proteins or lead to formation of reactive oxygen species (251). There is no accompanying rash, fever, or eosinophilia to suggest an immune mechanism (246), although increased eosinophils may be present in the liver, and at least one patient had a positive lymphocyte stimulation test (252). Individuals at risk cannot be identified at present and the toxicity is relatively infrequent with some 560 cases reported as possible cases to the Food and Drug Administration as of February 1999 (250). This prevalence of apparent toxicity is in the setting of an estimated one million patients having received the drug worldwide (250). There may be, however, some intrinsic toxicity from this drug at high doses, since at concentrations above 25 μM it was toxic to human hepatocytes in primary cultures (253). Subsequent studies, however, have shown that rat hepatocytes in tissue culture incubated for 24 h with 100 μM troglitazone showed essentially no toxic effects when bovine albumin (1–2 g/100 mL) was added (254)! By contrast in the same study, unbound troglitazone was toxic even at 20 μM. As troglitazone in serum is protein bound, studies that do not account for this (253) admittedly may have no relevance to the clinical setting. Other recent studies with perfused rat liver have suggested a cholestatic effect of the drug, possibly its sulfate moiety (141,254a), but such a selective impairment has not been generally reported in patients. In human hepatoma cells in vitro, troglitazone caused more cell injury than its derivatives, suggesting that the parent drug was the main culprit (254b). However, only concentrations much higher than those seen in patients' blood caused cell injury, and again, full consideration of drug binding in plasma does not appear to have been done. Future studies will need to mimic the actual concentrations of the drug (and its metabolites) in the liver of patients. That the toxicity is so uncommon and is not dose-dependent suggests that direct toxicity of the drug is not a primary mechanism of cell injury.

In premarketing studies, 1.9% of patients with elevated transaminases (vs. 0.6% for placebo) were identified, but this abnormality was reversible when the drug was stopped. Two patients became jaundiced, but they also recovered fully (246). Liver biopsies in two patients showed hepatocellular injury. It was only with the larger postmarketing surveillance that further evidence of liver injury was determined. Initially it was hoped that increasingly stringent monitoring of liver tests and discontinuation of therapy on detecting abnormal values would prevent hepatic injury. However, with the advent of two other drugs in the same class (pioglitazone and rosiglitazone), apparently without adverse hepatic effects, troglitazone was removed from the market.

Since the two above-mentioned new drugs in the thiazolidinedione class have some of the same structure as troglitazone, patients are monitored with liver tests to detect early hepatic dysfunction. Indeed two patients have been reported with presumed hepatic damage due to rosiglitazone (255,256). In one of these, in our view, the evidence for this is good (255). Interestingly, in both patients onset of liver damage was within only 3 weeks of start of therapy. Further postmarketing surveillance will be important. It is uncertain whether there will be cross-reactivity between prior hepatic damage from troglitazone and any subsequent use of the new drugs. At present, prior development of severe liver disease (i.e., jaundice) with troglitazone is considered a contraindication to therapy with the other thiazolidinedione agents (257,258). Even with milder injury, major caution would seem warranted to prevent any possible anamnestic (hypersensitivity) reaction. It is advised that in patients with mild prior liver disease (common in diabetes), both pioglitazone and rosiglitazone be used cautiously with early and frequent monitoring of tests (257,258). While underlying liver disease is not believed to enhance the risk of most hepatotoxic idiosyncratic reactions (259,260), detection of early drug-induced injury may be more difficult in this setting (259); hence this admonition seems reasonable. Very recently, however, a patient with prior severe troglitazone-induced hepatitis and recovery was retreated with rosiglitazone without recurrence of liver injury (261). Further information in this area will be of importance.

VI. GLUCOCORTICOIDS

The main adverse effect of corticosteroids on the normal liver may be deposition of fat (262). This information is based primarily on studies in experimental animals and apparently depends on increased flux of lipids from fat depots to the liver (263). This seldom is a clinical problem, except in the few cases where it appeared to lead to fat emboli to various organs (264).

Corticosteroids may also affect the diseased liver in a salutary manner. They decrease inflammation and necrosis, enhance albumin synthesis in patients with autoimmune hepatitis (265), and are beneficial in patients with severe (high discriminating index) alcoholic hepatitis (266). Corticosteroids have also been used in patients with hepatic sarcoidosis, assumed to be an autoimmune granulomatous process, and in selected patients with severe, hypersensitivity-type, drug reactions. The benefit of corticosteroids in these latter conditions is not established, but theoretically makes sense.

VII. ANTITHYROID DRUGS

A. General Comments

Thyroid hormones are synthesized by iodination of tyrosine residues on thyroglobulin within the lumen of thyroid follicles. The thyroglobulin is endocytosed and thyroxine (T_4) and triiodotyronine (T_3) are secreted. Synthesis and secretion of T_3 and T_4 are regulated by thyrotropin and influenced by plasma iodine. Thyroid hormones increase metabolism by modulating the actions of insulin, glucagon, glucocorticoids, and catecholamines. They also have a critical role in the growth and development of bones and the central nervous system. Thyroid hormones are degraded by deiodination, deamination, and conjugation with glucuronide and sulfate. This occurs mainly in the liver and the free and conjugated forms are excreted partly in the bile and partly in urine (267).

Hepatic dysfunction has been reported with a number of antithyroid medications in current use, but also may be seen with thyroid disease per se. Thus, patients with hyperthyroidism may rarely manifest increased transaminases, elevated bilirubin, as well as abnormal alkaline phosphatase, GGT, and even prothrombin time (268–270). Jaundice is rare (271). Hepatic dysfunction is especially evident when thyrotoxicosis causes congestive heart failure with hepatic congestion. Hypothyroidism also rarely increases transaminases (270). These intrinsic abnormalities in the liver due to thyroid disease must be differentiated from the adverse effects of antithyroid drugs.

B. Drug-Induced Injury

The five main agents used to treat hyperthyroidism are thiouracil, methylthiouracil, methimazole, carbimazole, and propylthiouracil. The former four drugs usually cause cholestasis (272,273), while propylthiouracil primarily affects hepatocellular function (274).

Severe cases of liver injury (i.e., jaundice) resulting from these agents are rare. They may develop within 1–3 months of starting therapy and may be accompanied by evidence of hypersensitivity with fever, rash, lymphadenopathy, and eosinophilia. Bone marrow depression and agranulocytosis may accompany the hepatic dysfunction (275–277), and may contribute to a fatal outcome. These features of hypersensitivity, in addition to an occasional positive response to the lymphocyte stimulation test in vitro (278,279), have suggested that the mechanism is likely to be one of idiosyncratic hypersensitivity. Moreover, minor increases of transaminase have been reported in as many as one-third of patients receiving propylthiouracil (280), and this seemed to abate despite continuation of the drug, albeit at a lower dose. This may then be similar to other agents (i.e., isoniazid) that may have some mild intrinsic toxicity that can then result in adaptation without injury, or in susceptible individuals may translate into clinically significant liver injury. The main issue, of course, is to be able to predict in advance which patients are susceptible to injury and in the absence of this to detect an early injury in the reversible stage. These two considerations are the main challenge in drug-induced liver injury, in general, and will require ongoing research for a possible solution.

DEDICATION

The authors dedicate this review to the late Hyman J. Zimmerman, whose encyclopedic knowledge, and enthusiasm for this field, has been a guide in our endeavors.

ACKNOWLEDGMENT

The authors greatly appreciate the help of Mrs. Anne Mundy in compiling this review.

REFERENCES

1. Goldfien A. The gonadal hormones and inhibitors. In: BG Katzung, ed. Basic and Clinical Pharmacology. 5th ed. Chap. 39. Norwalk, CT: Appleton & Lange, 1992:552–585.
2. Beato M. Gene regulation by steroid hormones. Cell 1989; 56:335–344.
3. Kalkhoff RK. Metabolic effects of progesterone. Am J Obstet Gynecol 1982; 142:735–738.
4. Bikle DD, Halloran BP, Harris ST, Portale AA. Progestin antagonism of estrogen-stimulated 1.25-dihydroxyvitamin D levels. J Clin Endocrinol Metab 1992; 75:519–523.
5. Elias H, Schwinner D. The hepatotoxic action of diethylstilbestrol with report of a case. Am J Med Sci 1945; 209:602.
6. Eisalo A, Jarvinen PA, Luukkainen T. Hepatic impairment during the intake of contraceptive pills: clinical trial with postmenopausal women. Br Med J 1964; 2:426–427.
7. Roman W, Hecker R. The liver toxicity of oral contraceptives, a critical review of the literature. Med J Aust 1968; 2:682–688.
8. Ticktin HE, Zimmerman HJ. Effects of a synthetic anabolic agent on hepatic function. Am J Med Sci 1966; 251:674–684.
9. Dalen E, Westerholm B. Occurrence of hepatic impairment in women jaundiced by oral contraceptives and their mothers and sisters. Acta Med Scand 1974; 195:459–463.
10. Haemmarli UP, Wyss HI. Recurrent intrahepatic cholestasis of pregnancy. Report of six cases, and review of the literature. Medicine (Baltimore) 1967; 46:299–321.
11. Holtzbach RT, Sivak DA, Braun WE. Familial recurrent intrahepatic cholestasis of pregnancy: a genetic study providing evidence for transmission of sex-limited, dominant trait. Gastroenterology 1983; 85:175–179.
12. Schaffner F. The effect of oral contraceptives on the liver. JAMA 1966; 198:1019–1021.
13. Lieberman DA, Keeffe EB, Stenzel P. Severe and prolonged oral contraceptive jaundice. J Clin Gastroenterol 1984; 6:145–148.
14. Metreau JM, Dhumeaux D, Berthelot P. Oral contraceptives and the liver. Digestion 1972; 7:318–335.
15. Farrell GC. Drug-induced cholestasis. In: Drug-Induced Liver Disease. Chap. 14. London: Churchill Livingstone, 1994:331.
16. Schiff ER, Sorrell MF, Maddrey WC, eds. Schiff's Diseases of the Liver. 8th ed. Vol. 3. Philadelphia: Lippincott-Raven, 1999:994.
17. Zimmerman HJ. In: Hepatotoxicity: The Adverse Effects of Drugs and Other Chemicals on the Liver. 2nd ed. Chap 20. Philadelphia: Lippincott Williams & Wilkins, 1999.
18. Phillips MJ, Poucell S, Oda M. Mechanisms of cholestasis. Lab Invest 1986; 54:593–608.
19. Perez V, Gorosdisch S, De Martire J, Nicholson R, Di Paola G. Oral contraceptives: long-term use produce fine structural changes in liver mitochondria. Science 1969; 165:805–807.
20. Gallagher TF Jr, Mueller MN, Kappas A. Estrogen pharmacology. IV. Studies of the structural basis for estrogen-induced impairment of liver function. Medicine (Baltimore) 1966; 45:471–479.
21. Zimmerman HJ, Lewis JH. Drug-induced cholestasis. Med Toxicol 1987; 2:112–160.
22. Stricker BHC. Hepatic injury by drugs and environmental agents. In: Arias M, Frenkel M, Wilson JHP, eds. The Liver Annual: a series of critical surveys of the international literature. Chap. 16. Amsterdam: Elsevier, 1986:419–482.
23. Mueller MN, Kappas A. Estrogen pharmacology. I. The influence of estradiol and estriol on hepatic disposal of sulfobromophthalein (BPS) in man. J Clin Invest 1964; 43:1905–1914.
24. Scherb J, Kirschner M, Arias I. Studies of hepatic excretory function: the effect of 17α-

ethyl-19-nortestosterone on sulfobromophthalein sodium (BSP) metabolism in man. J Clin Invest 1963; 42:404–408.

25. Gallagher TF Jr, Mueller MN, Kappas A. Estrogen pharmacology. IV. Studies on the structural basis for estrogen-induced impairment of liver function. Medicine 1966; 45:471–479.

26. Meyers M, Slikker W, Pascoe G, Vore M. Characterization of cholestasis induced by estradiol-17 beta-D-glucuronide in the rat. J Pharmacol Exp Ther 1980; 214:87–93.

27. Baker TS, Jennison KM, Kellie AE. The direct radioimmunoassay of oestrogen glucuronides in human female urine. Biochem J 1979; 177:729–738.

28. Adlercreutz H, Tikkanen MJ, Wichmann K, Svanborg A, Anberg A. Recurrent jaundice in pregnancy. IV. Quantitative determination of urinary and biliary estrogens, including studies in pruritus gravidarum. J Clin Endocrinol Metab 1974; 38:51–57.

29. Farrell GC. Drug-induced cholestasis. In: Drug-Induced Liver Disease. Chap. 14. London: Churchill Livingstone, 1994:332.

30. Chiarantine E, Arcangeli A, Mazzanti R, Romagnoli P, Moscarella S, Gentiline P. Ethinyl estradiol induced cholestasis. Morphological and functional aspects. In: P Gentilini, H Popper, S Sherlock, et al, eds. Problems in Intrahepatic Cholestasis. Second International Symposium on Intrahepatic Cholestasis, Florence (1978). Basel: S Karger, 1979:102–110.

31. Schwenk M, del Pino VL. Uptake of estrone sulfate by isolated rat liver cells. J Steroid Biochem 1980; 3:669–673.

32. Berr F, Simon FR, Reichen J. Ethynylestradiol impairs bile salt uptake and Na-K pump function of rat hepatocytes. Am J Physiol 1984; 147:G437–G443.

33. Meier PJ, Sztul ES, Reuben A, Boyer JL. Structural and functional polarity of canalicular and basolateral plasma membrane vesicles isolated in high yield from rat liver. J Cell Biol 1984; 98:991–1000.

34. Ruetz S, Fricker G, Hugentobler G, Winterhalter K, Kurz G, Meier PJ. Isolation and characterization of the putative canalicular bile salt transport system of rat liver. J Biol Chem 1987; 262:11324–11330.

35. Adachi Y, Kobayashi H, Mika Y, Kurumi Y, Shouji M, Kitano M, Yamamoto T. ATP-dependent taurocholate transport by rat liver canalicular membrane vesicles. Hepatology 1991; 14:655–659.

36. Nishida T, Gatmaitan Z, Che M, Arias IM. Rat liver canalicular membrane vesicles contain an ATP-dependent bile acid transport system. Proc Natl Acad Sci USA 1991; 8:6590–6594.

37. Lee JM, Frauner M, Soioka CJ, Stieger B, Meier PJ, Boyer JL. Expression of the bile salt export pump is maintained after chronic cholestasis in the rat. Gastroenterology 2000; 118: 163–172.

38. Klaassen CD. Watkins JB. Mechanisms of bile formation, hepatic uptake and biliary excretion. Pharmacol Rev 1984; 36:1–67.

39. Reichen J, Simon FR. Mechanisms of cholestasis. Int Rev Exp Pathol 1984; 26:231–274.

40. Tuchweber B, Weber A, Roy CC, Yousef IM. Mechanisms of experimentally induced intrahepatic cholestasis. Prog Liver Dis 1986; 8:161–178.

41. Schreiber AJ, Simon FR. Estrogen-induced cholestasis: clues to pathogenesis and treatment [review]. Hepatology 1983; 3:607–613.

42. Keeffe EB, Blankenship NM, Scharschmidt BF. Alteration of rat liver plasma membrane fluidity and ATPase activity by chlorpromazine hydrochloride and its metabolites. Gastroenterology 1980; 79:222–231.

43. Boelsterli UA, Rakhit G, Balazs T. SAMe modulates bile flow in estrogen-induced cholestasis. Hepatology 1983; 3:12–17.

44. Farrell GC. Drug-induced cholestasis. In: Drug-Induced Liver Disease. Chap. 14. London: Churchill Livingstone, 1994:334.

45. Bossard R, Stieger B, O'Neill B, Fricker G, Meier PJ. Ethinylestradiol treatment induces multiple canalicular membrane transport alterations in rat liver. J Clin Invest 1993; 91:2714–2720.

46. Huang L, Smit JW, Meijer DKF, Vore M. Mrp2 is essential for estradiol-17β(β-D-glucuronide)-induced cholestasis in rats. Hepatology 2000; 32:66–72.

47. Gumucio JJ, Valdivieso VD. Studies on the mechanism of the ethynylestradiol impairment of bile flow and bile salt excretion in the rat. Gastroenterology 1971; 61:339–344.

48. Stramentinoli G, Gualano M, Di Padova C. Effect of S-adenosyl-L-methionine on ethynylestradiol-induced impairment of bile flow in female rats. Experientia 1977; 33:1361–1362.

49. Davis RA, Kern F Jr, Showalter R, Sutherland E, Sinesky M, Simon FR. Alterations of hepatic Na$^+$, K$^+$-ATPase and bile flow by estrogen: effects on liver surface membrane lipid structure and function. Proc Natl Acad Sci USA 1978; 75:4130–4134.

50. Wolfhagen FHJ, Sternieri E, Hop WCS, Vitale G, Bertolotti M, Van Buren HR. Oral naltrexone treatment for cholestatic pruritus: A double blind placebo-controlled study. Gastroenterology 1997; 113:1264–1269.

51. Hoffman AF. Bile acid hepatotoxicity and the rationale of UDCA therapy in chronic cholestatic liver disease: some hypotheses. In: G Paumgartner, A Stiehl, L Barbara, E Roda, Eds. Strategies of the Treatment of Hepatobiliary Diseases. Dordrecht, The Netherlands: Kluwer Academic, 1990:13–33.

52. Boelsterli UA, Rakhit G, Balazs T. Modulation by S-Adenosyl-L-methionine of hepatic Na$^+$, K$^+$-ATPase, membrane fluidity and bile flow in rats with ethinyl estradiol-induced cholestasis. Hepatology 1983; 3:12–17.

53. Ribalta J, Reyes H, Gonzalez MC, Inglesias J, Arrese M, Poniachik J, Molina C, Segoiva N. S-adenosyl-L-methionine in the treatment of patients with intrahepatic cholestasis of pregnancy: a randomized, double-blind, placebo-controlled study with negative results. Hepatology 1991; 13:1084–1089.

54. Frezza M, Pozzato G, Chiesa L, Stramentinoli G, diPadova C. Reversal of intrahepatic cholestasis of pregnancy in women after high dose S-adenosyl-L-methionine administration. Hepatology 1984; 4:274–278.

55. Reyes H. The enigma of intrahepatic cholestasis of pregnancy: lessons from Chile. Hepatology 1982; 2:87–96.

56. Meng L-J, Reyes H, Axelson M, Palma J, Hernandez I, Ribalta J, Sjovall J. Progesterone metabolites and bile acids in serum of patients with intrahepatic cholestrasis of pregnancy: effect of ursodeoxycholic acid therapy. Hepatology 1997; 26:1573–1579.

57. Jacquemin E, Cresteil D, Manouvrier S, Boute O, Hadchouel M. Heterozygous nonsense mutation of the *MDR3* gene in familial intrahepatic cholestasis of pregnancy. Lancet 1999; 353:210–211.

58. Iglesias J, Galan G, Guerrero B, Herrera R, Mayorga L, Miller MF, Olguin O, Ovalle A, Pardo H, Silva O, Testa E, Varleta J, Veloso A, Prudencio E. Fetal maturity tests, resolution of labor and results concerning the newborn infant in 91 cases of intrahepatic cholestasis in pregnancy. Rev Chil Obstet Ginecol 1976; 41:278–284.

59. Rioseco AJ, Ivankovic MB, Manzur A, Hamed F, Kato SR, Parer JT, Germain AM. Intrahepatic cholestasis of pregnancy: a retrospective case-control study of perinatal outcome. Am J Obstet Gynecol 1996; 175:957–960.

60. Alsulyman OM, Ouzounian JG, Ames-Castro M, Goodwin TM. Intrahepatic choleastasis of pregnancy: Perinatal outcome associated with expectant management. Am J Obstet Gynecol 1996; 175:957–960.

61. Leslie KK, Reznikov L, Simon FR, Fennessey PV, Reyes H, Ribalta J. Estrogens in intrahepatic cholestasis of pregnancy. Obstet Gynecol 2000; 95:372–376.

62. Heikkinen J, Maentausta O, Ylustalo P, Janne O. Changes in serum bile acid concentrations during normal pregnancy, in patients with intrahepatic cholestasis of pregnancy and in pregnant women with itching. Br J Obstet Gynecol 1981; 88:240–245.

63. Agyogi T, Lowenstein LM. The effect of bile acids and renal ischemia on renal function. J Lab Clin Med 1968; 71:686–692.

64. Boston Collaborative Drug Surveillance Program. Surgically confirmed gallbladder disease,

venous-thromboembolism, and breast tumors in relation to postmenopausal estrogen therapy. N Engl J Med 1974; 290:15–19.

65. Leissner KH, Wedel H, Schersten T. Comparison between the use of oral contraceptives and the incidence of surgically confirmed gallstone disease. Scand J Gastroenterol 1977; 12:893–896.

66. Maringhini A, Ciambra M, Baccelliere P, Raimondo M, Orlando A, Tine F, Grasso R, Randazzo MA, Barresi L, Gullo D, Musico M, Pagliaro L. Biliary sludge and gallstones in pregnancy: incidence, risk factors, and natural history. Ann Intern Med 1993; 119:116–120.

67. Bennion LJ, Ginsberg RL, Gernick MB, Bennett PH. Effects of oral contraceptives on the gallbladder bile of normal women. N Engl J Med 1976; 294:189–192.

68. Henriksson P, Einarsson K, Eriksson A, Kelter U, Angelin B. Estrogen-induced gallstone formation in males: Relation to changes in serum and biliary lipids during hormonal treatment of prostatic carcinoma. J Clin Invest 1989; 84:811–816.

69. Kern F Jr, Everson GT, DeMark B, McKinley C, Showalter R, Erfling W, Braverman DZ, Szczepanik-Van Leeuwen P, Klein DP. Biliary lipids, bile acids and gall bladder function in the human female: effects of pregnancy and the ovulatory cycle. J Clin Invest 1981; 68:1229–1242.

70. Everson GT, McKinley C, Lawson M, Johnson M, Kern F Jr. Gallbladder function in the human female: effect of the ovulatory cycle, pregnancy and contraceptive steroids. Gastroenterology 1982; 82:711–719.

71. Edmondson HA. Tumors of the liver and intrahepatic bile ducts. In: Atlas of Tumor Pathology, Sect 7, Fasc 25. Washington, DC: AFIP, 1958:193–206.

72. Rooks JB, Ory HW, Ishak KG, Strauss LT, Greenspan JR, Hill AP, Tyler CW Jr. The Cooperative Liver Tumor Study Group. Epidemiology of hepatocellular adenoma: the role of oral contraceptive use. JAMA 1979; 242:644–648.

73. Benhamou JP. Diagnostic approach to a liver mass: diagnosis of an asymptomatic liver tumor in a young woman. J Hepatol 1996; 25(suppl):30–34.

74. Cherqui D, Rahmouni A, Charlotte F, Boulahdour H, Metreau JM, Meignan M, Fagniez PL, Zafrani ES, Mathieu D, Dhumeaux D. Management of focal nodular hyperplasia and hepatocellular adenoma in young women: a series of 41 patients with clinical, radiological, and pathological correlations. Hepatology 1995; 22:1674–1981.

75. Sturvetant FM. Oral contraceptives and liver tumors. In: KS Moghissi, ed. Controversies in Contraception. Baltimore: Williams & Wilkins, 1979:93–150.

76. Klatskin G. Hepatic tumors: possible relationship to use of oral contraceptives. Gastroenterology 1977; 73:386–394.

77. Edmondson HA, Henderson B, Benton B. Liver-cell adenomas associated with use of oral contraceptives. N Engl J Med 1976; 294:470–472.

78. Keefer WS Jr, Scott JC. Liver neoplasms and oral contraceptives. Am J Obstet Gynecol 1977; 128:448–454.

79. Kerlin P, Davis GL, McGill DB, Weiland LH, Adson MA, Sheedy PF 2d. Hepatic adenoma and focal nodular hyperplasia: clinical, pathologic, and radiologic features. Gastroenterology 1983; 84:994–1002.

80. Neuberger JM, Davis M, Williams R. Clinical aspects of oral contraceptive-associated liver tumors. In: M Davis, JM Tredger, R Williams, eds. Drug Reactions and the Liver. Bath, UK: Pittman Medical, 1981:271–283.

81. Rubin RA, Lichtenstein GR. Hepatic scintigraphy in the evaluation of solitary solid liver masses. J Nuclear Med 1993; 34:697–705.

82. Lubbers P, Ros P, Goodman Z, Ishak K. Accumulation of technetium-99m sulfur colloid by hepatocellular adenoma: scintigraphic-pathologic correlation. AJR 1987; 148:1105–1108.

83. De Carlis L, Pirotta V, Rondinara G, Sansalone CV, Colella G, Maione G, Slim AO, Rampaldi A, Cazzulani A, Belli L, Forti D. Hepatic adenoma and focal nodular hyperplasia: diagnosis and criteria for treatment. Liver Transplant Surg 1997; 3:160–165.

84. Mathieu D, Rahmouni A, Anglade MC, Falise B, Beges C, Gheung P, Mollet JJ, Vasile N. Focal nodular hyperplasia of the liver: Assessment with contrast-enhanced TurboFLASH MR imaging. Radiology 1991; 180:25–30.

85. Chung KY, Mayo-Smith WW, Saini S, Rahmouni A, Golli M, Mathieu D. Hepatocellular adenoma: MR imaging features with pathologic correlation. AJR 1995; 165:303–308.

86. Wanless I, Medline A. Role of estrogens as promoters of hepatic neoplasia. Lab Invest 1982; 46:313–320.

87. Eisenfeld AJ, Aten RF. Estrogen receptors and androgen receptors in the mammalian liver. J Steroid Biochem 1987; 27:1109–1118.

88. Masood S, West B, Barwick K. Expression of steroid hormone receptors in benign hepatic tumors: an immunocytochemical study. Arch Pathol Lab Med 1992; 116:1355–1359.

89. Bianchi L. Glycogen storage disease I and hepatocellular tumors. Eur J Pediatr 1993; 152(suppl 1):S63–S70.

90. Edmonson H, Reynolds T, Henderson B, Brenton B. Regression of liver cell adenomas associated with oral contraceptives. Ann Intern Med 1977; 86:180–182.

91. Klatskin G. Hepatic tumors: possible relationship to use of oral contraceptives. Gastroenterology 1977; 73:386–394.

92. Leese T, Farges O, Bismuth H. Liver cell adenomas. Ann Surg 1988; 208:558–564.

93. Gordon SC, Reddy KR, Livingston AS, Jeffers LJ, Schiff ER. Resolution of a contraceptive-steroid-induced hepatic adenoma with subsequent evolution into hepatocellular carcinoma. Ann Intern Med 1986; 105:547–549.

94. Shortell C, Schwartz S. Hepatic adenoma and focal nodular hyperplasia. Surg Gynecol Obstet 1991; 173:426–431.

95. Christensen SE, Andersen VR, Vilstrup H. A case of hepatoma in pregnancy associated with earlier oral contraception. Acta Obstet Gynecol Scand 1981; 60:519.

96. Molina EG, Schiff ER. Benign solid lesions of the liver. In: ER Schiff, MF Sorrell, WC Maddrey, eds. Schiff's Diseases of the Liver. 8th ed. Chap. 53. Philadelphia: Lippincott Raven Publishers, 1999:1245–1267.

97. Jenkins R, Johnson L, Lewis D. Surgical approach to benign liver tumors. Semin Liver Dis 1994; 14:178–189.

98. Eckhauser F, Knol J, Raper S, Thompson N. Enucleation combined with hepatic vascular exclusion in a safe and effective alternative to hepatic resection for liver cell adenoma. Am Surg 1994; 50:466–472.

99. Labrune P, Trioche P, Duvaltier I, Chevalier P, Odievre M. Hepatocellular adenomas in glycogen storage disease type I and III: a series of 43 patients and review of the literature. J Pediatr Gastroenterol Nutr 1997; 24:276–279.

100. Arsenault T, Johnson D, Gorman B, Burgart L. Hepatic adenomatosis. Mayo Clin Proc 1996; 71:478–480.

101. Wheeler PG, Melia W, Dubbins P, Jones B, Nunnerley H, Johnson P. Nonoperative arterial embolisation in primary liver tumors Br Med J 1979; 2:242–244.

102. Ault G, Wren S, Ralls PW, Reynolds TB, Stain SC. Selective management of hepatic adenomas. Am Surg 1996; 62:825–829.

103. Buhler H, Pirovino M, Akovbiantz A, Altorfer J, Weitzel M, Maranta E, Schmid M. Regression of liver cell adenoma: a follow up study of three consecutive patients after discontinuation of oral contraceptive use. Gastroenterology 1982; 82:775–782.

104. Foster J, Berman M. The malignant transformation of liver cell adenomas. Arch Surg 1994; 129:712–717.

105. Wanless I, Mawdsley C, Adams R. On the pathogenesis of focal nodular hyperplasia of the liver. Hepatology 1985; 5:1194–1200.

106. Wanless I. Micronodular transformation (nodular regenerative hyperplasia) of the liver: a report of 64 cases among 2500 autopsies and a new classification of benign hepatocellular nodules. Hepatology 1990; 11:787–797.

107. Weimann A, Ringe B, Klempnauer J, Lamesch P, Gratz KF, Prokop M, Maschek H, Tusch G, Pichlmayr R. Benign liver tumors: differential diagnosis and indications of surgery. World J Surg 1997; 21:982–991.

108. Flejou JF, Pignon JP, Le MG, Belghite J, Barge J, Bismuth H Benhamou JP. Liver cell adenoma, focal nodular hyperplasia and oral contraceptive use: a French case-control study in young women. Hepatology 1994; 20:S280A (abstr).

109. Pain JA, Gimson AE, Williams R, Howard ER. Focal nodular hyperplasia of the liver: results of treatment and options in management. Gut 1991; 32:524–527.

110. Mathieu D, Kobeiter H, Maison P, Rahmouni A, Cherqui D, Zafrani ES, Dhumeaux D. Oral contraceptive use and focal nodular hyperplasia of the liver. Gastroenterology 2000; 118: 560–564.

111. Ishak KG, Rabin L. Benign tumors of the liver. Med Clin North Am 1975; 59:995–1013.

112. Ndimbie OK, Goodman ZD, Chase RL, Ma CK, Lee MW. Hemangiomas with localized nodular proliferation: a suggestion on the pathogenesis of focal nodular hyperplasia. Am J Surg Pathol 1990; 14:142–150.

113. Haber M, Reuben A, Burrell M, Oliveris P, Salem RR, West AB. Multiple focal nodular hyperplasia of the liver associated with hemihypertrophy and vascular malformations. Gastroenterology 1995; 108:1256–1262.

114. Edmondson H, Henderson B, Benton B. Liver-cell adenomas associated with use of oral contraceptives. N Engl J Med 1976; 294:470–472.

115. Rogers JV, Mack LA, Freeny PC, Johnson ML, Sones PJ. Hepatic focal nodular hyperplasia: angiography, CT, sonography, and scintigraphy. AJR 1981; 137:983–990.

116. Stauffer JQ, Lapinski MW, Honold DJ, Myers JK. Focal nodular hyperplasia of the liver and intrahepatic hemorrhage in young women on oral contraceptives. Ann Intern Med 1975; 83:301–306.

117. Pain J, Gimson A, Wiliams R, Howard E. Focal nodular hyperplasia of the liver: results of treatment and options in management. Gut 1991; 24:345–350.

118. Di Stasi M, Caturelli E, De Sio I, Salmi A, Buscarini E, Buscarini L. Natural history of focal nodular hyperplasia of the liver: an ultrasound study. J Clin Ultrasound 1996; 24:345–350.

119. Cote C. Regression of focal nodular hyperplasia of the liver after oral contraceptive discontinuation. Clin Nucl Med 1997; 22:587–590.

120. Ishak KG. Benign tumors and pseudotumors of the liver. Appl Pathol 1988; 6:82–104.

121. Barrows GH, Christopherson WM. Human liver tumors in relation to steroidal usage. Environ Health Perspect 1983; 50:201–208.

122. Thalassinos NC, Lymberatos C, Hadjioannou J, Gardikas C. Liver-cell carcinoma after long-term estrogen-like drugs. Lancet 1974; 1:270.

123. O'Sullivan JP, Rosswick RP (letter). Oral contraceptives and malignant hepatic tumours. Lancet 1976; 1:1124–1125.

124. Vana J, Murphy GP. Primary malignant liver tumors: association with oral contraceptives. NY State J Med 1979; 79:321–325.

125. Tesluk H, Lawrie J. Hepatocellular adenoma. Its transformation to carcinoma in a user of oral contraceptives. Arch Pathol Lab Med 1981; 105:296–299.

126. Porter JB, Jick H, Ylvisaker JT. Malignant liver tumor associated with oral contraceptive use. Pharmacotherapy 1981; 1:160.

127. Littlewood ER, Barrison IG, Murray-Lyon IM, Paradinas FJ. Cholangiocarcinoma and oral contraceptives. Lancet 1980; 1:310–311.

128. Helling TS, Wood WG. Oral contraceptives and cancer of the liver: a review with two additional cases. Am J Med 1982; 77:504–508.

129. Shar SR, Kew MC. Oral contraceptives and hepatocellular carcinoma. Cancer 1982; 49:407–410.

130. Stanford JL, Ray RM, Thomas DB. Combined oral contraceptives and liver cancer: the WHO collaborative study of neoplasia and steroid contraceptives. Int J Cancer 1989; 43:254–259.

131. Neuberger J, Forman D, Doll R, Williams R. Oral contraceptives and hepatocellular carcinoma. Br Med J 1986; 292:1355–1357.

132. Henderson BE, Preston-Martin S, Edmondson HA, Peters RL, Pike MC. Hepatocellular carcinoma and oral contraceptives. Br J Cancer 1983; 48:437–440.

133. La Vecchia C, Negri E, Parazzini F. Oral contraceptives and primary liver cancer. Br J Cancer 1989; 59:460–461.

134. Palmer JR, Rosenberg L, Kaufman DW, Warshauer ME, Stolley P, Shapiro S. Oral contraceptives use and liver cancer. Am J Epidemiol 1989; 130:878–882.

135. Terpstra OT, ten Kate FJ, van Urk H. Long-term survival after resection of a hepatocellular carcinoma with lymph node metastasis and discontinuation of oral contraceptives. Am J Gastroenterol 1984; 79:474–478.

136. Forman D, Vincent TJ, Doll R. Cancer of the liver and the use of oral contraceptives. Br Med J 1986; 292:1357–1361.

137. Stubblefield PG. Oral contraceptives and neoplasia. J Reprod Med 1984; 29:524–529.

138. Brosens I, Johannisson E, Baulieu EE, Benagiano G, Cooke ID, Goldzicher JW. Oral contraceptives and hepatocellular carcinoma. Br Med J 1986; 292:1667–1668.

139. Persson I, Yuen J, Bergkvist L, Schairer C. Cancer incidence and mortality in women receiving estrogen-replacement therapy—long-term follow-up of a Swedish cohort. Int J Cancer 1996; 67:327–332.

140. Iverson D-E, Thoresen SO. Oral contraceptives and hepatocellular carcinoma. Br Med J 1986; 292:1668.

141. Kostrubsky VE, Vore M, Kindt E, Burliegh J, Rogers K, Peter G, Atlrogge D, Sinz MW. The effect of troglitazone biliary excretion on metabolite distribution and cholestasis in transporter-deficient rats. Drug Metab Disp 2001; 29:1561–1566.

142. Sontaniemi EA, Alvaikko MJ, Kaipainen WJ. Primary liver cancer associated with long-term oestrogen therapy. Ann Clin Res 1975; 7:287–289.

143. Rosinus V, Maurer R, Diethylstilbestrol-induced liver cancer. Schweiz Med Wochenschr 1981; 111:1139–1142.

144. Brooks JJ. Hepatoma associated with diethylstilbestrol therapy for prostatic carcinoma. J Urol 1982; 128:1044–1045.

145. Ham JM, Pirola RC, Crouch RL. Hemangioendothelial sarcoma of the liver associated with long-term estrogen therapy in a man. Dig Dis Sci 1980; 25:879–883.

146. Hoch-Ligeti C. Angiosarcoma of the liver associated with diethylstilbestrol. JAMA 1978; 240:1510–1511.

147. Monroe PS, Riddell RH, Siegler M, Baker AL. Hepatic angioscarcoma: possible relationship to long-term oral contraceptive ingestion. JAMA 1981; 246:64–65.

148. Maddrey WC. Hepatic vein thrombosis (Budd-Chiari syndrome): possible association with the use of oral contraceptives (review). Semin Liver Dis 1987; 7:32–39.

149. Valla D, Le MG, Poynard T, Zucman N, Rueff B, Benhamou JP. Risk of hepatic vein thrombosis in relation to recent use of oral contraceptives: a case-control study. Gastroenterology 1986; 90:807–811.

150. Valla D, Casadevall N, Lacombe C, Varet B, Goldwasser E, Franco D, Maillard JM, Pariente EA, Leporier M, Rueff B, et al. Primary myeloproliferative disorder and hepatic vein thrombosis. Ann Intern Med 1985; 103:329–334.

151. Zafrani ES, Pinaudeau Y, Dhumeaux D. Drug-induced vascular lesions of the liver. Arch Intern Med 1983; 143:495–502.

152. Minnema MC, Janssen HLA, Niermeijer P, deMan, RA. Budd-Chiari syndrome: Combination of genetic defects and the use of oral contraceptives leading to hypercoagulability. J Hepatol 2000; 33:509–512.

153. Orloff MJ, Daily PO, Orloff SL, Girard B, Orloff MS. A 27-year experience with surgical treatment of Budd-Chiari syndrome. Ann Surg 2000; 232:340–352.

154. Michl P, Bilzer M, Waggershauser T, Giilberg V, Rau GH, Reiser M, Gerbes AL. Successful

treatment of chronic Budd-Chiari syndrome with a transjugular intrahepatic portosystemic shunt. J Hepatol 2000; 32:516–520.

155. Reynolds TB. Budd-Chiari syndrome. In: L Schiff, ER Schiff, eds. Diseases of the Liver. 7th ed. Philadelphia: JB Lippincott, 1993:1091–1099.

156. Hobbs K. Hepatic hemangiomas. World J Surg 1990; 14:468–471.

157. Raufman JP, Miller DL, Gumucio JJ. Estrogen-induced zonal changes in rat liver sinusoids. Gastroenterology 1980; 79:1174–1177.

158. Schonberg LA. Peliosis hepatis and oral contraceptives. J Reprod Med 1982; 27:753–756.

159. Schenker S. Medical consequences of alcohol abuse: is gender a factor? Alcohol Clin Exp Res 1997; 21:179–181.

160. Deal SR, Gavaler JS. Are women more susceptible than men to alcohol-induced cirrhosis? Alcohol Health Res World 1994; 18:189–191.

161. Gavaler JS, Dorin AM. Increased susceptibility of women to alcoholic liver disease: artifactual or real? In: P Hall, ed. Alcoholic Liver Disease: Pathology and Pathogenesis. 2nd ed. London: Ed Arnold, 1995:123–137.

162. Schenker S, Bay MK. Medical problems associated with alcoholism. In: R Schrier, AS Fauci, eds. Advances in Internal Medicine. Vol. 43. Chicago: Mosby-Yearbook, 1998:27–48.

163. Becker V, Deis A, Sorensen TIA, Gronbock M, Borch-Johnson K, Muller CF, Schnohr P, Jensen G. Prediction of risk of liver disease by alcohol intake, sex and age: a prospective population study. Hepatology 1996; 23:1025–1029.

164. Iimuro Y, Frankenberg MU, Arteel GE, Bradford BU, Wall CA, Thurman RG. Female rats exhibit greater susceptibility to early alcohol-induced injury than males. Am J Physiol Gastrointest Liver Physiol 1997; 272:G1186–G1194.

165. Enomoto N, Schemmer P, Rivera CA, Bradford BU, Enomato A, Brenner DA, Thurman RG. Estriol sensitizes rat Kupffer cells by increasing permeability to gut-derived endotoxin. Gastroenterology 1999; 116:LO121 (abstr).

166. Ikejima K, Enomato N, Iimuro Y, Ikejima A, Fang D, Xu J, Forman DT, Brenner DA, Thurman RG. Estrogen increases sensitivity of hepatic Kupffer cells in endotoxin. Am J Physiol 1998; 274:G669–G676.

167. Thurman RG. II. Alcoholic liver injury involves activation of Kupffer cells by endotoxin [review]. Am J Physiol 1998; 275:G605–G611.

168. Grimbert S, Fisch C, Deschamps D. Effects of female sex hormones on mitochondria. Am J Physiol 1995; 268:G107–G115.

169. Grimbert S, Fromenty B, Fisch C. Decreased mitochondrial oxidation of fatty acids in pregnant mice. Hepatology 1993; 17:628–637.

170. Laine K, Palovaara S, Tapanainen P, Manninen P. Plasma tacrine concentrations are significantly increased by concomitant hormone replacement therapy. Clin Pharmacol Ther 1999; 66:602–608.

171. Patwardhan RV, Desmond PV, Johnson RF, Schenker S. Impaired elimination of caffeine by oral contraceptive steroids. J Lab Clin Med 1980; 95:603–608.

172. Mitchell MC, Hanew T, Meredith CG, Schenker S. Effects of oral contraceptive steroids on acetaminophen metabolism and elimination. Clin Pharmacol Ther 1983; 34:48–53.

173. Werner SC, Hanger FM, Kritzler RA. Jaundice during methyltestosterone therapy. Am J Med 1950; 8:325–331.

174. Pecking A, Lejolly JM, Najean Y. Liver toxicity of androgen therapy in aplastic anemia. Nouv Rev Fr Hematol 1980; 22:257–265.

175. Zimmerman HJ. Clinical and laboratory manifestations of hepatotoxicity. Ann NY Acad Sci 1963; 104:954–987.

176. Kosaka A, Takahashi H, Yajima Y, Tanaka M, Okamura K, Mizumoto R, Katsuta K. Hepatocellular carcinoma associated with anabolic steroids therapy: report of a case and review of the Japanese literature. J Gastroenterol 1996; 31:450–454.

177. Schaffner F, Popper H, Chesrow E. Cholestasis produced by the administration of norethandrolone. Am J Med 1959; 26:249–254.

178. Foss GL, Simpson SL. Oral methyltestosterone and jaundice. Br Med J 1959; 1:259–263.

179. Ishak KG, Zimmerman HJ. Hepatotoxic effects of the anabolic/androgenic steroids [review]. Semin Liver Dis 1987; 7:230–236.

180. Schaffner F, Popper H, Perez V. Changes in bile canaliculi produced by norethandrolone: electron microscopic study of human and rat liver. J Lab Clin Med 1960; 56:623–628.

181. Phillips MJ, Oda M, Funatsu K. Evidence for microfilament involvement in norethandrolone-induced intrahepatic cholestasis. Am J Pathol 1978; 93:729–744.

182. Schaffner F, Raisfeld IH. Drugs and the liver: a review of metabolism and adverse reactions [review]. Adv Intern Med 1969; 15:221–251.

183. Heaney RP, Whedon GD. Impairment of hepatic bromosulphalein clearance by two 17-substituted testosterones. J Lab Clin Med 1958; 52:169–175.

184. Leevy CM, Cherrick GR, Davidson CS. Observations of norethandrolone-induced abnormalities in plasma decay of sulfobromophthalein and indocyanine green. J Lab Clin Med 1961; 57:918–926.

185. Lennon HD. Relative effects of 17α-alkylated anabolic steroids on sulfobromophthalein (BSP) retention in rabbits. J Pharmacol Exp Ther 1966; 151:143–150.

186. Zimmerman HJ, Maddrey WC. Toxic and drug-induced hepatitis. In: L Schiff, ER Schiff, eds. Diseases of the Liver. 7th ed. Philadelphia: JB Lippincott, 1993:707–783.

187. Paumgartner G, Reichen J, von Bergmann K, Preisig R. Elaboration of hepatocytic bile [review]. Bull NY Acad Med 1976; 51:455–471.

188. Plaa GL, Priestly BG. Intrahepatic cholestasis induced by drugs and chemicals [review]. Pharmacol Rev 1976; 28:207–273.

189. Roberts RJ, Shriver SL, Plaa GL. Effect of norethandrolone on the biliary excretion of bilirubin in the mouse and rat. Biochem Pharmacol 1968; 17:1261–1268.

190. Gass GH, Umberger EJ. Lack of effect of two 17-substituted testosterones on hepatic sulfobromophthalein clearance in dogs. Toxicol Appl Pharmacol 1959; 1:545–547.

191. Somayaji BN, Paton A, Price JH, Harris AW, Flewett TH. Norethisterone jaundice in two sisters. Br Med J 1968; 2:281–283.

192. Farrell GC. Drug-induced cholestasis. In: Drug-Induced Liver Disease. Chap. 14. London: Churchill Livingstone, 1994:335.

193. Gilbert EF, DaSilva AQ, Queen DM. Intrahepatic cholestasis with fatal termination following norethandrolone therapy. JAMA 1963; 185:538–539.

194. Boyer JL. Androgenic-anabolic steroid associated peliosis hepatis in man—a review of 38 reported cases. Adv Pharmacol Ther 1978; 8:175–184.

195. Burger RA, Marcuse PM. Peliosis hepatis: report of case. Am J Clin Pathol 1952; 22:569–573.

196. Tsukamoto Y, Nakata H, Kimoto T, Noda T, Kuroda Y, Haratake J. CT and angiography of peliosis hepatis. Am J Roentgenol 1984; 142:539–540.

197. Nadell J, Kosek J. Peliosis hepatis. Twelve cases associated with oral androgen therapy. Arch Pathol Lab Med 1977; 101:405–410.

198. Lyon J, Bookstein JL, Cartwright CA, Romano A, Heeney DJ. Peliosis hepatis: diagnosis by magnification wedged hepatic venography. Radiology 1984; 150:647–649.

199. Westaby D, Williams R. Androgen and anabolic steroid-related liver tumors. In: M Davis, JM Tredger, R Williams, eds. Drug Reactions and the Liver. Bath, UK: Pittman, 1981:284–289.

200. Ishak KG. Hepatic neoplasms associated with contraceptive and anabolic steroids. Recent Results Cancer Res 1979; 66:73–128.

201. Lowdell CP, Murray-Lyon IM. Reversal of liver damage due to long term methyltestosterone and safety of non-17α-alkylated androgens. Br Med J 1985; 291:637.

202. McCaughan GW, Bilous MJ, Gallagher ND. Long-term survival with tumor regression in androgen-induced liver tumors. Cancer 1985; 56:2622–2626.

203. Bannister P, Sheridan P, Losowsky MS. Identification and characterization of the human hepatic androgen receptor. Clin Endocrinol 1985; 23:495–502.

204. Nagasue N, Ito A, Yukaya H, Ogawa Y. Androgen receptors in hepatocellular carcinoma and surrounding parenchyma. Gastroenterology 1985; 89:643–647.

205. Pelletier G, Frija J, Szekely AM, Clauvel JP. Adenoma of the liver in man. Gastroenterol Clin Biol 1984; 8:269–272.

206. Anthony PP. Hepatoma associated with androgenic steroids. Lancet 1975; 1:685–686.

207. Ching CK, Smith PG, Long RG. Tamoxifen-associated hepatocellular damage and agranulocytosis [letter]. Lancet 1992; 339:940.

208. Van Hoof M, Rahier J, Horsmans Y. Tamoxifen-induced steatohepatitis [letter]. Ann Intern Med 1996; 124:855–856.

209. Pratt DS, Knox TA, Erban J. Tamoxifen-induced steatohepatitis [letter]. Ann Intern Med 1996; 123:236.

210. Agrawal BL, Zelkowitz L. Bone "flare," hypercalcemia, and jaundice after tamoxifen therapy [letter]. Arch Intern Med 1981; 141:1240.

211. Blackburn AM, Amiel SA, Millis RR, Rubens RD. Tamoxifen and liver damage. Br Med J Clin Res Ed 1984; 289:288.

212. Cai Q, Bensen M, Greene R, Kirchner J. Tamoxifen-induced transient multifocal hepatic fatty infiltration. Am J Gastroenterol 200; 95:277–279.

213. Hamada N, Ogawa Y, Saibara T, Murata Y, Kariya S, Nishioka A, Terashima M, Inomata T, Yoshida S. Toremifene-induced fatty liver and NASH in breast cancer patients with breast-conservation treatment. Int J Oncol 2000; 17:1119–1123.

214. Olsson R, Tyllstrom J, Zettergren L. Hepatic reactions to cyclofenil. Gut 1983; 24:260–263.

215. Moller S, Iverson F, Franzmann MB. Flutamide-induced liver failure. J Hepatol 1990; 10:346–349.

216. Pescatore P, Hammel P, Durand F, Berthenu P, Beruau J, Huc D, Gerbal JL, Degott C, Benhamou JP. Fatal fulminant hepatitis induced by nilutamide (Anandron). Gastroenterol Clin Biol 1993; 17:499–501.

217. Blake JC, Sawyer AM, Dooley JS, Schouer PJ, McIntyre N. Severe hepatitis caused by cyproterone acetate. Gut 1990; 31:556–557.

218. Meijers WH, Willemse PH, Sleijfer DT, Mulder NH, Grond J. Hepatocellular damage by cyproterone acetate [letter]. Eur J Cancer Clin Oncol 1986; 22:1121.

219. Boue F, Coffin B, Delfraissay JF. Danazol and cholestatic hepatitis [letter]. Ann Intern Med 1986; 105:139–140.

220. Silva MO, Reddy KR, McDonald T, Jeffers LJ, Schiff ER. Danazol-induced cholestasis. Am J Gastroenterol 1989; 84:426–428.

221. Chevalier X, Awada H, Baetz A, Amor B. Danazol induced pancreatitis and hepatitis. Clin Rheumatol 1990; 9:239–241.

222. Babich MM, Pike I, Shiffman ML. Metformin-induced acute hepatitis. Am J Med 1998; 104:490–492.

223. Izumi T, Enomato S, Hosiyama K, Sasahara K, Stribukawa A, Nakagawa T, Sugiyama Y. Prediction of the human pharmacokinetics of troglitazone, a new and extensively metabolized antidiabetic agent, after oral administration, with an animal scale-up approach. J Pharmacol Exp Ther 1996; 277:1630–1641.

224. Yamazaki H, Shibata A, Suzuki M, Nakajima M, Shimada N, Guengerich FP, Yokoi T. Oxidation of troglitazone to a quinone-type metabolite catalyzed by cytochrome P-450 2C8 and P-450 3A4 in human liver microsomes. Drug Metab Dispos 1999; 27:1260–1266.

225. Ott P, Ranek L, Young MA. Pharmacokinetics of troglitazone, a PPAR-γ agonist, in patients with hepatic insufficiency. Eur J Clin Pharmacol 1998; 54:567–571.

226. Mezey E. Fatty liver. In: ER Schiff, MF Sorrell, WC Maddrey, eds. Schiff's Diseases of the Liver. 8th ed. Philadelphia: Lippencott-Raven, 1999:1185–1197.

227. Bacon BR, Farahvash MJ, Janney CG, Nauschwander-Tetri BA. Nonalcoholic steatohepatitis: an expended clinical entity. Gastroenterology 1994; 107:1103–1109.

228. Erbey JR, Silberman C, Lydick E. Prevalence of abnormal serum alanine aminotransferase levels in obese patients and patients with type 2 diabetes. Am J Med 2000; 109:588–590.

229. Zimmerman HJ. Hormonal derivatives and related drugs. In: HJ Zimmerman, ed. Hepatotoxicity. The Adverse Effects of Drugs and Other Chemicals on the Liver. 2nd ed. Philadelphia: Lippincott Williams & Wilkins, 1999:577.

230. Schneider HL, Hornbach KD, Kniaz JL, Efrusy ME. Chlorpropamide hepatotoxicity: report of a case and review of the literature. Am J Gastroenterol 1984; 79:721–724.

231. Ryder S, Sarokhan B, Shand D, Mullane JF. Human safety trail of tolrestat: an aldose reductase inhibitor. Drug Dev Res 1987; 11:131–143.

232. Gregory DH, Zaki GF, Sarcosi GA, Carey JB Jr. Chronic cholestasis following prolonged tolbutamide administration. Arch Pathol 1967; 84:194–201.

233. Nakao NL, Gelb AM, Stenger R, Siegel JH. A case of chronic liver disease due to tolazamide. Gastroenterology 1985; 89:192–195.

234. Wongpaitoon V, Mills PR, Russell RF, Patrick RS. Intrahepatic cholestasis and cutaneous bullae associated with glibenclamide therapy. Postgrad Med J 1981; 57:244–246.

235. Clarke BF, Campbell IW, Ewing DJ, Beveridge GW, MacDonald MK. Generalized hypersensitivity reaction and visceral arteritis with fatal outcome during glibenclamide therapy. Diabetes 1974; 23:739–742.

236. Rigberg LA, Robinson MJ, Espiritu C. Chlorpropamide-induced granulomas. A probable hypersensitivity reaction in liver and bone marrow. JAMA 1976; 235:409–410.

237. Creuzfeldt W. Oral antidiabetics. In: W Gerok, K Sickinger, eds. Drugs and the Liver. Stuttgart: FK Schattauer Verlag, 1975:366–373.

238. Sirek A, Sirek OV, Best CH. The toxic effect of carbutamide (BZ-55) in diabetic dogs. Diabetes 1957; 6:151–153.

239. Anderson RC, Worth HM, Harris PN. Toxicological studies on carbutamide. Diabetes 1957; 6:2–7.

240. Dunn M, Peters DH. Metformin: A review of its pharmacological properties and therapeutic use in non-insulin-dependent diabetes mellitus. Drug 1995; 49:721–749.

241. Chuckaree C, Yang SQ, Lin HZ, Diehl AM. Metformin improves nonalcoholic fatty liver disease in obese mice. Gastroenterology 2000; 118:A919.

242. Andrade RJ, Lucena MI, Rodriguez-Mendizabal M. Hepatic injury caused by acarbose [letter]. Ann Intern Med 1996; 124:931.

243. Diaz-Gutierrez FL, Ladero JM, Daiz-Rubio M. Acarbose-induced acute hepatitis [letter]. Am J Gastroenterol 1998; 93:481.

244. Carrascosa M, Pascual F, Aresti S. Acarbose-induced acute severe hepatotoxicity [letter]. Lancet 1998; 349:698–699.

245. Jagannath S, Rai R. Rapid onset of sulfulminant liver failure associated with troglitazone [letter]. Ann Intern Med 2000; 132:677.

246. Watkins PB, Whitcomb RW. Hepatic dysfunction associated with troglitazone [letter to the editor]. N Engl J Med 1998; 338:916–917.

247. Neuschwander-Tetri BA, Isley WL, Oki JC, Ramrakhiani S, Quiason SG, Phillips NJ, Brunt EM. Troglitazone-induced hepatic failure leading to liver transplantation. Ann Intern Med 1998; 129:38–41.

248. Gitlin N, Julie NL, Spurr CL, Lim KN, Juarbe HM. Two cases of severe clinical and histologic hepatotoxicity associated with troglitazone. Ann Intern Med 1998; 129:36–38.

249. Murphy EJ, Davern TJ, Shakil AO, Shick L, Masharani U, Chow H, Freise C, Lee WM, Bass NM, Acute Liver Failure Study Group. Troglitazone-induced fulminant hepatic failure. Dig Dis Sci 2000; 45:549–553.

250. Misbin RI. Troglitazone-associated hepatic failure [letter]. Ann Intern Med 1999; 130:330.

251. Bolton JL, Trush MA, Penning TM, Dryhurst G, Monks TJ. Role of quinones in toxicology. Chem Res Toxicol 2000; 13:135–160.

252. Shibuya A, Watanabe M, Fujita Y, Saigenji K, Kuwao S, Takahashi H, Takeuchi H. An autopsy case of Troglitazone-induced fulminant hepatitis. Diabetes Care 1998; 21:2140–2143.

253. Ramachandran V, Kostrubsky VE, Komoroski BJ, Zhang S, Dorko K, Esplen JE, Strom SC, Venkataramanan R. Troglitazone increases cytochrome P-450 3A protein and activity in primary cultures of human hepatocytes. Drug Metab Dispos 1999; 27:1194–1199.

254. Toyoda Y, Tsuchida A, Iwami I, Miwa I. Toxic effect of troglitazone on cultured rat hepatocytes. Life Sci 2001; 68:1867–1876.

254a. Preininger K, Stingl H, Englisch R, Furnsinn C, Graf J, Waldhausl W, Roden M. Acute triglitazone action in isolated perfused rat liver. Br J Pharmacol 1999; 126:372–378.

254b. Yamamoto Y, Nakajima M, Yamazaki H, Yokoi T. Cytotoxicity and apoptosis produced by troglitazone in human hepatoma cells. Life Sci 2001; 70:471–482.

255. Forman LM, Simmons DA, Diamond RH. Hepatic failure in a patient taking Rosiglitazone. Ann Intern Med 2000; 132:118–121.

256. Al-Salman J, Arjomand H, Kemp DG, Mittal M. Hepatocellular injury in a patient receiving Rosiglitazone. Ann Intern Med 2000; 132:121–124.

257. Actos (Proglitazone). In: Physicians' Desk Reference. 54th ed. 2000:3088.

258. Avandia (Rosiglitazone). In: Physicians' Desk Reference. 54th ed. 2000:2980.

259. Schenker S, Martin R, Hoyumpa AM. Antecedent liver disease and drug toxicity. J Hepatol 1999; 31:1098–1105.

260. Afterthoughts on hepatotoxicity (separate statement). In: HJ Zimmerman, ed. Hepatotoxicity. The Adverse Effects of Drugs and Other Chemicals on the Liver. Philadelphia: Lippincott Williams & Wilkins, 1999:744.

261. Lenhard MJ, Funk WB. Failure to develop hepatic injury from rosiglitazone in a patient with a history of troglitazone-induced hepatitis. Diabetes Care 2001; 24:168–169.

262. Itoh S, Igarashi M, Tsukada Y, Ichinoe A. Nonalcoholic fatty liver with alcoholic hyalin after long-term glucocorticoid therapy. Acta Hepato Gastroenterol 1977; 24:415–418.

263. Alpers DH, Sabesin SM, White HM. Fatty liver: biochemical and clinical aspects. In: L Schiff, ER Schiff, eds. Diseases of the Liver. 7th ed. Philadelphia: JB Lippncott, 1993:825–856.

264. Jones JP Jr, Engleman EP, Najarian JS. Systemic fat embolism after renal homotransplantation and treatment with corticosteroids. N Engl J Med 1965; 273:1453–1458.

265. Kirk AP, Jain S, Pocock S, Thomas HC, Sherlock S. Late results of the Royal Free Hospital prospective controlled trial of prednisolone therapy in hepatitis B surface antigen negative chronic active hepatitis. Gut 1980; 21:78–93.

266. Carithers RL, Herlong F, Diehl AM, Shaw EW, Combes B, Fallon HJ, Maddrey WC. Methyl prednisolone therapy in patients with severe alcoholic hepatitis. Ann Intern Med 1989; 110:685–690.

267. Brent GA. The molecular basis of thyroid hormone action. N Engl J Med 1994; 331:847–854.

268. Huang MJ, Liaw YF. Clinical association between thyroid and liver diseases. J Gastroenterol Hepatol 1995; 10:344–350.

269. Huang MJ, Li K, Wei JS, Wu S, Fan K, Liaw YF. Sequential liver and bone biochemical changes in hyperthyroidism: prospective controlled follow up study. Am J Gastroenterol 1995; 89:1071–1076.

270. Fong T, McHutchison JG, Reynolds TB. Hyperthyroid and hepatic dysfunction: a case series analysis. J Clin Gastroenterol 1992; 14:240–244.

271. Thompson NP, Leader S, Jamieson CP, Burnham WB, Burroughs AK. Reversible jaundice in primary biliary cirrhosis due to hyperthyroidism. Gastroenterology 1994; 106:1342–1343.

272. Kang H, Choi JD, Jung IG, Kim DW, Kim TB, Shin HK, Kim BT, Park CK, Yoo JY. A case of methimazole-induced acute hepatic failure in a patient with chronic hepatitis B carrier. Korean J Intern Med 1990; 5:69–73.

273. Wheeler D, Ayres JG, Skinner C. Carbimazole-induced jaundice. J Royal Soc Med 1985; 78:75–76.

274. Limaye A, Ruffola PR. Propylthiouracil-induced fatal hepatic necrosis. Am J Gastroenterol 1987; 82:152–154.

275. Pacini F, Sridama V, Refetoff S. Multiple complications of propylthiouracil treatment: granulocytopenia, eosinophilia, skin reaction and hepatitis with lymphocyte sensitization. J Endocrinol Invest 1982; 5:403–407.

276. Specht NW, Boehme EJ. Death due to agranulocytosis induced by methimazole therapy. JAMA 1952; 149:1010–1011.

277. Colwell AR Jr, Sando DE, Lang SJ. Propylthiouracil-induced agranulocytosis, toxic hepatitis, and death: report of a case. JAMA 1952; 148:639–641.

278. Hayashida CY, Duarte AJ, Sato AE, Yamoshiro-Kanashiro EH. Neonatal hepatitis and lymphocyte sensitization by placental transfer of propylthiouracil. J Endocrinol Invest 1991; 13: 937–941.

279. Jonas MM, Eidson MS. Propylthiouracil hepatotoxicity: two pediatric cases and review of the literature. J Pediatr Gastroenterol Nutr 1988; 7:776–779.

280. Liaw YF, Huang MJ, Fan KD, Li KL, Wu SS, Chen TJ. Hepatic injury during propylthiouracil therapy in patient with hyperthyroidism: a cohort study. Ann Intern Med 1993; 118:424–428.

28

Alternative Medicine, Vitamins, and Natural Hepatotoxins

GEORGES-PHILIPPE PAGEAUX and DOMINIQUE LARREY

Hôpital Saint Eloi and Montpellier School of Medicine, Montpellier, France

I. INTRODUCTION

Hepatic impairment resulting from the use of conventional drugs is widely acknowledged, but there is less awareness of the potential hepatotoxicity of alternative medicines such as herbal preparations, or vitamins, many of which are believed to be harmless and are commonly used for self-medication without supervision (1–5). There is a return to natural products occurring along with the ecological movement in industrialized countries, and patients are sometimes faced with new diseases with severe complications for which there is still no satisfying treatment, for instance the human immunodeficiency virus infection. Liver injury, including acute and chronic abnormalities and even cirrhotic transformation and liver failure, has been described after the ingestion of a wide range of herbal products and other botanical ingredients, such as mushrooms (6–11), and also from self-medication with vitamin A (12,13). A control of "natural" medicine utilization is appearing in many countries. Marketing authorization is given for plants considered efficient and innocuous. In most cases, the efficiency and safety are based more on a reputation acquired over centuries than on controlled trials and toxicity studies (11). There is another concern with natural botanical hepatotoxins, which comprise a wide range of agents that include fungal toxins (e.g., aflatoxin) and food-derived estrogens (3,4). This chapter summarizes the main herbal remedies and mushrooms known to be hepatotoxic, and also discusses vitamin A and botanical hepatotoxins.

II.   HERBAL REMEDIES

A.   Consumption of Herbal Medicines in Western Countries

As for other alternative medicines, the use of herbal remedies is increasingly attractive. In the United States, the marketing of herbs tripled between 1992 and 1996. The percentage of herbal medicine users in the United States is estimated to have increased from 2.5% in 1990 to 12% in 1998 representing a market of more than 5 billion dollars (4). For irritable bowel disease two North American inquiries showed a frequency of herb consumption as major treatment in 3–5%. Concerning liver disease, data remain limited. A first American study comprising about 100 patients showed a consumption frequency of 31% in patients with chronic liver disease (14). The second inquiry has recently been done on a prospective basis in outpatients seen for chronic liver disease. Herbal medicine consumption for more than 2 months was noted in 30% of 526 included patients (15).

B.   Diagnosis of Hepatotoxicity Caused by Herbal Remedies (11,16)

Hepatotoxicity of herbal remedies is particularly difficult to demonstrate. In addition to the usual difficulties observed to make a causal relationship between an adverse event and the intake of drug (absence of clinical specificity), one can observe additional difficulties such as frequent automedication and the reputation of safety so that the patient often forgets to mention herbal medicine ingestion to the physician. Other difficulties are related to the lack of control of safety in marketed products and to the complexity of herbal preparations in many cases. For instance, some Chinese preparations contain more than 10 different plants.

   In addition, there are specific risks contributing to the hepatotoxicity of herbal remedies (Table 1) and difficulties in making the diagnosis (Table 2).

C.   Main Plants

The medicinal plants reported to be toxic to the liver are listed in Table 3.

1.   Pyrrolizidine Alkaloids

The hepatotoxicity of these alkaloids, which are found in more than 350 plant species, has been known for more than 40 years. The main implicated species are: *Heliotroprium*, *Senecio*, and *Crotalaria* (17), and more recently, *Symphytum* (Comfrey) (18–20).

Table 1   Specific Risks Contributing to the Hepatotoxicity of Herbal Remedies

Misidentification of the plant
Selection of a wrong part of the plant
Inadequate storage
Contamination of the plant by various chemicals, heavy microorganisms
Adulteration during the processing
Mislabeling of the final product

Source: After ref. 11.

Table 2   Difficulties in Demonstrating the Hepatotoxicity
of Herbal Medicines

Absence of clinicopathological specificity
Relatively rare event
Frequent self-medication ⎫
Reputation of safety ⎬ Ingestion of plants remaining
Sale via Internet ⎭ unknown to the physician
Preparations containing numerous plants
Herbal preparations with unclear composition

Table 3   Medicinal Plants Reported To Be Toxic
to the Liver

Main plants or preparations
Pyrrolizidine alkaloids
  Crotalaria
  Senecio
  Heliotropium
  Symphytum officinale (comfrey)
Atractylis gummifera-L
Callilepsa laureola (impila)
Teucrium chamaedrys (germander)
Larrea tridentata (chaparral)
Cassia angustifolia (senna)
Chinese herbs
  Complex preparations used for skin diseases
  Lycopodium serratum (Jin Bu Huan)
  Ephedra (Ma Huang)
  Polygonum multiflora (Shou-Wu-Pian)
Plants containing pennyroyal oil
  Mentha pulegium
  Hedeoma pulegioïdes
Teucrium polium
Serenoa (saw palmetto)
Chelidonium majus (great celandine)
Azadirachta indica
Cathis edulis
Borago officinalis (borage)
Sassafras albidum (sassafras) hepatocarcinoma in animals
Plants with debated hepatotoxicity
Mistletoe
Valeriana officinalis (valerian)
Scutelleria (skullcap)
Piper methysticum (kava)

Pyrrolizidine poisoning is endemic in areas such as Africa and Jamaica, where toxic alkaloids are ingested as infusions, herbal teas, or decoctions or used as an enema (17). Contamination of flour by plants containing pyrrolizidine alkaloids has also caused epidemic intoxications in India and Afghanistan (15,16). Some cases have recently been observed in patients consuming toxic alkaloids in the form of herbal teas, capsules, or dietary supplements in Western countries (11).

The main liver injury induced by pyrrolizidine alkaloids is veno-occlusive disease (4,11). Pathological findings include a nonthrombotic occlusion of the lumen of small centrilobular veins in the absence of large hepatic vein lesions (11). This brings about hepatic congestion, which may lead to parenchymal necrosis. In some cases, fibrosis and even cirrhosis may develop. Different clinical subtypes have been described (11). The acute form is characterized by sudden abdominal pain, ascites, and hepatomegaly associated with markedly increased serum aminotransferase activities. Liver biopsy can reveal hemorrhagic centrilobular necrosis without inflammation due to acute centrilobular vein lesions. Limited lesions are usually followed by a complete recovery. When lesions are extensive, hepatic failure may occur, leading to death. In contrast, the chronic form insidiously develops and may mimic cirrhosis fully. One fatal case of veno-occlusive disease has been described in a newborn infant whose mother had been exposed to a plant containing pyrrolizidine alkaloids during pregnancy (21).

Hepatotoxicity of pyrrolizidine alkaloids is reproducible and dose-related in laboratory animals (11,22). It seems to be due to the biotransformation of unsaturated alkaloids into unstable, toxic metabolites, probably pyrrolic derivatives, by cytochrome P450 leading mainly to lesions of endothelial cells and, at a lesser extent, of hepatocytes (Fig. 1). This mechanism might explain the natural history of liver lesions observed in humans. Acute lesions seem to result from a short exposure to high doses of alkaloids, whereas chronic lesions appear to be related to prolonged exposure to small doses of pyrrolizidine

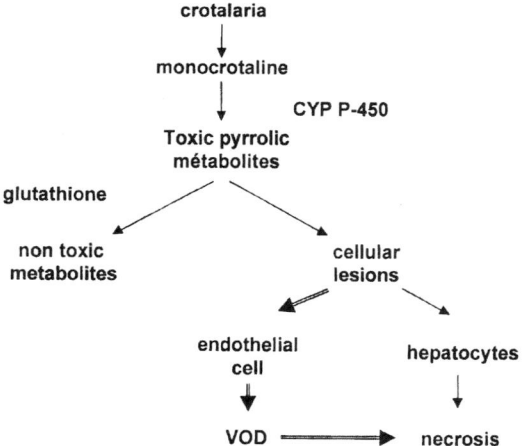

Figure 1 Hepatotoxicity mechanism of pyrrolizidine alkaloids. Crotalaria man toxins are oxidized into toxic metabolites in hepatocytes and endothelial cells. Endothelial cells are particularly sensitive having a limited stock of gluthathione which can provoke venoocclusive disease. Hepatocyte necrosis can further aggravate the extent of lesions. (From Ref. 22.)

alkaloids (11,22). However, exposure to a low dose for a short time also leads to liver injury (23).

2. *Atractylis gummifera*-L

The toxicity of this plant is well-known in Mediterranean countries (24). The intoxication is observed in children who use the white-yellowish substance secreted by the plant, which looks like glue, as chewing gum (11,24). *Atractylis gummifera* intoxication can also be caused by ingestion of the root extracts, used for their properties as an antipyretic, purgative and emetic, diuretic, and inducer of abortion, especially in North Africa (11,24). Toxicity can finally result from the botanical confusion between this plant and wild artichoke (11). Hepatocellular hepatitis generally occurs 24 h after ingestion and can be associated with hypoglycemia and renal failure (11,24,25). Fatal liver failure is frequent. The liver biopsy performed in rare cases revealed extensive hepatocyte necrosis. *Atractylis gummifera* hepatotoxicity is reproducible in experimental models and appears to be related to potassium atractylate and gummiferin, two compounds that inhibit mitochondrial oxidative phosphorylation and Krebs cycle.

Hypoglycemia is caused by inhibition of glycogen synthesis (11,26).

3. *Callepsis laureola* (Impila) (11)

Several cases of fatal fulminant hepatitis associated with tubular renal necrosis have been ascribed to this plant used as traditional medicine among Zulus from Natal. This plant contains compounds chemically related to potassium atractylate, which might explain its toxicity.

4. *Teucrium chamaedrys* (Germander)

Germander has been used for more than 2000 years for relieving fever and abdominal disorders as well as for its supposed diuretic, choleretic, and healing properties (6). Germander was given a marketing agreement as a traditional herbal medicine in 1986 in France as an adjuvant to weight control. Germander was rapidly incriminated in more than 30 cases of liver injury in France (6,27), mostly in middle-aged women. Germander was ingested at recommended doses (600–1600 mg/day), under various presentations: commercial herbal teas, capsules, or artisanal preparations. Liver injury was mainly characterized by mild to moderate acute cytolytic hepatitis occurring about 2 months after treatment was begun (6,27). However, fulminant hepatitis was observed in two patients, with a fatal course in one (28,29). Discontinuation of the treatment was followed by complete recovery within 2–6 months (27) except in the fatal case (28). In a few patients, the disease had a more insidious course and was discovered at the stage of chronic hepatitis and even cirrhosis, mostly in individuals with a long-lasting treatment or having a large consumption (29–31). In all the patients accidentally reexposed to germander, liver injury relapsed within a relatively short delay (6,27). A case of chronic cholangitis has been observed (16).

These observations led to extensive inquiries to determine whether toxicity was caused by the plant itself or by another source. Verifications showed neither misidentification of plant nor contamination with another plant nor contamination by insecticides and microorganisms nor failure in the manufacturing of capsules or tea bags (9). Germander hepatotoxicity has been reproduced in mice by using germander tea lyophilisate and was dose-dependent (32). The chemical composition of germander comprises furan-containing

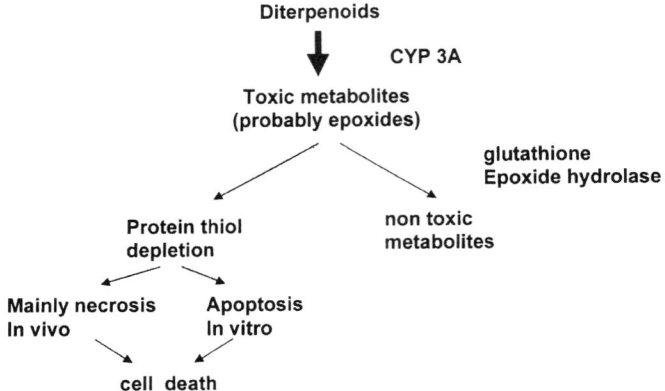

Figure 2 Germander hepatotoxicity—mechanism. Diterpenoids contained in germander are oxidized into toxic metabolites mainly by cytochromes P450 of family 3A. These metabolites can damage cellular structures thereby leading to cellular death through necrosis or apoptosis. (From Refs. 32–35.)

neoclerodane diterpenoids, saponins, glycosides, and flavonoids. Germander components have been shown to be oxidized by cytochrome P450 isoenzymes, in particular those of family 3A, into reactive metabolites. Interestingly, diterpenoids exhibit a chemical structure similar to that of other furano compounds, well known to produce cytochrome P450-mediated toxic metabolites (32). Studies in isolated rat hepatocytes have shown that formed reactive metabolites deplete glutathione and cytoskeleton-associated protein thiols and form plasma membrane blebs (33) (Fig. 2). Experimental data strongly support the belief that apoptosis can contribute to liver cell death (34,35). Finally, recent data suggest that the involved reactive metabolites derived from teucrin A could trigger hepatotoxicity through an immunoallergic reaction (36). Indeed, antimicrosomal epoxide hydrolase autoantibodies have been found in the sera of patients who drank germander teas for a long period of time (36). These antibodies were found to recognize teucrin A–alkylated epoxide hydrolase (36). Germander has been withdrawn from the market of herbal medicines in France and its free sale has been forbidden. However, it is still used in some other countries and new cases have recently been observed in Canada (37) and Belgium.

5. *Larrea tridentata* (Chaparral)

Chaparral is an evergreen desert shrub found mainly in the United States and Mexico. It has been used by native Americans and, now, by Western people for various ailments, bronchitis, common cold, rheumatic pain, stomach pain, snakebite, weight loss, and as antioxidant. More than 15 cases of liver injury have been collected by the Food and Drug Administration. Most cases were of acute hepatocellular or cholestatic hepatitis. Less frequently, fulminant hepatitis, cirrhosis, or cholangitis has been described (38,39).

6. *Cassia angustifolia* (Senna)

Senna, a plant used for its laxative properties, has been ascribed as causing one case of hepatitis in a patient ingesting high doses (40). Liver damage recurred after reexposure to the preparation containing extracts of senna. Hepatotoxicity might be caused by the laxative alkaloids, sennosides, which are the major substances of senna leaf and fruit. Sennosides are split into anthron in the intestine by intestinal bacteria. Anthron exhibits a chemical structure very close to that of danthron, a well-known hepatotoxic laxative (41).

7. Chinese Herbal Preparations

Chinese herbal medicines are widely used in Asian communities throughout the world. At least 7000 species of medicinal plants are used in China (42). Chinese herbs have been shown to have beneficial effects in eczema and atopic dermatitis (43,44). In these circumstances, several cases of acute hepatitis have been observed (45–47). The causal relationship between the exposure to Chinese herbal preparations and the occurrence of liver toxicity is strongly supported by a case of positive rechallenge (47). One case had a fatal course (47). Among the numerous plants present in these herbal remedies, the one responsible for liver toxicity has not yet been identified. Identification of the toxic substances is all the more difficult as Chinese herbal medicines are often adulterated with substituted herbs, heavy metals, and Western medicines (39). This difficulty is stressed by another preparation, Jin Bu Huan, that was recently incriminated (48,49). This herbal remedy (*Lycopodium serratum*), used for more than 1000 years as a sedative and analgesic in China, has been available in the United States for 15 years. Acute hepatitis has been observed in more than 15 patients after a mean duration of administration of 2 months. Readministration of Jin Bu Huan in two patients caused relapse of hepatitis (48–50). Hepatotoxicity mechanism is debated. It appears to be caused by levo-tetrahydropalmitine, the active ingredient of Jin Bu Huan, which exhibits some structural similarity with hepatotoxic pyrrolizidine alkaloids (11). The controversy results from the fact that the concentration of this compound was abnormally high in the preparation, suggesting a botanical misidentification and a mislabeling of the package (11,50).

Among Chinese herbs, *Ephedra* must be emphasized as this currently is a popular remedy. *Ephedra* species have a worldwide distribution and have a long history of use as a stimulant and for the management of bronchial disorders. Today, *Ephedra* continues to find a place in herbal preparations designed to relieve cold symptoms and to improve respiratory functions. The pharmacological effect is supported by ephedrine contained in *Ephedra*. One of the members of the genus *Ephedra*, *E. altissima*, yields several mutagenic *N*-nitrosamines under simulated gastric conditions. For example, *N*-nitrosephedrine causes metastasizing liver cell carcinoma in animals. However, the investigators noted that the potential for endogenous formation of these compounds following ingestion of the *Ephedra* infusions is extremely small (51).

8. Pennyroyal Oil (52)

This substance is provided by some mint species such as *Mentha pulegium* and *Hedeoma pulegioides*. These plants are particularly used in Hispanic populations to trigger abortion or menstruation and also to treat minor abdominal pain in children. Pennyroyal toxicity comprises seizures and mental disorders as well as acute hepatitis with fulminant course. The hepatotoxicity mechanism has been elucidated. Pennyroyal oil is mainly composed of pulegone (90%), a terpene oxidized by P450s into a reactive methofuran. Treatment consists of quickly administering *N*-acetylcysteine as for acetaminophen poisoning.

9. *Teucrium polium*

This plant, close to *Teucrium chamaedris*, has been proposed to treat moderate hypercholesterolemia. It has been involved in a fulminant hepatitis leading to liver transplantation (53)

10. Sereona

Sereona makes up the major part of a complex herbal preparation marketed with the name of Prostata, supposed to have antiandrogenic properties. A case of cholestatic hepatitis has been ascribed to this preparation (54).

11. *Chelidonium majus* (Greater Celandine)

This plant is being used in Europe for treating dyspepsia and gallstones. Several cases of liver injuries have been observed in Germany (55). Hepatotoxicity generally occurs within 4–12 weeks. The clinicopathological spectrum involves moderate to severe cholestasis, hepatocellular hepatitis with fibrosis in some cases, and acute cholangitis (55). The involved toxic agent remains unknown. Candidates include chelidonine, sanguinarien, berberine, and coptisine (55).

12. *Piper methysticum* (Kava)

Kava was initially used as a ritual narcotic compound in the South Pacific; it is now used to relieve anxiety. However, several cases of liver injury including fulminant hepatitis have recently been associated with kava use (56).

13. Other Plants

Oil extracts from *Azadirachza indica* seeds might cause microvesicular steatosis (11). *Cathis edulis* and *Borago officinalis* have been rarely ascribed as causing acute hepatitis. *Sassafras albidum* (Sassafras), used as a herbal tea in the United States, contains safrole, which has hepatocarcinogenic effects in animals (11). A prospective study performed in a health central laboratory in Sweden revealed that liver enzyme abnormalities were more frequent in patients who took herbal preparations. Liver abnormalities disappeared in the patients who stopped taking herbal preparations (57).

D. Other Plants with Debated Hepatotoxicity

1. *Viscus album* (Mistletoe)

Mistletoe has been proposed for treating asthma, epilepsy, and infertility. One case of hepatitis has been ascribed to a herbal preparation containing mistletoe and scutellaria (58). Liver injury relapsed after readministration of the same preparation. The role of mistletoe in this case has been controversial because the botanical composition of the preparation was not analyzed (59–61). Mistletoe hepatotoxicity therefore remains uncertain.

2. *Valeriana officinalis* (Valerian)

Several cases of acute hepatitis have been reported in patients taking herbal preparations for relieving stress, presented as tablets containing various extracts of plants, in particular valerian and, possibly, skullcap (11,62,63). In one patient, extensive fibrosis and liver failure with encephalopathy have been reported (62). However, there are no experimental data supporting the toxicity of valerian and the follow-up for the last 3 years does not confirm its hepatotoxicity.

III. MUSHROOMS

Mushroom poisoning is a common medical emergency in Western countries. Among more than 2000 species of mushrooms, approximately 50 are poisonous to humans. The overwhelming majority of lethal mushroom poisonings are attributable to the genus *Amanita*. *Lepiota* species may also cause the fatal phalloidian syndrome (9).

A. *Amanita* Poisoning

Of the three common amanita species—*A. phalloides*, *A. verna*, and *A. virosa*—*A. phalloides* has been held accountable for more than 90% of fatalities (8). *A. phalloides* exerts its hepatotoxicity through toxins. These toxins are cyclopeptides, among which eight amatoxins and seven phallotoxins have been isolated from *Amanita*. These toxins are heat stable, and therefore not destroyed by cooking. They have an enterohepatic circulation. The toxicity of phalloidin has been shown to reside in the thioamine bond of the sulfur atom of the indol ring (64). Clinically, this compound induces the initial symptoms of gastroenteritis. The cytotoxic effect of alpha-amanitin is due to an inhibition of ribonucleic acid polymerase II. This compound is responsible for severe liver, kidney, and brain damage that often leads to death (65).

Patients who consume mushrooms of the *Amanita* variety exhibit symptoms and signs that occur typically in three stages (66). There is an initial quiescent phase of 6–12 h following the meal, after which abdominal pain, nausea, vomiting, and watery diarrhea develop. This gives rise to a cholera-like syndrome that, in severe cases, can result in profound dehydration and hypotension. The second stage is characterized by clinical improvement that begins 24–48 h after ingestion and often masks the hepatic and renal deterioration that is occurring at that time: elevated transaminase and bilirubin level, prolonged prothrombin time, and elevated serum creatinine and blood urea nitrogen level. The transition into the third stage can occur quite suddenly and this final stage of the illness is characterized by fulminant hepatic failure with advancing encephalopathy and profound coagulopathy. Some evidence supports the hypothesis that neurological dysfunction may be due to a direct neurotoxic effect of alpha-amanitin, even though a similar association of confusion, seizure activity, visual disturbance, and coma can be seen with acute hepatic failure alone (8). Renal failure due to the hepatorenal syndrome and to the direct nephrotoxicity of alpha-amanitin may result in severe oliguria or anuria. Approximately 50% of patients have clinical or biochemical evidence of pancreatitis. The prognostic evaluation of these patients is exceedingly difficult. In a series of 205 patients, the mortality rate was 22% (8). The overall mortality rate of *Amanita* poisoning is estimated as 10–25%; with current supportive therapy, this has fallen to about 9% (8), but the greater availability of liver transplantation could further reduce this. Children under the age of 10 years have a higher risk of fatal intoxication than adults. Among those who develop hepatic encephalopathy, the mortality is very high. In less severe cases, recovery may occur but is often delayed for 2–3 weeks.

B. *Lepiota helveola* Poisoning

Fortunately, poisoning with *Lepiota helveola* is a rare clinical problem. Clinical consequences are similar to those of *A. phalloides*, as both species contain alpha-amanitin responsible for liver injury. Evolution occurs in three phases, and survival is rare in patients in whom hepatic coma develops. However, *Lepiota helveola* contains 3 150 µg of toxins per gram (dry weight), which is higher than the amount found in *A. phalloides* (2650 µg/g) (67). As soon as massive hepatic injury becomes evident, liver transplantation must be performed.

C. Mushroom Poisoning Therapy

The therapeutic goals can be summarized as follows: elimination of mushroom residues from the gastrointestinal tract, clearance of alpha-amanitin from blood and tissues, protection of the liver from the toxic effect of amanitin, and treatment of liver failure. At the early stage, the first principle of management is to refer every patient with gastroenteritis more than 6 h after mushroom ingestion to an intensive-care unit. First, gastric lavage is advocated, while aspiration of the duodenal content for 36 h can remove the large amount of mushroom toxin secreted in bile. Activated charcoal is administrated to absorb biliary excreted toxin, thereby promoting fecal excretion (8). Concerning protection of the liver from the toxic effects of amanitin, two pharmaceutical agents, penicillin G and silymarin, have been claimed to be therapeutically efficient (68,69). Penicillin G (40,000,000 U/24 h in adult patients) might produce protective effects by increasing renal excretion of amanitin and by inhibiting penetration of the toxin into the hepatocytes. Silymarin (20–50 mg/kg/24 h) might interrupt the enterohepatic circulation of amanitin and prevent the penetration of the toxin into the liver cells. However, there are no generally recognized medical treatment protocols for *Amanita* or *Lepiota helveola* poisoning. When hepatic coma develops, the chance of survival with medical therapy alone is practically nil (8,68). Therefore, these patients should be considered candidates for liver transplantation.

IV. VITAMIN A HEPATOTOXICITY

Vitamin A has been used for the treatment of xerophthalmia, hypogonadism, abnormal dark adaptation, biliary cirrhosis, chronic ileitis, or to prevent cancer. Hypervitaminosis A most often results from self-medication with vitamin A alone or polyvitamins containing from 25,000 to more than 100,000 IU retinol per tablet (70). Retinol is the main compound with vitamin A function, and these two terms are often used interchangeably. The hepatic disorders resulting from hypervitaminosis A vary from abnormal liver enzyme tests with minor histological changes to perisinusoidal fibrosis with noncirrhotic portal hypertension (71). The late stages can include cirrhosis.

A. Current Concept of Mechanisms

Vitamin A is a dose-dependent hepatotoxin, but the severity of hepatic changes depends also on the duration of exposure. Liver stellate cells are the main storage site of retinol in the body, and it is usual to relate vitamin A hepatotoxicity to activation of these cells. Acute or subacute intoxications related to consumption of high doses of vitamin A are responsible for hyperplasia and hypertrophy of liver stellate cells, responsible for early portal hypertension due to sinusoidal obstruction. The mechanism by which hypervitaminosis A produces cellular injury in the long term after acute intoxication or after chronic consumption of therapeutic doses of vitamin A is probably different. Indeed, it is well known that retinol is metabolized at the hepatocyte level to several metabolites, among them some polar metabolites with potential local toxicity (72). In animals models, pretreatment with vitamin A greatly enhances the hepatic toxicity of substances such as carbon tetrachloride, paracetamol, or endotoxins (73,74). Finally, retinol and retinoins play a major role in regulation of liver stellate cell differentiation, and in modulation of collagen synthesis by these cells (75). Thus, vitamin A toxicity in humans could be related either to an increased susceptibility to environmental factors because of interaction between vitamin and cytochrome P450 isoenzymes or to a direct toxicity of some polar metabolites modulated by exposition to environmental factors (12). Another characteristic of hypervitaminosis A is the chronicity of the fibrosis process initiated with vitamin consumption and not influenced by vitamin discontinuation. This is a result of a slow mobilization of hepatic stores.

B. Pathology

In less severe cases, the principal finding is the hypertrophy and proliferation of stellate cells (13). The other uniform feature is increased hepatic storage of vitamin A in stellate cells. This results in greenish autofluorescence after exposure to ultraviolet light (13). It is best observed in unstained frozen sections or in fresh tissue. Hyperplasia of stellate cells is massive in severe and acute forms of intoxication, and moderate in slight forms. In chronic intoxications, fibrosis, inflammatory infiltrate, cirrhosis, or, more uncommonly, peliosis has been described. Hepatocellular injury is indicated by microvesicular fatty change, which is usually minor, and by focal degeneration and necrosis.

C. Clinical Manifestations

The clinical and laboratory features of vitamin A−induced hepatotoxicity are listed in Table 4 (13,76). The characteristic clinical features are the relevant dietary and medication history and the nonspecific, protean manifestation of hypervitaminosis A. In cases of recent consumption of high doses of vitamin A, patients can present with portal hypertension, including ascites, edema, hepatomegaly, and splenomegaly. In patients with "therapeutic" consumption of vitamin A, clinical features are often minimal or nonspecific and fatigue is frequent. Uncommonly, patients present with complications of portal hypertension, including bleeding esophageal varices and hypersplenism. In the Geubel et al. series, portal hypertension with esophageal varices was present in 51% of cases (13). Liver test abnormalities are nonspecific. Vitamin A plasma levels may be normal in hypervitaminosis A (70). No laboratory investigations or clinical features can replace an appropriate history. Thus, specific inquiries about vitamins and other nonprescribed medications are essential

Table 4 Clinical and Laboratory Features of Vitamin A−Induced Hepatotoxicity

Abnormal liver tests	63%
Fatigue	34%
Hepatomegaly	47%
Splenomegaly	35%
Esophageal varices (bleeding in 100)	27%
Jaundice and ascites	12%
Hypersplenism	7%
Hemolytic anemia	2%

Source: After 41 cases reported by Geubel et al. (13).

in any patient with liver injury, particularly when the cause for hepatic damage is not readily apparent.

D. Management

In less severe cases, discontinuation of vitamin A ingestion leads to resolution of symptoms attributable to vitaminosis A, and gradual return of liver tests to normal (13). However, cessation of vitamin intake is not always associated with histological improvement (70). Among patients presenting with established cirrhosis or hepatic dysfunction, the prognosis is poor (13,70) and liver transplantation has been proposed (13). It must be emphasized that alcohol may potentiate liver injury, as has been shown in experimental models of interactive hepatotoxicity (12). Thus, avoidance of alcohol is advisable.

V. MICROCYSTIN TOXICITY

Microcystins are cyclic peptides that are potent liver toxins (77–79). Among this genus, *Microcystis aerugonisa* is a freshwater, bloom-forming cyanobacterium. Microcystins are common in inland waterways in Australia, in parts of the United States, in South America, especially Brazil, and in the Baltic Sea. Overgrowths are favored by stagnancy, hot weather, and increased concentrations of phosphate and other nutrients as the result of human contamination with fertilizers (76–78). Hepatotoxicity of microcystins occurs in domestic and wild animals. Animals die within hours to days after the initial exposure, often as the result of intrahepatic hemorrhage and hypovolemic shock (77). Microcystins cause liver injury through inhibition of protein phosphatases (78). The liver accumulates the toxins preferentially via an organic anion transporter and is their chief target organ. The liver rapidly removes the microcystins from the blood, but at potentially lethal doses clearance is reduced. Recently, a human parenteral exposure to microcystin has been reported in a hemodialysis center in Brazil (79). It was responsible for acute liver injury in 101 patients, 50 of whom died.

    Concerning treatment, the membrane-active antioxidant vitamin E and silymarin partly protect animals against microcystin hepatotoxicity (80).

VI. CONCLUSION

Alternative medicine and medicinal plant hepatotoxicity is often not recognized and the mechanisms of toxicity remain largely unknown. It is therefore important to better inform users, particularly because self-medication is frequent. It is also important to improve safety controls at the different stages from plant collection to distribution of the final product.

REFERENCES

1. Kassler WJ, Blanc P, Greenblatt R. The use of medicinal herbs by human immunodeficiency virus-infected patients. Arch Intern Med 1991; 151:2281–2288.
2. Huxtable RJ. The myth of beneficent nature: the risk of herbal preparations. Ann Intern Med 1992; 117:165–166.
3. Shaw D, Leon C, Kolev S, Murray V. Traditional remedies and food supplements: a 5-year toxicological study (1991–1995). Drug Safety 1997; 17:342–356.

4. Schuppan D, Jia JD, Brinkhaus B, Hahn EG. Herbal products for liver diseases: a therapeutic challenge for the new millennium. Hepatology 1999; 30:1099–1104.

5. Chan TYK, Critchley JAJH. Usage and adverse effects of Chinese herbal medicines. Hum Exp Toxicol 1996; 15:5–12.

6. Larrey D, Vial T, Pawels A, Castot A, Biour M, David M, Michel H. Hepatitis after germander (*Teucrium chamaedrys*) administration: another instance of herbal medicine hepatotoxicity. Ann Intern Med 1992; 117:129–132.

7. Venherweghem JL, Depierreux M, Tielemans C, Abramowicz D, Dratwa M, Jadoul M, Richard C, Vandervelde D, Verbeelen D, Vanhaelen-Fastre R, Vanhaelen M. Rapidly progressive interstitial renal fibrosis in young women: association with slimming regimen including Chinese herbs. Lancet 1993; 341:387–391.

8. Larrey D, Pageaux GP. Hepatotoxicity of herbal remedies and mushrooms. Semin Liver Dis 1995; 15:183–188.

9. Stickel F, Egerer G, Seitz HK. Hepatotoxicity of botanical. Public Health Nutr 2000; 3:113–124.

10. Kaplowitz N. Hepatotoxicity of herbal remedies: insights into the intricacies of plant-animal warfare and cell death. Gastroenterology 1997; 113:1408–1412.

11. Larrey D. Hepatotoxicity of herbal remedies. J Hepatol 1997; 26(suppl 1):47–51.

12. Leo MA, Liber CS. Alcohol, vitamin A, and β-carotene: adverse interactions, including hepatotoxicity and carcinogenicity. Am J Clin Nutr 1999; 69:1071–1085.

13. Geubel AP, de Galocsy C, Alves N, Rahier J, Dive C. Liver damage caused by therapeutic vitamin A administration: estimate of dose-related toxicity in 41 cases. Gastroenterology 1991; 100:1701–1709.

14. Flora K, Rosen HR, Benner KG. The use of naturopathic remedies for chronic liver disease. Am J Gastroenterol 1996; 12:2654–2655.

15. Detkova Z, Lefebvre A, Bastide C, Peladan N, Pageaux GP, Blanc P, Larrey D. Herbal medicines consumption for chronic liver disease and functional intestinal disorders: prospective study in 526 outpatients. Gastroenterology 2001; 120(suppl 1):A-228.

16. Larrey D. Drug-induced liver diseases. J Hepatol 2000; 32:77–88.

17. Smith LW, Culvenor CCJ. Plant sources of hepatotoxic pyrrolizidine alkaloids. J Nat Prod 1981; 44:129–152.

18. Weston CFM, Cooper BT, Davies JD, Levine DF. Veno-occlusive disease of the liver secondary to ingestion of comfrey. Br Med J 1987; 295:183.

19. Bach N, Thung SN, Schaffner F. Comfrey herb tea-induced hepatic veno-occlusive disease. Am J Med 1989; 87:97–99.

20. Ridker PM, McDermott V. Comfrey herb tea and hepatic veno-occlusive disease. Lancet 1989; 7:657–658.

21. Roulet M, Laurini R, Rivier L, Calame A. Hepatic veno-occlusive disease in newborn infant of a woman drinking tea. J Pediatr 1988; 112:433–436.

22. DeLeve LD, Wang X, Kuhlenkamp JF, Kaplowitz N. Toxicity of azathioprine and monocrotaline in murine sinusoidal endothelial cells and hepatocytes: the role of glutathione and relevance to hepatic venoocclusive disease. Hepatology 1996; 23:589–599.

23. Bensaude RJ, Monegier du Sorbier C, Jonville-Bera AP, Autret E, Ouyahya F, Metman EH. Maladie veino-occlusive après la prise de Seneçon (Hemoluol). Gastroenterol Clin Biol 1998; 22:363.

24. Georgiou M, Sianidou L, Hatzis T, Papadatos J, Koutselinis A. Hepatotoxicity due to *Atractylis gummifera*-L. Clin Toxicol 1988; 26:487–493.

25. Nogue S, Sanz P, Botey A, Esforzado N, Blanche C, Alvarez L. Insuffisance rénale aiguë due à une intoxication par le charbon à glu (*Atractylis gummifera*-L). Presse Med 1992; 21:130.

26. Hedili A, Warnet JM, Thevenin M, Martin C, Yacoub M, Claude JR. Ciochemical investigation of *Atractylis gummifera*-L hepatotoxicity in the rat. Arch Toxicol 1989; 13(suppl):312–315.

27. Castot A, Larrey D. Hépatites observées au cours d'un traitement par un médicament ou une tisane contenant de la germandrée petit-chêne. Bilan des 26 cas rapportés aux centres régionaux de pharmacovigilance. Gastroenterol Clin Biol 1992; 16:916–922.

28. Mostefa-Kara N, Pauwels A, Pines E, Biour M, Levy VG. Fatal hepatitis after herbal tea. Lancet 1992; 340:674.

29. Diaz D, Ferroudji S, Heran B, Barneon G, Larrey D, Michel H. Hépatite aiguë à la germandrée petit-chêne. Gastroenterol Clin Biol 1992; 16:1006.

30. Ben Yahia M, Mavier P, Metreau JM, Zafrani ES, Fabre M, Gatineau-Saillant G, Dhumeaux D, Mallat A. Hépatite chronique active et cirrhose induites par la germandrée petit-chêne à propos de trois cas. Gastroenterol Clin Biol 1993; 17:959–962.

31. Dao T, Peytier A, Galateau F, Valla A. Hépatite chronique cirrhogène à la germandrée petit-chêne. Gastroenterol Clin Biol 1993; 17:609–610.

32. Loeper J. Descatoire V, Letteron P, Moulis C, Degott C, Dansette P, Fau D, Pessayre D. Hepatotoxicity of germander in mice. Gastroenterology 1994; 106:464–472.

33. Lekehal M, Pessayre D, Lereau JM, Moulis C, Fouraste F. Hepatotoxicity of the herbal medicine germander. Metabolic activation of its furano diterpenoids by cytochrome P450 3A depletes cytoskeleton-associated protein thiols and forms plasma membrane blebs in rat hepatocytes. Hepatology 1996; 24:212–218.

34. Feldmann G, Moreau A, Fau D, Lekehal M, Farrel G, Pessayre D. Ultrastructural aspects of apoptosis in isolated rat hepatocytes treated by germander. J Hepatol 1996; 25:131.

35. Fau D, Lekehal M, Farrell G, Moreau A, Moulis C, Feldmann G, Haouzi D, Pessayre P. Diterpenoids from germander, an herbal medicine, induce apoptosis in isolated rat hepatocytes. Gastroenterology 1997; 113:1334–1336.

36. De Berardinis V, Moulis C, Maurice M, Beaune P, Pessayre D, Poupon D, Loeper J. Human microsomal epoxide hydrolase is the target of germander-induced autoantibodies on the surface of human hepatocytes. Mol Pharmacol 2000; 58:542–551.

37. Laliberté L, Villeneuve JP. Hepatitis after the use of germander, a herbal remedy. Can Med Assoc J 1996; 154:1689–1692.

38. Katz M, Saibil F. Herbal hepatitis subacute hepatic necrosis secondary to chapparal leaf. J Clin Gastroenterol 1990; 12:203–206.

39. Alderman S, Kailas S, Goldfarb S, Singaram C, Malone DG. Cholestatic hepatitis after ingestion of chaparral leaf: confirmation by endoscopic retrograde cholangiopancreatography and liver biopsy. J Clin Gastroenterol 1994; 19:242–247.

40. Beuers U, Splengler U, Pape GR. Hepatitis after chronic abuse of senna. Lancet 1991; 337: 372–373.

41. Tolman KG, Hammar S, Sannella JJ. Possible hepatotoxicity of Doxidan. Ann Intern Med 1976; 84:290–292.

42. Chan TYK, Chan JCN, Tomlinson B, Critchley AJH. Chinese herbal medicines revisited: a Hong Kong perspective. Lancet 1993; 342:1532–1534.

43. Davies KG, Pollock I, Steel HM. Chinese herbs for eczema. Lancet 1990; 336:177.

44. Sheehan MP, Rustin MH, Atherton DJ, Buckley C, Harris DJ, Brostoff J, Ostlere L, Dawson A, Harris DJ. Efficacy of traditional Chinese herbal therapy in adult atopic dermatitis. Lancet 1992; 340:13–17.

45. Sheehan MP, Atherton DJ. One year follow-up of children with atopic eczema treated with traditional Chinese medicinal plants. Br J Dermatol 1992; 127:13.

46. Graham-Brown R. Toxicity of Chinese herbal remedies. Lancet 1992; 340:673–674.

47. Perharic-Walton L, Murray V. Toxicity of Chinese herbal remedies. Lancet 1992; 340: 674.

48. Woolf GM, Petrovic LM, Rojter SE, Wainwright S, Vilamil FG, Katkov WN, Michieletti P, Wanless IR, Stermitz FR, Beck JJ, Vierling JM. Acute hepatitis associated with the Chinese herbal product Jin Bu Huan. Ann Intern Med 1994; 121:729–735.

49. Kaptchuk TP. Acute hepatitis associated with Jin Bu Huan. Ann Intern Med 1995; 122:636.

50. Horowitz RS, Feldhaus K, Dart RC, Stermitz FR, Beck JJ. The clinical spectrum of Jin Bu Huan toxicity. Arch Intern Med 1996; 156:899–903.

51. Tricker AR, Wacker CD, Preussmann R. 2-(*N*-nitroso-*N*-methylamino)propriophenone, a direct acting bacterial mutagen found in nitrosated Ephedra altissima tea. Toxicol Lett 1987; 38:45–50.

52. Bakerink JA, Gospe SM, Dimand RJ, Eldridge MW. Multiple organ failure after ingestion of pennyroyal oil form herbal tea in two infants. Pediatrics 1996; 98:944–947.

53. Mattei A, Rueay P, Samuell D, Feray C, Reynes M, Bismuth H. Liver transplantation for severe acute liver failure after herbal medicine (*Teucrium polium*) administration. J Hepatol 1995; 22:597.

54. Hamid S, Rotjer S, Vierling J. Protracted cholestatic hepatitis after the use of Prostata. Ann Intern Med 1997; 127:169–170.

55. Benninger J, Schneider HT, Schuppan D, Kirchner T, Hahn EG. Acute hepatitis induced by greater celandine (*Chelidonium majus*). Gastroenterology 1999; 117:1234–1237.

56. Russmann S, Lauterburg BH, Helbling A. Kava hepatotoxicity. Ann Intern Med 2001; 135: 68–69.

57. Carlsson C. Herbs and hepatitis. Lancet 1990; 336:1068.

58. Harvey J, Colin-Jones DG. Mistletoe hepatitis. Br Med J 1981; 282:186–187.

59. Fletcher Hyde F. Mistletoe hepatitis. Br Med J 1981; 282:739.

60. Farnsworth NR, Loub WD. Mistletoe hepatitis. Br Med J 1981; 283:1058.

61. Corrigan D. Phytotherapy. Int Pharm J 1987; 1:96–101.

62. Bagheri H, Broué P, Lacroix I, Larrey D, Olives JP, Vaysse P, Ghisolfi J, Montastruc JL. Fulminant hepatic failure after herbal medicine ingestion in children. Therapie 1998; 53:77–83.

63. Mennecier D, Saloum T, Dourthe PM, Bronstein JA, Thiolet C, Farret O. Hépatite aiguë et phytothérapie. Presse Méd 1999; 28:966.

64. Bartoloni ST, Omer F, Giannini A, et al. Amanita poisoning: a clinical–histological study of 64 cases of intoxication. Hepato-Gastroenterology 1985; 32:229–231.

65. Kroncke KY, Fricker G, Meier PJ, et al. Alpha-amanitin uptake into hepatocytes. J Biol Chem 1986; 261:12562–12567.

66. Alves A, Gouveia Ferreira M, Paulo J, Franca A, Carvalho A. Mushroom poisoning with *Amanita phalloides*—a report of four cases. Eur J Intern Med 2001; 12:64–66.

67. Piqueras J. Hepatotoxic mushroom poisoning: diagnosis and management. Mycopathologica 1989; 105:99–110.

68. Floersheim GL. Treatment of human amatoxin mushroom poisoning: myths and advances in therapy. Med Toxicol 1987; 2:1–9.

69. Klein AS, Hart J, Brems JJ, et al. *Amanita* poisoning: treatment and the role of liver transplantation. Am J Med 1989; 86:187–193.

70. Leo MA, Lieber CS. Hypervitaminosis A: a liver lover's lament. Hepatology 1988; 8:412–417.

71. Russel RM, Boyer JL, Bagheri SA, Hrubran Z. Hepatic injury from chronic hypertvitaminosis A resulting in portal hypertension and ascites. N Engl J Med 1974; 291:435–440.

72. Leo MA, Lasker JM, Raucy JL, Kim CI, Black M, Lieber C. Metabolism of retinol and retinoic acid by human liver cytochrome P450 IIC8. Arch Biochem Biophys 1989; 269:305–312.

73. Elsisi AE, Hall P, Sim WL, Earnest DL, Sipes IG. Characterization of vitamin A potentiation of carbon tetrachloride-induced liver injury. Toxicol Appl Pharmacol 1993; 119:280–288.

74. Rosengren RJ, Sauer JM, Hooser SB, Sipes IG. The interactions between retinol and five different hepatotoxicants in the Swiss Webster mouse. Fundam Appl Toxicol 1995; 25:281–292.

75. Sato T, Kato R, Tyson CA. Regulation of differentiated phenotype of rat hepatic lipocytes by retinoids in primary culture. Exp Cell Res 1995; 217:72–83.

76. De Groot AC. Dermatological drugs, topical agents and cosmetics. In: Meyler's Side Effects of Drugs. 14th ed. New York: Elsevier Science, 2000, pp. 447–480.

77. Rao PV, Bhattacharya R. The cyanobacterial toxin microcystin-LR induced DNA damage in mouse liver in vivo. Toxicology 1996; 114:29–36.

78. Runnegar M, Kaplowitz N. Microcystin uptake and inhibition of protein phosphatases. Toxicol Appl Pharmacol 1995; 134:264–272.

79. Jochimsen EM, Carmichael WW, An J, Cardo DM, Cookson ST, Holmes CEM, Antunes MB, De Melo Filho DA, Lyra TM, Barretto VST, Azevedo SMFO. Jarvis WR. Liver failure and death after exposure to microcystins at a hemodialysis center in Brazil. N Engl J Med 1998; 338:873–878.

80. Hermansky SJ, Stohs SJ, Eldeen ZM, Roche VF, Mereish KA. Evaluation of potential chemo-protectants against microcystin-LR hepatotoxicity in mice. J Appl Toxicol 1991; 11:65–73.

29

Occupational and Environmental Hepatotoxicity

KEITH G. TOLMAN

University of Utah School of Medicine, Salt Lake City, Utah, U.S.A.

I. INTRODUCTION

From the time of the Industrial Revolution through much of the twentieth century, man has ignored the conservation of his resources and the contamination of his environment and workplace. Thousands of chemicals exist in the workplace and environment. President Theodore Roosevelt in 1907 was the first political figure to recognize the importance of this contamination, stating: "Conservation of our natural resources and their proper use constitute the fundamental problem which underlies almost every other problem of our national life." Alice Hamilton, the first American physician to devote a career to industrial medicine, would comment in 1943: "American medical authorities had never taken industrial diseases seriously. . . . workers accepted the risk with fatalistic submissiveness as part of the price one must pay for being poor" (1). To this day, our solid waste tends to end up in the poor areas of our society because poor people have little political influence. Rachel Carson, in her enlightened book *Silent Spring*, first drew public attention to this problem (2). Forty years later, roughly 3000 chemicals are produced annually in quantities exceeding 1 million pounds. The National Research Council has concluded that 78% of these compounds lack minimal toxicity information (3) while the Environmental Defense Fund reported in 1997 that such data were lacking for 71% of chemicals produced in large quantity (4). As Robert F. Kennedy, Jr. commented during the William J. Taylor Executive Lecture Series at Westminster College in March 2000, "The most devastating impact of the free market is the suspension of laws that protect us." He would later say, "Investment in the environment is an investment in our infrastructure." Yet, as the late Dr. Hyman Zimmerman noted, "The issues have been clouded, however, by the incompleteness of the database, and the judgments are compromised by the efforts to balance the potential and proposed adverse effects of many pollutants against the important sociologic, economic and medical benefits. . . . Containment of the risks posed by environmental contamination requires systematic and coordinated epidemiologic, toxicologic and clinical studies to set the stage for the proper control measures" (5). A decade later, fewer than 30% of potentially toxic chemicals have been adequately tested and we have continuing exposure in the environment and workplace to known hepatotoxins such as vinyl chloride (6) and new exposures to yet-to-be-identified chemicals, as recently reported in petrochemical workers in Brazil (7,8).

II. TYPES OF INJURY

Virtually all types of liver disease may be mimicked by toxic exposure. Many chemicals in both the workplace and environment are capable of injuring the liver but rarely do so because the lungs and skin are more likely targets. The liver is typically a bystander organ or, more likely, acts to detoxify the foreign substance. Occasionally, the detoxification process goes awry leading to activation of toxic chemicals. This problem may be confounded by consumption of substances that enhance the toxicity of potential hepatotoxins, e.g., carbon tetrachloride and alcohol. The types of injury, examples of the substances involved, and their potential sources are identified in Table 1.

III. TYPES OF EXPOSURE

For exposure to occur, a chemical must be able to cross membrane barriers. The chemical structure and relative lipid solubility of the compound are the major determinants of absorption across membranes. The major routes of exposure to toxic chemicals are via the skin (dermal), gastrointestinal tract (ingestion), or lungs (inhalation). A parenteral route is also possible, although this is rare. Industrial exposure occurs primarily through inhalation and dermal exposure while environmental exposure occurs primarily through inhalation and ingestion. The route of exposure may affect the toxicity of the chemical. For example, if the compound is detoxified by the liver, exposure by inhalation may be more toxic than that by ingestion as the chemical will bypass the liver en route to the target organ. If, however, the liver activates a toxic chemical, exposure by ingestion may be more toxic.

Many inhaled compounds are toxic to the skin, lung, kidney, and bone marrow but hepatotoxic injury due to environmental pollutants appears to be rare (9). The liver, be-

Table 1 Types of Hepatic Injury

Type of injury	Examples	Exposure
Hepatocellular	Carbon tetrachloride	Household inhalation
	Tetrachloroethane	Industrial solvent
	Tetrachloroethylene	Dry-cleaning industry
	Dimethyl acetamide	Plastics and rubber industry
	Hydrochlorofluorocarbons	Refrigerants, solvents
	Vinyl chloride	Plastics industry
	Yellow phosphorus	Rat poison, firecrackers
	Poisonous mushrooms	Environmental
	Herbal preparations	Household
	2-Nitropropane	Paint coating, varnish remover
	DDT	Residual insecticide
Steatosis	Hypoglycin (Jamaican vomiting illness)	Accidental, unripe Akee fruit
	Toxic oil (rapeseed oil aniline)	Contaminated cooking oil
	Trinitrotoluene	Munitions industry
	Tetrachloroethane	Industrial solvent, chemical Manufacturing
Cholestasis	Toxic oil	
	Methylene dianiline (Epping jaundice)	Contaminated bread
	Paraquat	Residual herbicide Accidental/suicide
Subacute necrosis/ cirrhosis	Trinitrotoluene	Munitions industry
	Tetrachloroethane	Industrial solvent, chemical manufacturing
	Polychlorinated biphenyls	Residual, electrical soldering
Veno-occlusive disease	Pyrrolizidine alkaloids	Accidental plant ingestion
Hepatoportal sclerosis	Arsenic	Vintners
	Vinyl chloride	Plastics industry
Cirrhosis	Trinitrotoluene	Munitions industry
	Chlorinated hydrocarbons	Printing industry
	Arsenic	Vintners
	Trichloroethane	Solvent
Hepatocellular carcinoma	Aflatoxin B_1	Stored food contamination
	Arsenic	Vintners
Angiosarcoma	Vinyl chloride	Plastics industry

cause of its central role in detoxifying lipid soluble chemicals, is relatively spared. The risks are primarily hypothetical concerns for hepatocarinogenesis.

IV. MECHANISMS OF INJURY

Most chemicals exert their effect through selective targeting of specific tissue sites. The toxicity is a function of the ionization state, the specific interaction between the chemical and receptors on the target organ, and the organ's ability to metabolize the potentially toxic chemical. Most environmental and industrial toxins are highly lipid soluble and tend to become biocencentrated in body fat stores. They undergo metabolic transformation rather slowly. This allows them to exert their effects for prolonged periods. The polychlorinated biphenyls (PCBs) and vinyl chloride are good examples of such toxins that stay in the environment and the food chain for many years.

The ability of a chemical to enter a target cell is a function of the receptors on the cell and the ionization state of the chemical. Cell membranes are lipid bilayers and only chemicals in a nonionized and thus lipid-soluble state can enter the cell. The degree of ionization in solution is dependent upon the pH of the solution and the acidic dissociation constant (pKa) of the chemical. The pKa is the pH at which one-half of the compound is in the ionized state and one-half in the nonionized state. By convention this is expressed as the acidic pKa. For an acid, a low pKa indicates a strong acid and for a base a low pKa indicates a weak base. At a pH below the pKa, acids exist in the nonionized form while bases exist in the ionized form. Thus aspirin, a strong acid, exists in the nonionized state at gastric pH, as do nonsteroidal drugs, which for the most part are weak bases. Whenever there is a pH gradient across a membrane, a concentration gradient for the nonionized compound will exist. This is especially true in the stomach and kidneys. Thus aspirin at the acidic pH of the stomach is nonionized and tends to bioconcentrate across the cell membrane of the stomach but is excreted at high concentrations in alkaline urine.

Hepatic biotransformation usually converts lipid-soluble compounds to less toxic water-soluble compounds that can be eliminated. This process is usually protective to the host. However, it can go awry leading to the formation of toxic reactive metabolites. The biotransformation is mostly carried out by cytochrome P450–mediated oxidation in the microsomal enzyme system, a system that may be induced or inhibited by various compounds. Chemicals that either inhibit or induce this system may enhance or reduce the toxicity. This is the case with carbon tetrachloride (CCl_4) toxicity, which is worsened by alcohol, which accelerates the conversion of CCl_4 to a toxic reactive metabolite (10,11). Environmental interactions may also occur. For example, 2,3,7,8-tetrachlorodibenzo-*p*-dioxin is a potent inducer of aryl hydrocarbon hydroxylase, which metabolizes polycyclic aromatic hydrocarbons, which are ubiquitous in the environment (12), to potentially carcinogenic metabolites.

V. HEPATOTOXIC CHEMICALS

The National Institute for Occupational Safety and Health (NIOSH) has published a pocket guide to hazardous chemicals (13). A total of 667 industrial chemicals are listed of which 228 have reference to liver toxicity through either animal experimentation or clinical observation (13). The incidence and severity of liver toxicity, however, appear to be low and many of the chemicals are only of historical interest at this time. The most widely known are listed in Table 2.

VI. HALOGENATED AROMATIC HYDROCARBONS

Manufacturing of polychlorinated biphenyls (PCBs) was discontinued in 1977, but more than two decades later there is still concern. Their stability, resistance to biodegradation, and insolubility in water have allowed them to remain in the environment (14–16). They remain in wildlife and have entered the food chain including breast milk (17) in contaminated areas of the United States (as well as in Third World countries where polluting industries have moved in) (18).

Table 2 Most Widely Known Hepatotoxins

Chemical class	Use	Type of injury	Teratogenic	Carcinogenic
Halogenated aromatic hydrocarbons				
Polychlorinated biphenyls	Environmental contaminant (fish)	HCN	?	?
Chloronaphthalenes	Environmental contaminant (fish)	HCN	?	?
Chlorinated benzenes		HCN	?	?
Halogenated aliphatic hydrocarbons				
Carbon tetrachloride	Experimental hepatotoxin	Steatosis, HCN, ALF	?	Yes
1,1,2,2-Tetrachloroethane	Chemical manufacture	HCN	?	Yes
1,1,1-Trichloroethane	Varnish, solvent	HCN, steatosis	?	Yes
Chloroform	Pharmaceutical manufacture, sniffing	HCN, steatosis	?	Yes
Halothane	Anesthetic	HCN	?	Yes
Hydrochlorofluorocarbons (HCFC 123, HCFC 124)	Refrigerants, cleaning agents, solvents	HCN	?	Yes
Chlorinated ethylenes				
Vinyl chloride	Manufacture of PVC, plastics, food wrapping, ground water	Hepatic sclerosis	Yes	Yes
Vinylidine chloride	Manufacture of plastics		?	Yes
Trans-dichloroethylene	Solvent	Steatosis	?	
Cis-dichloroethylene	Solvent	Steatosis	?	
Trichloroethylene	Solvent, degreaser	Necrosis	?	Yes
Perchloroethylene	Solvent, dry cleaning, paint, pesticides, fluorocarbons	Steatosis, cirrhosis	?	Yes
N-substituted amides				
Dimethyl acetamide	Solvent, resins, polymers	HCN, J, steatosis	?	?
Dimethyl formamide	Solvent, resins, polymers	HCN, steatosis	?	?
Nitroaromatic compounds				
Dinitrobenzene		HCN	?	?
2,6-Dinitrotoluene		HCN, jaundice	?	Yes
Picric acid		HCN	?	?
Tetryl		HCN, steatosis	?	?
Trinitrotoluene (TNT)		HCN, jaundice	?	?

Table 2   Continued

Chemical class	Use	Type of injury	Teratogenic	Carcinogenic
Miscellaneous organics				
Diphenyl oxide		HCN		
Dimethylnitrosamine	Experimental	HCN	?	Yes
Methylene dianiline	Plastic	HCN, J		Yes
Pyridine	Solvent, chemical manu-facturing	HCN	?	?
Paraquat	Herbicide	HCN, chol		
Diquat	Herbicide	HCN	?	?
Miscellaneous inor-ganics				
Arsenic	Insecticide, miners, vineyard workers, ho-micide, experimental	Steatosis, HCN, AS		Yes
Beryllium	Experimental	Granulomas, zone 2 ne-crosis, ALT elevations, steatosis	?	Yes
Copper	Fungicide	Granulomas, AS		
Hydrazine	Rocket fuel	Steatosis, ALT elevations		
Alaphatic hydrocarbons				
Benzene				
Toluene	Glue sniffing	Steatosis		
Selenium	Semiconductors, photo-conductors	Steatosis, HCN	?	?

AS, angiosarcoma; ALF, acute liver failure; chol, cholestasis; J, jaundice; HCN, hepatocellular necrosis.

Their dielectric properties and noninflammability make PCBs highly desirable for high-voltage electrical apparatus. However, the exposure of workers has resulted in serious hepatic disease (19). Although PCBs are potent inducers of CYP 450 isoenzymes, which in turn are potential inducers of carcinogenic compounds, there is no convincing evidence that PCBs are hepatocarcinogenic (20). However, they also induce δ-aminolevulinic synthase, which probably accounts for the cases of porphyria cutanea tarda among those with occupational exposure.

Hepatic injury in humans has occurred as the result of industrial exposure or by accidental exposure to contaminated cooking oil (Yusho disease in Japan) (21). The level of exposure that occurs from residual amounts of PCBs in the environment does not appear to cause liver disease in humans (14–16). However, because these agents are such potent inducers of the CYP 450 system, there are continuing concerns about their potential enhancement of the hepatotoxic effects of other chemicals and drugs (22,23). In addition, PCBs have been shown to be carcinogenic in rodents (16). Studies of the environmental effects of PCBs, have been compromised by cross-contamination with dioxin, a well-known hepatotoxin in animals (12,24).

VII. HALOGENATED ALIPHATIC HYDROCARBONS

A. Carbon Tetrachloride

Carbon tetrachloride (CCl_4) is one of three classic hepatotoxins (the others are yellow phosphorus and toxic mushrooms) that cause acute hepatic and renal failure with hepatocellular necrosis and steatosis. In the early 1900s, CCl_4 was used as a vermifuge. Subsequently it was used as a solvent and in fire extinguishers resulting in household and industrial exposure (25). CCl_4 is no longer available in the United States other than as an experimental hepatotoxin. It is now largely of historical interest with no cases having been reported in the United States since 1985. Exposure typically occurred by inhalation of fumes during the cleaning of vats or by accidental ingestion in the household (25–27). It is now used in laboratories as an experimental hepatotoxin. It should not be forgotten, however, that in some parts of the world, CCl_4 is still used as an ingredient in fire extinguishers and refrigerants.

The toxicity of CCl_4 is mediated by a trichloromethyl radical generated by cytochrome P450 2E1. Cell membrane entry leads to lipid peroxidation, which inhibits triglyceride secretion with subsequent steatosis and necrosis (28). Fulminant hepatic failure ensues (29). The injury is potentiated by alcohol, which induces CYP 2E1 (30,31).

B. Tetrachloroethane

1,1,2,2-Tetrachloroethane is a chemical intermediate used in the manufacture of the solvents trichloroethylene and tetrachloroethane. Hepatotoxicity is characterized by hepatitis and has been reported in 25 patients (32). There has been one fatal case of a patient with cirrhosis and superimposed hepatitis (33). There is also a report of exposure in a penicillin-manufacturing facility where 50% of the workers developed abnormal liver chemistry tests over a 3-year period (34). Experimentally, fatty degeneration is seen in rodents (35).

C. Hydrochlorofluorocarbons

Hydrochlorofluorocarbons (HCFCs), specifically 1,1-dichloro-2,2,2-trifluoroethane (HCFC 123) and 1-chloro-1,2,2,2-tetrafluoroethane (HCFC 124), are being increasingly substituted for ozone-depleting chlorofluorocarbons (CFCs) (36). This was the result of a convention of international experts in June 1990, in Montreal, Canada where it was determined that depletion of the ozone layer was occurring as a result of release of active chlorine from CFCs. The potential health consequences of the ozone layer depletion created an urgent need for development of partially halogenated HFCAs, which are now used as refrigerants, cleaning agents, and industrial solvents as well as for foam blowing. The chemical structures of HCFC 123/124 are similar to that of halothane, an inhaled anesthetic known to cause hepatitis in susceptible individuals after repeated exposure. HCFCs 123/124 are metabolized through the same oxidative pathway to a reactive trifluoroacetyl halide that forms haptens (42). Animal studies, primarily in rats, have demonstrated some hepatotoxicity for HFCA 123, but not HFCA 124 (37–39). Acute exposure to HCFC 123 in guinea pigs has been demonstrated to be hepatotoxic (43). The toxicity is enhanced by glutathione depletion (44). Hepatic adenomas also have been seen in rats in subchronic studies. Dekant has emphasized the need for more research into the chronic effects and the mechanisms of injury (41). In 1997, Hoet et al. reported an "epidemic" of nine industrial workers who had reported accidental exposure to a mixture of HCFC 123/124 (40).

One of the workers developed a picture of "acute mixed hepatitis" with ALT, 1298 U/L; alkaline phosphatase, 303 U/L; prothrombin time, 51%; and bilirubin, 289 μmol/L. He recovered completely over the next 2 months and then relapsed when he returned to work. A liver biopsy showed hepatocellular coagulative necrosis and canalicular bile plugs in zone 3 with bridging necrosis. There was a moderate lymphoid infiltrate. Immunohistochemical staining demonstrated trifluoroacetyl protein adducts similar to those seen with halothane toxicity. Five of six HFCA 123/124–affected workers analyzed had antibodies to P58 and cytochrome P450 2E1, again similar to that seen with halothane hepatotoxicity. The current production of HCFCs is measured in kilotons per year but is expected to greatly increase owing to the ban on CFCs. The concerns about hepatotoxicity and possible carcinogenicity of HCFCs in humans raise questions about the risk-benefit ratio of the combined introduction of HCFCs and ban on CFCs.

VIII. CHLORINATED ETHYLENES

A. Tetrachloroethylene (Perchloroethylene)

Tetrachloroethylene is used primarily in the dry-cleaning industry and for textile processing. It is also used as an insulating fluid and in the production of fluorocarbons and, to a lesser extent, in the production of adhesives, aerosols, and paint. Most exposure occurs through inhalation and dermal contact as an industrial contaminant.

Liver injury, including cirrhosis, has been reported in workers with low-dose exposure over a 2–6-year period (45). Cases of accidental high-level exposure resulting in hepatotoxicity have also been reported (46–49). Tetrachloroethylene is hepatocarcinogenic in rodents (50).

IX. N-SUBSTITUTED AMIDES

A. Dimethylacetamide

N,N-Dimethylacetamide is a solvent used in the synthesis of resins and polymers. Jaundice has been seen in people repeatedly exposed to small amounts of the solvent (51). Workers monitored over a 2–10-year period have shown abnormal liver chemistries (52) while hepatitis after dermal exposure has been experienced by those employed in an acrylic manufacturing plant (53). As a result, biological monitoring of urinary metabolites is now recommended in exposed workers.

Fatty infiltration in dogs (54) and focal necrosis in rats (55) have been observed after high-dose experimental exposure.

B. Dimethylformamide

N,N-Dimethylformamide is a widely used solvent in the resin and polymer industries. It is also used in the manufacture of paint, film, and adhesives. Currently more than 100,000 workers per year are exposed to the solvent. Inhalation, ingestion, and dermal exposure all have been shown experimentally to lead to injury (56–61). Acute hepatitis is seen in rats (60) but there have been few occupational exposures resulting in tissue injury in humans (62,63). A relatively recent report, however, described cases of hepatic injury in a group of fabric workers with more than 1 year of exposure. Liver biopsies showed steatosis (64). There also have been scattered reports of mild hepatotoxicity (65–67).

X. CHLORPHENOXY COMPOUNDS

More than 15 isomers of chlorophenol are available for use as insecticides and pesticides. These include paraquat, chlordane, heptachlor, aldrin, dieldrin, lindane, and chlordecone (kepone) (59,69,70). While zonal necrosis and steatosis can occur with these compounds (71,72), there is little evidence of hepatotoxicity in humans, even when significant amounts are ingested. Ingestion of large quantities of DDT produces hepatic necrosis (73) but hepatic abnormalities are not usually seen among workers in DDT factories (74).

Experimental hepatocarcinogenesis has been shown for aldrin, amitrole, aramite, captan, chlorbenzilate, chlordane, chlordecone, DDT, dieldrin, heptachlor, lindane, mirex, and other pesticides (75–78). There is continuing concern about Agent Orange, a defoliant used in Vietnam. It is a mixture of the chlorophenoxy herbicides 2,4-dichlorophenoxyace-tic acid, 2,4,5-trichlorophenoxyacetic acid, and dioxin (79–81). Dioxin is a potent hepato-carcinogen. The chlorophenoxy compounds have been associated with porphyria cutanea tarda (82,83) but there is little evidence of hepatic injury. Nevertheless the latency period from exposure to development of tumors is measured in years in humans and this situation deserves continued monitoring.

A. Chlordecone (Kepone)

Chlordecone is a pesticide that attracted considerable attention in the lay press in the 1970s when workers at a small plant developed neurological and systemic symptoms (84,85). Contamination of an abutting structure and far-off waters was subsequently demonstrated (86–88). A year later chlordecone was still evident in the food chain (89).

Chlordecone is a relatively mild hepatotoxin with only slight biochemical and histo-logical changes noted despite high tissue levels in liver and other organs (84,90). Steatosis and mild necrosis have been seen in humans and animals. It is hepatocarcinogenic in mice and rats (84). It is a potent inducer of the CYP 450 system and has the ability to enhance the toxicity of CCl_4 and $CHCl_3$. Guzelian has demonstrated that treatment with cholestyramine enhances excretion of this agent (84).

The large body stores of chlordecone and its hepatocarcinogenicity in rats and mice raise concern about long-term safety but no evidence of hepatotoxicity in humans has appeared to date.

B. Paraquat

Paraquat is a toxic herbicide used as a crop defoliant and weed killer. Two fatal cases of hepatic injury were initially reported in 1966 (91). A number of cases have since been reported as the result of attempted suicide (91,92) or accidental ingestion (85). The case fatality rate is 50–70% but the cause of death is usually pulmonary from activated oxygen (94).

Patients present with severe vomiting, diarrhea, abdominal pain, and irritation of the oropharyngeal area. Hepatic manifestations, including jaundice, appear on the second or third day. Histological changes include hepatocellular necrosis followed by severe cho-langitis. Biochemical changes are mixed hepatocellular-cholestatic (95). Treatment con-sists of vigorous diuresis and intragastric administration of activated charcoal. There are also case reports crediting dexamethasone and cyclophosphamide with improving re-covery.

XI. SUMMARY

Contamination of the environment and workplace by toxic chemicals continues to pose some health hazard. The risk has become greatly reduced in terms of acute overt toxicity. The long-term effects, however, of low-level exposure in causing chronic liver disease and hepatic cancer remains a concern. The latency period from exposure to chronic liver disease and carcinoma is measured in years, yet the monitoring that is in place is confined to acute exposure without long-term monitoring of people who move from a potentially toxic environment. The discovery of latent injury in vinyl chloride workers (96) and of nonalcoholic steatohepatitis in workers and nearby residents of a petrochemical plant in Brazil (7,8) underscores the importance of monitoring and enhanced testing of potentially toxic chemicals. The science has been compromised by the paucity of biological models for chronic exposure and the persistence of often-conflicting medical, economic, social, and political priorities. Whether we will learn from the lessons of the past remains uncertain. It seems self-evident that a person's health is, in large part, a function of the health of his or her environment (97). As Kennedy said, "In a true free market, you clean up after yourself."

REFERENCES

1. Hamilton A. Exploring the Dangerous Trades. Boston: Little Brown, 1943:1.
2. Carson RI. Silent Spring. Cambridge: Riverside Press, 1962.
3. National Research Council. Toxicity Testing. Washington, DC: National Academic Press, 1984.
4. Roe D, Pease W, Horini K, et al. Toxic Ignorance: The Continuing Absence of Basic Health Testing for Top-Selling Chemicals in the United States. New York: Environmental Defense Fund, 1997.
5. Zimmerman HJ. Hepatotoxicity. Adverse Effects of Drugs and Other Chemicals on the Liver. New York: Appleton-Crofts, 1978:333.
6. Pirastu R, Combe P, Reggiani A, et al. Mortality from liver disease among Italian vinyl chloride monomer/polyvinyl chloride manufacturer. Am J Indust Med 1990; 17:155–156.
7. Cotrim HP, Freitas LA, Parana R, et al. Non alcoholic steatohepatitis (NASH) and environmental toxins: a liver disease in workers from an industrial area (abstr). Hepatology 1996; 24:337.
8. Cotrim HP, Parana R, Portugal M, et al. Non-alcoholic steatohepatitis (NASH) and industrial toxins: follow up of patients removed from one industrial area. Hepatology 1997; 26:149 (abstr).
9. Guzelian P. Hepatic injury due to environmental agents. Clin Lab Med 1984; 4:483–488.
10. Recknagel RO, Glende EA Jr, Dolak JH, et al. Mechanisms of carbon tetrachloride toxicity. Pharmacol Ther 1989; 43:139–154.
11. Zimmerman HJ. Effect of alcohol on other hepatotoxins. Alcohol Clin Exp Res 1986; 10:3–15.
12. Poland A, Kende A. 2,3,7,8-Tetrachlorodibenzo-p-dioxin: environmental contaminant and molecular probe. Fed Proc 1976; 35:2404–2411.
13. NIOSH. Pocket Guide to Chemical Hazards. U.S. Department of Health and Human Services Publication 94-116. U.S. Government Printing Office, 1994.
14. D'Itri FM, Kamrin MA, eds. PCBs: Human and Environmental Hazards. Woburn, MA: Butterworths, 1983.
15. Peakall DB, Lincer JL. Polychlorinated biphenyls: another long-life, widespread chemical in the environment. Bioscience 1970; 20:958.
16. Kimbrough RD. Human health effects of polychlorinated biphenyls (PCBs) and polybrominated biphenyls (PBBs). Annu Rev Pharmacol Toxicol 1987; 27:87–111.

17. Fries GF. The PBB episode in Michigan: an overall appraisal. Crit Rev Toxicol 1985; 16: 105–156.

18. La Dou J. The export of environmental responsibility [editorial]. Arch Environ Health 1994; 49:6–8.

19. Strauss N. Hepatotoxic effects following occupational exposure to halowax (chlorinated hydrocarbons). Rev Gastroenterol 1994; 11:381.

20. Goldstein JA, Friesen M, Scott TM, et al. Assessment of the contribution of the chlorinated dibenzo-p-dioxins and dibenzofurans to hexachlorobenzene-induced toxicity, porphyria, changes in mixed function oxygenases, and histopathological changes. Toxicol Appl Pharmacol 1978; 46:633–649.

21. Kuratsune M, Yoshimura T, Matzuzaka J, Yamaguchi A. Epidemiologic study on Yusho, a poisoning caused by ingestion of rice oil contaminated with a commercial brand of polychlorinated biphenyls. Environ Health Perspect 1972; 1:119–128.

22. Fouts JR. Interactions of chemicals and drugs to produce effects on organ function. In: DHK Lee, P Koten, eds. Multiple Factors in the Causation of Environmentally Induced Disease. New York: Academic Press, 1972:109–118.

23. Mitchell JR, Gillette JR. Drug-chemical interactions as a factor in environmentally induced disease. In: DHK Lee, P Koten, eds. Multiple Factors in the Causation of Environmentally Induced Disease. New York: Academic Press, 1972:119–131.

24. Poland A, Knutson JC. 2,3,7,8-Tetrachlorodibenzo-*p*-dioxin and related halogenated aromatic hydrocarbons: examination of the mechanism of toxicity. Annu Rev Pharmacol Toxicol 1982; 22:517–554.

25. Hardin BL Jr. Carbon tetrachloride poisoning—a review. Indust Med Surg 1954; 23:93–105.

26. Jennings RB. Fatal fulminant acute carbon tetrachloride poisoning. AMA Arch Pathol 1955; 59:269–284.

27. Von Oettingen WF. The Halogenated Hydrocarbons of Industrial and Toxicological Importance. Amsterdam: Elsevier, 1964.

28. Dianzani M. Biochemical aspects of fatty liver. In: RG Meeks, SD Harrison, RJ Bull, eds. Hepatotoxicity. Boca Raton, FL: CRC Press, 1991:327.

29. Recknagel RO, Glende EA Jr. Carbon tetrachloride hepatotoxicity: An example of lethal cleavage. CRC Crit Rev Toxicol 1973; 2:263–297.

30. Reichert D. Biological actions and interactions of tetrachloroethylene. Mutat Res 1983; 123: 411–429.

31. Reuber MD, Glover EL. Cirrhosis and carcinoma of the liver in male rats given subcutaneous carbon tetrachloride. J Natl Cancer Inst 1970; 44:419–427.

32. Ho SP, Phoon WH, Gan SL, Chan YK. Persistent liver dysfunction among workers at a vinyl chloride monomer polymerization plant. J Soc Occup Med 1991; 4:10–16.

33. Coyer HA. Tetrachloroethane poisoning. Indust Med 1944; 13:230–233.

34. Jeney E, Bartha F, Kondor L, Szendrei S. Prevention of industrial tetrachloroethane intoxication. Part 3. Egeszegtudmany 1967; 1:155–164.

35. Horiuchi K, Moriguchi S, Monimoto K, et al. Studies on industrial tetrachloroethane poisoning. Osaka City Med J 1962; 8:29–38.

36. WHO, Environmental Health Criteria 139. Partially Halogenated Chlorofluorocarbons (Ethane Derivatives). Geneva: WHO, 1992.

37. Malley LA, Carakostas M, Hansen JF, et al. Two-year inhalation toxicity study in rats with hydrochlorofluorocarbon 123. Fundam Appl Toxicol 1995; 24:101–104.

38. Urban G, Speerschneider P, Dekant W. Metabolism of the chlorofluorocarbon substitute 1,1-dichloro-2,2,2-trifluoroethane by rat and human liver microsomes: the role of cytochrome P_{450} 2E1. Chem Res Toxicol 1994; 7:170–176.

39. Malley, LA, Carakostas M, Elliott GS, et al. Subchronic toxicity and teratogenicity of 2-chloro-1,1,1,2-tetrafluoroethane (HCFA-124). Fundam Appl Toxicol 1996; 72:11–22.

40. Hoet P, Graf MLM, Bourdi M, et al. Epidemic of liver disease caused by hydrochlorofluorocarbons used as ozone-sparing substitutes of chlorofluorocarbons. Lancet 1997; 350:556–559.

41. Dekant W. Toxicology of chlorofluorocarbon replacements. Environ Health Perspect 1996; 104:75–83.

42. Harris JW, Jones JP, Martin JL, et al. Pentahaloethane-based chlorofluorocarbon substitutes and halothane: correlation of in vivo hepatic protein trichloroacetylation and urinary trifluoroacetic acid excretion with calculated enthalpies at activation. Chem Res Toxicol 1992; 5:420–752.

43. Marit GB, Didd DE, George ME, Vinegar A. Hepatotoxicity in guinea pigs following acute inhalation exposure to 1,1-dicloro-2,2,2-trifluoroethane. Toxicol Pathol 1994; 22:404–414.

44. Lind RC, Gandolfi AJ, Hall PD. Biotransformation and hepatotoxicity of HCFC-123 in the guinea pig: potentiation of hepatic injury by prior glutathione depletion. Toxicol Appl Pharmacol 1995; 134(1):175–181.

45. Lukaszewski T. Acute tetrachloroethylene fatality. Clin Toxicol 1979; 15:411–415.

46. Hake Cl, Stewart RD. Human exposure to tetrachloroethylene: Inhalation and skin contact. Environ Health Perspect 1977; 21:231–238.

47. Meckler LC, Phelps DK. Liver disease secondary to tetrachloroethylene exposure: a case report. JAMA 1966; 197:662–663.

48. Stewart RD. Acute tetrachloroethylene intoxication. JAMA 1969; 208:1490–1492.

49. Stewart RD, Gay HH, Erley DS, et al. Human exposure to tetrachloroethylene vapor. Arch Environ Health 1961; 2:516–522.

50. National Cancer Institute. Bioassay of Tetrachloroethylen+e for Possible Carcinogenicity. NCI TR 13. DHEW (NIH) Pub No. 77-813: NTIS Pub No PB-272-940. Springfield, VA: National Technical Service.

51. Johnson MD. Letter from Medical Director of Chemstrand Corporation to the TLV Committee, March 1961.

52. Corsi GC. Dimethylacetamide-induced occupational diseases with particular attention to hepatic function. Med Lav 1971; 62:28–30.

53. Spies GJ, Rhyne RH Jr, Evans RA, et al. Monitoring acrylic fiber workers for liver toxicity and exposure to dimethylacetamide. 1. Assessing exposure to dimethylacetamide by air and biological monitoring. J Occup Environ Med 1995; 37:1093–1101.

54. Kelly DP: Subchronic inhalation toxicity of dimethyl acetamide in rats. Toxicologist 1984; 4:65.

55. Horn HJ: Toxicology of dimethylacetamide. Toxicol Appl Pharmacol 1961; 3:12–24.

56. Clayton JW, Barnes JR, Hood DB, Schepers GWH. The inhalation toxicity of dimethylformamide (DMF). Am Indust Hyg Assoc J 1963; 24:144–154.

57. Craig DK, Weir RJ, Wagner W, Groth D. Subchronic inhalation toxicity of dimethylformamide in rats and mice. Drug Chem Toxicol 1984; 7:551–571.

58. Lundberg I, Lundberg S, Kronevi T. Some observations on dimethylformamide hepatotoxicity. Toxicology 1981; 22:1–7.

59. Wiles JS, Narcisse JK Jr. The acute toxicity of dimethylamides in several animal species. Am Indust Hyg Assoc J 1971; 32:539–545.

60. Kennedy GL Jr, Sherman H. Acute and subchronic toxicity of dimethylformamide and dimethylacetamide following various routes of administration. Drug Chem Toxicol 1986; 9:147–170.

61. Kennedy GL Jr. Biological effects of acetamide, formamide, and their monomethyl and dimethyl derivatives. Crit Rev Toxicol 1986; 17:129–182.

62. Massman W. Toxicological investigations on dimethylformamide. Br J Indust Med 1956; 13: 51–54.

63. Wang JD, Lai MY, Chen JS, Lin JM, Chiang JR, Shiau SJ, Chang WS. Dimethylformamide-induced liver damage among synthetic leather workers. Arch Environ Health 1991; 46:161–166.

64. Redlich CA, West AB, Flemming L, True LD, Cullen MR, Riely CA. Clinical and pathological

characteristics of hepatotoxicity associated with occupational exposure to dimethylformamide. Gastroenterology 1990; 99:748–757.

65. Potter HP. Dimethylformamide-induced abdominal pain and liver injury. Arch Environ Health 1973; 27:340–341.

66. Buylaert W, Calle P, De-Paep P, Verstraete A, Samyn N, Vogelaers D, Vandenbulcke M, Belpaire F. Hepatotoxicity of *N,N*-dimethylformamide (DMF) in acute poisoning with the veterinary euthanasia drug T-61. Hum Exp Toxicol 1996; 15:607–611.

67. Poelmans L, van-Besien B, VanGanse W, Deprez A. Toxic hepatitis due to dimethylformamide: case reports and literature review. Acta Clin Belg 1996; 51:360–366.

68. Hayes WJ Jr. Pesticides Studied in Man. Baltimore, MD: Williams & Wilkins, 1982.

69. Vettorazzi G. Toxicological decisions and recommendations resulting from the safety assessment of pesticide residues in food. CRC Crit Rev Toxicol 1975; 4:125–183.

70. Von Oettingen WF. The Halogenated Aliphatic, Olephinic, Cyclic, Aromatic, and Aliphatic-Aromatic Hydrocarbons Including the Halogenated Insecticides: Their Toxicity and Potential Dangers U.S. Dept. H.E.W. Washington, DC: U.S. Government Printing Office, 1995.

71. Folland DS, Schaffner W, Ginn HE, Crofford OB, McMurray DR. Carbon tetrachloride toxicity potentiated by isopropyl alcohol. JAMA 1976; 236(16):1853–1856.

72. Beloskurskaya GI, Korolchuk EI: Time course of the liver aspect enzymogram in workers engaged in phosphorus production and in patients with chronic phosphorus poisoning after hypobaric oygenation. Gigiens Trunda I Professionalye Zabolevani, July 11, 1984.

73. Smith NJ. Death following accidental ingestion of DDT. JAMA 1948; 136:469–471.

74. Siegers C-P, Oltmanns D, Younes M. Effect of alcohol and chronic liver disease on the metabolic disposal of acetaminophen in man. Hepatogastroenterology 1981; 28:304.

75. Tomatis L. The IARC program in the evaluation of carcinogenic risk of chemicals to man. Ann NY Acad Sci 1976; 271:396–409.

76. Timbrell JA, Scales MDC, Streeter AJ. Studies of hydrazine hepatotoxcity 2. Biochemical findings. J Toxicol Enviro Health 1982; 10(6):955–968.

77. Weisberger EK. Halogenated substances: Environmental and industrial materials. In: MAQ Khan, RH Stanton, eds. Toxicology of Halogenated Hydrocarbons: Health and Ecological Effects. New York: Pergamon Press, 1981:3–22.

78. Ecobichon DJ. Toxic effects of pesticides. In: CD Klaassen, ed. Cassarett and Doull's Toxicology: The Basic Science of Poisons. 5th ed. New York: McGraw-Hill, 1996:643–690.

79. Wade N. Viets and vets fear herbicide health effects: Vietnamese official brings concerns to Washington. Science 1979; 204(4395):870–873.

80. Sterling TD, Arundel A. Review of recent Vietnamese studies on the carcinogenic and teratogenic effects of phenoxy herbicide exposure. Int J Health Serv 1986; 16(2):265–278.

81. Council on Scientific Affairs of the AMA. The Health Effects of "Agent Orange" and Polychlorinated Dioxin Contaminants. Chicago: American Medical Association, 1981.

82. Jirasek L, Kalensky J, Huber K, Pazderovas, Lukas E. Choracne, porphyria cutanea tarda and other signs of intoxication by herbicides. Hautarzt 1976; 27(7):328–333.

83. Pazderova-Vejlupkova J, Nemcova M, Pickova J, et al. The development and prognosis of chronic intoxication by tetrachlorodibenzo-*p*-dioxin in men. Arch Environ Health 1981; 36:5–11.

84. Guzelian PS. Comparative toxicology of chlordecone (Kepone) in humans and experimental animals. Annu Rev Pharmacol Toxicol 1982; 22:89–113.

85. Blanke RV, Fariss MW, Griffith FD Jr, Guzelian PS. Analysis of chlordecone (Kepone) in biological specimens. J Anal Toxicol 1977; 1:57.

86. Huggett RJ, Bender ME. Kepone in the James River. Environ Sci Technol 1980; 14:918–923.

87. Huggett RJ, Nichols MM, Bender ME. Kepone contamination of the James River Estuary. Contam Sediments 1980; 1:33.

88. Sterrett FS, Boss CA. Careless Kepone. Environment 1977; 19:30.

89. The Kepone catastrophe. Washington Post, December 21, 1975.

90. Larson PS, Egle JR, Hennigar GR, Lane RW, Borzelleca JF. Acute, subchronic, and chronic toxicity of chloraecone. Toxicol Appl Pharmacol 1979; 48(1 pt 1):29–41.
91. Bullivant CM. Accidental poisoning by paraquat: report of two cases in man. Br Med J 1966; 5498:1272–1273.
92. Carson DJL, Carson ED. The increasing use of paraquat as a suicidal agent. Forensic Sci 1976; 7:151–160.
93. Anonymous. Paraquat poisoning. Lancet 1971; 2:1018–1019.
94. Bus JS, Aust SP, Gibson JE. Superoxide and singlet-oxygen-catalyzed lipid peroxidation as a possible mechanism for paraquat (methylviologen) toxicity. Biochem Biophys Res Commun 1974; 58:749.
95. Mullick FG, Ishak KG, Makabir R, Strobmeyer FW. Hepatic injury associated with paraquat toxicity in humans. Liver 1981; 1:209–221.
96. Thomas LB, Popper H, Berk PD, et al. Vinyl chloride-induced liver disease: from idiopathic portal hypertension (Banti's syndrome) to angiosarcomas. N Engl J Med 1975; 292:17–22.
97. Tolman KG, Sirrine R. Industrial hepatotoxicity. Clin Liver Dis 1998; 2(3):563–589.

30

Regulatory Perspectives

JOHN R. SENIOR

Food and Drug Administration, Rockville, Maryland, U.S.A.

I. INTRODUCTION

Injury to the liver caused by drugs or their metabolites is becoming recognized as an increasing concern for regulatory agencies, pharmaceutical companies, practicing physicians, and above all, for patients who take the drugs. This chapter will focus on regulatory

These comments are written from the perspective of the writer's past 7 years at the FDA as a reviewing medical officer for gastrointestinal drugs and advisor on drug safety, 11 years as an independent consultant to the pharmaceutical industry, a previous 5 years as a senior pharmaceutical company executive for clinical affairs worldwide, following 20 years as an investigator-practitioner-professor in academic gastroenterology/hepatology. They are not intended to provide a comprehensive description of the processes of drug development and review, marketing, and surveillance practiced by the industry and the FDA. The writer has selected points believed helpful and necessary for understanding by practicing and academic physicians, and by informed others. The comments do not reflect official Agency positions or policies, but represent the personal opinions of the writer based upon the diverse experiences mentioned.

aspects of this problem, but it is not just a problem for the Food and Drug Administration (FDA) or for other regulatory agencies in countries around the world. It is also a serious financial and public relations problem for the pharmaceutical companies that make and sell the drugs. It is both an ethical and a responsibility problem for the physicians who prescribe the drugs and advise patients about their concurrent use of other drugs, over-the-counter (OTC) medications, alcohol, and herbal or other dietary supplements. It is a confidence and survival problem for patients who trust in the safety of these drug products. It is a problem for all of us.

Although data are relatively sparse, Japan and Denmark have reported apparently increasing incidences of drug-induced liver injury in recent decades (1), and there is a sense that this is occurring elsewhere in Europe and North America (2). There are many reasons for this. People are taking more and more drugs, both under prescription and by personal choice of OTC remedies, in addition to alcohol and the so-called dietary or nutritional supplements not classified or regulated as drugs despite their obvious pharmacological effects, as well as exposure to environmental nondrug chemicals or agents.

Many or most of these xenobiotic substances are metabolized or cleared to varying extents by the vast array of enzymes and transport systems in the liver, and many of them induce changes in or inhibit those processes. The potential for drug-drug and drug-nondrug interactions rises steeply as the number of chemical agents increases. Perhaps as a consequence, drug-induced liver injury has become the leading cause for removal of approved drugs from the market (R. Temple, FDA, personal communication, "Hepatotoxicity Through the Years"), and for acute liver failure in patients evaluated at liver transplant centers in the United States, exceeding all other causes combined, mostly due to acetaminophen (3).

To better understand both the strengths and weaknesses of the processes that are used by the FDA in its attempts to protect patients by ensuring safety and effectiveness of approved medications, it may be of value and service to readers to summarize those processes briefly. They seem not to be well understood by most practicing or academic physicians, let alone by patients or the general public. We all need to think about these processes and ask how they might be improved to protect patients, particularly how especially susceptible patients might be identified and prevented from being exposed to the risks of drug-induced liver injury.

II. PRE- AND NONCLINICAL RESEARCH AND DEVELOPMENT

Potentially useful drugs have been identified by screening vast numbers of organic compounds for desired pharmacological activity and absence of toxicity, but recently more and more by molecular tailoring for binding affinities to specific target receptors. Candidate compounds may be synthesized to resemble approved drugs, but different enough to be patentable; or generated by computerized spatial modeling for effects at molecular binding sites; or purified from naturally occurring plant or animal sources following indications of effects from the crude material. Years of extensive preclinical study are needed for synthesis and purification of the new drug substance and to characterize physicochemical features, toxicology, and pharmacokinetics in animals, its metabolic pathways in both animals and humans, and induction/inhibition of metabolism of other drugs.

Most of the compounds screened in this initial research and development process are eliminated because of insufficient efficacy or excessive toxicity, and are never given

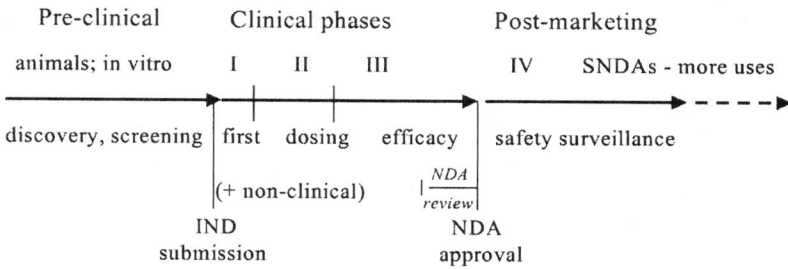

Figure 1 Scheme of development of new drugs, from discovery to established use, a process that takes many years.

to human subjects. This preclinical work usually precedes in most part the drug's study as an experimental product in humans, but may continue as supplemental but important nonclinical work concurrently with later clinical investigations. Final steps in the pre- or nonclinical phase, for still promising drug substances, include development of drug product formulations for ease of administration and acceptability, and the measurement of storage stability of the active components. This work is most often conducted by pharmaceutical companies, but may also be done by academic investigators. The process often takes from 6 to 10 years, from discovery to investigational new drug (IND) applications to approval of the new drug application (NDA), as outlined in Figure 1.

III. CONTROLLED CLINICAL TRIALS

As randomized, double-blinded, prospective, multiarmed clinical trials in humans have evolved over the past 50 years to become the "gold standard" for reducing unwanted biases and confounding (4), they have been classified by the FDA (5) and paraphrased by industry (6) into three phases for preapproval studies, and a fourth phase for additional studies after marketing. These phases are, in brief:

1. Initial introduction of the drug into humans, usually healthy volunteers or stable patients, to determine their tolerance to increasing doses, metabolism and pharmacokinetics, pharmacodynamic effects, and, particularly, safety of the drug in humans.
2. Limited controlled trials in patients, usually involving no more than several hundred persons, for evidence of effectiveness in treating their disease or disorder, dose determination, and safety.
3. Trials in expanded numbers and types of sick patients, for longer periods, using the final dosage form or formulation of drug product to be marketed if approved, for definitive efficacy testing and safety to obtain evidence sufficient to support claims for approval and labeling, in up to several thousands of patients of the type for whom the drug is intended to be prescribed.

4. Phase 4 studies may be negotiated at the time of approval to be carried out postmarketing to obtain further information about the drug's risks, optimal use, different regimens of administration, use in other patient populations or stages of disease than investigated previously, and use over longer times.

The Food, Drug, and Cosmetic Act of 1938 required that drug products be proved safe for use in patients. An amendment in 1962 required in addition that they be demonstrated by "adequate and well controlled trials" to be effective for treatment of the disease or disorder for which they are claimed to be indicated. Because these laws prohibit administration of FDA-unapproved drug products, exemptions from the laws are needed and may be granted to study and obtain data on investigational new drugs (INDs). According to federal regulations (7), applications for exemption from the law for INDs must be submitted for permission to initiate clinical trials. Applicants may be pharmaceutical companies intending eventually to commercialize successful new drugs or academic investigators who may wish to learn about and publish findings about the drug effects (and sometimes also to participate in financial rewards of the endeavors). Applications should include summaries of all preclinical information available, results of any human studies done abroad, and at least a first protocol for an initial clinical trial in humans. The FDA has 30 days to review the submitted application to determine whether the proposed trial appears reasonably safe to proceed, or to impose clinical hold if not. Failure of the FDA to communicate with the applicant within 30 days from receipt of the application may be taken as tacit permission to proceed. The emphasis of the review is on probable safety of giving the drug to humans.

In conducting investigational studies of new drug substances and drug products (the finished form of a tablet, capsule, solution to be given, including fillers, solvents, etc.), the sponsoring company or individual investigator incurs a number of responsibilities under IND regulations (6, §312.50–69). These include:

Review and approval of the initial plan for investigation and continuing studies by an institutional review board (IRB)

Careful record keeping and documentation (maintained for at least 2 years following approval for marketing)

Secure control of and accounting for the investigational drug product

Selection of qualified coinvestigators, and keeping them well informed

Operating only under written protocols, with informed consent of participants

Careful monitoring of the progress of the investigations

Prompt or immediate reporting of serious adverse events (life-threatening or fatal, causing or prolonging hospitalization, persistently disabling, causing genetic injury), especially unexpected fatal or life-threatening events (within 7 calendar days)

Annual (±60 days) reporting of findings, progress, participants under study or previously enrolled

Providing easy access to all study records to FDA inspectors

Information about the existence of or detail about the findings of studies conducted under IND regulations is confidential, not to be disclosed by the FDA unless previously reported or acknowledged publicly by the sponsor or investigator. However, the FDA will, upon request, disclose to a study participant a copy of their IND safety reports if any.

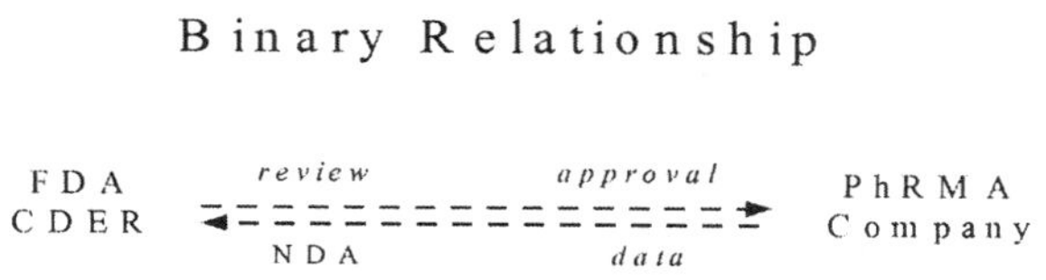

Binary Relationship

Figure 2   The two-way relationship between the FDA and a sponsoring pharmaceutical company, an increasingly interactive process.

During this clinical development process, there is a close interaction between the investigator or sponsoring company (usually one of the companies represented by the Pharmaceutical Research and Manufacturers of America, PhRMA) and members of the reviewing team of the appropriate FDA Division (see Figure 2). The 15 reviewing Divisions of the Center for Drug Evaluation and Research (CDER) of the FDA are organized by medical specialty (cardiorenal, pulmonary, oncologic, endocrine-metabolic, etc.) and grouped into five Offices for Drug Evaluation, each of which currently supervises sets of three Divisions. Applications for INDs are assigned for evaluation and review to the Division in which are located reviewers with the greatest expertise in the field of the disease to be treated and drug to be investigated.

IV.   NEW DRUG APPLICATION (NDA) REVIEW AND APPROVAL

When a sponsoring company or investigator has accumulated sufficient information about an investigational drug product, often determined in consultation with the FDA reviewing Division to which the IND had been assigned, it may prepare an NDA requesting review of the information by the chemists, pharmacologists-toxicologists, microbiologists, clinical pharmacologists, statisticians, and medical reviewers of that Division. The teams of reviewers and their supervisors in a Division are tasked to carry out a preliminary evaluation of the NDA submission within 60 days of its receipt to determine whether the submitted material appears sufficiently complete to permit substantive review. If so, the application is deemed as officially received and is filed as of 60 days after initial receipt. The date of filing of the NDA by the FDA (also called "Agency" in this chapter) starts a 180-day "clock" during which the FDA is required to review the application and send to the applicant a decision about whether the application is approved, is "approvable" provided certain issues are resolved, or is considered not approvable. In practice, this total 8-month period was seldom sufficient for the enormous work of NDA review, and more time was needed. However, additional funding and manpower were provided by the Prescription Drug User Fee Act of 1992 (PDUFA), and the succeeding Food and Drug Administration Modernization Act of 1997 (FDAMA). Total review times have shortened dramatically, from medians of 2–3 years to current medians of about 1 year for routine drugs and to less than 6 months for high-priority, urgently needed drugs.

Applications submitted for NDA review usually contain massive amounts of information, often hundreds of volumes of printed pages (each about 2 in. thick) or, in electronic form, hundreds of megabytes of information. It is customary to divide the submissions into sets of volumes or their electronic equivalents according to scientific discipline. These sets are assigned to one or more reviewers in that discipline (chemistry, microbiology, pharmacology-toxicology, clinical pharmacology, statistics, medicine). Individual reviewers prepare their work with varying degrees of interaction with reviewers in other disci-

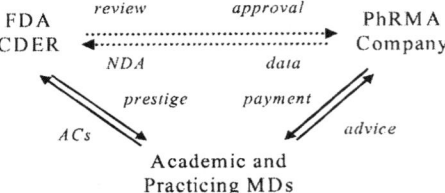

Figure 3 Expansion of the binary to a triangular interrelationship to include expert practicing and academic physicians as consultants.

plines and with supervising team leaders in each discipline. Completed reviews are discussed in the multidisciplinary NDA meetings; they are often exchanged, and sometimes combined medical-statistical reviews are prepared. The medical reviews usually incorporate salient findings or summaries from the reviews by other disciplines. Each review usually concludes with a recommendation for approval, as approvable with modification or additional information, or as not approvable, with reasons and justification. These recommendations are not binding on the decisions made by the Division or Office of CDER, but they carry considerable weight.

Before reaching final decisions, these units of the FDA may seek expert outside advice from academic and practicing consultants who serve 4-year terms on Advisory Committees to each of the CDER review Divisions, and from ad hoc consultants. Service on an FDA Advisory Committee (AC) is modestly recompensed, and travel expenses are paid, but the principal and most compelling incentives for the consultant are prestige and public service. The interrelationship between the Agency and the applicant (sponsoring company or investigator) thus is expanded to a trilateral set of interrelationships with physicians and others who are not in the employ of industry or government, but who are usually academic or practicing physicians or other specialists. However, the consultants who are sought and recruited to serve as AC members frequently belong to the same groups of people who serve as paid consultants to the pharmaceutical companies that commonly are the sponsors of new drug development (see Figure 3).

AC meetings are usually open to the public, and allow brief comments from interested patients, physicians, special interest groups, and others. Applicant companies and the FDA reviewing Division make summary presentations of data and points of view, with additional comments by consultants to the applicant. Members of the AC hear and discuss these presentations, and may appoint some of their members to make presentations as well. The ACs are often asked by the FDA to respond to, discuss, and vote upon specific questions concerning the NDA. Recommendations of ACs again are not binding on the Agency, but they carry great weight. Meetings of ACs frequently are very intense and dramatic public hearings, well covered by the press, and may be influential on the predicted valuation of the company perceived by stock analysts.

If the NDA is considered approvable, there will then be negotiations between the Agency and the applicant about the labeling language that describes exactly to whom the drug is to be given, its medical indication or use, its dose and regimen, warnings or precautions about adverse effects to be expected, and summaries of selected pharmacological and clinical information. The final approved labeling is used as the basis for allowable advertising and promotion, and for instructions to physicians and to patients as to how the drug product should be used. This labeling is printed in full in the *Physicians' Desk*

Tetrahedron of Interrelationships

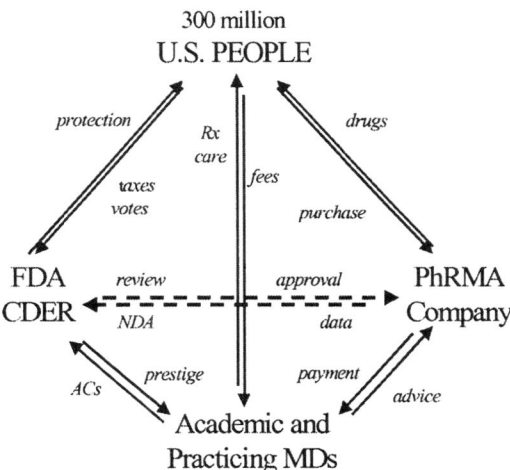

Figure 4   Inclusion of the people (patients, consumers, taxpayers) in the final processes of drug evaluation for approval.

Reference, now available on the internet. It should be understood that the labeling is not just a marketing or advertising piece written by the company that makes and sells the drug product. Every word in it must be negotiated, supported by data, justified, and agreed to by the FDA on behalf of the patients who will take the drug and the physicians who will prescribe it or recommend it (if OTC).

Thus, the process that began as an interaction between the FDA and the pharmaceutical company (in most cases) expanded into a second dimension to include expert consulting physicians who interact with both parties. Finally, it expanded further into a third dimension that included the patients or their representative spokespersons at AC meetings (see Figure 4). The people who will receive and pay for the drug are the same population who are taxpayers and voters who support the FDA, consumers who provide return-on-investment for the pharmaceutical companies, and who are patients of the consulting (and other) physicians. Including all the costs of research and development of unsuccessful candidate new drugs, the pharmaceutical industry estimates that it costs approximately $500 million to bring a new drug product to market (8).

V.   MARKETING AND SURVEILLANCE OF NEW DRUGS

Following approval of a new drug, the sponsoring company launches an active program of advertising, promoting, distributing, and selling it. Within the company, it is typical that the primary oversight of the product shifts from medical-scientific and regulatory efforts aimed at obtaining approval to marketing efforts aimed at maximizing sales, return-on-investment, and gaining market share. A natural dynamic tension exists between the backgrounds of training, experience, and viewpoints of conservative medical and aggressive marketing people. These two cultures often clash when unexpected new safety problems are discovered or confirmed after marketing, events that may dampen enthusiasm for the new drug product among prescribing physicians and their patients, and may generate concerns about meeting the predicted sales estimates among marketers.

Surveillance for safety of approved new drugs has depended on spontaneous reporting of unexpected or serious adverse reactions and events. Reports may be submitted by physicians, other health care personnel, patients, or family members, directly to FDA via MedWatch, or by reports to the manufacturer. Many reports are made verbally by physicians to company representatives during the latter's "detailing" office visits. Huge and ever-increasing numbers of such reports are being received each year, and are organized by the FDA into the large database of the Adverse Events Reporting System (AERS) administered by the Office of Drug Safety (ODS) of CDER. However, these reports depend on *voluntary* reporting, and probably represent a considerable underestimate of the true number, for many reasons, among which are:

> Inadequate follow-up or monitoring of patients, lack of data
> Failure of the patient to recognize the adverse event, or to report it to the physician
> Failure of the physician to appreciate the importance of the reaction
> Problem not believed severe enough to be "worth reporting"
> Erroneous attribution of the event to some cause other than the drug
> Reluctance to take the time to report the problem to the FDA or company, or procrastination
> Lack of reimbursement for the time taken to report
> A sense of guilt, for having caused harm to the patient
> Fear of lawsuit liability
> Denial that the new drug could be the cause
> Knowledge that others have reported such effects, and that it is not "news"
> Intent to publish the finding, and therefore keep it confidential
> Dislike/distrust of the "government"
> Other reasons peculiar to individual patients or doctors or other potential reporters

The proportion of spontaneously reported adverse events (AEs) is highly variable and uncertain, but is thought to be a substantial underestimate, ranging from 1% to 25% of the true number. It is difficult to estimate the number of patients exposed to the drug, to how much drug, and for how long. Therefore, nothing approaching a valid incidence rate of the problems can be assessed from spontaneous reports, since both numerator and denominator of the putative incidence rate are uncertain. Data from spontaneously reported AEs are often sketchy and incomplete, highly variable in quality, and frequently delayed in transmission. These factors make attribution of causality quite difficult, especially because of missing and unobtainable information. Nevertheless, the system is a very valuable and useful tool for detecting rare or unexpected problems not discovered during clinical trials or NDA review. The ODS group is developing ever more sophisticated programs to obtain information from the growing AERS database.

Once problems have been identified as probably or possibly drug induced, further options are available for confirming and clarifying the questions. Established clinical databases (such as Medicaid databases, the U.K. General Practice Research Database, etc.) may be interrogated for additional information. Nested case-control studies may provide information on risk factors that predispose certain patients to react adversely to a medication that is well tolerated by most people who can benefit from the treatment without the risk of serious AEs. However, such studies will not yield true incidence rates. Only by well-designed, large, prospective safety studies may these important findings be developed.

VI. DETECTION OF HEPATOTOXICITY BEFORE AND AFTER APPROVAL

Up to this point, the brief descriptions of drug development, review, approval, and post-marketing surveillance have been general, rather than directed specifically toward the problems of drug-induced injury to the liver. Unwanted liver effects may be seen with almost any class of drugs whose beneficial properties are intended for treating disorders of any organ or system. The liver is at increased risk because it plays such an important role in the metabolism, transport, activation-inactivation, or clearance of most drug substances. Therefore, it has become standard practice during drug development to screen for possible liver injury, beginning in the preclinical animal studies and continuing through all the clinical trials. Further, it is becoming increasingly more common for sponsors to investigate pathways of metabolism, and to perform studies using human hepatocytes and microsomal systems in vitro. With these methods, pharmacokinetics of metabolites, renal and nonrenal (mostly hepatobiliary-intestinal-fecal) clearances, and induction and inhibition of hepatic cytochrome P450 isozymes can be reported in the IND application packages, before the first human clinical trials are started.

Drugs that are clearly toxic to the liver or that produce toxic metabolites in studies with experimental animals are usually eliminated before ever being administered to humans. Even if a candidate drug is apparently safe in animal species tested, it is still not certain that the results may be extrapolated to humans. During clinical trials, drugs that cause elevations of serum enzymes (alanine aminotransferase, ALT; aspartate aminotransferase, AST; alkaline phosphatase, ALP; γ-glutamyl transferase, GGT) in substantial proportions of healthy volunteers or patients without prior liver disease are also very suspect and are likely to fail to be continued in clinical development. This is particularly true if hepatocellular injury (ALT or AST elevations) occurs, especially if the serum enzyme activities rise to 3 or 5 or 10 times the upper limit of the normal range (ULN), if the elevated enzyme levels remain persistently high, or if they become progressively more abnormal.

A useful observation, published by the late Hyman Zimmerman in the first edition of his book on drug-induced hepatotoxicity in 1978 (9), was that the combination of hepatocellular injury (transaminase activity elevations in the serum) and jaundice induced by a drug indicated a serious lesion, and that death from acute liver failure among patients showing that combination of abnormalities was at least 10%, and might be as high as 50% (see Table 1). Zimmerman and colleagues had observed earlier (10) that patients who showed jaundice in association with serum transaminase elevations after taking isoniazid had more severe subsequent outcomes. Zimmerman then applied this observation to several other drugs.

This observation was discussed also at the Fogarty International Center Conference on Hepatotoxicity (11) held in 1978 at the National Institutes of Health in Bethesda, Maryland, but it was not included in the final recommendations of the conference. The 1978 Fogarty Conference had been organized under the leadership of Dr. Robert Temple, Director of the Gastrointestinal Section of the U.S. Bureau of Drugs of the FDA, and Drs. William Summerskill and Nicholas Hightower, who had served as chairmen of its AC. The conference consensus clarified the distinction between tests of liver *function* and tests

Table 1 Estimated Case Fatality
Rate in Drug-Induced Acute
Hepatocellular Injury

Drug	Apparent fatality rate
α-Methyldopa	10%
Isoniazid	>10%
Iproniazid	15%
Phenytoin	>40%
Cinchophen	50%
Halothane	50%

Source: Data from ref. 9, Table 16.1, p. 351,
with permission.

that reflected liver *injury* without measuring liver function. Examples of liver *function* tests
were: bromsulfalein and indocyanine green dye (excretion), antipyrine and aminopyrine
(oxidation), serum bile acid and bilirubin concentrations (hepatic "clearance" of physiological substances), blood prothrombin, and serum albumin (protein synthesis). Tests of
liver *injury*—but not function—included activities of serum ALT and AST for hepatocellular injury, and serum ALP and GGT for cholestasis. It was the consensus of the conference that criteria for stopping a new drug in a person whose prior test results had been
normal included "markedly abnormal" results of serum AST or ALT more than 3 times
the ULN, ALP more than 1.5 times the ULN, and bilirubin more than 2 times the ULN,
at any time after starting administration of the drug. Although not specifically defined by
the Fogarty Conference of 1978, the combination of observed evidence of hepatocellular
injury to the liver and jaundice (as a measure of overall functional loss or severity) was
borne in mind by Dr. Temple in his oversight of new drug evaluations at the FDA. It was
also repeatedly observed by Dr. Zimmerman for another 21 years, and was mentioned
again in his second edition (2, p. 428) as the "gravity of hepatocellular jaundice" with a
case fatality rate ranging from 10 to 50%. Although too modest to claim it publicly even
up to the year of his death, Dr. Zimmerman agreed (personal communication, 1999) that
the rule still seemed valid.

A. "Hy's Rule" for Drug-Induced Hepatotoxicity

"Hy's rule" is that if both drug-induced hepatocellular injury and jaundice occur; that is,
when both transaminase and bilirubin elevations occur together in the absence of biliary
obstruction, mortality (or its surrogate, liver transplantation) of at least 10% may be expected among such patients.

Over the past several decades, hundreds of NDAs have been evaluated at CDER.
During this time Dr. Robert Temple noted that "Hy's rule" seemed to be a consistent
predictor if the combination of ALT elevation and jaundice had been seen in the preapproval clinical data from controlled trials. This predicted serious trouble to come in the
postmarketing phase of drug development when much larger numbers of patients would
be exposed to the drug. Of all causes for drug withdrawals from the market after approval
(see Table 2), hepatotoxicity has been the most common single cause (R. Temple, personal

Table 2 Hepatotoxicity: The Most Common
Single Adverse Effect Causing Major Drug
Problems (withdrawal or nonapproval)

Drug	Year
Iproniazid (Marsalid)	1956
Ibufenac (in Europe only)	1975
Ticrynafen (Selacryn)	1979
Benoxaprofen (Oraflex)	1982
Perihexilene (in France)	1985
Dilevalol (in Portugal, Ireland)	1990
Bromfenac (Duract)	1998
Troglitazone (Rezulin)	2000

Source: R. Temple, personal communication, 1999.

communication. "Hepatotoxicity Through the Years," at CDER course on "Drugs and the Liver: What They Do to Each Other," April 19, 1999 and November 15, 1999).

In addition, many other drugs have been restricted or limited in their use by requiring serial periodic monitoring of serum enzyme activities, or evaluation for prior liver disease or active injury before starting the drug. Other restrictions included severe warnings, or advising that drugs be stopped if the patient showed clinical symptoms or serological findings indicating liver dysfunction or injury. Examples of such drugs are: dantrolene, felbamate, labetalol, nicotinic acid, pemoline, tolcapone, valproic acid, and trovafloxacin.

Current labeling of drugs, as surveyed by searching the internet version of the *Physicians' Desk Reference*, disclosed 90 still-marketed drug entities whose labeling lists "acute liver failure" or "hepatic necrosis" as an adverse effect that has been reported in patients taking those drugs (M. Willy, Z. Li, FDA, personal communications). In a separate search, 124 drugs were found whose use is labeled as contraindicated in patients with a history of prior or currently active liver disease (actual terms used in the labeling: liver dysfunction, liver disease unspecified, history of jaundice, serum transaminase elevation, liver failure, hepatitis, unspecified cirrhosis, unspecified jaundice, autoimmune hepatitis). A total of 370 drugs were found whose labeling mentions adverse side effects of hepatic dysfunction or hepatitis, and many of these drugs have recommendations for monitoring serum enzyme levels at varying intervals and duration. These recommendations for labeling, warnings, and precautions have been suggested at various times, are variable in language and terminology, and usually have been based on opinions of consultants to the Agency. There is need for development of more consistent terminology for use in labeling, and for clinical data to support such recommendations.

Validation of "Hy's rule" is much needed, especially for its sensitivity and specificity, with clarification of whether the critical finding is appearance of clinical jaundice, or whether lesser elevations of serum bilirubin may be useful as part of the predictive combination of abnormal findings. Similarly, there is need to explore what degree of ALT elevation is most predictive, or whether the rate of change of those levels may be useful as a predictor of serious liver injury.

There has been no consistent method for assessing whether or not, or to what quantitative degree of likelihood, the drug suspected of causing hepatic injury or dysfunction is responsible. In clinical practice, even far more than during controlled clinical trials, there are often confounding potential causes for the observed test abnormalities or clinical findings. These may include other concurrently or previously administered drugs or chemicals, acute or chronic viral hepatitides, other liver diseases, and disorders of other body systems that may affect the liver (especially the cardiovascular system). Adequate data seldom are available to evaluate the spontaneously reported cases of possible drug-induced liver injury, and the delay in notification of them often makes impossible the prospective pursuit of such data. Proposals of quantitative scoring systems have been made by international panels of experts (12) but have not been generally accepted or widely used. More commonly, investigators are simply asked for their opinions as to whether the observed hepatotoxicity was definitely, probably, possibly, unlikely, or definitely not related to administration of the study drug. Paid consultants have also been asked to render their opinions on causality for reported cases, based on whatever information on each case may be available. Clearly there is need to develop a more valid consensus on this matter.

VII. IDIOSYNCRACY OR INTRINSICALLY HEPATOTOXIC DRUG?

Clear-cut intrinsic hepatotoxicity is relatively easy to detect and prevent. If a drug or chemical predictably causes liver injury in animals and in all persons exposed to enough of it, it is obviously a toxin or poison to the liver. Such chemicals, including carbon tetrachloride and white phosphorus, and drugs such as chloroform are known to be dangerous and are avoided or prohibited from use. Their toxicity is easily characterized as dose-related, predictable, occurring in all persons or animals exposed. However, such simplicity is not always the case. Certain individuals appear to be susceptible, or less resistant than most people, to agents such as ethyl alcohol, which does not cause severe liver injury or cirrhosis in all persons consuming it heavily and for a long time. The clinical problem comes when only a few, or even rare, individuals show hepatotoxicity to a drug that has not been found to cause liver injury in animals, even at relatively large doses, and nearly all patients who take it show no signs of liver injury. In such exceptional persons, hepatotoxicity is not predictable, and the severity of the reactions is not clearly related to the dose or duration of exposure; the adverse reaction in them is unexpected.

Some of the idiosyncratic hepatotoxic reactions may be due to genetic differences in metabolism; others may be related to nutritional deficiencies, or to other drugs or agents to which the person has been exposed. Still other differences may result from various acquired liver diseases, or to immunologically mediated differences. Both nature, in the form of the person's genetic makeup, and nurture, in the form of the experiences and vicissitudes of living, seem to affect the susceptibility of people to a given drug. The adjective "idiosyncratic" does not exactly mean either unpredictable or unexpected. Idiosyncrasy comes directly from three Greek words: *idios*, one's own; *syn*, together; *krasis*, mixing. "One's own mixing together" of traits and factors makes every individual unique, and potentially different in how that person will react or respond to a challenge such as a strange chemical substance. For most drugs, the risk factors are not well understood, and for most hepatotoxic reactions, the mechanisms are not well understood.

If a drug can be safely tolerated by 999 persons out of 1000, should it be called a poison or a hepatotoxic drug? The one person who cannot tolerate it, and who reacts with liver injury, is obviously different from the vast majority of people. Perhaps the focus of our efforts should be directed more to identifying the few exceptionally susceptible people, and preventing them from being exposed to a drug, than toward an effort at finding out which drugs are "toxic." The low incidence of these uncommon or rare, but sometimes

Table 3 Number of People Needed for >95% Chance of Observing at Least One Adverse Event

True incidence	Ordinary nonreactors	Number needed
1 in 10	0.9	29
1 in 100	0.99	299
1 in 1,000	0.999	2,995
1 in 10,000	0.9999	29,956

severe or fatal, hepatotoxic adverse events is at the core of why the painstaking and careful efforts at safety screening in the long drug development process sometimes fail.

Why cannot studies be done to detect these idiosyncratically different people? Consider the numbers. In the simple case of the chances that a hepatotoxic reaction may or may not occur, we can estimate what number will be needed to have 95% confidence that at least one such person will be found. The number needed is about three times the reciprocal of the incidence rate, if all such cases are detected (see Table 3).*

The epidemiological estimates in Table 3 have also been made by Stricker (13), with very slightly different figures, but all agree that approximately *three times* the reciprocal of the true incidence rate of patients will need to be observed, to have at least 95% confidence of finding at least one (the so-called "Rule of Three"). Many of the very serious, life-threatening hepatotoxic reactions to drugs have incidences on the order of 1 per 1000 to 1 per 10,000, and very large numbers of patients would need to be observed on drug and control agent to discover such rare reactions. Nevertheless, when popular drugs such as troglitazone (Rezulin) are approved and are given to millions of diabetic patients, such numbers are reached, and many cases of severe hepatotoxicity may be seen. It is not feasible to require that tens of thousands of patients be studied in controlled clinical trials before approval of a drug for clinical use and marketing. However, all of us must begin to realize and accept that current procedures cannot assure safety regarding such uncommon or rare adverse events. Spontaneous reporting systems can discover problems only after they have occurred, which they do quite well, but they cannot predict safety problems before they occur. To go beyond the limitations of spontaneous voluntary reporting, with all of its drawbacks, it may be necessary to consider and debate the wisdom of requiring large, prospective safety studies postmarketing. These might be considered if signals of sufficient strength of serious adverse effects are detected either during controlled trials or

---

* If we assume the chance of hepatotoxicity is 1 in 100 (0.01), then the chance of it not occurring will be 0.99. For n persons, the chances are given by $(0.01 + 0.99)^n$, which is recognizable as a binomial expression. For the simple case of $n = 3$, the expression expands to:

$$(0.01)^3 + 3(0.01)^2(0.99) + 3(0.01)(0.99)^2 + (0.99)^3$$

	0.000001 +	0.000297 +	0.029403 +	0.970299	
chance of seeing	3	2	1	0	cases

The chance of seeing at least one is the sum of the first three terms, 0.029701, which is equal to (1 − the last term); $1 - 0.970299 = 0.029701$. It can be shown that (1 − the last term) will always give the chance of seeing one or more (at least one) cases. If the true incidence rate, i, is 1 per 100, how many people would be needed for ≥95% chance of seeing at least 1? Obviously, 1 − the chance of not seeing any. This turns out to be 299 for $i = 0.01$: $(0.99)^{299} = 0.0495$ and $1 - 0.0495 = 0.9505$, or >95%.

NDA review, or by postmarketing surveillance. Clearly, there is need to develop consensus on a definition for "sufficient strength" of a clinical signal to justify action.

A great ethical difficulty lies in balancing the risks of severe toxicity for a very small number of patients against a benefit, however modest, for the vast majority of patients. If the disease being treated is trivial or cosmetic, or if considerably safer alternative treatments are available, then the decision may be easy, but often it is not.

VIII. DOES PREEXISTING LIVER DISEASE INCREASE THE RISK FOR DRUG-INDUCED HEPATIC INJURY?

This is really two questions, with perhaps different answers. If it is considered to mean "Does previous or currently active liver disease increase the risk of de novo idiosyncratic hepatic reactions to a new drug or chemical agent?" the answer may be no. Zimmerman (2, p. 430) maintained that "a stubborn misconception regarding susceptibility to hepatic injury has been the view that patients with preexisting liver disease are more likely than others to experience hepatic injury on exposure to drugs that cause liver damage. There has been virtually no evidence for this view." A similar view has been expressed by Schenker et al. (15), who wrote recently, "It seems evident that the presence of underlying liver disease should not promote this mechanism [unpredictable metabolic or immunologic] of injury." However, both Zimmerman and Schenker concede uncertainty, and admit the possibility of exceptions.

On the other hand, if the question were interpreted as "Does previous liver damage increase risk of poor outcome, slower recovery, or worse clinical effect because of the added damage?" the answer might be yes. Certainly, patients who have shown acute alcoholic hepatitis in the past and who have begun to show cirrhotic changes are more likely than the average alcoholic person both to react unfavorably again and to be at greater risk of liver failure if another bout of acute alcohol-induced liver injury occurs. Zimmerman conceded (2, p. 430) that "the addition of drug-induced hepatic injury to chronic liver disease would be troublesome." Schenker and colleagues (15, p. 1103) summarize the response to the question by saying, "Underlying liver disease should not be an automatic contraindication to the use of potentially hepatotoxic drugs. Rather, the patient needs to be followed more closely to detect any incipient incremental injury."

Easier said than done. Detection of drug-induced liver injury in patients with preexisting evidence of serum enzyme elevations due to their liver disease may be very difficult (W. Lee, personal communication, "Drug-Induced Liver Injury: The Threat Continues," at Medical Grand Rounds, University of Texas Southwestern Medical Center, June 8, 2000). Even with very frequent monitoring it may be exceedingly hard to distinguish between fluctuations of disease activity and new injury caused by the drug. It is also quite difficult to know when a drug should be stopped in such patients.

IX. DOES MONITORING PREVENT SERIOUS DRUG-INDUCED HEPATOTOXICITY?

Although monitoring of serum enzymes such as ALT activities may be encouraged by labeling, may be recommended by consultants, and may represent the easiest way to detect idiosyncratic drug-induced liver injury, it has by no means been proved to be effective. There is a practical limit to how often testing can be done. It is very costly to screen thousands of people repeatedly in the hope of catching one who may show an abnormality.

If the acute liver injury is rapid in onset, as it may be, it could well occur during the interval between tests. The true nature and extent of the liver damage is not proportional to the elevation in serum enzyme activity, and does not allow estimation of prognosis. The serum ALT is a fairly sensitive test for liver injury, but does not measure liver function at all. Other enzymes are no better indicators, although the serum AST may be elevated modestly when ALT is not in acute alcohol-induced liver injury. The ALP and GGT activities reflect cholestasis more than hepatocellular injury. However, serial monitoring of serum ALT is often the best that can be done to detect a drug-induced change early enough to stop the drug, nearly always the most important treatment. Only in special cases such as acetaminophen-induced liver injury is a real therapy available, in the form of *N*-acetylcysteine, which if given promptly may prevent serious damage to the liver. Labeling requirements for serum transaminase monitoring have had quite disappointing results, and there are few data showing that monitoring has prevented any cases of serious drug-induced liver injury by early detection and withdrawal of the offending agent. Compliance with labeling requirements to monitor for hepatotoxicity, even after repeated "Dear Doctor" letters and increasingly stringent labeling changes for a drug as well publicized as troglitazone (Rezulin), recently was found to be very poor [14].

It is not clear how closely or for how long patients should be monitored, what test or tests may be best to use, and how results should be interpreted. It is reasonable to suggest that finding a new elevation of serum enzyme activity in a patient who has started a new drug should lead to promptly confirming the finding. Also, intensive observation should commence, whether or not it is decided that the drug should be stopped. In cases of doubt it may be best to stop the drug and continue to observe the patient closely, to rule out alternative possible causes of the observed abnormalities, and to gather additional information [15,16].

There is no standard set of recommendations about management of a patient suspected of having a possible acute drug-induced liver injury, what information should be gathered, how quickly tests should be rechecked and how often these should be repeated, and whether or when a liver biopsy should or should not be done (W. Lee, personal communication; Medical Grand Rounds, June 8, 2000).

The use of rechallenge with the putative offending drug after patient recovery following withdrawal, or "dechallenge," is becoming increasingly less acceptable on safety and ethical grounds, even though it might provide powerful evidence imputing the drug as the causative agent. After a drug has caused hepatic injury and has been withdrawn, the onset of repeat injury is often faster and more severe [1,2,15,16], and the information may not be worth the risk unless that drug is vital to the patient's care, no satisfactory alternatives are available, and the risks are fully understood by both the physician and the patient. However, unintentional rechallenge history, from the pattern of drug exposure, is another matter that may provide extremely helpful information.

X. WHAT NEEDS TO BE DONE?

Throughout this chapter, an attempt has been made to set forth the problem of drug-induced liver injury as one for patients, physicians, and pharmaceutical companies, as well as for regulatory bodies. There is need for thoughtful consideration of the problems and complexities by persons from all these constituencies. They need to consider how they might work together to gather or provide data, solve problems, find answers and understanding, and improve processes that are now and have been working imperfectly.

More needs to be learned about the mechanisms of liver injury caused by drugs and their metabolites, the interactions between drugs and nondrug chemical substances, the role of genetic endowment, and the effects of life experiences on individual susceptibility. It is essential that we begin to recognize risk factors that should give pause to starting a given drug in a particular patient who may be different from most people who have shown that they tolerate the drug well. We need to develop consensus on the many things that we should be doing differently, to learn more, to eventually prevent drug-induced liver damage from increasing further, and to reduce its incidence.

REFERENCES

1. Farrell GC. Importance of drug-induced liver disease. In: Drug-Induced Liver Disease. Edinburgh: Churchill Livingstone, 1994:91–92.
2. Zimmerman HJ. Hepatotoxicity: The Adverse Effects of Drugs and Other Chemicals on the Liver. 2nd ed. Philadelphia: Lippincott Williams & Wilkins, 1999.
3. Ostapowicz G, Fontana RJ, Larson AM, Davern T, Lee WM, and the Acute Liver Failure Study Group. Etiology and outcome of acute liver failure in the USA: preliminary results of a prospective multi-center study. Hepatology 1999; 30:221A (abstr).
4. Friedman LM, Furberg CD, DeMets DL. Fundamentals of Clinical Trials. 3rd ed. St. Louis: Mosby, 1996.
5. Office of the Federal Register. §312.21 Phases of an investigation. 21 Code of Federal Regulations Ch. I (4-1-00 Edition), p. 63, and § 312.85 Phase 4 studies, p. 90.
6. Spilker B. Guide to Clinical Trials. Philadelphia: Lippincott-Raven Publishers, 1996.
7. Office of the Federal Register. Part 312: Investigational New Drug Application. 21 Code of Federal Regulations Ch. I (4-1-00 Edition), pp. 58–96.
8. Stolberg SG, Gerth J. In a drug's journey to market, discovery is just the first of many steps. New York Times, July 23, 2000.
9. Zimmerman HJ. Hepatotoxicity. The Adverse Effects of Drugs and Other Chemicals on the Liver. 1st ed. New York: Appleton-Century-Crofts, 1978. Chapter 16: Drug-induced liver disease.
10. Black M, Mitchell JR, Zimmerman HJ, Ishak KG, Epler GR. Isoniazid-associated hepatitis in 114 patients. Gastroenterology 1975; 69:289–302.
11. Davidson CS, Leevy CM, Chamberlayne EC, eds. Guidelines for Detection of Hepatotoxicity due to Drugs and Chemicals. [Fogarty Conference, 1978] NIH Publication No. 79-313. US Government Printing Office, Washington, DC 1979.
12. Bénichou C, Benhamou JP, Danan G, and International Consensus Meeting Participants. Criteria of drug-induced liver disorders. J Hepatol 1990; 11:272–276.
13. Stricker BHC. Epidemiology of drug-induced hepatic injury. In: BHCh Stricker, ed. Drug-Induced Hepatic Injury, 2nd ed. Amsterdam: Elsevier, 1992. Chap. 2.
14. Graham DJ, Drinkard CR, Shatin D, Tsong Y, Burgess MJ. Liver enzyme monitoring in patients treated with troglitazone. JAMA 2001; 286:831–833.
15. Schenker S, Martin RR, Hoyumpa AM. Antecedent liver disease and drug toxicity. J Hepatol 1999; 31:1098–1105.
16. Lee WM. Medical management of acute liver failure. In: WM Lee, R Williams, eds. Acute Liver Failure. Cambridge, UK: Cambridge University Press, 1997. Chap. 10.

Index

About the Editors

NEIL KAPLOWITZ is Brem Professor of Medicine, Director of the U.S.C. Research Center for Liver Disease, and Chief of the Division of Gastrointestinal and Liver Diseases, University of Southern California Keck School of Medicine, Los Angeles. The author or coauthor of more than 230 professional publications and editor of nine books, he is a Fellow of the American College of Gastroenterology, and a member of the American Association for the Study of Liver Disease and the American Gastroenterology Association, among others. He received the B.S. (1964) and M.D. (1967) degrees from New York University, New York.

LAURIE D. DELEVE is Associate Professor of Medicine at the University of Southern California Keck School of Medicine, Division of Gastrointestinal and Liver Diseases and the U.S.C. Research Center for Liver Disease, Los Angeles. The author or coauthor of more than 30 professional publications, she is a member of the American Gastroenterological Association, the Gastroenterology Research Group, and the American Association for the Study of Liver Disease. She received a B.S. (1976) and M.D. (1979) from Erasmus University of Rotterdam, The Netherlands, and a Ph.D. degree (1988) in pharmacology from the University of Toronto, Ontario, Canada.

ISBN 0-8247-0811-3

90000